Laboratory Tests
&
Diagnostic Procedures

Fourth Edition

Laboratory Tests & Diagnostic Procedures

Edited by

Cynthia C. Chernecky, PhD, RN, CNS, AOCN

Professor
Department of Nursing Science
School of Nursing
Medical College of Georgia
Augusta, Georgia

Barbara J. Berger, MSN, RN

Clinical Nurse Specialist
Southwest General Health Center
Partnering with University Hospitals Health System
Middleburg Heights, Ohio

SAUNDERS
An Imprint of Elsevier

ֽUNDERS

An Imprint of Elsevier Inc.

The Curtis Center
625 Walnut Street
Philadelphia, PA 19106-9884

NOTICE

Health science is an ever-changing field. Standard safety precautions must be followed, but as new research and clinical experience broaden our knowledge, changes in treatment and drug therapy may become necessary or appropriate. Readers are advised to check the most current product information provided by the manufacturer of each drug to be administered to verify the recommended dose, the method and duration of administration, and contraindications. It is the responsibility of the licensed prescriber, relying on experience and knowledge of the patient, to determine dosages and the best treatment for each individual patient. Neither the publisher nor the author assumes any liability for any injury and/or damage to persons or property arising from this publication.

Previous editions copyrighted 1993, 1997, 2001
International Standard Book Number 0-7216-0388-2

Executive Vice President, Nursing and Health Professions: Sally Schrefer
Executive Publisher: Darlene Como
Managing Editor: Brian Dennison
Publishing Services Manager: Catherine Albright Jackson
Project Manager: Mary G. Stueck
Designer: Amy Buxton

Printed in the United States of America

Last digit is the print number: 9 8 7 6 5 4 3 2 1

Contributors

Christine Alichnie, PhD, RN
Barbara J. Berger, MSN, RN
Cynthia C. Chernecky, PhD, RN,
   CNS, AOCN
Michelle Ficca, PhD, RN

Annette Gunderman, PhD, RN
Sharon Haymaker, PhD, RN
Marguerite J. Murphy, MS, RN
Timothy L. Wren, MS, RN

The Editors acknowledge the contributors to the Third Edition

John T. Benjamin, MD
Barbara J. Berger, MSN, RN
Amy Bieda, MSN, RN, CNP
Martha J. Bradshaw, PhD, RN
Wendy Gram Brick, MD
Russell E. Burgess, MD
Patricia A. Catalano, MSN, RN, CCRN
Cynthia C. Chernecky, PhD, RN,
   CNS, AOCN
Robyn DeGennaro, RN, CCRN
Michael E. Fincher, MD
Mark S. Green, MS, PA-C
Steve S. Lee, BSN, RN
Ronald W. Lewis, MD

Kathryn S. McLeod, MD
Shelli McLeod, BSN, RN-C, CCE
Marguerite J. Murphy, MS, RN
Carl E. Rosenberg, MD, MBA
William H. Salazar, MD
Robert R. Schade, MD
Judith Banks Stallings, BS, PA-C
Benjamin H. Taylor, Jr., MPAS,
   PA-C
Saundra L. Turner, EdD, RN-CS,
   FNP
Rachel Vaneck, MSN, RN, CNP
Kristy Woods, MD
Timothy L. Wren, MS, RN

Reviewers

Kenneth P. Miller, PhD, RN, CFNP,
   FAAN
David Nicolaou, MD, MS, FACEP
Eric Walsh, MD

Preface

We are pleased to announce the arrival of the fourth edition of *Laboratory Tests and Diagnostic Procedures*. The text is completely alphabetical, fully cross-referenced, and indexed. There is no need to know which body system is tested or whether the test uses blood or urine or is diagnostic to locate the test. The best advantage, we believe, is that all the information is complete and contained within one cover. There is no need to waste valuable time referring to multiple texts or flipping between sections to obtain test-specific information. Valuable features include designation of the most common tests used for diseases, conditions, or symptoms (Part One), norms throughout all age groups, drug and herbal and natural-remedy effects on test results, inclusion of medicolegal implications, panic levels and symptoms and emergency treatment for panic levels, dialysis implications for timing of blood draws or treating high levels, client and family teaching, risks of and contraindications for procedures, herbs that affect results of tests, and whether informed consent is needed. The content is basic enough for novices and complete enough for seasoned practitioners. It has significant value for both students and practitioners of medical technology, medicine, and nursing and is the kind of reference to use throughout one's career. It is appropriate for the many specialties within the professions, and it includes information from across the life span.

The text is organized into two parts. Part One is designed to help the practitioner confirm a suspected diagnosis or condition as well as to provide additional conditions that may demonstrate similar symptoms. The most common (or significant) tests or procedures used for the suspected diagnosis are indicated. Part Two lists the tests (laboratory tests including those for common medications and street drugs) and diagnostic procedures in alphabetical order with normal values; panic-level symptoms and treatment, including whether the substance is dialyzable; usage or conditions in which the values may be abnormal; and a concise description of the test and its significance. This edition also includes expanded information on consent requirements, risks and contraindications, client and family teaching, and the details of the test and client care, as well as integration of the most current scientific literature. Other features include the use of shading in Part Two for ease of use, reduction of blood sample volumes to the minimum amount required (to help avoid iatrogenic anemia), information on whether blood samples can be drawn during hemodialysis, expansion of age-specific norms, and improved quality-assurance information on factors that interfere with results. Finally, a comprehensive, international, up-to-date bibliography of specific resources is included to direct practitioners to additional information.

Other features of this edition include the newest tests in many fields. Cross-referencing of the test and procedure names includes associated acronyms to expedite the location of each. The index now includes a synthesis of diseases, tests, and procedures for the entire book in one place. The format of this text is the product of years of clinical practice and expertise. It has been written by practitioners *for* practitioners. The invaluable contributions of a large number of clinical experts and their contacts who freely shared the most up-to-date information about the tests, procedures, and medical conditions are a most valued feature of this edition.

The purpose of this text is to provide complete information to guide practitioners or students in the clinical care of patients. Applicability of information in a text of this type is relative. Although we have used reliable and current sources in the compilation of the book, variations in laboratory techniques and client conditions must be considered for interpretation. The normal and panic levels listed are not meant to be used as rigid separations of normal and abnormal but rather as guidelines for consideration within the context of individual client conditions and laboratory specifications.

We have provided information regarding procedures that may require separate consent forms, or those beyond the general institutional consent form. Certainly there is much variation among institutions regarding whether a consent form is necessary. At the minimum, oral consent is generally documented. We have provided what is general practice according to the literature and the experience of our expert contributors across the country. However, we caution that institutional protocols vary and should, of course, be consulted and followed. Regardless of whether formal consent is obtained, it is the responsibility of all health care professionals to educate clients undergoing *any* test or procedure. Teaching about the test or procedure must be tailored to the client's and the client's family's condition, language, comprehension, anxiety level, clinical goals, and other specific needs.

Most drugs in this text are listed by their generic names. This includes specific tests to determine drug levels in either blood or urine and includes within these tests names of drugs that may interfere with the test results. Generic names have been used to save valuable printed space and to avoid confusion attributable to multiple trade names. We must stress that, in judging possible drug interferences, the clinical evaluation of the client should remain primary in the process of interpreting test values. Clearly it is impractical to discontinue all medications to get a "pure value." If, however, a drug is known to cause severe interferences with the test results, it is clearly stated, and the drug should be discontinued when possible.

With concern about the transmission of bloodborne pathogens and in view of the content of this text, it is imperative to address the safe handling of specimens. In 1994, the Centers for Disease Control and Prevention (CDC) published "Standard Precautions," which include guidelines for isolation precautions in hospitals, designed to prevent the transmission of the hepatitis B virus and the human immunodeficiency virus (HIV). A condensed and current version of these recommendations is provided. Most institutions currently follow these guidelines in some version, and we recommend referral to individual institutional protocol.

Years of research and writing went into the completion of this text. It could not have been done without our many dedicated professional contributors, without the assistance and support of our editor Brian Dennison, and without the support of our families, friends, and professional colleagues. We know that we have acquired much knowledge through the process of writing and editing this book. We believe that the book is a valuable tool for all health care professionals.

      Cynthia C. Chernecky   **Barbara J. Berger**

Acknowledgments

It is with humble thanks that I dedicate this book to all those who have helped in its creation, support, and update and in particular to those who use it in their practice and education. This book has been a labor of love and continues to be used on both the national and international levels. I fully believe that an excellent clinical book on labs and diagnostics is what the clinical caregiver needs to give excellent care to persons who are ill and to all persons who have a right to disease prevention. This book was designed by clinical practitioners and is updated by experts in various fields who share their expertise so that the fulfillment of up-to-date excellent care can be sustained as a reality. There are others who, though they did not write, were supportive in ways that we can all understand—these are people who have integrity, caring souls, faith, and a sense of humor: my mother Olga, late father Edward Chernecky, godmother Helen Prohorik, godsons Jonathon Tarutis and Vincent Hunter, goddaughter Dawn Priscilla Payne, brother Dr. Richard Chernecky, nieces Ellie and Annie Chernecky, nephew Michael Chernecky, cousins Paula Smart, Karyn Tarutis, and Philip Prohorik, friends Elaine Calugar, Phyllis Skiba, Ursula Grimmett, David and Janice Douglass, Frankie Ekroyd, Molly Loney, Kim Black, colleagues Dr. Joyceen Boyle, Dr. Jean Brown, Dr. Mary Cooley, Pam Cushman, Dr. Leda Danao, Kitty Garrett, Beverly George-Gay, Dr. Rich Haas, Becki Hodges, Dr. Ann Kolanowski, Elisabeth Monti, Dr. Ruth McCorkle, Dr. Katherine Nugent, Dr. Linda Sarna, Dr. Geri Padilla, Lori Schumacher, Dr. Roma Williams, and those who keep me focused in life itself: Mother Thecla (Abbess), Mother Helena and Mother Seraphima of Saints Mary and Martha Orthodox Monastery in South Carolina, Priest Gregory and Presbytera Raisa Koo and Priest Antonio and Matushka Elizabeth Perdomo. It never fails to surprise me when I meet an Orthodox member of His Holy, Catholic, and Apostolic Church who has found true joy in that he or she has found the truth in the faith that we trace back to the time of Christ himself. I know from my life that the truth is worth the search.

To the universities that have shared their knowledge with me, I thank the University of Connecticut, Yale University, University of Pittsburgh, Clemson University, Case Western Reserve University, University of Wisconsin Oshkosh, and the University of California at Los Angeles.

As we continue in further editions of this book, I do not know what else to say about my coeditor, coauthor, friend, and colleague Barb Berger that I have not already said. We work well together, know how to laugh, know how to work hard, and have a commitment to care with an eye for quality research to make each and every edition packed with quality information and timely updates. This book is a massive project, and I could not have accomplished it without trust, equality, respect, and admiration, which is what Barb and I have for one another and why we make such a great team. Barb, you are one classy professional, a great role model, and maintain excellence as a clinical nurse, which adds not just to this book but to the discipline of nursing.

To all nurses, physicians, attorneys, and other health care professionals who give true meaning to this book by using it, we respect your comments and suggestions—after all we are all striving for the same goals in our respective services.

Cynthia (Cinda) Cecilia Chernecky

My thanks and gratitude for their meticulous attention to detail and sharing of their expertise go to current and past contributors and reviewers of this text. The format and types of information included have evolved over the years to meet the needs of today's busy professionals. For example, the designation of key tests for various diseases, conditions and symptoms is a direct response to feedback from our readers and is one of the newest features that set this book apart from others available. Thanks also go to our editor, Brian Dennison, for his good advice and helpfulness as we approached the completion of the manuscript. Thanks go to my husband, Stephan Berger, who shares my pride in this work and does more than his fair share keeping the home front running so that I can spend time working on the manuscript. My mother, Alice Adams, once again supported and encouraged my work on this fourth-edition text. Finally, thanks to Cinda Chernecky, my excellent coeditor and friend, who never fails to amaze me with her depth and breadth of knowledge and common sense.

Barbara J. Berger

How to Use This Book

This book contains two major sections: Part One is a selected alphabetical listing of diseases, conditions, and symptoms that will aid in the diagnosis and monitoring of illnesses. Part Two presents information on laboratory and diagnostic tests in alphabetical order, using a consistent, time-saving format.

PART ONE: DISEASES, CONDITIONS, AND SYMPTOMS
The purpose of this section is to assist practitioners in diagnosing and monitoring the progress of illness or wellness.

Part One is a selected alphabetical listing of diseases, conditions, and symptoms. Under each topic is a list of laboratory and diagnostic tests, also in alphabetical order. It is not expected that all the tests listed would necessarily be required or be abnormal for any one disease, condition, or symptom. Rather, any of the listed tests or a combination of tests would likely be performed to aid, confirm, monitor, or rule out that diagnosis or condition. Where appropriate, the tests and/or procedures considered diagnostic and/or significant in determining a diagnosis are highlighted with a star.

Additional Conditions includes other related diseases or conditions that should be considered when one is postulating the diagnosis above. Many of these additional conditions are, in fact, listed elsewhere in the section with their own battery of tests (see below).

PART TWO: LABORATORY TESTS AND DIAGNOSTIC PROCEDURES
The purpose of this section is to provide a comprehensive, concise, ready reference of practitioner "need-to-know" information about laboratory tests and diagnostic procedures. Features of this section, in format order, include:

- **Alphabetical list of laboratory tests and diagnostic procedures:** this saves you time in looking up any test. You will also find combined laboratory profiles listed such as CBC, CMP, and Chemistry Profile.
- **Norms** are listed for all known age groups and for all known units (i.e., national and international units). Also included are therapeutic peak and trough norms, toxic and panic levels, as well as associated signs, symptoms, and emergency treatment for overdose when applicable. Tests with toxic and/or panic levels include symptoms and treatment. Treatments listed are generally accepted treatments. The listing of these does not imply that some or all of them should be used. Selection of treatments must be based on the client's history and condition, as well as the history of the episode.
- **Usage** states the typical conditions or monitoring for which the diagnostic test or procedure is commonly used (i.e., cardiac catheterization).
- **Increased, Decreased** or **Positive, Negative** are categories to describe conditions that cause abnormal laboratory test results. Also listed, in alphabetical order, are medications and herbal and natural remedies that interfere with the laboratory results.

- **Description:** concise description of the test or procedure, including interpretation of results and significance for various conditions.
- **Professional Considerations** include seven types of information:
  1. **Consent, risks, and contraindications:** indicates whether a separate special consent form IS or IS NOT required. Where tests or procedures carry significant risks, the risks that should be explained to the client are included in a highlighted alert box. *Contraindications* are in a list of generally accepted conditions (in a highlighted alert box labeled *Risks*) in which the test or procedure should not be performed and *Relative Contraindications* in which the test or procedure should be modified, where applicable.
  2. **Preparation:** includes supplies needed, assessment for allergies, unusual scheduling requirements, procedural preparation requirements, such as establishing intravenous access, equipment/medications needed to treat anaphylaxis, and medicolegal handling.
  3. **Procedure:** gives step-by-step description of specimen collection or procedural steps, including client positioning and participation, and monitoring required during the procedure. Note: For blood samples, mini-volumes (1 to 3 mL) are listed for tests in which special manual tests may be run on smaller volumes for clients in whom blood preservation is essential. For pediatric clients, microtainers may be used, but volumes should equate to those specified in the text (e.g., two 1-mL sized microtainers would be needed for a 2-mL specimen). For clients not at risk for iatrogenic anemia as a result of frequent blood sampling, the quickest turnaround times are achieved with higher volumes, which enable automated testing.
  4. **Postprocedure care:** provides aftercare instructions regarding specimen handling, site dressing, activity restriction, vital signs, and post-sedation monitoring.
  5. **Client and family teaching:** includes instructions the client or family should be informed about, including precare, procedural care, aftercare, and monitoring as well as disease-specific information, time frame for test results, and follow-up recommendations.
  6. **Factors that affect results:** gives quality assurance information about items that will interfere with the accuracy of results, such as improper collection techniques, improper specimen handling, drugs and herbals that cause false-positive or false-negative results, and cross-reactivity of other diseases or conditions.
  7. **Other data:** provides selected information from current research that may not yet be generalizable but could be helpful in decision-making for individuals or groups of clients; recommendations for confirmatory testing if the results are positive; direction to other tests related to the same diagnosis or condition and known association between tests; and national guideline information and recommendations, when available.

Contents

Diffusing capacity for carbon
  monoxide, Diagnostic
Hepatitis B surface antigen, Blood
Lymphocyte subset enumeration,
  Blood
Mantoux skin test, Diagnostic
Oral mucosal transudate, Specimen
Pneumocystis immunofluorescent
  assay, Serum
Pulmonary function tests, Diagnostic
Single-photon emission computed
  tomography, Brain, Diagnostic
Skin, Mycobacteria, Culture
★T- and B-lymphocyte subset assay,
  Blood
Throat culture for *Candida albicans,*
  Culture
Toxoplasmosis serology, Serum

Additional Conditions
Anemia
Blood transfusion that is allogenic
Candidiasis
Cervical cancer
Coccidioidomycosis
Cryptococcosis
Cryptosporidium
Cytomegalovirus
Diarrhea
Drug abuse
Encephalopathy
Esophagitis
Hemophilia
Herpes simplex
Histoplasmosis
Hypocalcemia
Isosporiasis
Kaposi's sarcoma
Leukoencephalopathy, multifocal
Lymphoma
Meningitis
Mycobacterium tuberculosis
Pneumonia
Septicemia
Sexual promiscuity
Stomatitis
Thrombocytopenia
Toxoplasmosis of the brain
Washing syndrome caused by HIV

ACROMEGALY
(see also Hyperpituitarism)
Alkaline phosphatase, Serum
Alkaline phosphatase, Isoenzymes,
  Serum
Calcium, Total, Serum
Calcium, Urine
★Glucose, Blood
★Growth hormone, Blood

Hydroxyproline, Total, 24-H(
★Insulin-like growth factor-1, b
  Phosphorus, Serum

Additional Conditions
Adenomas
Bronchial carcinoids
Gangliocytomas
Intestinal carcinoids
Lung carcinoma

ACTINOMYCOSIS
Acid-fast stain, *Nocardia* species,
  Culture
★*Actinomyces,* Culture
★Biopsy, Anaerobic, Culture
Biopsy, Routine, Culture
Biopsy, Fungus, Culture
Body fluid, Anaerobic, Culture
  (Abscess)
Bronchial aspirate, Routine, Culture
Bronchial washing, Specimen,
  Diagnostic
Brushing cytology, Specimen,
  Diagnostic
Cervical-vaginal cytology, Specimen
Endometrium, Anaerobic, Culture
Foreign body, Routine, Culture
Histopathology, Specimen
Sputum fungus, Specimen
Wound culture

Additional Conditions
Lung abscess
Pelvic inflammatory disease
Sinus infection
Tooth extraction

ACUTE MYOCARDIAL INFARCTION
(see Myocardial infarction)

ACUTE RESPIRATORY DISTRESS SYNDROME (ARDS)
★Blood gases, Arterial, Blood
★Chest radiography, Diagnostic
Complete blood count, Blood
CO-oximeter profile, Blood
C-reactive protein, Serum
Oximetry, Diagnostic
Prothrombin time and international
  normalized ratio, Plasma
★Pulmonary artery catheterization,
  Diagnostic
Pulmonary function tests, Diagnostic
Sputum culture and sensitivity,
  Specimen

PART ONE

Diseases, Conditions, and Symptoms

ABDOMINAL AORTIC ANEURYSM

(see Aneurysm, Abdominal aortic; Aneurysm, Cerebral; or Aneurysm, Thoracic aortic)

ABORTION

Alpha-fetoprotein, Blood
Amniotic fluid, Alpha$_1$-fetoprotein, Specimen
Amniotic fluid, Chromosome analysis, Specimen
Amniotic fluid, Erythroblastosis fetalis, Specimen
Chorionic villi sampling, Diagnostic
Endometrium, Anaerobic, Culture
Estriol, Serum or 24-hour urine
Glucose tolerance test, Blood
★Histopathology, Specimen
★Human chorionic gonadotropin, Beta-subunit, Serum
★Pregnancy test, Routine, Serum and qualitative urine
Progesterone, Serum
Type and crossmatch, Blood

Additional Conditions

Ectopic pregnancy
Pelvic inflammatory disease

ABSCESS

Actinomyces, Culture
Biopsy, Anaerobic, Culture
★Biopsy, Fungus, Culture
★Body fluid, Anaerobic, Culture (Abscess)
Bronchial aspirate, Routine, Culture
Histopathology, Specimen
Magnetic resonance imaging, Diagnostic
Skin, *Mycobacterium,* Culture
Sputum, Routine, Culture
Wound, Culture
Wound, Fungus, Culture
Wound, *Mycobacterium,* Culture

Additional Conditions

Bronchiectasis
Dental problems
Empyema
Fever
Foreign body
Otitis media
Pelvic inflammatory disease
Postoperative
Rheumatic heart disease
Scarlet fever
Sepsis

Sinusitis
Systemic inflammatory response syndrome (SIRS)
Urinary tract infection

ACHLORHYDRIA

Acid perfusion test, Diagnostic
★Gastric analysis, Specimen
Gastrin, Serum
★Histopathology, Specimen
Intrinsic factor antibody, Blood
Pepsinogen-I antibody, Blood
pH, Urine
Schilling test, Diagnostic
Urinalysis, Urine
Vitamin B$_{12}$, Serum

Additional Conditions

Gastric cancer
Gastric ulcer
Peptic ulcer

ACIDOSIS

(see Metabolic acidosis or Respiratory acidosis)

ACNE VULGARIS

Biopsy, Anaerobic, Culture
★Histopathology, Specimen

Additional Conditions

Hormonal changes
Puberty
Stress

ACQUIRED IMMUNODEFICIENCY SYNDROME (AIDS)

★Acquired immunodeficiency syndrome evaluation battery, Diagnostic
Beta$_2$-microglobulin, Blood and 24-hour urine
Biopsy, Site-specific, Specimen
Bronchoscopy, Diagnostic
Cerebrospinal fluid, Routine, Cult and cytology
Chest radiography, Diagnostic
Cryptococcal antibody titer, Serum
Cryptococcal antigen titer, Cerebrospinal fluid, Specimen
Cryptococcal antigen titer, Serum
Cryptosporidium diagnostic procedures, Stool
Cytomegalovirus antibody, Seru

Additional Conditions
Aspiration of gastric contents
Chronic obstructive pulmonary disease
Hypoxemia
Multiple blood transfusions
Pancreatitis
Pneumonia
Pulmonary infiltrate
Sepsis
Severe acute respiratory syndrome
  (SARS)
Trauma

ADDISON'S DISEASE
Alkaline phosphatase, Serum
Alkaline phosphatase, Isoenzymes,
  Serum
★Calcium, Total, Serum
Calcium, Urine
★Cortisol, Plasma or serum
★Glucose, Blood
Growth hormone, Blood
Hydroxyproline, Total, 24-Hour urine
Insulin-like growth factor-I, Blood
Magnesium, Serum
Metyrapone test, Serum
Phosphorus, Serum

Additional Conditions
ACTH (adrenocorticotropic hormone)
  deficiency
Adrenoleukodystrophy
Amyloidosis
Adrenal hyperplasia
Anticoagulant therapy
Candidiasis (thrush)
Cushing syndrome
Diabetes mellitus
Hypogonadism
Hypoparathyroidism
Lymphoid hyperplasia
Metastasis, Breast or lung cancer
Pernicious anemia
Schmidt syndrome
Thyroiditis

ADENOVIRUS INFECTION
★Adenovirus antibody titer, Serum
★Adenovirus immunofluorescence,
  Diagnostic
Ocular cytology, Specimen
★Viral culture, Specimen

Additional Conditions
Acute hemorrhagic cystitis
Common cold
Nonstreptococcal pharyngitis

ADRENALECTOMY
★Cortisol, Serum
Magnesium, Serum

Additional Conditions
Adrenal adenoma
Adrenal carcinoma
Waterhouse-Friderichsen syndrome

**ADULT RESPIRATORY DISTRESS
SYNDROME**
(*see Acute respiratory distress
syndrome*)

AGRANULOCYTOSIS
Blood culture, Blood
★Bone marrow aspiration analysis,
  Specimen
★Complete blood count, Blood
Culture, Skin, Specimen
Culture, Urine
★Differential leukocyte count,
  Peripheral blood

Additional Conditions
Anemia
Leukemia
Myelodysplastic syndromes

AHAPTOGLOBINEMIA
★Haptoglobin, Serum

Additional Conditions
Disseminated intravascular
  coagulation
Hemolytic transfusion reaction
Sepsis

AIDS
(*see Acquired immunodeficiency
syndrome*)

ALBRIGHT SYNDROME
Alkaline phosphatase, Serum
Bone radiography, Diagnostic
★Hydroxyproline, Total, 24-Hour urine

Additional Conditions
Acromegaly
Cushing syndrome
Hyperthyroidism
Osteomalacia
Ovarian cysts

ALCOHOLISM

Alanine aminotransferase, Serum
Albumin, Serum, Urine, and 24-Hour
  urine
★Alcohol, Blood
Alkaline phosphatase, Serum
Alkaline phosphatase, Isoenzymes,
  Serum
Ammonia, Blood
Amylase, Serum and urine
Anion gap, Blood
Aspartate aminotransferase, Serum
Bilirubin, Direct, Serum
Bilirubin, Total, Serum
Blood gases, Arterial, Blood
Blood indices (MCV), Blood
Chemistry profile, Blood
Complete blood count, Blood
Differential leukocyte count,
  Peripheral blood
Electrolytes, Plasma or serum
Folic acid, Serum
Gamma-glutamyltranspeptidase,
  Blood
Glucose, Blood
Heavy metals, Blood and 24-Hour
  urine
Hepatitis C antibody, Serum
Hepatitis serologies
Histopathology, Specimen
Ketone bodies, Blood
Ketones, Semiquantitative, Urine
Lactate dehydrogenase, Blood
Lactate dehydrogenase, Isoenzymes,
  Blood
Lactic acid, Blood
Lipid profile, Blood
★Liver battery, Serum
Magnesium, Serum
5'-Nucleotidase, Blood
Occult blood, Stool, Diagnostic
Osmolality, Calculated test, Blood
Osmolality, Serum
Phosphorus, Serum
Platelet count, Blood
Prothrombin time and international
  normalized ratio, Plasma
Red blood cell morphology, Blood
Schilling test, Diagnostic
Sedimentation rate, Erythrocyte,
  Blood
★Toxicology, Volatiles group by GLC,
  Blood or urine
Transferrin, Carbohydrate-deficient,
  Serum
Transthyretin (Prealbumin), Serum
Triglycerides, Blood
Uric acid, Serum
★Vitamin B$_{12}$, Serum
Zinc, Blood

Additional Conditions
Alcohol withdrawal syndrome
Anemia
Brain encephalopathy
Bronchitis
Cardiopulmonary
Chronic obstructive pulmonary
  disease
Cirrhosis
Coronary artery disease
Depression
Dermatitis
Dysfunctional family
Esophageal varices
Gastric varices
Gastritis
Hepatomegaly
Hypertension
Hypertriglyceridemia
Hypocalcemia
Hypoglycemia
Hypomagnesemia
Hypophosphatemia
Impotence
Malabsorption
Malnutrition
Organic brain syndrome
Pancreatitis
Pancytopenia
Peptic ulcer disease
Pneumonia, aspiration
Portal hypertension
Seizures
Suicide
Thrombocytopenia
Tobaccoism

ALKALOSIS
(see Metabolic alkalosis or Respiratory alkalosis)

ALLERGIC REACTION
(see Hypersensitivity reaction)

ALZHEIMER'S DISEASE
Apolipoprotein E4 genotyping,
  Plasma
★Beta-amyloid protein 40/42, CSF
Bromides, Serum
Cerebrospinal fluid immunoglobulin
  G, Immunoglobulin G ratios and
  Immunoglobulin G index,
  Immunoglobulin G synthesis rate,
  Specimen
Cerebrospinal fluid, Oligoclonal
  bands, Specimen

Cerebrospinal fluid, Protein, Specimen
Cerebrospinal fluid, Routine analysis, Specimen
Ceruloplasmin, Serum
Computed tomography of the brain, Diagnostic
Copper, Serum
Copper, Urine
Heavy metals, Blood and 24-Hour urine
Magnetic resonance spectroscopy, Diagnostic
Positron emission tomography, Diagnostic
Protein electrophoresis, Cerebrospinal fluid, Specimen
★Single-photon emission computed tomography, Brain, Diagnostic
★Tau test, Cerebrospinal fluid
Toxicology screen, Blood or urine
Transthyretin (prealbumin), Serum

Additional Conditions
Dementia
Malnutrition
Organic brain syndrome
Poisoning

AMAUROSIS FUGAX
★Viscosity, Serum

Additional Conditions
Arteriosclerotic heart disease
Arteritis, Temporal
Cerebrovascular accident
Rheumatic heart disease
Sepsis
Transient ischemic attack

AMENORRHEA
Adrenocorticotropic hormone, Serum
Chromosome analysis, Blood
Cortisol, Plasma or serum
Cortisol, Urine
Estradiol, Serum
★Estrogens, Serum and 24-Hour urine
Estrogens, Nonpregnant, 24-Hour urine
★Follicle-stimulating hormone, Serum
Histopathology, Specimen
Hormonal evaluation, Cytologic, Specimen
17-Hydroxycorticosteroids, 24-Hour urine
Luteinizing hormone, Blood

PAP smear, Diagnostic
Pregnancy test, Routine, Serum and qualitative, Urine
Prolactin, Serum
Testosterone, Free, Bioavailable and total, Blood
★Thyroid-stimulating hormone, Blood
Thyroid test: Free thyroxine index, Serum

Additional Conditions
Acromegaly
Anorexia nervosa
Azotemia
Cushing syndrome
Excessive exercise
Galactorrhea
Herpes zoster
Hypothyroidism
Menstrual irregularity
Perimenopause
Pituitary tumor
Pregnancy
Renal failure
Stress

AMIKACIN
(see Aminoglycoside toxicity)

AMINOGLYCOSIDE TOXICITY
(see Amikacin and Gentamicin)
Amikacin sulfate, Blood
Beta$_2$-microglobulin, Blood
Beta$_2$-microglobulin, Urine
Bicarbonate, Serum
Blood gases, Arterial, Blood
Blood volume, Blood
Blood urea nitrogen/creatinine ratio, Blood
Creatinine clearance, Serum, Urine
★Creatinine, Serum
Creatinine, Urine (Spot)
Electrolytes, Urine
Gentamicin, Blood
Kidney ultrasonography, Diagnostic
Osmolality, Calculated test, Blood
Osmolality, Serum
Osmolality, Urine
Renal indices (Fractional excretion of sodium), Diagnostic
Sodium, Plasma, Serum or urine
Specific gravity, Urine
Tobramycin, Serum
Urinalysis, Urine

Additional Conditions
Deafness
Neuromuscular weakness
Renal dysfunction
Renal failure (acute)

AMPUTATION
(see Surgery, Preoperative; Surgery, Postoperative)

AMYLOIDOSIS
Bone marrow aspiration analysis, Specimen
Chemistry profile, Blood
Concentration test, Urine
Computed tomography of the body (HRCT), Diagnostic
Creatinine clearance, Serum, Urine
★Creatinine, Serum
Cytologic study of gastrointestinal tract, Diagnostic
D-Xylose absorption test, Diagnostic, Serum or urine
Globulin, Serum
★Histopathology, Specimen
Immunoelectrophoresis, Serum and urine
Leukocyte cytochemistry, Specimen
Liver biopsy, Diagnostic
Liver ^{131}I scan, Diagnostic
★Protein electrophoresis, Serum
Protein electrophoresis, Urine
Protein, Quantitative, Urine
Protein, Semiquantitative, Urine
Skin, Mycobacteria, Culture
Urea nitrogen, Plasma or serum
Urinalysis, Urine

Additional Conditions
Cardiomegaly
Cardiomyopathy
Carpal tunnel syndrome
Chronic renal failure
Endocrine gland abnormality
Intestinal obstruction
Macroglossia
Nephrotic syndrome
Peripheral neuropathy
Respiratory failure

AMYOTROPHIC LATERAL SCLEROSIS (ALS)
Biopsy, Site-specific (Muscle), Specimen
Creatine kinase, Serum
Creatinine clearance, Serum, Urine

★Electromyography and nerve conduction (electromyelogram) studies, Diagnostic
Magnetic resonance neurography, Diagnostic

Additional Conditions
Dementia
Neurologic diseases
Parkinsonism

ANAPHYLAXIS
(see Shock)

ANEMIAS
(see Aplastic, Dyserythropoietic, Folic acid, G6PD deficiency, Galactokinase deficiency, Heinz body, Hemolytic, Iron [hypochromic] deficiency, Megaloblastic, Pernicious, or Sickle cell anemias)

ANESTHESIA
(see also Surgery, Preoperative; Surgery, Postoperative)
ABO group and Rh type, Blood
Blood gases, Arterial, Blood
★Chest radiography, Diagnostic
★Complete blood count, Blood
Echocardiography, Diagnostic
Electrocardiography, Diagnostic
Electrolytes, Plasma or serum

Additional Conditions
Pregnancy, Cesarean birth
Surgery
Trauma

ANEURYSM
(see Aneurysm, Abdominal aortic; Aneurysm, Cerebral; Aneurysm, Thoracic aortic)

ANEURYSM, ABDOMINAL AORTIC
★Abdominal aorta ultrasonography, Diagnostic
Cardiac catheterization, Diagnostic
Chest radiography, Diagnostic
★Computed tomography of the body (Abdomen), Diagnostic
★Flat plate radiography of the abdomen, Diagnostic

Fluorescent treponemal antibody–absorbed double-stain test, Serum
Lipid profile, Blood
★Magnetic resonance angiography, Diagnostic
★Magnetic resonance imaging, Diagnostic
Rapid plasma reagin test, Blood
Venereal Disease Research Laboratory test, Serum

Additional Conditions
Aortitis
Arteriosclerosis
Congenital defects
Congestive heart failure
Hypertension
Local infection
Marfan syndrome
Pregnancy
Syphilis
Trauma

ANEURYSM, CEREBRAL
Activated partial thromboplastin time, Plasma
★Cerebral angiography, Diagnostic
★Cerebral computed tomography, Diagnostic
Cerebrospinal fluid, Protein, Specimen
Computed tomography of the body (HRCT), Diagnostic
Doppler ultrasonographic flow studies, Diagnostic (Transcranial)
★Magnetic resonance angiography, Diagnostic
★Magnetic resonance imaging (Brain), Diagnostic
Prothrombin time and international normalized ratio, Plasma

Additional Conditions
Arteriosclerosis
Congestive heart failure
Hypertension
Local infection
Seizure
Syphilis
Trauma

ANEURYSM, THORACIC AORTIC
★Chest radiography, Diagnostic
Fluorescent treponemal antibody–absorbed double-stain test, Serum
Lipid profile, Blood

★Magnetic resonance angiography, Diagnostic
★Pulmonary angiography, Diagnostic
Rapid plasma reagin test, Blood
Venereal Disease Research Laboratory test, Serum

Additional Conditions
Arteriosclerosis
Congestive heart failure
Hypertension
Local infection
Syphilis
Trauma

ANGINA PECTORIS
Anticardiolipin antibody, Serum
Antimyocardial antibody, Serum
Aspartate aminotransferase, Serum
Cardiac catheterization, Diagnostic
Computed tomography of the body (EBCT), Diagnostic
★Coronary intravascular ultrasonography, Diagnostic
Creatine kinase, Serum
Creatine kinase, Isoenzymes, Serum
D-Dimer test, Blood
Echocardiography, Diagnostic
★Electrocardiography, Diagnostic
Ergonovine provocation test, Diagnostic
Stress exercise test, Diagnostic
Heart scan, Diagnostic
Holter monitor, Diagnostic
Homocysteine, Plasma or urine
Lactate dehydrogenase, Isoenzymes, Blood
★Lipid profile, Blood
Positive emission tomography, Diagnostic
★Stress exercise test, Diagnostic
★Stress test, Pharmacologic, Diagnostic
Troponin I, Serum
Troponin T, Serum

Additional Conditions
Aortic stenosis
Cervical spine/disk disease
Diabetes mellitus
Gallbladder disease
Herpes zoster
Hypertension
Mitral valve prolapse
Myocardial infarction
Myocarditis
Peptic ulcer disease
Pericarditis
Peripheral vascular disease
Reflux esophagitis

Rheumatic fever
Thyrotoxicosis
Xanthelasma
Xanthomas

ANKYLOSING SPONDYLITIS
Antinuclear antibody, Serum
* C-reactive protein, Serum
Human leukocyte antigen B-27,
  Blood
* Immunoglobin G, Serum
Immunoglobulin M, Serum
Magnetic resonance imaging
  (Sacroiliac spine), Diagnostic
Protein electrophoresis, Serum
* Radiography (Bone), Diagnostic
Rheumatoid factor, Blood
* Sedimentation rate, Erythrocyte,
  Blood

Additional Conditions
Aortic insufficiency
Atrioventricular conduction defects
Diffuse idiopathic skeletal
  hyperostosis (DISH) syndrome
Herniated disc
Pulmonary fibrosis
Rheumatoid arthritis

ANOREXIA NERVOSA
* Estradiol, Serum
17-Hydroxycorticosteroids, 24-Hour
  urine
Low-density lipoprotein cholesterol,
  Blood
* Luteinizing hormone, Blood
Phenolphthalein test, Diagnostic
Potassium, Serum
Protein-bound iodine, Blood
Thyroid test: Free thyroxine index,
  Serum
* Thyroid test: Triiodothyronine, Blood
Thyroid test: Thyroxine, Blood
* Transthyretin (Prealbumin),
  Serum

Additional Conditions
Amenorrhea
Anovulation
Anxiety
Depression
Electrolyte disturbances
Endocrine disorders
Hypoglycemia
Hypotension
Malnutrition

ANOXIA
Apnea test, Diagnostic
Bicarbonate, Serum
* Blood gases, Arterial, Blood
Blood gases, Capillary, Blood
Blood gases, Venous, Blood
Carbon dioxide, Partial pressure, Blood
Carbon dioxide, Total content, Blood
Chest radiography, Diagnostic
Diffusing capacity for carbon
  monoxide, Diagnostic
Doppler ultrasonographic flow
  studies (Transcranial), Diagnostic
Electroencephalography, Diagnostic
Lactic Acid, Blood
Magnetic resonance angiography,
  Diagnostic
Magnetic resonance imaging,
  Diagnostic
* Oxygen saturation, Blood
Single-photon emission computed
  tomography, Brain, Diagnostic
Ultrasonography, Brain, Diagnostic

Additional Conditions
Anemia
Asthma
Carbon monoxide poisoning
Cerebral edema
Congestive heart failure
Diabetes mellitus
Emphysema
Empyema
Head trauma
Hepatic encephalopathy
Hypertension
Seizures

ANTHRAX
* Blood culture, Blood
Chest radiography, Diagnostic
Complete blood count, Blood
* Culture, Skin, Specimen
Differential leukocyte count,
  Peripheral blood
Gram stain, Diagnostic
Hypersensitivity pneumonitis
  serology, Blood

Additional Conditions
Cyanosis
Fever
Headache
Hemorrhagic meningitis
Nausea
Pneumonia
Sepsis
Shock
Vomiting

ANTIGENS
(see Immunoglobulin A)

ANXIETY
Blood gases, Arterial, Blood
Complete blood count, Blood
Electrocardiography, Diagnostic
Epinephrine, Blood
*Norepinephrine, Serum
Toxicology screen, Urine

Additional Conditions
Alcoholism
Depression
Drug abuse
Fever
Hyperventilation
Hypoxia
Mitral valve prolapse
Pain
Phobias
Sleep disturbances
Stress
Tachycardia

AORTIC ANEURYSM
(see Aneurysm, Abdominal aortic)

AORTIC VALVULAR STENOSIS
Blood gases, Arterial, Blood
Cardiac catheterization,
    Diagnostic
Chest radiography, Diagnostic
Digital subtraction angiography and
    transvenous-digital subtraction,
    Diagnostic
*Echocardiography, Diagnostic
Electrocardiography, Diagnostic
*Magnetic resonance angiography,
    Diagnostic
Transesophageal ultrasonography,
    Diagnostic

Additional Conditions
Angina
Cardiomegaly
Cardiomyopathy
Deep vein thrombosis
Dysrhythmias
Cerebrovascular accident
Congenital aortic narrowing
Myocardial infarction
Rheumatic fever
Syncope

AORTITIS
*Abdominal aortic ultrasonography,
    Diagnostic
*Complete blood count, Blood
Lipid profile, Blood
Rapid plasma reagin test, Blood
Venereal Disease Research Laboratory
    test, Serum

Additional Conditions
Endocarditis
Rheumatic heart disease
Scarlet fever
Sepsis
Syphilis

APLASTIC ANEMIA
*Bone marrow biopsy, Diagnostic
*Complete blood count, Blood
Differential leukocyte count,
    Peripheral blood
Mixed leukocyte culture, Specimen
Red blood cell morphology, Blood

Additional Conditions
Hypoplastic bone marrow
Leukemia
Pancytopenia
Systemic lupus erythematosus

APPENDICITIS
Blood culture, Blood
Body fluid, Anaerobic, Culture
    (Abscess)
*Complete blood count, Blood
*Differential leukocyte count,
    Peripheral blood
Histopathology (Postoperatively),
    Specimen
Infectious mononucleosis screening
    test, Blood
Occult blood, Stool
Urinalysis, Urine

Additional Conditions
Abscess
Acute pain, right lower quadrant
    (RLQ) abdomen
Amebiasis
Crohn's disease
Enteritis
Leukocytosis
Peritonitis

ARDS
*(see Acute respiratory distress
syndrome)*

ARRHYTHMIAS
(see Dysrhythmias)

ARTERIAL ISCHEMIC LEG ULCER
(see Peripheral vascular disease)

ARTERIAL OCCLUSION
(see Occlusion, Acute arterial)

ARTERIAL THROMBOSIS
(see Thrombosis)

ARTERIOSCLEROSIS
Activated partial thromboplastin time, Plasma
Anticardiolipin antibody, Serum
C-reactive protein, Blood
Cholesterol, Blood
Computed tomography of the body (EBCT), Diagnostic
★Coronary intravascular ultrasonography, Diagnostic
★Doppler ultrasonographic flow studies, Diagnostic
Electrocardiography, Diagnostic
High-density lipoprotein cholesterol, Blood
Homocysteine, Plasma or urine
★Lipid profile, Blood
Low-density lipoprotein cholesterol, Blood
Mean platelet volume, Blood
Prothrombin time and international normalized ratio, Plasma
Stress exercise test, Diagnostic
Stress plasma reagin, Pharmacologic, Diagnostic
Triglycerides, Blood

Additional Conditions
Arteriosclerotic heart disease
Arteriosclerosis obliterans
Coronary heart disease
Hypertension
Organic brain syndrome
Transient ischemic attack

ARTERIOSCLEROTIC HEART DISEASE
(see Arteriosclerosis)

ARTERITIS
★Biopsy, Site-specific (Temporal artery), Specimen
★Complete blood cell count, Blood
★Sedimentation rate, Erythrocyte, Blood

Additional Conditions
Anorexia
Atherosclerosis
Brain tumor
Headache
Multiple sclerosis
Transient ischemic attack
Vasculitis
Vision loss

ARTHRITIS
(see Osteoarthritis, Rheumatoid arthritis)

ASBESTOSIS
(see Industry-related diseases)

ASCITES
★Albumin, Serum, Urine and 24-Hour urine
Amylase, Serum and urine (Serum)
Body fluid analysis, Cell count, Specimen
★Body fluid cytology, Specimen
Flat-plate radiography of the abdomen (Kidneys, ureters, bladder), Diagnostic
Lipase, Serum
Liver battery, Serum
Paracentesis, Diagnostic
★Ultrasonography, Abdomen, Diagnostic

Additional Conditions
Alcoholism
Burns
Congestive heart failure
Cirrhosis
Esophageal/gastric varices
Hepatopulmonary syndrome
Hyponatremia
Malignancy
Malnutrition
Myxedema
Ovarian cancer
Pancreatitis
Peritonitis
Pleural effusion
Portal hypertension
Wilson's disease

ASHD/ARTERIOSCLEROTIC HEART DISEASE
(see Arteriosclerosis)

ASPIRATION PNEUMONIA
(see Pneumonia)

ASPIRIN POISONING
(see Poisoning, Salicylate)

ASTERIXIS
(see Liver failure)

ASTHMA
Acid perfusion test (Nocturnal asthma), Diagnostic
★ Allergen-specific IgE antibody, Serum
Bicarbonate, Serum
Blood gases, Arterial, Blood
Carbon dioxide, Partial pressure, Blood
Carbon dioxide, Total content, Blood
★ Chest radiography, Diagnostic
Complete blood count, Blood
Differential leukocyte count, Peripheral blood
Diffusing capacity for carbon monoxide, Diagnostic
Eosinophil count, Blood
Eosinophil peroxidase, Serum
Eosinophil smear (Fecal/nasal/sputum), Specimen
Hypersensitivity pneumonitis serology, Blood
Immunoglobulin E, Serum
Low-density lipoprotein cholesterol, Blood
Methacholine challenge test, Diagnostic
Ova and parasites, Stool
★ Pulmonary function tests, Diagnostic
Sputum cytology, Specimen
Theophylline, Blood

Additional Conditions
Allergies
Beta blockade
Bronchitis
Chronic obstructive pulmonary disease
Pneumonia

Pneumonitis
Pulmonary infection
Stress
Tachycardia

ATAXIA
Alcohol, Blood
Antistreptolysin-O titer, Serum
Benzodiazepines, Plasma and urine
★ Computed tomography, Brain, Diagnostic
Heavy metals, Blood and 24-Hour urine
Lead, Blood and urine
Magnesium, Serum
★ Oculoplethysmography, Diagnostic
Oculopneumoplethysmography, Diagnostic
Phenothiazines, Blood
Phenytoin, Serum
SCA gene test, Diagnostic
Streptozyme, Blood
Venereal Disease Research Laboratory test, Cerebrospinal fluid, Specimen

Additional Conditions
Aminoglycoside reaction
Aspirin toxicity
Brain tumor
Cerebrovascular accident
Labyrinthitis
Ménière's disease
Multiple sclerosis
Transient ischemic attack

ATELECTASIS
★ Blood gases, Arterial, Blood
★ Chest radiography, Diagnostic
Complete blood count, Blood

Additional Conditions
Chest trauma
Chronic obstructive pulmonary disease
Empyema
Neuromuscular disease
Pneumonia
Postoperative
Pulmonary embolism

ATHEROSCLEROSIS
(see Arteriosclerosis)

ATHLETE'S FOOT
★ Culture, Skin, Specimen

Additional Conditions
Cellulitis
Lymphadenitis
Lymphangitis

ATRIAL SEPTAL DEFECT
★Blood gases, Arterial, Blood
Cardiac catheterization, Diagnostic
Chest radiography, Diagnostic
★Echocardiography, Diagnostic
Electrocardiography, Diagnostic
Heart scan, Diagnostic
Pulmonary artery catheterization,
  Diagnostic
★Ventriculography, Diagnostic

Additional Conditions
Bundle branch block
Cleft mitral valve leaflet

AUSTRALIAN ANTIGEN
(see Hepatitis)

AUTOIMMUNE DISEASES
(see Amyloidosis, Ankylosing
spondylitis, Goodpasture
syndrome, Raynaud's disease,
Rheumatic fever, Rheumatoid
arthritis, Scleroderma, Sjögren
syndrome, Systemic lupus
erythematosus, or Vasculitis)

AZOTEMIA
Blood urea nitrogen/creatinine ratio,
  Blood
Calcium, Total, Serum
Chemistry profile, Blood
Creatinine clearance, Serum, Urine
★Creatinine, Serum
Creatinine, Urine (Spot)
★Electrolytes, Plasma or serum
Electrolytes, Urine
Flat-plate radiography of the
  abdomen (Kidneys, ureters,
  bladder), Diagnostic
Kidney ultrasonography (Kidneys,
  ureters, bladder), (Doppler)
  Diagnostic
Occult blood, Stool
Osmolality, Calculated test, Blood
Osmolality, Serum
Osmolality, Urine
Phosphorus, Serum
Phosphorus, Urine
Protein, Semiquantitative, Urine
★Urea nitrogen, Plasma or serum

Uric acid, Serum
Urinalysis, Urine

Additional Conditions
Amenorrhea
Anemia
Congestive heart failure
Hyperglycemia
Hyperparathyroidism
Hypertension
Hypothyroidism
Impotence
Infertility
Metabolic acidosis
Osteomalacia
Pericarditis
Pulmonary edema
Renal failure
Uremia

BACTEREMIA
(see Sepsis)

BACTERIAL ENDOCARDITIS
(see Endocarditis)

BELL'S PALSY
★Electromyography and nerve
  conduction studies, Diagnostic

Additional Conditions
Herpes simplex virus

BENIGN PROSTATIC HYPERTROPHY
Acid phosphatase, Serum
Alkaline phosphatase, Serum
Bicarbonate, Serum
Chemistry profile, Blood
Complete blood count, Blood
Electrolytes, Plasma or serum
Occult blood, Urine
Prostate-specific antigen, Blood
★Urinalysis, Urine

Additional Conditions
Uremia
Urinary retention
Incontinence
Impotence

BERGER'S DISEASE
Biopsy, Site-specific (Renal),
  Specimen

Creatinine clearance, 12- or 24-Hour
urine
★Immunoglobulin A, Serum
Intravenous pyelography, Diagnostic
★Urinalysis, Urine

Additional Conditions
Hematuria
Hypertension
Immune complex glomerulopathies
Proteinuria
Upper respiratory tract disease

BERIBERI
Chest radiography, Diagnostic
Electrocardiography, Diagnostic
Electromyography and nerve
conduction studies, Diagnostic
★Vitamin B_1, Serum or urine

Additional Conditions
Cardiomegaly
Congestive heart failure
Hepatomegaly
Korsakoff syndrome
Pulmonary edema
Tachycardia
Wernicke's encephalopathy

BERNARD-SOULIER SYNDROME
★Platelet adhesion test, Diagnostic
★Platelet aggregation, Blood
Platelet aggregation, Hypercoagulable
state, Blood
Platelet count, Blood
von Willebrand factor assay, Blood

Additional Conditions
Postoperative bleeding

BETA-GLUCURONIDASE SYNDROME
★Mucopolysaccharides, Qualitative,
Urine

Additional Conditions
Amyloidosis
Leukemia

BILIARY CALCULI
★Bile, Urine
Urobilinogen, Urine

Additional Conditions
Cholecystitis
Jaundice
Pancreatitis

BILIRUBINURIA
★Bile, Urine
Gallbladder and biliary system
ultrasonography, Diagnostic

Additional Conditions
Jaundice
Renal failure

BLACK LUNG DISEASE
(see Silicosis)

BLEPHARITIS
★Culture, Routine, Specimen (Eye
margin)

Additional Conditions
Herpes zoster
Seborrhea

BOTULISM
Body fluid, Anaerobic, Culture
(Abscess)
★Botulism, Diagnostic procedures,
Stool
Clostridium difficile toxin assay,
Stool
Complete blood count, Blood
★Culture, Stool, Specimen
Electromyography and nerve
conduction studies, Diagnostic

Additional Conditions
Fever
Gastritis
Paralytic ileus

BOWEL OBSTRUCTION
(see Obstruction)

BRADYCARDIA
★Complete blood count,
Blood
Creatine kinase, Isoenzymes,
Blood
Digitoxin, Serum
Digoxin, Serum
Disopyramide phosphate, Serum
Echocardiography, Diagnostic
★Electrocardiography, Diagnostic
★Electrolytes, Plasma or serum
Propranolol, Blood
Quinidine, Serum
Thyroid profile, Blood

Toxicology drug screen, Blood or urine
Troponin I, Serum

Additional Conditions
Atrioventricular heart block
Beta blockade
Calcium-channel blockade
Coronary artery disease
Infections, Severe
Jaundice
Myocardial infarction
Phenytoin, Rapid intravenous usage
Sick sinus syndrome
Sinus arrest

BRAIN ABSCESS
(see Abscess)

BRAIN CANCER
★Brain biopsy, Diagnostic
Computed tomography of the brain, Diagnostic
Electroencephalography, Diagnostic
Dual modality imaging, Diagnostic
★Magnetic resonance imaging, Diagnostic
Magnetic resonance spectroscopy, Diagnostic
Positron emission tomography, Diagnostic
Telomerase enzyme marker, Blood

Additional Conditions
Nausea
Personality changes
Seizures

BRAIN DEATH
Apnea test, Diagnostic
Autopsy, Diagnostic
Brain scan, Cerebral flow and pathology, Diagnostic
★Brainstem auditory evoked potential, Diagnostic
Carbon dioxide, Partial pressure, Blood
Cerebral angiography, Diagnostic
Doppler ultrasonographic flow studies (Transcranial), Diagnostic
★Electroencephalography, Diagnostic
Magnetic resonance angiography, Diagnostic
Magnetic resonance imaging, Diagnostic

Additional Conditions
Anoxia
Cerebral hemorrhage
Coma
Multiple system failure
Organ/tissue donation
Trauma

BRAIN TUMORS
★Brain biopsy, Diagnostic
Carcinoembryonic antigen, Serum
Cerebral angiography, Diagnostic
Cerebrospinal fluid, Protein, Specimen
Cerebrospinal fluid, Routine analysis, Specimen
★Computed tomography of the brain, Diagnostic
Doppler ultrasonographic flow studies, Diagnostic
Histopathology, Specimen
Homovanillic acid, 24-Hour urine
Ki-67 proliferation marker, Specimen
Magnetic resonance angiography, Diagnostic
★Magnetic resonance imaging (Diffusion-weighted), Diagnostic
Metanephrines, Total, 24-Hour urine and free plasma
Neuron-specific enolase, Serum
Octreotide scan, Diagnostic
Vanillylmandelic acid, Urine

Additional Conditions
Epilepsy
Hallucinations
Nausea
Personality changes
Seizures

BREAST CANCER
Alanine aminotransferase, Serum
Alkaline phosphatase, Serum
Alpha-fetoprotein, Blood
★Biopsy, Site-specific (Breast, lymph nodes), Specimen
BRCA (Breast cancer tumor suppressor genes) 1 and 2, Serum
Breast ultrasonography, Diagnostic
CA 15-3, Serum
CA 50, Blood
CA 125, Blood
CA 549, Blood
Calcitonin, Plasma or serum
Calcium, Total, Serum
Carcinoembryonic antigen, Serum
Cathepsin D, Serum

DNA ploidy, Specimen
Dual modality imaging, Diagnostic
Estradiol receptor and progesterone receptor in breast cancer, Diagnostic
Estrogen receptor assay, Tissue specimen
Follicle-stimulating hormone, Serum
HER-2/*neu* oncogene, Specimen
Ki-67 proliferation marker, Specimen
Liver battery, Serum
Magnetic resonance imaging, Diagnostic
Mammography, Diagnostic
Methotrexate, Serum
Mitogen-activated protein kinase, Specimen
Mucinlike carcinoma–associated antigen, Blood
Needle aspiration cytology (Breast cysts and abscesses), Diagnostic
Progesterone receptor assay, Specimen
Prolactin, Serum
Scintimammography, Diagnostic
★Stereotactic breast biopsy, Specimen
Telomerase enzyme marker, Blood

Additional Conditions
Chronic mastitis
Fibrocystic breast disease
Gynecologic cancer
Metastasis
Paget's disease, Breast

BRONCHITIS, ACUTE OR CHRONIC
Bicarbonate, Serum
Blood gases, Arterial, Blood
Blood gases, Venous, Blood
Bronchial aspirate, Fungus, Culture
Bronchial aspirate, Routine (Anaerobic), Culture
Bronchoscopy, Diagnostic
Carbon dioxide, Partial pressure, Blood
Carbon dioxide, Total content, Blood
★Chest radiography, Diagnostic
Chloride, Sweat, Specimen
Complete blood count, Blood
Low-density lipoprotein cholesterol, Blood
★Pulmonary function tests, Diagnostic
Sputum, Routine, Culture
Theophylline, Blood

Additional Conditions
Allergies
Chemical irritation
Chronic obstructive pulmonary disease
Upper respiratory infections

BRUCELLOSIS
Bone marrow aspiration analysis, Specimen
★Brucellosis agglutinins, Blood
★Brucellosis skin test, Diagnostic
Differential leukocyte count, Peripheral blood
Liver battery, Serum

Additional Conditions
Anemia
Fever
Joint pain
Lymphadenopathy
Splenomegaly

BUERGER'S DISEASE
(*see Thromboangiitis obliterans*)

BULIMIA
★Electrolytes, Plasma or serum
Electrolytes, Urine
Glucose, Fasting, Blood
★Phenolphthalein test, Diagnostic
Protein, Total, Serum

Additional Conditions
Alcoholism
Anxiety
Constipation
Dental caries
Depression
Electrolyte imbalance
Esophagitis
Malnutrition
Post-traumatic stress disorder
Upper gastrointestinal bleeding

BULIMOREXIA
(*see Anorexia nervosa or Bulimia*)

BURNS
Activated partial thromboplastin time, Plasma
Albumin, Serum, Urine and 24-Hour urine
Albumin/globulin ratio, Serum
Blood culture, Blood
Blood gases, Arterial, Blood

Blood urea nitrogen/creatinine ratio, Blood
Complete blood count, Blood
Culture, Routine, Specimen
D-Dimer test, Blood
★ Electrolytes, Plasma or serum
Electrolytes, Urine
Fibrinogen, Plasma
Hemoglobin, Plasma and qualitative, Urine
Occult blood, Urine
Osmolality, Calculated test, Blood
Osmolality, Serum
★ Protein, Total, Serum
Prothrombin time and international normalized ratio, Plasma
Pseudocholinesterase, Plasma

Additional Conditions
Alcoholism
Chemical irritant exposure
Diabetes mellitus
Dysrhythmias
Electrolyte imbalance
High-voltage injury
Psychiatric illness
Renal failure
Respiratory failure
Smoke inhalation

BURSITIS
Body fluid analysis, Cell count, Specimen
Radiography, Diagnostic

Additional Conditions
Gout
Rheumatoid arthritis

CABG
(see Coronary artery bypass graft)

CACHEXIA
(see Kwashiorkor or Marasmus)

CALCULI
(see Renal calculi or Biliary calculi)

CANCER
(see specific type of cancer and Ganglioneuroblastoma, Hodgkin's disease, Leukemia, Lymphoma, Metastasis, Neuroblastoma, or Wilms' tumor)

CANDIDIASIS
(see Thrush, Vaginitis)

CANNABIS DRUG ABUSE
(see Drug abuse)

CARBOHYDRATE-DEFICIENT GLYCOPROTEIN SYNDROME
★ Transferrin, Carbohydrate-deficient, Serum

Additional Conditions
Mental retardation
Psychomotor retardation
Thyroid disorder

CARBON MONOXIDE POISONING
Bicarbonate, Plasma
★ Blood gases, Arterial, Blood
★ Carbon monoxide, Blood
Carboxyhemoglobin, Blood
CO-oximeter profile, Blood
Diffusing capacity for carbon monoxide, Diagnostic
Electrocardiography, Diagnostic
Oximetry, Diagnostic

Additional Conditions
Coma
Hypoxia
Psychiatric illness

CARCINOMA
(see Cancer)

CARDIOGENIC SHOCK
(see Shock)

CARDIOMYOPATHY
Alanine aminotransferase, Serum
Aspartate aminotransferase, Serum
Cardiac enzymes/isoenzymes, Blood
Cardiac output, Diagnostic
Cardiac radiography, Diagnostic
★ Chest radiography, Diagnostic
Coronary intravascular ultrasonography, Diagnostic
Creatine kinase, Serum
★ Echocardiography, Diagnostic
Electrocardiography, Diagnostic
Electron microscopy (for Cardiomyopathy), Diagnostic

Histopathology, Specimen
Hydroxybutyrate dehydrogenase,
 Blood
Lactate dehydrogenase, Blood
Lactate dehydrogenase, Isoenzymes,
 Blood
Transesophageal ultrasonography,
 Diagnostic
Viral culture, Specimen

Additional Conditions
Congestive heart failure
Endocarditis
Familial trait
Hypertension, Chronic
Inflammatory processes
Neuromuscular disease
Radiation
Status post heart transplantation
Valvular regurgitation
Valvular stenosis
Ventriculography, Diagnostic
Viral infection

CARPAL TUNNEL SYNDROME
Electromyography and nerve
 conduction studies, Diagnostic
* Magnetic resonance neurography,
 Diagnostic

Additional Conditions
Alcoholism
Amyloidosis
Diabetes mellitus
Hyperparathyroidism
Leukemia
Myxedema
Rheumatoid arthritis
Sarcoidosis
Synovitis

CAT-SCRATCH DISEASE
* Biopsy, Site-specific (Lymph node),
 Specimen
Complete blood count, Blood
Differential leukocyte count,
 Peripheral blood
Lupus test, Blood
* *Rochalimaea henselae,* Antibody,
 Serum
Sedimentation rate, Erythrocyte,
 Blood
Skin test for hypersensitivity,
 Diagnostic

Additional Conditions
Encephalitis
Lymphadenopathy

CATARACTS
Galactokinase, Blood

Additional Conditions
Congenital abnormality
Diabetes mellitus
Trauma

CELIAC SPRUE
* Barium enema, Diagnostic
Complete blood count, Blood
Endomysial antibody, Serum
* Fecal fat, Quantitative, 72-Hour stool
Red blood cell size distribution
 width, Blood
Sigmoidoscopy, Diagnostic
* D-Xylose absorption test, Diagnostic,
 Serum

Additional Conditions
Enteritis
Gastric fistula
Lymphoma
Whipple's disease

CEREBRAL ANEURYSM
(see Aneurysm, Cerebral)

CEREBRAL ARTERIOVENOUS MALFORMATIONS
* Magnetic resonance angiography,
 Diagnostic

Additional Conditions
Congenital disease
Lung cancer
Polycythemia, Secondary

CEREBRAL INFARCTION
(see Cerebrovascular accident)

CEREBRAL INFECTIONS
(see Encephalitis or Meningitis)

CEREBRAL PALSY
Chloride, Serum
Computed tomography of the brain,
 Diagnostic
Electroencephalography, Diagnostic
Magnetic resonance imaging, Diagnostic
Pneumoencephalography, Diagnostic
* Potassium, Serum
* Sodium, Plasma, Serum or urine

Additional Conditions
Anemia
Cerebrovascular accident
Drug abuse
Hyperbilirubinemia
Meningitis
Rubella
Toxemia
Toxoplasmosis

CEREBROVASCULAR ACCIDENT (CVA)
Activated partial thromboplastin time, Plasma
Brain scan, Cerebral flow and pathology, Diagnostic
★Cerebral computed tomography, Diagnostic
Cerebrospinal fluid, Lactic acid, Specimen
Cerebrospinal fluid, Routine analysis, Specimen
Complete blood count, Blood
Computed tomography of the body (Spiral), Diagnostic
Differential leukocyte count, Peripheral blood
Doppler ultrasonographic flow studies (Carotid), Diagnostic
Electrolytes, Plasma or serum
Homocysteine, Plasma or urine
Magnetic resonance angiography, Diagnostic
★Magnetic resonance imaging (of brain) (Diffusion-weighted), Diagnostic
Magnetic resonance spectroscopy, Diagnostic
Platelet count, Blood
Prothrombin time and international normalized ratio, Plasma
Transesophageal ultrasonography, Diagnostic

Additional Conditions
Arteriosclerotic heart disease
Brain tumor
Cerebral aneurysm
Emboli
Hypertension
Seizure
Subdural hemorrhage

CERVICAL CANCER
★Cervical-vaginal cytology, Specimen
Colposcopy, Diagnostic
Conization of cervix, Diagnostic

Dual modality imaging, Diagnostic
Human papillomavirus in situ hybridization, Specimen
Ki-67 proliferation marker, Specimen
★Pap smear, Diagnostic
Pap smear, Ultrafast, Diagnostic
Tumor antigen 4, Blood and specimen
Telomerase enzyme marker, Blood
Thymidylate synthase, Specimen
Urinary chorionic gonadotropin peptide, Urine

Additional Conditions
Dysmenorrhea
Herpes virus

CERVICAL SPONDYLOSIS
Computed tomography of body (Spine), Diagnostic
★Magnetic-resonance imaging, Diagnostic
Radiography (Cervical disks of spine), Diagnostic

Additional Conditions
Myelopathy
Trauma to spine

CERVICITIS
★Cervical-vaginal cytology, Specimen
Chlamydia culture and group titer, Specimen (Culture)
Genital, *Neisseria gonorrhoeae*, Culture
Herpes virus antigen, Direct fluorescent antibody, Specimen
★Histopathology, Specimen
Human papillomavirus in situ hybridization, Specimen
Rapid plasma reagin test, Blood
Trichomonas preparation, Specimen
Urine culture and nucleic acid amplification tests for *Neisseria gonorrhoeae*, Urine
Urinary chorionic gonadotropin peptide, Urine
Venereal Disease Research Laboratory test, Serum

Additional Conditions
Abortion
Gonorrhea
Herpes virus
Syphilis

CHANCROID
★Genital, Bacillus *Haemophilus ducreyi*, Culture

Additional Conditions
Adenitis

Peptic ulcer disease
Sepsis

CHEST PAIN
*(see Angina Pectoris, Myocardial
infarction, Pleurisy, or Pneumonia)*

CHOLELITHIASIS
Alanine aminotransferase, Serum
Amylase, Serum
Bile fluid examination, Diagnostic
Bile, Urine
* Bilirubin, Serum
Chemistry profile, Blood
* Cholecystography radiography,
  Diagnostic
Chorionic villi sampling, Diagnostic
Endoscopic retrograde
  cholangiopancreatography,
  Diagnostic
Endoscopic ultrasonography,
  Diagnostic
Flat-plate radiography of the
  abdomen, Diagnostic
* Gallbladder and biliary system
  ultrasonography, Diagnostic
Histopathology, Specimen
Leucine aminopeptidase, Blood
Lipase, Serum
* Magnetic resonance
  cholangiopancreatography,
  Diagnostic
T-tube cholangiography
  (Postoperative), Diagnostic

Additional Conditions
Cholecystitis
Enteritis
Pregnancy

CHICKENPOX
Differential leukocyte count,
  Peripheral blood
* Varicella-zoster virus serology,
  Serum
* Tzanck test smear, Specimen

Additional Conditions
Herpes zoster
Leukopenia

CHLAMYDIA
Cervical-vaginal cytology, Specimen
* *Chlamydia* culture and group titer,
  Specimen (Culture)
Lymphogranuloma venereum titer,
  Blood
Ocular cytology, Specimen
Psittacosis titer, Blood

Additional Conditions
Keratoconjunctivitis
Lymphogranuloma venereum
Pneumonia
Proctitis
Vaginitis

CHRISTMAS DISEASE
(see Factor IX deficiency)

CHRONIC FATIGUE SYNDROME
* Dexamethasone suppression test,
  Diagnostic

Additional Conditions
Anemia
Autoimmune diseases
Depression
Mononucleosis
Multiple sclerosis

CHOLECYSTITIS
Amylase, Serum
* Bilirubin, Serum
Bilirubin, Urine
Cholecystography radiography,
  Diagnostic
Endoscopic retrograde
  cholangiopancreatography,
  Diagnostic
* Gallbladder and biliary system
  ultrasonography, Diagnostic
Gamma-glutamyltranspeptidase,
  Blood
Glucose, Serum (Random)
Histopathology, Specimen
Ornithine carbamoyltransferase,
  Blood

Additional Conditions
Gallstones
Pancreatitis

CHRONIC OBSTRUCTIVE
PULMONARY DISEASES
*(see Asthma, Bronchitis, or
Emphysema)*

CIRRHOSIS
Alanine aminotransferase, Serum
★Albumin, Serum, Urine and 24-Hour urine
Albumin/globulin ratio, Serum
Aldosterone, Serum and urine
Alkaline phosphatase, Heat stable, Serum
Alkaline phosphatase, Isoenzymes, Serum
Alkaline phosphatase, Serum
Alpha$_1$-antitrypsin, Serum
★Ammonia, Blood
Antimitochondrial antibody, Blood
Antinuclear antibody, Serum
Anti–smooth muscle antibody, Serum
Antithrombin III test, Diagnostic
Aspartate aminotransferase, Serum
★Bilirubin, Direct, Serum
Ceruloplasmin, Serum
Chemistry profile, Blood
Cold agglutinin titer, Serum
Copper, Serum or urine
Cryoglobulin, Qualitative, Serum
Endoscopic retrograde cholangiopancreatography, Diagnostic
Gamma-glutamyltranspeptidase, Blood
Hepatitis B surface antibody, Blood
Hepatitis B surface antigen, Blood
Histopathology, Specimen
Immunoglobulin M, Serum
Iron, Serum
Iron and total iron-binding capacity/transferrin, Serum
Lactate dehydrogenase, Blood
Lactate dehydrogenase, Isoenzymes, Blood
Leucine aminopeptidase, Blood
★Liver battery, Serum
Mucinlike carcinoma–associated antigen, Blood
5′-Nucleotidase, Blood
Ornithine carbamoyltransferase, Blood
★Prothrombin time and international normalized ratio, Plasma
Red blood cell morphology, Blood
Sodium, Serum
Urobilinogen, Urine
Zinc, Blood

Additional Conditions
Alcoholism
Anasarca
Ascites
Hepatitis
Jaundice
Osteomalacia

Pancreatitis
Pleural effusion
Varices

COARCTATION OF THE AORTA
Blood gases, Arterial, Blood
Cardiac catheterization, Diagnostic
★Chest radiography, Diagnostic
Echocardiography, Diagnostic
★Electrocardiography, Diagnostic

Additional Conditions
Dizziness
Endocarditis
Epistaxis
Hypertension

COCCIDIOIDOMYCOSIS
Body fluid, Anaerobic, Culture (Abscess)
Blood culture, Blood
Bone scan, Diagnostic
★*Coccidioides* serology, Blood or cerebrospinal fluid
★Culture, Routine, Specimen (Sputum, urine)
★Chest radiography, Diagnostic
Eosinophil count, Blood
Sedimentation rate, Erythrocyte, Blood

Additional Conditions
Conjunctivitis
Cervical adenopathy
Erythema nodosum multiforme
Fever
Friction rub
Pleural effusion
Pneumonia

COCCIDIOSIS
Acquired immunodeficiency syndrome evaluation battery, Diagnostic
Biopsy, Site-specific (Duodenum), Specimen
★*Coccidioides* serology, Blood or cerebrospinal fluid
Stool culture, Routine, Stool

Additional Conditions
Acquired immunodeficiency syndrome

COLD, COMMON
(*see also Rhinitis*)
Complete blood count, Blood
Viral culture, Specimen

Additional Conditions
Diarrhea
Enteritis
Fever
Sinusitis

COLITIS
(*see Ulcerative colitis*)

COLLAGEN DISEASES
(*see Arthritis, Autoimmune diseases,
Rheumatoid arthritis, Scleroderma,
Sjögren syndrome, or Systemic lupus
erythematosus*)

COLON CANCER
Brushing cytology, Specimen,
  Diagnostic
CA 19-9, Blood
CA 50, Blood
CA 72-4, Blood
Carcinoembryonic antigen, Serum
Colorectal cancer allelotyping for
  chromosomes 17p and 18q,
  Specimen and blood
Dual modality imaging, Diagnostic
Endoscopic ultrasonography,
  Diagnostic
*Histopathology, Specimen
Ki-67 proliferation marker, Specimen
K-*ras*, Blood or specimen
Mitogen-activated protein kinase,
  Specimen
Occult blood, Stool
Sedimentation rate, Erythrocyte,
  Blood
Telomerase enzyme marker, Blood
Thymidylate synthase, Specimen

Additional Conditions
Anemia
Ascites
Hypoalbuminemia
Hypokalemia
Low-fiber diet
Rectal bleeding

COLOSTOMY
(*see Ostomies*)

CONDYLOMA LATUM
*Condyloma latum, Vulvar or anal
  culture for cytology, Specimen

Additional Conditions
Gonorrhea
Human immunodeficiency virus
Syphilis

CONGENITAL HEART DISEASE
Magnetic resonance angiography,
  Diagnostic
*Magnetic resonance imaging,
  Diagnostic
Mean platelet volume, Blood
Oximetry, Pulse, Diagnostic

Additional Conditions
Bacterial endocarditis
Carcinoid syndrome
Marfan syndrome
Rheumatic valvular disease
Syphilis

CONGESTIVE HEART FAILURE
Alanine aminotransferase, Serum
Albumin, Serum, Urine and 24-Hour
  urine
Aspartate aminotransferase, Serum
Body fluid analysis, Cell count,
  Specimen
Cardiac enzymes/isoenzymes, Blood
*Chemistry profile, Blood
*Chest radiography, Diagnostic
Complete blood count, Blood
Comprehensive metabolic panel,
  Blood
Creatine kinase, Isoenzymes, Serum
Creatine kinase, Serum
Diffusing capacity for carbon
  monoxide, Diagnostic
Digitoxin, Serum
Digoxin, Serum
Disopyramide phosphate, Serum
Echocardiography, Diagnostic
*Electrocardiography, Diagnostic
Electrolytes, Plasma or serum
Electrolytes, Urine
Gamma-glutamyltranspeptidase,
  Blood
Heart scan, Diagnostic
Lactate dehydrogenase, Isoenzymes,
  Blood
Lidocaine, Serum
*Natriuretic peptides, Atrial, Brain,
  C-Type, Plasma
Osmolality, Calculated test, Blood
Osmolality, Serum

Osmolality, Urine
Positron emission tomography,
  Diagnostic
Procainamide, Serum
Propranolol, Blood
Protein, Quantitative, Urine
Sedimentation rate, Erythrocyte,
  Blood
Sodium, Plasma or serum
Thyroid profile, Blood
Transesophageal ultrasonography,
  Diagnostic
Troponin I, Serum
Urea nitrogen, Plasma or serum
Ventriculography, Diagnostic

Additional Conditions
Aortic dissection
Ascites
Cardiac disease
Dysrhythmias
Edema
Electrolyte imbalance
Hepatomegaly
Hypercholesterolemia
Hyperglycemia
Hypomagnesemia
Jaundice
Myocardial infarction
Myocarditis
Pleural effusion
Pulmonary hypertension
Renal disease
Rheumatic heart disease
Systemic hypertension
Valvular dysfunction

CONJUNCTIVITIS
Adenovirus immunofluorescence,
  Diagnostic
Chlamydia culture and group titer,
  Specimen (Culture)
★Conjunctivae, Routine, Culture
Ocular cytology, Specimen
Sjögren's antibodies, Blood

Additional Conditions
Allergies
Rheumatoid arthritis
Sjögren syndrome

**CONSTRICTIVE
PERICARDITIS**
(*see Pericarditis*)

CONVULSIONS
(*see Seizures*)

COPD
(*see Asthma, Bronchitis, or Emphysema*)

**CORONARY ARTERY BYPASS
GRAFT (CABG)**
Activated coagulation time,
  Automated, Blood
Blood gases, Arterial, Blood
Cardiac catheterization, Diagnostic
Cardiac output, Diagnostic
Coronary intravascular
  ultrasonography, Diagnostic

Additional Conditions
Angina
Coronary artery disease

CORONARY ARTERY DISEASE
(*see Arteriosclerosis*)

COUGH
Acid-fast bacteria, Culture and stain
  (Sputum)
★Chest radiography, Diagnostic
Sputum culture and sensitivity,
  Specimen
Sputum, Gram stain, Diagnostic

Additional Conditions
ACE inhibitor therapy
Allergies
Anticholinergic therapy
Acute respiratory distress syndrome
  (ARDS)
Asthma
Chronic obstructive pulmonary
  disease
Industry-related diseases
Lung cancer
Pneumonia

CRETINISM
(*see Hypothyroidism*)

CROHN'S DISEASE
Albumin, Serum
Anti-neutrophil cytoplasmic antibody
  screen, Serum
Barium enema, Diagnostic
Chemistry profile, Blood
★Colonoscopy, Diagnostic
Complete blood count, Blood
C-reactive protein, Serum
★Cytologic study of gastrointestinal
  tract, Diagnostic

Electrolytes, Plasma or serum
Fecal fat, Quantitative, 72-Hour stool
Flat-plate radiography of the
  abdomen, Diagnostic
Histopathology, Specimen
Muramidase, Serum
Occult blood, Stool
Oxalate, 24-Hour urine
Sedimentation rate, Erythrocyte,
  Blood
Small bowel series, Diagnostic
Vitamin B$_{12}$, Serum
Yersinia enterocolitica antibody, Blood

Additional Conditions
Amebiasis
Appendicitis
Anal-rectal fistula or abscess
Ankylosing spondylitis
Colitis
Granuloma
Ileitis
Intestinal obstruction
Malnutrition
Polyarthritis
Seizures
Stress

CUSHING SYNDROME
Adrenocorticotropic hormone, Serum
Aldosterone, Serum
Androstenedione, Serum
Calcitonin, Plasma or serum
Calcium, Urine
Chemistry profile, Blood
Chloride, Urine
Complete blood count, Blood
Computed tomography of the body
  (Kidney), Diagnostic
*Cortisol, Plasma or serum
*Cortisol, Urine
Creatinine, Serum
Creatinine, Urine
Differential leukocyte count,
  Peripheral blood
Electrolytes, Plasma or serum
Electrolytes, Urine
*Glucose, Blood
Glucose tolerance test, Blood
Histopathology, Specimen
17-Hydroxycorticosteroids, 24-Hour
  urine
17-Ketosteroids, Total, 24-Hour urine
*Low-density lipoprotein cholesterol,
  Blood
Magnetic resonance imaging,
  Diagnostic
Metyrapone test, Plasma
Renin activity, Plasma

Sodium, Serum or plasma
Testosterone, Free, Bioavailable and
  total, Blood

Additional Conditions
ACTH-secreting adenoma
Adrenal hyperplasia
Adrenal tumor
Alcoholism
Amenorrhea
Depression
Hyperglycemia
Hypertension
Hypothalamus lesion
Impotence
Nephrolithiasis
Osteoporosis
Ovarian cancer
Virilization

CVA
(see Cerebrovascular accident)

CYANOSIS
Bicarbonate, Serum
Blood gases, Capillary, Blood
*Blood gases, Venous, Blood
Carbon dioxide, Partial pressure,
  Blood
Carbon dioxide, Total content, Blood
Carboxyhemoglobin, Blood
Glucose, Blood
Heavy metal drug screen, Blood and
  24-Hour urine
5-Hydroxyindoleacetic acid,
  Quantitative, 24-Hour urine
Methemoglobin, Blood
Serotonin, Serum or blood

Additional Conditions
Anemia
Cardiac diseases
High-altitude sickness
Patent foramen ovale
Peripheral vascular disease
Polycythemia
Pulmonary diseases

CYSTECTOMY
Chemistry profile, Blood
*Complete blood count, Blood
Type and crossmatch, Blood
Urinalysis, Urine

Additional Conditions
Cholecystitis
Urinary carcinoma

CYSTIC FIBROSIS
Albumin, Serum
★Chloride, Sweat, Specimen
Chest radiography, Diagnostic
D-Xylose absorption test, Diagnostic, Serum or urine
Electrolytes, Plasma or serum
Fat, Semiquantitative, Stool
Liver battery, Serum
Pulmonary function tests, Diagnostic
Semen analysis, Specimen
Sputum, Routine, Culture
Trypsin, Plasma or serum
Trypsin, Stool
Vitamin E_1, Serum

Additional Conditions
Asthma
Atelectasis
Azoospermia
Biliary cirrhosis
Cholelithiasis
Chronic obstructive pulmonary disease
Cor pulmonale
Hemoptysis
Intussusception
Pancreatitis
Pneumonia
Pneumothorax
Steatorrhea

CYSTITIS
Body fluid, Routine, Culture (Urine)
Gram stain, Diagnostic (Urine)
Histopathology, Specimen
Nitrite, Bacteria drug screen, Urine
Occult blood, Urine
★Urinalysis, Urine
Urinalysis, Fractional, Urine
★Urine cytology, Urine
Urine, Fungus, Culture

Additional Conditions
Cervicitis
Cyclophosphamide medication
Pregnancy
Pyelonephritis
Urinary tract infection
Vaginitis

CYTOMEGALIC INCLUSION DISEASE
(see Cytomegalovirus)

CYTOMEGALOVIRUS
Acquired immunodeficiency syndrome evaluation battery, Diagnostic
Blood indices, Blood
Body fluid, Routine, Culture (Urine)
Brushing cytology, Specimen, Diagnostic
Chemistry profile, Blood
Complete blood count, Blood
Cytomegalic inclusion disease, Cytology, Urine
★Cytomegalovirus antibody, Serum
Differential leukocyte count, Peripheral blood
Heterophile agglutinins, Blood
Histopathology, Specimen
Infectious mononucleosis screening test, Blood
Red blood cell, Blood
Sputum cytology, Specimen
Toxoplasmosis, Rubella, Cytomegalovirus, Herpes virus serology, Blood
Urine cytology, Urine

Additional Conditions
Acquired immunodeficiency syndrome
Immunocompromised persons
Liver dysfunction
Massive blood transfusions
Pneumonia

DEAFNESS
(see Hearing disorders)

DECUBITI
Biopsy, Anaerobic, Culture
Biopsy, Routine, Culture
Blood culture, Blood
Culture, Routine, Specimen

Additional Conditions
Chronic bedrest
Malnutrition
Paralysis

DEEP VEIN THROMBOSIS (DVT)
Activated partial thromboplastin time, Plasma
Antithrombin III test, Diagnostic
Arteriography, Diagnostic
Color duplex ultrasonography, Diagnostic
Compression ultrasound, Diagnostic
Computed tomography of the body (Spiral), Diagnostic

D-dimer test, Plasma
*Doppler ultrasonographic flow
studies, Diagnostic
Factor V, (Leiden mutation), Blood
^{125}I-Labeled fibrinogen leg scan,
Diagnostic
Magnetic resonance angiography,
diagnostic
Plasminogen assay, Blood
Protein C, Blood
Protein S, Total and free, Blood
Prothrombin time and international
normalized ratio, Plasma
Soluble fibrin monomer complex,
Serum
*Venography, Diagnostic

Additional Conditions
Atherosclerosis
Chronic bedrest
Postoperative
Systemic lupus erythematosus

DEGENERATIVE ARTHRITIS
(see Cervical spondylosis)

DEGENERATIVE DISORDERS OF NERVOUS SYSTEM
(see Alzheimer's disease)

DEGENERATIVE JOINT DISEASE
(see Osteoarthritis)

DEHYDRATION
(see Hypovolemia)

DELIRIUM TREMENS
*Alcohol, Blood
Electrolytes, Plasma or serum

Additional Conditions
Alcoholism
Drug abuse
Seizures

DEMENTIA
Brain scan, Cerebral flow and
pathology, Diagnostic
*Chemistry profile, Blood
Chest radiography, Diagnostic
*Complete blood count, Blood

Computed tomography of the brain,
Diagnostic
Electroencephalography, Diagnostic
Electrolytes, Plasma or serum
Magnetic resonance imaging,
Diagnostic
*Magnetic resonance spectroscopy,
Diagnostic
*Thyroid profile, Blood
Vitamin B$_1$, Serum or urine
Vitamin B$_{12}$, Serum

Additional Conditions
Acquired immunodeficiency syndrome
Alzheimer's disease
Cerebrovascular accident
Hypothyroidism
Organic brain syndrome

DEMYELINIZATION
(see Multiple sclerosis)

DENGUE FEVER
Differential leukocyte count,
Peripheral blood
*Immune complex assay, Blood

Additional Conditions
Fever
Headache
Leukopenia
Rash

DEPRESSANT DRUG ABUSE
(see Drug abuse: Barbiturates,
Meprobamate, and Methaqualone)

DEPRESSION
Chromosome analysis, Blood
Cortisol, Plasma or serum
*Dexamethasone suppression test,
Diagnostic
Electroencephalography, Diagnostic
Selective serotonin reuptake
inhibitors, Blood
Serotonin, Serum or blood
Thyroid function testing, Blood

Additional Conditions
Alzheimer's disease
Anxiety
Chronic illness
Dementia
Insomnia
Schizophrenia

DERMATITIS
Allergen-specific IgE, Serum
Antinuclear antibody, Serum
Chromium, Serum
Complete blood count, Blood
Differential leukocyte count,
  Peripheral blood
Eosinophil count, Blood
Heavy metal screen, 24-Hour urine
★Histopathology, Specimen
Immunoglobulin E, Serum
Porphyrins, Quantitative, Blood
Skin, Fungus, Culture

Additional Conditions
Allergic reactions
Arthropod bite
Athlete's foot
Eczema
Herpes simplex or zoster
Impetigo
Kaposi's sarcoma
Malignant melanoma
Pemphigus
Pruritus
Psoriasis
Rash
Seborrhea
Skin cancer
Systemic lupus erythematosus
Tinea capitis
Tinea cruris

DIABETES, GESTATIONAL
★Glucose tolerance test, Blood

Additional Conditions
Pregnancy

DIABETES INSIPIDUS
Antidiuretic hormone, Serum
Chloride, Sweat, Specimen
★Concentration test, Urine
Creatinine, Serum
Cyclic adenosine monophosphate,
  Urine
Electrolytes, Plasma or serum
★Osmolality, Calculated test, Blood
Osmolality, Serum
Osmolality, Urine
★Sodium, Plasma or serum
★Sodium, Urine
Specific gravity, Urine

Additional Conditions
Amyloidosis, Renal
Breast cancer
Encephalitis

Hand-Schüller-Christian disease,
  Serum and urine
Lung cancer
Pyelonephritis
Sickle cell anemia
Sjögren syndrome
Syphilis
Tuberculosis

DIABETES MELLITUS
Anion gap, Blood
Body fluid, Routine, Culture (Urine)
Chemistry profile, Blood
Complete blood count, Blood
C-peptide, Serum
Creatinine clearance, Serum, Urine
Differential leukocyte count,
  Peripheral blood
Electrolytes, Plasma or serum
Electrolytes, Urine
Endomysial antibody, Serum
Fructosamine, Serum
Glucagon, Plasma
★Glucose, Blood
Glucose-monitoring machines,
  Diagnostic
Glucose, Qualitative,
  Semiquantitative, Urine
Glucose, Quantitative, 24-Hour urine
Glucose challenge test, Diagnostic
  (for gestational DM)
Glucose tolerance test, Blood
Glucose, 2-Hour postprandial, Serum
★Glycosylated hemoglobin, Blood
Insulin and insulin antibodies, Blood
Ketone bodies, Blood
Ketone, Semiquantitative, Urine
Lactic acid, Blood
Lipid profile, Blood
Magnesium, Serum
Magnetic resonance spectroscopy,
  Diagnostic
Osmolality, Urine
Potassium, Serum
Protein electrophoresis, Serum
Red blood cell, Blood
Triglycerides, Blood
Urinalysis, Urine
Urine, Fungus, Culture

Additional Conditions
Addison's disease
Atherosclerosis
Cancer
Cushing syndrome
Fanconi syndrome
Gangrene
Glucagonoma
Hemochromatosis

Liver disease
Obesity
Phenytoin medication
Pheochromocytoma
Pregnancy
Thiazide diuretic medications
Thyrotoxicosis

DIABETIC GLOMERULOSCLEROSIS
Creatinine clearance, Serum, Urine
Creatinine, Serum
Kidney biopsy, Specimen
*Protein, Quantitative, Urine
Urea nitrogen, Plasma or serum

Additional Conditions
Atherosclerosis
Diabetes insipidus
Diabetes mellitus
Scleroderma

DIABETIC KETOACIDOSIS (DKA)
*Anion gap, Blood
*Beta-hydroxybutyrate, Blood
*Blood gases (pH), Arterial, Blood
*Chemistry profile, Blood
Chest radiography, Diagnostic
*Complete blood count, Blood
Culture, Routine, Specimen (Urine)
Electrolytes, Plasma or serum
*Glucose, Serum
Osmolality, Serum
Phosphate, Serum
Potassium, Serum
Urea nitrogen, Plasma or serum

DIALYSIS, HEMO-
Activated coagulation time, Automated, Blood
Activated partial thromboplastin time, Plasma
Complete blood count, Blood
Creatinine, Serum
Electrolytes, Plasma or serum (Plasma)
Lee-White clotting time, Blood
Parathyroid hormone, Blood
Urea nitrogen, Plasma or serum

Additional Conditions
Diabetes mellitus
Heart failure
Hypercalcemia
Multiple myeloma

Nephrosis
Poisoning
Renal failure
Systemic lupus erythematosus
Uremia

DIALYSIS, PERITONEAL
Complete blood count, Blood
Creatinine, Serum
Electrolytes, Plasma
Urea nitrogen, Plasma or serum

Additional Conditions
Diabetes mellitus
Heart failure
Hypercalcemia
Multiple myeloma
Nephrosis
Poisoning
Renal failure
Systemic lupus erythematosus
Uremia

DIARRHEA
Albumin, Serum
Carotene, Serum
*Chemistry profile, Blood
Clostridial toxin, Serum
Clostridium difficile toxin assay, Stool
Cortisol, Plasma or serum
Cryptosporidium diagnostic procedures, Stool
D-Xylose absorption test, Diagnostic, Serum or urine
*Electrolytes, Plasma or serum
Entamoeba histolytica serologic test, Blood
Fat, Semiquantitative, Stool
Fecal fat, Quantitative, 72-Hour stool
Fecal leukocytes, Stool, Diagnostic
Gastrin, Serum
Glucagon, Plasma
Glucose, 2-Hour postprandial, Serum
Histopathology, Specimen
Homovanillic acid, 24-Hour urine
5-Hydroxyindoleacetic acid, Quantitative, 24-Hour urine
Magnesium, Serum
Mycoplasma titer, Blood
Occult blood, Stool
Osmolality, Calculated test, Blood
Osmolality, Serum
Osmolality, Urine
Ova and parasites, Stool

pH, Stool
Phenolphthalein test, Diagnostic
Reducing substances, Stool
Rotavirus antigen, Stool
Schilling test, Diagnostic
Serotonin, Serum or blood
Specific gravity, Urine
★Stool culture, Routine, Stool
Thyroid profile, Blood
Vasoactive intestinal polypeptide,
  Blood
Yersinia enterocolitica antibody,
  Blood

Additional Conditions
Acquired immunodeficiency
  syndrome
Anorexia nervosa
Botulism
Bulimia
Chlamydia
Cholera
Colitis
Colon cancer
Crohn's disease
Cytomegalovirus
Diabetes mellitus
Diverticulitis
Diverticulosis
Gastroenteritis
Giardiasis
Hepatitis
Hyperthyroidism
IgA deficiency
Kwashiorkor
Malabsorption
Marasmus
Medication side effect
Metabolic acidosis
Neisseria gonorrhoeae
Toxic shock syndrome
Transplant rejection
Traveler's diarrhea
Tube feeding

DIC
*(see Disseminated intravascular
coagulation)*

DIPHTHERIA
★Schick test for diphtheria, Diagnostic
Throat culture for *Corynebacterium
  diphtheriae,* Culture

Additional Conditions
Myocarditis
Neuritis
Proteinuria

DISACCHARIDE DEFICIENCIES
★D-Xylose absorption test, Diagnostic,
  Serum or urine
pH, Stool
★Reducing substances, Stool
Rotavirus antigen, Stool

Additional Conditions
Celiac disease
Colitis
Cystic fibrosis
Diarrhea
Giardiasis

**DISCOID LUPUS
ERYTHEMATOSUS**
(see Systemic lupus erythematosus)

**DISSEMINATED
INTRAVASCULAR
COAGULATION**
Activated coagulation time,
  Automated, Blood
★Activated partial thromboplastin
  time, Plasma
Antithrombin III test, Diagnostic
C3 proactivator, Serum
Clot retraction, Blood
★Complete blood count, Blood
★D-Dimer Test, Blood
Differential leukocyte count,
  Peripheral blood
Fibrin split products, Protamine
  sulfate test, Blood
Fibrinopeptide A, Blood
★Fibrinogen, Plasma
Fibrinogen breakdown products,
  Blood
Haptoglobin, Serum
Intravascular coagulation screen,
  Blood
Plasminogen assay, Blood
Protein C, Blood
Protein S, Total and free, Blood
★Prothrombin time and international
  normalized ratio, Plasma
Red blood cell morphology, Blood
★Soluble fibrin monomer complex,
  Serum
Thrombin time, Serum

Additional Conditions
Abortion, Septic
Acute respiratory distress
  syndrome
Amniotic fluid embolus
Anaphylaxis
Antibiotic therapy

Anticoagulant therapy
Blood transfusion reaction
Burns
Cancer
Head injury (penetrating)
Hemophilia
Hypothermia
Liver failure
Malnutrition
Massive transfusion
Obstetrical complications
Poisoning
Renal failure
Sepsis
Shock
Snake venom
Thrombocytopenia
Thrombolytic therapy
Trauma
Von Willebrand's disease

DIVERTICULITIS
Barium enema, Diagnostic
Blood indices, Blood
Colonoscopy, Diagnostic
Complete blood count, Blood
Differential leukocyte count,
   Peripheral blood
Fecal leukocytes, Stool, Diagnostic
Histopathology, Specimen
Occult blood, Stool
Red blood cell, Blood
*Sigmoidoscopy, Diagnostic

Additional Conditions
Abscess
Bowel obstruction
Constipation
Diarrhea
Sepsis

DIVERTICULOSIS
Barium enema, Diagnostic
Blood indices, Blood
Colonoscopy, Diagnostic
Complete blood count,
   Blood
Differential leukocyte count,
   Peripheral blood
Histopathology, Specimen
Occult blood, Stool
Red blood cell, Blood
*Sigmoidoscopy, Diagnostic

Additional Conditions
Bladder fistula
Constipation
Fever

DOWN SYNDROME
Amniotic fluid, Chromosome
   analysis, Specimen
Chorionic villi sampling, Specimen
*Chromosome analysis (#21
   Chromosome), Blood
Urinary chorionic gonadotropin
   peptide, Urine

Additional Conditions
Mental retardation

DRACUNCULIASIS
Culture, Skin, Specimen
Eosinophil count, Blood
Radiography, Diagnostic

Additional Conditions
Abscess
Pruritus
Tetanus

DROWNING, NEAR
*Blood gases, Arterial, Blood
Chest radiography, Diagnostic
Complete blood count, Blood
Computed tomography of the brain,
   Diagnostic
Drug screen, Blood
Electroencephalography, Diagnostic
Electrolytes, Plasma
Toxicology, Drug screen, Blood or
   urine

Additional Conditions
Alcoholism
Anaphylaxis
Brain death
Coma
Cyanosis
Drug abuse
Myocardial infarction
Pulmonary edema
Spinal cord injury

DRUG ABUSE
   *(Includes Cannabis, Depressants,
   Ethanol, Hallucinogenics, Narcotics,
   Stimulants)*
Acetaminophen, Serum
Alcohol, Blood
Barbiturates, Quantitative, Blood
Blood fungus, Culture
*Blood gases, Arterial, Blood
Cannabinoids (Marijuana, THC),
   Qualitative, Blood or urine
Carbamazepine, Blood

Chlordiazepoxide, Blood
Clonazepam, Blood
Cocaine, Blood
Cytologic study of gastrointestinal
  tract, Diagnostic
Diazepam, Serum
Ethchlorvynol, Blood
Ethosuximide, Blood
Fluorescent treponemal
  antibody–absorbed double-stain
  test, Serum
Flurazepam, Serum
Gamma-hydroxybutyric acid, Blood
  or urine
Glutethimide, Blood
Hepatitis B surface antigen, Blood
Lidocaine, Serum
Lithium, Serum
★Liver battery, Serum
Meprobamate, Blood
Methaqualone, Blood
Methotrexate, Serum
Methyprylon, Serum
Morphine, Urine
Phencyclidine, Qualitative, Urine
Phenobarbital, Plasma or serum
Phenothiazines, Blood
Phenytoin, Serum
Primidone, Serum
Propoxyphene, Blood
Rapid plasma reagin test, Blood
Salicylate, Blood
★Toxicology, Drug screen, Blood or
  urine
Toxicology, Volatiles group by GLC,
  Blood or urine
Tricyclic antidepressants, Plasma or
  serum

Additional Conditions
Acquired immunodeficiency syndrome
Alcoholism
Anxiety
Depression
Endocarditis
Insomnia
Malnutrition
Mitral valve prolapse
Rhabdomyolysis

DRUG WITHDRAWAL
(see Drug abuse)

DRY EYES
Ocular impression cytology,
  Specimen
★Schirmer tearing eye test, Diagnostic

Additional Conditions
Autoimmune disorders
Conjunctivitis
Kaposi's sarcoma
Keratitis
Ocular rosacea

**DUCHENNE'S MUSCULAR
DYSTROPHY**
Aldolase, Serum
Aspartate aminotransferase, Serum
Creatine kinase, Serum
Creatine kinase, Isoenzymes, Serum
★Muscle biopsy, Specimen

Additional Conditions
Dysrhythmias
Intellectual retardation
Skeletal deformity

DUODENAL ULCER
(see also Helicobacter pylori)
ABO group and Rh type, Blood
Barium swallow, Diagnostic
Complete blood count, Blood
★Esophagogastroduodenoscopy,
  Diagnostic
★Helicobacter pylori, Quick office
  serology, Serum and titer, Blood
Histopathology, Specimen
Pepsinogen I and pepsinogen II,
  Blood
Upper gastrointestinal series,
  Diagnostic

Additional Conditions
Bowel obstruction
Gastric cancer
Gastric ulcer
Gastritis
Hemorrhage
Hiatal hernia
Pancreatitis
Peptic ulcer

DWARFISM
(see Hypopituitarism)

DYSENTERY
★Entamoeba histolytica serologic test,
  Blood
Fecal leukocytes, Stool, Diagnostic
★Ova and parasites, Stool
Parasite drug screen, Stool
Stool culture, Routine, Stool

Additional Conditions
Arthritis
Dehydration
Diarrhea
Fever

DYSERYTHROPOIETIC ANEMIA
Blood indices, Blood
Bone marrow biopsy, Diagnostic
Complete blood count, Blood
Differential leukocyte count,
  Peripheral blood
Ham test, Diagnostic
Haptoglobin, Serum
Red blood cell, Blood
*Red blood cell morphology, Blood
Sucrose hemolysis test, Diagnostic

Additional Conditions
Hemoglobinuria
Leukopenia
Sepsis
Thrombocytopenia

DYSFIBRINOGENEMIA
Activated partial thromboplastin
  time, Plasma
Fibrin split products, Protamine
  sulfate test, Blood
*Fibrinogen, Plasma
Prothrombin time and international
  normalized ratio, Plasma
Thrombin time, Serum

Additional Conditions
Burns
Hypofibrinogenemia
Leukemia
Polycythemia vera
Syphilis
Thrombocytopenia

DYSMENORRHEA
Complete blood count, Blood
Dilatation and curettage, Diagnostic
*Estrogens, Serum and 24-Hour
  urine
Human chorionic gonadotropin,
  Serum
Iron, Serum
Laparoscopy, Diagnostic
Total iron-binding capacity, Serum
*Urinalysis, Urine

Additional Conditions
Endometriosis
Ovarian fibromas or cysts

Pelvic inflammatory disease
Submucous myoma

DYSPEPSIA
*Esophageal acidity test, Diagnostic
*Esophagogastroduodenoscopy,
  Diagnostic
Gastric analysis, Specimen
Gastric pH, Specimen

Additional Conditions
Gastric esophageal reflux disease
Gastritis
Hiatal hernia
Myocardial infarction
Peptic ulcer disease

DYSPHAGIA
Acid perfusion test, Diagnostic
*Esophageal manometry, Diagnostic

Additional Conditions
Foreign-object ingestion
Head and neck cancer
Laryngitis
Mucositis
Oral sexually transmitted disease
Pneumonia, Aspiration
Stomatitis

DYSPNEA
Bicarbonate, Serum
*Blood gases, Arterial, Blood
  Carbon dioxide, Partial pressure,
  Blood
  Carbon monoxide, Blood
  Carboxyhemoglobin, Blood
*Chest radiography, Diagnostic
*Complete blood count, Blood
  Diffusing capacity for carbon
  monoxide, Diagnostic
Heavy metals, Blood and 24-Hour
  urine
Methemoglobin, Blood
*Natriuretic peptides, Atrial, Brain,
  C-Type, Plasma
pCO_2, Blood

Additional Conditions
Anxiety
Cardiac disease
Chronic obstructive pulmonary disease
Congestive heart failure
Lung cancer
Obesity
Pulmonary edema
Severe acute respiratory syndrome
  (SARS)

DYSPROTEINEMIA
Blood indices, Blood
Bone marrow biopsy, Diagnostic
Chemistry profile, Blood
Complete blood count, Blood
Differential leukocyte count,
  Peripheral blood
Globulin, Serum
Immunoelectrophoresis, Serum and
  urine
Immunoglobulin A, Serum
Immunoglobulin D, Serum
Immunoglobulin E, Serum
Immunoglobulin M, Serum
Platelet aggregation, Blood
Platelet aggregation, Hypercoagulable
  state, Blood
★Protein electrophoresis, Serum
Protein electrophoresis, Urine
Red blood cell, Blood
★Urinalysis, Urine
Viscosity, Serum

Additional Conditions
Epistaxis
Gastrointestinal bleeding
Multiple myeloma
Purpura
Waldenström's macroglobulinemia

DYSRHYTHMIAS
Amiodarone, Plasma or serum
Bicarbonate, Serum
Blood gases, Arterial, Blood
Calcium, Total, Serum
Carbon dioxide, Partial pressure, Blood
Digitoxin, Serum
Digoxin, Serum
Disopyramide phosphate, Serum
★Electrocardiography, Diagnostic
Electrolytes, Plasma or serum
  (Plasma)
Electrophysiologic study, Diagnostic
Flecainide, Plasma or serum
Holter monitor, Diagnostic
Lidocaine, Serum
Magnesium, Serum
Natriuretic peptides, Atrial, Brain,
  C-Type, Plasma
Potassium, Serum
Procainamide, Serum
Propranolol, Blood
Quinidine, Serum
Signal-averaged electrocardiography,
  Diagnostic

Additional Conditions
Acid-base imbalance
Anemia

Anoxia
Anxiety
Cardiomyopathy
Cerebrovascular accident
Chest trauma
Chronic obstructive pulmonary
  disease
Congestive heart failure
Coronary artery disease
Digitalis toxicity
Emboli
Hepatomegaly
Hypertension
Hypoxia
Pacemaker failure
Pericarditis
Pheochromocytoma
Quinidine toxicity
Sepsis
Stress
Theophylline toxicity
Thyroid dysfunction
Trauma
Valvular disease
Vertigo

DYSURIA
Body fluid, Routine, Culture (Urine)
Chlamydia culture and group titer,
  Specimen (Culture)
Cytoscopy, Diagnostic
Nitrite, Bacteria drug screen, Urine
Occult blood, Urine
Trichomonas preparation, Specimen
★Urinalysis, Urine

Additional Conditions
Bladder infection
Prostate infection
Urinary tract infection

ECCHYMOSIS
(SPONTANEOUS)
★Activated partial thromboplastin
  time, Plasma
Bleeding time, Duke, Blood
Bleeding time, Ivy, Blood
Capillary fragility test (in vivo),
  Diagnostic
Factor VIII, Blood
Factor VIII R:Ag, Blood
Fibrinogen, Plasma
Fibrinogen breakdown products,
  Blood
Platelet aggregation, Blood; Platelet
  aggregation, Hypercoagulable state,
  Blood
★Platelet count, Blood

⋆Prothrombin time and international
normalized ratio, Plasma
Salicylate, Blood

Additional Conditions
Cancer
Chemotherapy drug usage
Disseminated intravascular
coagulation
Idiopathic thrombocytopenic
purpura
Leukemia

ECHINOCOCCOSIS
Bile fluid examination, Diagnostic
Cerebrospinal fluid, Cytology
specimen
Computed tomography of the body
(Abdomen, liver), Diagnostic
⋆Echinococcosis serologic test, Blood
Histopathology, Specimen

Additional Conditions
Cyst on the liver
Jaundice
Shock

ECLAMPSIA (TOXEMIA)
Activated partial thromboplastin time
and partial thromboplastin time,
Plasma
Albumin, 24-Hour urine
Complete blood count, Blood
Creatinine, Serum
D-Dimer test, Blood
Electrolytes, Plasma or serum
Glucose, Qualitative and
semiquantitative, Urine
Hematocrit, Blood
Liver battery, Diagnostic
Low-density lipoprotein cholesterol,
Blood
Prothrombin time and international
normalized ratio, Serum
⋆Protein, Quantitative, Urine
Sodium, Plasma, Serum
Urea nitrogen, Plasma or serum
Uric acid, Serum

Additional Conditions
Collagen disorder
Diabetes mellitus
Hydatidiform mole
Hypertension
Multiple pregnancy
Renal failure

ECTOPIC HYPERPARATHYROIDISM
Calcium, Ionized, Serum
⋆Calcium, Total, Serum
Calcium, Urine
Chemistry profile, Blood
⋆Parathyroid hormone, Blood
⋆Phosphorus, Serum
Phosphorus, Urine
Sputum cytology, Specimen

Additional Conditions
Hypercalcemia
Hypophosphatemia
Nephrolithiasis
Renal failure

ECTOPIC PREGNANCY
⋆Gynecologic ultrasound, Diagnostic
Histopathology, Specimen
Human chorionic gonadotropin,
Beta-subunit, Serum
Laparoscopy, Diagnostic
⋆Pregnancy test, Routine, Serum and
qualitative, Urine
Type and crossmatch, Blood (Screen)

Additional Conditions
Abdominal pain
Abortion
Amenorrhea
Appendicitis
Salpingitis
Shock
Urinary tract infection

ECZEMA
Allergen-specific IgE antibody, Serum
Eosinophil count, Blood
⋆Histopathology, Specimen
Immunoglobulin E, Serum

Additional Conditions
Allergic rhinitis
Asthma
Cataracts
Pruritus

EDEMA
Albumin/globulin ratio, Serum
Chemistry profile, Blood
⋆Electrolytes, Plasma
Magnetic resonance imaging,
Diagnostic
Osmolality, Serum
Osmolality, Urine
⋆Protein, Total, Serum

Additional Conditions
Cardiac diseases
Cellulitis
Deep vein thrombosis
High-altitude living
Kwashiorkor
Pulmonary disease

EFFUSIONS, ABDOMINAL
Body fluid, Amylase, Specimen
Body fluid, Anaerobic, Culture
Body fluid, Glucose, Specimen
Body fluid analysis, Cell count, Specimen
*Body fluid cytology, Specimen
Flat-plate radiography of the abdomen, Diagnostic
Gram stain (Effusion specimen), Diagnostic
*Paracentesis, Diagnostic
Sputum, Routine, Culture
Synovial fluid analysis, Diagnostic

Additional Conditions
Ascites
Empyema
Metastasis

EFFUSIONS, PERICARDIAL
Body fluid analysis, Specimen
Body fluid cytology, Specimen
*Chest radiography, Diagnostic
*Echocardiography, Diagnostic
Electrocardiography, Diagnostic
Pericardiocentesis, Diagnostic

Additional Conditions
Acquired immunodeficiency syndrome
Cancer
Chronic obstructive pulmonary disease
Congestive heart failure
Tachycardia
Trauma

EFFUSIONS, PLEURAL
*Blood gases, Arterial, Blood
Body fluid, Anaerobic, Culture
Body fluid, Glucose, Specimen
Body fluid analysis, Cell count, Specimen
Body fluid analysis, Specimen
Body fluid cytology, Specimen
*Chest radiography, Diagnostic
Computed tomography of the body (Lung), Diagnostic

Fluoroscopy, Diagnostic
Gram stain (Effusion specimen), Diagnostic
Sputum, Routine, Culture
Synovial fluid analysis, Diagnostic
Thoracentesis, Diagnostic

Additional Conditions
Ascites
Congestive heart failure
Empyema
Esophageal perforation
Lung cancer
Pulmonary emboli
Tuberculosis

EMBOLECTOMY
(*see Fat embolism or Pulmonary embolism*)

EMPHYSEMA
Alpha$_1$-antitrypsin, Serum
Bicarbonate, Serum
Blood gases, Arterial, Blood
Carbon dioxide, Partial pressure, Blood
Carbon dioxide, Total content, Blood
*Chest radiography, Diagnostic
Complete blood count, Blood
Diffusing capacity for carbon monoxide, Diagnostic
Digoxin, Serum
Electrolytes, Plasma or serum (Plasma)
Histopathology, Specimen
Low-density lipoprotein cholesterol, Blood
Natriuretic peptides, Atrial, Brain, C-Type, Plasma
*Pulmonary function tests, Diagnostic
Sputum cytology, Specimen
Theophylline, Blood

Additional Conditions
Asthma
Bronchitis
Cor pulmonale
Dyspnea
Pneumonia

EMPYEMA
Blood gases, Arterial, Blood
Body fluid, Anaerobic, Culture
Body fluid analysis (pH), Specimen

★Body fluid cytology, Specimen
Body fluid, Fungus, Culture
Body fluid, Mycobacteria, Culture
Body fluid, Routine, Culture
Chest radiography, Diagnostic
C-reactive protein, Serum
★Gram stain (Empyema specimen),
Diagnostic
Thoracentesis, Diagnostic

Additional Conditions
Acute respiratory distress syndrome
Chronic obstructive pulmonary disease
Lung abscess
Pleural effusion
Pneumonia

ENCEPHALITIS
California encephalitis virus titer,
Serum
Cerebrospinal fluid, Immunoglobulin
G, Immunoglobulin G ratios and
Immunoglobulin G index,
Immunoglobulin G synthesis rate,
Specimen
★Cerebrospinal fluid, Protein,
Specimen
★Cerebrospinal fluid, Routine analysis,
Specimen
Eastern equine encephalitis virus
titer, Specimen
Herpes virus antigen, Direct
fluorescent antibody, Specimen
Rubeola serology, Serum
St. Louis encephalitis virus serology,
Serum
Toxoplasmosis, Rubella,
Cytomegalovirus, Herpes virus
serology, Blood
Toxoplasmosis serology, Serum
Venezuelan equine encephalitis virus
serology, Serum
Viral culture, Specimen
Western equine encephalitis virus
serology, Serum

Additional Conditions
Fever
Herpes simplex virus
Infectious mononucleosis
Measles
Mumps
Poisoning
Polio
Rabies
Reye syndrome
Rubella
Sepsis
Vaccination-induced

ENCEPHALOPATHY
Ammonia, Serum
Cerebral angiography, Diagnostic
Chemistry profile, Blood
Computed tomography of brain,
Diagnostic
Electroencephalography, Diagnostic
Electrolytes, Plasma or serum
Doppler ultrasonographic flow
studies, Diagnostic
★Magnetic resonance imaging,
Diagnostic
Magnetic resonance spectroscopy,
Diagnostic
Urea nitrogen, Plasma or serum

ENDOCARDITIS
(see also Subacute bacterial
endocarditis)
Anti-DNA, Serum
Antinuclear antibody, Serum
★Blood culture, Blood
Blood culture with antimicrobial
removal device, Culture
Blood fungus, Culture
Blood indices, Blood
Clq immune complex detection,
Serum
C3 complement, Serum
C4 complement, Serum
Chemistry profile, Blood
Chest radiography, Diagnostic
Complement, Total, Serum
Complete blood count, Blood
C-reactive protein, Serum
Differential leukocyte count,
Peripheral blood
★Echocardiography, Diagnostic
Electrocardiography, Diagnostic
5-Hydroxyindoleacetic acid,
Quantitative, 24-Hour urine
Immune complex assay, Blood
Minimum bactericidal concentration,
Culture
Red blood cell, Blood
Rheumatoid factor, Blood
Schlichter test (Body fluid), Diagnostic
★Sedimentation rate, Erythrocyte,
Blood
Serotonin, Serum or blood
Teichoic acid antibody, Blood
Transesophageal ultrasonography,
Diagnostic
★Urinalysis, Urine

Additional Conditions
Abortion, Suction
Bacteremia
Coarctation of the aorta
Drug abuse, Intravenous
Myocarditis
Patent ductus arteriosus
Pulmonary emboli
Rheumatic fever
Status post-cardiac surgery
Tetralogy of Fallot
Valvular heart disease
Ventricular septal defect

ENDOCRINE TUMORS
*(see also Addison's disease, Cushing
syndrome, Hashimoto's thyroiditis,
Hyperparathyroidism,
Hyperpituitarism, Hyperthyroidism,
and Hypothyroidism)*
Computed tomography of the body,
  Diagnostic
Endoscopic ultrasonography, Diagnostic
Immunoperoxidase procedures,
  Diagnostic
*Magnetic resonance imaging,
  Diagnostic

Additional Conditions
Diabetes mellitus
Ulcerative colitis

ENDOMETRITIS
(ENDOMETRIOSIS)
Body fluid, Anaerobic, Culture
  (Abscess)
CA 125, Blood
Chlamydia culture and group titer,
  Specimen (Culture)
Endometrium, Anaerobic, Culture
Foreign body, Routine, Culture
Genital, *Candida albicans,* Culture
Genital, *Neisseria gonorrhoeae,* Culture
*Histopathology, Specimen
*Laparoscopy, Diagnostic

Additional Conditions
Acute pain
Dysmenorrhea
Infertility
Ovarian cancer
Salpingitis
Uterine myomas

ENTERIC FEVER
*Blood culture, Blood
  Complete blood count, Blood
  Stool culture, Routine, Stool

Additional Conditions
Diarrhea
Sepsis

EPIDIDYMITIS
Histopathology, Specimen
*Urinalysis, Urine

Additional Conditions
Acute pain
Urinary tract infection

EPIGLOTTITIS
Blood culture, Blood
*Culture, Routine, Specimen (Throat,
  nose)
Radiography of the skull, chest, and
  cervical spine (Cross-table neck
  radiography), Diagnostic
Culture for *Haemophilus* species,
  Sputum

Additional Conditions
Airway obstruction
Fever
Influenza B

EPILEPSY
Body fluid analysis, Cell count,
  Specimen (cerebrospinal fluid)
Brain scan, Cerebral flow and
  pathology, Diagnostic
Carbamazepine, Blood
Cerebrospinal fluid, Glucose,
  Specimen
Cerebrospinal fluid, Routine, Culture
  and cytology
Clonazepam, Blood
Computed tomography of the brain,
  Diagnostic
Diazepam, Serum
*Electroencephalography, Diagnostic
Ethosuximide, Blood
*Magnetic resonance imaging,
  Diagnostic
Mephenytoin, Blood
Methsuximide, Serum
Phenobarbital, Plasma or serum
Phenytoin, Serum
Primidone, Serum
Valproic acid, Blood

Additional Conditions
Abscess, Brain
Alcoholism
Brain tumor
Drug abuse

Encephalitis, Herpes
Ganglioneuroblastoma
Meningitis
Neuroblastoma
Peripheral vascular disease
Phenylketonuria
Syphilis
Trauma

EPISTAXIS
★Activated partial thromboplastin
   time, Plasma
Autoerythrocyte sensitivity test,
   Diagnostic
Bleeding time, Duke, Blood
Bleeding time, Ivy, Blood
★Complete blood count, Blood
Hematocrit, Blood
Hemoglobin, Blood
Platelet count, Blood
Red blood cell morphology,
   Blood
Thrombin time, Serum

Additional Conditions
Deviated nasal septum
Disseminated intravascular
   coagulation
Leukemia
Rhinitis
Thrombocytopenia
Trauma

EPSTEIN-BARR VIRUS
Complete blood count, Blood
Differential leukocyte count,
   Peripheral blood
★Epstein-Barr virus, Serology, Blood
Heterophile agglutinins, Blood
★Infectious mononucleosis screening
   test, Blood

Additional Conditions
Burkitt's lymphoma
Encephalitis
Hepatitis
Infectious mononucleosis
Myocarditis
Neuritis
Splenomegaly

ERECTILE DYSFUNCTION
Electromyography (of the penis),
   Diagnostic
Glucose, Blood

★Glycosylated hemoglobin Hb A_{1c},
   Blood
Lipid profile, Blood
Prolactin, Serum
Pulse volume recording of peripheral
   vasculature, Diagnostic
Testosterone, Free, Bioavailable and
   total, Blood

Additional Conditions
Alcoholism
Anxiety
Coronary artery disease
Depression
Herniated disk
Hyperlipidemia
Hyperprolactinemia
Hypertension
Hyperthyroidism
Hypogonadism, Compensated
   primary
Hypothyroidism
Liver disease
Medication side effects
Multiple sclerosis
Pelvic radiation
Pelvic surgery
Pelvic trauma
Peyronie's disease
Priapism
Renal failure
Smoking habit
Spinal cord injury
Stress
Vascular disease

ERYTHROBLASTOSIS FETALIS
★ABO group and Rh type, Blood
Amniotic fluid, Erythroblastosis
   fetalis, Specimen

Additional Conditions
Pregnancy

ESOPHAGEAL ATRESIA
WITH TRACHEOSEPTAL
FISTULA
★Blood gases, Arterial, Blood
★Esophagogastroduodenoscopy,
   Diagnostic
Flat-plate radiography of abdomen,
   Diagnostic

Additional Conditions
Congenital heart disease
Cyanosis
Pneumonitis

ESOPHAGEAL CANCER
Brushing cytology, Specimen, Diagnostic
CA 19-9, Blood
CA 72-4, Blood
Carcinoembryonic antigen, Blood
Dual modality imaging, Diagnostic
Endoscopic ultrasonography, Diagnostic
Esophageal radiography, Diagnostic
★Esophagogastroduodenoscopy, Diagnostic
★Histopathology, Specimen
Tumor antigen 4, Blood and specimen
Telomerase enzyme marker, Blood
Thymidylate synthase, Specimen
Washing cytology, Specimen

Additional Conditions
Esophageal varices
Esophagitis
Mallory-Weiss syndrome
Throat infection

ESOPHAGEAL VARICES
(see Varices)

ESOPHAGITIS
Biopsy, Fungus, Culture
Brushing cytology, Specimen, Diagnostic
Endoscopic ultrasonography, Diagnostic
Esophageal radiography, Diagnostic
★Esophagogastroduodenoscopy, Diagnostic
Herpes virus antigen, Direct fluorescent antibody, Specimen
Histopathology, Specimen

Additional Conditions
Acquired immunodeficiency syndrome
Asthma
Candida albicans
Cough
Cytomegalovirus
Herpes simplex
Hiatal hernia
Nasogastric tube irritation
Obesity
Pneumonia
Pregnancy
Raynaud's phenomenon

ETHYLENE GLYCOL POISONING
★Anion gap, Blood
Bicarbonate, Plasma
★Chemistry profile, Blood
★Electrolytes, Plasma or serum
Heavy metals, Blood
Osmolality, Calculated tests, Blood (Osmolar gap)
★Toxicology, Volatiles group by GLC, Blood or urine
Urea nitrogen, Plasma or serum

Additional Conditions
Alcoholism
Depression

ETOH
(see Alcoholism and Drug abuse)

FACTOR DEFICIENCY
Activated partial thromboplastin substitution test, Diagnostic
Activated partial thromboplastin time, Plasma
★Coagulation factor assay, Blood
Factor II, Blood
Factor V, Blood
Factor VII, Blood
Factor VIII, Blood
Factor VIII R:Ag, Blood
Factor IX, Blood
Factor X, Blood
Factor XI, Blood
Factor XII, Blood
Factor XIII, Blood
Factor, Fitzgerald, Plasma
Factor, Fletcher, Plasma
Fibrinogen, Plasma
Prothrombin time and international normalized ratio, Serum
Thrombin time, Serum
von Willebrand factor antigen, Blood
von Willebrand factor assay, Blood

Additional Conditions
Afibrinogenemia
Cancer
Disseminated intravascular coagulation
Hemophilia
Vitamin K deficiency

FACTOR IX DEFICIENCY (CHRISTMAS DISEASE)
Activated partial thromboplastin time, Plasma
Circulating anticoagulant, Blood

*Coagulation factor assay, Blood
Factor XII, Blood
Plasma recalcification time, Plasma
Prothrombin time and international normalized ratio, Plasma

Additional Conditions
Hemorrhage
Thrombosis

FACTOR V DEFICIENCY
*Coagulation factor assay, Blood
Factor V, Blood

Additional Conditions
Hemorrhage
Thrombocytopenia

FACTOR XIII DEFICIENCY
Activated partial thromboplastin time, Plasma
*Coagulation factor assay, Blood
Factor VIII, Blood
Factor VIII R:Ag, Blood
Plasma recalcification time, Plasma
Prothrombin time and international normalized ratio, Plasma
von Willebrand factor antigen, Blood
von Willebrand factor assay, Blood

Additional Conditions
Cirrhosis
Hemorrhage

FAILURE TO THRIVE
Blood gases, Arterial, Blood
*Complete blood count, Blood
Creatinine, Serum
Fat, Semiquantitative, Stool
Growth hormone, Blood
Ova and parasites, Stool
*Transthyretin (Prealbumin), Serum
Urea nitrogen, Plasma or serum
Urine, Culture and sensitivity, Urine

Additional Conditions
Alcohol abuse during pregnancy
Down syndrome
Drug abuse during pregnancy
Esophageal atresia
Galactosemia
Hypoxia

FANCONI SYNDROME
Anion gap, Blood
Alkaline phosphatase, Serum

Blood gases, Venous, Blood
Calcium, Urine
Chemistry profile, Blood
Complete blood count, Blood
Electrolytes, Plasma
Glucose, Semiquantitative, Urine
Ketone, Semiquantitative, Urine
pH, Urine
*Phosphorus, Serum
Phosphorus, Urine
Protein, Quantitative, Urine
Uric acid, Serum

Additional Conditions
Amyloidosis
Glycogen storage disease
Heavy metal poisoning
Osteomalacia
Renal tubular acidosis
Wilson's disease

FARMER'S LUNG
*Chest radiography, Diagnostic
*Hypersensitivity pneumonitis serology, Blood

Additional Conditions
Asthma
Bronchitis

FASCIOLIASIS
*Differential leukocyte count, Peripheral blood
Eosinophil count, Blood
Liver scan, Diagnostic

Additional Conditions
Fever
Hepatomegaly
Urticaria

FAT EMBOLISM
Bicarbonate, Serum
Blood gases, Arterial, Blood
Carbon dioxide, Total content, Blood
Chemistry profile, Blood
Complete blood count, Blood
Electrolytes, Plasma or serum
Lipase, Serum
*Radiography, Diagnostic
*Venography, Diagnostic

Additional Conditions
Anemia
Fractures, Long bones
Thrombocytopenia

FATIGUE
*(see also Cancer, Infectious
mononucleosis, Myasthenia gravis, and
Systemic lupus erythematosus)*
Alcohol, Blood
★ Complete blood count, Blood
Liver battery, Serum
Thyroid profile, Blood

Additional Conditions
Anemia
Cancer
Chronic obstructive pulmonary
disease
Fever of undetermined origin
Hypothyroidism
Sleep disorders

FATTY LIVER
(see Liver dysfunction)

FEBRILE DISEASES
(see Fever of undetermined origin)

FEMOROPOPLITEAL BYPASS
GRAFT
(see Anesthesia)

FETAL DISEASES
(see Pregnancy)

FEVER OF UNDETERMINED
ORIGIN (FUO)
Acid-fast stain, *Nocardia* species,
Culture
Anti-DNA, Serum
Antinuclear antibody, Serum
Biopsy, Mycobacteria, Culture
★ Blood culture, Blood
Blood culture with antimicrobial
removal device, Culture
Body fluid, Routine, Culture (Urine)
Bone marrow aspiration analysis,
Specimen
Borrelia burgdorferi C6 peptide
antibody, Serum
Chest radiography, Diagnostic
C-reactive protein, Serum
★ Differential leukocyte count,
Peripheral blood
Histopathology, Specimen
Malaria smear, Blood
Salmonella titer, Blood
Sedimentation rate, Erythrocyte, Blood

Additional Conditions
Cancer
Cat-scratch disease
Chickenpox
Lyme disease
Measles
Sepsis
Tick bite
Typhus
Urinary tract infection

FIBRINOLYSIS
D-Dimer test, Blood
Euglobulin clot lysis, Blood
Fibrinogen, Plasma
Fibrinogen breakdown products,
Blood
Intravascular coagulation screen,
Blood
★ Plasminogen assay, Blood

Additional Conditions
Cirrhosis
Disseminated intravascular
coagulation
Thrombolytic therapy

FIBRINOPENIA
Cryofibrinogen, Serum
★ Fibrinogen, Plasma
Intravascular coagulation screen,
Blood
Reptilase time, Serum
Thrombin time, Serum

Additional Conditions
Cirrhosis
Hemorrhage

FIBROCYSTIC BREAST
Estrogens, Serum and 24-Hour urine
Histopathology, Specimen
★ Mammography, Diagnostic
Nipple discharge cytology, Specimen
Scintimammography, Diagnostic

Additional Conditions
Acute pain
Breast cancer
Obesity

FLANK PAIN
Antegrade pyelography, Diagnostic
Complete blood count, Blood
Comprehensive metabolic panel,
Blood

Computed tomography, Diagnostic
Flat-plate radiograph of the
abdomen, Diagnostic
Intravenous pyelography, Diagnostic
★Kidney ultrasound, Diagnostic
Liver ultrasound, Diagnostic
Magnetic resonance urography,
Diagnostic
Nephrotomography, Diagnostic
★Urinalysis, Urine

Additional Conditions
Abdominal aortic aneurysm
Nephrolithiasis
Ureteral obstruction

FOLIC ACID ANEMIA (FOLATE DEFICIENCY ANEMIA)
Blood indices, Blood
Bone marrow biopsy, Diagnostic
Differential leukocyte count,
Peripheral blood
Folic acid, Red blood cell, Blood
★Folic acid, Serum
Lactate dehydrogenase, Isoenzymes,
Blood
Red blood cell, Blood
Red blood cell morphology
(Megalocyte), Blood
Schilling test, Diagnostic
Vitamin B_{12}, Serum

Additional Conditions
Alcoholism
Cachexia
Chronic hemolytic anemia
Dialysis
Exfoliative skin disease
Low-fiber diet
Pregnancy
Tropical sprue

FORBES-ALBRIGHT SYNDROME
★Prolactin, Serum

Additional Conditions
Amenorrhea
Galactorrhea
Hypogonadism
Impotence
Oligomenorrhea
Pituitary tumor

FRACTURES
★Bone radiography, Diagnostic
Complete blood count, Blood

Computed tomography of the body,
Diagnostic

Additional Conditions
Alcoholism
Drug abuse
Fat embolism
Metastasis
Osteoporosis
Paget's disease of the bone
Physical abuse
Trauma

FUNGAL INFECTIONS
Amphotericin B, Blood
Biopsy, Fungus, Culture
★Blood, Fungus, Culture
Bronchial aspirate, Fungus,
Culture
Cerebrospinal fluid, Fungus,
Culture
Fungal antibody screen, Blood
Genital, *Candida albicans,* Culture
★Skin, Fungus, Culture
★Sputum, Fungus, Culture
★Urine, Fungus, Culture
★Wound, Fungus, Culture

Additional Conditions
Acquired immunodeficiency syndrome
Cancer
Candidiasis (thrush)
Conjunctivitis
Status post transplantation

FUO
(see Fever of undetermined origin)

G6PD DEFICIENCY (GLUCOSE-6-PHOSPHATE DEHYDROGENASE)
Blood indices, Blood
Complete blood count, Blood
Differential leukocyte count,
Peripheral blood
Glucose-6-phosphate dehydrogenase,
Quantitative, Blood
★Glucose-6-phosphate dehydrogenase
screen, Blood
Haptoglobin, Serum
Red blood cell, Blood
Reticulocyte count, Blood

Additional Conditions
Anemia
Jaundice
Splenomegaly

G-CELL HYPERPLASIA
★Gastrin, Serum
★Histopathology, Specimen
 Immunoperoxidase procedures,
  Diagnostic
 Pepsinogen-I antibody, Blood

Additional Conditions
Stomach cancer
Ulcers

GALACTOKINASE DEFICIENCY
★Galactose, Screening test for
 galactosemia, Urine

Additional Conditions
Cataracts

GALACTORRHEA
★Nipple discharge cytology, Specimen
 Prolactin, Serum

Additional Conditions
Acromegaly
Myxedema
Thyrotoxicosis

GALACTOSEMIA
Galactokinase, Blood
★Galactose, Screening test for
 galactosemia, Urine
Galactose-1-phosphate, Blood
Galactose-1-phosphate uridyl
 transferase, Erythrocyte, Blood
Galactose-1-phosphate uridyl
 transferase, Qualitative, Blood
Glucose, Qualitative and
 semiquantitative, Urine

Additional Conditions
Cataracts
Cirrhosis
Failure to thrive
Mental retardation

GANGLIONEUROBLASTOMA
Bone marrow aspiration analysis,
 Specimen
Bone scan, Diagnostic
★Brain biopsy, Diagnostic
 Complete blood count, Blood
 Computed tomography of the brain,
  Diagnostic
 Histopathology, Specimen
 Homovanillic acid, 24-Hour urine

5-Hydroxyindoleacetic acid,
 Quantitative, 24-Hour urine
Metanephrines, Total, 24-Hour urine
 and free plasma
Magnetic resonance imaging, Brain,
 Diagnostic
★Magnetic resonance neurography,
 Diagnostic
★Magnetic resonance spectroscopy,
 Diagnostic
 Octreotide scan, Diagnostic
 Vanillylmandelic acid, Urine

Additional Conditions
Abdominal pain
Congenital heart disease
Diarrhea
Periorbital ecchymosis
von Recklinghausen's disease

GANGRENE
★Biopsy, Anaerobic, Culture
 Blood culture, Blood
 Blood indices, Blood
 Body fluid, Anaerobic, Culture
  (Abscess)
 Complete blood count, Blood
 Creatine kinase, Serum
 Differential leukocyte count,
  Peripheral blood
 Electrolytes, Plasma or serum
 Histopathology, Specimen
 Myoglobin, Qualitative, Urine
 Myoglobin, Serum
 Radiography, Diagnostic

Additional Conditions
Cholecystitis
Diabetes mellitus
Peripheral vascular disease
Sepsis
Trauma

GASTRIC CANCER
Biopsy, Site-specific, Specimen
CA 72-4, Blood
Carcinoembryonic antigen, Serum
Dual modality imaging, Diagnostic
Endoscopic ultrasonography,
 Diagnostic
★Gastroscopy, Diagnostic
 Helicobacter pylori, Quick office
  serology, Serum and titer, Blood
★Histopathology, Specimen
 Iron, Serum
 Mucinlike carcinoma–associated
  antigen, Blood
 Occult blood, Stool

Pepsinogen I and pepsinogen II, Blood
Telomerase enzyme marker, Blood
Thymidylate synthase, Specimen
Upper gastrointestinal series, Diagnostic

Additional Conditions
Anemia
Malnutrition
Metastasis

GASTRIC ULCER
ABO group and Rh type, Blood
Amylase, Serum
Brushing cytology, Specimen, Diagnostic
Complete blood count, Blood
Endoscopic ultrasonography, Diagnostic
Gastrin, Serum
⋆Gastroscopy, Diagnostic
Helicobacter pylori, Quick office serology, Serum and titer, Blood
⋆Histopathology, Specimen
Lipase, Serum
Occult blood, Stool
Pepsinogen I and pepsinogen II, Blood
Washing cytology, Specimen

Additional Conditions
Acute pain
Gastritis
Hemorrhage

GASTRINOMA
(see Zollinger-Ellison syndrome)

GASTRITIS
(see also Helicobacter pylori*)*
Brushing cytology, Specimen, Diagnostic
Campylobacter-like organism test, Specimen
Folic acid, Serum
Gastrin, Serum
⋆Gastroscopy, Diagnostic
Helicobacter pylori, Quick office serology, Serum and titer, Blood
⋆Histopathology, Specimen
Occult blood, Stool
Pepsinogen I and pepsinogen II, Blood
Schilling test, Diagnostic
Urea breath test, Diagnostic
Vitamin B$_{12}$, Serum

Additional Conditions
Alcoholism
Cytomegalovirus
Crohn's disease
Eosinophilia
Gastric ulcer
Ischemia
Sarcoidosis
Schistosomiasis
Syphilis
Tuberculosis

GASTROENTERITIS
Fecal leukocytes, Stool, Diagnostic
Meat fibers, Stool
⋆Stool culture, Routine, Stool

Additional Conditions
Acute pain
Fever
Immunocompromised persons
Malnutrition

GASTROESOPHAGEAL REFLUX
Acid perfusion test, Diagnostic
⋆Esophageal acidity test, Diagnostic
⋆Esophageal manometry, Diagnostic
Esophageal radiography, Diagnostic

Additional Conditions
Hiatal hernia
Stomach cancer

GASTROINTESTINAL BLEEDING
Autoerythrocyte sensitivity test, Diagnostic
Blood urea nitrogen/creatinine ratio, Blood
⋆Complete blood count, Blood
Esophagogastroduodenoscopy, Diagnostic
Occult blood, Stool
⋆Type and crossmatch, Blood (Screen)

Additional Conditions
Alcoholism
Ascites
Encephalopathy
Esophageal varices
Gastric varices
Gastritis
Hypovolemic shock
Ischemia
Mallory-Weiss syndrome
Peptic ulcer

Portal hypertension
Thrombocytopenia

GAUCHER'S DISEASE
Acid phosphatase, Serum
Bone marrow biopsy, Diagnostic
*Complete blood count, Blood
Magnetic resonance imaging,
  Diagnostic

Additional Conditions
Anemia
Hepatosplenomegaly
Leukopenia
Thrombocytopenia

GENITAL HERPES
*Herpes cytology, Specimen
*Herpes simplex antibody, Blood
Histopathology, Specimen
Rapid plasma reagin test, Blood
Viral culture, Specimen

Additional Conditions
Cervicitis
Gonorrhea
Syphilis
Urinary tract infection
Vaginitis
Vulvar cancer

GENTAMYCIN
(see Aminoglycoside toxicity)

GERMAN MEASLES
(see Rubella)

GIARDIASIS
Fecal leukocytes, Stool,
  Diagnostic
Histopathology, Specimen
*Ova and parasites, Stool
Washing cytology, Specimen

Additional Conditions
Acquired immunodeficiency syndrome
Diarrhea
Malabsorption syndrome

GLANZMANN'S DISEASE
*Bleeding time, Ivy, Blood
*Bleeding time, Mielke, Blood
Clot retraction, Blood

Platelet adhesion test (Venous
  blood), Diagnostic
Platelet aggregation, Blood
Platelet aggregation, Hypercoagulable
  state, Blood

Additional Conditions
Epistaxis
Menorrhagia

GLAUCOMA
*Tonometry test for glaucoma,
  Diagnostic

Additional Conditions
Acute pain
Visual blurring
Visual field loss

GLOMERULONEPHRITIS
Addis count, 12-Hour urine
Albumin/globulin ratio, Serum
Antideoxyribonuclease-B titer, Serum
Anti-DNA, Serum
Antihyaluronidase titer, Serum
Antistreptolysin-O titer, Serum
C1q immune complex detection,
  Serum
C3 complement, Serum
C3 proactivator, Serum
C4 complement, Serum
Chemistry profile, Blood
Complement components, Serum
Complement, Total, Serum
Creatinine clearance, Serum, Urine
Glomerular basement membrane
  antibody, Serum
Hepatitis B surface antigen, Blood
Immune complex assay, Blood
Intravenous pyelography, Diagnostic
Ki-67 proliferation marker, Specimen
Kidney biopsy, Specimen
Mean platelet volume, Blood
Occult blood, Urine
Protein electrophoresis, Serum
*Protein, Urine
Specific gravity, Urine
Streptozyme, Blood
Throat culture for group A
  beta-hemolytic streptococci, Culture
Urea nitrogen, Plasma or serum
*Urinalysis, Urine

Additional Conditions
Amyloidosis
Chickenpox
Colon cancer
Endocarditis

Goodpasture syndrome
Hepatitis
Kidney cancer
Leprosy
Lung cancer
Malaria
Measles
Melanoma
Pneumonia
Schistosomiasis
Scleroderma
Sickle cell disease
Syphilis
Systemic lupus erythematosus
Toxoplasmosis

GLUCAGONOMA
Chemistry profile, Blood
★Glucagon, Plasma
Glucose, Blood
Insulin and insulin antibodies, Blood

Additional Conditions
Hypoglycemia
Pheochromocytoma

GLYCOGEN STORAGE DISEASE
Bone marrow aspiration analysis,
   Specimen
★Glucose, Blood
Pregnancy test, Routine, Serum and
   qualitative, Urine
Glucose tolerance test, Blood
Glucose, 2-Hour postprandial, Serum
Histopathology, Specimen
Ketone bodies, Blood
★Ketones, Semiquantitative, Urine
Lipid profile, Blood
Uric acid, Serum

Additional Conditions
Ataxia
Congestive heart failure
Gout
Hepatomegaly
Hyperlipidemia
Hyperuricemia
Hypoglycemia

GLYCOGENOSIS
(see Glycogen storage disease)

GLYCOSURIA
★Glucose, Qualitative and
   semiquantitative, Urine

Glucose, Quantitative, 24-Hour urine
Glucose, 2-Hour postprandial, Serum
Glycosylated hemoglobin, Blood
Osmolality, Urine

Additional Conditions
Cancer
Diabetes mellitus
Obesity

GOITER
(see Hypothyroidism)

GONOCOCCAL INFECTION OF PHARYNX
Rapid plasma reagin test, Blood
★Throat culture for Neisseria
   gonorrhoeae, Culture

Additional Conditions
Pharyngitis

GONORRHEA
Chlamydia culture and group titer,
   Specimen (Culture)
Fluorescent treponemal
   antibody–absorbed double-stain
   test, Serum
Genital, Neisseria gonorrhoeae, Culture
Gram stain, Diagnostic (Urine)
★Neisseria gonorrhoeae smear,
   Specimen
Rapid plasma reagin test, Blood
Throat culture for Neisseria
   gonorrhoeae, Culture
Urine culture and nucleic acid
   amplification tests for Neisseria
   gonorrhoeae, Urine
★Venereal Disease Research Laboratory
   test, Serum

Additional Conditions
Cervicitis
Chlamydia
Conjunctivitis
Epididymitis
Human immunodeficiency virus
Prostatitis
Salpingitis
Syphilis
Trichomonas
Vaginitis

GOODPASTURE SYNDROME
Bronchial washing, Specimen,
   Diagnostic

Brushing cytology, Specimen,
  Diagnostic
Complete blood count,
  Blood
Creatinine, Serum
Creatinine, Urine
Electrolytes, Plasma or serum
Electrolytes, Urine
Eosinophil count, Blood
Glomerular basement membrane
  antibody, Serum
★ Kidney biopsy, Specimen
Occult blood, Urine
Protein, Quantitative, Urine
Protein, Semiquantitative, Urine
Sputum hemosiderin preparation,
  Specimen
★ Urinalysis, Urine
Washing cytology, Specimen

Additional Conditions
Glomerulonephritis
Hemodialysis
Hemoptysis
Hypoxia

GOUT
Body fluid analysis, Cell count,
  Specimen
Body fluid, Routine, Culture
Chemistry profile, Blood
Heavy metal screen, Blood and
  24-Hour urine
Mucin clot test, Specimen
Phosphorus, Serum
Synovial fluid analysis, Diagnostic
★ Uric acid, Serum
Uric acid, Urine

Additional Conditions
Anemia
Arthritis
Cancer
Chronic renal disease
Diabetes insipidus
Diabetic ketoacidosis
Glycogen storage disease
Hyperuricemia
Lead poisoning
Lesch-Nyhan syndrome
Multiple myeloma
Pruritus
Psoriasis
Sarcoma

GRANULOCYTIC LEUKEMIA
(see Leukemia)

GRANULOMAS
★ Liver ^{131}I scan, Diagnostic

Additional Conditions
Diabetes mellitus
Hypoxemia
Pulmonary infiltrates
Splenomegaly

GRAVES' DISEASE
(see Hyperthyroidism)

GROWTH HORMONE DEFICIENCY
Chromosome analysis, Blood
★ Growth hormone, Blood
Insulin-like growth factor-I, Blood
Zinc, Blood

Additional Conditions
Cushing syndrome
Dwarfism
Hashimoto's thyroiditis
Hypopituitarism
Rickets
Turner syndrome

GUILLAIN-BARRÉ SYNDROME
★ Cerebrospinal fluid, Routine analysis,
  Specimen
Electromyography and nerve
  conduction studies, Diagnostic
Heavy metal screen, Blood and
  24-Hour urine
Immunoglobulin G synthesis rate,
  Cerebrospinal fluid, Specimen
Magnetic resonance neurography,
  Diagnostic

Additional Conditions
Autoimmune diseases
Malnutrition
Viral disorder
Vitamin E deficiency

GYNECOMASTIA
Alcohol, Serum
Chemistry profile, Blood
★ Estradiol, Serum
Follicle-stimulating hormone,
  Serum
Histopathology, Specimen
★ Human chorionic gonadotropin,
  Beta-subunit, Serum

Liver battery, Serum
Prolactin, Serum
★Testosterone, Free, Bioavailable and
total, Blood

Additional Conditions
Addison's disease
Alcoholism
Cirrhosis
Hyperthyroidism
Hypogonadism
Puberty
Testicular tumors

HAEMOPHILUS INFLUENZAE INFECTION
Respiratory antigen panel,
Specimen
★Sputum for *Haemophilus* species,
Culture

Additional Conditions
Croup
Epiglottitis
Meningitis
Pneumonia

HAGEMAN FACTOR
Activated partial thromboplastin
time, Plasma
Coagulation factor assay, Blood
★Factor XII, Blood

Additional Conditions
Thrombocytopenia
Vasoconstriction

HAIRY CELL LEUKEMIA
Acid phosphatase, Serum
★Bone marrow biopsy, Diagnostic
Histopathology, Specimen
Leukocyte cytochemistry (Bone
marrow), Specimen
★Tartrate-resistant acid phosphatase,
Blood

Additional Conditions
Fatigue
Hepatomegaly
Pancytopenia
Splenomegaly

HALLUCINOGENS: LSD, MESCALINE, MDA, PCP, PSILOCYBIN
(see *Drug abuse*)

HAND-SCHÜLLER-CHRISTIAN DISEASE
Bone scan, Diagnostic
★Chest radiography, Diagnostic

Additional Conditions
Bronchiolitis
Dyspnea
Fever
Pneumothorax

HARTNUP DISEASE
★Indican, Urine

Additional Conditions
Dermatitis
Renal failure

HASHIMOTO'S THYROIDITIS
Histopathology, Specimen
Needle aspiration cytology (Thyroid),
Specimen
Thyroid peroxidase antibody, Blood
Thyroid antithyroglobulin antibody,
Serum
★Thyroid profile, Blood
★Thyroid-stimulating hormone, Blood

Additional Conditions
Goiter
Myxedema

HAY FEVER
Allergin-specific IgE, Serum
★Eosinophil count, Blood
Eosinophil peroxidase, Serum
Immunoglobulin E, Serum

Additional Conditions
Nasal polyps
Pruritus

HEAD AND NECK CANCER
Barium swallow, Diagnostic
★Biopsy, Site-specific, Specimen
CA 15-3, Serum
CA 50, Blood (Esophagus,
squamous)
Chest radiography, Diagnostic
★Computed tomography of the body
(Head and neck), Diagnostic
Dual modality imaging, Diagnostic
Esophageal radiography, Diagnostic
Magnetic resonance imaging,
Diagnostic

Telomerase enzyme marker, Blood or urine (Blood)
Transesophageal ultrasonography, Diagnostic

Additional Conditions
Alcoholism
Epstein-Barr virus
Iron deficiency
Malnutrition

HEAD INJURIES
Cerebrospinal fluid, Routine analysis, Specimen
Complete blood count, Blood
★ Computed tomography of the brain, Diagnostic
Doppler ultrasonographic flow studies (Transcranial), Diagnostic
Electroencephalography, Diagnostic
★ Magnetic resonance imaging, Diagnostic
Radiography of skull, chest, and cervical spine, Diagnostic

Additional Conditions
Coma
Concussion
Edema
Hematoma
Hemorrhage
Seizures
Shock
Trauma

HEADACHE
Carbon monoxide, Blood
Carboxyhemoglobin, Blood
Cerebrospinal fluid, Routine analysis, Specimen
Cold agglutinin screen, Blood
Cold agglutinin titer, Serum
Heavy metal screen, Blood and 24-Hour urine (Urine)
Methemoglobin, Blood
Mycoplasma titer, Blood
Rocky Mountain spotted fever serology, Blood
Viscosity, Serum

Additional Conditions
Allergies
Arteritis
Brain tumors
Concussion
Coughing
Depression
Encephalitis
Horner syndrome
Hypertension
Photophobia
Subarachnoid hemorrhage
Tension and stress

HEARING DISORDERS
Fluorescent treponemal antibody–absorbed double-stain test, Serum
★ Hearing test for loudness—recruitment, Diagnostic
Magnetic resonance imaging (functional), Diagnostic
★ Tuning fork test of Weber, Rinne, and Schwabach tests, Diagnostic

Additional Conditions
Aminoglycoside toxicity
Chemotherapy-induced
Diabetes mellitus
Hypothyroidism
Measles
Mumps
Otitis media
Renal failure
Syphilis
Tinnitus

HEART FAILURE
(*see Congestive heart failure*)

HEART-LUNG MACHINE
Activated coagulation time, Automated, Blood
Activated partial thromboplastin time, Plasma
Blood gases, Arterial, Blood
Complete blood count, Blood
Prothrombin time and international normalized ratio, Plasma

Additional Conditions
Chronic obstructive pulmonary disease
Coronary artery bypass graft (CABG), Surgery

HEART MURMUR
Cardiac radiography, Diagnostic
Echocardiography, Diagnostic
★ Electrocardiography, Diagnostic
Transesophageal ultrasonography, Diagnostic

Additional Conditions
Aortic stenosis
Mitral prolapse
Mitral stenosis
Patent ductus arteriosus

Pulmonic stenosis
Rheumatic fever
Scarlet fever
Tetralogy of Fallot
Tricuspid stenosis

HEART TRANSPLANT
(see Transplants)

HEAT STROKE
Calcium, Total, Serum
Complete blood count, Blood
* Electrocardiography, Diagnostic
* Electrolytes, Plasma or serum
Prothrombin time and international
   normalized ratio, Plasma
Urea nitrogen, Plasma or serum
Urinalysis, Urine

Additional Conditions
Hyperventilation
Myocardial infarction
Renal failure
Seizures

HEINZ BODY ANEMIA
Blood indices, Blood
Complete blood count, Blood
Differential leukocyte count,
   Peripheral blood
Glucose-6-phosphate dehydrogenase,
   Quantitative, Blood
Glucose-6-phosphate dehydrogenase
   screen, Blood
* Heinz body stain, Diagnostic
Hemoglobin electrophoresis, Blood
Hemoglobin, Unstable, Heat labile
   test, Blood
Hemoglobin, Unstable, Isopropanol
   precipitation test, Blood
Methemoglobin, Blood
Red blood cell, Blood
Red blood cell morphology, Blood
Reticulocyte count, Blood

Additional Conditions
G6PD deficiency
Hemoglobinemia
Hemoglobinuria
Hyperbilirubinemia
Jaundice

HELICOBACTER PYLORI
Campylobacter-like organism test,
   Specimen

Cytologic study of gastrointestinal
   tract, Diagnostic
Gastric acid analysis test,
   Diagnostic
Gastric analysis, Specimen
Gastroscopy or
   gastroduodenojejunoscopy,
   Diagnostic
Helicobacter pylori antigen test,
   Stool
* Helicobacter pylori, Quick office
   serology, Serum and titer, Blood
Immunoglobulin G, Serum
Pepsinogen I and pepsinogen II,
   Blood
Stool culture, Routine, Stool
Urea breath test, Diagnostic

Additional Conditions
Botulism
Colitis
Diarrhea
Peptic ulcer disease

HEMATURIA
Addis count, 12-Hour urine
Antideoxyribonuclease-B titer,
   Serum
Antihyaluronidase titer, Serum
Antistreptolysin-O titer, Serum
Body fluid, Routine, Culture (Urine)
Creatinine, Serum
Creatinine, Urine
Electrolytes, Plasma or serum
Electrolytes, Urine
Glomerular basement membrane
   antibody, Serum
Kidney biopsy, Specimen
Kidney stone analysis, Specimen
Myoglobin, Urine
* Occult blood, Urine
Streptozyme, Blood
Urea nitrogen, Plasma or serum
* Urinalysis, Urine
Urine cytology, Urine
Urine, Fungus, Culture
Urine, Mycobacteria, Culture

Additional Conditions
Bladder cancer
Disseminated intravascular
   coagulation
Glomerulonephrosis
Hemoglobinuria
Hemophilia
Renal disease
Sickle cell disease
Trauma
Urinary tract infection

HEMOCHROMATOSIS
Ferritin, Serum
Glucose, Blood
Glucose tolerance test, Blood
Hemosiderin stain, Urine
Histopathology, Specimen
★Iron, Serum
Iron stain, Bone marrow, Specimen
Liver battery, Serum
★Total iron-binding capacity, Serum

Additional Conditions
Congestive heart failure
Diabetes mellitus
Esophageal varices
Hepatomegaly
Hyperglycemia
Renal failure

HEMOFLAGELLATES
(see Trypanosomiasis)

HEMOGLOBIN C DISEASE
★Complete blood count, Blood
★Hemoglobin electrophoresis,
   Blood
Red blood cell morphology, Blood

Additional Conditions
Anemia
Jaundice
Retinopathy
Splenomegaly

HEMOLYTIC ANEMIA
★Bilirubin, Total, Serum
Complete blood count, Blood
Ham test, Blood
★Haptoglobin, Serum
Red blood cell morphology, Blood
★Reticulocyte count, Blood
Sedimentation rate, Erythrocyte,
   Blood
Urobilinogen, Urine

Additional Conditions
Burns
Disseminated intravascular
   coagulation
Drug reaction
G6PD deficiency
Malaria
Metastasis
Sickle cell disease
Transfusion reaction, Delayed or
   immediate
Vasculitis

HEMOPHILIA
Activated coagulation time,
   Automated, Blood
Activated partial thromboplastin
   time, Plasma
Aspirin tolerance test, Diagnostic
Circulating anticoagulant, Blood
Complete blood count, Blood
★Factor VIII, Blood
Factor VIII R:Ag, Blood
Occult blood, Urine
Plasma recalcification time, Plasma
Platelet aggregation, Hypercoagulable
   state, Blood

Additional Conditions
Acquired immunodeficiency
   syndrome
Hemorrhage
Thrombosis

HEMOPTYSIS
Activated partial thromboplastin
   time, Plasma
Bleeding time, Duke, Blood
Bleeding time, Ivy, Blood
Bronchial washing, Specimen,
   Diagnostic
★Bronchoscopy, Diagnostic
Brushing cytology, Specimen,
   Diagnostic
Complete blood count, Blood
★Chest radiography, Diagnostic
Computed tomography of the body
   (Lung), Diagnostic
Prothrombin time and international
   normalized ratio, Plasma
Sputum, Routine, Culture
★Sputum cytology, Specimen
Sputum, Mycobacteria, Culture and
   smear

Additional Conditions
Alveolar hemorrhage
Bronchitis
Esophageal varices
Lung cancer
Pneumonia
Tuberculosis

HEMORRHAGE
★Activated partial thromboplastin
   time, Plasma
Betke-Kleihauer stain, Diagnostic
Chemistry profile, Blood
★Complete blood count,
   Blood
D-Dimer Test, Blood

Hematocrit, Blood
Hemoglobin, Blood
Iron, Serum
Occult blood, Stool
Platelet count, Stool
★ Prothrombin time and international
   normalized ratio, Plasma
Sputum hemosiderin preparation,
   Specimen
Total iron-binding capacity, Serum
Type and crossmatch, Blood
Urinalysis, Urine

Additional Conditions
Aneurysm
Brain tumor
Burns
Cerebral hemorrhage
Cystitis
Disseminated intravascular
   coagulation
Esophageal varices
Hemophilia
Leukemia
Trauma
Ulcers

HEMORRHOIDS
Complete blood count, Blood
★ Proctoscopy, Diagnostic

Additional Conditions
Anal fissure
Anemia
Bowel incontinence
Colon cancer
Portal hypertension
Pregnancy
Rectal cancer

HEPATIC CIRRHOSIS
★ Liver biopsy, Diagnostic
Liver ultrasonography, Diagnostic

Additional Conditions
Alcoholism
Cystic fibrosis
Drug abuse
Peptic ulcers
Sjögren syndrome

HEPATIC COMA
(see also Hepatitis or Jaundice)
★ Albumin, Serum
★ Ammonia, Blood
Amylase, Serum
Antinuclear antibody, Serum

★ Bilirubin, Total, Serum
Cerebrospinal fluid, Routine, Culture
   and cytology
Cerebrospinal fluid, Glucose,
   Specimen
Cerebrospinal fluid, Protein,
   Specimen
Lactic acid, Blood
Urea nitrogen, Plasma or serum

Additional Conditions
Encephalitis
Heavy metal poisoning
Hepatorenal syndrome
Renal failure

HEPATIC ENCEPHALOPATHY
★ Ammonia, Blood
★ Liver battery, Serum
Liver biopsy, Diagnostic
★ Liver scan, Diagnostic
Liver ultrasonography, Diagnostic
Liver-spleen scan, Diagnostic
Magnetic resonance spectroscopy,
   Diagnostic
Paracentesis, Diagnostic
Ultrasonography, Liver, Diagnostic
★ Urea nitrogen, Plasma or serum

Additional Conditions
Gastrointestinal bleeding
Hypokalemia
Hypovolemia, After paracentesis
Metabolic acidosis
Sepsis

HEPATITIS
Acetaminophen, Serum
Alanine aminotransferase, Serum
Albumin/globulin ratio, Serum
Alkaline phosphatase, Isoenzymes,
   Serum
Alkaline phosphatase, Serum
Alpha-antitrypsin, Serum
Alpha-fetoprotein, Serum
Antimitochondrial antibody, Blood
Anti–smooth muscle antibody,
   Serum
Aspartate aminotransferase, Serum
★ Bilirubin, Direct, Serum
Bilirubin, Indirect, Serum
C1q immune complex detection,
   Serum
C3 complement, Serum
C4 complement, Serum
Chemistry profile, Blood
Cytomegalovirus antibody, Serum
Epstein-Barr virus, Serology, Blood

Gamma-glutamyltranspeptidase, Blood
Hepatitis A antibody, IgM and IgG, Blood
Hepatitis B core antibody, Blood
Hepatitis B e antibody, Serum
Hepatitis B e antigen, Blood
Hepatitis B surface antibody, Blood
Hepatitis B surface antigen, Blood
Hepatitis C antibody, Serum
Hepatitis C genotype, Serum
Hepatitis delta antibody, Serum
★Hepatitis serologies
Histopathology, Specimen
Lactate dehydrogenase, Isoenzymes, Blood
★Liver battery, Serum
Liver biopsy, Diagnostic
Liver scan, Diagnostic
Liver ultrasonography, Diagnostic
Lupus test, Blood
Methotrexate, Serum
5'-Nucleotidase, Blood
Ornithine carbamoyltransferase, Blood
Protein electrophoresis, Serum
Prothrombin time and international normalized ratio, Plasma
Salicylate, Blood
Toxoplasmosis serology, Serum
Urobilinogen, Urine

Additional Conditions
After transfusion of blood
Alcoholism
Amenorrhea
Anemia, Hemolytic
Cirrhosis
Drug abuse
Hepatic coma
Hyperuricemia
Hypocholesterolemia
Jaundice
Pruritus

HEPATOMAS
Liver ^{131}I scan, Diagnostic
★Liver ultrasonography, Diagnostic

Additional Conditions
Cirrhosis
Endocrine syndrome
Immunoglobulin changes

HEPATOMEGALY
Liver biopsy, Diagnostic
★Liver ultrasonography, Diagnostic

Additional Conditions
Alcohol abuse
Cirrhosis
Esophageal varices
Leukemia
Neoplastic disease
Portal hypertension

HERPES SIMPLEX (COLD SORE, FEVER BLISTER)
Herpes simplex antibody, Blood
★Herpes virus antigen, Direct fluorescent antibody, Specimen
★Tzanck test smear, Specimen

Additional Conditions
Encephalitis
Keratitis
Ophthalmitis
Stress
Varicella-zoster virus infection

HERPES VIRUS INFECTION
Bronchial washing, Specimen, Diagnostic
Brushing cytology, Specimen, Diagnostic
Cervical-vaginal cytology, Specimen
★Herpes cytology, Specimen
Herpes simplex antibody, Blood
Oral cavity cytology, (Scrape) Specimen
Sputum cytology, Specimen
Toxoplasmosis, Rubella, Cytomegalovirus, Herpes virus serology, Blood
Tzanck smear, Specimen
Varicella-zoster virus serology, Serum
Viral culture, Specimen

Additional Conditions
Cervicitis
Glaucoma
Leukemia
Stomatitis
Varicella-zoster virus infection

HERPES ZOSTER (SHINGLES)
★Varicella-zoster virus serology, Serum

Additional Conditions
Chickenpox
Fever
Hodgkin's disease
Leukemia
Lymphoma
Monkeypox

HIATAL HERNIA
Barium swallow, Diagnostic
*Esophageal radiography, Diagnostic
Upper gastrointestinal series,
  Diagnostic

Additional Conditions
Dysphagia

HIRSCHSPRUNG'S DISEASE
*Barium enema, Diagnostic
Histopathology, Specimen

Additional Conditions
Abdominal pain
Constipation
Vomiting

HIRSUTISM (HYPERTRICHOSIS)
Androstenedione, Serum
*Dehydroepiandrosterone sulfate,
  Serum
17-Hydroxycorticosteroids, 24-Hour
  urine
*17-Hydroxyprogesterone, Blood
17-Ketosteroids, Total, 24-Hour urine
Pregnanetriol, Urine
Prolactin, Serum
*Testosterone, Free, Bioavailable and
  total, Blood

Additional Conditions
Amenorrhea
Cushing syndrome
Hypertension
Hypokalemia
Obesity
Ovarian tumor
Postmenopausal effect

HISTOPLASMOSIS
Amphotericin B, Blood
Biopsy, Fungus, Culture
Blood, Fungus, Culture
Body fluid, Fungus, Culture
Bone marrow biopsy, Diagnostic
Bronchial aspirate, Routine, Culture
Bronchial aspirate, Fungus, Culture
Bronchial washing, Specimen,
  Diagnostic
Brushing cytology, Specimen,
  Diagnostic
Cerebrospinal fluid, Fungus, Culture
Chest radiography, Diagnostic
Complement fixation, Serum
Flucytosine, Serum
Fungal antibody screen, Blood

Histopathology, Specimen
*Histoplasmosis serology, Blood
Needle aspiration cytology, (Lung)
  Specimen
Platelet count, Blood
Sputum cytology, Specimen
Sputum, Fungus, Culture

Additional Conditions
Anemia
Chronic obstructive pulmonary
  disease
Diarrhea
Fever
Hepatosplenomegaly
Immunosuppression
Pneumonia

HODGKIN'S DISEASE
Biopsy, Site-specific, Specimen
Body fluid cytology, Specimen
Bone marrow biopsy, Diagnostic
Chemistry profile, Blood
Chromosome analysis, Blood
Complete blood count, Blood
C-reactive protein, Serum
Cryoglobulin, Qualitative, Serum
Differential leukocyte count,
  Peripheral blood
D-Xylose absorption test, Diagnostic,
  Serum or urine
Globulin, Serum
*Histopathology, Specimen
Immunoelectrophoresis, Serum and
  urine
Immunoglobulin A, Serum
Immunoglobulin G, Serum
Immunoglobulin M, Serum
Immunoperoxidase procedures (for
  antigens), Diagnostic
Leukocyte cytochemistry,
  Specimen
*Lymph node biopsy, Specimen
Lymphocyte subset enumeration,
  Blood
Muramidase, Serum and urine
Needle aspiration cytology, (Mass)
  Specimen
Platelet count, Blood
Pneumocystis immunofluorescent
  assay, Serum
Protein electrophoresis, Serum
Protein electrophoresis, Urine
T- and B-lymphocyte subset assay,
  Blood
Terminal deoxynucleotidyltransferase,
  Bone marrow
Uric acid, Serum

Additional Conditions
Cat-scratch disease
Fever
Infectious mononucleosis
Lymphadenopathy
Night sweats

HORMONAL THERAPY
Estrogen receptor and progesterone
   receptor in breast cancer,
   Diagnostic
Progesterone receptor assay,
   Specimen

Additional Conditions
Breast cancer
Endometrial cancer
Postmenopause
Prostate cancer

HUMAN PAPILLOMAVIRUS
★Human papillomavirus, Specimen

Additional Conditions
Acquired immunodeficiency
   syndrome
Chancroid
Chlamydia
Gonorrhea
Granuloma inguinale
Herpesvirus hominis II
Human immunodeficiency virus
Lymphogranuloma venereum
Syphilis

HUMORAL IMMUNE DEFICIENCY
Globulin, Serum
★Immunoelectrophoresis, Serum and
   Urine
Immunoglobulin A, Serum
Immunoglobulin G, Serum
Immunoglobulin M, Serum
Protein electrophoresis, Serum
★T- and B-lymphocyte subset assay,
   Blood

Additional Conditions
Lymphoma
Multiple myeloma
Thymoma

HUNTER SYNDROME
★Mucopolysaccharides, Qualitative,
   Urine

Additional Conditions
Rheumatic fever
Rheumatoid arthritis
Scleroderma
Sjögren syndrome
Systemic lupus erythematosus

HURLER SYNDROME
Differential leukocyte count,
   Peripheral blood
Fibroblast skin culture
★Mucopolysaccharides, Qualitative,
   Urine
S mucopolysaccharide turnover,
   Diagnostic

Additional Conditions
Corneal blurring
Deafness
Hepatosplenomegaly
Mental retardation
Myocarditis

HYALINE MEMBRANE DISEASE
★Alpha$_1$-antitrypsin, Serum
★Amniotic fluid analysis, (Pulmonary
   surfactant) Specimen
Bicarbonate, Serum
Blood gases, Arterial, Blood
Blood gases, Capillary, Blood
Carbon dioxide, Partial pressure, Blood
Chest radiography, Diagnostic

Additional Conditions
Diabetes mellitus in pregnancy
Premature infants weighing between
   1000 and 1500 g

HYDATIDIFORM MOLE
Histopathology, Specimen
★Human chorionic gonadotropin,
   Beta-subunit, Serum
Obstetric ultrasonography, Diagnostic
Protein, Quantitative, Urine

Additional Conditions
Eclampsia
Hyperthyroidism
Nausea and vomiting
Uterine bleeding

HYDRATION
Chemistry profile, Blood
★Complete blood count, Blood
★Electrolytes, Plasma or serum

Electrolytes, Urine
Osmolality, Serum
Osmolality, Urine
Parathyroid hormone, Blood
Sodium, Plasma, Serum or urine

Additional Conditions
Chemotherapy
Postoperative
Preoperative

HYDRONEPHROSIS
Body fluid, Routine, Culture (Urine)
Complete blood count, Blood
Computed tomography of the body
  (Kidney), Diagnostic
★Creatinine, Serum
Creatinine clearance, Serum, Urine
Electrolytes, Plasma or serum
Electrolytes, Urine
Intravenous pyelography, Diagnostic
★Kidney ultrasonography, Diagnostic
Magnetic resonance imaging,
  Diagnostic
Prostate-specific antigen, Serum
Urea nitrogen, Plasma or serum
Urinalysis, Urine
Urine cytology, Urine

Additional Conditions
Pyelonephritis
Ureteral obstruction

HYPERALDOSTERONISM
★Aldosterone, Serum and urine
Chemistry profile, Blood
Electrolytes, Plasma
Electrolytes, Urine
Histopathology, Specimen
Kidney profile, Specimens
Osmolality, Calculated test, Blood
Osmolality, Serum
Osmolality, Urine
★Potassium, Serum
Renin activity, Plasma
Sodium, Plasma, Serum or urine

Additional Conditions
Cirrhosis
Congestive heart failure
Conn syndrome
Headache
Hypernatremia
Hypertension
Hypokalemia
Metabolic alkalosis
Polydipsia
Polyuria

HYPERALIMENTATION
Albumin, Serum
Albumin/globulin ratio, Serum
Blood, Fungus, Culture
Chemistry profile, Blood
Electrolytes, Plasma
Foreign body, Routine, Culture
Glucose, Blood
Lipid profile, Blood

Additional Conditions
Anorexia nervosa
Cachexia
Cancer
Catatonia
Coma
Malnutrition

HYPERBARIC OXYGENATION
Blood gases, Arterial, Blood

Additional Conditions
Divers' bends
Gangrene
Sepsis

HYPERBILIRUBINEMIA
Alanine aminotransferase, Serum
Aspartate aminotransferase, Serum
★Bilirubin, Total, Serum

Additional Conditions
Cholestasis
Crigler-Najjar syndrome
Dubin-Johnson syndrome
Gilbert syndrome
Jaundice
Rotor syndrome

HYPERCALCEMIA
Albumin, Serum
Alkaline phosphatase, Serum
Anion gap, Blood
Blood urea nitrogen/creatinine ratio,
  Blood
★Calcium, Total, Serum
Calcium, Urine
Cyclic adenosine monophosphate,
  Serum and urine
Magnesium, Serum
Parathyroid hormone, Blood
★Phosphorus, Serum
Phosphorus, Urine
Vitamin D_3, Plasma or serum

Additional Conditions
Acromegaly
Cancer
Hyperparathyroidism
Hypophosphatemia
Immobilization
Metastasis to bone
Multiple myeloma
Paget's disease of bone
Sarcoidosis

HYPERCAPNIA
Bicarbonate, Serum
★Blood gases, Arterial, Blood
Blood gases, Capillary, Blood
Blood gases, Venous, Blood
Carbon dioxide, Blood
Chest radiography, Diagnostic
pH, Blood
Pulmonary function tests,
    Diagnostic

Additional Conditions
Anesthesia
Chronic obstructive pulmonary
    disease
Congestive heart failure
Dysrhythmias
Kyphoscoliosis
Myocardial infarction
Poisoning
Respiratory acidosis
Stroke

HYPERCHOLESTEROLEMIA
Cholesterol, Blood
Glucose, Blood
High-density lipoprotein cholesterol,
    Blood
Low-density lipoprotein cholesterol,
    Blood
★Lipid profile, Blood
Phospholipids, Serum
Thyroid profile, Blood
Triglycerides, Blood
Uric acid, Serum

Additional Conditions
Atherosclerosis
Hypercalcemia
Hypertension
Hyperuricemia
Hypoalbuminemia
Myocardial infarction
Obesity

HYPERGLUCAGON SYNDROME
★Glucagon, Plasma

Additional Conditions
Addison's disease
Cirrhosis
Hypopituitarism

HYPERGLYCEMIA
Chemistry profile, Blood
Cortisol, Plasma or serum
Glucagon, Plasma
★Glucose, Blood
Glucose-monitoring machines,
    Diagnostic
Glucose tolerance test, Blood
Glucose, 2-Hour postprandial, Serum
Glycosylated hemoglobin, Blood
Growth hormone, Blood
Insulin and insulin antibodies, Blood
Ketone bodies, Blood
Urinalysis, Urine

Additional Conditions
Cancer
Diabetes mellitus
Metabolic syndrome

HYPERGLYCEMIC HYPEROSMOLAR NONKETOTIC COMA (HHNK)
Blood gases (pH), Arterial, Blood
Chemistry profile, Blood
Complete blood count, Blood
Creatinine, Serum
Creatinine, Urine
Electrolytes, Plasma or serum
Electrolytes, Urine
★Glucose, Blood
★Osmolality, Serum
Osmolality, Urine
Urea nitrogen, Plasma or serum

Additional Conditions
Acute infection
Diabetes mellitus, Type 2
Renal failure
Steroid use
Stress
Trauma

HYPERINSULINISM
C-peptide, Serum
★Insulin and insulin antibodies, Blood

Additional Conditions
Hypoglycemia
Insulinoma

HYPERKALEMIA
Aldosterone, Serum and urine
Calcium, Total, Serum
Chemistry profile, Blood
★ Electrocardiography, Diagnostic
Electrolytes, Plasma
Glucose, Blood
Magnesium, Serum
★ Potassium, Serum
Potassium, Urine

Additional Conditions
Acidosis
Dehydration
Hypercapnia
Hyperlipoproteinemia
Poisoning
Renal failure

HYPERLIPOPROTEINEMIA
Cholesterol, Blood
★ Lipid profile, Blood
Triglycerides, Blood

Additional Conditions
Alcoholism
Atherosclerosis
Glycogen storage disease
Hepatic disease
Hypercholesterolemia
Hypothyroidism
Metabolic syndrome
Myocardial infarction
Pancreatitis

HYPERMAGNESEMIA
Anion gap, Blood
Calcium, Total, Serum
Electrolytes, Plasma
★ Magnesium, Serum
Magnesium, 24-Hour urine

Additional Conditions
Adrenal insufficiency
Antacid abuse (containing magnesium)
Apnea
Burns
Cathartic abuse
Diabetic ketoacidosis
Hypothyroidism
Hypoxia
Rhabdomyolysis
Trauma

HYPERNATREMIA
Cholesterol, Blood
★ Electrolytes, Plasma or serum
Electrolytes, Urine
Glucose, Blood
Glucose, Quantitative, 24-Hour urine
Osmolality, Serum
★ Sodium, Plasma or serum
Triglycerides, Blood

Additional Conditions
Dehydration
Diabetes insipidus
Diabetic ketoacidosis
Hyperglycemic hyperosmolar nonketotic coma
Hypotension
Tachycardia

HYPERPARATHYROIDISM
Alkaline phosphatase, Serum
Amylase, Serum and urine (Serum)
Calcitonin, Plasma or serum
★ Calcium, Total, Serum
Calcium, Urine
Chemistry profile, Blood
Cyclic adenosine monophosphate, Serum and urine
Histopathology, Specimen
Magnesium, Serum
Osteocalcin, Plasma or serum
★ Parathyroid hormone, Blood
Phosphorus, Serum
Phosphorus, Urine

Additional Conditions
Adrenal gland(s) cancer
Hypercalcemia
Hypertension
Pancreatic cancer
Pituitary cancer
Renal failure
Thyroid cancer
Uremia
Vitamin D deficiency

HYPERPHOSPHATEMIA
Calcium, Total, Serum
Creatinine, Serum
Electrolytes, Plasma or serum
★ Phosphorus, Serum

Additional Conditions
Burns
Cathartic abuse
Cytotoxic drugs
Hypoparathyroidism
Renal failure
Rhabdomyolysis

HYPERPITUITARISM (ACROMEGALY OR GIGANTISM)
Adrenocorticotropic hormone, Serum
Alkaline phosphatase, Isoenzymes, Serum
Alkaline phosphatase, Serum
Calcium, Total, Serum
Calcium, Urine
Follicle-stimulating hormone, Serum
Glucose, Blood
★Growth hormone, Blood
Hydroxyproline, Total, 24-Hour urine
Insulin-like growth factor-I, Blood
Luteinizing hormone, Blood
Phosphorus, Serum
Prolactin, Serum
Thyroid function tests, Blood

Additional Conditions
Adenomas
Amenorrhea
Headaches
Lung cancer

HYPERSENSITIVITY (ALLERGIC) REACTION
Esophinophil peroxidase, Serum
Immunoglobulin E, Serum
Skin test for hypersensitivity, Diagnostic

Additional Conditions
Allergy to hairdressing chemicals
Allergy to latex gloves
Asthma
Dermatitis
Eczema

HYPERTENSION
Aldosterone, Serum or urine
Angiotensin-converting enzyme, Blood
Blood urea nitrogen/creatinine ratio, Blood
Catecholamines, Fractionation free, Plasma
Catecholamines, Urine
★Chemistry profile, Blood
Complete blood count, Blood
Creatinine clearance, Serum, Urine
Creatinine, Serum
★Electrolytes, Plasma or serum
Electrolytes, Urine
Mean platelet volume, Blood
Metanephrines, Total, 24-Hour urine and free plasma
Potassium, Serum
Protein, Quantitative, Urine

Renin activity, Plasma
Sodium, Plasma or serum
Urea nitrogen, Plasma or serum
★Uric acid, Serum
★Urinalysis, Urine
Vanillylmandelic acid, Urine

Additional Conditions
Emboli
Emphysema
Encephalopathy
Left ventricular heart disease
Metabolic syndrome
Obesity
Oral contraception usage
Pericarditis
Pheochromocytoma
Polycythemia
Pregnancy
Renal disease
Stroke
Vasculitis

HYPERTHERMIA
Blood culture, Blood
Chest radiography, Diagnostic
Chloride, Serum
Complete blood count, Blood
Creatine kinase, Serum
★Differential leukocyte count, Peripheral blood
Lactic acid, Blood
Myoglobin, Urine
Potassium, Serum
Sodium, Plasma or serum

Additional Conditions
Anesthesia
Fever of undetermined origin
Liver abscess
Myocardial infarction
Neuroleptic malignant syndrome
Pulmonary emboli
Rheumatic fever
Sarcoidosis
Seizures
Sepsis
Systemic lupus erythematosus

HYPERTHYROIDISM (THYROTOXICOSIS)
Albumin, Serum
Calcium, Total, Serum
Chemistry profile, Blood
Cholesterol, Blood
Endomysial antibody, Serum
Human leukocyte antigen B-27, Blood

Hydroxyproline, Total, 24-Hour urine
Magnesium, Serum
Mean platelet volume, Blood
Thyroid antithyroglobulin antibody,
 Serum
Thyroid function tests, Blood
Thyroid peroxidase antibody, Blood
Thyroid scan, Diagnostic
★Thyroid-stimulating hormone, Blood
Thyroid-stimulating hormone,
 Immunoglobulins, Blood
Thyroid-stimulating hormone,
 Sensitive assay, Blood
Thyroid test: Free thyroxine index,
 Serum
Thyroid test: Thyroid hormone
 binding ratio, Blood
★Thyroid test: Thyroxine, Blood
Thyroid test: Thyroxine free, Serum
★Thyroid test: Triiodothyronine,
 Blood
Triglycerides, Blood

Additional Conditions
Graves' disease
Hydatidiform mole
Jodbasedow disease
Plummer's disease
Pregnancy
Tachycardia

HYPERVENTILATION
(see Respiratory alkalosis)

HYPERVOLEMIA
(see Overhydration)

HYPOCALCEMIA
Calcium, Ionized, Blood
★Calcium, Total, Serum
Calcium, Urine
Creatinine, Serum
Magnesium, Serum
Parathyroid hormone, Blood
★Phosphorus, Serum
Vitamin D, Plasma or serum

Additional Conditions
Burns
Hyperphosphatemia
Hypomagnesemia
Hypoparathyroidism
Liver failure
Malabsorption
Massive infusion therapy
Pancreatitis

Renal failure
Rhabdomyolysis
Sepsis
Steroid use
Thyroid cancer
Tumor lysis
Vitamin D deficiency

HYPOCHROMIC ANEMIA
(see Iron deficiency anemia)

HYPOGLYCEMIA
Cortisol, Plasma or serum
C-peptide, Serum
Glucagon, Plasma
★Glucose, Blood
Glucose-monitoring machines,
 Diagnostic
Glucose tolerance test, Blood
Insulin and insulin antibodies,
 Blood
Tolbutamide tolerance test,
 Diagnostic
Urinalysis, Urine

Additional Conditions
After gastrectomy surgery
Alcoholism
Bulimia
Hyperinsulinism
Malnutrition
Pancreatic cancer

HYPOGONADISM
(see also Erectile Dysfunction)
★Luteinizing hormone, Blood
Mendelian inheritance in genetic
 disorders, Diagnostic
Prolactin, Serum
★Testosterone, Free, Bioavailable and
 total, Blood
★Thyroid Function Tests, Blood

Additional Conditions
Androgen receptor abnormalities
Androgen synthesis defects
Genetic disorders
Steroid abuse

HYPOKALEMIA
Aldosterone, Serum and urine
Digitoxin, Serum
Digoxin, Serum
★Electrolytes, Plasma or serum
Electrolytes, Urine

pH, Blood
★Potassium, Serum
Potassium, Urine
Renin activity, Plasma

Additional Conditions
Alcoholism
Bartter syndrome
Burns
Cushing syndrome
Diarrhea
Fanconi's anemia
Hypomagnesemia
Laxative abuse
Malabsorption
Poisoning
Renal disease

HYPOMAGNESEMIA
Calcium, Total, Serum
Electrolytes, Plasma or serum
Electrolytes, Urine
★Magnesium, Serum
Magnesium, 24-Hour urine
Phosphorus, Serum

Additional Conditions
Alcoholism
Aminoglycoside use
Diabetic ketoacidosis
Diarrhea
Digitalis use
Diuretic use
Hyperaldosteronism
Hypercalcemia
Hyperthyroidism
Hypothyroidism
Malabsorption
Pancreatitis
Renal failure

HYPONATREMIA
Cholesterol, Blood
Cortisol, Plasma or serum
Creatinine, Serum
Creatinine, Urine
★Electrolytes, Plasma or serum
Electrolytes, Urine
Osmolality, Calculated tests, Blood
  (Osmolar gap)
Osmolality, Serum
Osmolality, Urine
★Sodium, Plasma, Serum or urine
Triglycerides, Blood

Additional Conditions
Abscess
Adrenocorticoid deficiency

Burns
Cirrhosis
Congestive heart failure
Diuresis
Hypoproteinemia
Hypothyroidism
Nephrosis
Pancreatitis
Peritonitis
Pneumonia
Renal disease
Syndrome of inappropriate
  antidiuretic hormone secretion
Tuberculosis

HYPOPARATHYROIDISM
Alkaline phosphatase, Serum
Calcium, Calculated ionized, Serum
Calcium, Ionized, Serum
★Calcium, Total, Serum
Calcium, 24-Hour urine
Chemistry profile, Blood
Cyclic adenosine monophosphate,
  Serum and urine
★Magnesium, Serum
Parathyroid hormone, Blood
★Phosphorus, Serum
Phosphorus, Urine
Uric acid, Serum
Vitamin D_3, Plasma or serum

Additional Conditions
Addison's disease
Candidiasis
Diabetes mellitus
Hypomagnesemia
Pernicious anemia
Radiation to the neck
Thyroidectomy

HYPOPHOSPHATEMIA
★Calcium, Total, Serum
Chloride, Serum
Magnesium, Serum
★Phosphorus, Serum
Sodium, Plasma, Serum or urine

Additional Conditions
Acromegaly
Chemotherapy treatment
Hyperglycemia
Hyperparathyroidism
Hypervitaminosis D
Hypokalemia
Hypomagnesemia
Laxative abuse
Malnutrition
Renal failure

Steroid therapy
Stress

Myxedema
Raynaud's disease

HYPOPHYSECTOMY
Complete blood count, Blood
Luteinizing hormone, Blood
Type and crossmatch, Blood
Urinalysis, Urine

Additional Conditions
Acromegaly
Diabetes mellitus

HYPOPITUITARISM (DWARFISM)
Adrenocorticotropic hormone, Serum
Chromosome analysis, Blood
Follicle-stimulating hormone, Serum
*Growth hormone, Blood
Insulin-like growth factor-I, Blood
Luteinizing hormone, Blood
Zinc, Blood

Additional Conditions
Craniopharyngiomas
Headaches
Visual acuity loss

HYPOTENSION
Aldosterone, Serum and urine
Catecholamines, Fractionation free, Plasma
Catecholamines, Urine
Sodium, Plasma or serum

Additional Conditions
Adrenal insufficiency
Left ventricular dysfunction
Myocardial infarction
Shock

HYPOTHERMIA
Computed tomography of the brain, Diagnostic
Lactic acid, Blood
*Specific gravity, Urine
Urea nitrogen, Plasma or serum
Urinalysis, Urine

Additional Conditions
Alcoholism
Cardiovascular disease
Frostbite
Hypopituitarism
Malnutrition
Mental retardation

HYPOTHYROIDISM (CRETINISM)
(see also Myxedema)
Alkaline phosphatase, Serum
Chemistry profile, Blood
Chloride, Sweat, Specimen
Cholesterol, Blood
Complete blood count, Blood
Creatine kinase, Serum
Lactate dehydrogenase, Blood
Lactate dehydrogenase, Isoenzymes, Blood
Lipid profile, Blood
Red blood cell morphology, Blood
Sodium, Plasma or serum
Thyroid peroxidase antibody, Blood
Thyroid antithyroglobulin antibody, Serum
Thyroid function tests, Blood
*Thyroid-stimulating hormone, Blood
Thyroid-stimulating hormone, Filter paper, Blood
Thyroid test: Free thyroxine index, Serum
Thyroid test: Thyroid hormone binding ratio, Blood
*Thyroid test: Thyroxin, Blood
Thyroid test: Thyroxin, Free, Serum

Additional Conditions
Amenorrhea
Constipation
Deafness
Goiter
Myxedema
Thyroiditis
Umbilical hernia

HYPOVOLEMIA
Albumin/globulin ratio, Serum
Anion gap, Blood
Blood volume, Blood
Complete blood count, Blood
Creatinine, Serum
Creatinine, Urine
*Electrolytes, Plasma or serum
Electrolytes, Urine
Osmolality, Serum
*Osmolality, Urine
Potassium, Serum
Protein, Total, Serum
Sodium, Plasma or serum
*Specific gravity, Urine
Type and crossmatch, Blood
Urinalysis, Urine

Additional Conditions
Ascites
Bowel obstruction
Burns
Dehydration
Diabetic ketosis
Hemorrhage
Hypotension
Peritonitis
Shock
Tachycardia
Trauma

HYPOXIA
Bicarbonate, Serum
★Blood gases, Arterial, Blood
 Carbon dioxide, Total content, Blood
 Chest radiography, Diagnostic
 Diffusing capacity for carbon
  monoxide, Diagnostic
 Doppler ultrasonographic flow studies
  (Lower extremities), Diagnostic
★Oxygen saturation, Blood
 Ventilation-perfusion lung scan,
  Diagnostic

Additional Conditions
Acidosis and acidemia
Anemia
Carbon monoxide poisoning
Chronic obstructive pulmonary disease
Head trauma
Lung cancer
Pneumonia
Pulmonary embolus
Seizures
Severe acute respiratory syndrome
 (SARS)

HYSTERECTOMY
★Complete blood cell count, Blood
 Dilatation and curettage, Diagnostic
 Gynecologic ultrasonography,
  Diagnostic
 Hysteroscopy, Diagnostic
 Obstetric ultrasonography, Diagnostic
 Pap smear, Diagnostic
 Potassium, Serum
 Prothrombin time and international
  normalized ratio, Plasma
 Sodium, Plasma, Serum or urine
★Type and crossmatch, Blood

Additional Conditions
Menorrhagia
Uterine cancer
Uterine fibroids

IDIOPATHIC THROMBOCYTOPENIC PURPURA (ITP)
★Bleeding time, Duke, Blood
★Bleeding time, Ivy, Blood
 Bone marrow biopsy, Diagnostic
 Capillary fragility test,
  Diagnostic
 Complete blood count, Blood
 Differential leukocyte count,
  Peripheral blood
 Histopathology, Specimen
 Mean platelet volume, Blood
 Platelet antibody, Blood
★Platelet count, Blood
 Red blood cell, Blood

Additional Conditions
Epistaxis
Hemorrhage
Menorrhagia
Thrombocytopenia

ILEAL CONDUIT
(*see Ostomies*)

ILEITIS
(*see Crohn's disease*)

IMMUNODEFICIENCY
 Acquired immunodeficiency
  syndrome evaluation battery,
  Diagnostic
 Blood culture, Blood
 Bone marrow aspiration analysis,
  Specimen
 C3 complement, Serum
 C4 complement, Serum
 Chest radiography, Diagnostic
 Complement, Total, Serum
 Complete blood count, Blood
 Cytomegalic inclusion disease,
  Cytology, Urine
 Cytomegalovirus antibody, Serum
★Differential leukocyte count,
  Peripheral blood
 Hepatitis B core antibody, Blood
 Herpes cytology, Specimen
 Immunoglobulin A, Serum
 Immunoglobulin D, Serum
 Immunoglobulin E, Serum
 Immunoglobulin G, Serum
 Immunoglobulin M, Serum
 Lymph node biopsy, (Tissue)
  Specimen

Lymphocyte subset enumeration,
Blood
Mantoux skin test, Diagnostic
Nocardia culture, All sites,
Specimen
Oral cavity cytology, Specimen
Oral mucosal transudate,
Specimen
Pneumocystis immunofluorescent
assay, Serum
Protein electrophoresis, Serum
Rapid plasma reagin test, Blood
★T- and B-lymphocyte subset assay,
Blood
Toxoplasmosis serology, Serum

Additional Conditions
Acquired immunodeficiency syndrome
Ataxia-telangiectasia
Cancer
Congenital immunologic defects
Cytomegalovirus
Diabetes mellitus
Drugs that suppress bone marrow
Eczema
Hodgkin's disease
Human immunodeficiency virus
Infectious process
Liver failure
Renal failure
Sarcoidosis
Sepsis
Silicone hypersensitivity
Splenectomy
Status post transplantation
Steroid use
Thrombocytopenia

IMMUNOGLOBULIN A DEFICIENCY
★Immunoglobulin A, Serum
Immunoglobulin A antibodies,
Serum

Additional Conditions
Ataxia-telangiectasia

IMPETIGO
Culture, Skin, Specimen (Bullae
for group A beta-hemolytic
streptococci or *Staphylococcus
aureus*)
Gram stain, Diagnostic

Additional Conditions
Fever
Pruritus

IMPOTENCE
Acid phosphatase, Serum
Alkaline phosphatase, Serum
Complete blood count, Blood
Drug screen, Blood
★Glucose, Blood
Glucose, 2-Hour postprandial, Serum
Polysomnography, Diagnostic
Prolactin, Serum
Prostate-specific antigen, Blood
Pulse volume recording of peripheral
vasculature, Diagnostic
Testosterone, Free, Bioavailable and
total, Blood

Additional Conditions
Acromegaly
Addison's disease
Alcoholism
Arteriosclerosis
Depression
Diabetes mellitus
Drug usage
Endocrine disorders
Hyperthyroidism
Klinefelter syndrome
Multiple sclerosis
Peripheral vascular disease
Pernicious anemia
Spinal cord injury
Syphilis
Vascular diseases

INDIGESTION
(*see Dyspepsia*)

INDUSTRY-RELATED DISEASES
Blood gases, Arterial, Blood
Bronchoscopy, Diagnostic
★Chest radiography, Diagnostic
Chloride, Serum
★Complete blood count, Blood
Computed tomography of the body
(HRCT) (Lungs), Diagnostic
Potassium, Serum
Lupus test, Blood
Sedimentation rate, Erythrocyte, Blood
Sodium, Plasma, Serum or urine
Sputum cytology, Specimen

Additional Conditions
Asbestosis
Berylliosis
Byssinosis
Coal miner's pneumoconiosis
Siderosis
Silicosis
Talc pneumoconiosis

INFARCTION
(*see Cerebral, Myocardial, or Renal infarction*)

INFECTION
(*see Pulmonary infection, Sepsis, or Urinary tract infection*)

INFECTIOUS MONONUCLEOSIS
Alkaline phosphatase, Serum
Antinuclear antibody, Serum
Aspartate aminotransferase, Serum
Bilirubin, Total, Serum
Chemistry profile, Blood
Complete blood count, Blood
Cytomegalovirus antibody, Serum
Differential leukocyte count, Peripheral blood
★Epstein-Barr virus serology, Blood
Heterophile agglutinins, Blood
Lactate dehydrogenase, Blood
Lactate dehydrogenase, Isoenzymes, Blood
Liver battery, Serum
★Monospot screen, Blood
Ornithine carbamoyltransferase, Blood
Smooth muscle antibody, Blood
Tartrate-resistant acid phosphatase, Blood
Toxoplasmosis serology, Serum
Uric acid, Serum

Additional Conditions
Encephalitis
Epstein-Barr virus
Fever
Hepatitis
Hyperuricemia
Myocarditis
Splenectomy
Thrombocytopenia

INFERTILITY
Cervical culture
Chromosome analysis, Blood
Dilation and curettage, Diagnostic
Biopsy, Site-specific, Specimen (Endometrium)
Estradiol, Serum
Estrogens, Serum and 24-Hour urine
Follicle Stimulating Hormone, Serum
★Gynecologic ultrasonography, Diagnostic
Histopathology, Specimen
Hysterosalpingography, Diagnostic
Hysteroscopy, Diagnostic
★Infertility screen, Specimen
Laparoscopy, Diagnostic
Luteinizing hormone, Blood
Mercury, Blood and urine
Progesterone, Serum
Prolactin, Serum
Rubin's test, Diagnostic
★Semen analysis, Specimen
Sims-Huhner test, Diagnostic
Testosterone, Blood

Additional Conditions
Amenorrhea
Azoospermia
Endometriosis
Peritubal adhesions
Sperm immobilization

INFLAMMATION
Complete blood count, Blood
Computed tomography (Site-specific), Diagnostic
C-reactive protein, Serum
★Differential leukocyte count (Neutrophils), Peripheral blood
Sedimentation rate, Erythrocyte, Blood

Additional Conditions
Abscess
Appendicitis
Arthritis
Bronchitis
Cellulitis
Cholecystitis
Conjunctivitis
Diverticulitis
Epiglottitis
Myocarditis
Pelvic inflammatory disease
Sinusitis
Spider bites
Tonsillitis

INFLUENZA
(*see also Haemophilus influenzae*)
Cold agglutinin titer, Serum
Culture, Routine, Specimen (Sputum)
Influenza A and B titer, Blood
Respiratory antigen panel, Specimen
★Viral culture, Specimen

Additional Conditions
Bronchitis
Fever
Headache

Otitis media
Pneumonia
Reye syndrome
Sinusitis

INSECTICIDE POISONING
★Pseudocholinesterase, Plasma

Additional Conditions
Dysrhythmias
Seizures

INSOMNIA
Cortisol, Plasma or serum
Electroencephalography, Diagnostic
17-Hydroxycorticosteroids, 24-Hour
  urine
Oximetry, Diagnostic
Polysomnography, Diagnostic
Tryptophan, Plasma

Additional Conditions
Alcoholism
Depression
Drug abuse
Rheumatoid arthritis
Sleep disorders
Stress

INSULINOMA
Adrenocorticotropic hormone, Serum
C-peptide, Serum
Electrolytes, Plasma
Gastrin, Serum
Glucagon, Plasma
★Glucose, Blood
Histopathology, Specimen
Human chorionic gonadotropin,
  Beta-subunit, Serum
Insulin and insulin antibodies,
  Blood
Tolbutamide Tolerance Test,
  Diagnostic
Vasoactive intestinal polypeptide,
  Blood

Additional Conditions
Adenomas
Anxiety
Hypoglycemia
Islet cell cancer
Whipple's disease

INTERMITTENT CLAUDICATION
(see Peripheral vascular disease)

INTERVERTEBRAL DISK ABNORMALITIES
★Magnetic resonance imaging,
  Diagnostic

Additional Conditions
Muscle strain
Neuropathy
Scoliosis
Spinal cord compression

INTOXICATION
Alcohol, Blood
Anion gap, Blood
Bromides, Serum
Cannabinoids, Qualitative, Blood or
  urine
Drug screen, Blood
Osmolality, Calculated tests, Blood
  (Osmolar gap)
Osmolality, Serum
pH, Blood
★Toxicology, Drug screen, Blood or
  urine
★Toxicology, Volatiles group by GLC,
  Blood or urine

Additional Conditions
Ascites
Ataxia
Delirium tremens
Encephalopathy
Hepatomegaly

INTRACEREBRAL HEMORRHAGE
(see Hemorrhage)

INTRACRANIAL PRESSURE
Antidiuretic hormone, Serum
Cerebrospinal fluid, Routine analysis,
  Specimen
★Computed tomography of the brain,
  Diagnostic
Electrolytes, Plasma or serum
  (Plasma)
Specific gravity, Urine

Additional Conditions
Brain tumor
Cerebral hemorrhage
Papilledema
Trauma

INTRACRANIAL TUMORS
(see Brain tumors)

INTRADUCTAL PAPILLOMA (BREAST)
*Histopathology, Specimen
Mammography, Diagnostic
Nipple discharge cytology, Specimen

Additional Conditions
Breast cancer
Paget's disease, Breast

INTUSSUSCEPTION
*Barium enema, Diagnostic
Flat-plate radiograph of abdomen, Diagnostic
Occult blood, Stool

Additional Conditions
Bowel obstruction
Colon tumor
Rectal bleeding

IRON DEFICIENCY ANEMIA (UNCOMPLICATED)
Complete blood count, Blood
Ferritin, Serum
*Iron, Serum
*Iron and total iron-binding capacity/transferrin, Serum
Reticulocyte count, Blood

Additional Conditions
Gastrointestinal bleeding
Hemoglobinuria
Malignancy
Menorrhagia
Pregnancy

ISCHEMIC HEART DISEASE
(see Angina pectoris)

ISLET CELL TUMORS
(see Insulinoma)

JAUNDICE
Amylase, Serum
*Bilirubin, Serum (Total and direct)
Coombs', Direct, Serum
Coombs', Indirect, Serum
Endoscopic retrograde cholangiopancreatography, Diagnostic
Gallbladder and biliary system ultrasonography, Diagnostic
Galactose, Screening test for galactosemia, Urine
Gamma-glutamyltranspeptidase, Blood
Hepatitis A antibody IgM and IgG, Blood
Hepatitis B surface antigen, Blood
Hepatitis C genotype, Serum
Histopathology, Specimen
Infectious mononucleosis screening test, Blood
Leptospira serodiagnosis, Blood
Leucine aminopeptidase, Blood
Lipase, Serum
*Liver battery, Serum
Liver biopsy, Diagnostic
Liver scan, Diagnostic
Liver ultrasonography, Diagnostic
Magnetic resonance cholangiopancreatography, Diagnostic
Malaria smear, Blood
Ornithine carbamoyltransferase, Blood
Phenobarbital, Plasma or serum
Red blood cell enzyme deficiency screen, Blood
Urobilinogen, Urine

Additional Conditions
Alcoholism
Anemia
Cirrhosis
Crigler-Najjar syndrome
Gilbert syndrome
Hepatitis
Infectious mononucleosis
Liver cancer
Lymphoma
Pancreatitis
Sarcoidosis
Wilson's disease

JOCK ITCH
(see Tinea cruris)

KAPOSI'S SARCOMA
Acquired immunodeficiency syndrome evaluation battery, Diagnostic
*Biopsy, *Mycobacterium*, Culture
Cytomegalovirus antibody, Serum
Ocular cytology, Specimen
Oral mucosal transudate, Specimens
T- and B-lymphocyte subset assay, Blood

Additional Conditions
Acquired immunodeficiency syndrome
Fever
Gingivitis

KERATITIS
Ocular cytology, Specimen

Additional Conditions
Herpes simplex virus

KETOACIDOSIS
Alcohol, Blood
★Anion gap, Blood
Blood indices, Blood
★Chemistry profile, Blood
★Complete blood count, Blood
Differential leukocyte count,
Peripheral blood
Electrolytes, Plasma
★Glucose, Blood
Ketone bodies, Blood
Ketone, Semiquantitative, Urine
Magnesium, Serum
Osmolality, Serum
Osmolality, Urine
pH, Blood
Phosphorus, Serum
Potassium, Serum
Red blood cell, Blood
Salicylate, Blood
Urea nitrogen, Plasma or serum
Urinalysis, Urine

Additional Conditions
Diabetes mellitus
Infectious process
Myocardial infarction
Trauma

KIDNEY
(see Renal)

KIDNEY STONE
Calcium, Total, Serum
Calcium, Urine
Chemistry profile, Blood
Computed tomography, Diagnostic
Creatinine clearance, Serum, Urine
Cystine, Qualitative, Urine
Electrolytes, Urine
Flat-plate radiograph of the
abdomen, Diagnostic
Histopathology, Specimen
Intravenous pyelography, Diagnostic
★Kidney stone analysis, Specimen
Kidney ultrasonography, Diagnostic
Magnesium, Serum
Magnesium, Urine
Magnetic resonance urography,
Diagnostic
Occult blood, Urine

Oxalate, 24-Hour urine
pH, Urine
Phosphorus, Urine
Sodium, Urine
Uric acid, Serum
Uric acid, Urine
Urinalysis, Urine

Additional Conditions
de Toni-Franconi defect
Hyperparathyroidism
Hypervitaminosis D
Metastasis to bone
Nephritis
Osteoporosis
Renal tubular acidosis
Urinary tract infection

KIMMELSTIEL-WILSON DISEASE
Creatinine, Serum
Creatinine clearance, Serum, Urine
★Kidney biopsy, Specimen
Protein, Urine
Urea nitrogen, Plasma or serum

Additional Conditions
Diabetes mellitus
Diabetic nephropathy
Glomerulonephritis
Hypertension
Nephrosis

KLINEFELTER SYNDROME
Biopsy, Site-specific (Testes),
Specimen
Estradiol, Serum
★Follicle-stimulating hormone, Serum
17-Ketosteroids, Total, 24-Hour urine
★Luteinizing hormone, Blood
Oral cavity cytology, Specimen
★Semen analysis, Specimen
Testosterone, Free, Bioavailable and
total, Blood

Additional Conditions
Azoospermia
Gynecomastia
Sterility

KWASHIORKOR
★Albumin, Serum
Amylase, Serum
Carotene, Serum
Cholesterol, Blood
Complete blood count, Blood
Lipase, Serum
Phospholipids, Serum

Protein electrophoresis, Serum
★Protein, Total, Serum
Triglycerides, Blood
Trypsin, Plasma or serum

Additional Conditions
Anorexia nervosa
Depression
Fistula draining
Malabsorption
Malnutrition
Nephrosis

LACTOSE INTOLERANCE
★D-Xylose absorption test, Diagnostic,
Serum or urine

Additional Conditions
Malabsorption

LAMBERT-EATON MYASTHENIC SYNDROME
★Striational antibody, Specimen

Additional Conditions
Guillain-Barré syndrome
Muscle disease
Myasthenia gravis
Oat cell carcinoma of the lung

LEAD POISONING
Lead mobilization test, 24-Hour
urine
Complete blood count, Blood
Coproporphyrin, Urine
Erythrocyte protoporphyrin, Blood
Heavy metal screen, Blood and
24-Hour urine
★Lead, Blood and urine
Radiography of long bones (for
increased density), Diagnostic
Red blood cell, Blood
Thyroid function tests, Blood

Additional Conditions
Anorexia
Diarrhea
Emphysema
Failure to thrive
Headache
Seizures

LEGIONNAIRES' DISEASE
Alkaline phosphatase, Serum
★Biopsy, Site-specific, Specimen
(Lung)

Brushing cytology, Specimen,
Diagnostic
Chest radiography, Diagnostic
Histopathology, Specimen
★*Legionella antigen,* Urine
★*Legionella pneumophila,* Culture
Legionella pneumophila, Culture, IgM
titer, Blood
Legionella pneumophila, Direct FA
smear, Specimen (Lung)
Legionnaires' disease antibodies,
Blood
★Sputum cytology, Specimen

Additional Conditions
Emphysema
Endocarditis
Pericarditis

LEPROSY (HANSEN'S DISEASE)
★Acid-fast bacteria, Culture and stain
Biopsy, Site-specific, Specimen
Histopathology, Specimen
Immune complex assay, Blood
Protein, Total, Serum

Additional Conditions
Anemia
Epistaxis
Keratitis
Neuritis
Systemic lupus erythematosus
Tattoos

LEPTOSPIROSIS
Alanine aminotransferase, Serum
Bacterial serology, Blood
Blood culture, Blood
Electrolytes, Plasma or serum
Electrolytes, Urine
★*Leptospira* culture, Urine
★*Leptospira* serodiagnosis, Blood

Additional Conditions
Fever
Headache
Hypotension
Meningitis
Myocarditis
Renal failure
Sepsis
Weil syndrome

LEUKEMIA
Blood culture, Blood
★Bone marrow biopsy, Diagnostic

Chest radiography, Diagnostic
Complete blood count, Blood
Cryoglobulin, Qualitative, Serum
*Differential leukocyte count, Peripheral blood
Immunoelectrophoresis, Serum and urine
Methotrexate, Serum
T- and B-lymphocyte subset assay, Blood
Sudan Black B stain, Diagnostic
T- and B-lymphocyte subset assay, Blood
Tartrate-resistant acid phosphatase, Blood
Terminal deoxynucleotidyl transferase, Blood or bone marrow
Vitamin B_{12}, Serum
Xanthuric acid, Urine
Zinc, Blood

Additional Conditions
Bone marrow transplant
Candidiasis
Epistaxis
Fever
Graft-versus-host disease
Joint pain
Pneumonia
Sepsis

LEUKOCYTOSIS
*Bone marrow biopsy, Diagnostic
*Complete blood count, Blood
*Differential leukocyte count, Peripheral blood
Electrolytes, Plasma or serum

Additional Conditions
Abscess
Infection, Acute
Leukemia
Seizure
Sepsis

LEUKOPENIA
Blood fungus, Culture
Bone marrow biopsy, Diagnostic
Chest radiography, Diagnostic
*Complete blood count, Blood
Culture, Routine, Specimen (Blood, ulcerative lesions, urine)
*Differential leukocyte count, Peripheral blood

Foreign body, Routine, Culture (Catheters or venous access devices)
Lymph node biopsy, Specimen

Additional Conditions
Agranulocytosis
Anemia
Hodgkin's disease
Malaria
Schistosomiasis
Splenomegaly
Thrombocytopenia
Typhoid
Viral infections

LEUKORRHEA
*Cervical-vaginal cytology, Specimen
Complete blood count, Blood
Urinalysis, Urine

Additional Conditions
Menstruation
Trichomoniasis

LICE
*Arthropod identification, Specimen

Additional Conditions
Fever
Typhus

LIVER ABSCESS
Activated partial thromboplastin time, Plasma
Alanine aminotransferase, Serum
Albumin, Serum
Alkaline phosphatase, Serum
Bilirubin, Direct, Serum
Bilirubin, Total, Serum
Blood culture, Blood
Leucine aminopeptidase, Blood
Liver battery, Serum
Liver biopsy, Diagnostic
Liver scan, Diagnostic
*Liver ultrasonography, Diagnostic
Prothrombin time and international normalized ratio, Plasma

Additional Conditions
Anemia
Chest pain, Acute
Diarrhea
Fever
Leukocytosis
Sepsis

LIVER CANCER

Alpha-fetoprotein, Blood
Computed tomography of the body
  (Liver), Diagnostic
Dual modality imaging, Diagnostic
Ki–67 proliferation marker,
  Specimen
Leucine aminopeptidase, Blood
Liver battery, Serum
★Liver biopsy, Diagnostic
Liver scan, Diagnostic
Liver ultrasonography, Diagnostic
5′-Nucleotidase, Serum
Ornithine carbamoyltransferase,
  Blood
Telomerase enzyme marker, Blood

Additional Conditions

Ascites
Cachexia
Hepatitis
Hepatomegaly
Jaundice

LIVER DYSFUNCTION

Alanine aminotransferase, Serum
Alkaline phosphatase, Serum
Antimitochondrial antibody, Serum
Antinuclear antibody, Serum
Bilirubin, Total, Serum
Ceruloplasmin, Serum
Gamma-glutamyltranspeptidase,
  Blood
Hepatitis serologies, Serum
Leucine aminopeptidase, Blood
★Liver battery, Serum
Liver biopsy, Diagnostic
Liver scan, Diagnostic
Liver ultrasonography, Diagnostic
5′-Nucleotidase, Blood
Ornithine carbamoyltransferase,
  Blood
Prothrombin time and international
  normalized ratio, Plasma
Striational antibody, Specimen

Additional Conditions

Amyloidosis
Cirrhosis
Galactosemia
Hepatitis
Jaundice
Liver abscess
Liver cancer
Sarcoidosis
Schistosomiasis
Syphilis
Tuberculosis
Weil syndrome

LIVER FAILURE

Alanine aminotransferase, Serum
Albumin, Serum
Albumin/globulin ratio, Serum
Alkaline phosphatase, Serum
★Ammonia, Blood
Amylase, Serum
Blood culture, Blood
★Creatinine, Serum
Creatinine, Urine
Electrolytes, Plasma or serum
Electrolytes, Urine
Globulin, Serum
Hepatitis serologies, Serum
Leucine aminopeptidase, Blood
Lipase, Serum
★Liver battery, Serum
Liver ultrasonography, Diagnostic
5′-Nucleotidase, Blood
Paracentesis, Diagnostic
Protein, Total, Serum
Prothrombin time and international
  normalized ratio, Plasma
Toxicology, Drug screen, Blood or urine
Urea nitrogen, Plasma or serum

Additional Conditions

Alcoholism
Cancer
Cirrhosis
Hepatitis
Hyperbilirubinemia
Jaundice
Sepsis
Wilson's disease

LUNG CANCER

Alpha$_1$-antitrypsin, Serum
CA 15-3, Blood
CA 50, Blood
★Biopsy, Site-specific (Lung), Specimen
Bone scan, Diagnostic
Brain scan, Cerebral flow and
  pathology, Diagnostic
Bronchial washing, Specimen,
  Diagnostic
Bronchoscopy, Diagnostic
Brushing cytology, Specimen,
  Diagnostic
CA 15-3, Serum
CA 50, Blood
Chest radiography, Diagnostic
Complete blood count, Blood
Computed tomography of the body
  (Spiral) (Lung), Diagnostic
Dual modality imaging, Diagnostic
Mediastinoscopy, Diagnostic
Mucinlike carcinoma–associated
  antigen, Blood

Neuron-specific enolase, Serum
Pulmonary function tests, Diagnostic
Sputum cytology, Specimen
Striational antibody, Specimen
Telomerase enzyme marker, Blood
Thoracentesis, Diagnostic
Tumor antigen 4, Blood and
  specimen

Additional Conditions
Anemia
Anorexia
Chronic obstructive pulmonary
  disease
Gynecomastia
Hypercalcemia
Hypoxia
Industry-related diseases
Pleural effusion
Syndrome of inappropriate
  antidiuretic hormone secretion

LUPOID HEPATITIS
*Lupus panel, Blood

Additional Conditions
Chronic fatigue syndrome
Liver disease

LUPUS ERYTHEMATOSUS
Antinuclear antibody, Serum
Circulating anticoagulant, Blood
Complete blood count, Blood
*Lupus panel, Blood
Lupus test, Blood
Protein electrophoresis, Serum
Protein, Total, Serum
Rheumatoid factor, Blood
Sedimentation rate, Erythrocyte,
  Blood

Additional Conditions
Leukopenia
Proteinuria
Renal failure

LYME DISEASE
Borrelia burgdorferi C6 peptide
  antibody, Serum
Immunoglobulin G, Serum
Immunoglobulin M, Serum
*Lyme disease antibody, Blood

Additional Conditions
Fever
Headache
Joint pain

Meningitis
Myopericarditis
Tick bite

LYMPHADENITIS
Blood culture, Blood
Lymph node biopsy, Specimen

Additional Conditions
Abscess
Cellulitis
Fever
Lymphoma
Sepsis

LYMPHANGITIS
Blood culture, Blood
Culture, Routine, Specimen

Additional Conditions
Abscess
Cat-scratch disease
Thrombophlebitis

**LYMPHOGRANULOMA
VENEREUM**
Chlamydia group titer, Serum
*Histopathology, Specimen
Lymphogranuloma venereum titer,
  Blood

Additional Conditions
Arthritis
Conjunctivitis
Fever
Headache
Proctitis

LYMPHOMA
Biopsy, Site-specific, Specimen
Calcium, Total, Serum
Complete blood count,
  Blood
Cytologic study of gastrointestinal
  tract, Diagnostic
Differential leukocyte count,
  Peripheral blood
*Lymph node biopsy, Specimen
Mediastinoscopy, Diagnostic
O-Banding (CSF proteins), Serum
Phosphorus, Serum
Platelet count, Blood
Potassium, Serum
Tartrate-resistant acid phosphatase,
  Blood

Terminal
 deoxynucleotidyl-transferase, Blood
 or Bone marrow
Uric acid, Serum
Xanthuric acid, Urine

Additional Conditions
Fever
Lymphadenopathy
Night sweats

MACROGLOBULINEMIA
(*see Waldenström's macroglobulinemia*)

MALABSORPTION
Calcium, Total, Serum
Carotene, Serum
★ D-Xylose absorption test, Diagnostic,
 Serum or urine
Fat, Semiquantitative, Stool
★ Fecal fat, Quantitative, 72-Hour stool
Folic acid, Serum
Glucose tolerance test, Blood
Glucose, 2-Hour postprandial, Serum
Lipid profile, Blood
Magnesium, Serum
Phosphorus, Serum
Protein, Total, Serum
Pyridoxal 5′-phosphate, Plasma
Sigmoidoscopy, Diagnostic
Sodium, Plasma, Serum or urine
Transferrin, Serum
Trypsin, Plasma or serum
Trypsin, Stool
Vitamin B_{12}, Serum
Vitamin C, Plasma or serum

Additional Conditions
Anemia
Celiac sprue
Crohn's disease
Diarrhea
Hematuria
Hypoalbuminemia
Hypokalemia
Hyponatremia
Osteomalacia
Tropical sprue
Ulcerative colitis
Whipple's disease

MALARIA
Alanine aminotransferase, Serum
Alkaline phosphatase, Serum
Bilirubin, Total, Serum
Blood indices, Blood

Cold agglutinin titer, Serum
Complement, Total, Serum
Complete blood count, Blood
Differential leukocyte count,
 Peripheral blood
Electrolytes, Plasma or serum
Glucose, Blood
Liver battery, Serum
★ Malaria smear, Blood
Parasite screen, Blood
Platelet count, Blood
Protein electrophoresis, Serum
Red blood cell morphology, Blood
Rheumatoid factor, Blood

Additional Conditions
Anemia
Diaphoresis
Fever
Headache
Leukopenia
Mosquito bite
Pulmonary edema
Urinary tract infection

MALIGNANT HYPERTENSION
(*see Hypertension*)

MALNUTRITION
(*see Kwashiorkor and Marasmus*)

MANIC-DEPRESSIVE PSYCHOSIS
Complete blood count, Blood
★ Cortisol, Plasma or serum
Electrolytes, Plasma or serum
★ Lithium, Serum
Valproic acid, Blood

Additional Conditions
Alcoholism
Anorexia nervosa
Catatonia
Head injury
Suicide

MARASMUS
Albumin, Serum
Blood urea nitrogen/creatinine ratio,
 Blood
Complete blood count, Blood
Protein electrophoresis, Serum
★ Protein, Total, Serum
★ Transthyretin (Prealbumin), Serum
Vitamin B_6, Plasma

Additional Conditions
Growth retardation
Hepatomegaly
Lymphocyte depletion

MARFAN SYNDROME
Bone scan, Diagnostic
*Echocardiography, Diagnostic
Hydroxyproline, Total, 24-Hour
  urine
Magnetic resonance imaging,
  Diagnostic

Additional Conditions
Abortion, Spontaneous
Endocarditis
Kyphoscoliosis
Mitral valve prolapse
Myopia

MAROTEAUX-LAMY SYNDROME
*Mucopolysaccharides, Qualitative,
  Urine

Additional Conditions
Dysrhythmias
Mental retardation

MEASLES
(see Rubella and Rubeola)

MEGALOBLASTIC ANEMIA
Blood indices, Blood
*Bone marrow biopsy, Diagnostic
Complete blood count, Blood
Differential leukocyte count,
  Peripheral blood
*Folic acid, Serum
Folic acid, Red blood cells, Blood
Gastric analysis, Specimen
Gastric pH, Specimen
Gastrin, Serum
Intrinsic factor antibody, Blood
Lactate dehydrogenase, Blood
Lactate dehydrogenase, Isoenzymes,
  Blood
Pepsinogen-I antibody, Blood
Platelet count, Blood
Red blood cell morphology, Blood
Reticulocyte count, Blood
Schilling test, Diagnostic
Type and crossmatch, Blood
  (Screen)
Vitamin B_{12}, Serum

Additional Conditions
Alcoholism
Hyperbilirubinemia
Leukocytosis
Malnutrition
Pernicious anemia
Vitamin B_{12} deficiency

MELANOMA
*Biopsy, Site-specific, Specimen
Bone marrow aspiration analysis,
  Specimen
Chest radiography, Diagnostic
Computed tomography of the body
  (Melanoma site), Diagnostic
Computed tomography of the brain,
  Diagnostic
Histopathology, Specimen
Liver battery, Serum
Melanin, Urine
TA90 Immune complex assay, Serum

Additional Conditions
Pruritus
Sunburn

MÉNIÈRE'S DISEASE
Cerebrospinal fluid, Protein,
  Specimen
*Hearing test for loudness—
  recruitment, Diagnostic

Additional Conditions
Head trauma
Syphilis
Tinnitus
Vertigo

MENINGITIS
Blood culture, Blood
*Cerebrospinal fluid, Cytology,
  Specimen
Cerebrospinal fluid, Fungus,
  Culture
Cerebrospinal fluid, Mycobacterium,
  Culture
Cerebrospinal fluid, Routine analysis,
  Specimen
Complete blood count, Blood
Computed tomography of brain,
  Diagnostic
Coxsackie A or B virus titer, Blood
Cryptococcal antigen titer, Serum
Cryptococcal antigen titer,
  Cerebrospinal fluid, Specimen
Cryptococcus antibody titer, Serum

Differential leukocyte count,
Peripheral blood
Gastric aspirate, Routine, Culture
Herpes cytology, Specimen
Leptospira serodiagnosis, Blood
Magnetic resonance imaging,
Diagnostic
O-Banding (CSF proteins), Plasma
Sodium, Plasma, Serum or urine
Sputum for *Haemophilus* species,
Culture
Toxoplasmosis, Rubella,
Cytomegalovirus, Herpes virus
serology, Blood
Viral culture, Specimen

Additional Conditions
Acquired immunodeficiency syndrome
Arthritis
Fever
Headache
Hydrocephalus
Influenza
Myocarditis
Nephritis
Pneumonia
Seizures
Sepsis

MENOPAUSE
Biopsy, Site-specific (Endometrium),
Specimen
Bone scan, Diagnostic
Estradiol, Serum
*Estrogens, Serum
Estrogens, Nonpregnant, 24-Hour
urine
Follicle-stimulating hormone, Serum
Hormonal evaluation, Cytologic,
Specimen
17-Ketosteroids, Total, 24-Hour urine
Luteinizing hormone, Blood

Additional Conditions
Dyspareunia
Hot flashes
Night sweats
Osteoporosis

MENORRHAGIA (HYPERMENORRHEA)
Activated partial thromboplastin
time, Plasma
*Complete blood count, Blood
Cortisol, Plasma or serum
Estrogens, Serum and 24-Hour urine
Prothrombin time and international
normalized ratio, Plasma

Additional Conditions
Endometriosis
Hypothyroidism
Menopause
Uterine cancer

MENSTRUATION
Estrogens, Serum and 24-Hour urine
Follicle-stimulating hormone, Serum
Luteinizing hormone, Blood

Additional Conditions
Anemia
Menorrhagia
Pneumothorax

METABOLIC ACIDOSIS
Beta-hydroxybutyrate, Blood
*Blood gases, Arterial, Blood
*Chemistry profile, Blood
Creatinine, Serum
Dinitrophenylhydrazine test,
Diagnostic
Electrolytes, Plasma
Glucose, Blood
Osmolality, Calculated tests, Blood
(Osmolar gap)
Osmolality, Serum
Salicylate, Blood
Toxicology, Drug screen, Blood or
urine
Toxicology, Volatiles group by GLC,
Blood or urine
Urea nitrogen, Plasma or serum
Urinalysis, Urine

Additional Conditions
Alcoholic ketoacidosis
Anoxia
Carbon monoxide poisoning
Dehydration
Diabetic ketoacidosis
Ethylene glycol poisoning
Leukemia
Malnutrition
Maple syrup urine disease
Methanol poisoning
Renal failure
Seizures
Shock

METABOLIC ALKALOSIS
*Blood gases, Arterial, Blood
Electrolytes, Plasma
Potassium, Serum
Urinalysis, Urine

Additional Conditions
Hypovolemia
Renal insufficiency
Vomiting

METABOLIC SYNDROME
C-reactive protein, Blood
★Lipid profile, Blood
Triglycerides, Blood
Uric acid, Serum

Additional Conditions
Adrenal dysfunction
Diabetes mellitus
Hypertension
Hypothyroidism
Obesity

METAL POISONING
Arsenic, Blood
Arsenic, Urine
Cadmium, Serum and 24-Hour urine
Chemistry profile, Blood
Chromium, Serum
Chromium, Urine
★Heavy metals, Blood and 24-Hour
  urine
Lead, Blood or urine
Lithium, Serum
Mercury, Blood
Mercury, 24-Hour urine
Thallium, Serum or 24-Hour urine
Urinalysis, Urine
Zinc, Blood

Additional Conditions
Ataxia
Coma
Dehydration
Diarrhea
Papilledema
Pulmonary edema
Renal failure
Shock
Vomiting

METASTASIS
Acid phosphatase, Serum
Adrenocorticotropic hormone, Serum
Alkaline phosphatase, Serum
Alkaline phosphatase, Heat stable,
  Serum
Alkaline phosphatase, Isoenzymes,
  Serum
Alpha-fetoprotein, Blood
Body fluid cytology, Specimen
Bone marrow biopsy, Diagnostic

Bone scan, Diagnostic
Bronchial washing, Specimen,
  Diagnostic
Brushing cytology, Specimen,
  Diagnostic
CA 15-3, Serum (Breast metastasis)
Calcium, Total, Serum
Carcinoembryonic antigen, Serum
Cathepsin D, Specimen
Cerebrospinal fluid, Cytology,
  Specimen
Cervical-vaginal cytology, Specimen
Chemistry profile, Blood
Complete blood count, Blood
Computed tomography of the body
  (Site-specific, Spiral), Specimen
Differential leukocyte count,
  Peripheral blood
Electrolytes, Plasma or serum
Estrogen receptor and progesterone
  receptor in breast cancer, Diagnostic
Gamma-glutamyltranspeptidase, Blood
Gastrin, Serum
Histopathology, Specimen
Human chorionic gonadotropin,
  Beta-subunit, Serum
Magnetic resonance imaging,
  Diagnostic
Magnetic resonance spectroscopy,
  Diagnostic
Mucinlike carcinoma–associated
  antigen, Blood
Needle aspiration, Diagnostic
5′-Nucleotidase, Blood
Ocular cytology, Specimen
Parathyroid hormone, Blood
Progesterone receptor assay,
  Specimen
Serotonin, Serum or blood
Sputum cytology, Specimen
Urine cytology, Urine
Washing cytology, Specimen

Additional Conditions
Anemia
Ascites
Confusion
Congestive heart failure
Dyspnea
Hepatomegaly
Hypercalcemia
Hyperglycemia
Pain, Chronic
Peripheral edema
Splenomegaly

METRORRHAGIA
Cortisol, Plasma or serum
★Estrogens, Serum and 24-Hour urine

Additional Conditions
Cervical cancer
Uterine cancer

MICROCYTIC ANEMIA
Bone marrow aspiration analysis,
  Specimen
Ferritin, Serum
Fetal hemoglobin, Blood
Heavy metal screen, 24-Hour urine
Hemoglobin A$_2$, Blood
Hemoglobin electrophoresis, Blood
Iron, Serum
Lead, Blood and urine
*Red blood cell morphology, Blood
Reticulocyte count, Blood
Total iron-binding capacity, Serum

Additional Conditions
Dysphagia
Glossitis
Hyperferremia
Thalassemia

MIGRAINE HEADACHES
Arteriography, Diagnostic
Cerebrospinal fluid, Glucose,
  Specimen
Cerebrospinal fluid, Routine analysis,
  Specimen
Cerebrospinal fluid, Protein,
  Specimen
Computed tomography of the body
  (Cervical spine), Diagnostic
Computed tomography of the brain,
  Diagnostic
Electroencephalography, Diagnostic
Lumbar puncture, Diagnostic
Magnetic resonance imaging,
  Diagnostic
Pneumoencephalography,
  Diagnostic
Radiography of skull, chest, and
  cervical spine, Diagnostic

Additional Conditions
Anorexia
Diplopia
Photophobia
Stress
Vomiting

MITRAL STENOSIS
*Echocardiography, Diagnostic
Transesophageal ultrasonography,
  Diagnostic
Ventriculography, Diagnostic

Additional Conditions
Atrial mass
Congestive heart failure (right-side of
  heart)
Cor pulmonale
Pulmonary edema
Pulmonary hypertension

MITRAL VALVE REGURGITATION
*Echocardiography, Diagnostic
Pulmonary artery catheterization,
  Diagnostic
Transesophageal ultrasonography,
  Diagnostic

Additional Conditions
Endocarditis
Marfan syndrome

MONGOLOIDISM
(see Down syndrome)

MONILIASIS
(see Thrush, Vaginitis)

MONKEYPOX
*Biopsy, Site-specific, Specimen (Lesion)
*Culture, Routine, Specimen
  (Oropharynx, tonsillar area)

Additional Conditions
Herpes zoster
Measles
Smallpox

MONONUCLEOSIS
(see Infectious mononucleosis)

MORQUIO SYNDROME
*Mucopolysaccharides, Qualitative,
  Urine

Additional Conditions
Dysrhythmias
Mental retardation

MULTIPLE MYELOMA
Acid phosphatase, Serum
Albumin, Serum
*Bence Jones protein, Urine
Bone marrow aspiration analysis,
  Specimen

Bone scan, Diagnostic
Calcium, Total, Serum
Complement components, Serum
Immunoelectrophoresis, Serum
and urine
Sedimentation rate, Erythrocyte, Blood
T- and B-lymphocyte subset assay,
Blood
Urinalysis (for protein), Urine

Additional Conditions
Anemia
Hypercalcemia
Osteoporosis
Pathologic fractures
Renal failure

MULTIPLE SCLEROSIS
Cerebrospinal fluid, Immunoglobulin
G, Specimen
Cerebrospinal fluid, Myelin basic
protein, Specimen
★Cerebrospinal fluid, Oligoclonal
bands, Specimen
Cerebrospinal fluid, Protein, Specimen
Cerebrospinal fluid, Protein
electrophoresis, Specimen
Cerebrospinal fluid, Routine analysis,
Specimen
Human leukocyte antigen B-27, Blood
★Magnetic resonance imaging
(diffusion-weighted), Diagnostic
Magnetic resonance spectroscopy,
Diagnostic
O-Banding (CSF proteins), Plasma
Somatosensory evoked potential,
Diagnostic

Additional Conditions
Diplopia
Neuritis
Numbness
Vertigo
Visual blurring
Weakness

MUMPS
★Mumps antibody, Blood

Additional Conditions
Meningoencephalitis
Orchiitis
Pancreatitis
Salivary gland inflammation

MUSCULAR DYSTROPHY
(see also Duchenne's muscular dystrophy)
Aldolase, Serum

Aspartate aminotransferase, Serum
Catecholamines, Fractionation free,
Plasma
Creatine, Urine
Creatine kinase, Serum
Creatine kinase, Isoenzymes, Serum
Creatinine, Serum
Electromyography and nerve
conduction studies, Diagnostic
Lactate dehydrogenase, Blood
Metanephrines, Total, 24-Hour urine
and free plasma
★Muscle biopsy, Specimen
Myoglobin, Serum and qualitative,
Urine

Additional Conditions
Cataracts
Diabetes mellitus
Dysrhythmias
Myotonia
Testicular atrophy

MYASTHENIA GRAVIS
Acetylcholine receptor antibody,
Serum
Cerebrospinal fluid,
Immunoglobulin G ratios and
immunoglobulin G index, Specimen
★Electromyography and nerve
conduction studies, Diagnostic
(Electromyography)
Human leukocyte antigen B-27,
Blood
Metanephrines, Total, 24-Hour urine
and free plasma
Pulmonary function tests, Diagnostic
(Spirometry)
Striational autoantibody,
Specimen
Thyroid peroxidase antibody,
Blood
Thyroid profile, Blood

Additional Conditions
Diplopia
Guillain-Barré syndrome
Ptosis
Thyrotoxicosis

MYCOSES
Gastric cytology, Specimen
Sputum cytology, Specimen

Additional Conditions
Abscess
Dyspnea

MYOCARDIAL CONDUCTION DEFECT

Cardiac enzymes/isoenzymes, Blood
Chemistry profile, Blood
Creatine kinase, Serum
Creatine kinase, Isoenzymes, Serum
Digitoxin, Serum
Digoxin, Serum
* Electrocardiography, Diagnostic
Electrolytes, Plasma or serum
* Electrophysiologic study, Diagnostic
Lactate dehydrogenase, Blood
Lactate dehydrogenase, Isoenzymes, Blood
Lidocaine, Serum
Procainamide, Serum
Propranolol, Serum
Quinidine, Serum
Signal-averaged electrocardiography, Diagnostic
Toxicology, Drug screen, Blood or urine

Additional Conditions
Beta blockade
Calcium-channel blockade
Congestive heart failure

MYOCARDIAL INFARCTION

Activated coagulation time, Automated, Blood
Activated partial thromboplastin time, Plasma
Anticardiolipin antibody, Serum
Antimyocardial antibody, Serum
Aspartate aminotransferase, Serum
Basic metabolic panel, Blood
Cardiac catheterization, Diagnostic
* Cardiac enzymes/isoenzymes, Blood
Cardiac output, Diagnostic
Chemistry profile, Blood
Chest radiography, Diagnostic
Coronary intravascular ultrasonography, Diagnostic
Creatine kinase, Isoenzymes, Serum
Creatine kinase, Serum
D-Dimer test, Blood
Digitoxin, Serum
Digoxin, Serum
Disopyramide phosphate, Serum
Echocardiography, Diagnostic
* Electrocardiography, Diagnostic
Glucose, Blood
Heart scan, Diagnostic
Hydroxybutyrate dehydrogenase, Blood
Lactate dehydrogenase, Blood
Lactate dehydrogenase, Isoenzymes, Blood
Lidocaine, Serum

Low-density lipoprotein cholesterol, Blood
Magnesium, Serum
Myoglobin, Qualitative, Urine and serum
Persantine-Sestamibi stress test and scan, Diagnostic
P-selectin, Plasma
Positron emission tomography, Diagnostic
Procainamide, Serum
Propranolol, Blood
Prothrombin time and international normalized ratio, Plasma
Quinidine, Serum
Signal-averaged electrocardiography, Diagnostic
Stress exercise test, Diagnostic
Stress test, Pharmacologic, Diagnostic
Thyroid-stimulating hormone, Sensitive assay, Blood
* Troponin I, Serum
* Troponin T, Serum

Additional Conditions
Angina pectoris
Aortic stenosis
Atherosclerosis
Chest wall trauma
Congestive heart failure
Diabetes mellitus
Dissecting aortic aneurysm
Duodenal ulcer
Esophageal spasm
Esophagitis
Gallbladder disease
Hiatal hernia
Hypercholesterolemia
Hypertension
Hypertriglyceridemia
Hyperuricemia
Hypoalbuminemia
Hyponatremia
Metabolic acidosis
Mitral valve prolapse
Muscular strain
Peptic ulcer
Pericarditis
Pulmonary embolus
Shock
Stress
Thrombosis
Vasculitis

MYOCARDITIS

Antimyocardial antibody, Serum
Antinuclear antibody, Serum
Antistreptolysin-O titer, Serum

Aspartate aminotransferase, Serum
Blood culture, Blood
Blood indices, Blood
Cardiac enzymes/isoenzymes, Blood
Complete blood count, Blood
★Coxsackie A or B virus titer, Blood
Creatine kinase, Isoenzymes, Serum
Creatine kinase, Serum
Differential leukocyte count,
    Peripheral blood
Echocardiography, Diagnostic
★Electrocardiography, Diagnostic
Histopathology, Specimen
Transesophageal ultrasonography,
    Diagnostic

Additional Conditions
Congestive heart failure
Q fever
Rocky mountain spotted fever
Toxoplasmosis
Trichinosis
Typhus
Vasculitis

MYOCLONUS
Computed tomography of the brain,
    Diagnostic
Electroencephalography, Diagnostic
★Magnetic resonance imaging,
    Diagnostic

Additional Conditions
Creutzfeldt-Jakob disease
Encephalopathy
Epilepsy
Ramsay-Hunt syndrome
Seizures

MYXEDEMA (HYPOTHYROIDISM)
Alkaline phosphatase, Serum
Chemistry profile, Blood
Chloride, Sweat, Specimen
Cholesterol, Blood
Complete blood count, Blood
Creatine kinase, Serum
Creatine, Urine
Differential leukocyte count,
    Peripheral blood
Electrocardiography, Diagnostic
Electrolytes, Plasma or serum
Lactate dehydrogenase, Blood
Lactate dehydrogenase, Isoenzymes,
    Blood
Lipid profile, Blood
Red blood cell morphology, Blood
Sodium, Plasma or serum
Thyroid peroxidase antibody, Blood

Thyroid antithyroglobulin antibody,
    Serum
★Thyroid function tests, Blood
Thyroid-stimulating hormone,
    Blood
Thyroid-stimulating hormone,
    Sensitive assay, Blood
Thyroid test: Free thyroxine index,
    Serum
Thyroid test: Thyroid hormone
    binding ratio, Blood
Thyroid test: Thyroxine, Blood
Thyroid test: Thyroxine free, Serum

Additional Conditions
Anemia
Bradycardia
Coma
Constipation
Fatigue
Hoarseness
Infection
Menorrhagia
Sepsis
Thyroiditis
Thyrotoxic periodic paralysis

NARCOLEPSY
(see Sleep disorders)

NARCOTICS
(see Drug abuse)

NEOPLASIA
(see Tumors)

NEPHRECTOMY
Aspartate aminotransferase, Serum
Complete blood count, Blood
Creatinine, Serum
Erythropoietin, Serum
Lactate dehydrogenase, Blood
Type and crossmatch, Blood
Urea nitrogen, Plasma or serum
Urinalysis, Urine

Additional Conditions
Glomerulonephritis
Kidney cancer
Pyelonephritis

NEPHRITIS
Anti-DNA, Serum
Body fluid, Routine, Culture (Urine)
★Creatinine, Urine

Kidney ultrasonography, Diagnostic
Electrolytes, Urine

Additional Conditions
Dyspnea
Gout
Hemoptysis

NEPHROLITHIASIS
Body fluid, Routine, Culture (Urine)
Calcium, Total, Serum
Calcium, Urine
Chemistry profile, Blood
Creatinine clearance, Urine
Cystine, Qualitative, Urine
* Electrolytes, Plasma or serum
Histopathology, Specimen
* Kidney ultrasonography, Diagnostic
Kidney stone analysis, Specimen
Magnesium, Serum
Magnesium, 24 Hour urine
* Occult blood, Urine
Oxalate, Urine
pH, Urine
Phosphorus, Urine
* Uric acid, Serum
Uric acid, Urine
Urinalysis, Urine

Additional Conditions
Fanconi syndrome
Gouty arthritis
Nephrocalcinosis
Osteoporosis
Renal tubular acidosis
Sarcoidosis

NEPHROSCLEROSIS
Complete blood count, Blood
Creatinine, Serum
Urea nitrogen, Plasma or serum
* Urinalysis, Urine

Additional Conditions
Hypertension
Papilledema
Renal failure

NEPHROSIS
Albumin, Serum
Antinuclear antibody, Serum
C3 complement, Serum
C4 complement, Serum
Creatinine, Serum
Creatinine clearance, Serum, Urine
Kidney biopsy, Specimen
Kidney ultrasonography, Diagnostic

* Protein electrophoresis, Serum
Urea nitrogen, Plasma or serum
* Urinalysis, Urine

Additional Conditions
Amyloidosis
Glomerulonephritis

NEPHROTIC SYNDROME
Albumin, Serum
Albumin/globulin ratio, Serum
Cholesterol, Blood
Creatinine clearance, Serum, Urine
Electrolytes, Plasma or serum
Electrolytes, Urine
Glucose tolerance test, Blood
Glucose, 2-Hour postprandial, Serum
Kidney biopsy, Specimen
Kidney ultrasonography, Diagnostic
* Lipid profile, Blood
Phosphorus, Serum
Protein electrophoresis, Serum
Protein electrophoresis, Urine
Protein, Semiquantitative, Urine
Protein, Total, Serum
Sodium, Urine
Transferrin, Serum
Triglycerides, Blood
Urea nitrogen, Plasma or serum
* Urinalysis, Urine

Additional Conditions
Acquired immunodeficiency
  syndrome
Amyloidosis
Edema
Glomerulonephritis
Heavy metal poisoning
Hepatitis B
Human immunodeficiency virus
Hyperlipidemia
Hypoalbuminemia
Syphilis
Systemic lupus erythematosus

NEUROBLASTOMA
Bone scan, Diagnostic
Computed tomography of the body
  (Abdomen and chest), Diagnostic
* Homovanillic acid, 24-Hour urine
Magnetic resonance imaging,
  Diagnostic
Magnetic resonance spectroscopy,
  Diagnostic
* Neuron-specific enolase, Serum
Octreotide scan, Diagnostic
* Vanillylmandelic acid, Urine

Additional Conditions
Diarrhea
Malabsorption
von Recklinghausen's disease

NEURODEGENERATION
*Magnetic resonance spectroscopy,
  Diagnostic

Additional Conditions
Amyotrophic lateral sclerosis
Multiple sclerosis

NEUROFIBROMATOSIS
*Biopsy, Site-specific (Skin, Nerves),
  Specimen

Additional Conditions
Bone cysts
Glioma
Hydrocephalus
Pheochromocytoma
Sarcoma
Scoliosis

NEUROGENIC PULMONARY EDEMA
(see Pulmonary edema)

NEUROPATHY
*Electromyography and nerve
  conduction studies, Diagnostic
Electron microscopy (for nerve
  tissue), Diagnostic
Folate, Serum
Glucose, Blood
Glucose, 2-Hour postprandial,
  Serum
Histopathology, Specimen
Lead, Blood
Magnetic resonance neurography,
  Diagnostic
Nerve biopsy, diagnostic
Protoporphyrin, Free erythrocyte,
  Blood
Vitamin B_{12}, Serum
Vitamin E_1, Serum

Additional Conditions
Alcoholism
Amyloidosis
Cancer
Charcot-Marie-Tooth disease
Diabetes mellitus
Guillain-Barré syndrome

Leprosy
Multiple myeloma
Rheumatoid arthritis
Sarcoidosis
Uremia

NEUROSYPHILIS
(see Syphilis)

NIEMANN-PICK DISEASE
*Sphingomyelinase, Diagnostic

Additional Conditions
Hepatosplenomegaly
Lymphadenopathy

NONTROPICAL SPRUE
(see Celiac sprue)

OBESITY
C-reactive protein, Blood
*Cholesterol, Blood
*Glucose, Blood
Insulin, Blood
Insulin-like growth factor-I, Blood
Melanocyte-stimulating hormone,
  Urine
Thyroid test: Thyroxine, Blood
*Thyroid test: Triiodothyronine,
  Blood

Additional Conditions
Asthma
Cerebrovascular accident
Diabetes mellitus
Hypercholesterolemia
Hyperlipidemia
Hypertension
Metabolic syndrome

OBSTRUCTION, BOWEL
Alanine aminotransferase, Serum
Alkaline phosphatase, Serum
Amylase, Serum and urine
Aspartate aminotransferase, Serum
Barium enema, Diagnostic
Chloride, Serum
Complete blood count, Blood
Differential leukocyte count,
  Peripheral blood
Doppler ultrasonographic flow
  studies, Diagnostic
*Flat-plate radiograph of the
  abdomen, Diagnostic

Occult blood, Stool
Potassium, Serum
Sigmoidoscopy, Diagnostic
Sodium, Plasma or serum
Urinalysis, Urine

Additional Conditions
Colon cancer
Constipation
Hirschsprung's disease
Paralytic ileus

OBSTRUCTIVE JAUNDICE
(*see Jaundice*)

OCCLUSION, ACUTE ARTERIAL
Activated partial thromboplastin
   time, Plasma
★Arteriography, Diagnostic
Blood gases, Arterial, Blood
Complete blood count, Blood
Glucose, Blood
Magnetic resonance angiography,
   Diagnostic
Prothrombin time and international
   normalized ratio, Plasma

Additional Conditions
Arteriosclerosis
Buerger's disease
Lymphedema
Raynaud's disease
Syphilis
Thrombosis
Trauma

ORGANIC BRAIN SYNDROME
Adrenocorticotropic hormone, Serum
Calcium, Total, Serum
Glucose, Blood
★Potassium, Serum
Red blood count, Serum
Thyroid-stimulating hormone,
   Blood

Additional Conditions
Alzheimer's disease
Amyotrophic lateral sclerosis
Anxiety
Cognitive impairment
Dementia
Depression
Drug withdrawal
Hydrocephalus
Multiple sclerosis
Thyrotoxicosis
Wilson's disease

ORTHOSTATIC HYPOTENSION
Catecholamines, Fractionation free,
   Plasma
Complete blood count, Serum
Cortisol, Serum

Additional Conditions
Addison's disease
Aldosteronism
Dehydration
Diabetes mellitus
Gastrointestinal bleeding
Pheochromocytoma

OSTEOARTHRITIS
Body fluid cytology, Specimen
★Bone radiography, Diagnostic
   (Spine)
Bone scan, Diagnostic
Culture, Routine (Synovial fluid),
   Specimen
Histopathology, Specimen
Mucin clot test (Synovial fluid),
   Specimen
Synovial fluid analysis, Diagnostic
★Radiography of long bones,
   Diagnostic

Additional Conditions
Metastasis from cancer
Multiple myeloma
Osteoporosis
Rheumatoid arthritis

OSTEOMALACIA
★Alkaline phosphatase, Serum
Bone scan, Diagnostic
★Calcium, Total, Serum
Calcium, Urine
★Parathyroid hormone, Blood
★Phosphorus, Serum
Vitamin D_3, Plasma or serum

Additional Conditions
Hyperparathyroidism
Hypocalcemia
Hypokalemia
Renal tubular nephrosis
Rickets

OSTEOMYELITIS
Blood culture, Blood
Complete blood count, Blood
Differential leukocyte count,
   Peripheral blood
★Radiography of the body (Affected
   area), Diagnostic

★Sedimentation rate, Erythrocyte,
  Blood

Additional Conditions
Drug abuse
Fever
Pain in bone
Thrombosis

OSTEOPOROSIS
Bone scan, Diagnostic
★Bone densitometry, Diagnostic
Bone ultrasonometry, Diagnostic
Calcium, Total, Serum
Cortisol, Plasma or serum
Estradiol, Serum
Estrogens, Serum
Glucose, Blood
Osteocalcin, Plasma or serum
Phosphorus, Serum
Prolactin, Serum
Protein electrophoresis, Urine

Additional Conditions
Anorexia nervosa
Backache
Bone pain
Cushing syndrome
Hypopituitarism
Leukemia
Malabsorption
Menopause
Multiple myeloma

OSTOMIES
Chloride, Serum
Complete blood count, Blood
Potassium, Serum
Sodium, Plasma, Serum or urine
Type and crossmatch, Blood
Urinalysis (from ileal conduit),
  Urine

Additional Conditions
Bladder cancer
Colon cancer
Colitis
Crohn's disease
Obstruction, Intestine

OTITIS MEDIA
Biopsy, Anaerobic, Culture
Complete blood count, Blood
Ear, Routine, Culture
Gamma globulin, Plasma
Sputum for *Haemophilus* species,
  Culture

Additional Conditions
Cholesteatoma
Mastoiditis
Meningitis
Upper respiratory infection

OVARIAN CANCER
CA 15-3, Blood
CA 72-4, Blood
★CA 125, Blood
Dual modality imaging, Diagnostic
Mucinlike carcinoma–associated
  antigen, Blood
Obstetric ultrasonography, Diagnostic
Osteopontin, Serum
Prostasin, Serum
Telomerase enzyme marker, Blood
Urinary chorionic gonadotropin
  peptide, Urine

Additional Conditions
Ascites
Back pain

OVARIAN FUNCTION TESTS
Androstenedione, Serum
★Estradiol, Serum
Estrogens, Serum and 24-Hour
  urine
★Follicle-stimulating hormone, Serum
Hormonal evaluation, Cytologic,
  Specimen
17-Hydroxyprogesterone, Blood
17-Ketosteroids, Total, 24-Hour
  urine
★Luteinizing hormone, Blood
Pregnanetriol, Urine
★Progesterone, Serum

Additional Conditions
Abscess, Ovarian
Dysmenorrhea
Hirsutism
Ovarian cancer

OVARIAN HYPERSTIMULATION SYNDROME
Activated partial thromboplastin
  time, Plasma
Alanine aminotransferase, Serum
Albumin, Serum
Alkaline phosphatase, Serum
Aspartate aminotransferase, Serum
Bilirubin, Indirect (Unconjugated),
  Serum
Blood gases, Arterial, Blood

Body fluid analysis, Cell count, Specimen
Body fluid cytology, Specimen
Chest radiography, Diagnostic
Complete blood count, Blood
C-reactive protein, Serum
Creatinine, Serum
Differential leukocyte count, Peripheral blood
Doppler ultrasonographic flow studies, Diagnostic
Electrolytes, Plasma or serum
Estradiol, Serum
Gamma-glutamyltranspeptidase, Blood
Gram stain (Effusion specimen), Diagnostic
★Gynecologic ultrasonography, Diagnostic
Paracentesis, Diagnostic
Pregnancy test (hCG), Routine, Serum
Prothrombin time and international normalized ratio, Plasma
Thoracentesis, Diagnostic
Urea nitrogen, Plasma or serum

Additional Conditions
Appendicitis
Ectopic pregnancy
Ovarian torsion
Pelvic inflammatory disease
Ruptured ovarian cyst
Tuboovarian abscess

OVERDOSE
(see Poisonings)

OVERHYDRATION
Albumin, Serum
★Complete blood count, Blood
★Osmolality, Serum
Osmolality, Urine
Protein, Total, Serum
Sodium, Plasma or serum
Urinalysis, Urine

Additional Conditions
Ascites
Congestive heart failure
Renal failure
Syndrome of inappropriate antidiuretic hormone secretion

OVULATION
★Progesterone, Serum

Additional Conditions
Infertility

PAGET'S DISEASE, BONE
Acid phosphatase, Serum
★Alkaline phosphatase, Serum
★Bone radiography, Diagnostic
Calcium, Total, Serum
Calcium, Urine
★Hydroxyproline, Total, 24-Hour urine
Osteocalcin, Plasma or serum
Phosphorus, Urine

Additional Conditions
Bone pain
Fractures
Kyphosis

PAGET'S DISEASE, BREAST
★Biopsy, Site-specific (Breast), Specimen
Mammography, Diagnostic

Additional Conditions
Pruritus
Ulceration

PAIN, ABDOMINAL
★Acute abdominal series, Diagnostic
Amylase, Serum
★Complete blood count, Blood
Computed tomography of the body (Abdomen), Diagnostic
Electrolytes, Plasma or serum
★Flat-plate radiograph of the abdomen, Diagnostic
Glucose, Blood
Lipase, Serum
Liver battery, Serum
Potassium, Serum
Sedimentation rate, Erythrocyte, Blood
Sodium, Plasma or serum
Urinalysis, Urine

Additional Conditions
Abscess
Appendicitis
Ascites
Cholelithiasis
Colitis
Colon cancer
Menstruation
Paralytic ileus
Pelvic inflammatory disease
Q fever

PAIN, ACUTE
*Complete blood count, Blood
Glucose, Blood
Radiography, Diagnostic
Sedimentation rate, Erythrocyte,
    Blood
Urinalysis, Urine

Additional Conditions
Aneurysm
Migraine headache
Trauma
Tumor

PAIN, BACK
Bone radiography, Diagnostic
Calcium, Total, Serum
Complete blood count, Blood
Magnetic resonance imaging,
    Diagnostic
Magnetic resonance neurography,
    Diagnostic
Myelography, Diagnostic
Phosphorus, Serum
Red blood cell morphology, Blood
Rheumatoid factor, Blood
Sedimentation rate, Erythrocyte,
    Blood
Urinalysis, Urine

Additional Conditions
Arthritis
Disk degeneration, Spine
Metastasis
Osteomyelitis
Ovarian cancer
Prostatitis
Vascular aneurysm

PAIN, CHEST
(*see Angina pectoris, Myocardial
infarction, Pleurisy, or Pneumonia*)

PAIN, CHRONIC
Complete blood count, Blood
C-reactive protein, Serum
Magnetic resonance neurography,
    Diagnostic
Platelet count, Blood
Radiography, Diagnostic
Rheumatoid factor, Blood
Sedimentation rate, Erythrocyte,
    Blood
Serotonin, Serum or blood
Sickle cell test, Blood
Urea nitrogen, Plasma or serum
Urinalysis, Urine

Additional Conditions
Arthritis
Cancer
Disk degeneration, Spine
Fibromyalgia
Nerve root irritation and
    compression
Reflex sympathetic dystrophy
Sickle cell anemia

PAIN, MUSCLE AND BONE
Aspartate aminotransferase, Serum
Bone scan, Diagnostic
Calcium, Total, Serum
Complete blood count, Blood
Creatine kinase, Serum
Muscle biopsy, Specimen
Phosphorus, Serum
Thyroid test: Thyroxine, Blood
Thyroid test: Triiodothyronine,
    Blood
Uric acid, Serum

Additional Conditions
Cerebral palsy
Hypothyroidism
Muscular dystrophy
Poliomyelitis

PAIN, VASCULAR
Activated partial thromboplastin
    time, Plasma
Cerebrospinal fluid, Routine analysis,
    Specimen
Complete blood count, Blood
Doppler ultrasonic flow studies,
    Diagnostic
Glucose, Blood
Platelet count, Blood
Prothrombin time and international
    normalized ratio, Plasma
Urinalysis, Urine

Additional Conditions
Atherosclerosis
Peripheral vascular disease
Thrombosis
Vasculitis

PALPITATIONS, HEART
Alcohol, Blood
Blood gases, Arterial, Blood
Cholesterol, Blood
Complete blood count, Blood
Creatine kinase, Serum
Echocardiography, Diagnostic
*Electrocardiography, Diagnostic

Stress test, Diagnostic
Thyroid test: Thyroxine, Blood
Thyroid test: Triiodothyronine, Blood

Additional Conditions
Anemia
Anxiety
Cardiomyopathy
Dysrhythmias
Exercise
Syncope
Thyrotoxicosis

PANCREATIC CANCER
Amylase, Serum and urine, and
    Amylase clearance
CA 19-9, Blood
CA 50, Blood
★Computed tomography of body
    (Pancreas), Diagnostic
Dual modality imaging, Diagnostic
Endoscopic retrograde
    cholangiopancreatography,
    Diagnostic
★Endoscopic Ultrasonography,
    Diagnostic
Glucose, Blood
K-*ras*, Blood or specimen
Laparoscopy, Diagnostic
Lipase, Serum
★Magnetic resonance
    cholangiopancreatography,
    Diagnostic
Occult blood, Stool
Pancreatic secretory trypsin inhibitor,
    Diagnostic
★Pancreas ultrasonography, Diagnostic
Telomerase enzyme marker, Blood
Urobilinogen, Urine

Additional Conditions
Abdominal pain
Diabetes mellitus
Diarrhea
Jaundice
Thrombophlebitis

PANCREATIC CHOLERA
★Amylase, Serum and urine
★Lipase, Serum
Vasoactive intestinal polypeptide,
    Blood

Additional Conditions
Anemia
Diabetes mellitus
Hypoaminoacidemia
Skin rash

PANCREATIC ISLET CELL LESION
Gastrin, Serum
Glucagon, Plasma
Insulin and insulin antibodies, Blood
★Vasoactive intestinal polypeptide,
    Blood

Additional Conditions
Anemia
Diabetes mellitus
Hypochlorhydria
Malabsorption

PANCREATIC TRAUMA
★Amylase, Serum
Complete blood count, Blood
Glucose, Blood
★Lipase, Serum
Peritoneal fluid analysis, Specimen
Type and crossmatch, Blood (Screen)
Urinalysis, Urine

Additional Conditions
Anemia
Hyperglycemia
Jaundice

PANCREATITIS
Alcohol, Serum
★Amylase, Serum and urine and
    Amylase clearance
Blood indices, Blood
Body fluid, Amylase, Specimen
Calcium, Total, Serum
Carotene, Serum
Chemistry profile, Blood
Complete blood count, Blood
Computed tomography, Diagnostic
C-Reactive protein, Serum
Differential leukocyte count,
    Peripheral blood
Endoscopic retrograde
    cholangiopancreatography,
    Diagnostic
Endoscopic ultrasonography,
    Diagnostic
Gamma-glutamyltranspeptidase,
    Blood
Glucose, Blood
Histopathology, Specimen
Leucine aminopeptidase, Blood
★Lipase, Serum
Lipid profile, Blood
Magnesium, Serum
Magnetic resonance
    cholangiopancreatography,
    Diagnostic

Methemoglobin, Blood
Pancreatic secretory trypsin inhibitor,
  Diagnostic
Pancreas ultrasonography,
  Diagnostic
Protein electrophoresis, Serum
Secretin test for pancreatic function,
  Diagnostic
Soluble fibrin monomer complex,
  Serum
Triglycerides, Blood
Trypsin, Plasma or serum
Trypsin, Stool
Trypsinogen-2, Urine

Additional Conditions
Alcoholism
Hypercalcemia
Hyperglycemia
Hyperlipidemia
Hyperuricemia
Hypoalbuminemia
Pleural effusion
Trauma, Abdominal
Vasculitis

PANIC DISORDER
Computed tomography of the brain,
  Diagnostic
Echocardiography, Diagnostic
Electrocardiography, Diagnostic
Stress exercise test, Diagnostic
Upper gastrointestinal series,
  Diagnostic

Additional Conditions
Alcoholism
Depression
Drug abuse
Mitral valve prolapse
Phobias
Tachycardia
Sleep disorders

PARALYTIC ILEUS
Chloride, Serum
Electrolytes, Plasma or serum
*Flat-plate radiograph of abdomen,
  Diagnostic
Sodium, Plasma or serum

Additional Conditions
Abdominal pain
Hemorrhage
Pancreatitis
Peritonitis
Spinal cord injury

PARKINSON'S DISEASE
Haloperidol, Serum
Phenothiazines, Blood
Reserpine, Serum
*Single-photon emission computed
  tomography, Brain, Diagnostic

Additional Conditions
Brain tumor
Carbon monoxide poisoning
Drug-related tremors
Seborrhea
Tremors

PAROXYSMAL HYPERTENSION
(see Pheochromocytoma)

PATENT DUCTUS ARTERIOSUS
*Blood gases, Arterial, Blood
  Cardiac catheterization, Diagnostic
*Chest radiography, Diagnostic
*Echocardiography, Diagnostic
  Electrocardiography, Diagnostic
  Transesophageal ultrasonography,
    Diagnostic

Additional Conditions
Left ventricular failure
Pulmonary hypertension

PATERNITY TESTING
Banding in genetic disorders,
  Diagnostic
Red blood cell enzyme deficiency
  screen, Blood
*Human leukocyte antigen typing,
  Blood

PELVIC INFLAMMATORY
DISEASE (PID)
Actinomyces, Culture
Biopsy, Anaerobic, Culture
Biopsy, *Mycobacterium,* Culture
Body fluid, Anaerobic, Culture
Chlamydia culture and group titer,
  Specimen (Culture)
Endometrium, Anaerobic, Culture
Fluorescent treponemal
  antibody–absorbed double-stain
  test, Serum
Genital, *Candida albicans,* Culture
Genital, *Neisseria gonorrhoeae,*
  Culture
*Histopathology, Specimen
*Laparoscopy, Diagnostic
  Obstetric ultrasonography, Diagnostic

Pap smear, Diagnostic
Sedimentation rate, Erythrocyte,
  Blood
Venereal Disease Research Laboratory
  test, Serum
Wound culture

Additional Conditions
Abdominal pain
Abscess
Cervical cancer
Chlamydia
Dysmenorrhea
Endometriosis
Gonorrhea
Infertility
Salpingitis

PEMPHIGUS
Brushing cytology, Specimen,
  Diagnostic
Fibroblast skin culture
★Histopathology, Specimen
Immunofluorescence, Skin biopsy,
  Specimen
Oral cavity cytology, (Scrape)
  Specimen
Pemphigus antibodies, Blood

Additional Conditions
Pneumonia
Septicemia
Shock
Toxemia

PEPTIC ULCER
ABO group and Rh type, Blood
Amylase, Serum and urine
Brushing cytology, Specimen,
  Diagnostic
Campylobacter-like organism test,
  Specimen
Complete blood count, Blood
Gastric analysis, Specimen
Gastric pH, Specimen
Gastrin, Serum
★Gastroscopy, Diagnostic
★*Helicobacter pylori*, Quick office
  serology, Serum
Helicobacter pylori titer, Blood
Histopathology, Specimen
Lipase, Serum
Occult blood, Stool
Pepsinogen I and pepsinogen II,
  Blood
Type and crossmatch, Blood
Urea breath test, Diagnostic
Washing cytology, Specimen

Additional Conditions
Burns
Duodenal ulcer
Epigastric pain
Gastric ulcer
Gastrinoma
Gastritis
Stress
Zollinger-Ellison syndrome

PERICARDITIS
Anti-DNA, Serum
Antinuclear antibody, Serum
Body fluid, Routine, Culture
Chest radiography, Diagnostic
Coxsackie A or B virus titer, Blood
C-reactive protein, Serum
★Echocardiography, Diagnostic
Electrocardiography, Diagnostic
Histopathology, Specimen
Pericardiocentesis, Diagnostic
Sedimentation rate, Erythrocyte,
  Blood

Additional Conditions
Aortic murmur
Congestive heart failure
Dysrhythmias
Mitral valve murmur
Myocardial infarction
Neoplastic disease
Radiation therapy
Tachycardia
Trauma
Uremia

PERIPHERAL NEUROPATHY
★Electromyography and nerve
  conduction studies, Diagnostic
  (Electromyography)
Glucose, Blood
Glucose, 2-Hour postprandial, Serum
Glutethimide, Blood
Heavy metals, Blood and 24-Hour
  urine
Histopathology, Specimen
Magnetic resonance neurography,
  Diagnostic
Nerve biopsy, Diagnostic

Additional Conditions
Arteritis
Brachial plexopathy
Brain tumor
Diabetes mellitus
Guillain-Barré syndrome
Leprosy
Rheumatoid arthritis

Sarcoidosis
Uremia

PERIPHERAL VASCULAR DISEASE (PVD)
Ankle-brachial index, Diagnostic
Antiphospholipid antibodies, Serum
Cholesterol, Blood
*Doppler ultrasonographic flow studies, Diagnostic
Prothrombin time and international normalized ratio, Plasma
Pulse volume recording of peripheral vascular disease, Diagnostic

Additional Conditions
Arteriosclerosis
Hypercholesterolemia
Hyperlipidemia
Obesity

PERITONITIS
Body fluid, Amylase, Specimen
Body fluid, Anaerobic, Culture
Body fluid, Fungus, Culture
Body fluid, Mycobacteria, Culture
Body fluid, Routine, Culture
Body fluid analysis, Cell count, Specimen
*Body fluid cytology, Specimen
Cerebrospinal fluid, Lactic acid, Specimen
Complete blood count, Blood
C-reactive protein, Serum
Flat-plate radiograph of the abdomen, Diagnostic
Genital, *Candida albicans,* Culture
Genital, *Neisseria gonorrhoeae,* Culture
Histopathology, Specimen
Lactic acid, Blood
Lactate dehydrogenase, Blood
Magnetic resonance imaging, Diagnostic
Paracentesis, Diagnostic
Sedimentation rate, Erythrocyte, Blood

Additional Conditions
Abscess
Ascites
Burns
Cirrhosis
Diabetic ketosis
Paralytic ileus
Sepsis

PERNICIOUS ANEMIA
Blood indices, Blood
Bone marrow biopsy, Diagnostic
Complete blood count, Blood
Cytologic study of gastrointestinal tract, Diagnostic
Differential leukocyte count, Peripheral blood
Folic acid, Red blood cells, Blood
Folic acid, Serum
Gastrin, Serum
*Intrinsic factor antibody, Blood
Lactate dehydrogenase, Blood
Lactate dehydrogenase, Isoenzymes, Blood
Pepsinogen I and pepsinogen II, Blood
Pepsinogen-I antibody, Blood
Platelet count, Blood
Reticulocyte count, Blood
Red blood cell morphology, Blood
*Schilling test, Diagnostic
*Vitamin B_{12}, Serum
Vitamin B_{12}, Unsaturated binding capacity, Serum

Additional Conditions
Autoimmune thyroid disease
Crohn's disease
Diabetes mellitus (Type 1)
Gastrectomy
Gastritis
Graves' disease
IgA deficiency
Rheumatoid arthritis

PERTUSSIS
(*see Whooping cough*)

PHARYNGITIS
Adenovirus immunofluorescence, Diagnostic
Antideoxyribonuclease-B titer, Serum
Antihyaluronidase titer, Serum
Antistreptolysin-O titer, Serum
*Complete blood count, Blood
*Culture, Routine, (Throat, Nose) Specimen
Differential leukocyte count, Peripheral blood
Infectious mononucleosis screening test, Blood
Throat culture for *Candida albicans,* Culture
Throat culture for *Corynebacterium diphtheriae,* Culture

Throat culture for group A
  beta-hemolytic streptococci, Culture
Throat culture for *Neisseria
  gonorrhoeae,* Culture
★Throat culture, Routine, Culture
Viral culture, Specimen

Additional Conditions
Acquired immunodeficiency syndrome
Diphtheria
Epiglottitis
Epstein-Barr virus
Tonsillitis

PHENYLKETONURIA (PKU) DISEASE
★Guthrie test for phenylketonuria,
  Diagnostic
Phenistix test, Diagnostic
Phenylalanine, Blood

Additional Conditions
Eczema
Mental retardation
Seizures

PHEOCHROMOCYTOMA
Calcitonin, Plasma or serum
★Catecholamines, Fractionation free,
  Plasma
Homovanillic acid, 24-Hour urine
★Metanephrines, Total, 24-Hour urine
  and free, Plasma
★Vanillylmandelic acid, Urine

Additional Conditions
Aortic aneurysm
Cerebrovascular accident
Headache
Hyperparathyroidism
Hypertension
Hypotension
Neurofibromatosis
Tachycardia
Thyroid cancer

PHLEBITIS
(see Thrombophlebitis)

PID
(see Pelvic inflammatory disease)

PINWORM
★Parasite screen, Stool

Additional Conditions
Enuresis
Insomnia
Pruritus
Urinary tract infection

PITUITARY
*(see Addison's disease or Cushing
syndrome)*

PKU DISEASE
(see Phenylketonuria)

PLEURAL EFFUSION
(see Effusions, Pleural)

PLEURISY
Biopsy, Routine, Culture
Blood culture, Blood
Blood gases, Arterial, Blood
★Chest radiography, Diagnostic
Complete blood count, Blood
Coxsackie A or B virus titer, Blood
Histopathology, Specimen
Sputum, Routine, Culture

Additional Conditions
Ascites
Congestive heart failure
Meningitis
Myocarditis
Pericarditis
Pneumothorax

PNEUMOCONIOSIS
(see Black lung disease)

PNEUMONIA
Blood culture, Blood
Blood gases, Arterial, Blood
★Chest radiography, Diagnostic
★Complete blood count, Blood
Electrolytes, Plasma or serum
Legionella pneumophila, Direct
  fluorescent antibody smear, Specimen
Mycoplasma enzyme immunoassay,
  Blood
Mycoplasma titer, Blood
Pulmonary function tests, Diagnostic
Respiratory antigen panel, Specimen
Sputum, Routine, Culture
Viral culture, Specimen

Additional Conditions
Acquired immunodeficiency
  syndrome
Anemia
Aspiration
Chronic obstructive pulmonary disease
Endocarditis
Fever
Hemoptysis
Immunosuppression
Lung cancer
Pleural effusion
Right ventricular failure
Sepsis
Severe acute respiratory syndrome
  (SARS)

PNEUMOTHORAX
Blood gases, Arterial, Blood
★Chest radiography, Diagnostic
Complete blood count, Blood
Sputum cytology, Specimen

Additional Conditions
Chronic obstructive pulmonary
  disease
Cyanosis
Cystic fibrosis
Dyspnea
Hemothorax
Trauma
Tuberculosis

POISONINGS
Acetaminophen, Serum
Anion gap, Blood
Bicarbonate, Plasma
Blood gases, Arterial, Blood
Carbon monoxide, Blood
Cyanide, Blood
Heavy metals, Blood and 24-Hour
  urine
Lead, Blood and urine
Morphine, Urine
Salicylate, Blood
★Toxicology, Drug screen, Blood or
  urine

Additional Conditions
Coma
Cyanosis
Depression
Dysrhythmias
Hypertension
Hypotension
Metabolic acidosis
Seizures
Suicidal ideation and gesture

POLIO
(*see Poliomyelitis*)

POLIOMYELITIS (POLIO)
★Poliomyelitis I, II, III titer, Blood
Viral culture, Specimen

Additional Conditions
Diarrhea
Fever
Headache
Meningitis
Stiff neck
Tremors

POLYCYSTIC OVARIAN DISEASE
Estrogens, Serum and 24-Hour urine
★Follicle-stimulating hormone, Serum
Follicle-stimulating hormone, Urine
★Luteinizing hormone, Blood
Obstetric ultrasonography, Diagnostic
Testosterone, Free, Bioavailable and
  total, Blood

Additional Conditions
Diabetes mellitus, Type 2
Endometrial hyperplasia
Hirsutism
Infertility
Ovarian cancer
Pelvic inflammatory disease
Uterine fibroids

POLYCYTHEMIA VERA
Bilirubin, Serum (Total)
Blood volume, Blood
Bone marrow biopsy, Diagnostic
★Complete blood count, Blood
^{51}Cr–red blood cell survival, Blood
Leukocyte alkaline phosphatase, Blood
Red blood cell morphology, Blood
Vitamin B_{12}, Unsaturated binding cap-
  acity, Serum

Additional Conditions
Dizziness
Headache
Hypertension
Obesity
Splenomegaly
Tinnitus

POLYURIA
★Glucose, Blood
Glucose, 2-Hour postprandial, Serum
Urinalysis, Urine

Additional Conditions
Diabetes insipidus
Fanconi syndrome
Hypercalcemia
Hyperparathyroidism
Renal tubular acidosis

POSTOPERATIVE
(see Surgery)

PREECLAMPSIA
(see Pregnancy-induced hypertension)

PREGNANCY
Amniocentesis and amniotic fluid
analysis, Diagnostic
Chorionic villi sampling, Diagnostic
D-Dimer test, Blood
Fetal fibronectin, Specimen
Fetal monitoring, External,
Diagnostic
Fetal monitoring, Internal, Diagnostic
Fetoscopy, Diagnostic
Foam stability test, Amniotic fluid
Fructosamine, Serum
Glucose challenge test, Diagnostic
Glucose tolerance test, Blood
Hematocrit, Blood
Hemoglobin, Blood
Human chorionic gonadotropin,
Beta-subunit, Serum
Mendelian inheritance in genetic
disorders, Diagnostic
Obstetric ultrasonography, Diagnostic
P-selectin, Plasma
★Pregnancy test, Routine, Serum and
qualitative, Urine
Protein, Urine
Thyroid peroxidase antibody, Blood

Additional Conditions
Amenorrhea
Anemia
HELLP syndrome
Hyperglycemia
Nausea
Preeclampsia
Rubella
Syphilis

PREGNANCY-INDUCED HYPERTENSION
Activated partial thromboplastin
time, Plasma
★Chemistry profile, Blood

Complete blood count, Blood
Kidney biopsy, Specimen
★Liver battery, Serum
Magnesium, Serum
★Platelet count, Blood
Pregnancy test, Routine, Serum and
qualitative, Urine
Pregnanetriol, Urine
★Protein, Urine (24-Hour)
Prothrombin time and international
normalized ratio, Plasma
Sodium, Plasma or serum
★Uric acid, Serum
Urinalysis, Urine

Additional Conditions
Diabetes mellitus
Edema
HELLP syndrome
Hydatidiform mole
Hypertension
Nephritis
Pregnancy
Renal disease

PREOPERATIVE
(see Surgery)

PRIMARY ESSENTIAL HYPERTENSION
(see Hypertension)

PROSTATE CANCER
Acid phosphatase, Serum
CA 15-3, Blood
Dual modality imaging, Diagnostic
Mitogen-activated protein kinase,
Specimen
Prostatic acid phosphatase, Blood
Prostate ultrasonography,
Diagnostic
Prostatic acid phosphatase, Blood
★Prostate-specific antigen, Blood
Telomerase enzyme marker, Blood or
urine

Additional Conditions
Anemia
Hematuria
Hydronephrosis
Hyperglycemia
Hypoalbuminemia
Hypophosphatemia
Metastasis to bone
Uremia
Urinary tract infection

PROSTATITIS
Body fluid, Routine, Culture (Urine)
Blood culture, Blood
★Complete blood count, Blood
Urinalysis, Urine
Urinalysis, Fractional, Urine

Additional Conditions
Chlamydia
Dysuria
Gonorrhea
Tuberculosis
Urinary tract infection

PRURITUS
Culture, Skin, Specimen
Toxicology, Drug screen, Blood

Additional Conditions
Dermatitis
Iron deficiency anemia
Obstructive biliary disease
Psychiatric disturbances
Uremia

PSITTACOSIS
Chlamydia culture and group titer,
    Specimen (Culture)
Cold agglutinin screen, Blood
Complement fixation, Serum
★Complete blood count,
    Blood
Protein, Quantitative, Urine
Sedimentation rate, Erythrocyte,
    Blood

Additional Conditions
Epistaxis
Fever
Headache
Pneumonitis

PSORIASIS
Culture, Skin, Specimen
★Histopathology, Specimen

Additional Conditions
Candidiasis
Onychomycosis
Rheumatoid arthritis
Streptococcal infection of the
    pharynx

PULMONARY EDEMA
Albumin, 24-Hour urine
Blood gases, Arterial, Blood

Blood urea nitrogen/creatinine ratio,
    Blood
★Chest radiography, Diagnostic
Complete blood count, Blood
Digoxin, Serum
Electrolytes, Plasma or serum
Electrolytes, Urine
Sputum cytology, Specimen

Additional Conditions
Congestive heart failure
Cyanosis
Mitral valve stenosis
Myocardial infarction
Ventricular septal defect

PULMONARY EMBOLISM
Activated partial thromboplastin
    time, Plasma
Antithrombin III test, Diagnostic
Blood gases, Arterial, Blood
Chemistry profile, Blood
Complete blood count, Blood
Computed tomography of the body
    (Spiral, EBCT), Diagnostic
Electrocardiography, Diagnostic
★Lung scan, Perfusion and ventilation,
    Diagnostic
Plasminogen assay, Blood
★Pulmonary angiography, Diagnostic
Sedimentation rate, Erythrocyte,
    Blood
Venography, Diagnostic

Additional Conditions
Atrial fibrillation
Congestive heart failure
Deep vein thrombosis
Dyspnea
Hemoptysis
Hip fracture
Hypoxemia
Immobility
Lung cancer
Myocardial infarction
Obesity
Pregnancy
Respiratory alkalosis
Shock
Stroke
Surgery
Syncope
Trauma
Vascular disease

PULMONARY INFECTION
Blood culture, Blood
Blood gases, Arterial, Blood

★Chest radiography, Diagnostic
★Complete blood count, Blood
Sputum, Routine, Culture

Additional Conditions
Chronic obstructive pulmonary
disease
Industry-related diseases
Lung cancer
Pleural effusion
Pneumonia
Tuberculosis

PULMONIC STENOSIS
Blood gases, Arterial, Blood
Cardiac catheterization, Diagnostic
★Chest radiography, Diagnostic
★Electrocardiography, Diagnostic

Additional Conditions
Atrial septal defect
Cardiomyopathy
Dyspnea
Heart murmur, Systolic

PYELONEPHRITIS
Body fluid, Routine, Culture
(Urine)
Chemistry profile, Blood
Complete blood count, Blood
Creatinine clearance, Urine
Electrolytes, Plasma or serum
Nitrite, Bacteria screen, Urine
★Urinalysis, Urine

Additional Conditions
Chlamydia
Cystitis
Gonorrhea
Trichomonas
Ureteral obstruction
Urethritis
Urinary tract infection

PYREXIA
★Blood culture, Blood
Body fluid, Routine, Culture
(Urine)
Creatine kinase, Isoenzymes, Serum
Culture, Routine, Specimen
(Sputum)

Additional Conditions
Leukemia
Neuroleptic malignant syndrome
Pneumonia
Sepsis

Q FEVER
Complete blood count, Serum
Differential leukocyte count,
Peripheral blood
Liver battery, Serum
★Weil-Felix agglutinins, Blood

Additional Conditions
Abdominal pain
Encephalopathy
Headache
Hepatitis
Pneumonitis

RABIES
★Animals and rabies Negri bodies,
Brain tissue, Specimen
Fluorescent rabies antibody, (Brain
tissue) Specimen

Additional Conditions
Paresthesia
Seizures

RAPE TRAUMA
★Acid phosphatase, Vaginal swab
★Blood group antigen of semen,
Vaginal swab
Body fluid, Amylase, Specimen
Cervical culture for Neisseria
gonorrhoeae, Culture
Chlamydia culture and group titer,
Specimen (Culture)
Gamma-hydroxybutyric acid, Blood
or urine
★Motile sperm, Wet mount, Diagnostic
Pap smear, Diagnostic
Precipitin test against human sperm
and blood, Vaginal swab
★Pregnancy test, Routine, Serum and
qualitative, Urine
Sims-Huhner test, Diagnostic
Syphilis, Serum
Trichomonas preparation, Specimen
★Venereal Disease Research Laboratory
test, Serum

Additional Conditions
Acquired immunodeficiency syndrome
Anxiety
Chlamydia
Depression
Gonorrhea
Pregnancy
Trichomoniasis

RAT-BITE FEVER
★Biopsy, Site-specific (Bite site),
Specimen

Complete blood count, Blood
Differential leukocyte count,
  Peripheral blood
Fluorescent treponemal
  antibody–absorbed double-stain
  test, Serum

Additional Conditions
Arthritis
Fever
Headache
Lymphangitis
Splenomegaly

RAYNAUD'S DISEASE
Antinuclear antibody, Serum
Cold agglutinin titer, Serum
*Cryoglobulin, Qualitative, Serum
Extractable nuclear antigen, Serum

Additional Conditions
Arteriosclerosis
Carpal tunnel syndrome
Cyanosis
Gangrene
Rheumatoid arthritis
Systemic lupus erythematosus

RECTAL CANCER
(see Colon Cancer)

RENAL CALCULI
Body fluid, Routine, Culture (Urine)
Calcium, Total, Serum
*Kidney ultrasonography, Diagnostic
Phosphorus, Serum
Uric acid, Serum
Urinalysis, Urine

Additional Conditions
Back pain, Acute
Gout
Urinary tract infection

RENAL CELL CANCER
*Biopsy, Site-specific (Kidney),
  Specimen
Computed tomography of the body
  (Kidney), Diagnostic
Dual modality imaging, Diagnostic
Intravenous pyelography, Diagnostic
Kidney ultrasonography, Diagnostic
Nephrotomography, Diagnostic
Renal angiography, Diagnostic
Telomerase enzyme marker, Urine

Additional Conditions
Anemia
Fever
Hematuria
Hypercalcemia
Hypoglycemia

RENAL FAILURE
Beta$_2$-microglobulin, Blood and
  24-Hour urine
Bicarbonate, Serum
Chemistry profile, Blood
Complete blood count, Blood
*Creatinine, Serum
Creatinine clearance, Serum, Urine
*Electrolytes, Plasma or serum
Electrolytes, Urine
Globulin, Serum
Homocysteine, Plasma or urine
Immunoelectrophoresis, Serum and
  urine
Intravenous pyelography, Diagnostic
Inulin clearance test, Diagnostic
Kidney biopsy, Specimen
Magnesium, Serum
Magnetic resonance angiography,
  Diagnostic
Magnetic resonance imaging,
  Diagnostic
Mean platelet volume, Blood
Myoglobin, Qualitative, Urine
Myoglobin, Serum
pH, Blood
Phosphorus, Serum
Potassium, Serum
Protein, Semiquantitative, Urine
Protein, Urine (Quantitative,
  24-Hour)
Retrograde pyelography, Diagnostic
Technetium-penta acetic acid
  clearance, Diagnostic
Transferrin, Serum
*Urea nitrogen, Plasma or serum
Uric acid, Serum
Urinalysis, Urine

Additional Conditions
Aminoglycoside toxicity
Blood transfusion incompatibility
Burns
Dehydration
Disseminated intravascular
  coagulation
Hypertension
Leptospirosis
Liver failure
Multiple myeloma
Myocardial infarction
Peritonitis

Poisoning
Toxic shock syndrome

RENAL HYPERTENSION
*Aldosterone, Serum and urine
Arteriography, Diagnostic
Chloride, Serum
Color duplex ultrasonography,
   Diagnostic
Intravenous pyelography, Diagnostic
Potassium, Serum
Renal function tests, Diagnostic
Renal indices, Diagnostic
*Renin activity, Plasma
Renocystogram, Diagnostic
   (Captopril renography)
Sodium, Plasma, Serum or urine

Additional Conditions
Atherosclerosis
Posttransplantation surgery
Renal stenosis

RENAL INFARCTION
Chemistry profile, Blood
Creatine kinase, Serum
Creatine kinase, Isoenzymes, Serum
*Histopathology, Specimen
Kidney ultrasonography, Diagnostic
Lactate dehydrogenase, Blood
Lactate dehydrogenase, Isoenzymes,
   Blood
Urinalysis, Urine

Additional Conditions
Abscess
Kidney cancer
Renal failure
Renal hypertension
Trauma

RENIN HYPERTENSION
(see Renal hypertension)

RESPIRATORY ACIDOSIS
Bicarbonate, Plasma
*Blood gases, Arterial, Blood
Chest radiography, Diagnostic
Complete blood count, Blood
Electrolytes, Plasma or serum
Urinalysis, Urine

Additional Conditions
Acute respiratory distress syndrome
Congestive heart failure

Chronic obstructive pulmonary
   disease
Hypercapnia
Hypoxemia
Kyphoscoliosis
Myocardial infarction
Shock

RESPIRATORY ALKALOSIS
*Blood gases, Arterial, Blood
Calcium, Total, Serum
Chest radiography, Diagnostic
Lung scan, Perfusion and ventilation,
   Diagnostic
Potassium, Serum
Urinalysis, Urine

Additional Conditions
Acute respiratory distress syndrome
Anxiety
Asthma
Congestive heart failure
Liver disease
Pneumonia
Pregnancy
Pulmonary emboli

RESPIRATORY FAILURE
Alpha$_1$-antitrypsin, Serum
Bicarbonate, Plasma
Blood culture, Blood
*Blood gases, Arterial, Blood
Chest radiography, Diagnostic
Complete blood count, Blood
Culture, Routine, Specimen
   (Sputum)
Differential leukocyte count,
   Peripheral blood
Electrolytes, Plasma or serum
Lung scan, Perfusion and ventilation,
   Diagnostic
Pulmonary artery catheterization,
   Diagnostic
Pulmonary function tests, Diagnostic
Sputum, Routine, Culture

Additional Conditions
Acute respiratory distress syndrome
Botulism
Chronic obstructive pulmonary
   disease
Congestive heart failure
Guillain-Barré syndrome
Myasthenia gravis
Pneumonia
Pneumothorax
Poliomyelitis
Pulmonary edema

Pulmonary embolus
Severe acute respiratory syndrome
(SARS)
Spinal cord injury

RESTLESS LEGS SYNDROME
(see Sleep disorders)

REYE SYNDROME
Activated partial thromboplastin
time, Plasma
Alanine aminotransferase, Serum
★Ammonia, Blood
Aspartate aminotransferase, Serum
Bilirubin, Direct, Serum
Creatinine, Serum
Glucose, Blood
Histopathology, Specimen
★Liver battery, Serum
Liver biopsy, Diagnostic
Lumbar puncture, Diagnostic
Prothrombin time and international
normalized ratio, Plasma
Toxicology, Drug screen, Blood or
urine
Urea nitrogen, Plasma or serum

Additional Conditions
Bronchitis
Encephalopathy
Hepatic failure
Hypoglycemia
Myocarditis
Otitis media
Pericarditis
Pneumonia
Sinusitis
Thrombophlebitis

RHABDOMYOLYSIS
Cocaine, Blood
Creatine kinase, Isoenzymes, Serum
Muscle biopsy, Specimen
★Myoglobin, Qualitative, Urine
★Myoglobin, Serum

Additional Conditions
Dermatomyositis

RHEUMATIC FEVER
Antideoxyribonuclease-B titer, Serum
★Antistreptolysin-O titer, Serum
C-reactive protein, Serum
Mean platelet volume, Blood
Streptozyme, Blood

Additional Conditions
Cardiomegaly
Congestive heart failure
Mitral valve stenosis
Pericarditis

RHEUMATOID ARTHRITIS
(see also Osteoarthritis)
Anti-neutrophil cytoplasmic antibody
screen, Serum
Anti-DNA, Serum
Antinuclear antibody, Serum
Antistreptolysin-O titer, Blood
Body fluid, Routine, Culture
C4 complement, Serum
Chemistry profile, Blood
Complement components, Serum
Complement, Total, Serum
C-reactive protein, Serum
Extractable nuclear antigen, Serum
Genital, *Candida albicans,* Culture
Genital, *Neisseria gonorrhoeae,* Culture
Human leukocyte antigen B-27,
Blood
Immune complex assay, Blood
Lupus test, Blood
Mean platelet volume, Blood
Mucin clot test (Synovial fluid),
Specimen
Protein electrophoresis, Serum
★Rheumatoid factor, Blood
Sedimentation rate, Erythrocyte,
Blood
Sjögren's antibodies, Blood
Synovial fluid analysis, Diagnostic
Uric acid, Serum
Uric acid, Urine

Additional Conditions
Amyloidosis
Lymphadenopathy
Pericarditis
Pleural effusion
Raynaud's phenomenon
Splenomegaly
Vasculitis

RHINITIS
Allergen-specific IgE, Serum
Computed tomography of the body
(Sinuses), Diagnostic
Eosinophil count, Blood
Sinus radiography, Diagnostic

Additional Conditions
Nasal polyps
Osteomyelitis
Sinusitis

RICKETS
(see Osteomalacia)

RINGWORM (TINEA CAPITIS)
*Culture, Skin (Scalp for Microsporum
  audouinii), Specimen

Additional Conditions
Lymphadenopathy
Pruritus

ROCKY MOUNTAIN SPOTTED FEVER
Complete blood count, Blood
Differential leukocyte count,
  Peripheral blood
*Rocky Mountain spotted fever
  serology, Serum

Additional Conditions
Coma
Fever
Headache
Rash

RUBELLA (GERMAN MEASLES)
Immunoglobulin M, Serum
*Rubella serology, Serum and specimen
Toxoplasmosis, Rubella,
  Cytomegalovirus, Herpes virus
  serology, Blood
Viral culture, Specimen

Additional Conditions
Adenitis
Fever
Lymphadenopathy
Monkeypox
Pregnancy

RUBEOLA
Differential leukocyte count,
  Peripheral blood
Histopathology, Specimen
Lymph node biopsy, Specimen
*Rubeola serology, Serum

Additional Conditions
Fever
Monkeypox
Rash

SALMONELLOSIS
Blood culture, Blood
Complete blood count, Blood

Differential leukocyte count,
  Peripheral blood
Febrile agglutinins, Serum
*Salmonella titer, Blood
Stool culture, Routine, Stool

Additional Conditions
Bacteremia
Enterocolitis
Fever
Typhoid

SANFILIPPO SYNDROME
*Mucopolysaccharides, Qualitative,
  Urine
S mucopolysaccharide turnover,
  Diagnostic

Additional Conditions
Dysrhythmias
Mental retardation

SARCOIDOSIS
Bronchial washing, Specimen,
  Diagnostic
Brushing cytology, Specimen,
  Diagnostic
*Chest radiography, Diagnostic
Computed tomography of the body
  (HRCT), Diagnostic
Diffusing capacity for carbon
  monoxide, Diagnostic
*Histopathology, Specimen
Ki-67 proliferation marker,
  Specimen
Liver biopsy, Diagnostic
Liver ^{131}I scan, Diagnostic
Mediastinoscopy, Diagnostic
Muramidase, Serum and urine
Nerve biopsy, Diagnostic
Sputum cytology, Specimen

Additional Conditions
Arthritis
Dyspnea
Fever
Hepatosplenomegaly
Lymphadenopathy
Pleural effusion
Sinusitis

SARCOMA
*Biopsy, Site-specific (Bone),
  Specimen
Bone scan, Diagnostic
Computed tomography of the body
  (Bone), Diagnostic

Magnetic resonance imaging,
  Diagnostic

Additional Conditions
Bowel obstruction
Osteomyelitis
Paralytic ileus

SARS
(see Severe acute respiratory syndrome)

SCABIES
★Culture, Skin (Scrapings for ova or
  mites), Specimen

Additional Conditions
Malnutrition
Pyoderma
Pruritus

SCARLET FEVER
★Antistreptolysin-O titer, Serum
Throat culture for group A
  beta-hemolytic streptococci, Culture

Additional Conditions
Fever
Tonsillitis
Vomiting

SCHISTOSOMIASIS
Complete blood count, Blood
Differential leukocyte count,
  Peripheral blood
Eosinophil count, Blood
Liver battery, Serum
Liver biopsy, Diagnostic
Liver-spleen scan, Diagnostic
★Ova and parasite, Stool
★Urinalysis, Urine

Additional Conditions
Bladder cancer
Diarrhea
Nephrotic syndrome
Renal failure

SCHIZOPHRENIA, CHRONIC
Iron, Serum
Tricyclic antidepressants, Plasma or
  serum

Additional Conditions
Catatonia
Dementia

Hallucinations
Seizures

SCIATICA
Complete blood count, Blood
Computed tomography of the body
  (Spine), Diagnostic
Differential leukocyte count,
  Peripheral blood
Electromyography and nerve
  conduction studies
  (Electromyography), Diagnostic
Magnetic resonance imaging,
  Diagnostic
Magnetic resonance neurography,
  Diagnostic
Radiography of the body (Spine),
  Diagnostic

Additional Conditions
Cancer
Herniated disk
Infection
Low back pain
Metastasis
Spondylolisthesis
Trauma

SCLERODERMA
Antinuclear antibody, Serum
D-Xylose absorption test, Diagnostic,
  Serum or urine
Histopathology, Specimen
★Scleroderma antibody, Blood

Additional Conditions
Diverticulitis
Dysphagia
Pericarditis
Polyarthralgia
Pulmonary fibrosis
Pulmonary hypertension
Raynaud's phenomenon
Telangiectasia

SCURVY
Capillary fragility test, Diagnostic
★Vitamin C, Plasma or serum

Additional Conditions
Anemia
Gingivitis
Malnutrition

SECONDARY HYPERTENSION
(see Hypertension)

SEIZURES
Alcohol, Blood
Blood gases, Arterial, Blood
Brain scan, Cerebral flow and
  pathology, Diagnostic
Brain ultrasonography, Diagnostic
Calcium, Blood
Carbon monoxide, Blood
Carboxyhemoglobin, Blood
Cerebral computed tomography,
  Diagnostic
Cerebrospinal fluid, Glucose,
  Specimen
Cerebrospinal fluid, Routine analysis,
  Specimen
Chemistry profile, Blood
Chlordiazepoxide, Blood
Chromium, Serum
Clonazepam, Blood
Cocaine, Blood
Complete blood count, Blood
Creatine kinase, Serum
Diazepam, Serum
★Electroencephalography,
  Diagnostic
Electrolytes, Plasma or serum
Ethosuximide, Blood
Flurazepam, Serum
Glucose, Blood
Heavy metals, 24-Hour urine
Ketone bodies, Blood
Ketones, Semiquantitative, Urine
Lidocaine, Serum
Magnesium, Serum
Mephenytoin, Blood
Methsuximide, Serum
Neuron-specific enolase, Serum
Osmolality, Serum
Phenobarbital, Plasma or serum
Phenytoin, Serum
Primidone, Serum
Pseudocholinesterase, Plasma
Sodium, Plasma, Serum or urine
Theophylline, Blood
Thiocyanate, Blood
Thiocyanate, Urine
Toxicology, Drug screen, Blood or
  urine
Valproic acid, Blood
Vitamin B_6, Plasma

Additional Conditions
Alcoholism
Brain tumor
Carbon monoxide poisoning
Cerebrovascular accident
Drug abuse
Epilepsy
Hysteria
Poisoning

SENILE DEMENTIA
(*see Dementia*)

SEPSIS
★Blood culture, Blood
Body fluid, Anaerobic, Culture
  (Abscess)
★Body fluid (Urine), Routine, Culture
Complete blood count, Blood
Culture, Routine, Specimen
Differential leukocyte count,
  Peripheral blood
Electrocardiography, Diagnostic
Foreign body, Routine, Culture
Urinalysis, Urine

Additional Conditions
Abscess
Arthritis
Bacteremia
Cancer
Empyema
Toxic shock syndrome
Urinary tract infection

SERUM SICKNESS
C1q immune complex detection,
  Serum
C3 complement, Serum
C4 complement, Serum
Heterophile agglutinins, Blood
Immune complex assay, Blood

Additional Conditions
Anaphylaxis
Arthritis
Fever
Hepatitis B
Lymphadenopathy
Urticaria

SEVERE ACUTE RESPIRATORY SYNDROME (SARS)
Blood culture, Blood
Bronchoscopy, Diagnostic
★Chest radiography, Diagnostic
Calcium, Blood
Complete blood count, Blood
Computed tomography of the body
  (Chest), Diagnostic
Creatine kinase, Serum
★Gram stain (Sputum), Diagnostic
Influenza A and B titer, Blood
Lactate dehydrogenase, Blood
Legionella pneumophilia culture, IgM
  titer, Blood

Oximetry, diagnostic
Respiratory antigen panel, Specimen
★Severe acute respiratory
   syndrome–associated coronavirus
   antibody and reverse transcriptase
   polymerase chain reaction tests,
   Specimen (NOTE: experimental as of
   print date; consult www.cdc.gov for
   updated test information)
★Viral culture, (Nasopharynx, stool)
   Specimen

Additional Conditions
Acute respiratory distress syndrome
   (ARDS)
Influenza
Legionella
Pneumonia
Respiratory syncytial virus

SEXUAL ASSAULT
(*see Rape trauma*)

SEXUALLY TRANSMITTED DISEASE
(*see Acquired immunodeficiency
syndrome, Chancroid, Chlamydia,
Gonorrhea, Human papillomavirus,
Lymphogranuloma venereum, and
Syphilis*)

SHINGLES
(*see Herpes zoster*)

SHOCK
Activated partial thromboplastin
   time, Plasma
Aspartate aminotransferase, Serum
Blood culture, Blood
★Blood gases, Arterial, Blood
Blood urea nitrogen/creatinine ratio,
   Blood
★Complete blood count, Blood
Creatinine, Serum
Electrolytes, Plasma or serum
Glucose, Blood
Lactic acid, Blood
Osmolality, Serum
Potassium, Serum
Prothrombin time and international
   normalized ratio, Plasma
Pulmonary artery catheterization,
   Diagnostic
Urinalysis, Urine

Additional Conditions
Anaphylaxis
Bacteremia
Burns
Coronary artery disease
Drug overdose
Dysrhythmias
Electrolyte imbalance
Gastrointestinal bleeding
Hypovolemia
Myocardial infarction
Myocarditis
Pancreatitis
Pulmonary hypertension
Sepsis
Status post-cardiac surgery
Status post-cardiopulmonary
   resuscitation
Toxic shock syndrome
Transfusion reaction
Trauma

SIADHS
(*see Syndrome of inappropriate
antidiuretic hormone secretion*)

SICKLE CELL ANEMIA
C3 proactivator, Serum
D-Dimer (for crisis), Blood
Fetal hemoglobin, Blood
Hemoglobin electrophoresis, Blood
★Sickle cell test, Blood

Additional Conditions
Acute pain
Cardiomegaly
Jaundice
Splenomegaly

SIGMOIDOSCOPY
Complete blood count, Blood
Potassium, Serum
Sodium, Plasma or serum

Additional Conditions
Hemorrhage
Polyps in colon/rectum
Tumor of colon/rectum

SILICOSIS
★Chest radiography, Diagnostic
Pulmonary function tests, Diagnostic

Additional Conditions
Dyspnea
Tuberculosis

SINUSITIS
Body fluid, Anaerobic, Culture, (Abscess)
Complete blood count, Blood
★Culture, Routine, Specimen (Nose)
Histopathology, Specimen
Immunoglobulin A, Serum
Sedimentation rate, Erythrocyte, Blood
Sinus radiography, Diagnostic
Tomography of paranasal sinuses, Diagnostic

Additional Conditions
Influenza
Pneumonia
Respiratory infection

SJÖGREN SYNDROME
Antinuclear antibody, Serum
Blood indices, Blood
Complete blood count, Blood
Differential leukocyte count, Peripheral blood
Extractable nuclear antigen, Serum
Histopathology, Specimen
Immune complex assay, Blood
Protein electrophoresis, Serum
Red blood count, Serum
Rheumatoid factor, Blood
★Sjögren's antibodies, Blood

Additional Conditions
Cirrhosis
Hashimoto's thyroiditis
Polymyositis
Pulmonary fibrosis
Rheumatoid arthritis
Scleroderma
Systemic lupus erythematosus
Xerostomia

SLEEP DISORDERS
(see also Insomnia)
Oximetry, Diagnostic
Polysomnography, Diagnostic

Additional Conditions
Aging
Congestive heart failure
Epilepsy
Seizures

SPIDER BITES
★Arthropod identification, Specimen
Complete blood count, Blood

Additional Conditions
Anaphylaxis
Seizures

SPINAL CORD INJURY
Activated partial thromboplastin time, Plasma
Calcium, Total, Serum
Cerebral computed tomography, Diagnostic
★Magnetic resonance imaging, Diagnostic
Phosphorus, Serum
Prothrombin time and international normalized ratio, Plasma
Uric acid, Serum
Urinalysis, Urine

Additional Conditions
Brown-Séquard syndrome
Depression
Hypotension
Hypoxia
Spinal cord compression

SPLENOMEGALY
Alanine aminotransferase, Serum
Aspartate aminotransferase, Serum
Bone marrow biopsy, Diagnostic
★Complete blood count, Blood
Computed tomography of the body (Abdomen), Diagnostic
Immunoperoxidase procedures (for antigens), Diagnostic
Liver battery, Serum
Platelet count, Blood
Spleen scan, Diagnostic
★Spleen ultrasonography, Diagnostic
Sputum, Mycobacteria, Culture and smear

Additional Conditions
Cancer
G6PD deficiency
Histoplasmosis
Infectious mononucleosis
Leukemia
Metastasis
Polycythemia vera
Sarcoidosis
Sickle cell anemia

STATUS EPILEPTICUS
Cerebral computed tomography, Diagnostic
★Electroencephalography, Diagnostic

Phenobarbital, Plasma or serum
Phenytoin, Serum
Valproic acid, Blood

Additional Conditions
Alcoholism
Brain tumor
Trauma

STEATORRHEA
★Fat, Semiquantitative, Stool

Additional Conditions
Whipple's disease

STEIN-LEVENTHAL SYNDROME
(see Polycystic ovarian disease)

STERILITY
(see Infertility)

STIMULANT DRUG ABUSE
(see also Drug abuse)
Amphetamines, Blood
Cocaine, Blood
Methylphenidate, Serum
Phenmetrazine, Blood

Additional Conditions
Alcoholism
Depression
Stress

STOMATITIS
★Complete blood count, Serum
Differential leukocyte count,
  Peripheral blood
Glucagon, Plasma
T- and B-lymphocyte subset assay,
  Blood
Throat culture for Candida albicans,
  Culture
Tzanck smear, Specimen

Additional Conditions
Acquired immunodeficiency
  syndrome, Diagnostic
Cancer
Candidiasis
Herpes simplex virus
Immunosuppression after
  transplantation
Malnutrition
Steroid and steroid inhaler use

STRESS
Adrenocorticotropic hormone, Serum
Aldosterone, Serum
Cortisol, Plasma or serum

Additional Conditions
Anxiety
Dermatitis
Hypertension
Myocardial infarction
Stroke

STRESS ULCER
(see Peptic ulcer)

STROKE
(see Cerebrovascular accident)

SUBACUTE BACTERIAL ENDOCARDITIS (SBE)
Blood culture, Blood
Blood indices, Blood
C3 complement, Serum
C4 complement, Serum
Complement, Total, Serum
★Complete blood count, Blood
C-reactive protein, Serum
Differential leukocyte count,
  Peripheral blood
Echocardiography, Diagnostic
★Sedimentation rate, Erythrocyte,
  Blood
Teichoic acid antibody, Blood
Transesophageal ultrasonography,
  Diagnostic
★Urinalysis, Urine

Additional Conditions
Disseminated intravascular
  coagulation
Drug abuse
Valvular stenosis

SUBARACHNOID HEMORRHAGE
Cerebrospinal fluid, Routine analysis,
  Specimen
Computed tomography of the brain,
  Diagnostic
Lumbar puncture, Diagnostic
★Magnetic resonance imaging,
  Diagnostic

Additional Conditions
Cerebral aneurysm
Cerebrovascular accident
Trauma

SUNSTROKE
(see Heat stroke)

SURGERY, POSTOPERATIVE
Activated partial thromboplastin
time, Plasma
Blood gases, Arterial, Blood
Chloride, Serum
*Complete blood count, Blood
D-Dimer test, Blood
Glucose, Blood
Platelet count, Blood
Potassium, Serum
Prothrombin time and international
normalized ratio, Plasma
Sodium, Plasma or serum
Urea nitrogen, Plasma or serum
Urinalysis, Urine

Additional Conditions
Bacteremia
Emboli
Hypoxemia
Pneumonia
Sepsis
Thrombosis

SURGERY, PREOPERATIVE
Activated partial thromboplastin
time, Plasma
Carbon dioxide, Partial pressure,
Blood
*Chest radiography, Diagnostic
Chloride, Serum
*Complete blood count, Blood
Creatinine, Serum
Differential leukocyte count,
Peripheral blood
Electrocardiography, Diagnostic
Electrolytes, Plasma or serum
Glucose, Blood
Pregnancy test, Routine, Serum and
qualitative, Urine
Type and crossmatch, Blood
Urea nitrogen, Plasma or serum
Urinalysis, Urine

Additional Conditions
Aneurysm
Appendicitis
Cancer
Cholecystitis
Coronary artery disease
Intestinal obstruction
Peripheral vascular disease
Trauma

SYNCOPE
Carotid phonoangiography,
Diagnostic
*Doppler ultrasonographic flow
studies (Carotid), Diagnostic
Echocardiography, Diagnostic
*Electrocardiography, Diagnostic
Oculoplethysmography, Diagnostic
Oculopneumoplethysmography,
Diagnostic
*Tilt table test, Diagnostic

Additional Conditions
Aortic stenosis
Atherosclerosis
Atrioventricular block
Cardiomyopathy
Hypotension
Neurogenic syncope
Pulmonary stenosis
Sick sinus syndrome
Vasovagal syncope

SYNDROME OF INAPPROPRIATE ANTIDIURETIC HORMONE SECRETION
*Antidiuretic hormone, Serum
Electrolytes, Plasma or serum
Electrolytes, Urine
Osmolality, Serum
Osmolality, Urine
*Sodium, Plasma, Serum or urine
Specific gravity, Urine
Urea nitrogen, Plasma or serum
Uric acid, Serum

Additional Conditions
Bronchogenic cancer
Hyponatremia
Leukemia
Myocardial infarction
Myxedema
Pancreatic cancer

SYPHILIS
Automated reagin testing,
Diagnostic
Fluorescent treponemal antibody–
absorbed double-stain test,
Serum
Hemagglutination treponemal test for
syphilis, Serum
Microhemagglutination–*Treponema
pallidum* test, Serum

Rapid plasma reagin test, Blood
*Venereal Disease Research Laboratory
test, Serum
Venereal Disease Research Laboratory
test, Cerebrospinal fluid, Specimen

Additional Conditions
Acquired immunodeficiency syndrome
Aortitis
Hepatitis
Lymphadenopathy
Meningitis
Pregnancy

SYSTEMIC LUPUS ERYTHEMATOSUS (SLE)
Anti-DNA, Serum
Antinuclear antibody, Serum
C3 complement, Serum
C4 complement, Serum
Complete blood count, Blood
C-reactive protein, Serum
Fibrinopeptide A
Fluorescent treponemal antibody–
absorbed double-stain test, Serum
Immune complex assay, Blood
*Lupus panel, Blood
Lupus test
Magnetic resonance spectroscopy,
Diagnostic
Platelet count, Blood
Viscosity, Serum

Additional Conditions
Arthritis
Leukopenia
Photosensitivity
Rash
Renal disease
Stomatitis
Thrombocytopenia

TAY-SACHS DISEASE
*Amniocentesis, Diagnostic
Galactose-1-phosphate, Blood

Additional Conditions
Blindness
Dementia
Mental retardation

TENSION
(see Headache)

TESTICULAR CANCER
Alpha-fetoprotein, Blood
*Biopsy, Site-specific (Testes),
Specimen

Computed tomography of the body
(Retroperitoneum), Diagnostic
Dual modality imaging, Diagnostic
Human chorionic gonadotropin,
Beta-subunit, Serum
Telomerase enzyme marker, Blood or
urine

Additional Conditions
Atrophic testes
Cryptorchid testes
Gynecomastia
Hydrocele
Leukemia
Virilization

TETANY
Calcium, Total, Serum
Calcium, Urine
*Chemistry profile, Blood
*Electrolytes, Plasma or serum
Magnesium, Serum

Additional Conditions
Anxiety
Hyperaldosteronism
Hypocalcemia
Hypoparathyroidism
Osteomalacia
Rickets

TETRALOGY OF FALLOT
Blood gases, Arterial, Blood
Cardiac catheterization, Diagnostic
*Chest radiography, Diagnostic
*Electrocardiography, Diagnostic
Hematocrit, Blood
Hemoglobin, Blood
Iron, Serum
Red blood count, Serum

Additional Conditions
Cyanosis
Emboli
Hypoxia
Polycythemia

THALASSEMIA
Chorionic villi sampling, Specimen
*Complete blood count, Blood
*Ferritin, Serum
Fetal hemoglobin, Blood
*Hemoglobin electrophoresis, Blood
Iron and total iron-binding
capacity/transferrin, Serum

Additional Conditions
Anemia
Cardiomyopathy
Hypogonadism
Jaundice
Splenomegaly

THORACIC AORTIC ANEURYSM
(see Aneurysm)

THROMBOANGIITIS OBLITERANS
*Arteriography, Diagnostic

Additional Conditions
Peripheral vascular disease
Thrombosis

THROMBOCYTOPENIA
*Bone marrow biopsy, Diagnostic
Capillary fragility test, Diagnostic
Complete blood count, Blood
Folic acid, Serum
Liver battery, Serum
Mean platelet volume, Blood
Occult blood, Urine
Platelet antibody, Blood
*Platelet count, Blood
Potassium, Serum
Red blood cell morphology, Blood
Vitamin B_{12}, Serum

Additional Conditions
Acquired immunodeficiency syndrome
Alcoholism
Anemia
Cancer
Disseminated intravascular coagulation
Drug effect
Hypersplenism
Idiopathic thrombocytopenia purpura
Leukemia
Sepsis
Severe acute respiratory syndrome (SARS)

THROMBOPHLEBITIS
Activated partial thromboplastin time, Plasma
Circulating anticoagulant, Blood
Protein C, Blood
Protein S, Total and free, Plasma
*Prothrombin time and international normalized ratio, Plasma
Venography, Diagnostic

Additional Conditions
Cancer
Congestive heart failure
Pulmonary embolism
Systemic lupus erythematosus
Trauma
Varicose veins

THROMBOSIS
Activated partial thromboplastin time, Plasma
Antiphospholipid antibodies, Serum
Antithrombin III test, Diagnostic
D-Dimer test, Blood
Doppler ultrasonographic flow studies, Diagnostic
Factor V, Blood (Leiden mutation)
Fibrinogen, Plasma
Hemoglobin, Blood
Lung scan, Perfusion and ventilation, Diagnostic
Magnetic resonance angiography, Diagnostic
Magnetic resonance imaging, Diagnostic
Protein C, Blood
Protein S, Total and free, Plasma
*Prothrombin time and international normalized ratio, Plasma
Soluble fibrin monomer complex, Serum
Urinalysis, Urine
Venography, Diagnostic

Additional Conditions
Aneurysm
Cancer
Dysfibrinogenemia
Peripheral vascular disease
Ulcerative colitis

THRUSH (CANDIDIASIS, MONILIASIS)
Complete blood count, Blood
Oral cavity cytology, Specimen
Throat culture for *Candida albicans*, Culture
Vaginal culture

Additional Conditions
Acquired immunodeficiency syndrome
Cancer
Fever
Immunosuppression
Leukemia
Lymphadenopathy
Steroid and steroid inhaler use

THYROID
(see Goiter, Hyperthyroidism, Hypothyroidism)

THYROID CANCER
★Biopsy, Site-specific (Thyroid), Specimen
Dual modality imaging, Diagnostic
Electrolytes, Plasma or serum
Neuron-specific enolase, Serum
Telomerase enzyme marker, Blood
Thyroid scan, Diagnostic
Thyroid ultrasonography, Diagnostic

Additional Conditions
Goiter
Thyroiditis

THYROIDECTOMY
Calcium, Total, Serum
Cholesterol, Blood
Complete blood count, Blood
Phosphorus, Serum
Thyroid test: Thyroxine, Blood
Thyroid test: Triiodothyronine, Blood
Type and crossmatch, Blood

Additional Conditions
Hypoparathyroidism

THYROTOXICOSIS
(see Hyperthyroidism)

TIA
(see Transient ischemic attack)

TIC DOULOUREUX (TRIGEMINAL NEURALGIA)
Complete blood count, Blood
Magnetic resonance angiography, Diagnostic
Phenytoin, Serum
Platelet count, Blood
Tegretol, Serum

Additional Conditions
Acute facial pain
Brain tumor
Multiple sclerosis

TINEA CAPITIS
(see Ringworm)

TINEA CRURIS
Culture, Skin, Specimen

Additional Conditions
Candidiasis
Dermatitis
Pruritus

TINNITUS
Cerebral angiography, Diagnostic
Cerebral computed tomography, Diagnostic
★Hearing test for loudness— recruitment, Diagnostic
Salicylate, Blood
★Tuning fork test of Weber, Rinne, and Schwabach tests, Diagnostic

Additional Conditions
Aneurysm
Carotid occlusion
Otitis media

TONSILLITIS
★Complete blood count, Blood
Differential leukocyte count, Peripheral blood
★Throat culture for group A beta-hemolytic streptococci, Culture

Additional Conditions
Epiglottitis
Esophagitis
Infectious mononucleosis
Myocarditis
Pharyngitis
Scarlet fever

TOXEMIA
(see Pregnancy-induced hypertension)

TOXIC SHOCK SYNDROME
★Bilirubin, Total, Serum
Blood culture, Blood
★Chemistry profile, Blood
Chloride, Serum
★Complete blood count, Blood
Creatinine, Serum
Genital, Routine (for Staphylococcus aureus), Culture
Glucose, Blood
Obstetric ultrasonography, Diagnostic
pH, Blood

Potassium, Serum
Prothrombin time and international
   normalized ratio, Plasma
Rocky Mountain spotted fever
   serology, Serum
Sodium, Plasma or serum
Urea nitrogen, Plasma or serum
Urinalysis, Urine
Vaginal culture (for *Staphylococcus
   aureus*)

Additional Conditions
Conjunctivitis
Diarrhea
Erythroderma
Fever
Hypotension
Postpartum
Vomiting

TRANSFUSION REACTION
Antibody identification, Red blood
   cell, Blood
Blood culture, Blood
Coombs', Direct, Serum
Coombs', Direct IgG, Serum
Haptoglobin, Serum
Hemoglobin, Plasma and qualitative,
   Urine
Hemosiderin, Urine
Immunoglobulin A antibodies, Serum
Occult blood, Urine
★Transfusion reaction work-up,
   Diagnostic

Additional Conditions
Chills
Disseminated intravascular coagulation
Dyspnea
Fever
Graft-versus-host disease
Headache
Hypotension
Renal failure
Sepsis
Shock

TRANSIENT ISCHEMIC ATTACK (TIA)
Activated partial thromboplastin
   time, Plasma
★Carotid doppler, Diagnostic
Cerebral angiography, Diagnostic
★Cerebral computed tomography,
   Diagnostic
Cholesterol, Blood
Oculoplethysmography, Diagnostic

Oculopneumoplethysmography,
   Diagnostic
Ophthalmodynamometry, Diagnostic
Protein electrophoresis, Serum
Prothrombin time and international
   normalized ratio, Plasma
Single-photon emission computed
   tomography, Brain, Diagnostic
Triglycerides, Blood
Viscosity, Serum

Additional Conditions
Aortic stenosis
Atherosclerosis
Atrial fibrillation
Carotid stenosis
Diplopia
Dizziness
Hypotension
Stroke

TRANSPLANT (BONE MARROW, CORNEA, HEART, LIVER, KIDNEY)
Blood culture, Blood
Blood gases, Arterial, Blood
Calcium, Total, Serum
Carbon dioxide, Partial pressure,
   Blood
Carbon dioxide, Total content, Blood
Chloride, Serum
★Complete blood count, Blood
Computed tomography, Diagnostic
Creatinine, Serum
Diffusing capacity for carbon
   monoxide, Diagnostic
Hepatitis C genotype, Diagnostic
Human leukocyte antigen typing, Blood
Magnetic resonance imaging,
   Diagnostic
Mixed leukocyte culture, Specimen
Potassium, Serum
Renocystography, Diagnostic
Sodium, Plasma or serum
★Type and crossmatch, Blood
Urea nitrogen, Plasma or serum

Additional Conditions
Aplastic anemia
Cancer
Cardiac failure
Corneal eye trauma
Graft-versus-host disease
Insulin-dependent diabetes
Leukemia
Liver failure
Lung failure
Renal failure

TRANSPLANT REJECTION
Activated partial thromboplastin
time, Plasma
Alanine aminotransferase, Serum
Aspartate aminotransferase, Serum
Blood gases, Arterial, Blood
Bone marrow biopsy, Diagnostic
Complete blood count, Blood
Creatinine, Serum
Differential leukocyte count,
Peripheral blood
Muramidase, Serum and urine
Platelet count, Blood
Prothrombin time and international
normalized ratio, Plasma
Urea nitrogen, Plasma or serum

Additional Conditions
Candidiasis
Congestive heart failure
Diarrhea
Graft-versus-host disease
Hemorrhage
Renal failure
Sepsis

TRANSPOSITION OF THE GREAT ARTERIES
★Blood gases, Arterial, Blood
Cardiac catheterization, Diagnostic
★Chest radiography, Diagnostic
Echocardiography, Diagnostic
Electrocardiography, Diagnostic
Platelet count, Blood
Red blood count, Serum

Additional Conditions
Cardiomegaly
Congestive heart failure
Cyanosis

TREMOR
Calcium, Ionized, Blood
★Cerebral computed tomography,
Diagnostic
Electroencephalography, Diagnostic
Electrolytes, Plasma or serum
Glucose, Blood

Additional Conditions
Alzheimer's disease
Brain tumor
Encephalopathy
Gilles de la Tourette syndrome
Huntington's disease
Multiple sclerosis
Parkinson's disease
Spinal cord trauma

TREPONEMA PALLIDUM
(see Syphilis)

TRICHINOSIS
Aldolase, Serum
Eosinophil count, Blood
Muscle biopsy, Specimen
Muscle profile, Specimen
Parasite screen, Blood
★Trichinosis serology, Serum

Additional Conditions
Conjunctivitis
Diarrhea
Dyspnea
Edema
Encephalitis
Fever
Muscle pain
Myocarditis
Nephritis
Photophobia
Pneumonia

TRICHOMONAS
(see Vaginitis)

TRICUSPID ATRESIA
★Blood gases, Arterial, Blood
Cardiac catheterization, Diagnostic
Chest radiography, Diagnostic
★Echocardiography, Diagnostic
Electrocardiography, Diagnostic
★Transesophageal ultrasonography,
Diagnostic

Additional Conditions
Cor pulmonale
Cyanosis
Dyspnea
Polycythemia

TRIGEMINAL NEURALGIA
(see Tic douloureux)

TRYPANOSOMIASIS
African trypanosomiasis, Blood
Malaria smear, Blood
Microfilaria, Peripheral blood
Parasite screen, Blood
★Trypanosomiasis serologic test, Blood

Additional Conditions
Ascites
Edema

Fever
Hepatosplenomegaly
Lymphadenopathy
Myocarditis

TUBAL PREGNANCY
(see Ectopic pregnancy)

TUBERCULOSIS (TB), PULMONARY
*Acid-fast bacteria, Culture and stain (Sputum)
*Chest radiography, Diagnostic
Computed tomography of the body (HRCT), Diagnostic
Immunoglobulin G, Serum
Liver ^{131}I scan, Diagnostic
*Mantoux skin test, Diagnostic
Muramidase, Serum and urine
Urinalysis (for kidney tuberculosis), Urine

Additional Conditions
Acquired immunodeficiency syndrome, Diagnostic
Anorexia
Fever
Pleural effusion
Urinary tract infection

TULAREMIA
Bacterial serology, Blood
Blood culture, Blood
Brucellosis agglutinins, Blood
Complete blood count, Blood
Differential leukocyte count, Peripheral blood
Febrile agglutinins, Serum
*Tularemia agglutinins, Serum
Weil-Felix agglutinins, Blood

Additional Conditions
Enteritis
Fever
Headache
Lymphadenopathy
Ulceration of lesion

TUMORS
Alkaline phosphatase, Serum
Alpha-fetoprotein, Blood
Bone marrow biopsy, Diagnostic
CA 15-3, Serum
CA 50, Blood
Carcinoembryonic antigen, Serum
Cervical-vaginal cytology, Specimen

Chest radiography, Diagnostic
Chromosome analysis, Blood
Complete blood count, Blood
Estradiol receptor and progesterone receptor in breast cancer, Diagnostic
HER-2/*neu* oncogene, Specimen
*Histopathology, Specimen
Immunoperoxidase procedures, Diagnostic (for antigens)
Ki-67 proliferation marker, Specimen
Magnetic resonance imaging, Diagnostic
Mucinlike carcinoma–associated antigen, Blood
Myelography, Diagnostic
Needle aspiration, Diagnostic
Occult blood, Stool
Sputum, Routine, Culture
Sputum cytology, Specimen
Urinalysis, Urine
Vanillylmandelic acid, Urine

Additional Conditions
Acquired immunodeficiency syndrome
Acute pain
Anorexia
Cancer
Dyspnea
Leukemia
Metastasis
Pneumonia

TURNER SYNDROME
*Chromosome analysis, Blood
Follicle-stimulating hormone, Serum
Glucose, Blood
Luteinizing hormone, Blood
Oral cavity cytology, Specimen

Additional Conditions
Amenorrhea
Coarctation of the aorta
Diabetes mellitus
Infertility
Mental retardation
Osteoporosis
Thyroiditis

TYPHOID
Febrile agglutinins, Serum
Salmonella titer, Blood
*Stool culture (for *Salmonella*), Routine, Stool

Additional Conditions
Bradycardia
Diarrhea

Headache
Leukopenia
Splenomegaly

TYPHUS
Complement fixation, Serum
Febrile agglutinins, Serum
★Typhus titer, Blood
Weil-Felix agglutinins, Blood

Additional Conditions
Chills
Fever
Headache

ULCERS
(see Decubiti, Duodenal, or Peptic)

ULCERATIVE COLITIS
Albumin, Serum
Anti-neutrophil cytoplasmic antibody
  screen, Serum
Aspartate aminotransferase, Serum
Barium enema, Diagnostic
Calcium, Total, Serum
★Colonoscopy, Diagnostic
Complete blood count, Blood
Creatinine, Serum
Cytologic study of gastrointestinal
  tract, Diagnostic
Histopathology, Specimen
Lactate dehydrogenase, Blood
★Occult blood, Stool
Ova and parasites, Stool
Phosphorus, Serum
Stool, Routine, Culture
Urea nitrogen, Plasma or serum
Uric acid, Serum

Additional Conditions
Anemia
Constipation
Diarrhea
Fever
Hemorrhoids
Hypoproteinemia

UNSTABLE ANGINA
(see Angina pectoris)

UREMIA
Activated coagulation time, Blood
★Anion gap, Blood

Bleeding time, Duke, Ivy, or Mielke,
  Blood
Creatinine, Serum
Creatinine clearance, Serum, Urine
★Electrolytes, Plasma or serum
Electrolytes, Urine
Liver battery, Serum
Neuron-specific enolase, Serum
★Platelet count, Blood
★Renal function test, Diagnostic
★Urea nitrogen, Plasma or serum
Urinalysis, Urine

Additional Conditions
Anemia
Gastrointestinal bleeding
Glomerulonephritis
Hypertension
Hyponatremia
Neuropathy
Renal failure

URETERAL STENTS
Activated partial thromboplastin
  time, Plasma
Body fluid, Routine, Culture (Urine)
Complete blood count, Blood
Creatinine, Serum
Prothrombin time and international
  normalized ratio, Plasma
Urea nitrogen, Plasma or serum
Urinalysis, Urine

Additional Conditions
Bladder cancer
Prostate cancer

URETEROSIGMOIDOSTOMY
Calcium, Total, Serum
Chloride, Serum
★Complete blood count, Blood
Potassium, Serum
Prothrombin time and international
  normalized ratio, Plasma
Type and crossmatch, Blood
Urinalysis, Urine

Additional Conditions
Colon cancer
Metastasis

URINARY TRACT INFECTION
★Body fluid, Routine, Culture
  (Urine)
Complete blood count, Blood
Differential leukocyte count,
  Peripheral blood

Foreign body (Indwelling catheter),
Routine, Culture
Urinalysis, Urine

Additional Conditions
Abscess
Cystitis
Diabetes mellitus
Pregnancy
Prostatitis
Pyelonephritis
Tuberculosis
Urethritis

UTERINE CANCER
*Biopsy, Site-specific (Uterus),
Specimen
Dilatation and curettage, Diagnostic
Computed tomography of the body,
Diagnostic
Dual modality imaging, Diagnostic
Obstetric ultrasonography, Diagnostic
Pap smear, Diagnostic
Telomerase enzyme marker, Blood

Additional Conditions
Diabetes mellitus
Menorrhagia
Obesity
Polycystic ovarian syndrome

VAGINAL CANCER
*Biopsy, Site-specific (Vagina),
Specimen
Colposcopy, Diagnostic
Dual modality imaging, Diagnostic
Obstetric ultrasonography,
Diagnostic
Pap smear, Diagnostic
Telomerase enzyme marker, Blood
Thymidylate synthase, Specimen

Additional Conditions
Cervical cancer
Endometriosis
Polyps
Vaginitis

VAGINITIS
*Cervical-vaginal cytology, Specimen
Chlamydia culture and group titer,
Specimen (Culture)
Genital, *Candida albicans*, Culture
Genital, *Neisseria gonorrhoeae*,
Culture
Glucose, Blood
Herpes cytology, Specimen

Neisseria gonorrhoeae smear,
Specimen
Rapid plasma reagin test, Blood
Trichomonas preparation, Specimen
Urinalysis, Urine
Venereal Disease Research Laboratory
test, Serum

Additional Conditions
Candidiasis
Chlamydia
Dysuria
Gonorrhea
Pruritus
Toxic shock syndrome
Trichomonas

VARICELLA
(see Chickenpox)

VARICES (ESOPHAGEAL, LEG)
Calcium, Total, Serum
Complete blood count, Blood
*Endoscopic ultrasound, Diagnostic
(Esophageal varices)
Esophagogastroduodenoscopy,
Diagnostic (Esophageal varices)
Occult blood, Stool
Potassium, Serum

Additional Conditions
Acute pain
Alcoholism
Edema
Hemorrhage

VASCULITIS
Antineutrophil cytoplasmic antibody
screen, Serum
Eosinophil count, Blood
*Histopathology, Specimen
Immunofluorescence, Skin biopsy,
Specimen
Nerve biopsy, Diagnostic
Raji cell assay, Blood
Rheumatoid factor, Blood
Sedimentation rate, Erythrocyte,
Blood

Additional Conditions
Alcoholism
Anemia
Hepatitis B
Hypertension
Urticaria
Wegener's granulomatosis

VENOUS STASIS ULCER
(see Ulcers)

VENTRICULAR SEPTAL DEFECT
* Blood gases, Arterial, Blood
  Cardiac catheterization, Diagnostic
* Chest radiography, Diagnostic
* Echocardiography, Diagnostic
  Electrocardiography, Diagnostic

Additional Conditions
Cardiac murmur
Congestive heart failure
Pulmonary hypertension
Systolic heart thrill

VERTIGO
(see also Tinnitus)
Alcohol, Blood
Blood gases, Arterial, Blood
Carbon dioxide, Blood
Cerebral computed tomography,
  Diagnostic
Complete blood count, Blood
Magnesium, Serum

Additional Conditions
Brain tumor
Infection (ear)
Labyrinthitis
Ménière's disease
Nystagmus
Tinnitus
Trauma to the head

VIRAL HEPATITIS
(see Hepatitis)

VIRILIZATION
* Androstenedione, Serum
  Dehydroepiandrosterone sulfate,
    Serum and 24-Hour urine
* Estrogens, Serum and 24-Hour urine
  17-Hydroxycorticosteroids, 24-Hour
    urine
  17-Hydroxyprogesterone, Serum
  17-Ketosteroids, Total, 24-Hour urine
  Pregnanetriol, Urine
* Testosterone, Free, Bioavailable and
    total, Blood

Additional Conditions
Acromegaly
Choriocarcinoma
Hirsutism
Pregnancy

VOMITING
Blood gases, Arterial, Blood
* Chloride, Serum
* Potassium, Serum
* Sodium, Plasma or serum
  Urinalysis, Urine

Additional Conditions
Ascites
Bulimia
Cancer
Diabetic acidosis
Gastroenteritis
Increased intracranial pressure
Intestinal obstruction
Malnutrition
Ménière's disease
Migraine
Pancreatitis
Paralytic ileus
Pregnancy
Uremia

VON WILLEBRAND'S DISEASE
Aspirin tolerance test, Diagnostic
Bleeding time, Ivy, Blood
Factor VIII, Blood
Factor VIII R:Ag, Blood
Platelet aggregation, Blood; Platelet
  aggregation, Hypercoagulable state,
  Blood
* von Willebrand factor antigen,
    Blood
* von Willebrand factor assay, Blood

Additional Conditions
Epistaxis
Gastrointestinal bleeding
Gingivitis
Menorrhagia

WALDENSTRÖM'S MACROGLOBULINEMIA
Bone marrow biopsy, Diagnostic
Cryoglobulin, Serum
* Immunoelectrophoresis, Serum and
    urine
  Immunofluorescence, Skin biopsy,
    Specimen
  Protein electrophoresis, Serum
  Red blood count, Serum

Additional Conditions
Anemia
Fatigue
Gastrointestinal bleeding
Hepatosplenomegaly
Lymphadenopathy

Nausea
Raynaud's phenomenon
Retinal hemorrhage
Vertigo

WEGENER'S GRANULOMATOSIS
*Antineutrophil cytoplasmic antibody
screen, Serum

Additional Conditions
Human immunodeficiency virus
Talc granulomatosis

WEIL SYNDROME
(*see Leptospirosis*)

WHIPPLE'S DISEASE
*Biopsy, Site-specific (Pancreas),
Specimen
Cytologic study of gastrointestinal
tract, Diagnostic
D-Xylose absorption test, Diagnostic,
Serum or Urine
Electron microscopy, Diagnostic (for
small bowel mucosa, Macrophage
laden)
Histopathology, Specimen

Additional Conditions
Abdominal pain
Diarrhea
Fever
Gastrointestinal bleeding
Lymphadenopathy
Malabsorption
Steatorrhea

WHOOPING COUGH
*Bordetella pertussis, Culture

Additional Conditions
Anorexia
Lymphocytosis

WILMS' TUMOR
*Chromosome analysis (Deletion
of 11p), Blood
Computed tomography of the body
(Abdomen), Diagnostic
*Histopathology, Specimen
Intravenous pyelography,
Diagnostic

Additional Conditions
Abdominal pain
Anemia
Hematuria
Hypertension
Metastasis

WILSON'S DISEASE
Ceruloplasmin, Serum
*Copper, Serum

Additional Conditions
Anemia
Ascites
Cirrhosis
Hepatitis
Jaundice
Splenomegaly

WOUNDS
Biopsy, Anaerobic, Culture
Biopsy, Routine, Culture
Body Fluid, Anaerobic, Culture
Gram stain (Wound specimen),
Diagnostic
Nocardia culture, All sites, Specimen
Wound culture
Wound, Fungus, Culture
Wound, Mycobacteria, Culture

Additional Conditions
Abscess
Burns
Diabetes mellitus
Fever
Kaposi's sarcoma
Sepsis
Trauma

XEROSTOMIA
Antinuclear antibody, Serum
Complete blood count, Blood
Differential leukocyte count,
Peripheral blood
Extractable nuclear antigen, Serum
Histopathology, Specimen
Immune complex assay, Blood
Protein electrophoresis, Serum
Rheumatoid factor, Blood
Sedimentation rate, Erythrocyte,
Blood
Sjögren's antibodies, Blood

Additional Conditions
Cancer
Dehydration

Postoperative procedure
Sjögren syndrome
Stomatitis

Jaundice
Photophobia
Tachycardia (Initially)

YAWS
Bone scan, Diagnostic
* Culture, Skin, Specimen

Additional Conditions
Lymphadenopathy
Rheumatism
Ulcerations of skin

YELLOW FEVER
* Bilirubin, Total, Serum
Bilirubin, Urine
Differential leukocyte count,
  Peripheral blood
Electrocardiography, Diagnostic
* Electrolytes, Plasma or serum
Gastric analysis, Specimen
Urinalysis, Urine
Viral culture (Group B arbovirus),
  Specimen

Additional Conditions
Bradycardia (Late effect)
Delirium
Gastrointestinal bleeding
Headache
Hypotension

ZOLLINGER-ELLISON SYNDROME
Chloride, Serum
Esophagogastroduodenoscopy,
  Diagnostic
Fat, Semiquantitative, Stool
Gastric analysis, Specimen
* Gastrin, Serum
Octreotide scan, Diagnostic
* Pepsinogen I and pepsinogen II,
  Blood
Pepsinogen-I antibody, Blood
Potassium, Serum
Sodium, Plasma or serum

Additional Conditions
Abdominal pain, Acute
Diarrhea
Hemorrhage
Hypercalcemia
Intestinal obstruction
Pancreatic tumor
Peptic ulcer

ZOSTER
(see Herpes zoster)

PART TWO

Laboratory Tests and Diagnostic Procedures

ABDOMINAL AORTA ULTRASONOGRAPHY (ABDOMINAL AORTA ECHOGRAM, ABDOMINAL AORTA ULTRASOUND), DIAGNOSTIC

Norm. Negative for presence of aneurysm. Normal cross-sectional diameter of adult aorta (maximum internal diameter) varies from 3 cm at the xiphoid to about 1 cm at the bifurcation. Transverse and vertical diameters should be the same. Measurements should be taken at various points down the length of the aorta. Any significant increase in diameter toward the feet (caudally) is abnormal. Ultrasound underestimates the anteroposterior diameter (mean, 2.16 mm) and transverse diameter (mean, 4.29 mm) of the abdominal aorta.

Usage. Localization, measurement, and monitoring of abdominal aortic aneurysm; follow-up evaluation of surgical graft and aortic attachment after surgery for aneurysm; and detection of abdominal aortic atherosclerosis or thrombus. May be indicated in clients with pulsatile abdominal mass, poor circulation of the legs, recent abdominal trauma, and suspected idiopathic aortitis.

Description. Evaluation of the structure, size, and position of the abdominal aorta and branches (celiac trunk and renal, superior mesenteric, and common iliac arteries) by the creation of an oscilloscopic picture from the echoes of high-frequency sound waves passing over the anterior portion of the trunk (acoustic imaging). The time required for the ultrasonic beam to be reflected back to the transducer from differing densities of tissue is converted by a computer to an electrical impulse displayed on an oscilloscopic screen to create a three-dimensional picture of the abdominal aorta and branches. Ultrasonography allows measurement of the luminal diameter of the aorta. A narrowed lumen would indicate atherosclerosis or thrombus, whereas a wider-than-normal lumen with an irregular border may indicate aneurysm. Scattered internal echoes within the aneurysm may indicate an internal clot. A double lumen may indicate a tear in the wall of the abdominal aorta. Surgical grafts from aneurysm repair appear as bright echo reflections.

Professional Considerations
1. Consent form NOT required.
2. Preparation:
   A. This test should be performed before intestinal barium tests or else after the barium is cleared from the system (with allowance of several days for clearance).
   B. An enema may be prescribed to be given before the ultrasonogram is taken.
   C. The client should wear a gown.
   D. Obtain ultrasonic gel or paste.
3. Procedure:
   A. Client is positioned supine on a procedure table.
   B. The abdomen is covered with conductive gel.
   C. A lubricated transducer is passed slowly along the abdomen at 1-cm intervals along the transverse and then longitudinal lines, covering the area between the xiphoid process and the symphysis pubis. If dissection is suspected, real-time techniques can be used more specifically to locate the site.
   D. Photographs are taken of the oscilloscopic images.
   E. Procedure takes less than 60 minutes.
4. Postprocedure care:
   A. Cleanse skin of ultrasonic gel.
5. Client and family teaching:
   A. Eat a low-residue diet the day before the ultrasonogram is taken, fast from food and fluids after midnight before the test, and refrain from smoking.
   B. Lie as still as possible during the procedure, which is painless and carries no risks.
   C. Results are normally available within 24 hours.
6. Factors that affect results:
   A. Dehydration interferes with adequate contrast between organs and body fluids.
   B. Intestinal barium or gas obscures results by preventing proper transmission and deflection of the high-frequency sound waves.
   C. The more abdominal fat present, the greater is the attenuation (reduction in sound-wave amplitude and intensity), which interferes with the clarity of the picture.

D. Aorta may be displaced by scoliosis, a retroperitoneal mass, or the para-aortic lymph nodes; in some clients, these can mimic an aneurysm.

7. Other data:
   A. There is some evidence that aneurysms <4 cm in diameter may be safely followed by ongoing monitoring and any aneurysm >4 cm in diameter should be considered for surgery.

ABDOMINAL PLAIN FILM
(see Flat-plate radiography of abdomen, Diagnostic)

ABETA
(see Beta-amyloid protein, CSF)

ABG
(see Blood gases, Arterial, Blood)

ABI
(see Ankle-brachial index, Diagnostic)

ABO GROUP and Rh TYPE, BLOOD

Norm. Specific to each individual.

Usage. Blood transfusion therapy, erythroblastosis fetalis, paternity determinations, pregnancy, and preoperatively.

Description. The ABO blood group is the phenotype of a client's blood resulting from genetic inheritance. The four most common phenotypes are A, B, AB, and O, referring to the type of antigen present on the surface of red blood cells. Rh type refers to whether an Rh antigen is present (Rh positive) or absent (Rh negative) on the surface of a client's red blood cells. Routine testing usually involves only the $Rh_0(D)$ antigen. If an Rh-negative client receives Rh-positive blood, he or she will develop Rh antibodies, and future Rh-positive transfusions may cause a transfusion reaction. In pregnancy, antibodies from an Rh-negative mother may hemolyze fetal erythrocytes in a fetus that has inherited the Rh-positive

antigen from the father (erythroblastosis fetalis, or hemolytic disease of the newborn). This test determines the specific ABO phenotype and Rh type by determining which A and B red blood cell antigens are present as well as whether the $Rh_0(D)$ antigen is present.

Professional Considerations
1. Consent form NOT required.
2. Preparation:
   A. Assess client for history of recent blood transfusion reaction, which can result in a positive antibody screen and require further testing. Write affirmative history on blood bank requisition.
   B. Tube: Red topped, red/gray topped, or gold topped, 1 or 2 tubes.
3. Procedure:
   A. Ask the client to state full name and compare with the client's name band. Label the sample tube and laboratory requisition with the client's name, identification number, date, time, and initials and sign it. Some institutions require additional data.
   B. Draw one or two 10-mL blood samples, depending on institutional requirements.
4. Postprocedure care:
   A. Some institutions require application of a blood band to the client's wrist. The blood bank identification numbers should match the identification numbers on any blood bag used for transfusion for the client.
5. Client and family teaching:
   A. Results are normally available within 24 hours.
6. Factors that affect results:
   A. Hemolyzed specimen invalidates results.
   B. Specimen drawn from extremity into which blood or dextran is infusing invalidates results.
   C. Drugs causing a false-positive Rh test include levodopa, methyldopa, and methyldopate hydrochloride.
   D. Abnormal plasma proteins, cold autoagglutinins, positive direct antiglobulin test, and in some cases bacteremia may interfere with results.
7. Other data:
   A. The test must be performed within 48 hours of specimen collection.

B. Amerindians are blood group O. Incompatible platelet products that are transfused can cause acute intravascular hemolysis and ventricular tachycardia.
C. ABO incompatibility is a significant prognostic risk factor in allogeneic bone marrow transplant for acute myelogenous leukemia or myelodysplastic syndrome.

D. Group B is associated with the incidence of cardiac cancer in males and cancer in the upper third of the esophagus.
E. Group A is common for myocardial infarction and angina pectoris while group O is least common for these.

ABSCESS, ANAEROBIC CULTURE
(see Body fluid, Anaerobic culture)

ACA
(see Antiphospholipid antibody, Serum)

ACCU-CHEK, DIAGNOSTIC
(see Glucose monitoring machines, Diagnostic)

ACE
(see Angiotensin-converting enzyme, Blood)

ACETAMINOPHEN, SERUM

Norm. 2 months – 10 years (received > 60 mg APAP/kg/d) = 0-23 mg/mL.

	4 HOURS AFTER LAST DOSE	SI UNITS
Therapeutic level	10-30 µg/mL	66-199 µmol/L
Toxic level	>150 µg/mL	>990 µmol/L
Panic level (hepatotoxicity)	>200 µg/mL	>1320 µmol/L

Overdose Symptoms and Treatment

Symptoms. Occur in four stages.
Stage I (ingestion to 24 hours) Gastrointestinal irritation, pallor, lethargy, diaphoresis, metabolic acidosis, and coma (massive ingestion with serum concentration >800 µg/mL have been reported, but coma is usually attributed to a coingestant such as alcohol).
Stage II (24 to 48 hours) Increased serum hepatic enzymes, right upper quadrant abdominal pain, possible decreased renal function.

Stage III (72 to 96 hours) Increased AST, increased ALT, nausea, vomiting, jaundice, lethargy, confusion, coma, coagulation disorders, possible decreased renal function.
Stage IV (4 days to 2 weeks) Clinical symptoms subside; laboratory values return to baseline.

Treatment:
Note: Treatment choice(s) depend on client history and condition and episode history.
1. Establish and maintain adequate airway, respiratory, and circulatory function.

2. If client is obtunded or unconscious, appropriate doses of thiamine, dextrose, and naloxone must be considered.
3. Gastric decontamination: In one study, rapid complete bowel lavage with 4 g of polyethylene glycol electrolyte solution was shown to significantly reduce serum acetaminophen levels. In another, use of activated charcoal prevented acetaminophen absorption when given within 60 minutes of acetaminophen ingestion. Syrup of ipecac may be used to induce emesis for recent ingestion, but it must be used with extreme caution. Ondansetron can be used to manage vomiting if acetaminophen ingestion occurred within the previous 8 hours.
4. Oral administration of N-acetylcysteine (Mucomyst by Mead Johnson) for suspected toxic doses (>7.5 g). Mucomyst is most likely to be effective when given within 16 hours after acetaminophen ingestion.
5. Laboratory monitoring: Urine toxicology screen, hepatic profile q 24 hours × 3-4 days, BUN, Cr, serum electrolytes, serum acetaminophen concentration level 4 hours after ingestion.
6. Coingestion of other substances that delay gastric emptying is an indication for serial measurement to detect late-rising acetaminophen levels.
7. Chronic alcohol intake enhances acetaminophen hepatotoxicity.
8. Hemodialysis WILL but peritoneal dialysis will NOT remove acetaminophen.

Usage. Drug abuse, hepatitis, monitoring for toxicity during acetaminophen therapy, overdose, poisoning, and suicide.

Description. Acetaminophen is a p-aminophenol derivative that has antipyretic (direct action on hypothalamus) and moderate analgesic actions. It is absorbed by the gastrointestinal tract and metabolized by liver microsomes. Half-life is 1 to 4 hours with peak blood levels reached in 30 minutes to 1 hour. Used for headache, fever, and relief of pain in clients who cannot tolerate aspirin or those with peptic ulcers or bleeding disorders. It is the drug of choice (antipyretic/analgesic) in children 13 years of age and younger because of the possible development of Reye syndrome associated with aspirin. In adults, ingestion of >4 g/d can be hepatotoxic.

Professional Considerations
1. Consent form NOT required.
2. **Preparation:**
   A. Tube: Red topped, red/gray topped, gold topped, or lavender topped.
   B. Do NOT draw during hemodialysis.
   C. Document times of ingestion and sample collection on lab requisition.
3. **Procedure:**
   A. Draw a 1-mL blood sample.
4. **Postprocedure care:**
   A. None.
5. **Client and family teaching:**
   A. Results are normally available within 24 hours.
   B. If overdose is suspected, prepare client and family for necessary supportive treatment described above.
   C. If activated charcoal was given for elevated levels, client should drink 4 to 6 glasses of water each day for 2 days to prevent constipation. Activated charcoal will also cause stools to be black for a few days.
6. **Factors that affect results:**
   A. Cardiovascular, hepatic, gastrointestinal, or renal dysfunction can alter drug absorption and elimination.
   B. Toxic levels of acetaminophen positively interfere with glucose-monitoring machine results.
   C. Draw two samples, 4 hours apart to determine half-life of acetaminophen.
7. **Other data:**
   A. Acetaminophen is present in many medicines: Anacin3, Datril, Liquiprin, Panadoe, Panex, paracetamol, Phenaphen, Tempra, and Tylenol.

B. Acetaminophen used with aspirin and caffeine alleviates migraine headache pain.
C. Premedication with acetaminophen does not significantly lower the incidence of non-hemolytic transfusion reactions.

ACETONE, SERUM
(see Ketone bodies, Blood or Toxicology, Volatiles group by GLC, Blood or Urine)

ACETONE, URINE

Norm. Keto-Diastix or Multistix: Negative. Quantitative 0.3-2.0 mg/dL.

Usage. Differentiation of diabetic coma and insulin shock, evaluation of glucose control in diabetics, preadmission screening, pregnancy, screening for ketoacidosis, increased in ethanol hangover, increased in ingested denatured alcohol, and monitoring for occupational exposure to isopropyl alcohol.

Description. Acetone is a byproduct of fat and fatty acid metabolism that provides a source of cellular energy for cells when glucose stores are exhausted or when glucose is prevented from entering cells because of lack of insulin. Acetone entering the bloodstream is almost completely metabolized in the liver. When acetone is formed at a faster-than-normal rate, it is excreted in the urine.

Professional Considerations
1. Consent form NOT required.
2. Preparation:
   A. Obtain a 50-mL, clean urine container and acetone testing strips or tablets.
   B. Client should empty the bladder 30 minutes before specimen collection time and then drink a glass of water.
   C. For specimens obtained from an indwelling urinary catheter, also obtain a catheter clamp, a sterile 10-mL syringe and needle, and an alcohol wipe.
3. Procedure:
   A. Obtain a 20-mL double-voided urine specimen in a clean container.

B. Specimens from catheter: Clamp the catheter tubing for 15 minutes to allow urine to accumulate above the sample port. Cleanse the sample port with an alcohol wipe and allow to dry. Aspirate 20-mL urine from the sample port, using a sterile syringe and needle. Collect only fresh urine that has accumulated above the sample port. Unclamp the catheter tubing.
C. Dip the Keto-Diastix, Multistix, or other acetone testing material in fresh urine and hold the strip horizontally for 15 seconds.
D. Compare the color of the ketone patch on the strip with the color chart on the Keto-Diastix or Multistix container.
E. Alternative method using Acetest tablets: Place a drop of urine on an Acetest tablet and wait 30 seconds. Compare the color with the Acetest color chart.
4. Postprocedure care:
   A. None.
5. Client and family teaching:
   A. Results are immediately available.
6. Factors that affect results:
   A. Fasting or dieting may cause acetone to appear in the urine.
   B. Use of acetone tablets that are darkened invalidates results.
   C. Drugs that may cause false-positive results include captopril, levodopa, paraldehyde, and phenazopyridine hydrochloride.
7. Other data:
   A. Refrigerate the specimen if the test cannot be performed within 1 hour of collection.
   B. In a recent study, ratings on scales of well-being and acute symptoms correlated significantly with the concentration of acetone in urine after acute airborne acetone exposure.
   C. See also *Ketone, Semiquantitative, Urine.*

ACETYLCHOLINE RECEPTOR ANTIBODY, SERUM

Norm. ≤0.03 nmol/L.

Usage. Diagnosis and clinical monitoring of myasthenia gravis, Lambert-Eaton myasthenic syndrome, small cell lung carcinoma.

Description. In clients with myasthenia gravis, this antibody interferes with the binding of acetylcholine to receptor sites on the muscle membrane, thus preventing muscle contraction. Assays for acetylcholine receptor antibodies are positive in 85%-90% of clients with acute myasthenia gravis and are replacing the Tensilon test as a diagnostic aid for this condition. However, this assay is less sensitive for Lambert-Eaton myasthenic syndrome diagnosis.

Professional Considerations
1. Consent form NOT required.
2. Preparation:
   A. Tube: Red topped, red/gray topped, or gold topped.
   B. List on the laboratory requisition any recent immunosuppressive drug therapy the client received.
3. Procedure:
   A. Draw a 2-mL blood sample.
4. Postprocedure care:
   A. None.
5. Client and family teaching:
   A. Results may not be available for several days.
6. Factors that affect results:
   A. False-positive results may be caused by D-penicillamine.
   B. Decrease in titer may be caused by intravenous immunoglobulin (IVIg) therapy.
7. Other data:
   A. Undetectable titer occurs in 33.4% of clients who have only ocular myasthenia gravis.
   B. See also *Tensilon test, Diagnostic*.

ACETYLSALICYLIC ACID
(see Salicylate, Blood)

ACID-FAST BACTERIA, CULTURE AND STAIN

Norm. Negative.

Usage. Acquired immunodeficiency syndrome (AIDS); suspected *Helicobacter pylori*, intestinal parasites, leprosy, mycobacteriosis, or tuberculosis; and differentiation of tuberculosis from carcinoma and bronchiectasis.

Description. *Mycobacterium tuberculosis* is a rod-shaped bacterium that resists decolorizing chemicals after staining, a property termed "acid-fastness." *M. tuberculosis* is transmitted most commonly by the airborne route to the lungs, where it survives well, causes areas of granulomatous inflammation, and, if not dormant, causes cough, fever, and hemoptysis. Acid-fast bacterium *M. avium-intracellulare* is a common cause of infection in clients with AIDS. Culture of sputum is necessary to confirm the diagnosis of tuberculosis and for sensitivity studies for drug therapy. The sensitivity of sputum smears, however, is only 50% for tuberculosis.

Professional Considerations
1. Consent form NOT required.
2. Preparation:
   A. Obtain three small, sterile containers.
   B. See *Client and family teaching*.
3. Procedure:
   A. Aerosolized therapy before sputum collection may stimulate sputum production and produce a better specimen.
   B. When tuberculosis is suspected, collect three daily, early-morning sputum, deep-cough specimens in a sterile container.
   C. When leprosy is suspected, obtain smear from nasal scrapings or biopsy from lesions and place in sterile container.
4. Postprocedure care:
   A. Provide mouth care.
5. Client and family teaching:
   A. Perform oral hygiene before giving specimens to reduce chances of contamination.
   B. Deep coughs are necessary to produce sputum, rather than saliva. To produce the proper specimen, take several breaths in, without fully exhaling each, and then expel sputum with a "cascade cough."
6. Factors that affect results:
   A. Antituberculous drug therapy may cause negative results because of inhibition of growth of *M. tuberculosis*.
   B. A high–carbon dioxide atmosphere for growth may increase the number of positive cultures.
   C. Culture medium containing glycerin accelerates growth.
7. Other data:
   A. Culture results may take 3-8 weeks.

B. The most prevalent intestinal parasites in cancer clients diagnosed by acid-fast stain are *Entamoeba histolytica/Entamoeba dispar* (8.5%), *Giardia lamblia* (3.1%), *Strongyloides stercoralis* (0.6%), and *Cryptosporidium parvum* (0.3%).

ACID-FAST STAIN, *NOCARDIA* SPECIES, CULTURE

Norm. Negative.

Usage. Aids in diagnosis of Behçet's disease, mycetoma, *Nocardia brasiliensis*, and nocardiosis of the respiratory tract found in persons with systemic lupus erythematosus and nocardial thyroiditis.

Description. *Nocardia* is an aerobic, gram-positive, filamentous branching bacterium that segments into reproductive bacillary fragments. It is weakly acid fast and found outdoors in decayed matter, soil, grass, and straw and enters the body primarily through inhalation of contaminated dust. The type species, *Nocardia asteroides,* and *N. brasiliensis, N. farcinica, N. otitidiscaviarum, N. nova,* and *N. transvalensis* cause a variety of diseases in both normal and immunocompromised humans and animals. The *N. asteroides* species causes primary skin lesions, visceral infections (most commonly abscesses of the lungs, brain, and subcutaneous tissue), and sometimes disseminated infections in humans.

Professional Considerations
1. Consent form NOT required.
2. Preparation:
   A. Obtain a sterile scalpel or spatula, or a sterile needle and syringe, and both anaerobic and aerobic culture media.
3. Procedure:
   A. Obtain a scraping from a skin lesion or an aspirate of an abscess using sterile technique.
   B. Inoculate both aerobic and anaerobic culture media with the specimen.
   C. Aerobic culture media of beef infusion broth or thioglycolate broth may be used.
   D. Initial incubation at temperatures from 38°-45°C should be used.

E. Examine cultures for growth beginning at 48 hours and recheck daily for 2 weeks.
4. Postprocedure care:
   A. Apply dry sterile dressing to site.
5. Client and family teaching:
   A. Avoid application of creams or lotions to sample site and allow site to remain open to air for healing.
   B. At least 2-3 days are required for growth and results.
6. Factors that affect results:
   A. Nocardia growth may be mistaken for nontuberculous *Mycobacterium* when a *Mycobacterium* culture medium is used.
7. Other data:
   A. Common specimens include pus, tissue, body fluid, and sputum.
   B. Final reports may take 10 days.

ACIDIFIED SERUM TEST, BLOOD
(*see Ham test, Blood*)

ACID PERFUSION (BERNSTEIN) TEST, DIAGNOSTIC

Norm. No burning or pain after saline or acidic infusions.

Usage. Differentiation between chest pain caused by a cardiac disorder and chest pain caused by esophagitis. Not commonly used by cardiologists; more often used by gastroenterologists. Aids diagnosis of gastroesophageal reflux as a cause of nocturnal asthma or hiatal hernia and in Barrett's esophagus. This test is obsolete if 24-hour esophageal pH monitoring is available.

Description. Saline and then acidic solutions are slowly perfused through a nasogastric tube into the stomach. Clients with esophagitis caused by relaxation of the lower esophageal sphincter usually experience burning or pain after the perfusion of acidic solution but not after the saline solution. Gastroesophageal reflux has been found to occur in some clients with nocturnal asthma. Such clients show an exacerbation of asthmatic symptoms when this test is performed.

Professional Considerations
1. Consent form NOT required.

Risks
Exacerbation of asthma in asthmatics. Complications of nasogastric tube insertion include bleeding, dysrhythmias, esophageal perforation, laryngospasm, and decreased mean pO_2.

Contraindications
Cardiac disorders; esophageal varices.

2. **Preparation:**
   A. Obtain nasogastric tube, tape, gel, glass of water, and a liter each of normal saline solution and 0.1 N hydrochloric acid (HCl) solution.
   B. See *Client and family teaching.*
3. **Procedure:**
   A. Mark a nasogastric tube at 12 inches from the distal tip.
   B. Insert the nasogastric tube into the stomach and aspirate stomach contents.
   C. Withdraw the nasogastric tube until the 12-inch mark is at the tip of the nares. This ensures that the tube tip is located in the esophagus.
   D. Perfuse normal saline into the nasogastric tube at 60-120 drops per minute. Assess for discomfort after 10 minutes.
   E. Connect 0.1 N HCl solution piggybacked onto the normal saline line. Close the clamp on the normal saline and open the line on the HCl solution at a rate of 60-120 drops per minute for 30 minutes or until the client

spontaneously complains of discomfort or when assessed every 10 minutes.
   F. At the first sign of discomfort, clamp the HCl and open the normal saline line until the client experiences no further pain or burning.
   G. Clamp and remove the nasogastric tube.
4. **Postprocedure care:**
   A. An antacid may be necessary if discomfort continues after the test.
5. **Client and family teaching:**
   A. Fast and do not smoke for 12 hours before the test.
   B. Antacids should not be ingested within 24 hours before the test.
   C. The test involves insertion of a tube through the nose into the stomach. The insertion may be uncomfortable and cause a pressure-like feeling or cause you to gag and cough. You will be asked to take sips of water and swallow to make tube insertion easier.
   D. The test may reproduce the pain in 20% of clients, but this will help differentiate the cause of the pain, and the discomfort will be temporary.
6. **Factors that affect results:**
   A. None found.
7. **Other data:**
   A. This procedure has been used in some studies to monitor the effect of gastroesophageal reflux on air exchange.
   B. See also *Esophageal acidity test, Diagnostic; Esophageal manometry, Diagnostic.*

ACID PHOSPHATASE, SERUM
Norm:

METHOD		SI UNITS
Bodansky	0.5-2 U/L	2.7-10.7 IU/L
King-Armstrong	0.1-5 U/L	0.2-8.8 IU/L
Bessey-Lowery-Brock	0.1-0.8 U/L	1.7-13.4 IU/L
Gutman	0.1-2 U/L	

Increased. Bone fracture, cancer with bone metastasis, Gaucher's disease, hairy cell leukemia (leukemic reticuloendotheliosis), hepatitis (viral), hyperparathyroidism, hypophosphatemia, idiopathic thrombocytopenic purpura (with bone marrow megakaryocytes), jaundice (obstructive), Laënnec's cirrhosis, leukemia (myelogenous), multiple myeloma, osteogenesis imperfecta, Paget's disease (advanced), partial translocation trisomy 21, prostate cancer, prostatic infarction, prostatic surgery or trauma, renal impairment (acute), sickle cell crisis, thrombo-cythemia, thrombocytosis, thromboem-bolism, and thrombophlebitis. Drugs include anabolic steroids.

Decreased. No clinical significance. Drugs include fluorides.

Description. Acid phosphatase is one of a group of enzymes located prima-rily in the prostate gland and prostatic secretions. Smaller amounts are found in the bone marrow, spleen, liver, kid-neys, and blood components such as erythrocytes and platelets. Isoenzymes of acid phosphatase include prostatic isoenzyme and erythrocytic isoen-zyme. Used in diagnosing and moni-toring treatment response of prostate cancer.

Professional Considerations
1. Consent form NOT required.
2. Preparation:
    A. Tube: Red topped, red/gray topped, or gold topped.
3. Procedure:
    A. Collect a 1-mL blood sample.
4. Postprocedure care:
    A. Send the specimen to the labora-tory immediately.

B. Separate the serum, add 0.01 mL of 20% acetic acid per milliliter of serum, and refrigerate if the test is not performed immediately.
5. Client and family teaching:
    A. Results may not be available for several days.
6. Factors that affect results:
    A. Hemolysis or specimens received more than 15 minutes after col-lection invalidate results.
    B. False-negative results may be attributable to fluorides, oxalates, or phosphates.
    C. False-positive results may be attributable to clofibrate.
    D. Elevated levels may be caused by rectal examination, prostatic mas-sage, or urinary catheterization within 2 days before the test.
7. Other data:
    A. This test is more helpful for diag-nosis in advanced prostate cancer than in early prostate cancer.
    B. Use of prostate-specific acid phosphatase as a tumor marker for prostate cancer is being replaced by *Prostate-specific anti-gen, Serum.*
    C. See also Prostatic acid phos-phatase, Blood.

ACID PHOSPHATASE, TARTRATE-RESISTANT, BLOOD
(see Tartrate-resistant acid phosphatase, Blood)

ACID PHOSPHATASE, VAGINAL SWAB

Norm. Method: Dilution with a substrate of thymolphthalein monophosphate.
  <5: Normal vaginal secretions.
  <7: Inconclusive.
 7-50: Highly suggestive of coitus within the prior 36 hours.
  50: Confirmation of recent coitus.

Usage. Rape trauma work-up.

Description. Acid phosphatase is one of a group of enzymes located pri-marily in the prostate gland and pros-tatic secretions, with smaller amounts found elsewhere in the body. Normal vaginal secretions contain only low levels of acid phosphatase. Because acid phosphatase is found in such high concentrations in semen, its isolation in high levels from vaginal

fluid in cases of suspected rape is strong evidence that coitus occurred recently.

Professional Considerations
1. Consent form NOT required unless specimen may be used as legal evi-dence.
2. Preparation:
    A. Obtain speculum, cotton wool swab supplied in a sexual offense kit, and sterile container.

3. **Procedure:**
   A. If the specimen may be used as legal evidence, have the specimen collection witnessed.
   B. Position the client in the dorsal lithotomy position and drape for privacy and comfort.
   C. Gently scrape the walls of the vagina with a plain cotton wool swab until it is saturated.
   D. Place the swab in a sterile container.
4. **Postprocedure care:**
   A. Write the client's name, the date, the exact time of collection, and the specimen source on the laboratory requisition. Sign and have the witness sign the laboratory requisition.
   B. Transport the specimen to the laboratory immediately in a sealed plastic bag marked as legal evidence. All clients handling the specimen should sign and mark the time of receipt on the laboratory requisition.
5. **Client and family teaching:**
   A. Provide repeated and thorough explanation of the purpose and process of specimen collection.
   B. Follow-up: Survivors of sexual assault should be referred to appropriate crisis counseling agencies as well as gynecologic follow-up. Facilitate referral if desired by client.
   C. Referral for HIV testing should be reviewed and offered to all sexual assault victims.
   D. Preventive treatment for *Chlamydia,* gonorrhea, and syphilis should be provided to all survivors of sexual assault.
   E. The option of postcoital contraceptive should be reviewed with all survivors of sexual assault.
6. **Factors that affect results:**
   A. Vaginal swabs for acid phosphatase should be collected as soon as possible after the assault. Swabs have the highest chance of being positive when collected within 5 hours of the assault and are least likely to be positive after 12 hours. By 48 hours, normal vaginal levels are usually found.
   B. Negative results may be obtained if the assailant was sexually dysfunctional or has had a vasectomy or if the client bathed, douched, or defecated after the assault.
   C. This test cannot identify the perpetrator.
   D. Contamination of the vagina or the specimen with substances other than semen or normal vaginal substances may cause false-positive results.
7. **Other data:**
   A. Negative results caused by a long delay between the occurrence of the assault and collection of the vaginal specimen are sometimes used by defense attorneys as evidence that a rape did not occur.
   B. Although swabs may also be taken of other body orifices for evidence of acid phosphatase, they rarely yield positive results when taken more than 5 hours after the sexual assault occurred.
   C. A spot test, intended for field use outside of the lab, is currently being tested. A test swab is covered with the moistened specimen, and characteristic color changes in the swab indicate positive or negative presence of acid phosphatase. Vaginal washings should be evaluated within 24 hours of deposition. Results are independent of sperm count.
   D. See also *Blood group antigen of semen, Vaginal swab; and Precipitin test against human sperm and blood, Vaginal swab.*

ACID SCHIFF STAIN
(see *Periodic Acid–Schiff stain, Specimen*)

ACOUSTIC IMMITTANCE TESTS, DIAGNOSTIC

Norm. Normal acoustic immittance.

Tympanogram. The tympanogram recording shows a symmetric, shallow upslope and downslope free of notches or peaks with middle ear pressure of −100 to +100 dPa.

Pure-Tone Reflex Threshold:

Transbrainstem	70-100 dB HL
Ipsilateral	3-12 dB HL
Reflex decay	< ½ baseline/ 10 seconds

Usage. Assessment of middle ear and tympanic membrane functioning; identification of location of middle ear lesions; and differential diagnosis of brainstem lesions and hearing loss.

Description. The acoustic immittance tests measure middle ear functioning and locate abnormalities by tympanometry and measurement of acoustic reflexes. Tympanometry assesses stiffness of the middle ear by measuring admittance (that is, how much impedance exists to the flow of sound into the ear). Lower than normal admittance can be caused by cerumen, the presence of fluid in the middle ear, or a perforated tympanic membrane. Higher than normal admittance results when ear scarring is present. Measurement of acoustic reflexes reveals how well the stapedius muscle responds to the delivery of sound against it. Poor or no acoustic reflexes can indicate hearing loss or neurologic or stapedius muscle damage or lesions.

Professional Considerations
1. Consent form NOT required.

Risks
Infection.

Contraindications
May be contraindicated in clients with accidental head injuries or suspected labyrinthine fistula or in those who have recently undergone ear surgery.

2. **Preparation:**
   A. Obtain admittance meter; recorder; probe with tips, cuffs, and silicone putty; otoscope; and audiometer.

B. See *Client and family teaching.*
3. **Procedure:**
   A. Cleanse the bores of the ear probe with wire. Calibrate the admittance meter. Inspect the ear canal, and remove any impacted cerumen.
   B. Lift the auricle up and out, and insert the admittance meter's cuffed probe into the external auditory canal until a pressure of −200 dPa is achieved, indicating an adequate seal.
   C. Admittance measurement: Admittance recordings are made in response to air-pressure changes made by the meter.
   D. Acoustic reflex measurement: Measure acoustic reflexes when a 500- to 4000-Hz tone is sent into either ear. Perform ipsilateral measurement in the stimulated ear. You may perform contralateral (transbrainstem) measurement by sending the tone into the opposite ear.
   E. Reflex-threshold measurement: Measure the reflex threshold by sending progressively louder tones into the ear in 10-dB increments until a reflex occurs and then decreasing the decibels in smaller steps until the lowest level that elicits a reflex is identified.
   F. Reflex-decay measurement: Measure the reflex decay by sending a 10-second tone equal to the reflex threshold plus 10 dB into the contralateral ear and comparing the degree of initial, 5-second, and 10-second reflexes.
4. **Postprocedure care:**
   A. Cleanse the ear probe.
5. **Client and family teaching:**
   A. Avoid moving, talking, or swallowing during the test. The test involves transmitting into the ear loud tones, which may be uncomfortable but will not damage the ear.
6. **Factors that affect results:**
   A. The most accurate results are obtained when the air seal remains continuous. Silicone putty may be used around the circumference of the canal to help maintain the seal.

B. Cerumen or silicone putty clogging the probe may cause the tympanogram to show as a flat waveform.

7. **Other data:**
   A. Prevalence of hearing loss is 46% for persons over 66 years of age, is greater in males than in females, and increases with age.

ACQUIRED IMMUNODEFICIENCY SYNDROME EVALUATION BATTERY (AIDS EVALUATION BATTERY), DIAGNOSTIC

Norm. Negative AIDS battery, nonreactive.

Antigen Detection by Serology. Negative for HIV antigens.

Antibody Detection. Negative for HIV antibodies.

LYMPHOCYTE SUBSET ENUMERATION	
Total	1500-4000/mL
B cells	65-475/mL
OKT-3 cells	875-1900/mL
OKT-4 cells (CD4)	450-1400/mL
OKT-8 cells	190-725/mL
OKT-4:OKT-8 ratio	1-3.5
Beta$_2$-microglobulin	<2 mg/mL (<170 nmol/L, SI units)

Usage. Used often in combination with cultures and for confirmation of opportunistic infection to help diagnose acquired immunodeficiency syndrome (AIDS).

Description. AIDS is caused by human immunodeficiency virus (HIV), a cytoplasmic retrovirus of the human T-cell leukemia and lymphoma virus family that reproduces and infects, even when antibodies against the virus are present. There are several strains. All attack a subgroup of T lymphocytes known as "helper" T cells, which are important in cell-mediated immunity. AIDS causes immunosuppression and susceptibility to infection with opportunistic organisms such as *Pneumocystis carinii, Candida albicans, Cryptococcus neoformans, Mycobacterium, Toxoplasma gondii, Cryptosporidium,* and herpes simplex. The predominant modes of transmission of HIV are believed to be (1) direct contact between the blood of an uninfected person and the blood of an infected person and (2) sexual and body fluid transmission. The incubation period may be as short as 6 days and as long as several years.

HIV is now the leading cause of death in men 25-40 years of age, the sixth leading cause of death worldwide in adolescent males 15-24 years, and the fourth leading cause of death in women 25-44 years. It is estimated that 42 million people worldwide, including 980,000 North Americans are HIV infected (WHO, 12/2002). In 2002, 3.1 million people died of HIV/AIDS and AIDS-related diseases.

Persons may be infected with the human immunodeficiency virus for several years without becoming symptomatic when the virus enters a nonreplicating latent period. When the virus begins actively replicating, the person may develop AIDS. At 2-6 weeks after infection, clients may develop a viral-like illness consisting of fever, sweats, fatigue, malaise, lymphadenopathy, sore throat, and sometimes splenomegaly. Clients may remain asymptomatic for months to years, depending on the progression of the disease.

In 1993, the CDC expanded the AIDS surveillance case definition to include all HIV-infected persons who have <200 CD4+ T lymphocytes/μL or a CD4+ T lymphocyte percentage of total lymphocytes <14. This expansion includes the addition of three clinical conditions: pulmonary tuberculosis, recurrent pneumonia, and invasive cervical cancer. As the number of CD4+ T lymphocytes decreases, the risk and severity of opportunistic illnesses increase. Measures of CD4+ T lymphocytes are used to guide clinical and therapeutic management of HIV-infected persons. Antimicrobial prophylaxis and antiretroviral therapies have been shown to be most effective within certain levels of immune dysfunction.

The AIDS evaluation battery results are often considered with other diagnostic tests for opportunistic infection such as body fluid culture and cytology, central nervous system tomography, bronchoscopy, and biopsy to complete the clinical picture description before diagnosis is made. The AIDS evaluation battery comprises the following tests: blood and body fluid cultures, antigen detection by serology, antibody detection, confirmatory antibody detection methods, and tests for immunologic status evaluation and $beta_2$-microglobulin. No test that by itself confirms HIV infection has yet been developed.

Blood and body fluid cultures have been found to show positive results in some persons soon after infection with HIV. Although difficult to do, isolation of HIV has been accomplished in concentrated peripheral blood lymphocytes and body fluids. However, a negative result does not rule out infection (see *Blood culture, Blood; Body fluid, Routine, Culture*).

Antigen detection by serology methods may be positive for the viral antigen (frequently p24 core protein, HIV core antigen) from 1-2 weeks up to about 1 month after infection with the virus. The antigen is detectable during acute (initial) infection, undetectable as the virus becomes latent, and again detectable as the infection progresses. The enzyme-linked immunosorbent assay (ELISA) is used for screening for HIV. Detection of HIV antibody by ELISA must be confirmed by Western blot. Alternative diagnosis may be made by viral culture, by antigen detection, or by HIV DNA or RNA polymerase chain reaction (PCR). Quantitative virology using quantitative RNA PCR or branched-chain DNA (bDNA) has become a popular method to access viral load in staging clients or for therapeutic monitoring. Maternal antibodies may be present in infants until 18 months of age; therefore CD4 counts, viral culture, or PCR followed by antibody detection after 18 months must be performed to diagnose HIV in infants.

Studies indicate that the frequency of false-positive tests in a low-prevalence population with both the ELISA and Western blot is about 0.0007%, and the frequency of false-negative results in a high-prevalence population is about 0.3%. The usual cause of false-negative tests is testing in the time between transmission and seroconversion, a period that rarely lasts longer than 3 months. When the results are positive, it is recommended that repeat testing be done for those with no likely risk factors, and those who report positive results from an anonymous test site. Periodic tests are suggested for clients with negative results who continue to practice high-risk behaviors.

Confirmatory antibody detection methods include the Western blot, immunofluorescence, radioimmunoprecipitation, and ELISA tests that detect antibodies to genetically engineered HIV proteins. The Western blot and immunofluorescence methods have similar sensitivities. Immunofluorescence results are obtained more quickly but are less reliable than those of the Western blot. Radioimmunofluorescence is more sensitive than the Western blot but is not widely used because of the technical difficulty of the procedure. Newer ELISA tests are able to pinpoint the specific HIV antibody present in serum when one incubates the serum first with specific HIV proteins and then a tagged, anti-immunoglobulin enzyme and measures the amount of substrate hydrolyzed by the antigen-antibody reaction.

Quantitative testing for HIV p24 antigen may provide a surrogate marker for disease progression: however, this antigen usually disappears from the blood during the asymptomatic phase. The PCR for the detection of HIV DNA or RNA has been extensively used in the research setting and proven extremely valuable.

A few alternative detection methods are actively being studied. Two home test kits for HIV detection (Direct Access Diagnostics and ChemTrak) are under review by the FDA. There are currently two FDA-licensed rapid tests: SUDS (Murex) and Recombigen latex agglutination assay (Cambridge Biotech). These tests are attractive for use in areas such as emergency rooms, autopsy rooms, and STD clinics.

Tests for immunologic status evaluation include lymphocyte subset enumeration, T-lymphocyte and B-lymphocyte subset assays, and skin tests with known antigens for the person such as *Candida* or mumps; these often demonstrate normal results until the later stages of infection. As T-lymphocyte helper cells (OKT-4 cells) become infected by the human immunodeficiency virus, their numbers decrease. Levels of suppressor T cells (OKT-8 cells) may remain normal or increase as virus activity progresses. Lymphocyte counts decrease as immune function decreases. False-negative results from known antigen skin tests indicate that the client's immune function is compromised.

Beta$_2$-microglobulin is an amino acid peptide component of lymphocyte HLA complexes that increases in the serum in inflammatory conditions and when lymphocyte turnover increases, as when T-lymphocyte helper (OKT-4) cells are attacked by HIV. Rising levels may also be caused by conditions other than HIV. Although beta$_2$-microglobulin levels usually rise with HIV infection, the levels do not always correlate with the stages of the infection (see *Beta$_2$-microglobulin, Blood and 24-hour urine*).

CD4+ T-lymphocyte test results alone should not be used as a surrogate marker for HIV or AIDS. A low CD4+ T-lymphocyte count without a positive HIV test result will not be reportable, since other conditions may be the cause. Health care providers must ensure that persons who have a CD4+ T-lymphocyte count of <200/μL are HIV infected before initiating treatment for HIV disease.

Professional Considerations

1. Consent form IS required because of area-specific legal regulations. Testing should be voluntary with appropriate counseling before and after informed consent.
2. Preparation:
   A. Clarify the type of tube needed for lymphocyte subset enumeration if the Becton Dickinson Immunocytology Systems method is not used.
   B. Tube: Red topped, red/gray topped, gold topped, or lavender topped.

3. Procedure:
   A. Antigen detection by serology, antibody detection, and confirmatory antibody detection method: Draw a 5-mL venous blood sample.
   B. Lymphocyte subset enumeration (Becton Dickinson Immunocytology Systems method): Completely fill two lavender-topped tubes with venous blood. Label one tube for complete blood count and the other tube for lymphocyte subset enumeration.
   C. Beta$_2$-microglobulin: Draw a 10-mL venous blood sample in a lavender-topped tube.
4. Postprocedure care:
   A. Either leave reusable equipment in the client's room or dispose of the equipment in the room.
5. Client and family teaching:
   A. Explain the purpose of the test, the procedure for collection, and the results to the client.
   B. Two days are required for the Western blot.
   C. Assess client understanding of safe sex practices and provide counseling as needed.
   D. CDC National AIDS hotline: 1-800-342-AIDS.
6. Factors that affect results:
   A. Antibody results may be negative up to 35 months after infection because of viral latency.
   B. False-positive ELISA results may be caused by HLA antibody reaction with specific proteins in certain test kits. False-negative ELISA results may occur in a small proportion of clients with HIV-1 infection and in some children infected with HIV in utero.
   C. Falsely depressed lymphocyte counts may be caused by steroids and general anesthetics.
   D. Beta$_2$-microglobulin results are invalidated if the person has undergone a scan involving the administration of radioactive dyes within 1 week before the test.
7. Other data:
   A. Legal restrictions exist and vary regarding HIV testing and reporting of results.
   B. Demonstration of homogeneous B or T lymphocytes is helpful in prognosis and therapeutic plan-

ning of malignant lymphoprolif-erative disorders.

C. In a recent study at the National Institute of Allergy and Infectious Diseases, in a small number of HIV-infected clients, infusions of an immune system protein signif-icantly increased levels of the infection-fighting white blood cells normally destroyed during HIV infection.

D. Begin antiretroviral therapy before CD4 cells drop below 200/μL.

E. Progression of cytomegalovirus retinitis occurs in 17% with low CD4 cell count.

F. The Genie assay is faster, less costly, and yields fewer indeterminate results in detecting HIV-1 antibod-ies than the Western blot method.

G. Miller V et al. (2002) showed that independent predictors to progres-sion include CD4 <50 cells/mm^3, *Pneumocystis carinii* pneumonia prophylaxis, low hemoglobin lev-els, and high virus load.

H. Total viral load can sometimes be assessed to help monitor the impact of treatment.

I. See also *T- and B-lymphocyte sub-set assay, Blood; Beta$_2$-microglobu-lin, Blood and 24-Hour urine;* and *Oral mucosal transudate, Specimen.*

ACTH STIMULATION TEST, DIAGNOSTIC

Norm. 17-OHCS levels increase by two to four times between the first and second 24-hour urine collection.

Usage. Definitive diagnosis of Addi-son's disease and adrenal adenoma.

Description. Adrenocorticotropic hormone (ACTH) is secreted by the pituitary gland and acts on the adrenal cortex to cause release of adrenal hormones. This test measures blood cortisol and urinary 17-hydroxycorti-costeroids (17-OHCS) before and after an infusion of ACTH. It is diagnostic of Addison's disease when an infusion of ACTH fails to cause an increase in cor-tisol or 17-OHCS, urinary metabolites of plasma cortisol. A small response occurs in those with high mortality in the ICU and in older clients.

Professional Considerations

1. Consent form NOT required.

2. **Preparation:**

   A. To prevent hypersensitivity reac-tions when using biologic rather than synthetic ACTH, give 0.5 mg dexamethasone orally before the test.

   B. Obtain a 3-L container with 10 mL of concentrated hydrochlo-ric acid (HCl) preservative.

   C. Write starting time of collection on the laboratory requisition.

   D. The test can be performed at any time of the day.

3. **Procedure:**

   A. Discard the first morning-urine specimen.

   B. Save all urine voided for 24 hours in a refrigerated, clean, 3-L con-tainer to which 10 mL of concen-trated HCl have been added. Doc-ument the quantity of urine output during the collection period. Include urine voided at the end of the 24-hour period.

   C. Begin a second 24-hour urine col-lection.

   D. During the second collection, infuse 24 U of ACTH in 500 mL of normal saline intravenously over 8 hours.

4. **Postprocedure care:**

   A. Record the total 24-hour output on the laboratory requisition and send the entire specimen to the laboratory.

5. **Client and family teaching:**

   A. Save all urine voided in the 24-hour period, and urinate before defecating to avoid loss of urine. If any urine is accidentally discarded, discard the entire spec-imen and restart the collection the next day.

6. **Factors that affect results:**

   A. Maintenance steroids that must be given during the testing period should be in the form of small doses of dexamethasone to avoid false elevation of 17-OHCS in the urine.

7. **Other data:**

   A. The test should be repeated in 24 hours if pituitary deficiency is suspected. Pituitary insufficiency would be evident by a gradual but small response to the ACTH stim-ulation test during the second test.

B. The ACTH stimulation test is useful for identifying adrenal insufficiency; however, it is not sensitive or specific for clients suspected of having secondary adrenal insufficiency or those with recent pituitary injury.

ACTINOMYCES, CULTURE

Norm. Negative.

Positive. Abscess, actinomycosis, pelvic inflammatory disease, and root canal infection.

Description. A slow-growing, gram-positive, non–acid-fast bacillus that is anaerobic to microaerophilic and shows up in variable lengths and shapes on a Gram stain. *Actinomyces israelii* is a part of the normal oral flora in many people. Possibly because of mouth trauma or infection, it sometimes becomes invasive, forms draining sinus tracts, and becomes a chronic, suppurative disease called "actinomycosis" that spreads by direct extension. The characteristic lesion is a hard, red, nontender nodule that eventually begins draining. The *Actinomyces* organisms are also found in the vaginal smears of a small percentage of women in whom intrauterine devices have been inserted.

Professional Considerations
1. Consent form NOT required.
2. **Preparation:**
   A. Obtain a sterile cotton swab and culture media.
3. **Procedure:**
   A. Swab the drainage (pus from lesion, sinus tract, or fistula; or sputum or tissue biopsy material).
   B. Inoculate the drainage into thioglycolate medium and streak it onto brain-heart infusion agar plates.
   C. Incubate anaerobically for 2 weeks or more.
4. **Postprocedure care:**
   A. Apply a dry sterile dressing as needed.
   B. Send the specimen to the laboratory immediately.
5. **Client and family teaching:**
   A. Results will not be available for at least 14 days.
   B. Treatment for actinomycosis usually includes drainage of lesions and penicillin or tetracycline drug therapy.
6. **Factors that affect results:**
   A. Do NOT refrigerate or store the specimen.
7. **Other data:**
   A. Some tissue damage from actinomycosis is irreversible.

ACTIVATED COAGULATION TIME (ACT), AUTOMATED, BLOOD

Norm. Varies, depending on the type of system in use and the type of test reagent or activator. There are currently two commercially available systems for analyzing ACT by automation: ACT II by Medtronic Hemotec Inc. and Hemochron by International Technidyne Corporation.

HEMOCHRON SYSTEM		
TUBE	RANGE IN SECONDS	ACT II
TCA510 and FTCA510	105-167	Multiple methods are available for
K-ACT and FTK-ACT	91-151	measuring ACT values; thus, values
P214/215	110-182	should be evaluated according to
S412	186-306	reference levels of the individual
		machine and test tube used. The ACT II
		machine has an overall range of 0-999.

Usage. Commonly used for heparin anticoagulation monitoring during bypass surgery, percutaneous transluminal coronary angioplasty (PTCA), interventional radiology, neonatal extracorporeal membrane oxygenation (ECMO), hemofiltration, hemodialysis, and critical and telemetry care.

Increased. Afibrinogenemia, circulating anticoagulants, dysproteinemia, factor deficiency (V, VIII, IX, X, XI, or XII), fibrinolysis, hemophilia, hemorrhagic disease of the newborn, hypofibrinogenemia, hypoprothrombinemia, leukemia, and liver disease. Drugs include antithrombin III, aprotinin, heparin calcium, heparin sodium (including blood obtained from an introducer with a heparin-coated pulmonary artery catheter), and warfarin.

Description. Measures the ability of the blood to clot. Fresh whole blood is added to a test tube containing an activator (diatomaceous earth, glass particles, or kaolin) and timed for the formation of a clot. The ACT is more sensitive to the effects of factor VIII deficiency and heparin than whole-blood clotting time is. The ACT test has become a mainstay in monitoring heparin anticoagulation during invasive procedures and is the preferred method for monitoring high-level anticoagulation. The ACT is quick, reliable, and easy and can be performed at the bedside. Disadvantages of the ACT are operator variability and differences between the two commercially available systems.

Professional Considerations
1. Consent form NOT required.
2. **Preparation:**
   A. Obtain a tube with a designated activator for the specific ACT test. May be drawn from indwelling venous blood line, extracorporeal blood line port, direct venipuncture, or vacuum draw. Do not obtain blood from a heparinized access line, an indwelling heparinized lock, or a hemodialysis line.
   B. Obtain two 5-mL syringes.
3. **Procedure** (if using the ACT II system, see instructions below before obtaining client sample):
   A. *Indwelling venous line sampling:* With the first syringe, withdraw and discard 5 mL of blood. Attach the second syringe and withdraw a 3-mL blood sample.
   Venipuncture sampling: With the first syringe, withdraw and discard 2 mL of blood. Attach the second syringe and withdraw a 3-mL sample.

Hemochron System
   B. Dispense exactly 2 mL of blood into the test tube (note: tubes P214/P215 require only 0.4 mL of blood). At the same time, depress the start-button timer on the machine. Close the tube and agitate it briskly 10 times.
   C. Insert the test tube into the Hemochron machine port and rotate clockwise until green light indicator lights. Await the result, which will be displayed in the number of seconds required to obtain coagulation on the Hemochron screen.

Act II System
   A. Prewarm the cartridge in the ACT heat block for 3 minutes.
   B. Gently tap or shake the cartridge to resuspend the activator.
   C. Inject the client sample into channel 2 and then channel 1 of the cartridge, filling to between the lines (<1 mL).
   D. Place the cartridge in the instrument and pull the actuator cover forward. The instrument will sound an audible alert when the end point is reached. (*Note:* The instrument has two readout displays. The Channel 1 result is of ACT without heparin; the Channel 2 result is of ACT with the influence of heparin.)
4. **Postprocedure care:**
   A. If the test is performed at the client's bedside, document on the client's medical record the result of the test, time, date, machine number, tube type or number, site of draw, and rate of infusion in units per hour if the client is receiving IV heparin.
5. **Client and family teaching:**
   A. Results are normally available within a few minutes.
6. **Factors that affect results:**
   A. Tests may be affected by hemodilution, poor operator technique, inadequate reagent-to-specimen mixture, improper storage of test kits, cardioplegic solutions, hypothermia, platelet dysfunction, hypofibrinogenemia, other coagulopathies, and certain medications.
   B. In acute coronary cases, such as unstable angina and acute myocardial infarction, baseline

ACTs may be lower and heparin requirements higher, reflecting a thrombogenic state.

C. Heparinase-I (Neutralase) restores activated coagulation time in clients undergoing coronary artery surgery, as an alternative to protamine.

7. **Other data:**
A. Test cartridges available for the ACT II system: LR ACT, RACT, HR ACT, PT, GPC, and HTC. Test cartridges available for the Hemochron system are listed above under *Norms.*
B. Heparin requirements as well as baseline ACTs vary from client to client, and so ACT determinations allow a quick titration of the effective heparin dose.
C. Therapeutic ACT values depend on several factors: type of ACT system, type of test tube and reagent, type of procedure being performed, clinical condition of client, and clinical preference of physician.
D. HemoTec and Hemochron ACT measurements cannot be used interchangeably.

ACTIVATED PARTIAL THROMBOPLASTIN SUBSTITUTION TEST, DIAGNOSTIC

Norm. Normal factors VIII, IX, X, XI, and XII.

Usage. Helps identify single factor deficiencies causing prolonged partial thromboplastin time, including factors VIII, IX, XI, and XII.

Description. A differential activated partial thromboplastin time (APTT) method that identifies which factor deficiency or deficiencies are present when APTT is prolonged. Known reagents for each factor are systematically added to the client's blood sample. A factor is determined to be deficient when the substitution produces a normal APTT.

Professional Considerations
1. Consent form NOT required.
2. **Preparation:**
A. Tubes: Red topped and blue topped.

B. Preschedule the test with the laboratory.
3. **Procedure:**
A. Draw 2-3 mL of blood into a red-topped tube and discard. Completely fill a blue-topped tube with the blood sample.
4. **Postprocedure care:**
A. Hold pressure over the venipuncture site for 5 minutes if the client is receiving heparin therapy. Observe the site closely for development of hematoma.
B. Write the collection time on the laboratory requisition.
C. Refrigerate the specimen until the test is completed.
5. **Client and family teaching:**
A. Results are normally available within 24 hours.
6. **Factors that affect results:**
A. Failure to discard the first few milliliters of blood drawn may contaminate the specimen with tissue thromboplastin, which can activate coagulation.
B. Failure to completely fill the tube with blood may cause falsely prolonged results.
C. Hematocrit over 50% may cause falsely prolonged results, and hematocrit under 20% may cause falsely decreased results.
D. Drawing the sample from a line being kept open with a heparin flush will cause falsely prolonged results.
E. Reject hemolyzed specimens and specimens received more than 2 hours after collection.
F. Anticoagulant therapy within 2 weeks before the test invalidates results.
7. **Other data:**
A. Useful only with single-factor deficiencies.
B. See also *Activated partial thromboplastin time and partial thromboplastin time, Plasma.*

ACTIVATED PARTIAL THROMBOPLASTIN TIME (APTT) AND PARTIAL THROMBOPLASTIN TIME (PTT), PLASMA

Note: Activated partial thromboplastin time (APTT) is the current method of this test, which is still commonly referred to as "PTT".

Norm. Standardized times should be reported by each laboratory because results depend on the type of activator used. In general, standards are less than 35 seconds and vary 20-36 seconds.

Premature infants	<120 seconds
Newborn	<90 seconds
Infants	24-40 seconds
Children	24-40 seconds
Adult panic level	>70 seconds

Therapeutic Heparin Therapy Levels

Acute coronary artery disease	60-70 seconds
Peripheral vascular disease with embolism	60-70 seconds

Panic Level Symptoms and Treatment

Symptoms. Prolonged bleeding, hematoma at venipuncture site, cerebrovascular accident, hemorrhage, shock.

Treatment:
Note: Treatment choice(s) depend on client history and condition and episode history.
Assess heparin therapy.
Administer protamine sulfate (usual dose of 1 g of protamine sulfate for every 100 units of heparin).
Monitor vital signs.
Monitor for neurologic changes every hour until levels are within desired range.

Increased. *Major causes:* genetic or acquired deficiency of blood clotting factors IX, X, XI, or XII and with factor V or II deficiencies.

Deficiencies are usually below 30-40% normal levels for clotting factors to produce increased APTT and bleeding tendencies as seen in hemophilia A. Associated with deficiencies of HMW kininogen and Fletcher factor, prekallikrein. Also occurs with abruptio placentae, afibrinogenemia, cardiac surgery, hypothermia, cirrhosis, disseminated intravascular coagulation, dysfibrinogenemia, fibrinolysis, Fitzgerald factor deficiency (severe), in clients receiving hemodialysis, hemorrhagic disease of the newborn, hypofibrinogenemia, liver disease, hypoprothrombinemia, presence of circulating antico-

agulants, lupus anticoagulant, and von Willebrand's disease.

Drugs include alcohol, antistreplase (a thrombolytic agent) bishydroxycoumarin (excess therapy), chlorpromazine, codeine, eptifibatide, heparin calcium, heparin sodium, phenothiazines, salicylates, warfarin administration, and valproic acid.

Decreased. May occur with abnormalities of Fletcher factor, which are not associated with bleeding and in which thromboemboli may occur. A shortened aPTT (less than or equal to control) on presentation in clients with chest pain is associated with increased risk of acute MI.

Description. Partial thromboplastin time (PTT) evaluates how well the coagulation sequence is functioning by measuring the amount of time it takes for recalcified, citrated plasma to clot after partial thromboplastin is added to it. The PTT is abnormal in 90% of coagulation defects and screens for deficiencies and inhibitors of all factors except VII and XIII. Most commonly used to monitor effectiveness of heparin therapy and to screen for disorders of coagulation. When commercial activating materials are used to standardize the test, the PTT is called the APTT, or activated partial thromboplastin time.

Professional Considerations
1. Consent form NOT required.
2. Preparation:
   A. For intermittent heparin dosing, the sample should be drawn 1 hour before the next dose. A baseline APTT may not be needed before heparin therapy unless disease is suspected.
   B. Tube: 2.7- or 4.5-mL blue-topped tube, a control tube, and a waste tube or syringe.
   C. Do NOT draw specimens during hemodialysis.
   D. Do NOT draw specimens from a closed-loop blood sampling system in an arterial line that uses heparin flush solution.
3. Procedure:
   A. Withdraw 2 mL of blood into a syringe or vacuum tube. Remove the syringe or tube, leaving the needle in place. Attach a second syringe, and draw a blood sample

quantity of 2.4 mL for a 2.7-mL tube, or 4.0 mL for a 4.5-mL tube. Collect the sample without trauma.

4. Postprocedure care:
   A. If the test cannot be performed within 2 hours after specimen collection, separate and freeze the plasma.
   B. Transport the specimen to the laboratory immediately.
5. Client and family teaching:
   A. Surgery may need to be postponed if the results are prolonged.
   B. Bleeding precautions for prolonged values include the following: use a soft toothbrush; use an electric razor; avoid aspirin or aspirin products; avoid constipation; wear loose clothing; avoid intramuscular injections.
   C. Watch for and report signs of bleeding: bruising, petechiae, blood in stool/urine/sputum, bleeding from invasive lines, bleeding gums, abnormal or excessive vaginal bleeding.
   D. Many herbs can cause bleeding effects. For this reason, do not take any herbal preparations or natural remedies without receiving your doctor's approval.
6. Factors that affect results:
   A. Do NOT draw samples from an arm into which heparin is infusing.
   B. Failure to completely fill the tube will alter the results.
   C. If you are drawing samples from an arterial line with a heparin-flush pressure bag, at least 10 mL of blood must be withdrawn before the PTT sample is drawn.
   D. Failure to discard the first 1 to 2 mL of traumatic venous draw may result in a falsely decreased APTT.
   E. A false-normal PTT may occur if factor levels are deficient but not less than 25-30% of normal.
   F. Factor I (fibrinogen) deficiency may not be detectable unless levels are <100 mg/dL.
   G. Hematocrit >55% may cause falsely prolonged results. The test should be redrawn in a tube furnished by the laboratory that has had the concentration or amount of citrate adjusted for the elevated hematocrit level.
   H. Freezing the sample will decrease the test sensitivity to lupus anti-

coagulant and to deficiencies of XII, XI, HMW kininogen, and prekallikrein.
   I. Herbs or natural remedies that may increase PTT include *dan[1] shen[1]* (red-ginseng, *Salvia miltiorrhiza*), *dang[1]gui[1]* [variants: *tangkuei, dong quai*] (*Angelica sinensis*) (in clients receiving warfarin concurrently), feverfew (*Tanacetum parthenium*), *Ginkgo biloba,* ginger, ginseng.
7. Other data:
   A. Protamine sulfate, 1 mg, will reverse the effects of 100 U of heparin.
   B. Hemophilia A has increased APTT with normal PT and bleeding time.
   C. Hemophilia B is diagnosed by increased APTT with normal or increased PT and direct assay of levels of factor IX.
   D. APTT is not helpful in the diagnosis of hemophilia type.
   E. APTT and PT are both increased with prothrombin and HMW kininogen and prekallikrein deficiencies.
   F. Age, sex, and ABO blood group may have an influence on the APTT in normal clients.

ACTIVATED PARTIAL THROMBOPLASTIN TIME
(*see Partial thromboplastin time, Plasma*)

ACTIVATED PROTEIN C RESISTANCE TEST
(*see Protein C, Blood*)

ACUTE ABDOMINAL SERIES, DIAGNOSTIC

Norm. Requires individual interpretation.

Usage. Differential diagnosis of the cause of acute abdomen. Some examples are abdominal aortic aneurysm dissection, abscess, acute cholecystitis, acute ischemia, acute pancreatitis, appendicitis, bile duct obstruction, bowel strangulation, choledocholithiasis, gastric outlet obstruction, perforated abdominal viscus, peritonitis, pyelonephritis, ruptured ectopic pregnancy, *Salmonella* enterocolitis, and ureteral obstruction. Also useful for identifying the presence and location of (a) foreign body(ies).

Description. The acute abdomen is characterized by the abrupt onset of abdominal pain, distention, diminished or absent bowel sounds, and sometimes guarding. Causes of these symptoms may be many, and the disorder within the abdomen is hidden. In addition to a routine external physical assessment, seven routes of diagnostic work-up are used. Less invasive testing is usually performed first.

Laboratory studies include coagulation studies, hemoglobin and hematocrit tests, and blood volume determinations to rule out internal bleeding, leukocyte differential to determine whether an infectious or inflammatory process is present, amylase level to rule out pancreatic and other pathologic conditions, liver panels to rule out a hepatic disorder, blood urea nitrogen and creatinine determinations and urinalysis to rule out urinary tract infection, and stool examination to rule out *Salmonella*. Fine-needle aspiration cytologic testing provides clues to the type of process occurring.

Plain-film radiography is taking a radiograph without the use of an injected radiopaque agent. Plain-film radiography of the abdomen may identify compression fractures, intestinal obstruction, metastasis, perforated abdominal viscus, pancreatic calcification, and renal calculi.

Contrast radiography involves injection of a radiopaque agent into the vascular space. The contrast agent enhances the appearance of organ and vascular lumens and thus is more likely to reveal a pathologic condition than is plain film radiography. Vascular contrast examinations of the abdominal area such as intravenous pyelography help identify lumbar aortic aneurysms, urinary tract trauma, lesions, or other disorders.

Intestinal contrast examinations such as barium enema, oral cholecystogram, and upper gastrointestinal series may identify colonic lesions or perforation but should not be performed when obstruction is suspected. They may also rule out appendicitis.

Ultrasonography may help diagnose acute abscesses, cholecystitis, Crohn's disease, dilated bile duct, hepatic cancer, hepatic or splenic hematoma, spleno-megaly, hydronephrosis, intussusception, pancreatitis, pancreatic pseudocyst, pancreatic carcinoma, urinary tract obstruction, and the presence of foreign bodies.

Computed tomography helps identify, differentiate, and evaluate hepatic, pancreatic, renal, and retroperitoneal abscesses, fluid accumulations, masses and cysts, and pancreatitis.

Nuclear medicine studies help identify intra-abdominal abscesses, sites of gastrointestinal bleeding, hematoma, and areas of abnormal tissue metabolism. Nuclear medicine scans may also help to rule out cholecystitis.

In extremely acute situations and when findings from any combination of the above tests are inconclusive, surgical exploration of the abdomen may be required.

Professional Considerations
1. Consent form NOT required.

Risks
Allergic reaction to radiographic dye or nuclear medicine radiopharmaceutical for applicable tests (itching, hives, rash, tight feeling in the throat, shortness of breath, bronchospasm, anaphylaxis, death), renal toxicity.

Contraindications
Previous allergy to radiographic dye, iodine, or seafood or radionuclide for those tests involving injections; renal insufficiency.

Precautions
During pregnancy, risks of cumulative radiation exposure to the fetus from this and other previous or future imaging studies must be weighed against the benefits of the procedure. Although formal limits for client exposure are relative to this risk-benefit comparison, the United States Nuclear Regulatory Commission requires that the cumulative dose equivalent to an embryo/fetus from *occupational* exposure not exceed 0.5 rem (5 mSv). Radiation dose to the fetus is proportional to the distance of the anatomy studied from the abdomen and decreases as pregnancy progresses. For pregnant clients, consult the Radiologist/Radiology Department to obtain estimated fetal radiation exposure from this procedure.

2. **Preparation:**
   A. No preprocedural care is required for plain-film radiography.
   B. Intestinal contrast examinations often require clear liquids the day before the test and cathartics with or without cleansing enemas before the test. However, this requirement may be waived for a client with acute abdominal symptoms.
   C. Have emergency equipment readily available for tests involving injection of radionuclide or dye.

3. **Procedure:**
   A. Plain-film radiography: The client is positioned in supine, upright, oblique, and lateral decubitus positions, and radiographic films are taken from various angles. The best results are not obtained from portable films, especially in obese clients. The films should be taken in the radiology department, where the most powerful radiography is available, whenever possible. The lateral decubitus position is used for clients who are unable to stand, and the radiograph is taken horizontally across the table. A "kidneys, ureters, bladder film (KUB)" includes the majority of the abdomen and is taken from an anteroposterior angle. An anteroposterior scout film is used both before an intravenous pyelogram and in combination with an upright abdominal film for suspected intestinal obstruction. Subdiaphragmatic free air from perforated abdominal viscus may be identified with an upright abdominal film or an upright chest film.
   B. Vascular contrast examinations: Radiographic dye is injected into an arm vein, and oblique films of the abdomen are taken 15 minutes later. A left posterior oblique position may help identify a lumbar aortic aneurysm because the position enhances visualization by rotating the aorta off of the spine. Arteriography and venography may also help identify blood vessel abnormalities such as aneurysm, hemorrhage, or occlusion.
   C. Intestinal contrast examination: The client is placed in a Sims' position. Barium with or without air is instilled into the lower gastrointestinal tract, and radiographic films are taken. In upper gastrointestinal series, the client must swallow barium, and radiographic films are then taken. Oral cholecystography is a fluoroscopic study in which films of the gallbladder and ducts are taken after administration of a fat stimulus.
   D. Ultrasonography: The client is positioned on the side or supine, and a series of high-frequency sound waves are transmitted into the abdomen. The echoes reflected from the differing tissue densities are converted by a gel-coated transducer to form patterns of the abdominal structures on an oscilloscope screen.
   E. Computed tomography: The client is placed in a supine position on a platform table that moves the client through a circular computed tomography scanner. As several transverse films are taken, differing tissue densities are calculated based on varying absorption of the x rays. Findings may indicate the need for further computed tomography after the administration of contrast medium.
   F. Nuclear medicine studies: At varying intervals after the intravenous injection of a radioactive tracer, scintigraphic scans, which detect areas of increased concentration of the tracer at sites of a pathologic condition, are taken of the abdominal area.

4. **Postprocedure care:**
   A. Fluids should be encouraged after studies involving the administration of radiopaque dyes or barium.
   B. Cathartics may be prescribed after studies involving the administration of barium.

5. **Client and family teaching:**
   A. Explain the purpose of each test as appropriate, the procedure for the test, and the results. See individual test listings for specific client teaching.

6. **Factors that affect results:**
   A. The presence of gastrointestinal barium negates the value of plain-film radiography, vascular con-

trast examinations, ultrasonography, computed tomography, and nuclear medicine scintigraphy and so should be performed last.
7. Other data:
   A. See also *Barium enema, Diagnostic; Radiography of the abdomen, Flat-plate radiography of the abdomen, Diagnostic; Intravenous pyelogram, Diagnostic; Upper gastrointestinal series, Diagnostic; Computed tomography of the body, Diagnostic.*
   B. Health care professionals working in a nuclear medicine area must follow federal standards set by the Nuclear Regulatory Commission. These standards include precautions for the handling of the radioactive material and the monitoring of potential radiation exposure.
   C. Some extra-abdominal conditions that may cause acute abdominal pain include pneumonia, pulmonary or myocardial infarction, and pericarditis. Other conditions that may cause symptoms of acute abdomen include acute intermittent porphyria, diabetic neuropathy, heavy metal poisoning, sickle cell disease, and tabes dorsalis.

ADDIS COUNT, 12-HOUR URINE

Norm:

Erythrocytes	0-5,000/mm^3
Leukocytes	0-500,000/mm^3
Casts	1,000,000/mm^3

Increased. Glomerulonephritis and hematuria.

Description. When subclinical glomerulonephritis is suspected, an Addis count on a 12-hour urine specimen may demonstrate increased erythrocytes and leukocytes and increased rates of cast excretion in amounts too small to be detected in a random urine specimen examined microscopically. The count is performed on the sediment from a portion of the 12-hour collection.

Professional Considerations
1. Consent form NOT required.
2. Preparation:
   A. Obtain a 1- or a 2-L bottle that has been rinsed in formalin.

3. Procedure:
   A. The clean-catch urine technique must be used to decrease the risk of specimen contamination. See clean-catch collection instructions in *Body fluid, Routine, Culture.*
   B. Keep the specimen container refrigerated during and after specimen collection. For catheterized specimens, keep the drainage bag on ice and empty it into the collection container hourly.
4. Postprocedure care:
   A. Send the entire 12-hour urine specimen to the laboratory.
5. Client and family teaching:
   A. Do not drink any fluids throughout the collection period.
   B. Collect a clean-catch urine sample according to the technique above if this collection method is used.
6. Factors that affect results:
   A. Hematuria, pyuria, or a contaminated specimen will cause falsely elevated results.
7. Other data:
   A. This test is not usually necessary when a thorough history and renal work-up are done.
   B. An approximate Addis count can be performed on a first-morning voided specimen after a 16-hour fast from fluids and food.

ADENOVIRUS ANTIBODY TITER, SERUM

Norm. Negative. Results require interpretation with consideration of the site of the specimen correlated with clinical symptoms.

Current Adenovirus Infection. Fourfold rise in titer.

Increased. Adenovirus infection, respiratory failure, or graft failure in lung-transplanted clients. Gene therapy with replication-deficient adenoviral vector-mediated herpes simplex virus-thymidine kinase.

Description. A group of virus types responsible for upper respiratory disease, hemorrhagic cystitis, and epidemic keratoconjunctivitis. The mode of transmission is by direct or indirect contact. Measurement of adenovirus antibody titers is the test of choice for detection of current adenovirus infections. Results are reported as the highest dilution of serum that completely neutralizes the virus.

Professional Considerations

1. Consent form NOT required.
2. Preparation:
   A. Tube: Red topped, red/gray topped, or gold topped.
3. Procedure:
   A. Draw a 2-mL blood sample no later than 5-7 days after onset of symptoms.
   B. After allowing the specimen to clot at room temperature, centrifuge and separate the serum into a separate vial.
   C. Draw a convalescent sample in 14-21 days.
4. Postprocedure care:
   A. Mark the tube label and laboratory requisition with "acute phase" or "convalescent phase" for the first and second specimens, respectively.
5. Client and family teaching:
   A. Return in 2-3 weeks to have the convalescent sample drawn.
6. Factors that affect results:
   A. Reject hemolyzed or frozen specimens.
   B. Specimens may be stored several weeks at 4-6° C.
   C. Antibody titers for both specimens should be performed by the same laboratory.
7. Other data:
   A. This test is nonspecific for the type of adenovirus present.

ADENOVIRUS IMMUNOFLUORESCENCE, DIAGNOSTIC

Norm. Negative.

Usage. Adenovirus infection, conjunctivitis, hemorrhagic cystitis, and pharyngitis.

Description. A group of virus types responsible for upper respiratory disease, hemorrhagic cystitis, and epidemic keratoconjunctivitis. The mode of transmission is by direct or indirect contact. Direct immunofluorescence is performed for adenovirus group antigen on a swab or scraping.

Professional Considerations

1. Consent form NOT required.
2. Preparation:
   A. Obtain a sterile microbiologic swab or scraper and viral transport media. For a tracheal specimen, obtain a sputum trap and a suction cannula.
3. Procedure:
   A. *Upper respiratory disease, nasopharyngeal specimen:* Advance a curved swab through the nares to the posterior pharyngeal wall and leave it in place for 10 seconds. Remove the swab.
   B. *Pharyngeal specimen:* In a well-lit location with the client's head tilted back and the mouth open, depress the tongue with a tongue blade. Have the client say "Ah." Swab the posterior pharyngeal wall with a curved wire swab from one side to the other. Swab any lesions or drainage noted. Remove the swab without touching it to any other portions of the oropharynx or mouth.
   C. *Tracheal specimen:* Obtain a 1- to 3-mL sample of tracheal aspirate by oral or nasotracheal suction directly into a sterile sputum trap.
   D. *Hemorrhagic cystitis:* Swab or scrape urethral discharge (or a vesicle lesion visualized by cystoscopy). Alternatively, using a small platinum loop, scrape the inside of the anterior urethra.
   E. *Keratoconjunctivitis:* Do not rinse the eye or apply medication to the conjunctiva before specimen collection. Swab or scrape the inflamed surface of the inner, lower conjunctiva or the inner canthus of the eye.
4. Postprocedure care:
   A. Place the swab or scraping in viral transport media or a tightly capped tube containing 2 mL of 1% bovine serum albumin or veal infusion broth.
   B. Refrigerate the specimen.
5. Client and family teaching:
   A. Sampling should be painless.
6. Factors that affect results:
   A. Failure to send the specimen to the laboratory immediately or to immediately chill the sample.
7. Other data:
   A. This test is nonspecific for the type of adenovirus present.

ADRENOCORTICOTROPIC HORMONE (ACTH, CORTICOTROPIN), SERUM

Norm:

		SI UNITS
0800 hours, peak	25-100 pg/mL	25-100 ng/L
1800 hours, trough	0-50 pg/mL	0-50 ng/L

Increased. Addison's disease, ectopic ACTH syndrome, pituitary adenoma, pituitary Cushing's syndrome, primary adrenal insufficiency, and stress. Drugs include amphetamine sulfate, calcium gluconate, corticosteroids, estrogens, ethanol, lithium carbonate, and spironolactone.

Decreased. Primary adrenocortical hyperfunction (caused by tumor or hyperplasia) and secondary hypoadrenalism. Drugs include CPH 82, a non-steroid antirheumatic drug.

Description. ACTH is an anterior pituitary hormone that stimulates cortisol and androgen production by the adrenal gland. Diurnal variations of ACTH are typical, with peak levels occurring from 0600 to 0800 and trough levels occurring from 1800 to 2300.

Professional Considerations
1. Consent form NOT required.
2. Preparation:
   A. Tube: Plastic green topped or plastic lavender topped, and ice water slush.
   B. See *Client and family teaching.*
3. Procedure:
   A. Draw a 1-mL blood sample at 0600. Repeat the sampling at 1800 if trough levels are needed.
   B. Place the specimen in ice-water slush.
4. Postprocedure care:
   A. Write the collection time on the laboratory requisition.
   B. Transport the specimen to the laboratory immediately. The specimen should be frozen within 15 minutes if it will not be spun and tested within the first hour.
5. Client and family teaching:
   A. Consume a low-carbohydrate diet for 48 hours before the test.
   B. Avoid physical and emotional stress for 12 hours before the test.
   C. For peak and trough levels, two samples are required at different times of the day because the blood levels fluctuate throughout the day.
   D. Results may take several days.
6. Factors that affect results:
   A. Reject specimens received more than 60 minutes after collection.
   B. Values increase within 90 seconds of traumatic, repeated, or prolonged venipuncture.
   C. Menstruation cycle, pregnancy, and radioactive scanning within 7 days affect ACTH levels.
7. Other data:
   A. The ACTH stimulation test must be performed to confirm the diagnosis of Addison's disease.

ADT
(see Respiratory Antigen Panel, Specimen)

AFB SMEAR
(see Sputum, Mycobacteria, Culture and smear)

AFP
(see Alpha-fetoprotein, Blood)

AFRICAN TRYPANOSOMIASIS, BLOOD

Norm. Negative. No parasites identified.

Positive. African trypanosomiasis (African sleeping sickness).

Description. Also known as sleeping sickness, African trypanosomiasis is a vector-borne parasitic infection indigenous to tropical Africa caused in humans by the bite of a tsetse fly of the genus *Glossina*. Symptoms include a chancre at the site of the bite, progressing to headache, fever, insomnia, anemia, rash, and lymph node swelling. After inoculation, trypanosomes invade all body organs. CNS symptoms appear in disease stage II. The course of the disease may run months to years and is frequently fatal with treatment and always fatal without treatment.

Professional Considerations

1. Consent form NOT required.
2. Preparation:
   A. Obtain an alcohol wipe, lancet, and capillary tube.
3. Procedure:
   A. Perform this procedure in the early afternoon, again at night, and when fever spikes occur.
   B. Cleanse the pad of the index or second finger with the alcohol wipe and allow the pad to dry.
   C. Perform a finger stick and fill the capillary tube completely with blood. Quickly seal the capillary tube.
4. Postprocedure care:
   A. Write on the laboratory requisition the name of the parasite suspected and the place(s) and date(s) of recent travel.
5. Client and family teaching:
   A. Results are normally available within 24 hours.
6. Factors that affect results:
   A. Reject clotted specimens.
   B. Transport the capillary tube to the laboratory immediately for thick and thin smears to be performed before blood clots form.
7. Other data:
   A. Person-to-person transmission of African trypanosomiasis is possible either by direct contact with infected blood or from mother to fetus. Pentamidine and suramin are used for early-stage disease, depending on the causative organism. Melarsoprol is the drug of choice for late-stage treatment. Eflornithine is better tolerated but difficult to administer and Nifurtimox is cheap and can be administered orally but is not fully validated yet for use in humans.
   B. See also *Trypanosomiasis serologic test, Blood; Parasite screen, Blood.*

AHI
(see Polysomnography, Diagnostic)

AIDS EVALUATION BATTERY
(see Acquired immunodeficiency syndrome evaluation battery, Diagnostic; T- and B-lymphocyte subset assay; T- and B-lymphocyte subset assay, Blood)

AIR TONOMETRY
(see Tonometry test for glaucoma, Diagnostic)

ALA
(see Antiphospholipid antibody, Serum)

ALANINE AMINOTRANSFERASE (ALT, ALANINE TRANSAMINASE, SGPT), SERUM

Norm:

Adult Females	4-19 U/L or 10-30 Karmen units/mL or 317 nKat/L
Adult Males	7-30 U/L or 14-50 Karmen units/mL or 500 nKat/L
Children	
<12 months	≤54 U/L
1-2 years	3-37 U/L
2-8 years	3-30 U/L
8-16 years	3-28 U/L

Increased. Anorexia nervosa, biliary tract obstruction, brain tumor, cerebrovascular accident (increased after 1 week), cirrhosis, congestive heart failure (with liver damage), delirium tremens, dermatomyositis, dysrhythmias, Gaucher's disease, hepatic cancer, hepatic damage, hepatitis (viral, toxic), hyperglycemia, hypertension, hypercholesterolemia, hyperlipidemia, hypertriglyceridemia, infectious mononucleosis, intramuscular injections, intestinal infarction, liver passive congestion, local irradiation injury, muscle injury (caused by electroshock, infection, seizure, or trauma), muscular dystrophy, myocardial infarction, myoglobinuria, Niemann-Pick disease, obesity, pancreatitis (acute), polymyositis, postoperatively (intestinal surgery), pulmonary infarction, renal infarction, Reye syndrome, rhabdomyolysis, and shock with liver damage. Drugs include allopurinol, ampicillin, anabolic steroids, aspirin, barbiturates, bromocriptine mesylate, captopril, chlordiazepoxide, chlorpromazine hydrochloride, cincophen, deferiprone, diphenylhydantoin, fosinopril, and heparin (bovine, porcine). Herbal or natural remedies include chaparral tea (or misspelled chapparel tea, *Larrea tridentata*), *Echinacea,* pennyroyal. Herbal or natural remedies that have the potential to cause hepatotoxicity and elevate values include akee fruit (ackee, *Blighia sapida*), *Atractylis gummifera,* Azadirachta indica (see *margosa*), *Berberis vulgaris* (barberry), *Callilepsis laureola* (blazing star, *Liatris spicata*), chaparral tea (*Larrea tridentata*), cocaine, comfrey ("knitbone," *Symphytum officinale*), *Crotalaria* (bush tea), cycasin (a toxin from a *Cycas* species of sago palm of Guam), *Echinacea,* germander (genera *Teucrium* and *Veronica*; do not confuse with "safe skullcap", a name often falsely used in selling germander), *Heliotropium* (germander, valerian), *jin^1 bu^2 huan^4* ("gold-inconvertible", Jin Bu Huan Anodyne Tablets, patent medicine with misidentified constituents: essence of *t'ienchi [tianqi]* flowers, "Notoginseng"; also *kombucha*; also *Lycopodium serratum,* or club moss), *ma^{2}huang^2* (Ephedra), *margosa* (Melia azadirachta, *Azadirachta indica*), *maté* tea (Ilex paraguayensis), *mistletoe, pennyroyal, sassafras, Senecio, skullcap* (*Scutellaria*; do not confuse with "unsafe germander"), syo-saiko-to (xiao^3 chai^{2}hu^2 tang^1, 'minor *Bupleurum* combination'), *Teucrium polium* (golden germander), and valerian (*Valeriana officinalis,* garden heliotrope).

Decreased. Steatosis in clients with hepatitis C and weight loss. Herbal or natural remedy is Chinese fructus schizandrae sinensis (*wu^{3}wei^{4}zi^3,* 'five flavors herb', *Schisandra chinensis* [Turcz.] Baill.).

Description. Alanine aminotransferase (ALT) is an enzyme primarily produced by the liver and found in certain body fluids (such as bile, cerebrospinal fluid, plasma, and saliva) and in the heart, liver, kidneys, pancreas, and skeletal muscle. It acts as a catalyst in the transamination reaction that is necessary for amino acid production. This test is most commonly used to evaluate liver injury, where levels may rise to as much as 50 times normal range. The ALT levels are analyzed with aspartate aminotransferase (AST) levels to evaluate the degree of liver injury and to confirm a hepatic cause of AST increase. After the early stage of liver injury, ALT levels surpass AST levels. Serial measurements help track the course of hepatitis. This test may also be used by blood banks to screen for hepatitis in samples of donor blood.

Professional Considerations
1. Consent form NOT required.
2. **Preparation:**
   A. Tube: Red topped, red/gray topped, or gold topped.
   B. List medications taken by the client within the last 3 days on the laboratory requisition.
   C. Do NOT draw during hemodialysis.
3. **Procedure:**
   A. Draw a 1-mL blood sample.
4. **Postprocedure care:**
   A. The specimen may be refrigerated but not frozen.
5. **Client and family teaching:**
   A. Results are normally available within 12 hours.
6. **Factors that affect results:**
   A. Hemolysis causes unreliable results.
   B. Drugs that may cause falsely increased results include erythromycin, opiates, oxacillin sodium (Prostaphlin), and ampicillin (Polycillin).
   C. Falsely decreased results may occur in beriberi, diabetic ketoacidosis, hemodialysis (chronic), liver disease (severe), and uremia or with coffee ingestion.
   D. Herbal or natural remedies that may cause falsely decreased results include coffee (*Coffea*).
   E. Serial norms generally vary by less than 10 U/L in the same healthy client.
7. **Other data:**
   A. Older names for this test were glutamate-pyruvate transaminase and glutamic pyruvic transaminase.

ALBUMIN, SERUM, URINE, AND 24-HOUR URINE

Norm. Nephelometric, calorimetric, and (combined) nephorimetric.

		SI UNITS
Serum		
Adult	3.5-5.0 g/dL	35-50 g/L
>60 years	3.4-4.8 g/dL	34-48 g/L
Average at rest	0.3 g/dL	3 g/L
Urine		
Adult at rest	2-80 mg/24 hours	0.002-0.08 g/day
Adult ambulatory	<150 mg/24 hours	<0.15 g/day
Child, <10 years	<100 mg/24 hours	<0.10 g/day

Increased in Serum. Dehydration, diarrhea, Hodgkin's disease, meningitis, metastatic carcinomatosis, multiple myeloma, myasthenia, neoplasms, nephrosis, nephrotic syndrome, non-Hodgkin's lymphoma, osteomyelitis, peptic ulcer, pneumonia, polyarteritis nodosa, pregnancy, protein-losing enteropathy, rheumatic fever, rheumatoid arthritis, sarcoidosis, scleroderma, sprue, steatorrhea, stress, systemic lupus erythematosus, trauma, tuberculosis, ulcerative colitis, uremia, vomiting, and water intoxication. Drugs include sulfobromophthalein (Bromsulphalein), cytotoxic agents, and oral contraceptives.

Increased in Urine. Acute tubular necrosis, amyloid disease, anemia (severe), Bartter syndrome, Butler-Albright syndrome, Bright's disease, cardiac disease, central nervous system lesions, cerebrovascular accident, convulsions, cystitis, diabetes insipidus (nephrogenic), diabetic nephropathy, diphtheria, drug reaction, epididymitis, exercise, Fanconi syndrome, fever, galactosemia, glomerular lesion, glomerulonephritis, glomerulosclerosis, Goodpasture syndrome, heavy metal poisoning, hyperthyroidism, idiopathic thrombocytopenic purpura, intestinal obstruction, leukemia, liver disease, membranous nephropathy, multiple myeloma, nephritis, nephrosclerosis, nephrotic syndrome, pneumonia, poisoning (arsenic, carbon tetrachloride, ether, lead, mercury, mustard, opiates, phenol, phosphorus, propylene glycol, sulfosalicylic acid, turpentine), polycystic kidney disease, prostatitis, pyelonephritis (bacterial, chronic, hypertensive), renal radiation, renal tubular acidosis,

renal vein thrombosis, scarlet fever, septicemia, streptococcal infection, subacute bacterial endocarditis, systemic lupus erythematosus, toxemia of pregnancy, tumor (abdominal, bladder, renal pelvis), typhoid fever, and Wilson's disease. Drugs include amphotericin B, ampicillin, ampicillin sodium, aspirin, bacitracin, barbiturates, cephaloridine, corticosteroids, gentamicin sulfate, gold, kanamycin, mercurial diuretics, neomycin sulfate, phenylbutazone, and polymyxin B.

Decreased in Serum. Acute infection, ascites, alcoholism, beriberi, bone fractures, brucellosis, burns, cholecystitis, cirrhosis, congenital analbuminemia, congestive heart failure, Crohn's disease, cystic fibrosis, dementia, diabetes mellitus, edema, essential hypertension, glomerulonephritis, hemorrhage, hepatitis (viral), Hodgkin's dementia, disease, hyperthyroidism, infection, liver diseases, systemic lupus erythematosus (SLE), leukemia (lymphatic, monocytic, and myelogenous), lymphoma, macroglobulinemia, malnutrition, malabsorption syndrome, meningitis, metastatic carcinomatosis, multiple myeloma, myasthenia, myocardial infarction, neoplasms, nephrosis, nephrotic syndrome, osteomyelitis, peptic ulcer, pneumonia, polyarteritis nodosa, pregnancy, protein-losing enteropathy, rheumatic fever, rheumatoid arthritis, sarcoidosis, scleroderma, sprue, steatorrhea, stress, surgery, trauma, tuberculosis, ulcerative colitis, uremia, and water intoxication. Drugs include ampicillin, asparaginase, fluorouracil, and oral contraceptives.

Decreased in Urine.
Not clinically significant.

Description. Albumin is one of the two main protein factions of blood. It functions in maintaining oncotic pressure and in transportation of bilirubin, fatty acids, drugs, hormones, and other substances that are insoluble in water. Protein is normally almost completely reabsorbed by the kidneys and undetectable in the urine. Therefore the presence of detectable albumin, or protein, in urine is indicative of abnormal renal function.

Professional Considerations
1. Consent form NOT required.
2. **Preparation:**
   A. Tube: Red topped, red/gray topped, or gold topped for serum albumin.
   B. Do NOT draw specimen during hemodialysis.
   C. Obtain a 3-L specimen container without preservative for 24-hour urine albumin and write the beginning time of specimen collection on the container.
   D. Obtain a clean specimen container for the spot urine specimen.
   E. See *Client and family teaching.*
3. **Procedure:**
   A. *Serum:* Draw a 1-mL blood sample from an extremity that does not have intravenous fluids infusing into it (to avoid hemodilution and falsely low results). Avoid prolonged application of the tourniquet.
   B. *24-hour urine:* Collect all urine voided in a 24-hour period and refrigerate. For catheterized clients, keep the collection bag on ice, and empty it hourly into the collection container.
   C. *Spot urine collection* may also be collected.
4. **Postprocedure care:**
   A. Document the quantity of urine output and the ending time for the collection period on the laboratory requisition.
5. **Client and family teaching:**
   A. Consume a low-fat diet the day of the test.
   B. Empty the bladder before starting 24-hour urine collection.
   C. Save all urine voided in the 24-hour period, and urinate before defecating to avoid loss of urine. If any urine is accidentally discarded, discard the entire specimen and restart the collection the next day.
6. **Factors that affect results:**
   A. The results are invalid if the measurement is performed on plasma rather than serum.
   B. Bromsulphalein testing within 2 days before specimen collection invalidates serum results.
   C. Values are higher when upright or ambulatory. Serum values are higher after hemodialysis caused by fluid overload.
   D. Falsely elevated urine results may be caused by contamination of the specimen with pus, menstrual blood, or vaginal discharge.
   E. One study found a diurnal variation in urinary albumin levels in clients with insulin-dependent diabetes. Levels significantly increased between 2400 and 0800.
7. **Other data:**
   A. A 24-hour urine collection for measuring protein loss may be helpful in clients with low serum albumin levels.

ALCOHOL (ETHANOL), BLOOD

Norm. Negative.

		SI UNITS
Negative	0 mg/dL	0 mmol/L
Intoxication	>100 mg/dL	>22 mmol/L
Coma	>300 mg/dL	>65.1 mmol/L
Panic level	350-800 mg/dL	76.0-174.0 mmol/L

Ethyl Alcohol (Ethanol) Poisoning Overdose Symptoms and Treatment

Symptoms:

<50 mg/dL	Muscular incoordination
50-100 mg/dL	Worsening incoordination of movement
100-150 mg/dL	Mood and behavior changes
150-200 mg/dL	Delayed reactions
200-300 mg/dL	Ataxia, double vision, nausea, vomiting
300-400 mg/dL	Amnesia, dysarthria, hypothermia
400-700 mg/dL	Respiratory failure, coma, death possible

Treatment:
Note: Treatment choice(s) depend on client history and condition and episode history.
Support oxygenation and protect airway.
Monitor for dehydration. Administer fluids as needed.
Hemodialysis WILL remove ethanol but is seldom necessary unless levels rise above 300 mg/dL. During hemodialysis, levels drop an average of 62 mg%/hour.

Increased. Alcohol ingestion; concomitant use of alcohol and certain drugs (antihistamines, barbiturates, chlordiazepoxide, cyproheptadine, diazepam, glutethimide, guanethidine, isoniazid, meprobamate, opiates, phenytoin, tranquilizers); ethylene glycol poisoning; and ingestion of liniments, shaving lotion, astringents, elixirs, fluid extracts, tinctures, and cough medicines.

Description. Alcohol (ethanol) is a central nervous system depressant with anesthetic and diuretic effects that is taken orally by clients. Ethanol is also used to treat methanol poisoning, and may be used prophylactically to prevent alcohol withdrawal symptoms from occuring.

Professional Considerations
1. Consent form NOT required unless the specimen may be used as legal evidence.
2. Preparation:
   A. Tube: Red topped, red/gray topped, gold topped, black topped, or lavender topped.
   B. Do NOT draw during hemodialysis.
   C. If a specific type of alcohol measurement is desired (methanol, isopropanol, ethylene glycol), list the specific alcohol on the laboratory requisition.

D. Screen client for the use of herbal preparations or natural remedies such as kavakava (*Piper methysticum*) or ginseng.
3. Procedure:
   A. If the specimen is being collected for legal evidence, have the collection witnessed.
   B. Cleanse the venipuncture site with povidone-iodine solution and allow it to dry.
   C. Draw a 3-mL blood sample.
4. Postprocedure care:
   A. If the specimen may be used for legal evidence, include the exact time of specimen collection on the tube label and sign and have the witness sign the laboratory requisition. Transport the specimen to the laboratory in a sealed plastic bag labeled as legal evidence. Each person handling the specimen should sign and record the time of receipt on the laboratory requisition.
5. Client and family teaching:
   A. Results are normally available within 24 hours.
   B. Refer clients with intentional overdose for crisis intervention.
   C. Referrals to appropriate rehabilitation centers and therapeutic community programs should be offered to all addicted clients who may be interested.

6. Factors that affect results:
  A. Cleansing the venipuncture site with an alcohol wipe may cause false-positive results.
7. Other data:
  A. Tolerance to alcohol's effects may develop in chronic alcoholics. Therefore, normally lethal levels may not lead to death in these clients.
  B. Positive blood alcohol is associated with higher trauma severity in road accidents.
  C. In hypothermia, the degree of ketosis is inversely proportional to blood ethanol concentration.
  D. Men have significantly higher alcohol elimination rates compared to women.
  E. Food intake increases alcohol elimination rates.
  F. Only blood alcohol (rather than urine alcohol) levels are acceptable as legal evidence in most countries.
  G. Postmortem alcohol levels may differ from sites including hematomas, blood, urine, and stomach contents.
  H. Kavakava (*Piper methysticum*), an herbal or natural remedy anxiolytic, potentiates the effects of ethanol.
  I. Ginseng (*Panax* spp.) increases alcohol clearance by increasing the activity of alcohol dehydrogenase and aldehyde dehydrogenase.
  J. See also *Isopropyl alcohol, Blood; Toxicology, Volatiles group by GLC, Blood or urine.*

ALDOLASE, SERUM

Norm:

		SI UNITS
Adult		
Ambulatory	1.0-7.5 U/L (30° C)	0.02-0.13 μKat/L
Bed rest	0.3-3.0 U/L (30° C)	0.005-0.05 μKat/L
Children		
Newborn to 24 months	3.4-11.8 U/L (37° C) or up to 4 times the adult level	0.06-0.20 μKat/L
25 months to 16 years	1.2-8.8 U/L (37° C) or up to 2 times the adult levels	0.02-0.15 μKat/L

Increased. Anemia (megaloblastic, hemolytic), burns, cancer, cirrhosis, congestive heart failure, crushing injury, dermatomyositis, Duchenne muscular dystrophy, eosinophilic fasciitis, erythroblastosis fetalis, hepatic necrosis, hepatitis (acute viral), hepatoma, jaundice (obstructive), lead intoxication, leukemia (chronic granulocytic), liver metastasis, lymphoma, metastasis, mononucleosis (infectious), muscle trauma, muscular dystrophy, myocardial infarction (acute), myopathy, Niemann-Pick disease, pancreatitis (acute), pericarditis (hemorrhagic), polycythemia vera, polymyositis, prostate cancer, pulmonary infarction, skeletal muscle disease, surgical trauma, and trichinosis. Drugs include aminocaproic acid (large doses), carbenoxolone, chlorinated insecticides, clofibrate, corticotropin, cortisone acetate, cyclophosphamide (high dose), labetalol, organophosphorus insecticides, and thiabendazole.

Decreased. Not clinically significant. Drugs include phenothiazines (when aldolase values are initially high in schizophrenics).

Description. An enzyme found throughout the body but in highest concentrations in skeletal muscle tissue. Because aldolase rises during active skeletal muscle disease, its measurement helps track the progress of diseases, such as progressive muscular dystrophy.

Professional Considerations
1. Consent form NOT required.
2. **Preparation:**

A. Tube: Red topped, red/gray topped, or gold topped.
B. See *Client and family teaching.*
3. **Procedure:**
   A. Draw a 2-mL blood sample.
4. **Postprocedure care:**
   A. Place the sample on ice for immediate transport to the laboratory.
5. **Client and family teaching:**
   A. Avoid strenuous exercise for 12 hours before sampling.
   B. Results are normally available within 24 hours.
6. **Factors that affect results:**
   A. Reject hemolyzed specimen to avoid falsely elevated results.
   B. Recent intramuscular injections may elevate results.
7. **Other data:**
   A. Although norms are not established for aldolase isoenzymes A, B, and C, one study (Asaka et al. 1994) found that serum aldolase A/B ratios increased in clients with cancer with normal GPT levels and decreased in clients with liver disease.
   B. Measurement of aldolase A and gamma-enolase together provides information directly relevant to prognosis in cases of renal cell carcinoma.
   C. May be useful indicator of disease activity in eosinophilic fasciitis (EF).

ALDOSTERONE, SERUM AND URINE

Norm: Norms assume an average sodium diet (3 g/day)

PERIPHERAL BLOOD	SERUM	SI UNITS
Supine	3-60 ng/dL	0.14-1.9 nmol/L
Upright		
Adult female		
Pregnant	18-100 ng/dL	0.5-2.8 nmol/L
Nonpregnant	5-30 ng/dL	0.14-0.8 nmol/L
Adult male	6-22 ng/dL	0.17-0.61 nmol/L
Adrenal Vein	200-800 ng/dL	5.54-2.22 nmol/L
Child		
1 week-12 months	1-160 ng/dL	0.03-4.43 nmol/L
1-3 years	5-60 ng/dL	0.14-1.7 nmol/L
3-11 years	5-70 ng/dL	0.14-1.9 nmol/L
11-15 years	<5-50 ng/dL	<0.14-1.4 nmol/L

URINE		SI UNITS
Normal urine	2-26 mg/24 hours	5.6-73 nmol/day

		URINARY ALDOSTERONE	
URINARY SODIUM	PLASMA RENIN	µg/DAY	nmol/DAY
<30 nmol/day	5-24 Al/mL/hour	35-80	97-220
20-50 nmol/day	2-7 Al/mL/hour	13-33	36-91
50-100 nmol/day	1-5 Al/mL/hour	5-24	14-66
100-150 nmol/day	0.5-4 Al/mL/hour	3-19	8-53
150-200 nmol/day	<0.5 Al/mL/hour	1-16	3-44
200-250 nmol/day	<0.5 Al/mL/hour	1-13	3-36

Increased in Serum and Urine. Adrenal tumor (aldosterone-producing adenoma), aldosteronism (primary, secondary), bilateral adrenal hyperplasia, cirrhosis, congestive heart failure, Conn syndrome, hemorrhage, hypertension (essential, >140/90 mm Hg), hyponatremia, hypovolemia, idiopathic cyclic edema, nephrosis (lower nephron), nephrotic syndrome, and renovascular hypertension. Drugs that increase serum levels include angiotensin-converting enzyme (ACE) inhibitors, estrogens, corticotropin, diuretics that promote sodium excretion, laxatives that are abused, some oral contraceptives, and potassium. Drugs that increase urine levels include angiotensin, deoxycorticosterone, diuretics (loop, thiazide), etiocholanolone, oral contraceptives, and steroids.

Decreased in Serum and Urine. Addison's disease, preeclampsia, primary hypoaldosteronism, salt-wasting syndrome, septicemia, stress, and toxemia of pregnancy. Herbal or natural remedy is licorice. Drugs that decrease serum levels include aminoglutethimide, ACE inhibitors, deoxycorticosterone, etomidate, fludrocortisone, heparin (after several days of continuous therapy), indomethacin, methyldopa, and saralasin. Drugs that decrease urine levels include aminoglutethimide, clonidine, deoxycorticosterone, fludrocortisone, glucocorticoids, labetalol, heparin, methyldopa, metyrapone, and propranolol.

Description. Aldosterone is a mineralocorticoid secreted by the adrenal cortex that functions in blood pressure and body fluid regulation. It acts on the renal distal tubules, causing increased resorption of sodium and water and increased excretion of potassium.

Professional Considerations
1. Consent form NOT required.
2. **Preparation:**
   A. The client should rest in a supine position for 8-12 hours. The sample should be drawn before noon.
   B. Tube: Red topped, red/gray topped, gold topped; lavender topped, or green topped for serum collection.
   C. For urine test, obtain a 3-L container (to which 10 g of boric acid have been added) and a 100-mL specimen container for urinary sample.
   D. See *Client and family teaching.*
3. **Procedure:**

   Serum Test
   A. Collect 2.5-mL blood sample for serum aldosterone.

   Urine Test
   A. Discard the first morning-urine specimen.
   B. Collect all urine voided in a 24-hour period in a refrigerated container to which 10 g of boric acid have been added. Include

urine voided at the end of the 24-hour period. For catheterized clients, keep the drainage bag on ice and empty the urine into the collection container hourly.
   C. At the end of 24 hours, mix the urine gently and collect a 100-mL aliquot in a clean container.
4. **Postprocedure care:**
   A. Note total 24-hour urine volume on the laboratory requisition and the aliquot container label.
   B. Transport the 24-hour and aliquot samples to the laboratory immediately.
5. **Client and family teaching:**
   A. Follow a 3-g/day sodium diet for 2 weeks if not contraindicated by medical condition.
   B. Avoid physical or psychologic stress throughout the collection period.
   C. Save all urine voided in the 24-hour period, urinate before defecating to avoid loss of urine, and avoid contaminating the specimen with feces or soiled tissue. If any urine is accidentally discarded, discard the entire specimen and restart the collection the next day.
   D. Results may not be available for several days.
6. **Factors that affect results:**
   A. Radioactive scans within 7 days before urine collection invalidate the results.
   B. Hemolysis invalidates the serum results.
   C. Decreased kidney perfusion may cause increased aldosterone and renin values.
   D. Levels may be suppressed in clients with insulin-dependent diabetes mellitus.
   E. An upright client position for serum collection invalidates the results. Changes in urine aldosterone are not affected by body position.
7. **Other data:**
   A. Serum electrolyte and renin levels should be measured before this test.

ALDOSTERONE SUPPRESSION TEST, DIAGNOSTIC

Norm. <5 ng/dL (<0.14 nmol/L SI units).

Primary Aldosteronism. >10 ng/ dL (>0.2777 nmol/L SI units).

Usage. Definitive diagnosis of primary aldosteronism, which is also common in clients with essential hypertension.

Description. Aldosterone is a mineralocorticoid secreted by the adrenal cortex that functions in blood pressure and body fluid regulation. It acts on the renal distal tubule, where it increases resorption of sodium and water at the expense of increased potassium excretion. Levels are affected by body position and sodium and potassium levels. The aldosterone suppression test measures aldosterone levels before and after an infusion of saline. In primary aldosteronism, the saline infusion fails to suppress aldosterone levels as much as it suppresses the levels in a normal client.

Professional Considerations
1. Consent form NOT required.

Risks
Volume overload, hypertension, myocardial ischemia, congestive heart failure.

Contraindications
The serum test is contraindicated in clients with congestive heart failure.

2. Preparation:
   A. The client should be positioned upright for 2 hours and then lie in a recumbent position from the onset of the test until second specimen is drawn at the completion of the infusion.
   B. Tubes: Two red topped, red/gray topped, gold topped, green topped, or lavender topped.
   C. Obtain 2 L of 0.9% saline and a 24-hour urine collection container to which 10 g of boric acid have been added.
3. Procedure:

   Serum Collection
   A. Draw a 2.5-mL blood sample for the baseline aldosterone level.
   B. Infuse 2 L of normal saline intravenously over a 4-hour period to the recumbent client.
   C. Draw a final 2.5-mL blood sample for aldosterone level.

   Urine Collection
   A. Discard the first morning-urine specimen.
   B. Collect all urine voided in a 24-hour period in a refrigerated

container to which 10 g of boric acid have been added. Include urine voided at the end of the 24-hour period. For catheterized clients, keep the drainage bag on ice and empty the urine into the collection container hourly.
   C. At the end of 24 hours, mix the urine gently and collect a 100-mL aliquot in a clean container.
4. Postprocedure care:
   A. Note the collection site and the time on all laboratory requisitions and blood tubes. For the urine sample, write the total 24-hour urine volume on the laboratory requisition and the aliquot container label.
   B. Transport each specimen to the laboratory immediately after collection.
5. Client and family teaching:
   A. The test takes several hours. Bring reading material or other diversional item.
   B. Results are normally available within 24 hours.
6. Factors that affect results:
   A. Reject hemolyzed specimens.
   B. Radioactive scans within 7 days before urine collection invalidate results.
   C. Cimetidine, but not omeprazole, inhibits test results.
7. Other data:
   A. Insulin resistance occurs with primary hyperaldosteronism.

ALKALINE PHOSPHATASE, HEAT STABLE, SERUM

Norm. Interpreted by laboratory. Results are reported in the percentage of alkaline phosphatase that is heat stable. Residual activity >30% favors hepatic origin and <30% favors bone origin (see *Description*).

Usage. Aids in differentiation of the source of increased alkaline phosphatase activity. Decreased in premature uterine contractility in women in second trimester. Diagnosis and treatment monitoring for breast cancer, squamous cell carcinoma of the head and neck, and leukemia.

Description. Alkaline phosphatase is an enzyme normally found in bone, liver, intestine, and placenta that rises during periods of bone growth (osteoblastic activity), liver disease, and bile duct obstruction. It is made up of bone, liver, and placental and intestinal isoenzymes that can be separated by heat fractionation. Liver and placental alkaline phosphatase isoenzymes are heat stable, and bone isoenzyme is inactivated by heat. Greater than 30% of the alkaline phosphatase being heat stable is suggestive of activity of liver origin, whereas <30% being heat stable is suggestive of activity of bone origin.

Professional Considerations
1. Consent form NOT required.
2. **Preparation:**
   A. Tube: Red topped, red/gray topped, or gold topped.
   B. Do NOT draw during hemodialysis.
3. **Procedure:**
   A. Draw a 1-mL blood sample.
4. **Postprocedure care:**
   A. Transport the specimen to the laboratory immediately for testing or for spinning and refrigeration.
5. **Client and family teaching:**
   A. The client may be asked to fast for 10-12 hours.
   B. Results may take several days.
6. **Factors that affect results:**
   A. Reject hemolyzed specimens.
   B. Hepatotoxic drugs within 12 hours before specimen collection invalidate the test.
   C. Failure to fast before the test may result in falsely elevated levels.
   D. Specimens left at room temperature may result in falsely elevated levels.
   E. *Echinacea* taken for 8 weeks or longer may cause hepatotoxicity.
7. **Other data:**
   A. Postmenopausal females have slightly increased total alkaline phosphatase and a low percentage of heat-stable fraction, indicating osseous origin.

ALKALINE PHOSPHATASE, ISOENZYMES, SERUM
(*see Alkaline phosphatase, Serum*)

ALKALINE PHOSPHATASE, SERUM

Norm:

TOTAL ALKALINE PHOSPHATASE		SI UNITS
King-Armstrong Method		
Adults, 20-60 years	4.5-13 U/dL	32-92 U/L
Elderly	Slightly higher	
Newborn	5-15 U/dL	36-107 U/L
Premature newborn	1.5-2 times adult value	
Children: Values remain high until epiphyses close		
1 month	10-30 U/dL	71-213 U/L
3 years	10-20 U/dL	71-142 U/L
10 years	15-30 U/dL	107-213 U/L
Bodansky Method		
Adults, 20-60 years	2-4 U/dL	10.7-21.5 U/L
Elderly	Slightly higher	
Children	5-14 U/dL	27-75 U/L
Bessey-Lowrey-Brock Method		
Adults, 20-60 years	0.8-2.3 U/dL	13.3-38.3 U/L
Elderly	Slightly higher	
Bowers and McComb Method		
Females		
1-12 years	<350 U/L	<5.95 µKat/L
Puberty: Values may triple		
>15 years	25-100 U/L	0.43-1.70 µKat/L

TOTAL ALKALINE PHOSPHATASE, SERUM—cont'd

Males

1-12 years	<350 U/L	<5.95 µKat/L
12-14 years	<500 U/L	<8.50 µKat/L
Puberty: Values may triple		
>20 years	25-100 U/L	0.43-1.70 µKat/L

HEAT INACTIVATION METHOD	ISOENZYME NORMS (ISOENZYME INACTIVATED AFTER 16 MINUTES AT 55°C)	
	PERCENTAGE	FRACTION
Liver isoenzyme	50-700	0.50-0.70
Bone isoenzyme	90-100	0.90-1.00
Intestinal isoenzyme	50-600	0.50-0.60
Placental isoenzyme		
Trimester 1 to 1 month postpartum	50% of total	

Increased Biliary Isoenzyme. Biliary cirrhosis, biliary duct obstruction, cholangiar obstruction (in hepatitis), and cholestasis.

Increased Bone Isoenzyme. Bone cancer accompanied by bone formation, bone growth or healing, familial hyperphosphatemia, familial osteoectasia, Gaucher's disease, growth hormone overproduction, hyperparathyroidism, hyperthyroidism, leukemia of bone marrow, lymphoma, malabsorption, myositis ossificans, Niemann-Pick disease, osteoblastic metastases, osteogenesis imperfecta, osteomalacia, osteoporosis, osteogenic sarcoma, Paget's disease, polyostotic fibrous dysplasia, renal osteodystrophy, and rickets.

Increased Intestinal Isoenzyme. Gastrointestinal disease, clients with blood type O or B (some), pancreatic duct obstruction, pancreatic cancer, splenic infarction, steatorrhea (idiopathic), and ulcer (perforated).

Increased Liver I Isoenzyme. Impaired enzyme metabolism, liver congestion, hepatic carcinoma, hepatotoxic drugs, jaundice (obstructive), pregnancy, and vasculitis.

Increased Liver II Isoenzyme. Hepatitis (infectious, viral), parenchymal cell damage.

Increased Placental Isoenzyme. Pregnancy (late).

Increased Total Alkaline Phosphatase. May also be caused by alcoholism, carbohydrate ingestion (large quantities), children, cholelithiasis in persons with sickle cell disease, diabetes mellitus, Fanconi syndrome, fat ingestion, fibrous dysplasia, histiocytosis, Hodgkin's disease, hyperalimentation, hyperparathyroidism (with bone disease), hyperthyroidism, hypophosphatemia, kidney tissue rejection, liver abscess, liver disease, lung cancer, lymphoma, mononucleosis (infectious), multiple myeloma, myocardial infarction, osteosarcoma, primary biliary cirrhosis, pulmonary infarction, renal infarction, rheumatoid arthritis, rickets, sarcoidosis, and sickle cell crisis. Drugs include acetohexamide, albumin, allopurinol, aluminum nicotinate, amitriptyline, ampicillin, anabolic steroids, androgens, asparaginase, aspirin, aurothioglucose, azothioprine, baclofen, barbiturates, bromocriptine mesylate, carbamazepine, carmustine, cephaloridine, chlordiazepoxide, chlorpromazine hydrochloride, chlorpropamide, cholestyramine resin, cimetidine, cincophen, clindamycin, clonazepam, colchicine, ergosterol, erythromycin, estrogens, floxuridine, flurazepam, fosinopril, gold sodium, *n*-hydroxyacetamide, imipramine, imipramine pamoate, indomethacin, isoniazid, lincomycin, meclofenamate sodium, methyldopa, methyldopate hydrochloride, methyltestosterone, metoprolol tartrate, minoxidil, mithramycin, naproxen sodium, niacin, nifedipine, nitrofurantoin, novobiocin, oral contraceptives, oxacillin sodium, oxyphenisatin, papaverine hydrochloride, penicillamine, pertofrane, phenobarbital, phenothiazines, phenylbutazone, phenytoin, procainamide hydrochloride, propranolol, propylthiouricil, rifampin, salicylates, sulfamethoxazole, sulfisoxazole, sulfisoxazole acetyl, sulfobromophthalein sodium, tetracycline, thiomalate, thiothixene, thyroid hormone replacement, tolazamide, tolbutamide, tolmetin sodium, valproic acid, and vitamin D.

Decreased. Anemia (pernicious), blood transfusions (massive), celiac disease, cretinism, hypophosphatasia, hypothyroidism, malnutrition, milk-alkali syndrome (Burnett syndrome), nephritis (chronic), osteolytic sarcoma, scurvy, vitamin D intoxication, and zinc depletion. Drugs include aminobiphosphonate (Neridronate), edetate disodium, fluorides, oxalates, phosphates, and propranolol.

Description. Alkaline phosphatase is an enzyme found in bone, liver, intestine, and placenta that rises during periods of bone growth (osteoblastic activity), liver disease, and bile duct obstruction. It is made up of bone, liver, placental, biliary, and intestinal isoenzymes that can be separated by electrophoresis. Alkaline phosphatase isoenzymes should be measured for any client who has an elevated alkaline phosphatase level.

Professional Considerations
1. Consent form NOT required.
2. Preparation:
   A. Tube: Red topped, red/gray topped, or gold topped.
   B. See *Client and family teaching.*
3. Procedure:
   A. Draw a 1-mL blood sample.
4. Postprocedure care:
   A. Transport the specimen to the laboratory for immediate testing or for spinning and refrigeration.
5. Client and family teaching:
   A. Client may be asked to fast for 10-12 hours.
   B. Results are normally available within 24 hours.
6. Factors that affect results:
   A. Reject hemolyzed specimens.
   B. Hepatotoxic drugs within 12 hours before collection invalidate the test.

C. Falsely elevated results may be caused by failure to fast before the test or by specimens left at room temperature.
D. *Echinacea* taken for 8 weeks or longer may cause hepatotoxicity.
7. **Other data:**
   A. Isoenzymes are required to interpret the contributing source (liver, bone, placenta) of elevated total alkaline phosphatase.
   B. At least 2 days are required for isoenzyme results.
   C. Differentiation of bone and liver isoenzyme is difficult, because both are derived from a single gene. A monoclonal antibody assay that may aid in differentiation of liver and bone isoenzyme is being tested.

ALLERGEN-SPECIFIC IgE, SERUM

Norm. <2% of serum immunoglobulins.

Adults	<41 U/mL
Children	
Neonate	<12 U/mL
1-3 years	<10 U/mL
4-6 years	<24 U/mL
7-8 years	<46 U/mL
9-12 years	<116 U/mL
13-14 years	<63 U/mL

Increased. Allergic rhinitis, asthma (exogenous), anaphylaxis, atopic dermatitis, atopic eczema, *Echinococcus* infestation, eczema, hay fever, hookworm disease, latex allergy, schistosomiasis, and visceral larva migrans. Drugs include aminophenazone, anticonvulsants, asparaginase, hydralazine hydrochloride, oral contraceptives, and phenylbutazone.

Decreased. Asthma (endogenous), pregnancy, and radiation therapy. Drugs include methotrexate.

Description. Immunoglobulin E is a protein produced in the bone marrow that functions as an antibody in response to antigen stimulation in hypersensitivity reactions. IgE levels are influenced by the nature of the allergen, length of exposure to the allergen, symptomatic responses, and hyposensitization treatments. The test is performed by radioimmunoassay.

Professional Considerations

1. Consent form NOT required.
2. **Preparation:**
   A. Tube: Red topped, red/gray topped, or gold topped.
   B. List vaccinations, immunizations, and tetanus antitoxin received within the previous 6 months on the laboratory requisition.
   C. List the blood products the client received within 6 weeks before the test on the laboratory requisition.
3. **Procedure:**
   A. Draw a 3-mL blood sample.
4. **Postprocedure care:**
   A. Transport the specimen to the laboratory immediately.
5. **Client and family teaching:**
   A. Fast, except for water, 12-14 hours before the test.
   B. Results are normally available within 24 hours.
   C. Refer the client with elevated IgE levels and allergic symptoms to an allergist for more specific testing and guidance on potential treatments and environmental reduction of allergens.
6. **Factors that affect results:**
   A. A delay in testing invalidates results.
   B. Results are invalidated if the client has undergone a scan using a radioisotope within 1 week before the test.
7. **Other data:**
   A. This test is often used to accompany a negative radioallergosorbent test (RAST) to assess for reactivity to untested allergens.
   B. A newer serum test under investigation to determine its sensitivity is the multiple antigen simultaneous test (MAST), which can simultaneously detect allergies to up to 3.5 allergens in one serum sample.
   C. See also *Allergen-specific IgE antibody, Serum; Skin test for hypersensitivity, Diagnostic.*

ALLERGEN-SPECIFIC IgE ANTIBODY (RAST TEST, RADIOALLERGOSORBENT TEST, ALLERGY SCREEN), SERUM

Norm. Negative.

ImmunoCAP FEIA method. <0.35 kU/L.

Pharmacia CAP system:

	ASYMPTOMATIC CLIENTS	SYMPTOMATIC ALLERGY
Perennial allergens	≤10.7 kU/L	>10.7 kU/L
Seasonal allergens	≤8.4 kU/L	>8.4 kU/L
All allergens	≤11.7 kU/L	>11.7 kU/L

Results Reported by Allergen Scores on 0-4 Scale:

0	No IgE detected
1	Borderline
2-4	Increasing levels of IgE

Modified RAST

CLASS	COUNTS	SIGNIFICANCE
	0-749	No specific IgE activity
1	750-1600	Borderline activity
2	1601-3600	Low positive
3	3601-8000	Moderate positive
4	8001-18,000	High positive
5	18,001-40,000	Very high positive
6	>40,000	Extreme high positive

Usage. Helps with differential diagnosis of allergies (especially food allergies of the immediate type), atopic asthma, natural rubber latex allergies, psoriasis, and monitoring of treatment for specific allergies.

Description. This test measures the amount of IgE directed against specific allergens by binding a specific antigen to a carrier substance and allowing it to react with a specific IgE antibody in the client's blood sample. The amount of bound IgE is then measured. The test is used to identify allergies to foods, grasses, weeds, trees, molds, epidermals, insects, and miscellaneous substances such as house dust, insulin, latex, and silk. An advantage of this test is that one can obtain the information without causing an allergic reaction because the allergen is introduced into the blood sample rather than into the body.

Professional Considerations
1. Consent form NOT required.
2. Preparation:
   A. Tube: Red topped, red/gray topped, or gold topped.
3. Procedure:
   A. Draw a 2-mL blood sample.
4. Postprocedure care:
   A. Transport the specimen to the laboratory for immediate spinning, serum separation, and refrigeration of serum.
5. Client and family teaching:
   A. Results may take several days.
6. Factors that affect results:
   A. IgE levels are influenced by the nature of the allergen, length of exposure to the allergen, symptomatic responses, and hyposensitization treatments.
   B. Results are invalidated if the client received radioactive dyes within 7 days before the test.
   C. False-positive results may be caused by high IgE levels (>3000 U/mL) attributable to parasitic infection.
7. Other data:
   A. This test correlates 80-85% with subcutaneous skin testing and is more specific.
   B. A total IgE level should also be obtained. If the RAST test is negative but total IgE level is ele-

vated, the allergen may not be one for which the RAST test can be used.
   C. The oral challenge test (OCT) is still the standard of critical comparison often used in the diagnosis of food allergy according to a 1994 study by Roger et al.
   D. See also *Allergen-specific IgE, Serum; Skin test for hypersensitivity, Diagnostic.*

ALLERGY SCREEN
(see Allergin-specific IgE antibody, Serum)

ALLERGY SKIN TEST
(see Skin test for hypersensitivity, Diagnostic)

ALPHA₁-ANTITRYPSIN, SERUM

Norm. 80-260 mg/dL (0.8-2.6 g/L, SI units).

Increased. Alzheimer's disease, cholangiocarcinoma, emphysema, hepatitis, hepatocholangiocarcinoma, hyaline membrane disease, hypercholesterolemia, infection, inflammation (acute, chronic), liver disease (chronic), neoplasm, pregnancy, sepsis, systemic lupus erythematosus, and ulcerative colitis. Drugs include estrogens, oral contraceptives, and steroids.

Decreased. Congenital alpha₁-antitrypsin deficiency, chronic obstructive pulmonary disease, emphysema, and liver disease (chronic) and in newborns (transient).

Description. A major faction of alpha₁-globulin protein detected by serum protein immunoelectrophoresis. Alpha₁-antitrypsin functions in protection of body fluids by preventing release of protease by dying cells. The test is used to screen for clients at high risk for emphysema and liver disease associated with a congenital absence of the protein. Other uses for this test include nonspecific detection of inflammatory, infectious, and necrotic processes.

Professional Considerations
1. Consent form NOT required.
2. **Preparation:**
   A. Tube: Red topped, red/gray topped, or gold topped.
   B. See *Client and family teaching*.
3. **Procedure:**
   A. Draw a 1-mL blood sample.
4. **Postprocedure care:**
   A. Freeze the specimen.

5. **Client and family teaching:**
   A. The client with hypercholesterolemia or hyperlipemia should fast 8-10 hours.
   B. Results are normally available within 24 hours.
6. **Factors that affect results:**
   A. Reject hemolyzed specimens.
7. **Other data:**
   A. Levels may also be measured in amniotic fluid.

ALPHA-FETOPROTEIN (AFP), BLOOD

Norm. Tumor marker <8.5 ng/mL

		SI UNITS
Nonpregnant Female	0-10 ng/mL	0-10 µg/L
Pregnant		
2 months	<75 ng/mL	<75 µg/L
3 months	<130 ng/mL	<130 µg/L
4 months	<210 ng/mL	<210 µg/L
5 months	<300 ng/mL	<300 µg/L
6 months	<400 ng/mL	<400 µg/L
7 months	<450 ng/mL	<450 µg/L
8 months	<450 ng/mL	<450 µg/L
9 months	<400 ng/mL	<400 µg/L
Immediately postpartum	<375 ng/mL	<375 µg/L
Adult Males	0-10 ng/mL	0-10 µg/L
Children	0-30 ng/mL	0-30 µg/L
Full-term infant	41,687 ng/mL	41,687 µg/L
Premature infant	158,125 ng/mL	158,125 µg/L
180-720 days of life	87 ng/mL	87 µg/L
2-year-old child	8 ng/mL	8 µg/L

Increased. Ataxia telangiectasia, cirrhosis, gonadal teratoblastoma, cancer (embryonal, hepatoblastoma, hepatocellular, lung, pancreatic with liver metastases, malignant teratoma of ovary or testes, gastric with liver metastases, biliary system, germ cell tumors), hemangioendothelioma, hepatitis (acute, chronic, neonatal), liver metastasis from gastric cancer, pregnancy (with fetal neural tube defects, multiple fetuses, fetal distress, fetal death, intrauterine death, duodenal atresia, omphalocele), pure seminoma, spontaneous abortion, spontaneous preterm birth in pregnant women 24-28 weeks of gestation, tetralogy of Fallot (or Turner syndrome), tyrosinemia, and ulcerative colitis.

Decreased. Has been associated with Down syndrome when less than 0.25 times the normal median, associated with high birth weight with very low second-trimester levels.

Description. A globulin protein secreted by liver cells during hepatic cell multiplication and found in high amounts in fetal plasma. Highest adult amounts are found during pregnancy and in primary hepatic cancer. Maternal levels should be measured initially at 15-18 weeks of gestation as a screening method for fetal neural tube defects. Confirmatory testing (for levels greater than 0.5-2.5 times the normal median) should be repeated in 7 days. For positive confirmatory test, ultrasonography and amniotic fluid AFP measurement should be performed.

Professional Considerations
1. Consent form NOT required.
2. **Preparation:**

A. Tube: Red topped, red/gray topped, or gold topped.
B. List on the laboratory requisition: maternal weight, maternal race, week of gestation, and any history of diabetes mellitus.
3. **Procedure:**
A. Draw a 1-mL blood sample from the mother.
4. **Postprocedure care:**
A. Apply a dry, sterile dressing over the amniocentesis site.
5. **Client and family teaching:**
A. Results may take several days.
6. **Factors that affect results:**
A. Normal levels are affected by the mother's age, weight, and number of fetuses present.
B. Reject hemolyzed specimens.
C. Results are invalid if the client has undergone a radioisotope scan within the previous 2 weeks.
7. **Other data:**
A. AFP testing may also be performed on amniotic fluid to detect neurologic congenital defects and Down syndrome.

Serum AFP measurement is believed to increase accuracy of antenatal detection of Down syndrome from 35% to 67%, but its accuracy can be affected by maternal weight, smoking history, and diabetes mellitus and by whether the gestational age of the fetus is correctly estimated.
B. AFP is not a screening test for cancer.
C. AFP is insensitive for the diagnosis of hepatocellular carcinoma in African-Americans.

ALT
(see Alanine aminotransferase, Serum)

ALTERNATE PATHWAY FACTOR B, SERUM
(see C3 proactivator, Serum)

AMA
(see Antimitochondrial antibody, Blood)

AMIKACIN SULFATE, BLOOD

Norm:

		SI UNITS
Therapeutic peak	20-25 mg/L or µg/mL	34-43 µmol/L
Toxic peak	>35 mg/L or µg/mL	>60 µmol/L
Therapeutic trough	5-10 mg/L or µg/mL	9-17 µmol/L
Toxic trough (adult)	>10 mg/L or µg/mL	>17 µmol/L
Toxic trough (child)	>5 ng/mL	>9 µmol/L

Toxic Level Symptoms and Treatment

Symptoms. Ototoxicity, nephrotoxicity.

Treatment:
Note: Treatment choices depend on client history and condition and episode history.
Stop drug.
Monitor amikacin levels.
Serum BUN and creatinine every day.
Eighth cranial nerve assessments every day.
Both hemodialysis and peritoneal dialysis WILL remove amikacin.

Increased. Aminoglycoside toxicity and impaired renal function.

Decreased. Subtherapeutic levels in client treated with aminoglycoside.

Description. Amikacin is a semisynthetic aminoglycoside antibiotic derived from kanamycin and effective against gram-negative and gram-positive organisms. It is excreted by glomerular filtration, with a half-life of 1.9-2.8 hours. Peak and trough levels should be monitored throughout therapy. Toxicity is possible at trough levels. Steady-state levels are reached after 10-15 hours. Effective in the treatment of ventilator-associated pneumonia and gram-positive bacteremia in childhood.

Professional Considerations
1. Consent form NOT required.
2. Preparation:
   A. Tube: Red topped, red/gray topped, or gold topped.
   B. Do NOT draw during hemodialysis.
   C. Write the time, dose, and route of the most recent dose on the laboratory requisition.
3. Procedure:
   A. Draw a 1-mL blood sample.
4. Postprocedure care:
   A. None.
5. Client and family teaching:
   A. Results are normally available within 24 hours.
6. Factors that affect results:
   A. Cross-reactivity may occur with concomitant antibiotic therapy (cephalosporin, chloramphenicol, clindamycin, kanamycin, penicillin, tetracycline, tobramycin).
7. Other data:
   A. Potentially nephrotoxic, irreveribly ototoxic, and neurotoxic.
   B. Creatinine clearance should be monitored every day for clients receiving amikacin.
   C. Hypoalbuminemia correlates strongly with amikacin nephrotoxicity.

AMINO ACID SCREEN, BLOOD
(*see Dinitrophenylhydrazine test, Diagnostic*)

AMINOPHYLLINE, BLOOD
(*see Theophylline, Blood*)

AMIODARONE, PLASMA OR SERUM

Norm. Negative.

		SI UNITS
Therapeutic level	0.5-2.5 µg/mL	0.8-3.9 µmol/L
Panic level	>2.5 µg/mL	>3.9 µmol/L

For samples tested >24 hours after collection, see *Factors that affect results.*

Panic Level Symptoms and Treatment

Symptoms. Bronchial asthma, heart failure, hepatic dysfunction, hyponatremia, jaundice, pulmonary fibrosis (irreversible), syndrome of inappropriate antidiuretic hormone, thyrotoxicosis.

Treatment:
Note: Treatment choice(s) depend on client history and condition and episode history.
Respiratory and hemodynamic support.
Discontinue medication.
Continuous ECG monitoring to identify reappearing dysrhythmias and bradycardia.
Transcutaneous pacemaker (prophylactically for sinus arrest).
Induce emesis (cautiously) with syrup of ipecac if soon after ingestion. Tap water or warm saline lavage may be added.
Administer activated charcoal, saline or sorbitol cathartic.
Hemodialysis and peritoneal dialysis will NOT remove amiodarone.

Usage. Monitoring for therapeutic levels during amiodarone therapy.

Description. Amiodarone is a fat-soluble, Class III antidysrhythmic, with several mechanisms of action, including (weak) negative inotropic activity coupled with compensatory vasodilatation, prolongation of cardiac tissue refractory period, depression of sinus node automaticity, and slowing of atrioventricular node conduction. It is used to treat clients with a history of life-threatening dysrhythmias that are not controllable by other drugs and after a myocardial infarction for symptomatic or sustained ventricular dysrhythmias. Because amiodarone is fat soluble, with a long half-life, it takes up to 4 weeks to reach steady-state levels and will remain in the fat-storage sites of the body long after it is discontinued. Amiodarone is metabolized and excreted primarily by the liver. This drug's potentially life-threatening side effects (acute hepatitis, pulmonary toxicity, bronchiolitis obliterans, pulmonary fibrosis) necessitate close monitoring of blood levels as well as clear and specific client teaching about side effects.

Professional Considerations
1. Consent form NOT required.
2. **Preparation:**
   A. Tube: Red topped, red/gray topped, or gold topped.
   B. MAY be drawn during hemodialysis.
3. **Procedure:**
   A. Draw the specimen before the dose, or at least 12 hours after the last dose.
   B. Draw a 1-mL blood sample.
4. **Postprocedure care:**
   A. None.
5. **Client and family teaching:**
   A. Results may not be available for several days.

B. If activated charcoal was given for elevated levels, the client should drink 4-6 glasses of water each day for 2 days to prevent constipation. Activated charcoal will also cause stools to be black for a few days.
6. **Factors that affect results:**
   A. Height and weight have not been shown to affect plasma concentrations.
   B. Amiodarone levels in stored specimens decrease over time. One study recommends the following correction factors for stored values:

Time Sample Stored Before Testing	Correction Factor
24 hours	Add 8% to obtained value
48 hours	Add 16% to obtained value
72 hours	Add 19% to obtained value
7 days	Add 23% to obtained value
14 days	Add 32% to obtained value

7. **Other data:**
   A. Amiodarone minor side effects include (usually reversible) corneal and skin micro deposits of the drug, causing grayish coloring of the sclera and skin, photosensitivity, and neuromuscular weakness. Side effects may take several months to appear.
   B. Any concurrent digoxin dose should be reduced during amiodarone therapy.
   C. Increases in serum creatinine may be related to the drug itself.

AMITRIPTYLINE
(see Tricyclic antidepressants, Plasma or serum)

AMMONIA (NH₃), BLOOD AND URINE

Norm. Norms vary by specific laboratory.

		SI UNITS
Plasma		
Adult	15-45 µg/dL	11-32 µmol/L
Newborn	90-150 µg/dL	64-107 µmol/L
First 2 weeks	79-129 µg/dL	56-92 µmol/L
Child	40-80 µg/dL	28-57 µmol/L

Continued

AMMONIA, BLOOD AND URINE—cont'd

		SI UNITS
Urine		
Spot	36-750 µg/dL	20-500 µmol/L
24-hour		
Adult	140-1500 mg/N/24 hours	10-107 mmol/N/24 hours
Infant	560-2900 mg/N/24 hours	40-207 mmol/N/24 hours

ARTERIAL BLOOD IN UREMIC PERSONS

Adult before hemodialysis	98.32 mg/dL
Adult after hemodialysis	63.18 mg/dL

VENOUS BLOOD IN UREMIC PERSONS

Adult before hemodialysis	71.70 mg/dL
Adult after hemodialysis	58.05 mg/dL

Hepatic Encephalopathy Symptoms and Treatment

Symptoms. (Symptoms do not correlate well with blood levels.) Asterixis, ataxia, coma, confusion, drowsiness, seizures, sluggish speech, somnolence, stupor.

Treatment:

Note: Treatment choice(s) depend on client history and condition and episode history.

Lactulose nasogastrically or rectally. Both hemodialysis and peritoneal dialysis WILL remove NH_3.

Increased. Alzheimer's, azotemia, carbamoyl phosphate synthetase I deficiency (CPSID), cirrhosis, coma (diabetic, hepatic), congestive heart failure, erythroblastosis fetalis, esophageal varices (hemorrhagic), exercise, hepatic encephalopathy, hepatitis (acute), pneumonia, portacaval shunt, premature infant (with neurologic abnormalities), Reye syndrome, and shock. Drugs include acetazolamide, ammonium salts, asparaginase, chlorothiazide, heparin calcium, heparin sodium, methicillin sodium, neomycin, thiazide diuretics, urea, and valproic acid.

Decreased. Hypertension (essential, malignant) and renal failure.

Description. Ammonia is a waste product from nitrogen breakdown during protein metabolism. It is metabolized by the liver and excreted by the kidneys as urea. Elevated levels caused by hepatic dysfunction may lead to encephalopathy.

Professional Considerations
1. Consent form NOT required.
2. **Preparation:**
   A. Tube: Refrigerated gray topped, lavender topped, or heparinized green topped.
   B. Do NOT draw during hemodialysis.
   C. See *Client and family teaching.*
   D. Notify laboratory personnel that a blood sample for ammonia level will be arriving.
3. **Procedure:** Samples should preferably be taken from arterial or earlobe capillary blood because ammonia metabolism in muscle causes increased levels in venous blood.
   A. *Arterial sampling:* Draw a 1-mL blood specimen.
   B. *Capillary sampling:* Using a lancet, completely fill a capillary tube with blood from the earlobe.
   C. *Venous sampling:* Leaving a tourniquet in place no more than 15 seconds, draw a 1-mL blood specimen. If a syringe is used for blood collection, uncap the tube and transfer the blood into it without using the needle. Tilt the tube back and forth to mix the contents.
4. **Postprocedure care:**
   A. Place the specimen in an ice-water bath.

B. Transport the specimen to the laboratory immediately.
5. **Client and family teaching:**
   A. Fast, except for water, and refrain from smoking for 8-10 hours before sampling.
   B. Avoid stress and strenuous exercise for several hours before sampling.
6. **Factors that affect results:**
   A. Green-topped tubes containing ammonium-heparin should not be used.

B. Reject hemolyzed specimens.
C. A delay in processing the specimen may cause falsely elevated results.
D. A high-protein diet may increase levels.
7. **Other data:**
   A. Ammonia levels are NOT reliable indicators of impending hepatic coma.
   B. Liver transplant corrects hyperammonemia.

AMNIOCENTESIS AND AMNIOTIC FLUID ANALYSIS, DIAGNOSTIC

Routine Analysis
Color: Colorless, straw-colored, or clear to milky.

		SI UNITS
Acetylcholinesterase	Negative	
Alpha$_1$-fetoprotein:		
12 weeks of gestation	≤42 µg/mL	
14 weeks of gestation	≤35 µg/mL	
16 weeks of gestation	≤29 µg/mL	
18 weeks of gestation	≤20 µg/mL	
20 weeks of gestation	≤18 µg/mL	
22 weeks of gestation	≤14 µg/mL	
30 weeks of gestation	≤3 µg/mL	
35 weeks of gestation	≤2 µg/mL	
40 weeks of gestation	≤1 µg/mL	
Normal values may also be reported in multiples of the median (MOM) or 0.5-3.0 MOM.		
Bilirubin:		
Trimesters 1 and 2	≤0.074 mg/dL	≤1.2 µmol/L
40 weeks of gestation	≤0.024 mg/dL	≤0.4 µmol/L
Calcium	4 mEq/L	4 mmol/L
Carbon dioxide	16 mEq/L	16 mmol/L
Chloride	102 mEq/L	102 mmol/L
Creatinine:		
≤27 weeks of gestation	0.8-1.1 mg/dL	72-99 µmol/L
30-34 weeks of gestation	1.1-1.8 mg/dL	99-162 µmol/L
35-40 weeks of gestation	1.8-4.0 mg/dL	162-360 µmol/L
Estriol:		
Trimesters 1 and 2	≤9 µg/dL	≤309 nmol/L
Term	≤59 µg/dL	≤2023 nmol/L
Glucose	30 mg/dL	2 mmol/L
Lecithin:		
<35 weeks of gestation	6-9 mg/dL	
≥35 weeks of gestation	15-20 mg/dL	
Lecithin/sphingomyelin (L/S) ratio:		
Immaturity	≤1.5	
Borderline maturity	1.6-1.9	
Maturity	2.0-4.0	
After maturity	≥4.1	
Meconium	Negative	
pH:		
Trimesters 1 and 2	7.12-7.38	7.12-7.38
Term	6.91-7.43	6.91-7.43
Potassium	4.9 mEq/L	4.9 mmol/L
Sodium	133 mEq/L	133 mmol/L

		SI UNITS
Sphingomyelin	4-6 mg/dL	
Total protein	2.5 g/dL	25 g/L
Urea:		
Trimesters 1 and 2	12-24 mg/dL	
Term	19-42 mg/dL	
Uric acid:		
Trimesters 1 and 2	2.76-4.68 mg/dL	0.17-0.28 mmol/L
Term	7.67-12.13 mg/dL	0.46-0.72 mmol/L

ABNORMALITIES THAT MAY BE FOUND ON ROUTINE ANALYSIS

Abnormal Color	Possible Cause
Yellow	Caused by fetal bilirubin, erythroblastosis fetalis
Green	Caused by meconium, breech presentation, fetal death, defecation, distress, hypoxia, intrauterine growth retardation, status post maturity, vagal stimulation
Red	Caused by presence of blood, intrauterine hemorrhage
Port wine	Acute fetal distress, abruptio placentae
Brown	Oxidized hemoglobin, maternal tissue trauma, fetal death, fetal maceration

			SI UNITS
Abnormal Bilirubin			
Fetal involvement	0.10-0.28 mg/dL	= 1 +	1.6-4.5 μmol/L
Later fetal involvement	0.29-0.36 mg/dL	= 2 +	4.7-5.8 μmol/L
Fetal distress	0.47-0.95 mg/dL	= 3 +	7.6-15.4 μmol/L
Fetal death	>0.95 mg/dL	= 4 +	>15.4 μmol/L

		SI UNITS
Abnormal Creatinine		
35-40 weeks of gestation:		
Large muscle mass, possible diabetes	>2 mg/dL	>180 μmol/L
Low birth weight	<2 mg/dL	<180 μmol/L

Increased Alpha$_1$-fetoprotein. Anencephaly, cleft lip and palate, cystic fibrosis, duodenal atresia, esophageal atresia, fetal bladder neck obstruction with hydronephrosis, fetal death, meningomyelocele, multiple pregnancy, nephrosis (congenital), neural tube defects, spina bifida, omphalocele, and Turner syndrome.

Increased Bilirubin. Anencephaly, erythroblastosis fetalis, hemolytic disease of the newborn, hydrops fetalis, intestinal obstruction, and Rh sensitization.

Increased Lamellar Bodies in Amniotic Fluid. Respiratory distress syndrome.

Positive Acetylcholinesterase. Neural tube abnormalities that allow cerebrospinal fluid (which contains acetylcholinesterase) to leak into the amniotic sac.

Positive Meconium. Fetal distress.

Decreased Alpha$_1$-fetoprotein. Not applicable.

Decreased Bilirubin. Not clinically significant.

Decreased Creatinine. Fetal lung immaturity.

Chromosome Analysis. Interpretation required.

Description. Detection of fetal jeopardy or genetic disease and determination of fetal maturity. *Amniocentesis* is a 20- to 30-minute procedure in which an aspiration of amniotic fluid is taken transabdominally and usually performed after week 12 of gestation. In routine analysis, amniotic fluid is examined for levels of calcium, chloride, carbon dioxide, creatinine, estriol, glucose, pH, potassium, sodium, protein, urea, uric acid, and culture and for genetic defects, chromosomal studies, detection of fetal jeopardy or distress (by color, bilirubin) and to measure lung maturity (by L/S ratio) and age (by creatinine of the fetus). *Alpha₁-fetoprotein* is a globulin protein secreted by the yolk sac and by fetal liver cells during hepatic cell multiplication. The highest amounts are found during pregnancy and in hepatic cancer. Measurement is usually performed from week 16 to 20 to help identify fetal neural abnormalities, gastroesophageal atresia, and nephrosis. *Chromosome analysis* of amniotic fluid cells is performed by examination of karyotyped cells for genetic abnormalities such as Down syndrome, Tay-Sachs disease, and other inborn errors of metabolism. Amniotic fluid is examined for color and bilirubin level for detection of fetal jeopardy or distress caused by hemolysis of fetal red blood cells. Erythroblastosis fetalis occurs when maternal antibodies attack fetal red blood cells, causing fetal anemia. This occurs when the mother's blood contains the Rh factor that reacts with fetal erythrocyte antigens. The test is usually performed at gestation week 24 or later and can help determine the need for intrauterine fetal blood transfusion. After the 35th week of pregnancy, the phospholipid levels of lecithin and sphingomyelin change in a predictable pattern that indicates the level of maturity of fetal lungs. Lecithin rises and sphingomyelin decreases as the fetal lungs mature.

Professional Considerations
1. Consent form IS required.

Risks
Bleeding, intrauterine death, premature labor, spontaneous abortion.

Contraindications
Abruptio placentae, incompetent cervix, placenta previa, and a history of premature labor.

2. **Preparation:**
   A. Obtain an amniocentesis tray, surgical scrub solution, a light-protected container, and povidone-iodine solution. Also obtain RhoGAM for Rh-negative mothers.
   B. Obtain maternal vital signs. Auscultate baseline fetal heart tones.
   C. Note the estimated date of conception and week of gestation on the laboratory requisition.
   D. Procedure should be performed in a darkened room if the specimen will be tested for bilirubin.
   E. See *Client and family teaching.*
3. **Procedure:**
   A. The position of the fetus and a pocket of amniotic fluid are determined using ultrasound and palpation, with the mother in a supine position.
   B. The mother's abdominal area is cleansed with surgical scrub solution and povidone-iodine and allowed to dry.
   C. The aspiration site is draped to demarcate a sterile field.
   D. The mother is instructed to place her hands behind her head, and the aspiration site is anesthetized with 1 mL of 1% or 2% lidocaine intradermally and subcutaneously.
   E. A 20- to 22-gauge, 5-inch-long spinal needle with a stylet is inserted through the abdominal wall into the intrauterine cavity, and the stylet is withdrawn.
   F. About 7-15 mL of amniotic fluid is aspirated through the spinal needle into a syringe, and the needle is withdrawn. Use a 20-mL amniotic fluid sample for direct genetic analysis for the four most common mutations responsible for Tay Sachs disease.
4. **Postprocedure care:**
   A. Apply a dry sterile dressing to the aspiration site.
   B. Inject 2-5 mL of amniotic fluid into a light-protected (foil-covered or amber) test tube to test for bilirubin. Inject 5-10 mL of amniotic fluid into a sterile, siliconized glass container or a polystyrene container for culture and genetic and other studies (AFP). Specimens to be transported to another site for testing should be packed in a cool, insulated container to maintain a temperature of 2°-5°C.

Freezing temperatures should be avoided.

C. Obtain the mother's vital signs. Auscultate fetal heart tones for changes from the baseline value.

D. The mother should rest on her right side for 15-20 minutes after the procedure.

E. RhoGAM may be prescribed for Rh-negative mothers.

F. Transport the amniotic fluid specimen to the laboratory immediately and refrigerate.

5. **Client and family teaching:**

A. Empty your bladder immediately before the procedure if gestation is 21 weeks or more. You must have a full bladder during the procedure if gestation is 20 weeks or less.

B. It is important to lie motionless throughout the procedure. You may experience a strong contraction with the needle insertion.

C. Chromosome analysis results may take up to 4 weeks.

D. After the procedure, notify the physician for cramping, abdominal pain, unusual vaginal drainage/fluid loss, fever, chills, dizziness, or more or less than the usual amount of fetal activity.

E. Inform the client with abnormal genetic findings of choices regarding pregnancy and pregnancy termination. Also refer the client for genetic counseling before future attempts to become pregnant.

6. **Factors that affect results:**

A. Reject frozen or clotted specimens.

B. Inadvertent aspiration of maternal urine can be ruled out by testing the specimen for blood urea nitrogen (BUN) and creatinine. Urine BUN is >100 mg/dL, whereas amniotic fluid is well under 100 mg/dL. Urine creatinine is usually >80 mg/dL, whereas amniotic fluid creatinine is usually ≤4 mg/dL.

C. Nonsiliconized glass containers for routine analysis may result in cell adherence on the sides of the container.

D. Amniotic fluid testing must be performed within 3 days of collection.

E. Amniocentesis should be performed between weeks 24 and 28 when one is checking for hemolytic disease of the newborn and Rh sensitization.

F. Falsely low bilirubin levels may result from failure to protect the specimen from light.

G. Specimens contaminated with blood should be tested for fetal hemoglobin to determine whether the blood is of maternal or fetal origin. Fetal blood contamination results in falsely high bilirubin levels. Fetal or maternal blood will interfere with measurements of fetal lung maturity and amniotic fluid constituents that are also constituents of plasma, such as protein, potassium, and glucose.

H. Creatinine levels are affected by maternal creatinine clearance and maternal creatinine levels. A concurrent maternal serum creatinine should be drawn. Maternal serum to amniotic fluid creatinine should be about 2:1.

I. Elevated AFP results may be caused by contamination of the specimen with fetal blood.

J. Small and closed neural tube defects may not cause elevated AFP levels.

K. Accurate L/S ratio measurement is not possible if the specimen is contaminated with blood (fetal or maternal) or meconium.

7. Other data:

A. Direct karyotyping of placental villi samples obtained by needle aspiration has been found to yield faster results than amniotic fluid chromosome analysis. (See *Chorionic villi sampling, Diagnostic*.)

B. Chromosomal aberration has been found in 4.6% of fetuses in women over 38 years of age, the most common being trisomy 21 (62%), Klinefelter syndrome (11%), and Edward syndrome (trisomy 18) (11%).

C. For diamniotic twin pregnancies, each amniotic sac should be sampled.

D. Early amniocentesis is feasible from 11 weeks of gestation and can be performed for the usual indications as an alternative to chorionic villus sampling. Results are available in less than 1 week using cytogenetic techniques.

E. Prenatal cystic fibrosis profile may be performed by polymerase chain reaction (PCR) for mutations (F508, R553X, g551D, g542X, n1303K, and w1282X).

F. Amniotic fluid neuron-specific enolase is useful as a marker for neonatal neurologic injury.

G. Amniotic fluid in the third trimester can be obtained to measure insulin levels in women with gestational diabetes mellitus.

AMNIOTIC FLUID, ALPHA$_1$-FETOPROTEIN, SPECIMEN
(see Amniocentesis and amniotic fluid analysis, Diagnostic)

AMNIOTIC FLUID, CHROMOSOME ANALYSIS, SPECIMEN
(see Amniocentesis and amniotic fluid analysis, Diagnostic)

AMNIOTIC FLUID, ERYTHROBLASTOSIS FETALIS, SPECIMEN
(see Amniocentesis and amniotic fluid analysis, Diagnostic)

AMNIOTIC FLUID ANALYSIS, SPECIMEN
(see Amniocentesis and amniotic fluid analysis, Diagnostic)

AMOXAPINE
(see Tricyclic antidepressants, Plasma or serum)

AMPHETAMINES, BLOOD

Norm. Negative.

| DRUG | NORMAL RANGES DURING THERAPY | | | SI UNITS |
	ng/mL	µg/mL	mg/L	nmol/L
Amphetamine sulfate	20-120	0.02-0.12		150-900
Toxic level	>200		>2	>1500
Chlorphentermine	100-400	0.10-0.40		750-3000
Diethylpropion	1-10	0.001-0.010		7.5-75
Ephedrine	50-100	0.05-0.10		375-750
Fenfluramine	30-300	0.03-0.30		225-2250
Methamphetamine	10-50	0.01-0.05		75-375
Toxic level	>500		>5	>3750
p-Methoxyamphetamine	<200	<0.2		<1500
Methylenedioxy-amphetamine	<400	< 0.4		<3000
Toxic level	>400		>4	>3000
Phendimetrazine	30-250	0.03-0.25		225-1875
Phenmetrazine	60-250	0.06-0.25		450-1875
Toxic level	>400		>4	>3000
Phentermine	30-90	0.03-0.09		225-675
Phenylpropanolamine	50-100	0.05-0.10		375-750
Tranylcypromine	10-100	0.01-0.10		75-750

Toxic Levels Symptoms and Treatment

Symptoms. Psychoses, tremors, convulsions, insomnia, tachycardia, dysrhythmias, impotence, cerebrovascular accident, and respiratory collapse.

Treatment:

Note: Treatment choice(s) depend on client history and condition and episode history.

1. Use gastric lavage or induce vomiting (with extreme caution) if within 4 hours of ingestion. (Induction of vomiting is contraindicated in clients with no gag reflex or with central nervous system depression or excitation.)
2. Give a slurry of activated charcoal 1 g/kg (minimum 30 g), followed by a magnesium citrate cathartic.
3. Amphetamine excretion may be accelerated by acidification of the urine with ammonium chloride 1-2 g intravenously or ascorbic acid 0.5-1.5 g orally every 4-6 hours to keep urine pH <5.5.
4. Increase fluids to keep urine output at 3-6 mL/kg/hour.
5. Consider using mannitol or furosemide to force diuresis (efficacy of acid diuresis has not been clearly established).
6. Both hemodialysis and peritoneal dialysis WILL remove amphetamines.
7. Barbiturates may counteract amphetamine stimulant effects and chlorpromazine (Thorazine) may help control the symptoms of an overstimulated central nervous system.

Increased. Stimulant drug abuse or use.

Description. Amphetamines are sympathomimetic amines that act on the cortex and reticular activating system of the brain to stimulate the release and block the reabsorption of norepinephrine and dopamine. They cause mood elevation and wakefulness and decrease the perception of fatigue through stimulation of the heart and central nervous system. They are rapidly absorbed from the gastrointestinal tract and reach all tissues but concentrate in the central nervous system and are excreted by the

kidneys. Half-lives vary depending on the individual drug. Synonyms include bennies, crystal, ice, pep pills, speed, uppers, and wake-ups. Side effects include multiple visceral aneurysms, cognitive deficits, hypertension, hyponatremia, jaw clenching, lack of appetite, loss of sexual interest, impaired gait, inability to concentrate, hepatic toxicity, memory problems, renal failure, and disseminated intravascular coagulation (DIC) (especially from MDMA/ecstasy). Blood amphetamine levels are used for monitoring the appropriateness of dosage regimen and for detection of amphetamine abuse.

Professional Considerations
1. Consent form NOT required.
2. Preparation:
   A. Tube: Lavender topped.
   B. Assess for a history of drug abuse.
   C. Do NOT draw during hemodialysis.
3. Procedure:
   A. Draw a 5-mL blood sample.
4. Postprocedure care:
   A. None.
5. Client and family teaching:
   A. Results are normally available within 4 hours.
   B. If activated charcoal was given for elevated levels, drink 4-6 glasses of water each day for 2 days to prevent constipation. Activated charcoal will also cause stools to be black for a few days.
   C. Referrals to appropriate rehabilitation centers and therapeutic community programs should be offered to all addicted clients.
6. Factors that affect results:
   A. High concentrations of beta-phenethylamine, a blood product formed from the decomposition of protein, may mask a low amphetamine level.
7. Other data:
   A. Toxicity in children occurs over a wide range of doses.
   B. Abrupt discontinuation may cause psychotic symptoms.
   C. See also *Toxicology drug screen, Blood; Toxicology drug screen, Urine.*

AMPHOTERICIN B, BLOOD

Norm. Negative.

Therapeutic Levels. 1-2 µg/mL (1-2.2 µmol/L, SI units).

Potential toxicity beyond therapeutic levels.

Toxic Levels Symptoms and Treatment

Symptoms. Acute tubular necrosis, coagulopathies, hearing loss, hypotension, ventricular fibrillation, coagulopathies.

Treatment:
Note: Treatment choice(s) depend on client history and conditions and episode history.
Treat symptoms and provide supportive therapy as needed until levels decrease.
Prepare the client for the possibility of permanent loss of hearing or renal function.
Hemodialysis and peritoneal dialysis will NOT remove amphotericin significantly.

Usage. Evaluating serum level of amphotericin B and assessing for toxic levels in clients with fever, chills, nausea, or bone marrow suppression.

Description. A potent nephrotoxic antifungal antibiotic ineffective against bacteria, viruses, or rickettsias. Peak levels occur 60-120 minutes after intravenous administration; half-life is 24 hours. Over a 7-day period 40% is excreted in the urine. Effective to treat fungal keratitis, mucormycosis, and prototothecosis.

Professional Considerations
1. Consent form NOT required.
2. Preparation:
   A. Tube: Red topped, red/gray topped, or gold topped.
   B. Do NOT draw during hemodialysis.
3. Procedure:
   A. Draw a 5-mL blood sample.
4. Postprocedure care:
   A. None.
5. Client and family teaching:
   A. Results are normally available within 24 hours.
6. Factors that affect results:
   A. Draw the specimen from an extremity that does not have amphotericin B infusing into it.
7. Other data:
   A. Transfusing platelets at least 2 hours after amphotericin-B infusion has been completed decreases

the detrimental effects on transfused platelet recovery and survival.
   B. Rapid infusion of amphotericin-B can cause hyperkalemia.

AMSLER GRID TEST, DIAGNOSTIC

Norm. The lines are clearly visualized and appear straight. A black dot is visualized in the center of the grid. No distortions of the lines is seen. No blank spots are seen other than within each square.

Usage. Detection of macular edema, macular blind spots, scotoma.

Description. An optical screening test using a grid of intersecting lines with a black dot in the center. The visual acuity of the macular portion of the retina can be affected by macular edema, causing distortions of the lines, or by scotomas, causing blind spots, which make the grid appear to the client as having blank areas.

Professional Considerations
1. Consent form NOT required.
2. Preparation:
   A. Obtain an Amsler grid and an eye occluder (eye patch, hand held, or occluding eyeglasses).
3. Procedure:
   A. With one eye covered, have the client view the Amsler grid at his or her usual reading distance.
   B. Ask whether the black dot is visible, whether the complete square grid is visible when looking at the dot, whether the lines are perfectly straight, and whether any of the lines are blurred or look as though they are moving.
   C. Ask if there are any blank areas on the grid, other than within each square. Have the client draw what he or she sees if the answer to any of the questions is yes.
   D. Repeat the test for the other eye.
4. Postprocedure care:
   A. Refer the client to a specialist if necessary.
5. Client and family teaching:
   A. The test takes less than 30 minutes.
6. Factors that affect results:
   A. Performing this test before retinal examination with an ophthalmoscope and fundus examination or refraction test avoids falsely abnormal results caused by retinal

bleaching from the bright light or loss of focusing ability.
7. Other data:
   A. An abnormal test indicates the need for more specific testing such as fluorescein angiography.

B. Amsler grid reports have poor validity and cannot be accurately interpreted for use in the clinical diagnosis of retinal defects or overall ocular disease.

AMYLASE, SERUM AND URINE AND AMYLASE CLEARANCE

Norm:

URINE

Mayo clinic method	10-80 amylase U/hour
Somogyi method	26-950 U/24 hours
Beckman method	1-17 U/hour

SERUM		SI UNITS
Somogyi method	50-180 U/dL	92-330 U/L
Beckman method		20-125 U/L
Over 70 years of age		20-160 U/L
Panic level	Three times the upper limit of normal	

AMYLASE CLEARANCE	2%-5%
Macroamylasemia	Decreased (usually <1%) or normal clearance
Pancreatitis	Increased clearance

Increased. Abdominal aortic aneurysm (ruptured), acute exacerbation of chronic pancreatitis, ampulla of Vater obstruction, cerebral trauma, cholecystitis (acute), choledocholithiasis, common bile duct obstruction, diabetic ketoacidosis, ectopic pregnancy, empyema (gallbladder), fructose malabsorption, hyperthyroidism, intestinal obstruction with strangulation, intra-abdominal abscess, lung cancer, macroamylasemia, mesenteric thrombosis, mumps, pancreatic duct obstruction, pancreatic cancer, pancreatitis (acute), perforated intestine, perforated ulcer, peritonitis, salivary gland disease (acute, duct obstruction, suppurative inflammation), spasm of sphincter of Oddi, surgery (postoperative upper abdominal, peripancreatic), trauma (pancreas, spleen), tuberculosis. Drugs include aspirin, opiates, propofol, radiographic dyes, and thiazides. Herbs or natural remedies include *vinho abafado* (augmented Port wine, Brazil).

Decreased. Alcoholic liver disease, alcoholism, burns (severe), cachexia, cirrhosis, cystic fibrosis (advanced), hepatic abscess, hepatic cancer, hepatitis, pancreatic cancer, pancreatitis (acute fulminant, advanced chronic), poisoning, renal dysfunction, thyrotoxicosis (severe), and toxemia of pregnancy. Drugs include glucose and fluorides.

Description. An enzyme produced by the pancreas and salivary glands that aids digestion of complex carbohydrates. It is excreted by the kidneys. In acute pancreatitis, serum amylase starts rising at about 2 hours after the onset, peaks at about 24 hours, and returns to normal in 2-4 days after the onset. Urine amylase will be elevated from several hours after the onset until 7-10 days after the onset. Because urine amylase levels remain elevated longer than serum amylase levels do, they are useful for providing evidence of pancreatitis after serum amylase has returned to normal levels.

Amylase clearance is reported in a ratio in proportion to creatinine clearance. This amylase clearance–creatinine clearance ratio helps determine whether hypermacroamylasemia is secondary to pancreatitis (see norms).

Amylase clearance = (urine amylase concentration) × (serum creatinine concentration)/(serum amylase concentration) × (urine creatinine concentration)

Amylase rises and falls in tandem with lipase in acute pancreatitis but is a less specific marker than lipase for this condition.

Professional Considerations
1. Consent form NOT required.
2. **Preparation:**
   A. Obtain a urine container without preservatives, including toluene or acetic acid preservatives, in sizes as follows: 1-L size, 2- or 6-hour collection; 2-L size, 8- or 12-hour collection; 3-L size, 24-hour collection.
   B. Tube: Red topped, red/gray topped, or gold topped.
   C. List medications taken in the past 24 hours on the laboratory requisition.
   D. Screen client for the use of herbal preparations or natural remedies such as *vinho abafado*.
3. **Procedure:**
   A. Discard the first morning-voided urine specimen.
   B. Collect a timed urine specimen over 2, 6, 8, 12, or 24 hours in a refrigerated or iced container without preservatives or to which toluene or acetic acid has been added. For catheterized clients, keep the drainage bag on ice and empty the urine into the collection container hourly.
   C. Encourage fluid intake throughout the collection period if not contraindicated.
   D. For serum collection, draw a 1-mL sample at least 2 hours after a meal and before treatment has begun.
4. **Postprocedure care:**
   A. List the beginning and ending times of urine specimen collection on the laboratory requisition.
   B. Send the urine specimen to the laboratory and refrigerate.
5. **Client and family teaching:**
   A. For the urine test, save all urine voided in the 2-, 6-, 8-, 12-, or 24-hour period. Urinate before defecating to avoid loss of urine and to avoid contaminating the specimen with feces or toilet tissue. If any urine is accidentally discarded, discard the entire specimen and restart the collection the next day.
   B. Do not drink alcohol for 24 hours before sampling.
6. **Factors that affect results:**
   A. Urine amylase determinations should not be performed on females during menstruation.

B. Results reported in U/mL give an inaccurate picture because they are influenced by the varying urine volumes, depending on the length of the collection period.
C. Reject hemolyzed specimens.
D. Drugs that may falsely elevate results of serum amylase include aminosalicylic acid, asparaginase, azathioprine, bethanechol, bethanechol chloride, chloride salts, cholinergics, corticosteroids, corticotropin, cyproheptadine hydrochloride, ethacrynic acid, ethyl alcohol (large quantities), fluoride salts, furosemide, indomethacin, loop diuretics, mercaptopurine, methacholine, narcotic analgesics, oral contraceptives, pancreozymin, rifampin, sulfasalazine, and thiazide diuretics.
E. Falsely decreased results of serum amylase may be caused by citrates and oxalates.
F. Massive hemorrhagic pancreatic necrosis may cause so much pancreatic cell destruction that amylase cannot be produced, resulting in no elevation in serum amylase.
G. Contamination of the serum specimen with saliva will cause falsely elevated results.
H. Serum lipemia or hypertriglyceridemia may result in falsely low or spuriously normal serum amylase results.
I. Results are invalidated if the specimen is drawn <72 hours after cholecystography with radiopaque dyes.
J. Falsely high serum amylase results may be caused by renal failure.
K. There can be pronounced fluctuation in serum amylase, ranging from 115% to 1160% in clients with macroamylasemia, and this fluctuation may cause confusion in differentiating macroamylasemia from other causes of hyperamylasemia.
L. Baseline levels increase during pregnancy.
7. **Other data:**
   A. Macroamylasemia causes a high serum but normal urine amylase.
   B. Urine amylase does not produce falsely high results with renal failure as serum amylase does.
   C. Normal serum amylase may occur in pancreatitis, especially chronic pancreatitis and severe necrotizing pancreatitis.

ANA, SERUM
(see *Antinuclear antibody, Serum*)

ANAEROBIC CULTURE
(see *Body fluid, Anaerobic culture*)

ANCA, SERUM
(see *Antineutrophil cytoplasmic antibody screen, Serum*)

ANDROSTENEDIONE, SERUM

Norm:

		SI UNITS
Adult female	85-275 ng/dL	3.0-9.6 nmol/L
Postmenopausal	30-140 ng/dL	1.0-4.8 nmol/L
Adult male	70-205 ng/dL	2.6-7.2 nmol/L
Cord blood	30-150 ng/dL	1.0-5.2 nmol/L
Premature newborn	80-446 ng/dL	2.8-15.6 nmol/L
Newborn	20-290 ng/dL	0.7-10.1 nmol/L
Female children		
1-3 months	15-25 ng/dL	0.5-0.9 nmol/L
3-5 months	10-15 ng/dL	0.3-0.5 nmol/L
Male children		
1-3 months	20-45 ng/dL	0.7-1.6 nmol/L
3-5 months	10-40 ng/dL	0.3-1.4 nmol/L
Panic level (all ages)	>1000 ng/dL	>34.9 nmol/L

Usage. Nonspecific evaluation of androgen production in female hirsutism.

Increased. Alzheimer's, congenital adrenal hyperplasia, Cushing syndrome, hirsutism, recurrent miscarriages, Stein-Leventhal disease (polycystic ovarian disease), and tumor (adrenal, ovarian). Herbs or natural remedies include Siberian ginseng.

Decreased. Decreases with age in men and potential factor in pathogenesis of bone loss.

Description. A metabolite of dehydroepiandrosterone sulfate (DHEA-S) produced in the ovaries and the adrenal gland that is converted to testosterone in peripheral tissues. Peak levels occur in the early morning and low levels in the late afternoon. After puberty, levels rise and peak around 20 years of age. Elevation is one of several causes of female hirsutism, which is characterized by a male hair-growth pattern. Very elevated levels are suggestive of the presence of a virilizing tumor.

Professional Considerations
1. Consent form NOT required.
2. **Preparation:**
   A. Schedule the test at least 7 days before or after a female client's menstruation.
   B. Tube: Red topped, red/gray topped, or gold topped.
   C. Screen client for the use of herbal preparations or natural remedies, such as Siberian ginseng.
   D. See *Client and family teaching.*
3. **Procedure:**
   A. Draw a 2-mL blood sample. Draw between 0600 and 0900 for peak levels.
4. **Postprocedure care:**
   A. Place the specimen on ice.
   B. Transport the specimen to the laboratory immediately for spinning and freezing of serum.

5. Client and family teaching:
   A. Fast for 8 hours before sampling.
   B. Test must be drawn 1 week before or after menstruation to avoid falsely elevated values.
6. Factors that affect results:
   A. Results are invalidated if the client has undergone a scan involving radioactive dyes within 1 week before specimen collection.
7. Other data:
   A. Plasma levels do not correlate well with the severity of symptoms.
   B. Lymphocytes found in breast cancer tissue convert androstenedione.

ANGEL DUST
(see Phencyclidine, Qualitative, Urine)

ANGIOCARDIOGRAPHY PROCEDURE, DIAGNOSTIC
(see Cardiac catheterization, Diagnostic)

ANGIOGRAM (ANGIOGRAPHY), DIAGNOSTIC
(see Arteriogram, Cardiac catheterization, Cerebral angiogram, Pulmonary angiogram, or Renal angiogram, Diagnostic)

ANGIOGRAPHY, CEREBRAL CORONARY
(see Cerebral angiogram, Diagnostic)

ANGIOTENSIN-CONVERTING ENZYME (ACE), BLOOD

Norm:

		SI UNITS
Adults	13-25 kU/L	221-425 µKat/L
Clients under 19 years have higher ACE levels		

Increased. Arthritis (rheumatoid), bronchitis, cervical adenitis, cirrhosis (nonalcoholic), connective tissue disease, fungal diseases, Gaucher's disease, histoplasmosis, Hodgkin's disease, hypercalcemia, hyperthyroidism (untreated), Langerhans cell histiocytosis, leprosy, myeloma, non-Hodgkin's lymphoma, pulmonary embolus, pulmonary fibrosis, sarcoidosis (active), and scleroderma.

Decreased. Acute respiratory distress syndrome, coccidioidomycosis, diabetes mellitus, farmer's lung, hypothyroidism, pulmonary neoplasm (advanced), severe illness, and tuberculosis. Drugs include cadmium, captopril, estrogen (replacement therapy), L-arginine, and steroids.

Description. An enzyme found mainly in lung epithelial cells and in smaller amounts in blood vessels and renal tissue that converts angiotensin I to angiotensin II, a vasopressor that also stimulates the adrenal cortex to produce aldosterone. High levels of ACE are strongly correlated with pulmonary sarcoidosis.

Professional Considerations
1. Consent form NOT required.
2. Preparation:
   A. Write the client's age on the laboratory requisition.
   B. Tube: Red topped, red/gray topped, gold topped, or green topped.
   C. See *Client and family teaching.*
3. Procedure:
   A. Draw a 2-mL blood sample.
4. Postprocedure care:
   A. Transport the specimen to the laboratory immediately. Freeze the specimen and store it in dry ice if the test is not performed immediately.
5. Client and family teaching:
   A. Fast for 12 hours before sampling.
6. Factors that affect results:
   A. Reject hemolyzed or lipemic specimens.
   B. A delay in testing or failure to freeze the specimen if not tested immediately may cause falsely low results.
7. Other data:
   A. ACE is useful in evaluating the effectiveness of therapy and in confirming clinical status.

ANH
(see Natriuretic peptides, Plasma)

ANIMALS AND RABIES, SERUM
(see Fluorescent rabies antibody, Specimen)

ANIMALS AND RABIES NEGRI BODIES, BRAIN TISSUE, SPECIMEN

Norm. Negative.

Positive. Rabies.

Description. A postmortem histologic examination of the brain tissue of an animal suspected to have rabies, usually performed after the animal has bitten a human. Rabies produces Negri bodies, a specific and diagnostic lesion of the central nervous system that contains inclusion bodies in the cytoplasm of the nerve cells. Animal specimen examination is the only method to identify rabies because there is no laboratory or diagnostic test to identify the disease in humans until after symptoms appear (listed below). Diagnosis in humans is based on history and symptoms. Symptoms may appear 10 days to a year after the bite but more commonly appear in humans 2-8 weeks later.

Professional Considerations
1. Consent form NOT required.
2. **Preparation:**
   A. Obtain a container and ice or dry ice.
   B. Prepare for the examination by wearing protective clothing, a face shield, and heavy rubber gloves.
3. **Procedure:**
   A. The animal is killed and decapitated. The head is sealed in a watertight metal container and refrigerated as follows: with regular ice if the specimen will be examined within 24 hours; with dry ice if the specimen will be examined after 24 hours.
   B. Thin-tissue impressions are made from the medulla, the cerebellum, and Ammon's horn of the hippocampus; immersed for 5 seconds in Seller's stain and then in tap water; and examined under high magnification. Negri bodies appear as cherry red, sharply defined, spherical, oval, or elongated bodies containing dark blue-staining granules.
4. **Postprocedure care:**
   A. Include a detailed history of the date of human exposure, the method of exposure, the names and addresses of the client(s) exposed, the animal's owners, the species and breed of animal, whether it died or was killed, and its vaccination history, if known.
   B. The bitten human should be monitored for the development of signs of rabies, which include laryngeal spasm when drinking water, restless behavior, hyperreactivity or convulsions with increased sensory input, neuromuscular twitching, tachypnea/hyperventilation, hydrophobia, and excess salivation.
5. **Client and family teaching:**
   A. Client and family should observe for signs of rabies (listed above) for the next 12 months. Notify the physician immediately if symptoms appear.
   B. Have pets vaccinated against rabies.
   C. If a bite occurs, clean the wound quickly with a disinfectant to kill any rabies virus in the wound.
   D. The family should follow universal precautions in handling any items from the client that have been contaminated with saliva until a year has passed without symptoms.
6. **Factors that affect results:**
   A. Inability to obtain animal or brain tissue.
7. **Other data:**
   A. The likelihood of Negri body development increases with the length of time the animal lives after acquiring rabies. Therefore, Negri bodies may not always be present.
   B. Results should be confirmed by mouse inoculation intracerebrally with the animal's brain tissue.
   C. The only method of preventing rabies is animal vaccination.
   D. Rabies is a reportable disease in most areas, as are animal bites.

ANION GAP, BLOOD

Norm:

		SI UNITS
With K⁺ in the equation	12-20 mEq/L	12-20 mmol/L
Without K⁺ in the equation		
Adults	8-16 mEq/L	8-16 mmol/L
Child < age 3	10-14 mEq/L	10-14 mmol/L
Child > age 3	10-18 mEq/L	10-18 mmol/L
Norm using Beckman E4A or CX5 analyzers		3-11 mmol/L

Increased. Acidosis, cancer, carbon monoxide poisoning, chronic renal failure, cyanide poisoning, dehydration, heart disease, heatstroke, hypertension, hypocalcemia, hypomagnesemia, metabolic acidosis caused by diabetic ketoacidosis (because of acetone, beta-hydroxybutyrate ketone content), ethyl alcohol ketoacidosis, ethylene glycol poisoning, lactic acidosis, methanol poisoning, multiple acyl-CoA dehydrogenase deficiency, renal failure, salicylate overdose, and uremia. Drugs include acetaminophen (alone or in combination with oxycodone), acetazolamide, ammonium chloride, antihypertensives, carbenicillin, corticosteroids, 5% dextrose in water (prolonged infusion), diazoxide, dimercaprol, ethacrynic acid, ethyl alcohol (ethanol), ethylene glycol, formaldehyde, fructose, furosemide, hippuric acid, hydrogen sulfide, iodine, iron, isoniazid, metformin, methenamine mandelate, nalidixic acid, nitrates, nitrites, oral phosphosoda, oxalic acid, paraldehyde, penicillins, phenformin, propofol (infusion 100 μg/kg/min), salbutamol, salicylates, sodium bicarbonate, sodium nitroprusside, sorbitol, streptozotocin, sulfur (elemental), thiazides, ticarcillin, toluene, xylitol, and any drug that may result in hypotension with reduced tissue perfusion or renal failure.

Decreased. Bromism (from cough medications, very low–to–negative anion gap caused by halide ion falsely measured as chloride), hyperdilution, hypercalcemia, hypermagnesemia, hypoalbuminemia, (causes a decrese in amount of anions not measured) (1 gm/dL drop in serum albumin correlation with a 2.5 mEq/L decrease in anion gap), hyponatremia, hypophosphatemia, multiple myeloma, (causes abnormal cations called paraproteins), polyclonal gammopathy, proteinuric

hypertension from pregnancy, Waldenström's macroglobulinemia. Drugs include alkalis, ammonium chloride, boric acid, bromides, chlorpropamide, cholestyramine, cortisone acetate, corticotropin, hypercalcemia, hyperkalemia, hypermagnesemia, lithium carbonate (toxicity) (causes very low–to–negative anion gap because of excess unmeasured cation) magnesium-containing antacids, phenylbutazone, polymyxin B, oxyphenbutazone, sodium chloride (large amounts intravenously), tromethamine, and vasopressin. Herbal or natural remedies include licorice.

Description. A calculation of the difference between the major cations and the major anions in the blood that helps determine the cause of metabolic acidosis. The two formulas used to determine the anion gap are:

$$Anion\ gap = (Na^+) - (Cl^- + HCO_3^-)$$

or

$$Anion\ gap = (Na^+ + K^+) - (Cl^- + HCO_3^-)$$

Anion gap is simply a term used to signify the amount of unmeasured anions in the blood plasma. The anion "gap" is created on paper because the formula excludes some anions (such as proteins, organic acids, phosphates, sulfates and cations (such as calcium and magnesium and, sometimes, potassium). If all possible types of anions and cations were used in the formula, instead of only those above, the answer would be zero, because the body's homeostatic mechanisms ensure electrochemical balance in the plasma. The formula's result has different implications, depending on whether the answer is positive or negative. A negative anion gap is less common than an elevated anion gap.

Professional Considerations
1. Consent form NOT required.

2. **Preparation:**
   A. Tube: Red topped, red/gray topped, or gold topped.
   B. Do NOT draw during hemodialysis.
3. **Procedure:**
   A. Draw a 10-mL blood sample.
4. **Postprocedure care:**
   A. None.
5. **Client and family teaching:**
   A. Not applicable.
6. **Factors that affect results:**
   A. Metabolic acidosis may exist with a normal anion gap, as when bicarbonate is lost in body fluids and chloride is retained in the following conditions: hyperchloremic acidosis, renal tubular acidosis, biliary or pancreatic fistulas, and ileal loop hypofunctioning.
   B. Iodine absorption from wounds packed with povidone-iodine solution may cause falsely low results.
   C. Reject hemolyzed specimens.
7. **Other data:**
   A. Normal anion gap can occur with diarrhea, hyperalimentation, renal tubular acidosis, and ureterostomies.
   B. Treatment for an anion gap acidosis is to correct the cause. Sodium bicarbonate 1-2 mEq/kg has been used in some cases.
   C. See also *Ketone bodies, Blood* and *Beta-hydroxybutyrate, Blood.*

ANKLE-BRACHIAL INDEX (ABI), DIAGNOSTIC

Norm:

PRESSURE INDEX	INTERPRETATION
≥0.86	Normal
0.75-0.85	Mild occlusive disease
0.50-0.75	Intermittent claudication
0.30-0.50	Severe disease: rest pain may occur; pregangrenous state
0.20-0.30	Poor probability for tissue healing or limb viability unless compensation by collateral blood flow occurs
<0.20	Ischemic or gangrenous extremities

Usage. Assessment of arterial blood flow in clients with peripheral vascular disease; monitoring postoperative flow in the lower extremities after vascular surgery such as femoral bypass or after aortofemoral bypass from iliac occlusion; assessment of severity of peripheral vascular disease; predicting carotid artery stenosis. Cilostazol (Pletal) increases ABI at rest.

Description. The ABI is a mathematically calculated ratio of the systolic pressure at a pulse point in a lower extremity with peripheral vascular disease as compared to the systolic pressure of the brachial artery. The index provides a quick, noninvasive assessment of how much arterial blood is perfusing the extremity. Typically an ABI that increases by at least 0.15 (15%) after vascular surgery indicates that the surgery was successful. A baseline in women with an ABI of <0.60 indicates significantly higher probability of developing severe disability for walkingspecific outcomes such as walking a quarter of a mile.

Professional Considerations
1. Consent form NOT required.
2. **Preparation:**
   A. Obtain a dual-frequency Doppler ultrasonograph, a marker, two sphygmomanometers, and ultrasonic gel.
3. **Procedure:**
   A. Client is positioned supine.
   B. The femoral, popliteal, dorsalis pedis, and posterior tibial pulse points in both lower extremities are palpated and identified with a marker.
   C. The sphygmomanometer cuff is placed proximally to the marked site. If the flow is being assessed at the knee, the cuff is placed proximally to the popliteal pulse. If the flow is being assessed at the ankle, the cuff is placed proximally to the ankle.
   D. Ultrasonic gel is placed over the marked site (popliteal or posterior tibial or dorsalis pedis), and the Doppler flow signal is identified.
   E. With the Doppler in place, the sphygmomanometer cuff is inflated until the Doppler flow signal disappears.
   F. The cuff is slowly deflated, and the pressure at which the Doppler tone is again audible is noted and recorded.
   G. The brachial systolic blood pressure in both arms is measured with a Doppler scanner, and the

highest pressure is selected for use in the ABI calculation.

H. The ABI ratio is calculated with the following equation:

$$ABI = \frac{\text{Lower extremity pressure from step F}}{\text{Brachial Doppler systolic pressure}}$$

4. **Postprocedure care:**
   A. Wipe the ultrasonic gel from the skin and remove the sphygmomanometer cuff.
   B. If performing serial ABI measurements postoperatively, notify the physician for a decrease in ABI of at least 0.15 (15%) or for the loss of a previously palpable pulse or audible Doppler tone.
5. **Client and family teaching:**
   A. This test is painless.
   B. This measurement helps estimate how much blood is flowing to the leg and foot.
6. **Factors that affect results:**
   A. Values may be inconsistent if the same arm is not used for every brachial pressure measurement.
   B. Immediate postoperative hypotension and low body temperature may necessitate use of a Doppler scanner to locate pulse tones because pulses may not be palpable.
7. **Other data:**
   A. The ABI is a good predictor of survival in clients with peripheral vascular disease. Those with ABIs less than 0.30 have significantly poorer survival than clients with ABIs 0.31-0.91.
   B. The Transfer Function Index (TFI) has been shown to be superior to ABI in detecting vascular grafts at risk for failing. See *Pulse volume recording of peripheral vasculature, Diagnostic.*
   C. See also *Doppler ultrasonographic flow studies, Diagnostic.*

ANP
(*see Natriuretic peptides, Plasma*)

ANTEGRADE PYELOGRAPHY, DIAGNOSTIC

Norm. The selected ureter fills from the renal pelvis to the urinary bladder.

Normal renal pelvic, ureteral, and urinary bladder contours are demonstrated radiographically after the injection of radiopaque contrast material.

Usage. Most commonly requested in clinical scenarios where ureteral obstruction is suspected but cannot be diagnosed effectively by intravenous pyelography (IVP) or cystoscopy and retrograde pyelography. Used in detection of synchronous tumor of the upper urinary tract, ureteropelvic laceration after blunt body trauma, ileal conduit stenosis. Frequently performed with the placement of percutaneous nephrostomy tubes in the treatment of urinary tract obstruction and analysis of ureteral stent placement.

Description. Antegrade pyelography is an invasive radiographic procedure in which radiocontrast material is injected percutaneously into the renal pelvis. The flow of the contrast material is then observed as it progresses into the ureter and urinary bladder. Hydronephrosis or obstruction of the flow of the radiocontrast material into the urinary bladder is diagnostic of urinary tract obstruction and may be suggestive of the need to place a percutaneous nephrostomy tube.

Professional Considerations
1. Consent form IS required.

Risks
Allergic reaction to the radiocontrast material or anesthetic agents, bleeding (bladder clots, hematuria, perinephric hematoma), bowel perforation, infection, laceration of the renal collecting system with resulting urine leaks, pneumothorax.

Contraindications
Allergy to radiocontrast material, hemorrhagic diathesis.

Precautions
During pregnancy, risks of cumulative radiation exposure to the fetus from this and other previous or future imaging studies must be weighed against the benefits of the procedure. Although formal limits for client exposure are relative to this risk-benefit comparison, the United States Nuclear Regulatory Commission requires that the cumulative dose equivalent to an embryo/fetus from *occupational* exposure not exceed 0.5 rem (5 mSv). Radiation dose to the fetus is

proportional to the distance of the anatomy studied from the abdomen and decreases as pregnancy progresses. For pregnant clients, consult the Radiologist/Radiology Department to obtain estimated fetal radiation exposure from this procedure.

2. **Preparation:**
   A. This test is generally performed by a urologist or an interventional radiologist in an area equipped with fluoroscopy or ultrasound equipment.
   B. A formal assessment to rule out hemorrhagic diathesis (PT, PTT, bleeding time, platelet count) as well as baseline determination of hematocrit and hemoglobin is advisable. A baseline urinalysis is also often obtained. It is useful to determine if the client will permit transfusion in the event of hemorrhage. If not, it may be necessary to reconsider the procedure.
   C. Orders may include a 4-hour fast from food and a sedative.
   D. Vital signs (blood pressure, pulse, respiratory rate) immediately before the procedure are indicated.

3. **Procedure:**
   A. In the fluoroscopy or sonography suite, the position of the renal pelvis is demonstrated radiographically. A posterior vertical approach to the kidney is usually selected.
   B. The flank over the renal pelvis is prepped with an iodine solution, and sterile drapes are applied to create a sterile field.
   C. A 22-gauge needle is advanced into the renal pelvis under fluoroscopic or ultrasonographic guidance. Once within the collecting system, urine samples can be obtained and radiocontrast material injected to confirm location of the needle tip within the renal pelvis.
   D. At this point, a guidewire is advanced through the needle allowing placement of larger introducer needles or urostomy catheters, or both types. Further radiocontrast material can be injected to complete the antegrade pyelogram procedure.

4. **Postprocedure care:**
   A. Frequent determination of the vital signs is indicated in the immediate postprocedure period. Vital signs are generally obtained at 15-minute intervals for the first hour after the procedure and then at frequent intervals as specified by the physician performing the test.
   B. Close monitoring of the urine output and observation for the development of hematuria are important. The client may have a nephrostomy bag as well as a Foley catheter bag after the pyelography so that separate records of each output source may be necessary.
   C. Serial determinations of hematocrit, hemoglobin, creatinine, and serum electrolytes may be indicated.
   D. If nephrostomy tubes have been placed, dressing checks and changes may be needed.
   E. New fluid and antibiotic orders may need to be executed after the pyelography procedure.

5. **Client and family teaching:**
   A. The need to frequently monitor vital signs and urine output should be discussed.
   B. Gross hematuria is not unusual after this procedure and a relatively small amount of blood will produce red urine. The client should be reassured that this development generally is to be expected and does not necessarily indicate an unfavorable outcome.
   C. Special positioning of the client may be required because of the nephrostomy tubes, and this should be explained to the client.

6. **Factors that affect results:**
   A. Postprocedure bleeding or infection.
   B. Hematuria resulting in clotting of nephrostomy tubes.
   C. Formation of bladder clots causing pain and diminished urine output.
   D. Accelerated urine output after nephrostomy tube placement (postobstructive diuresis) resulting in volume depletion (hypotension, tachycardia, electrolyte abnormalities).

7. **Other data:**
   A. Intravenous pyelography, CT scan, and nuclear magnetic resonance scanning are noninvasive alternative diagnostic modalities useful in the evaluation of urinary tract obstruction.
   B. Renal insufficiency is a relative contraindication for the adminis-

tration of intravenous radiocontrast material but is not a contraindication for antegrade or retrograde pyelography.
C. See also *Retrograde pyelography, Diagnostic.*

ANTHRAX
(see Blood culture, Blood)

ANTIBODY IDENTIFICATION, RED CELL, BLOOD

Norm. Requires interpretation.

Usage. Identification of the specific nature of antibodies detected with more general antibody screens (indirect Coombs' testing). Found in clients who are homozygous for sickle cell disease.

Description. Irregular antibodies are usually detected in clients who have had prior exposure to foreign antigens through blood transfusions or pregnancy. The presence of these irregular antibodies may cause transfusion reactions and hemolytic disease of the newborn. The exact antibody is identified when the client's serum is combined with a panel of red blood cell samples, each containing a known antigen. This test is typically performed in a blood bank.

Professional Considerations
1. Consent form NOT required.
2. Preparation:
   A. Tube: One lavender topped and one red topped, red/gray topped, or gold topped.
   B. Note the client's age, medications, past transfusions of blood products, and number of pregnancies on the laboratory requisition.
3. Procedure:
   A. Draw a 7-mL blood sample in the lavender-topped tube.
   B. Draw a 10-mL blood sample in the red-topped, red/gray-topped, or gold-topped tube.
4. Postprocedure care:
   A. None.
5. Client and family teaching:
   A. Results are normally available within 24 hours.
6. Factors that affect results:
   A. Reject hemolyzed specimens.

7. **Other data:**
   A. Identification of cold-reacting antibodies reactive at −30° C may require the use of a blood warmer during transfusion.
   B. Anti-D and anti-C antibodies are associated with most neonatal morbidity.

ANTICARDIOLIPIN ANTIBODY
(see Antiphospholipid antibody, Serum)

ANTIDEOXYRIBONUCLEASE B TITER (ANTI-DNASE B, STREPTODORNASE), SERUM

Norm:
Adult	<85 Todd U/mL
Child <7 years	<60 Todd U/mL
Child ≥7 years	<170 Todd U/mL

Increased. Anorexia nervosa, Tourette syndrome, glomerulonephritis (poststreptococcal), pharyngitis (streptococcal), poststreptococcal reactive arthritis (PSReA), pyodermic skin infections, rheumatic fever (acute).

Description. Deoxyribonuclease B is an antigen produced by group A streptococci. The anti-DNase B test detects antibodies to deoxyribonuclease B, which appear when a client has a poststreptococcal infection. The levels increase after a client recovers from a group A streptococcal infection and thus are a reliable indicator of recent hemolytic streptococcal infection.

Professional Considerations
1. Consent form NOT required.
2. Preparation:
   A. Tube: Red topped, red/gray topped, or gold topped.
   B. List drug therapy and previous vaccinations on the laboratory requisition.
   C. Transport the specimen to the laboratory immediately. Spin and refrigerate the specimen if not tested immediately.
3. Procedure:
   A. Draw a 5-mL blood sample.
4. Postprocedure care:
   A. None.
5. Client and family teaching:
   A. Results are normally available within 48 hours.

6. Factors that affect results:
   A. Reject hemolyzed specimens.
   B. False-negative results may occur in hemorrhagic pancreatitis.
7. Other data:
   A. This test is more sensitive to streptococcal pyoderma than the antistreptolysin-O (ASO) test.
   B. Anti–zymogen antibody titers are a better marker for streptococcal infection associated with acute glomerulonephritis.

ANTIDIURETIC HORMONE (ADH), SERUM

Norm:

SERUM OSMOLARITY (mOsm/kg)	ADH LEVEL (pg/mL)	SI UNITS (pmol/L)
270-280	<1.5	<1.4
280-285	<2.5	<2.3
285-290	1-5	0.9-4.6
290-295	2-7	1.9-6.5
295-300	4-12	3.7-11.1

Increased. Acute intermittent porphyria, cancer (brain, intrathoracic nonpulmonary cancer, gastrointestinal cancer, gynecologic cancer, breast cancer, prostate cancer, sarcoma), cerebrovascular disease, cerebral infection, diabetes insipidus (nephrogenic), ectopic production from neoplasm, Guillain-Barré syndrome, meningitis (tuberculous), pneumonia, syndrome of inappropriate antidiuretic hormone secretion (SIADHS) (caused by malignant tumors, CNS disorders, intrathoracic infections, positive- pressure ventilation), and tuberculosis (pulmonary). Drugs include anesthetics, antipsychotics, barbiturates, carbamazepine, chlorothiazide, chlorpropamide, cisplatin, clofibrate, cyclophosphamide, desmopressin, furosemide, estrogens, lithium, melphalan, morphine sulfate and other narcotic analgesics, oxytocin citrate, oxytocin injection, psychotropic drugs, thiazides, tolbutamide, tricyclic antidepressants and vidarabine, vinblastine, and vincristine sulfate.

Decreased. Enuresis, nephrotic syndrome, pituitary diabetes insipidus, and psychogenic polydipsia. Drugs include alcohol, demeclocycline, ethyl alcohol, lithium carbonate, and phenytoin sodium.

Description. A hormone produced by the hypothalamus and stored and released from the posterior lobe of the pituitary gland in response to increased serum osmolarity. Acts to maintain body water balance through regulation of sodium and potassium and vascular smooth muscle control. Release of ADH is inhibited by decreased serum osmolarity.

Professional Considerations
1. Consent form NOT required.
2. Preparation:
   A. See *Client and family teaching*.
   B. Tube: Lavender topped, made of plastic rather than glass.
   C. Notify laboratory personnel that a specimen for ADH measurement will be arriving shortly.
3. Procedure:
   A. Draw a 5-mL blood sample.
4. Postprocedure care:
   A. Write the collection time on the laboratory requisition.
   B. Transport the specimen to the laboratory for spinning within 10 minutes of collection.
5. Client and family teaching:
   A. Fast and refrain from stress and strenuous activity for 12 hours before the test.
   B. Results are normally available in about 5 days.
6. Factors that affect results:
   A. Reject specimens received more than 10 minutes after collection.
   B. Elevated ADH levels may be caused by physical and psychologic stress and positive-pressure mechanical ventilation. Highest levels are obtained at night. Pain, stress, exercise, and elevated blood osmolality will each cause increased secretion.
   C. Decreased ADH levels may be caused by negative-pressure mechanical ventilation, recumbent position, hypoosmolar blood, and hypertension.
   D. Results are invalidated if the specimen is drawn within 1 week after the client has undergone a scan using radioactive dye.
   E. Glass causes degradation of ADH.
7. Other data:
   A. None.

ANTI-DNA, SERUM

Norm:
Negative: 0-0.9 mg of native
DNA/mL of plasma,
or   <70 IU/mL
Borderline SLE   70-200 IU/mL

Increased. Autoimmune disorder
(1-2.5 mg/mL), myasthenia gravis,
rheumatoid arthritis, sclerosis (systemic), Sjögren syndrome, systemic
lupus erythematosus (SLE) nephritis,
SLE (active = 10-15 mg/mL; remission =
1-2.5 mg/mL) and non-Hodgkin's lymphoma. Drugs include estrogen.

Description. Detects the presence of
antibodies to native deoxyribonuclease
that indicate autoimmune activity. The
test may be used to monitor the progression (increasing levels) and remission (decreasing levels) of SLE.

Professional Considerations
1. Consent form NOT required.
2. Preparation:
   A. Tube: Red topped, lavender topped,
   or gray topped (depending on specific laboratory requirements).
3. Procedure:
   A. Draw a 2-mL blood sample.
4. Postprocedure care:
   A. None.
5. Client and family teaching:
   A. Results may not be available for
   several days if testing is not performed on site.
6. Factors that affect results:
   A. Results are invalid if the specimen is drawn less than 1 week
   after the client received a scan
   using radioactive dye.
   B. Procainamide and hydralazine
   can induce anti-DNA antibodies.
7. Other data:
   A. In the past it was unnecessary to
   test clients with negative antinuclear antibodies (ANA). However,
   there exists a group of ANA-
   negative lupus clients who have
   elevated anti-DNA levels.
   B. In SLE, immune complexes of
   anti-DNA may be deposited in the
   brain, heart, kidneys, and synovial
   tissue.

ANTI-DNASE B
(see Antideoxyribonuclease B titer, Serum)

ANTIGEN DETECTION TEST
(see Respiratory Antigen Panel, Specimen)

ANTIHEMOPHILIA FACTOR, BLOOD
(see Factor VIII, Blood)

ANTIHYALURONIDASE (AH) TITER, SERUM

Norm. <128 U/mL
A fourfold increase between acute and
convalescent samples is significant,
regardless of the magnitude of the titer.

Increased. Recent group A streptococcal disease, glomerulonephritis (acute),
and rheumatic fever (acute).

Description. Hyaluronidase is an extracellular enzyme antigen produced by
group A beta-hemolytic streptococci.
This test measures levels of antibodies to
hyaluronidase that appear in clients who
are recovering from group A beta-
hemolytic streptococcal infections. Levels increase after a client recovers from
a group A beta- hemolytic streptococcal
infection (about the second week of
infection) and fall 3-5 weeks after infection. Levels are thus a reliable indicator of
recent infection from this cause.

Professional Considerations
1. Consent form NOT required.
2. Preparation:
   A. Tube: Red topped, red/gray
   topped, or gold topped.
   B. List drug therapy and all previous
   vaccinations on the laboratory
   requisition.
3. Procedure:
   A. Draw a 5-mL blood sample.
4. Postprocedure care:
   A. Transport the specimen to the
   laboratory immediately. Spin and
   refrigerate the specimen if not
   tested immediately.
5. Client and family teaching:
   A. Return in 1-3 weeks for convalescent samples to be drawn.
6. Factors that affect results:
   A. Reject hemolyzed specimens.
   B. Drugs that may cause falsely suppressed results include antibiotics
   and corticosteroids.

C. Falsely elevated results may occur in the presence of hyperlipoproteinemia.
7. **Other data:**
    A. A better test than the antistreptolysin-O (ASO) test for detecting antibodies in acute glomerulonephritis, which follows a streptococcal pyoderma.

ANTI-La/SS-B TEST, DIAGNOSTIC

Norm. Negative.

Usage. Differential diagnosis of systemic lupus erythematosus (SLE), Sjögren syndrome, and mixed connective tissue disease.

Positive. Antinuclear antibody (ANA)–negative lupus, congenital heart block, neonatal lupus, Sjögren syndrome. Drugs include terbinafine.

Description. Anti-La/SS-B is an autoantibody characteristically found in high titers in clients with primary Sjögren syndrome or Sjögren syndrome with (SLE). The SS-B(La) are antibodies directed against ribonucleic acid (RNA) protein particles that are a cofactor in RNA polymerase III. Although electrophoresis is the most sensitive method for detecting anti-La/SS-B, immunodiffusion is the method most commonly used.

Professional Considerations
1. Consent form NOT required.
2. **Preparation:**
    A. Tube: Red topped, red/gray topped, or gold topped.
3. **Procedure:**
    A. Draw a 7-mL blood sample.
4. **Postprocedure care:**
    A. Transport the specimen to the laboratory for immediate spinning.
5. **Client and family teaching:**
    A. Results may not be available for several days if testing is not performed on site.
6. **Factors that affect results:**
    A. None found.
7. **Other data:**
    A. This test is less sensitive but more specific for primary Sjögren syndrome than the anti-Ro/SS-A test.
    B. The presence of both anti-La/SS-B and anti-Ro/SS-A antibodies is generally associated with a milder disease of SLE.

C. Clients who are positive for antinuclear antibody and who have SS-A but not SS-B are likely to have nephritis.

ANTIMICROSOMAL ANTIBODY
(see Thyroid Peroxidase Antibody, Blood)

ANTIMITOCHONDRIAL ANTIBODY (AMA), BLOOD

Norm. Negative at 1:5 to 1:10 dilution.

Suggestive of primary biliary cirrhosis	>1:20
Probable primary biliary cirrhosis	>1:80
Diagnostic of primary biliary cirrhosis	>1:160

Increased. Acute cholestatic hepatitis, autoimmune diseases, carbon monoxide poisoning, chronic active hepatitis (20% of clients), cryptogenic cirrhosis, gastric adenocarcinoma, hepatitis C, jaundice (drug induced), myasthenia gravis, and primary biliary cirrhosis.

Decreased or Absent. Autoimmune cholangitis, drug-induced cholestatic jaundice, extrahepatic obstructive biliary disease, status post liver transplantation for primary biliary cirrhosis, sclerosing cholangitis, and viral hepatitis.

Description. An immunofluorescent test that detects and measures autoimmune immunoglobulins (antibodies) to mitochondria that attack organs, which then expend large amounts of energy. A majority of clients with primary biliary cirrhosis have antimitochondrial antibodies. This test is usually performed with the test for anti–smooth muscle antibodies to aid in differentiating primary biliary cirrhosis and chronic active hepatitis from diffuse, extrahepatic biliary obstruction and other liver diseases.

Professional Considerations
1. Consent form NOT required.
2. **Preparation:**
    A. See Client and family teaching.
    B. Tube: Red topped, red/gray topped, or gold topped.
3. **Procedure:**
    A. Draw a 2-mL blood sample.

4. Postprocedure care:
   A. Transport the specimen to the laboratory for immediate spinning.
5. Client and family teaching:
   A. Fast for 8 hours before sampling.
   B. Results may not be available for several days if testing is not performed on site.
6. Factors that affect results:
   A. Reject hemolyzed specimens.
   B. Results are unreliable for clients using oxyphenisatin.
   C. False-positive results may occur in clients with syphilis.
7. Other data:
   A. Although titers over 1:80 are strongly suggestive for primary biliary cirrhosis, liver biopsy is recommended.

ANTIMYOCARDIAL ANTIBODY, SERUM

Norm. Negative.

Positive. Cardiomyopathy (idiopathic), Dressler syndrome, fibrosis (endomyocardial), status after myocardial infarction, myocarditis, pericarditis (idiopathic), postcardiac injury syndrome (PCIS), pleural fluid analysis, postpericardiotomy syndrome, post-thoracotomy syndrome, rheumatic fever, rheumatic heart disease, systemic lupus erythematosus, and thoracic injury.

Description. Antimyocardial antibody is an antibody to an organ-specific antigen in myocardial tissue that causes autoimmune damage to the heart and may be detected in serum before the appearance of clinical symptoms. The myocardial antigenic determinant is also believed to be a characteristic of streptococci because the antibodies may appear in rheumatic fever or after a streptococcal infection. This test uses an indirect immunofluorescence method by treatment of extracts of animal cardiac tissue with the client's serum and observation for the development of antigen-antibody immune complexes. Positive results are reported in titers of the lowest dilution at which the immune complexes can be detected, and decreasing titers correlate with response to treatment. This test is used in the detection of an autoimmune cause for the above-listed conditions and for monitoring therapeutic response to treatment for the above-listed conditions.

Professional Considerations
1. Consent form NOT required.
2. Preparation:
   A. Tube: Red topped, red/gray topped, or gold topped.
3. Procedure:
   A. Draw a 5-mL blood sample.
4. Postprocedure care:
   A. Transport the specimen to the laboratory for immediate spinning.
5. Client and family teaching:
   A. Results are normally available within 48 hours.
6. Factors that affect results:
   A. No factors known to affect results.
7. Other data:
   A. Myocardial antibodies do not usually occur in clients with coronary insufficiency alone but do occur in clients who also have had a myocardial infarction.
   B. Pleural fluid can be analyzed for antimyocardial antibody to determine postcardiac injury syndrome (PCIS) and help exclude other diagnoses.

ANTINEUTROPHIL CYTOPLASMIC ANTIBODY SCREEN (ANCA, CYTOPLASMIC NEUTROPHIL ANTIBODIES), SERUM

Norm:

	SCREEN	TITER
p-ANCA	Negative	<1:40
c-ANCA	Negative	<1:40

Usage. Helps diagnose conditions in which vasculitis is suspected. p-ANCA is used for clients with inflammatory bowel or liver disease.

Increased c-ANCA. Human immunodeficiency virus, microscopic polyangitis, Wegener's granulomatosis.

Increased p-ANCA. Churg-Strauss syndrome, Crohn's disease, Felty's syndrome, hepatitis (50%-80% of clients, chronic), systemic lupus erythematosus (SLE), microscopic polyangitis, primary sclerosing cholangitis (72%-80% of clients), rheumatoid arthritis, ulcerative colitis 72%-80% of clients).

Description. Neutrophils are very active in the body's immune defenses by releasing proteolytic enzymes to phagocytose bacteria. In conditions characterized by necrotizing vasculitis, Antineutrophil cytoplasmic antibodies (ANCA) are present. ANCA are autoimmune antibodies directed against the lysosomal enzymes in neutrophil granules. ANCA occur in two patterns. The p-ANCA (perinuclear) antibody pattern is similar to that of antinuclear antibodies. The c-ANCA (classical) antibody pattern is present in 90% of persons with Wegener's granulomatosis. This test is the only test available for the diagnosis of vasculitis, a condition in which endothelial inflammation in blood vessels leads to organ damage. The test is first done as an indirect immunofluorescence screen in certain conditions, followed by an ELISA test to confirm positives.

Professional Considerations
1. Consent form IS required.
2. **Preparation:**
   A. Tube: Red-topped.
3. **Procedure:**
   A. Collect a 3-ml blood sample.
4. **Postprocedure care:**
   A. Deliver specimen to the laboratory. Separate and refrigerate serum until testing.
5. **Client and family teaching:**
   A. Results are not usually available for 3-5 days.
6. **Factors that affect results:**
   A. Both IgM and IgG antibodies must be tested to avoid a false negative result.
   B. Results are unreliable if formalin is used to fix the slides.
   C. Immunofluorescence titers usually, but do not always decrease with remission.
   D. Reject hemolyzed of lipemic specimen.
7. **Other data:**
   A. The cANCA sensitivity and specificity for Wegener's granulomatosis are (90%) and (80%).
   B. p-ANCA is also known as "UC-ANCA" and "X-ANCA".

ANTINUCLEAR ANTIBODY (ANA), SERUM

Norm. Negative at 1:20 dilution.

Positive. Autoimmune pancreatitis, autoimmune thyroid disease, cancer (hepatic or pulmonary), dermatopolymyositis, hepatitis (chronic active, lupoid), mixed connective tissue disease, myasthenia gravis, polymyositis, pulmonary fibrosis (idiopathic), Raynaud syndrome, rheumatoid arthritis, scleroderma, some healthy older adults, systemic lupus erythematosus (SLE), systemic sclerosis, and Sjögren syndrome. Drugs include beta-adrenergic blockers, carbamazepine, lovastatin, methyldopa, nitrofurantoin sodium, penicillamine, and tocainide.

Description. Antinuclear antibodies are antibodies the body produces against its own DNA and nuclear material that cause tissue damage and characterize autoimmune diseases. Highest titers occur in SLE. The immunofluorescent procedure results in four characteristic staining patterns, which help differentiate the type of connective tissue disease. These patterns and their specificities include the *homogeneous* pattern specific for SLE and other connective diseases; the *peripheral* pattern specific for SLE; the *speckled* pattern specific for mixed connective disease, SLE, Sjögren syndrome, polymyositis, dermatomyositis, and scleroderma; and the *nucleolar* pattern specific for scleroderma and Sjögren syndrome. These patterns, however, are not diagnostic of the various diseases. If positive results are obtained, the *anti*-DNA test should be performed to aid differentiation of SLE.

Professional Considerations
1. Consent form NOT required.
2. **Preparation:**
   A. Tube: Red topped, red/gray topped, or gold topped.
   B. List drug therapy on the laboratory requisition.
   C. See *Client and family teaching.*
3. **Procedure:**
   A. Draw a 2-mL blood sample.
4. **Postprocedure care:**
   A. Transport the specimen to the laboratory for immediate spinning.
5. **Client and family teaching:**
   A. Fast for 8 hours before sampling.
   B. Results may not be available for several days if testing is not performed on site.
6. **Factors that affect results:**
   A. Reject hemolyzed specimens.
   B. False-negative results may be caused by drug therapy with corticosteroids.

C. Drugs that may cause false-positive results from a drug-induced syndrome resembling SLE include acetazolamide, aminosalicylic acid, carbidopa, chlorothiazide, chlorpromazine, clofibrate, diphenylhydantoin, ethosuximide, gold salts, griseofulvan microsize, griseofulvan ultramicrosize, hydralazine hydrochloride, hydroxytryptophan, isoniazid, mephenytoin, methyldopa, methyldopate hydrochloride, methylthiouracil, methysergide maleate, oral contraceptives, penicillin, phenylbutazone, phenytoin, primidone, procainamide hydrochloride, propylthiouracil, quinidine gluconate, quinidine polygalacturonate, quinidine sulfate, reserpine, streptomycin sulfate, sulfadimethoxine, sulfonamides, tetracyclines, thiouracil, and trimethadione.
D. Pregnancy or therapeutic exposure to UV radiation can increase ANA levels.

7. **Other data:**
   A. The peroxidase method may be used, but patterns are not obtained.
   B. In children with musculoskeletal or dermatologic disease, the prognosis of children who have positive ANA test results in the absence of autoimmune conditions is excellent.
   C. Persons over 60 years of age have a 20% chance of a positive test.
   D. Up to one third of first-degree relatives of clients with SLE have a positive ANA, though they are healthy.

ANTI-PARIETAL CELL ANTIBODY, BLOOD
(see Parietal cell antibody, Blood)

ANTIPHOSPHOLIPID ANTIBODY (APA), SERUM

Norm. Negative.

Positive. Antiphospholipid (Hughes syndrome), anticardiolipin syndrome (primary, secondary), Behçet's disease, cerebral palsy, chorea, diabetic muscle infarction, epilepsy, essential thrombocythaemia, giant cell arteritis, human immunodeficiency virus (HIV), in vitro fertilization and embryo transfer failures, moyanoya, polymyalgia rheumatica, preeclampsia, renal allograft failure, retinal occlusive vasculopathy, syphilis, temporal arteritis, thrombosis (systemic venous), varicella zoster virus infection. Drugs include minocycline.

Description. Antiphospholipid antibodies (APA) constitute a family of immunoglobulins active against phospholipids. Phospholipids are complex triglyceride esters containing long-chain fatty acids, phosphoric acid, and nitrogenous bases. The group includes fatty compounds, such as lecithin, found in animal and plant cells. The APA family is composed of the anticardiolipin antibodies (ACA), lupus anticoagulant (LA), and antibodies that cause biologic false-positive results in syphilis serologic tests. ACA and LA have been described as occurring in thromboses, autoimmune disease, infectious diseases, and neoplastic disease. An APA syndrome that occurs during pregnancy includes loss of the fetus, systemic thromboses, and thrombocytopenia. The pathophysiology of fetal loss is not clearly known, but several theories have been suggested. Clients with APA syndrome are treated with long-term oral anticoagulation.

Professional Considerations
1. Consent form NOT required.
2. **Preparation:**
   A. Tube: Red topped, red/gray topped, or gold topped.
3. **Procedure:**
   A. Draw a 1-mL blood sample.
4. **Postprocedure care:**
   A. None.
5. **Client and family teaching:**
   A. Results are normally available within 48 hours.
   B. This test detects antibodies that bind to fatty substances in your body. It helps identify an illness called "antiphospholipid syndrome," or "anticardiolipin syndrome," in which the blood clots faster than normal. It is important to identify and treat this syndrome because it can lead to a greater risk for fetal death and a higher incidence of stroke, heart attack, and blindness.
6. **Factors that affect results:**
   A. Levels vary, depending on which commercial kit is used for this

test, because the assays are not yet standardized.

7. **Other data:**
   A. In women with previous fetal loss who have received prophylactic treatment during subsequent pregnancy, the live birth rate is 70%. Treatment has included antiplatelet drugs, immunosuppressives, and/or anticoagulants including combination therapy with aspirin and heparin.
   B. Antiphospholipid antibodies are found in pediatric clients with SLE who have thrombotic events.

ANTIPLATELET ANTIBODY
(see Platelet antibody, Blood)

ANTIRIBONUCLEOPROTEIN TEST, DIAGNOSTIC
(see Anti-RNP test, Diagnostic)

ANTI-RNP TEST (ANTIRIBONUCLEOPROTEIN TEST, EXTRACTABLE NUCLEAR ANTIGEN), DIAGNOSTIC

Norm. Negative.

Usage. Assists in differentiating the type of autoimmune disease occurring. Highest titers (≥1:10,000) are suggestive of mixed connective tissue disease such as Raynaud's phenomenon. Positive in cytomegalovirus infection, neonatal lupus erythematosus, Sjögren syndrome, systemic lupus erythematosus.

Description. An antinuclear antibody present in autoimmune disease detected by an immunofluorescent procedure. Immunofluorescence results in characteristic staining patterns that help differentiate the type of connective tissue disease occurring. Anti-RNP antibodies are associated with a speckled pattern and occur in almost all clients with mixed connective tissue syndrome and about one fourth of clients with scleroderma and discoid and systemic lupus erythematosus. High titers are usually accompanied by clinical symptoms of mixed connective tissue disease.

Professional Considerations
1. Consent form NOT required.

2. **Preparation:**
   A. Tube: Red topped, red/gray topped, or gold topped.
   B. See *Client and family teaching.*
3. **Procedure:**
   A. Draw a 2-mL blood sample.
4. **Postprocedure care:**
   A. Transport the specimen to the laboratory for immediate spinning.
5. **Client and family teaching:**
   A. Fast for 8 hours before sampling.
   B. Results may not be available for several days if testing is not performed on site.
6. **Factors that affect results:**
   A. Reject hemolyzed specimens.
   B. False-negative results may be caused by drug therapy with corticosteroids.
   C. Drugs that may cause false-positive results caused by a drug-induced syndrome resembling systemic lupus erythematosus (SLE) include acetazolamide, aminosalicylic acid, carbidopa, chlorothiazide, chlorpromazine, clofibrate, diphenylhydantoin, ethosuximide, gold salts, griseofulvan microsize, griseofulvan ultramicrosize, hydralazine, hydrochloride, hydroxytryptophan, isoniazid, mephenytoin, methyldopa, methyldopate hydrochloride, methylthiouracil, methysergide maleate, oral contraceptives, penicillin, phenylbutazone, phenytoin, primidone, procainamide hydrochloride, propylthiouracil, quinidine gluconate, quinidine polygalacturonate, quinidine sulfate, reserpine, streptomycin sulfate, sulfadimethoxine, sulfonamides, tetracyclines, thiouracil, and trimethadione.
7. **Other data:**
   A. Titer is determined by counterimmunoelectrophoresis (CIE).

ANTI-Ro/SS-A TEST, DIAGNOSTIC

Norm. Negative.

Positive. ANA-negative lupus, complete congenital heart block, neonatal lupus, polymyositis/dermatomyositis, and Sjögren syndrome.

Description. Anti-Ro/SS-A is an autoantibody to the cytoplasmic RNA Ro antigen characteristically found in high titers in clients with primary Sjögren syndrome or Sjögren syndrome with systemic lupus erythematosus (SLE). Although electrophoresis is the most sensitive testing method for detection of these antibodies, the most common method used is immunodiffusion. This test is used in the differential diagnosis of SLE, Sjögren syndrome, and mixed connective tissue disease.

Professional Considerations
1. Consent form NOT required.
2. Preparation:
   A. Tube: Red topped, red/gray topped, or gold topped.
3. Procedure:
   A. Draw a 2-mL blood sample.
4. Postprocedure care:
   A. Send the specimen to the laboratory for immediate spinning.
5. Client and family teaching:
   A. Results may not be available for several days if testing is not performed on site.
6. Factors that affect results:
   A. No known factors affect results.
7. Other data:
   A. This test is more sensitive but less specific for primary Sjögren syndrome than the anti-La/SS-B test.
   B. The presence of both anti-La/SS-B and anti-Ro/SS-A antibodies is generally associated with a milder form of SLE.
   C. Clients who are positive for antinuclear antibody and who have SS-A but not SS-B are likely to have nephritis.
   D. African-Americans are at increased risk for presence of anti-Ro antibodies and SLE.

ANTI-Sm TEST (EXTRACTABLE NUCLEAR ANTIGEN), DIAGNOSTIC

Norm. Negative.

Usage. Assists in differentiating the type of autoimmune disease occurring. The presence of antibodies specific against Sm is strongly suggestive of systemic lupus erythematosus (SLE). Increases are seen in arthritis, heart-related diseases, Raynaud's phenomenon, and SLE.

Description. An antinuclear antibody active against acidic nuclear proteins, present in autoimmune disease detected by an immunofluorescent procedure. Immunofluorescence results in characteristic staining patterns that help differentiate the type of connective tissue disease occurring. Anti-Sm antibodies are associated with a speckled pattern and occur in clients with mixed connective tissue syndrome and in about one fourth of clients with scleroderma, discoid lupus erythematosus, and SLE.

Professional Considerations
1. Consent form NOT required.
2. Preparation:
   A. Tube: Red topped, red/gray topped, or gold topped.
   B. See *Client and family teaching*.
3. Procedure:
   A. Draw a 2-mL blood sample.
4. Postprocedure care:
   A. Send the specimen to the laboratory for immediate spinning.
5. Client and family teaching:
   A. Fast for 8 hours before sampling.
   B. Results may not be available for several days if testing is not performed on site.
6. Factors that affect results:
   A. Reject hemolyzed specimens.
   B. False-negative results may be caused by drug therapy with corticosteroids.
   C. Drugs that may cause false-positive results arising from a drug-induced syndrome resembling SLE include acetazolamide, aminosalicylic acid, carbidopa, chlorothiazide, chlorpromazine, clofibrate, diphenylhydantoin, ethosuximide, gold salts, griseofulvan microsize, griseofulvan ultramicrosize, hydralazine hydrochloride, hydroxytryptophan, isoniazid, mephenytoin, methyldopa, methyldopate hydrochloride, methylthiouracil, methysergide maleate, oral contraceptives, penicillin, phenylbutazone, phenytoin, primidone, procainamide hydrochloride, propylthiouracil, quinidine gluconate, quinidine polygalacturonate, quinidine sulfate, reserpine, streptomycin sulfate, sulfadimethoxine, sulfonamides, tetracyclines, thiouracil, and trimethadione.
7. Other data:
   A. There is a clinical association of this antibody titer with vasculitis.

B. Not useful as a screening test for lupus.

ANTI–SMOOTH MUSCLE ANTIBODY, SERUM

Norm. Negative at titer <1:20.

Increased. Asthma (intrinsic) (positive at titer <1:10), biliary cirrhosis (positive at titer 1:10–1:40), autoimmune hepatitis, chronic active (lupoid) hepatitis (majority of clients) (positive at titers of 1:80–1:320), cryptogenic cirrhosis (rare), hepatocellular carcinoma, malignancies, mononucleosis (infectious with liver damage), pancreatitis (autoimmune), tumors (infiltrative), viral hepatitis (acute) (positive at titer <1:10), yellow fever, and in clients 50-70 years of age. Drug includes minocycline.

Description. An immunofluorescent test that detects and measures autoimmune immunoglobulins (antibodies) to smooth muscle that appear in chronic active hepatitis and also in response to damaged liver cells. This test is usually performed with the test for antimitochondrial antibodies as an aid in differentiating primary biliary cirrhosis and chronic active hepatitis from diffuse, extrahepatic biliary obstruction and other liver diseases.

Professional Considerations
1. Consent form NOT required.
2. **Preparation:**
   A. Tube: Red topped, red/gray topped, or gold topped.
   B. See *Client and family teaching.*
3. **Procedure:**
   A. Draw a 2-mL blood sample.
4. **Postprocedure care:**
   A. Send the specimen to the laboratory for immediate spinning.
5. **Client and family teaching:**
   A. Fast for 8 hours before sampling.
   B. Results may not be available for several days if testing is not performed on site.
6. **Factors that affect results:**
   A. Reject hemolyzed specimens.
   B. Antinuclear antibody impairs interpretation of results.
7. **Other data:**
   A. This test is not diagnostic. A liver biopsy is recommended.
   B. Low titers may occur with infectious mononucleosis, rheumatoid arthritis, liver disease, and malignancies.

ANTISPERM ANTIBODIES, SPECIMEN
(see Infertility screen, Specimen)

ANTISTREPTOCOCCAL ENZYME
(see Antistreptolysin-O titer, Serum)

ANTISTREPTOLYSIN-O (ASO) TITER, SERUM
Norm:

Adults	<166 Todd U/mL
	or <270 IU/mL
Children	
<2 years	<50 Todd U/mL
2-5	<100 Todd U/mL
5-19	<200 Todd U/mL

A fourfold rise in titer between acute and convalescent specimens is diagnostically significant.

Increased. Acute poststreptococcal endocarditis, acute poststreptococcal glomerulonephritis (500-5000 Todd U/mL), pediatric autoimmune neuropsychiatric disorders associated with streptococcal infections (PANDAS), reactive arthritis, rheumatic fever (inactive is <250 Todd U/mL; active is 500-5000 Todd U/mL), scarlet fever, recent streptococcal disease (small elevations), scarlet fever, Sydenham's chorea, Tourette syndrome.

Decreased. Not clinically significant. Levels may decrease with antibiotic therapy.

Description. Antibody to the streptolysin-O enzyme produced by Lancefield group A beta-hemolytic streptococci. These titers rise about 7 days after infection, peak at 3-5 weeks, and then gradually return to baseline level over the next 6-12 months. Because ASO titers remain elevated in clients with poststreptococcal infections, the test is used to determine whether symptoms such as joint pains, rheumatic fever, or glomerulonephritis are of a poststreptococcal disease origin.

Professional Considerations
1. Consent form NOT required.

2. **Preparation:**
   A. Tube: Red topped, red/gray topped, or gold topped.
3. **Procedure:**
   A. Draw a 1-mL blood sample.
   B. Draw a repeat titer in 10-14 days.
4. **Postprocedure care:**
   A. Send the specimen to the laboratory for immediate spinning.
5. **Client and family teaching:**
   A. Repeated ASO titers every 10-14 days are recommended. When poststreptococcal disease occurs, titers begin to rise 1 week after the initial streptococcal infection and peak 2-4 weeks later; 6 months to 1 year is required for postinfection levels to return to the baseline level.
   B. Results may not be available for several days if testing is not performed on site.
6. **Factors that affect results:**
   A. Reject hemolyzed specimens.
   B. Falsely suppressed results may be caused by nephrotic syndromes, antibody deficiency syndromes, or drug therapy with corticosteroids or antibiotics.
   C. Falsely elevated results may be caused by contaminated serum, hyperbetalipoproteinemia, hypercholesterolemia, hyperglobulinemia, lipemic serum, or liver disorders.
   D. The persistent presence of an antibody from a previous but not recent infection may mildly increase titers. Only very high titers are indicators of recent infection (such as adult, >250 Todd U; child, >333 Todd U).
7. **Other data:**
   A. Up to 20% of clients with poststreptococcal glomerulonephritis may have normal titers. The anti-DNase-B test is recommended to improve specificity.
   B. See also *Antihyaluronidase titer, Serum; Streptozyme, Blood.*

ANTITHROMBIN III (AT-III) TEST, DIAGNOSTIC

Norm:

		SI UNITS
Plasma	21-30 mg/dL	210-300 mg/L
	85-115% of standard	0.85-1.15
	>50% of control value	
Serum	15-35% lower than plasma values	
Immunologic	17-30 mg/dL	
Functional	80-130%	

Increased. Factor deficiency (V, VII), hemophilia (A, B), hepatitis (acute), inflammation, jaundice (obstructive), menstruation, nephrotic syndrome, renal transplantation, vitamin K deficiency. Drugs include anabolic steroids, androgens, bishydroxycoumarin, gemfibrozil, oral contraceptives (containing progesterone), progesterone, and warfarin sodium.

Decreased. Alcoholic liver disease, arteriosclerosis, burns, cardiovascular disease, cerebrovascular accident, carcinoma, cirrhosis, congenital antithrombin III deficiency, deep vein thrombosis, Dengue shock syndrome, diabetes mellitus (type II), disseminated intravascular coagulation, hepatic disease (abscess, hepatitis), homocystinuria, hypercoagulation, liver failure (chronic), liver transplantation, malignancy (extensive), malnutrition, nephrotic syndrome, status post partial hepatectomy, postoperatively, post partum, preeclampsia, pulmonary embolism, septicemia, thromboembolism, venoocclusive disease (VOD). Drugs include estrogens, fibrinolytics, gestodene, heparin calcium, heparin sodium, L-asparaginase, methylprednisolone, and oral contraceptives (containing estrogen).

Description. A naturally occurring protein, IgG (immunoglobulin), probably synthesized by the liver, that inhibits coagulation through inactivation of thrombin and other factors. The action of AT-III is catalyzed by heparin. Hereditary AT-III deficiency is an autosomal dominant disease that predisposes clients to venous thrombosis and heparin resistance.

Professional Considerations
1. Consent form NOT required.
2. Preparation:
   A. Tube: 2.7-mL blue topped or 4.5-mL blue topped.
   B. See *Client and family teaching.*
3. Procedure:
   A. Draw 2.4 mL of blood for a 2.7-mL tube or 4.0 mL of blood for a 4.5-mL tube.
4. Postprocedure care:
   A. Send the specimen to the laboratory for immediate spinning.
5. Client and family teaching:
   A. Fast, except for water, for 10-12 hours before testing.
6. Factors that affect results:
   A. Reject hemolyzed or lipemic specimens.
   B. Results are normally available within 3-5 days.

7. Other data:
   A. Levels of 50%-75% indicate moderate risk for thrombosis, whereas levels under 50% indicate significant risk for thrombosis.
   B. A low level in clients taking warfarin indicates that the warfarin is not working effectively.
   C. AT-III is positively correlated to hematoma volume in hypertensive intracerebral hemorrhage (HICH).

ANTITHYROGLOBULIN ANTIBODY
(*see Thyroid antithyroglobulin antibody, Serum*)

ANTITHYROID MICROSOMAL ANTIBODY
(*see Thyroid Peroxidase Antibody, Blood*)

APEXCARDIOGRAPHY, DIAGNOSTIC

Norm. Normal a wave, c point, e point, o point, rf wave, f point, sf wave, and stasis.

CARDIAC ABNORMALITIES	CHANGES THAT MAY BE FOUND IN APEXCARDIOGRAPHIC RECORDING
Aortic valve stenosis	Large a wave; apical impulse occurring late in systole
Atrial fibrillation	Absent a wave; steepened slope of rf wave
Cardiac failure	Apical impulse occurring late in systole
Coronary artery disease	Apical impulse occurring late in systole
Mitral regurgitation	Steepened slope of rf wave
Mitral stenosis	Absent a wave; shallow slope of rf wave
Hypertension	Large a wave; apical impulse occurring late in systole
Idiopathic hypertrophic	Large a wave subaortic stenosis
Left ventricular aneurysm	Apical impulse occurring late in systole
Myocardial ischemia or	Apical impulse occurring late in systole infarction
Pericarditis	Steepened slope of rf wave

Usage. Helps diagnose heart abnormalities and arterial hypertension. In conjunction with phonocardiography, helps to identify heart sounds.

Description. Apexcardiography is a method to transfer cardiac movement and pulsations into electrical energy by a transducer and produce a graphic recording of waveforms that characterize the status of the heart. The test takes less than ½ hour to perform.

Professional Considerations
1. Consent form NOT required.
2. Preparation:
   A. Remove jewelry and any metal objects.
   B. The client should disrobe above the waist.
3. Procedure:
   A. The client is placed in a left oblique position, and electrocardiographic limb leads are applied. The transducer tip, covered with

electroconductive gel, is strapped in place in contact with the point of maximum impulse at the apex of the heart.
  B. Apexcardiographic recordings are made as the client lies motionless and performs isometric hand-clenching exercises, which increase systemic vascular resistance.
4. Postprocedure care:
  A. Remove transducer and limb leads. Cleanse the electroconductive gel off the transducer and off the client's chest.
5. Client and family teaching:
  A. The test is painless.
  B. Slow, even respirations promote the most accurate test results. You should not talk or move during the procedure.
  C. You will be asked to isometrically clench your fists, which means clenching them and then squeezing them and holding them tightly shut.
6. Factors that affect results:
  A. See above under *Norms*.
  B. Implantable metal devices in the chest wall, such as venous access devices, do not interfere with the test as long as leads are not placed directly over the metal device.
7. Other data:
  A. None.

APNEA HYPOPNEA INDEX
(*see Polysomnography, Diagnostic*)

APNEA TEST, DIAGNOSTIC

Norm:

Negative test (absence of brain death).
Spontaneous respiratory effort occurs after mechanical ventilation is stopped.

Positive test (presence of brain death).
Absence of spontaneous respiratory effort throughout test (up to 8 minutes for adults and up to 15 minutes for pediatrics), $Paco_2$ ≥60 mm Hg or 20 mm Hg higher than baseline value.

Usage. Determination of the absence (or presence) of spontaneous breathing when one is testing for brain death; evaluation of the intracranial hemodynamic status in carotid occlusive disease.

Description. The apnea test is part of a neurologic evaluation that tests for the respiratory reflex in clients suspected of having brain death. It is performed with a full neurologic examination, clinical history that includes a central nervous system event, and other confirmatory tests to determine brain death. Brain death is the term used when the entire brain, including the brainstem, has irreversibly stopped functioning. Brain death cannot be determined in clients receiving neuromuscular blockers, or with low core-body temperatures (such as ≤32.2° C).

Professional Considerations
1. Consent form NOT required.
2. Preparation:
  A. Obtain and document baseline $Paco_2$ value.
  B. Determine if client meets requirements for apnea testing
    i. Pco_2 ≥40 mm Hg
    ii. Mean arterial pressure (MAP) >54 mm Hg
    iii. Positive fluid balance in previous 6 hours
    iv. Absence of the possibility of acute drug or alcohol intoxication
    v. Absence of the presence of any centrally acting drugs that could depress respiration
  C. Obtain a pulse oximeter, ice, oxygen T-piece, and arterial blood gas kit.
3. Procedure:
  A. Position pulse oximetry probe on client. Set heart rate, blood pressure, and respiratory rate alarms. Monitor all throughout the test.
  B. Preoxygenate client with 100% oxygen × 10 minutes.
  C. Remove client's gown or clothing from the chest and abdominal area to allow visualization of respiratory muscle efforts.
  D. Discontinue mechanical ventilation. Apply oxygen through a T-piece at 6 L/min. Monitor for spontaneous respiratory effort.
    i. If no respiratory effort is noted after 5-8 minutes, obtain an arterial blood gas sample and restart mechanical ventilation.
    ii. Observe chest for spontaneous respirations or any respiratory effort.

iii. Discontinue the test if any of the following occur:
(1) Presence of spontaneous respiratory effort
(2) Hemodynamic instability
E. Test is repeated at least 6-12 hours later.
4. Postprocedure care:
A. Document procedure, including methodology, length of apneic time, baseline and ending $Paco_2$ values, stability of vital signs, and apneic status.
B. For positive tests, request organ donation, as and when appropriate.
5. Client and family teaching:
A. Organ and tissue donation rates are higher when families or significant others receive a careful and thorough explanation of the concept of brain death.
6. Factors that affect results:
A. $Paco_2$ rises approximately 3 mm Hg each minute while the client is apneic and not receiving mechanical ventilation.
B. Results must be interpreted with extreme caution in clients with brain injury. Caution should be used in determining the brain death when the cause of the brain injury is not known and in high cervical spine fracture in which there is damage to the spinal cord.
C. Posturing may make detection of respiratory effort impossible.
7. Other data:
A. The neurologic examination in brain death reveals the absence of spontaneous reflexes, absence of response to pain, and absence of brainstem reflexes, including the respiratory reflex.
B. Complications known to have occurred during this test include pneumothorax, pneumoperitoneum, and cardiac arrest.

APOLIPOPROTEIN A-I (APOPROTEIN-A, APO-A), PLASMA

Norm. Values 5%-10% higher in African-Americans.

AGE	FEMALE		MALE	
	mg/dL	SI UNITS g/L	mg/dL	SI UNITS g/L
Adult				
20-29 years	80-184	0.80-1.84	81-153	0.81-1.53
30-39 years	83-187	0.83-1.87	79-155	0.79-1.55
40-49 years	93-181	0.93-1.81	100-140	1.00-1.40
50-59 years	76-204	0.76-2.04	81-169	0.81-1.69
60-65 years	122-214	1.22-2.14	86-166	0.86-1.66
Child				
Birth	38-106	0.38-1.06	41-93	0.41-0.93
0.5-4 years	60-148	0.60-1.48	67-163	0.67-1.63
5-7 years	90-151	0.90-1.51	92-151	0.92-1.51
8-9 years	94-151	0.94-1.51	96-151	0.96-1.51
10-11 years	92-151	0.92-1.51	96-151	0.96-1.51
12-13 years	83-146	0.83-1.46	88-151	0.88-1.51
14-15 years	96-146	0.96-1.46	85-139	0.85-1.39
16-17 years	96-151	0.96-1.51	83-146	0.83-1.46

CORONARY ATHEROSCLEROTIC RISK	APOLIPOPROTEIN B/A RATIO	
	FEMALE	MALE
Average risk	0.6	0.7
Twice average risk	0.9	0.9
Three times average risk	1.0	1.0

Increased. Not clinically significant. Familial hyperalphalipoproteinemia. Drugs include carbamazepine, chlorinated hydrocarbons, clofibrate, deflazacort, estrogen, ethyl alcohol, exercise, gemfibrozil, hormone replacement therapy of conjugated estrogen and medroxyprogesterone or 17-beta-estradiol/desogestrel, lovastatin, niacin, oral contraceptives (containing estrogen), phenobarbital, phenytoin, pravastatin, simvastatin, weight-reduction diet. Ingestion of beef increases apolipoprotein A-I.

Decreased. Alzheimer's disease, atherosclerosis, cholestasis, coronary artery disease, diabetes mellitus (poorly controlled), hepatectomy, hepatocellular abnormalities, hypertriglyceridemia, hypoalphalipoproteinemia, ischemic coronary disease, lipoprotein lipase cofactor deficiency, myocardial infarction, nephrotic syndrome, polycystic ovary syndrome (PCOS), renal failure (chronic), stroke. Drugs include androgens, beta-adrenergic receptor blocking agents, diuretics, probucol, progestins, and synthroid.

Description. An inherited alpha$_1$-globulin that is the major protein component (70%) of high-density lipoprotein (HDL). It is synthesized in the liver and small intestine and is essential for the transport of peripheral cholesterol to the liver for eventual excretion. Calculation of the ratio of apolipoprotein A-1 to apo-lipoprotein B and plasma levels of apo A-I are the strongest predictors, more useful than HDL cholesterol, for identifying clients at risk for coronary artery disease.

Professional Considerations
1. Consent form NOT required.
2. Preparation:
   A. Tube: Red topped, red/gray topped, or gold topped.
   B. Several testing methods are used to measure apolipoprotein A-1. Clarify the proper blood-drawing procedure with the individual laboratory.
   C. See *Client and family teaching.*
3. Procedure:
   A. Draw a 1-mL blood sample.
4. Postprocedure care:
   A. None.
5. Client and family teaching:
   A. Fast for 12 hours before testing.
   B. Refrain from smoking for 4 hours before testing.
   C. A ratio of apolipoprotein A to apolipoprotein B is sometimes used to predict coronary heart disease.
6. Factors that affect results:
   A. Reject hemolyzed or lipemic specimens.
   B. Apolipoprotein A-1 levels rise during acute illness.
   C. Levels are decreased in smokers and in clients who consume high-carbohydrate or high–polyunsaturated fat diets.
7. Other data:
   A. Apolipoprotein levels remain stable after acute ischemic stroke.

APOLIPOPROTEIN B (APOPROTEIN B, APO B), PLASMA

Norm:

AGE	FEMALE mg/dL	FEMALE SI UNITS g/L	MALE mg/dL	MALE SI UNITS g/L
Adult	86-159	0.86-1.59	96-174	0.96-1.74
Child				
Birth	11-31	0.11-0.31	11-31	0.11-0.31
0.5-4 years	23-75	0.23-0.75	23-75	0.23-0.75
5-7 years	49-110	0.49-1.10	47-106	0.47-1.06
8-9 years	53-132	0.53-1.32	49-105	0.49-1.05
10-11 years	54-121	0.54-1.21	52-110	0.52-1.10
12-13 years	46-110	0.46-1.10	46-113	0.46-1.13
14-15 years	41-108	0.41-1.08	44-103	0.44-1.03
16-17 years	41-96	0.41-0.96	48-139	0.48-1.39

CORONARY ATHEROSCLEROTIC RISK	APOLIPOPROTEIN B/A RATIO	
	FEMALE	MALE
Average risk	0.6	0.7
Twice average risk	0.9	0.9
Three times average risk	1.0	1.0

Increased. Acute illness, Alzheimer's disease, angina pectoris, anorexia nervosa, cigarette smokers, coronary heart disease (premature), Cushing syndrome, diabetes mellitus, dysglobulinemia, hepatic disease and obstruction, hypercalcemia (infantile), hyperlipemia (familial combined), hypothyroidism, myocardial infarction, nephrotic syndrome, porphyria, pregnancy, renal failure, sexual ateliotic dwarfism, sphingolipodystrophies, stress (emotional), and Werner syndrome.

Decreased. Anemia (chronic), alphalipoprotein deficiency, heterozygous hypobetalipoproteinemia, hepatocellular dysfunction, hyperlipoproteinemia (type I), hyperthyroidism, joint inflammation, lecithin-cholesterol acyltransferase deficiency, lipoprotein lipase cofactor deficiency, malabsorption, malnutrition, myeloma, pulmonary disease (chronic), Reye syndrome, stress (acute physical), weight-reduction diet. Drugs include xenical (Orlistat), levothyroxine (Synthroid).

Description. A beta-globulin that is the major protein component of low-density lipoprotein (LDL) and is also found in very-low-density lipoprotein (VLDL). Functions in cholesterol synthesis and is required for the secretion into plasma of intestinal and hepatic triglyceride-rich lipoproteins. There are two Apo B glycoproteins, Apo B-48 and Apo B-100, which have different molecular weights. Apo B-48 is produced in the small intestine and Apo B-100 is produced in the liver. Calculation of the ratio of apolipoprotein A-1 to apolipoprotein B is believed to be more useful than LDL cholesterol for identifying clients at risk for atherosclerosis.

Professional Considerations
1. Consent form NOT required.
2. Preparation:
   A. Tube: Red topped, red/gray topped, or gold topped.

B. Several testing methods are used to measure apolipoprotein B. Clarify the proper blood-drawing procedure with the individual laboratory.
C. See *Client and family teaching.*
3. Procedure:
   A. Draw a 1-mL blood sample.
4. Postprocedure care:
   A. None.
5. Client and family teaching:
   A. Fast for 12 hours before testing.
   B. A ratio of apolipoprotein A to apolipoprotein B is sometimes used to predict coronary heart disease.
6. Factors that affect results:
   A. Reject hemolyzed or lipemic specimens.
   B. Apolipoprotein B levels rise during acute illness.
7. Other data:
   A. Garlic has no effect on apolipoprotein levels.

APOLIPOPROTEIN E-4 (APO E-4) GENOTYPING, PLASMA

Norm. APO E-4 allele is not present.

Usage. Helps identify risk for, but cannot confirm Alzheimer's disease, as the disease also occurs in those not carriers or homozygotes. Genotyping more recently piloted for determination of risk of developing Alzheimer's disease through the National Institutes of Health. NOT useful for monitoring disease progression.

Description. Alzheimer's disease, the most common form of dementia, is characterized by the presence of senile plaques and neurofibrillary tangles. Two forms of Alzheimer's disease are known to exist. The majority (90%-95%) are termed, "late onset," with the remaining 5%-10% termed, "early onset." The apolipoprotein (APO) E-4 allele is an important genetic risk factor for late onset Alzheimer's disease, occurring more than twice as often in those with Alzheimer's disease as in control groups. The exact mechanism by which the APO E-4 allele contributes to the development of Alzheimer's disease is not known, but there is some evidence that its action contributes to the development of plaques and neurofibrillary tangles, as well as to the loss of brain tissue volume. Carriers of the APO E-4 allele can have up to a 2.9 times greater chance and homozygotes can have up to a 15 times greater chance than noncarriers of developing Alzheimer's disease.

Professional Considerations

1. Consent form IS required due to experimental nature of current usage.
2. Preparation:
   A. Tube: Green topped.
3. Procedure:
   A. Draw a 4-mL blood sample.
4. Postprocedure care:
   A. None.
5. Client and family teaching:
   A. Results are normally available in 1-2 weeks.
   B. Refer the client with abnormal results for genetic counseling.
6. Factors that affect results:
   A. Heparin in the specimen collection tube must be sodium heparin.
7. Other data:
   A. This test is currently available for research and experimental purposes.

APTT

(see Activated partial thromboplastin time and partial thromboplastin time, Plasma)

ARSENIC, BLOOD

Norm:

		SI UNITS
Whole blood		
Normal	2-23 µg/L	0.03-0.31 µmol/L
Chronic poisoning	100-500 µg/L	1.33-6.65 µmol/L
Acute poisoning	>600 µg/L	>7.98 µmol/L
Serum	1.7-1.54 µg/L	0.02-0.20 µmol/L

Acute Poisoning Symptoms and Treatment

Symptoms. Abdominal pain, nausea, vomiting, bloody diarrhea, and thirst progressing to dehydration and fluid and electrolyte imbalance, hematuria, metallic taste, pain (gastrointestinal), renal failure, jaundice, hypoxia, convulsions, coma, and respiratory and cardiovascular collapse. May lead to death.

Treatment:
Note: Treatment choice(s) depend on client history and condition and episode history.
Induction of emesis
Lavage GI tract
Saline cathartic
Penicillamine chelation
Dimercaprol (BAL)
Support hemodynamic status
Replace blood lost to GI hemorrhage
Both hemodialysis and peritoneal dialysis WILL remove arsenic

Chronic Poisoning Symptoms and Treatment

Symptoms. Abnormal erythropoiesis and myelopoiesis, alopecia (thinning of hair), anemia, basophilic stippling, delirium, diarrhea, gastrointestinal symptoms, hepatomegaly, hyperkeratosis of palms of hands and soles of feet, leukopenia, macular hypopigmentation, Mee's lines, metallic taste, peripheral neuropathy, rain drop like skin pigmentation changes and scaling, and thrombocytopenia.

Treatment:
Note: Treatment choice(s) depend on client history and condition and episode history.
Avoid exposure to arsenic.
Remove household sources of arsenic (described below).

Increased. Arsenic poisoning and heavy metal poisoning, peripheral vascular disease. Herbs or natural remedies include Korean herbal medicines usually prescribed for hemorrhoids, powdered blend of folk remedies of Hmong people from Thailand, and Indian ethnic remedies for treatment of congenital retinoblastoma.

Decreased. Not clinically significant.

Description. Arsenic is a trace element found in all human tissues that may become elevated when occupational, environmental (coal burning), or intentional exposure occurs. Sixty-three percent of ingested arsenic is excreted in the urine. Arsenic is found environmentally in well water and as an ingredient of pesticides, paints, treated wood, cosmetics, and antiprotozoal medications. Arsenic inhibits sulfhydryl enzyme systems required for cellular metabolism. Blood specimens are used for rapid confirmation of acute poisoning and blood levels are transitory. Workplace exposure or chronic ingestion is associated with skin, lung and other cancers.

Professional Considerations
1. Consent form NOT required unless the specimen may be used for legal evidence.
2. **Preparation:**
   A. Tube: Black topped or green topped (whole blood) or red topped, red/gray topped, or gold topped (serum).
   B. Do NOT draw during hemodialysis.
   C. Screen client for the use of herbal preparations or natural remedies

such as Korean red or white ginseng (*Panax*).
3. **Procedure:**
   A. The specimen should be collected and labeled in the presence of a witness if it may be used for legal evidence.
   B. Draw a 20-mL blood sample.
4. **Postprocedure care:**
   A. Note the exact time of specimen collection, along with the client's name, date, contents, and your signature on the tube label and laboratory requisition.
   B. Have the witness sign the laboratory requisition.
   C. Transport the specimen to the laboratory in a sealed plastic bag labeled as legal evidence if that is the case. Have each person handling the specimen write his or her name and time of receipt of the specimen on the laboratory requisition.
5. **Client and family teaching:**
   A. For intentional poisoning, refer the client and family for crisis intervention.
   B. For chronic poisoning, the client should be taught to remove household sources of arsenic (described above).
6. **Factors that affect results:**
   A. A diet rich in seafood may elevate the blood level.
7. **Other data:**
   A. Arsenic is easily transferred to a fetus.

ARSENIC, HAIR OR TOENAILS, SPECIMEN

Norm:

		SI UNITS
Hair		
Normal levels	20-60 µg/100 g	<8.7 nmol/g
Chronic poisoning	>100 µg/100 g	>13.4 nmol/g
Nails		
Normal levels	20-60 µg/100 g	<8.7 nmol/g
Chronic poisoning	90-180 µg/100 g	12-24 nmol/g

Poisoning Level Symptoms and Treatment. See *Arsenic, Blood.*

Increased. Arsenic poisoning and industrial or environmental exposure to arsenic. Blackfoot disease.

Decreased. Not clinically significant.

Description. A common heavy metal poison that combines with intracellular proteins and is rapidly removed from the blood (63% excreted in the urine). Arsenic, a trace element found in all human tissues, may become elevated when occupational (treated wood), environmental, or intentional usage occurs. It is found environmentally as an ingredient of pesticides, paints, cosmetics, and antiprotozoal medications. Arsenic inhibits sulfhydryl enzyme systems required for cellular metabolism. Because it can be found in keratin, specimens of hair and nail are used to pinpoint chronic exposure to arsenic.

Professional Considerations
1. Consent form NOT required.
2. **Preparation:**
   A. Obtain scissors or nail clippers.
3. **Procedure:**
   A. *Hair:* Hair samples must contain the root end and the distal end. Collect 0.5 g of hair (preferably pubic hair). Ensure privacy when obtaining a pubic hair sample.
   B. *Nails:* Clip the end of all 10 toenails. Collect a total of 0.5 g of nails (preferably toenails). Place the specimens in a clean, dry envelope or heavy metal-free plastic container.
4. **Postprocedure care:**
   A. Transport the samples to the laboratory as soon as possible.

5. **Client and family teaching:**
   A. For chronic poisoning, client should be taught to remove household sources of arsenic (described above).
6. **Factors that affect results:**
   A. A diet rich in seafood may raise levels.
7. **Other data:**
   A. Arsenic in toenails represents deposition of arsenic for 6 months.
   B. The earliest detection of excess arsenic in hair is 2 weeks after a dose of arsenic and may persist for months or years.
   C. A 10-fold increase in well water concentrations is reflected in a twofold increase in toenail concentration.
   D. After exposure to arsenic, white strips about 1 mm wide extend across the entire base of the nails and contain very high concentrations of arsenic.
   E. Symptoms of chronic toxicity include fatigue, weakness, diarrhea, weight loss, dermatitis, and nausea progressing to paralysis, encephalopathy, renal and hepatic damage, and respiratory tract inflammation.

ARSENIC, URINE

Norm:

		SI UNITS
Normal	5-50 μg/24 hours	0.067- 0.665 μmol/d
Chronic poisoning	50-5000 μg/L	0.67-66.50 μmol/L
Acute poisoning	>1000 μg/L	>13.3 μmol/L

Poisoning Level Symptoms and Treatment. See *Arsenic, Blood.*

Increased. Alcohol intake, arsenic poisoning, and metal poisoning.

Decreased. Not clinically significant.

Description. A common heavy metal poison that combines with intracellular proteins and is rapidly removed from the blood (63% excreted in the urine). Arsenic, a trace element found in all human tissues, may become elevated when occupational (treated wood),

environmental, or intentional usage occurs. It is found environmentally as an ingredient of pesticides, paints, cosmetics, and antiprotozoal medications. Arsenic inhibits sulfhydryl enzyme systems required for cellular metabolism. Urine specimens are used for rapid confirmation of acute poisoning and monitoring ongoing exposure.

Professional Considerations
1. Consent form NOT required unless the specimen may be used as legal evidence.
2. **Preparation:**
   A. Obtain a 3-L container without preservatives.

3. **Procedure:**
   A. The specimen should be collected and labeled in the presence of a witness if it may be used for legal evidence.
   B. Collect a 24-hour urine sample in a 3-L container without preservatives.
   C. Discard the first morning-urine specimen.
   D. Save all urine voided for 24 hours in a refrigerated, clean, 3-L container without preservatives. Document the quantity of urine output during the collection period. Include urine voided at the end of the 24-hour period. For catheterized clients, keep the drainage bag on ice and empty the urine into the collection container hourly.
4. **Postprocedure care:**
   A. Note the exact beginning and ending times of urine collection, along with the client's name, date, contents, and your signature on the container and laboratory requisition.
   B. Have a witness sign the laboratory requisition.
   C. Transport the entire specimen to the laboratory in a sealed plastic bag labeled as legal evidence, if that is the case. Have each person handling the specimen write his or her name and the time of receipt of the specimen on the laboratory requisition.
5. **Client and family teaching:**
   A. Save all urine voided in the 24-hour period, and urinate before defecating to avoid loss of urine. If any urine is accidentally discarded, discard the entire specimen and restart the collection the next day.
   B. For chronic poisoning, the client should be taught to remove household sources of arsenic (described above).
6. **Factors that affect results:**
   A. A diet rich in seafood may show elevated concentration levels in the urine as high as 500-1500 mg/L with no apparent signs of toxicity.
7. **Other data:**
   A. Hyperbilirubinemia and increased serum ALP found in conjunction with arsenic in the urine.

B. Urinary arsenic levels slightly higher in males (36-541 nmol/L) than females (21-475 nmol/L).
C. Children exposed to high levels of arsenic in drinking water have a health risk.

ART
(see Automated reagin test, Diagnostic)

ARTERIAL BLOOD GASES
(see Blood gases, Arterial, Blood)

ARTERIOGRAM, DIAGNOSTIC

Norm. Even filling of the arteries with radiographic dye. The artery walls show progressive narrowing without abrupt occlusions, isolated bulging or narrow areas. No evidence of leakage of the dye into tissues, which would indicate hemorrhage. No evidence of vascular anomalies. No displacement of vessels.

Usage. Aids diagnosis of arterial occlusion, aneurysm, abnormal vascular development, hemorrhage and transitory ischemia attacks (TIAs). Helps identify areas of arterial narrowing caused by plaque buildup, degree of stenosis after myocardial infarction (MI), tumor, or vascular abnormalities. Useful preoperatively to help identify potential failing arterial bypass grafts.

Description. An arteriogram is a radiographic examination of arteries through which radiographic contrast medium is flowing. The arteries are assessed for abnormalities in blood flow, such as narrowing or outpouching of the walls, and for collateral circulation.

Professional Considerations
1. Consent form IS required.

Risks
Aphasia, cerebrovascular accident, dysrhythmias, embolus, endocarditis, hematoma, hemiplegia, hemorrhage, infection, MI, paresthesia, allergic reaction to dye (itching, hives, rash, tight feeling in the throat, shortness of

breath, bronchospasm, anaphylaxis, death), renal toxicity.

Contraindications

Anticoagulant therapy, bleeding disorders, thrombocytopenia, dehydration, uncontrolled hypertension, previous allergy to radiographic dye, iodine, or shellfish, renal insufficiency, and pregnancy (if iodinated contrast medium is used, because of radioactive iodine crossing the blood-placental barrier).

2. **Preparation:**
   A. See *Client and family teaching.*
   B. Obtain baseline CBC, PT/PTT, and APTT values.
   C. Remove all jewelry and metal objects.
   D. The client should void just before the procedure.
   E. Obtain baseline vital signs, and mark peripheral pulses.
   F. Have emergency equipment readily available for anaphylaxis and cardiac arrest.

3. **Procedure:**
   A. Client is placed supine on the radiograph table.
   B. A maintenance intravenous line is started.
   C. The peripheral pulses are marked, and the extremity is immobilized.
   D. The femoral or brachial artery area is located and cleansed with povidone-iodine solution and allowed to dry, and the surrounding area is covered with a sterile drape.
   E. A local anesthetic (1%-2% lidocaine) is injected intradermally and subcutaneously over the artery.
   F. The femoral or brachial artery is punctured with a large-bore needle. A wire is passed through the needle and the needle removed over the guidewire.
   G. The catheter is then inserted into the artery over the guidewire, and placement is confirmed by fluoroscopy.
   H. The catheter is advanced under fluoroscopy to a location depending on the area to be examined, and radiographic dye is injected.
   I. Several rapid radiographic pictures are taken of the artery and its branches during and after dye injection.
   J. The catheter is removed, and sterile gauze is applied immediately,

with pressure, to the site for at least 15 minutes.

4. **Postprocedure care:**
   A. Apply pressure dressing to arterial puncture site.
   B. The client remains on bed rest with the affected extremity immobilized for 12 hours.
   C. Assess the site and dressing for hematoma or bleeding; the distal pulses for presence and strength; and color, motion, temperature, and sensation of the affected extremity every 15 minutes × 4, every half hour × 4, then every hour × 4, and then every 4 hours.
   D. Apply pressure for at least 15 minutes if bleeding occurs.
   E. Encourage oral intake of fluids if not contraindicated.

5. **Client and family teaching:**
   A. If the abdominal vasculature is to be examined, a cathartic may be administered 1 day before the test and a tap-water enema may be given on the morning of the test.
   B. Consume clear liquids only for 24 hours and fast from food and fluids for 8 hours before the test.
   C. It is normal to experience a brief flushing sensation and possibly nausea when the dye is injected, but the feeling will pass quickly.
   D. It is important to lie still throughout the procedure.
   E. Bed rest and frequent site and extremity checks are performed as standard postprocedure care.
   F. In women who are breast-feeding, formula should be substituted for breast milk for 1 or more days after the procedure.

6. **Factors that affect results:**
   A. Movement of the client during filming may obscure the pictures.

7. **Other data:**
   A. Clients with cardiomegaly need to be monitored carefully during this procedure or assessed to see if this procedure is fundamentally necessary.
   B. Odds of receiving this test are lower for Hispanics when compared to non-Hispanic White counterparts (Elixhauser et al., 2002).
   C. See also *Cardiac catheterization, Cerebral angiogram, Pulmonary angiogram,* or *Renal angiogram, Diagnostic.*

ARTHROGRAPHY, DIAGNOSTIC

Norm. Intact soft-tissue structures of the joint. Absence of lesions, fractures, or tears.

Usage. Detection of damage to joint connective tissue and structures (that is, adhesions, tears, fractures). Specific for full-thickness triangular fibrocartilage tears, rotator cuff tears, and ankle ligament visualization. Ganglion cyst.

Description. Arthrography involves fluoroscopic and radiographic examination of a joint after air or radiographic dye is injected into it. Arthrography provides better visualization of the connective tissue of joints than routine radiography. It is most commonly used to view the knees and shoulders but may also be performed on other joints such as the ankle, hip, wrist, or temporomandibular joint.

Professional Considerations
1. Consent form IS required.

Risks
Allergic reaction to dye (itching, hives, rash, tight feeling in the throat, shortness of breath, bronchospasm, anaphylaxis, death), renal toxicity; bleeding, hematoma, or infection at injection site.

Contraindications
Previous allergy to iodine, seafood, or radiographic dye; pregnancy; active rheumatoid arthritis; infection of the joint to be studied; pregnancy (if iodinated contract medium is used, because of crossing the blood-placental barrier).

2. **Preparation:**
    A. Obtain a sterile arthrography tray, povidone-iodine solution, and 1%-2% lidocaine.
    B. Have emergency equipment readily available.
    C. See *Client and family teaching.*
3. **Procedure:**
    A. The skin is cleansed with povidone-iodine solution and allowed to dry.
    B. A local anesthetic (1%-2% lidocaine) is injected subdermally and subcutaneously around the site to be punctured.
    C. A needle is inserted into the joint space, and a small amount of contrast dye is injected through it as

placement is checked under fluoroscopy.
    D. After correct placement is confirmed, the remainder of the dye is injected and the needle withdrawn.
    E. The extremity may be moved briefly through a range of motion, and then several fluoroscopic films are taken of the joint in different positions.
4. **Postprocedure care:**
    A. Minimize use of the joint for 12 hours.
    B. For knee arthrography, an elastic wrap should be worn over the knee for 3-4 days.
5. **Client and family teaching:**
    A. Fast from food and fluids for 8 hours before the procedure.
    B. Some mild pain and pressure will be felt during the procedure, but local anesthesia will be used to keep these sensations tolerable.
    C. Postarthrography edema and tenderness occur frequently for 1-2 days and may be treated with ice packs and mild analgesia. Symptoms lasting more than 2 days necessitate a physician's assessment.
    D. If air injection was used, it is normal to feel crepitus in the joint for up to 2 days, because air remains in the joint space until it dissolves into the tissues. The air causes a popping or cracking sensation when the joint moves.
6. **Factors that affect results:**
    A. Fluid in the joint space decreases the quality of the films caused by dilution of the dye. If present, it should be aspirated before dye injection.
7. **Other data:**
    A. Arthrography is 100% specific and 85% sensitive for detection of full-thickness triangular fibrocartilage tears.
    B. MRI and arthrography have a similar diagnostic and therapeutic effect.

ARTHROPOD IDENTIFICATION, SPECIMEN

Norm. Requires interpretation.

Usage. Insect bites.

Description. There are over 1 million species in the phylum Arthropoda, including flies, mosquitos, fleas, lice, itch mites (producing scabies), mites, maggots, bedbugs, spiders, cockroaches, termites, ticks, bees, wasps, and scorpions. Specimens are usually presented for identification after a human has been bitten by or infested with them. Arthropod bites may cause a variety of wheals, rashes, or anaphylactic reactions in humans.

Professional Considerations
1. Consent form NOT required.
2. **Preparation:**
   A. Obtain alcohol wipes, tweezers, and a container of 70% alcohol.
3. **Procedure:**
   A. Capture and preserve the arthropod in a sealed container of 70% alcohol. If the arthropod is a tick, rub the tick and site with an alcohol wipe. Then, holding the tick close to the skin with tweezers, pull the tick straight out and apply gentle pulling, without twisting, until the tick lets loose from the skin.
   B. Wash fly larvae in water and then boil for a few minutes before placing in 70% alcohol.
4. **Postprocedure care:**
   A. Transport the specimen to the laboratory.
5. **Client and family teaching:**
   A. For an arthropod bite or sting, swelling and itching can be controlled by placement of a cold washcloth or towel over the site for 20 minutes once per hour. Change to warm washcloths after 1-2 days.
   B. Pain can be reduced by application of a paste of water and baking soda to the site for 5-10 minutes.
   C. Itching can be controlled with calamine lotion.
   D. Use insect repellant whenever venturing into grassy or wooded areas.
   E. The main concern with flea bites is secondary infection. Therefore keep fingernails short to avoid scratching. Bathe in a tub of water filled with 1 kg of starch, apply calamine lotion to skin, and take antihistamines as prescribed. If an infection develops, antibiotics such as neomycin or polymyxin may be prescribed.
   F. For head lice:
      i. To avoid transmitting head lice:
         a. Do not allow your head to come into close proximity with that of another person.
         b. During active infestation, rinse hairbrushes and combs off after use, to wash away any lice. Avoid sharing hair brushes or combs, because they may forcibly remove healthy head lice, which can reinfest for up to 24 hours.
      ii. It is not necessary to wash or "disinfest" clothing or linen. This advice is common, but mistaken, and applies only to clothing lice, which are found only on clothes and not on the body. Healthy head lice do not disperse except when scraped off (such as by combing) or when moving directly to another person's head. Shedding on linen occurs only when they are dying.
6. **Factors that affect results:**
   A. None.
7. **Other data:**
   A. Spiders: Two venomous spiders are the brown recluse and the black widow spider, which are more common in the southern United States. The redleg spider of Florida may also produce symptoms of poisoning. Treatment includes slow intravenous administration of 10 mL of 10% calcium gluconate and a muscle relaxant such as diazepam. A commercially prepared antivenom for the black widow, though rarely needed, is available in vials of 6000 U diluted in 2.5 mL of sterile water and given intramuscularly or intravenously.
   B. A generalized systemic reaction to bee, wasp, and ant stings is believed to be IgE mediated. Treatment includes epinephrine hydrochloride 1:1000, 0.3-0.5 mL for an adult and 0.01 mL/kg for a child, prednisone orally to reduce swelling, and diphenhydramine hydrochloride, 25-50 mg orally, to relieve itching. "Killer bees" envenomation can cause acute tubular necrosis and death.

C. Lice or itch mites (producing scabies) frequently found in hair on the head or on the hands, feet, and pubic hair require a thorough application of gamma-benzene hexachloride (Kwell, GBH) cream or lotion. Since GBH is toxic, it is questionable whether it should be used for young children or pregnant women. Some references recommend treatment only if a live louse is found.

D. The puss caterpillar, found in the southeastern United States, especially Texas and Florida, can cause shocklike signs and symptoms, as well as skin necrosis, edematous infiltration, and major fibrinogenolysis. Treatment includes immediate removal of the stinger. This may be followed by slow intravenous administration of 10 mL of 10% calcium gluconate and a muscle relaxant such as diazepam.

E. Mosquitoes are known carriers of yellow fever.

F. Dust mites are retained, thereby increasing allergy symptoms, by larger carpet surfaces, fluorocarbon-treated fibers, and carpets with low pile.

ARTHROSCOPY, DIAGNOSTIC

Norm. Internal anatomy of the joint space is undisturbed. Synovial fluid is clear. Synovial membranes are not erythematous. There are no free-floating materials within the joint space.

Usage. Diagnostic use of the procedure is mainly to determine the cause of chronic arthritic complaints that cannot be established with serologic tests. The therapeutic use of the procedure involves the treatment of various acute and chronic arthritic conditions (including the management of septic arthritis and the treatment of torn ligaments) that would otherwise require arthrotomy.

Description. A diagnostic and therapeutic procedure involving the insertion of an arthroscope into a joint that provides direct visualization of the joint space to the physician without the requirement of surgical exposure of the joint (arthrotomy). In addition to the arthroscope, an irrigation cannula and various small resection instruments can be introduced into the joint space during the procedure. Total intravenous anesthesia with propofol and alfentanil or remifentanil does not affect the risk of postoperative nausea and vomiting. Joints that are frequently studied with this procedure include the knee, shoulder, wrist, and (occasionally) the temporomandibular joint. Neurovascular complications are the most serious and devastating complications of this procedure.

Professional Considerations
1. Consent form IS required.

Risks
Bleeding (hemarthrosis), infection, allergic reaction to the local or general anesthetic agent(s) to be used during the procedure.

Contraindications
History of bleeding diathesis, history of allergic reaction to anesthetic agents to be used during the procedure, severe arthritis resulting in narrowing of the joint space that would preclude insertion of the required instruments, cellulitis over the joint to be studied.

2. Preparation:
   A. Preoperative determination of the vital signs is indicated.
   B. The surface over the joint to be studied is shaved and prepped with an iodine solution.
   C. If the procedure is to be performed with the client under general anesthesia, anesthetic premedication may be given and the client is taken to the operating room where a general anesthetic agent is administered.
   D. If the procedure is to be performed with the client under local anesthesia, the client may need to be properly positioned. (As an example, arthroscopy of the knee is at times performed with the client in a sitting position.)
3. Procedure:
   A. If the procedure is to be performed with the client under local anesthesia, infiltration of the skin over the joint is performed with a local anesthetic agent (lidocaine).
   B. The joint space is infiltrated with the local anesthetic agent.

C. If the joint to be studied is located in an extremity, a proximal tourniquet is occasionally applied.
D. A small incision is made, and the irrigation cannula is passed into the joint space. The joint space is irrigated and distended with irrigation solution (saline).
E. The arthroscope is placed into the joint space through a second incision. The internal structures of the joint are visualized.
F. If arthroscopic surgery is to be performed, insertion of various arthroscopic surgical cannulae can be performed through a third incision.
G. At the end of the procedure the instruments are removed from the joint, and the incisions are closed with sutures or Steri-strip tape.
H. Various dressings are applied. In the case of knee arthroscopy an Ace wrap is often used.
I. The pneumatic cuff is then deflated.

4. **Postprocedure care:**
A. Postoperative determination of the vital signs and a dressing check are indicated.
B. Frequent reevaluation of the dressing and the joint may be needed. The physician supervising the care of the client should be informed if bleeding, swelling of the joint ,or leakage of synovial fluid is noted.
C. Postoperative analgesic medications and antibiotic agents may be ordered by the physician supervising the test.
D. A program of physical therapy may be required, although frequently the client may resume normal activity within 24 hours of the procedure.

5. **Client and family teaching:**
A. A general preoperative orientation to the procedure and postoperative care plan is indicated.
B. The client and family will need instruction in any physical therapy routines or mobility limitations imposed by the procedure.
C. Orientation as to the nature and prognosis of the disease process diagnosed by the arthroscopy may be indicated.
D. An ice pack may help ease postprocedure pain. Use a towel between the ice pack and the joint.
E. Use crutches for 5-7 days when walking.

F. Do not exercise the joint more than normal activity for 5-6 weeks after the procedure if surgery was performed.
G. Call the physician if edema continues more than 3 days or if fever over 101° F (38.3° C) or increased knee pain develops.

6. **Factors that affect results:**
A. Client cooperation during arthroscopy performed with the client under local anesthesia is essential.
B. Severe arthritis-producing deformity of the joint space may limit the effectiveness of the procedure.
C. Postoperative complications such as bleeding or infection may limit the effectiveness of arthroscopic surgical procedures.

7. **Other data:**
A. Wrist arthroscopy is ideal for evaluating intra-articular soft-tissue injuries.
B. The cause of various types of chronic arthritis can frequently be determined with radiographic or serologic tests without the need to perform arthroscopy.
C. The increasing availability of smaller arthroscopic instruments has resulted in a growing trend to perform these procedures with the client under local anesthesia and in an office (rather than a hospital) setting.

ASA
(see Salicylate, Blood)

ASA, SPECIMEN
(see Infertility screen, Specimen)

ASCORBIC ACID, SERUM
(see Vitamin C, Plasma or Serum)

ASCUS
(see Pap smear, Diagnostic)

ASM ANTIBODY
(see Anti–smooth muscle antibody, Serum)

ASO TITER, SERUM
(see Antistreptolysin-O titer, Serum)

ASPARTATE AMINOTRANSFERASE (AST, ASPARTATE TRANSAMINASE, SGOT), SERUM

Norm:

		SI UNITS
Adult Females		
Under 61 years	8-20 U/L	0.14-0.34 μKat/L
	10-40 Karmen units/mL	8-20 U/L
Over 60 years	10-20 U/L	0.17-0.34 μKat/L
Adult Males		
Under 61 years	8-20 U/L	0.14-0.34 μKat/L
	10-40 Karmen units/mL	8-20 U/L
Over 60 years	11-26 U/L	0.19-0.44 μKat/L
Children		
Newborn	25-75 U/L	0.43-1.28 μKat/L
Infants	15-60 U/L	0.26-1.02 μKat/L
2-5 months	20-50 U/L	0.34-0.85 μKat/L
1 year	16-35 U/L	0.27-0.60 μKat/L
5 years	19-28 U/L	0.32-0.48 μKat/L
8-12 years	15-40 U/L	0.26-0.68 μKat/L
12-14 years	15-35 U/L	0.26-0.60 μKat/L
14-16 years	15-30 U/L	0.26-0.51 μKat/L

Increased. Acute myocardial infarction (rises 6-12 hours after injury, peaks at 18-24 hours, and returns to normal within 1 week; average increases are about fourfold; large infarcts may cause increases up to 15-fold), alcoholism, anorexia nervosa (emaciated multi organ disorders), calcium dust inhalation, cerebral infarction, cirrhosis, diabetes mellitus, hepatitis (viral preicteric phase), HELLP syndrome, intestinal injury, intramuscular injections, irradiation injury, Lassa fever, lead, lipemia, liver disease, liver necrosis postlaparoscopic cholecystectomy, metal poisoning, musculoskeletal diseases, myoglobinuria, pancreatitis (acute), polymyositis/dermatomyositis, pulmonary infarction, renal infarction, toxic shock syndrome, trauma. Drugs include allopurinol, aluminum nicotinate, amantadine, ampicillin, anabolic steroids, androgens, ascorbic acid, asparaginase, aspirin (value returns to normal within 48 hours of ingestion), azaserine, baclofen, barbiturates, bethanechol chloride, bromocriptine mesylate, captopril, carmustine, carbenicillin, carbon tetrachloride, cardiotonic glycosides, cephalothin sodium, chlordiazepoxide, chloroquine, chlorpromazine hydrochloride, cholinergics, cholestyramine resin, cincophen, clindamycin, clofibrate, cloxacillin, codeine, colchicine, cortisone, cyclacillin, cycloserine, desipramine, dicumarol, digitalis, diphenylhydantoin, disopyramide phosphate, erythromycin, ethionamide, ethyl biscoumacetate, floxuridine, flurazepam, flutamide, fosinopril, gentamicin sulfate, griseofulvin, guanethidine analogs, hydralazine, n-hydroxyacetamide, ibufenac, isoniazid, lincomycin, lorazepam, meperidine, methotrexate, methyldopa, metoprolol tartrate, mithramycin, morphine, nafcillin, nalidixic acid, narcotics, niacin, nifedipine, nitrofurantoin, oral contraceptives, oxacillin, *para*-aminosalicylic acid, phenothiazines, placebo, polycillin, procainamide hydrochloride, propranolol, propylthiouracil, prostaphlin, pyrantel pamoate, pyrazinamide, pyridoxine, rifampin, salicylates, sulfamethizole, sulfamethoxypyridazine, theophylline, tetracycline, thiabendazole, thiothixene, thyroid hormone, tolbutamide, tolmetin sodium, troleandomycin, valproic acid, vitamin A, and vitamin B_6. Herbal or natural remedies include chaparral tea (or misspelled chapparel tea, *Larrea tridentata*), *Echinacea*, pennyroyal. Herbal or natural remedies that have the potential to cause hepatotoxicity and elevate values include akee fruit (ackee, *Blighia sapida*), Atractylis gummifera, Azadirachta indica (see margosa), *Berberis vulgaris* (barberry), *Callilepsis laureola* (blazing star, *Liatris spicata*), chaparral tea (*Larrea tridentata*), cocaine, comfree ("knitbone," *Symphytum*), *Crotalaria* (bush tea), cycasin (a toxin from a *Cycas* species of sago palm of Guam), *Echinacea*, germander (genera Teucrium and Veronica; do not confuse with safe skullcap, a name often falsely used in selling germander), *Heliotropium* (germander, valerian), jin^{1}bu^{2}huan^4 ('gold-inconvertible', Jin Bu Huan Anodyne Tablets, patent medicine with misidentified constituents: essence of t'ienchi [tianqi] flowers, "Noto-ginseng"; also kombucha; also *Lycopodium serratum,* or club moss; but with plant alkaloid levo-tetrahydropalmatine, a potent neuroactive substance), ma^{2}huang^2 (*Ephedra*), margosa (*Melia azadirachta, Azadirachta indica*), maté tea (*Ilex paraguayensis*), mistletoe, pennyroyal, sassafras, skullcap (*Scutellaria; do not confuse with unsafe germander*), syo-saiko-to (xiao^3 chai^{2}hu^2 tang^1, 'minor Bupleurum combination'), *Teucrium polium* (golden germander), and valerian (*Valeriana officinalis, garden heliotrope*).

Decreased. Beriberi, diabetic ketoacidosis, hemodialysis (chronic), liver disease, and uremia (all conditions cause false decreases). Drugs include metronidazole, and trifluoperazine. Herbal or natural remedies include Chinese *fructus schizandrae sinensis* (wu^3 wei^{4}zi^3, coffee (*Coffea*) [in alcoholics], "five flavors herb," *Schisandra chinensis* [Turcz.] Baill.).

Description. A catalytic enzyme found primarily in the heart, liver, and muscle tissue. AST is found in two distinct forms or isoenzymes. c-AST is located in cytoplasm, and m-AST is found in mitochondria. Increases in the serum total AST level occur any time there is serious damage to cells. In addition, AST may be found in complex with IgA in hepatic cancer. AST is also evaluated in comparison with alanine aminotransferase (ALT) to serially monitor liver damage.

Professional Considerations
1. Consent form NOT required.
2. Preparation:
   A. Tube: Red topped, red/gray topped, or gold topped.
   B. Do NOT draw during hemodialysis.

3. **Procedure:**
   A. Draw a 1-mL, nontraumatic blood sample.
4. **Postprocedure care:**
   A. Handle the specimen carefully, avoiding hemolysis.
5. **Client and family teaching:**
   A. Results are normally available within 12 hours.
6. **Factors that affect results:**
   A. Hemolysis of the specimen may cause falsely increased values.
   B. Echinacea taken for 8 weeks or longer may cause hepatotoxicity.
7. **Other data:**
   A. There are no conditions that result in a true decrease in AST. All decreases listed are false decreases.
   B. Bloodletting reduces serum aminotransferase in persons with chronic hepatitis C and iron overload.

ASPERGILLUS ANTIBODY, SERUM

Norm. Negative <1:8. Suspicious infection: Fourfold rise in paired serum specimens. (Isolation does not prove pathogenesis for opportunistic fungi.)

Increased. Allergic bronchopulmonary aspergillosis, hypersensitivity to *Aspergillus,* immunodeficiency, leukemia, and pulmonary aspergilloma.

Description. *Aspergillus* species are saprophytic, opportunistic fungi that can grow on soil and organic materials and often become airborne in large numbers. Over 200 strains exist and may colonize the human body (respiratory tract, skin, nails, ear canal, burns) and become pathogenic in immunosuppressed clients, when they invade human tissue. or when a client becomes sensitized to the organism. In this test, an indirect Coombs' test is performed to identify the presence of *Aspergillus* antibody.

Professional Considerations
1. Consent form NOT required.
2. **Preparation:**
   A. Verify whether the client received antifungal skin testing within the last few weeks. Write the dates and names of such tests on the laboratory requisition.
   B. Tube: Red topped, red/gray topped, or gold topped.

3. Procedure:
   A. Collect a 10-mL blood sample as soon as possible after infection is suspected. Label the specimen as the acute sample.
   B. Repeat the test in 2-3 weeks and label the specimen as the convalescent sample.
4. Postprocedure care:
   A. Transport the specimen to the laboratory promptly and refrigerate at 25° C for no longer than 9 hours.
5. Client and family teaching:
   A. Return in 2-3 weeks for the convalescent sampling.
   B. Amphotericin B is used to treat aspergillosis.
6. Factors that affect results:
   A. False-negative results may occur in immunosuppressed clients.
   B. False-positive results may be caused by recent fungal antigen skin tests.
7. Other data:
   A. Five percent of clients without pulmonary aspergillosis or *Aspergillus* allergy will have *Aspergillus* antibodies.
   B. Identification requires that *Aspergillus* be directly identified in body tissues or fluids, be isolated in multiple specimens, and be identified by microscopic observation of characteristic conidial formation.
   C. The lysis-centrifugation method of culturing is the most sensitive method for detecting molds that cause fungemia. Blood cultures for *Aspergillus* are helpful in diagnosing an *Aspergillus* infection only when repeated lysis-centrifugation tests can distinguish between specimen contamination and pathogenesis based on the number of colonies appearing.
   D. A biopsy is required to diagnose invasive aspergillosis.

ASPIRIN, BLOOD
(see Salicylate, Blood)

ASPIRIN TOLERANCE TEST (ASA TOLERANCE TEST, BLEEDING TIME ASPIRIN TOLERANCE TEST), DIAGNOSTIC

Norm. Requires interpretation. Normal baseline Ivy bleeding time is 2-7 minutes. One study demonstrated bleeding time in normal clients to increase from 2.5 to 4.2 minutes at 2 hours after aspirin ingestion. Bleeding time should return to baseline level by 96 hours after aspirin ingestion.

Increased. Bernard-Soulier syndrome, collagen vascular disease, Cushing's disease, disseminated intravascular coagulation, Glanzmann's thrombasthenia, gray platelet syndrome, hypersplenism, thrombocytopenia with immunosuppression, and von Willebrand's disease. Drugs include anticoagulants (oral), aspirin, indomethacin, and phenylbutazone. Herbs or natural remedies that may inhibit platelet activity include feverfew *(Tanacetum parthenium)*, *Ginkgo biloba*, garlic, ginger, ginseng.

Decreased. Drugs include 1-deamino-8-D-arginine vasopressin (DDAVP).

Description. The Ivy bleeding time test is performed before and after aspirin ingestion to evaluate the drug's effect on platelet function. In normal clients, aspirin ingestion has minimal influence on bleeding time.

Professional Considerations
1. Consent form NOT required for most laboratories.

Risks
Bleeding, ecchymoses, hematoma.

Contraindications
In clients who require upper-extremity restraints, have edematous or very cold arms, or are prone to keloid formation. This test should not be performed if there are contraindications to placing or inflating a blood pressure cuff on the arm (casts, rash, arteriovenous fistula). Other contraindications include platelet count <50,000/mm^3, severe bleeding disorders, skin infectious diseases, senile skin changes, or medications containing acetyl groups, such as those containing aspirin, within the previous 5 days.

2. Preparation:
   A. See *Client and family teaching.*
   B. Obtain povidone-iodine solution, a blood pressure cuff, a lancet, a stopwatch, and filter paper.

3. **Procedure:**
   A. Cleanse the volar aspect of the forearm with povidone-iodine and allow it to dry completely.
   B. Place the blood pressure cuff on the upper arm and inflate to 40 mm Hg.
   C. Make two small incisions 2-3 mm deep on the prepared site. Start timing with the stopwatch.
   D. Remove blood from the wound with filter paper every 15 seconds until bleeding stops. Stop timing with the stopwatch.
   E. If bleeding time is more than 10 minutes, do not proceed further because this test would be contraindicated.
   F. Administer 10 grains (adults) or 5 grains (children weighing less than 32 kg) of aspirin orally.
   G. Repeat steps 3A through 3E after 2 hours.
4. **Postprocedure care:**
   A. If bleeding time is normal, apply a Band-Aid to the site. If bleeding time is prolonged, apply a pressure bandage to the site.
   B. Assess the site(s) for bleeding every 5 minutes for ½ hour. Observe for signs of site infection until healed.
5. **Client and family teaching:**
   A. Do not take aspirin for 5 days before this test.

B. Bring reading material or some other diversion because the test takes 2-3 hours.
6. **Factors that affect results:**
   A. The most sensitive and reproducible measurements may be those taken from a horizontal incision.
7. **Other data:**
   A. The depth of the puncture with the lancet is difficult to standardize and results in poorly reproducible bleeding times.

AST
(see Aspartate aminotransferase, Serum)

AT-III TEST
(see Antithrombin III test, Diagnostic)

ATRIAL NATRIURETIC HORMONE
(see Natriuretic peptides, Plasma)

ATRIAL NATRIURETIC PEPTIDE
(see Natriuretic peptides, Plasma)

AUDIOMETRY TEST (PURE TONE AUDIOMETRY AND SPEECH AUDIOMETRY), DIAGNOSTIC

Norm:

Adult	0-25 dB HL hearing sensitivity
Child	0-15 dB HL hearing sensitivity
Word-discrimination score:	Client is able to repeat list of spoken words with 90% accuracy.

Usage. Delineation of type and amount of hearing loss (that is, conductive, sensorineural, or mixed), rehabilitation monitoring post cochlear implant or poststapedectomy, diagnosis of glue ear (otitis media with effusion).

Description. *Pure tone audiometry* is a hearing test using an audiometer that sends tones into the client's ear and vibrations through the bone. It measures the frequencies at which the client is able to hear 50% or more of the tones.

The test is able to detect defects in air conduction (conductive hearing loss) through the use of tones or defects in air *and* bone conduction (sensorineural hearing loss) through the use of vibrations to help identify the amount and type of hearing loss present. *Speech audiometry* is a hearing test that determines the client's speech-reception threshold and word-discrimination score by measuring the number of words the client can repeat after they are heard when delivered through earphones at precise decibel intensities. Speech audiometry helps differentiate between conductive and sensorineural hearing loss.

Professional Considerations

1. Consent form NOT required.
2. **Preparation:**
   A. See *Client and family teaching.*
   B. Ensure that the external auditory canal is free of impacted cerumen.
   C. Obtain an audiometer, earphones, a vibrator for bone-conduction testing, and an otoscope.
3. **Procedure:**
   A. A plastic tube may be inserted into the external auditory canal to maintain the canal's patency during testing with earphones.
   B. The earphones are placed over the ears and fastened in place.
   C. A preliminary tone is demonstrated for the client to become familiar with the test.
   D. The ear not being tested is masked with audiometer noise to prevent crossover interference and subsequent inaccurate estimation of hearing loss.
   E. *Air conduction testing:* The better ear is tested first. The client is instructed to give a signal each time a tone is heard. Starting with 1000 Hz, tones are delivered to the ear, decreasing by increments of 10 dB until a negative response is obtained. Tone levels are then increased in smaller increments and then decreased until the air conduction threshold level is obtained. The air conduction threshold level is the lowest hertz level at which the client is able to hear two out of three tones. This procedure is then repeated several times, starting with a different tone level each time (such as 2000, 4000, 8000, 1000, 500, and finally 250 Hz). The second ear is then tested in the same way. Finally, retesting is performed on each ear to determine test/retest reliability. Acceptable variation for retesting for each ear must be within 5 dB above or below the initial test result. Graphic recordings are made of the threshold levels.
   F. *Bone conduction testing:* The better ear is tested first. After removal of the earphones, the bone conduction vibrator is held on the mastoid process of the ear. Starting from 250 Hz, tones are delivered to the ear, with decrements at 10 dB until a negative response is obtained. Tone levels are then increased in smaller increments and then decreased until the bone conduction threshold level is obtained. The bone conduction threshold level is the lowest hertz level at which the client is able to hear two out of three tones. This procedure is then repeated several times, starting with a different tone level each time (500, 1000, 2000, and finally 4000 Hz). The second ear is then tested in the same way. Finally, retesting is performed on each ear to determine test/retest reliability. Acceptable variation for retesting for each ear must be within 5 dB above or below the initial test result. Graphic recordings are made of the threshold levels.
   G. *Speech reception threshold measurement:* Two-syllable, familiar, spoken words are delivered through the earphones. The client is asked to repeat each word. The speech reception threshold is the decibel level at which the client is able to restate correctly at least half the words.
   H. *Word discrimination score:* One-syllable, familiar, phonetically balanced words are delivered through the earphones at 30 dB higher than the client's own speech reception threshold. The client is asked to repeat each word. Clients with conductive hearing loss will have a normal word discrimination score. Those with sensorineural hearing loss will have a lower than normal score.
   I. *Amount-of-hearing-loss calculation:* The amount of hearing loss, called the "pure tone average" (PTA), is calculated by averaging the air conduction threshold levels. *Mild* hearing loss demonstrates a PTA of 26-40 dB. *Moderate* hearing loss demonstrates a PTA of 41-55 dB. *Moderately severe* hearing loss demonstrates

a PTA of 56-70 dB. *Severe* hearing loss demonstrates a PTA of 71-90 dB. Profound hearing loss demonstrates a PTA of over 90 dB.

J. *Type-of-hearing-loss calculation:* The type of hearing loss is interpreted by examination of the relationship between the air conduction threshold levels and the bone conduction threshold levels at the different frequencies. In sensorineural hearing loss, both thresholds are depressed to about the same degree. In conductive hearing loss, only the air conduction thresholds are depressed. In mixed hearing loss, both thresholds are depressed, but air conduction threshold levels are more depressed than bone conduction threshold levels.

4. **Postprocedure care:**
   A. Cleanse the earphones and otoscope with antiseptic.

5. **Client and family teaching:**
   A. Stay in an environment free of extremely loud noises for 16 hours before the test.

6. **Factors that affect results:**
   A. Testing should be performed in a very quiet environment for the most accurate results.
   B. The client should not be able to see the examiner because changes in tone level are made. Signals should be delivered in a nonrhythmic pattern.
   C. The client must be able to distinguish between the pure tones and tinnitus or vibrotactile stimulation.
   D. Test/retest differences of more than 10 dB may be caused by unreliable equipment.
   E. The use of plastic tubes to maintain external auditory canal patency should be noted on the audiogram.
   F. Low levels of serum estradiol can impede hearing sensitivity in pure tone audiometry results in postmenopausal women.

7. **Other data:**
   A. See also *Acoustic immittance tests, Diagnostic.*
   B. There is higher prevalence of hearing impairment in persons with diabetes, cognitive impairment, or low education levels or in those who use alcohol or smoke.

AUTOERYTHROCYTE SENSITIVITY TEST, DIAGNOSTIC

Norm. Negative.

Usage. Aids differential diagnosis of the cause of spontaneous bruising and swelling.

Description. The rare autoerythrocyte sensitization syndrome (AESS) (Gardner-Diamond syndrome or psychogenic purpura) is characterized by the appearance of sudden, spontaneous, and severe inflammatory purpura preceded by sensations of pain or burning at the site. It occurs most often in women, often with psychiatric disorders and normal coagulation studies. The bruising characteristically occurs in groups on the extremities and often at times of stress. The syndrome's cause is unknown, but some evidence points to an autoimmune sensitization to erythrocyte stroma because intradermal injection of the client's own red blood cells stimulates development of ecchymosis. There is also some evidence for psychogenic cause. This test helps differentiate self-mutilation from AESS. In a positive test, self-mutilation may be ruled out as the cause of the bruising.

Professional Considerations
1. Consent form IS required.

Risks
Bleeding.

Contraindications
In clients with known bleeding disorders or abnormal coagulation studies.

2. **Preparation:**
   A. Obtain alcohol wipes, a tourniquet, three needles, and two syringes.

3. **Procedure:**
   A. Draw a 1-mL blood sample, and place a fresh needle on the syringe.
   B. Cleanse a thigh site that is free of purpura with an alcohol wipe and allow it to dry. Inject 0.1 mL of the client's own whole blood

intradermally into the thigh site. Mark the site by drawing a circle around it. A more specific method is to use 0.1 mL of the client's own washed erythrocyte stroma for the injection.

C. Cleanse a site on the other thigh that is free of purpura with an alcohol wipe and allow it to dry. Inject 0.1 mL of 0.9% saline intradermally into the cleansed site as a control. Mark the site by drawing a circle around it.

D. A positive reaction is manifest by the development of painful, edematous erythema at the site of the blood injection, with no reaction at the control site.

4. Postprocedure care:
   A. Assess the sites of injection for reaction, including pain, edema, and erythema.

5. Client and family teaching:
   A. This test helps determine if a process in the body is the cause of bruises for which a reasonable cause cannot be found.

6. Factors that affect results:
   A. None.

7. Other data:
   A. Autoerythrocyte sensitization syndrome may also include positive anticardiolipin antibodies.

AUTOMATED REAGIN TESTING (ART), DIAGNOSTIC

Norm. Negative.

TITER	INTERPRETATION
Nonreactive	Negative
≤1:8	False positive
1:9–1:32	Primary-stage syphilis (requiring interpretation)
>1:32	Secondary-stage syphilis

Positive. Syphilis. (See *Factors that affect results* for biologic false-positive results.)

Description. A nonspecific, nontreponemal test used for syphilis screening and monitoring of response to therapy in the postchancre period of the primary stage and in the secondary stage when treponemal antibodies are more difficult to detect. When *Treponema pal-*

lidum, the causative agent of syphilis, invades human tissue, reagin is produced and can be isolated from 7 to 21 days after the appearance of the chancre. Results are reported as the highest titer that produces a positive reaction.

Professional Considerations
1. Consent form NOT required.
2. Preparation:
   A. Tube: Red topped, red/gray topped, or gold topped.
   B. See *Client and family teaching.*
3. Procedure:
   A. Draw a 5-mL blood sample.
4. Postprocedure care:
   A. None.
5. Client and family teaching:
   A. Do not drink alcohol for 24 hours before testing.
   B. Weekly testing for 2 months is recommended before syphilis can be ruled out.
   C. If testing positive:
      i. Notify all sexual contacts from the last 90 days (if early stage) to be tested for syphilis.
      ii. Syphilis can be cured with antibiotics. These may worsen the symptoms for the first 24 hours.
      iii. Do not have sex for 2 months and until after repeat testing has confirmed that the syphilis is cured. Use condoms after that for 2 years. Return for repeat testing every 3-4 months for the next 2 years to make sure the disease is cured.
      iv. Do not become pregnant for 2 years because syphilis can be transmitted to the fetus.
      v. If left untreated, syphilis can damage many body organs, including the brain, over several years.
6. Factors that affect results:
   A. Reject hemolyzed specimens.
   B. False-negative results may occur before the appearance of the chancre in the initial stage of syphilis or during the tertiary stage.
   C. False-negative results may be caused by ingestion of alcohol within 24 hours before specimen collection.
   D. Biologic false-positive results lasting up to 6 months may be

caused by bejel, chickenpox, DPT immunization, hepatitis (infectious), malaria, measles, mononucleosis (infectious), pneumonia (atypical, pneumococcal), scarlet fever, smallpox vaccination, subacute bacterial endocarditis, or tuberculosis.

E. Biologic false-positive results lasting more than 6 months may be caused by hyperglobulinemia, leprosy, leptospirosis, periarteritis nodosa, pinta, rheumatic fever, rheumatoid arthritis, systemic lupus erythematosus, thyroiditis, *Vaccinia*, or yaws.

7. **Other data:**
   A. Suspected false-positive results should be followed by repeat testing at 3, 6, and 9 months.

AUTOPROTHROMBIN IIA
(*see Protein C, Blood*)

AUTOPSY, DIAGNOSTIC

Norm. Requires interpretation.

Usage. Determination of cause and manner of death, reporting of contagious diseases, quality assurance, teaching, and legal purposes.

Description. A postmortem examination and dissection of a corpse. The procedure is usually performed by two pathologists and an assistant.

Professional Considerations
1. Consent form IS required.
2. **Preparation:**
   A. After death, determination should be made whether the circumstances of death require that the coroner be notified. Coroner's cases usually include unexpected death, death within 24 hours of admission to a hospital, death while under anesthesia, suspected homicides or suicides, accidental or violent deaths, deaths of clients with contagious disease, or any death occurring under unusual circumstances or involving the public interest. If any of these conditions apply, the coroner should be called by the

physician for a determination of the need for an autopsy. If the coroner determines that an autopsy is required, the family should be notified, but next-of-kin permission is not needed.

B. Autopsy may also be performed without next-of-kin permission when it is necessary to complete the death certificate or when the deceased client has given consent before death.

C. When the need for an autopsy is determined, other than for coroner's cases, next-of-kin permission must be obtained by means of a signature on the consent form or possibly by a witnessed telephone conversation between the physician and the next of kin. Guidelines vary depending on area laws and institution.

D. All invasive lines, tubes, and devices should be left intact in the body.

E. Obtain an autopsy knife with a blade, a scalpel with a disposable blade, toothed forceps, forceps with serrated tips, a medium-long knife with a blade, a long knife with a blade, scissors with one pointed and one blunt blade, scissors with two blunt blades, scissors for cutting bones, intestinal scissors (enterotome), scissors with long curved blades, a 1-mm probe, a metal metric rule, a costotome, rib shears, intestinal clamps, a vibratory saw with large blades, an amputating saw, a band saw, a hammer with a hook, a chisel, bone-cutting forceps, a meter stick, a body scale, an organ scale, balances, a ladle, a graduate, sea sponges, pans with fixative, pan and pail containers, a large container for fixation of gross organs in solution, fixing solution, string, needles, abrasive whetstone and oil, and a slicing machine.

F. Obtain containers for the samples for toxicologic studies, culture, or cytologic tests.

G. Make sure that the autopsy-permit name and identification number correspond to the name and identification number on the client's body. If there are no tags on the body, have the nurse, physician, or relative identify the body.

H. Wear a mask, an eye or face shield, gloves, and a plastic apron.

3. **Procedure:**

A. *Recording:* The sequence of events and findings of autopsy are recorded either by concurrently written notes or by a foot-operated dictation machine. Descriptions of the body and organs, including condition, arrangement, and weight of the organs, are made and recorded as the dissection is performed.

B. *Sequence:* The sequence of the autopsy may vary. In cases in which a specific cause of death is suspected, the appropriate body cavity for that cause may be opened first. A usual autopsy proceeds in the following order: external examination; incision of the skin, ribs, and sternoclavicular joints; examination of thoracic and abdominal cavities; removal and examination of the organs of the trunk (thymus, heart, lungs, mediastinal lymph nodes, spleen, intestines, diaphragm, liver, gallbladder, pancreas, stomach, duodenum, rectum, spermatic cords, testes, adrenals, uterus, ovarian tubes, ovaries, bone marrow [sternal, vertebral, femoral], neck organs, bones, joints, and muscles); and removal and examination of the organs of the cranium and spine (brain, eyes, ears, paranasal sinuses, pituitary gland, spinal cord, and spinal root ganglia).

C. *Content of assessment:* In the external examination, the body is observed and palpated, and the length, size, and weight are measured. Rigor mortis, edema, and jaundice are noted. The head, lymph nodes, and genitalia are assessed. A Y incision is then made on the torso, and the thoracic and abdominal cavities are assessed. The arrangement and status of the organs and the presence of adhesions, excess fluid, or gas is noted. As they are excised, the weight, size, and contents of the organs and blood vessels are assessed. Biopsy specimens, sections, and smears may be taken throughout the process. The organs of the cranium and spine are then assessed. An incision is made from ear to ear over the vertex of the cranium, and the scalp is separated from the skull with a scalpel. The anterior portion of the scalp is pulled down over the forehead and face. After the skull is opened with a saw and the top portion removed, the brain is removed and placed in 10% formalin. Biopsy specimens of the brain are taken if a virus is suspected. The remainder of the head organs are removed and examined. Formalin is injected into the eyes before removal. The spinal cord is then removed and examined for lesions. Complete organs or portions of organs may be fixed in solution for later reference. An alternative method is to remove the trunk organs in one block, with examination of organs on a dissecting table.

4. **Postprocedure care:**

A. The body is cleansed, and the incisions are sewn. The body may or may not be embalmed at this point.

5. **Client and family teaching:**

A. Autopsy incisions will not be visible should an open-casket wake be held.

B. Durable "power of attorney for health care" does NOT apply after death.

6. **Factors that affect results:**

A. A routine hospital autopsy should be interrupted and the coroner notified if any unexpected findings that may be of traumatic origin are encountered.

7. **Other data:**

A. The order of authority for granting permission for an autopsy is normally spouse, adult child, parent, adult sibling, other relative, and any other person accepting responsibility for burial of the body. This order may vary by area laws.

B. Be aware of religious considerations concerning autopsy.

C. There is a 44% discordance rate between clinical and autopsy diagnosis of malignant neoplasms.

BACTERIAL SEROLOGY, BLOOD

Norm. Requires interpretation.

Usage. Suspected bacterial infections. Most commonly, legionellosis, leptospirosis, *Mycoplasma*, *Rickettsia* (typhus fever, spotted fever, scrub typhus, trench fever, and Q fever), staphylococcosis, streptococcosis, and *Yersinia*. Adult-onset Still's disease.

Description. An indirect method of identifying blood bacterial infections by assessment of the host response (antibody production) to the invading microorganism. Results may be reported qualitatively (positive, negative) or quantitatively (titers) and should be interpreted in consideration of the predictive value of the specific test. Bacterial serologic testing produces faster results than cultures of some organisms that take several weeks to grow.

Professional Considerations
1. Consent form NOT required.
2. Preparation:
   A. Tube: Red topped, red/gray topped, or gold topped.
   B. See *Client and family teaching*.
3. Procedure:
   A. Two blood samples, 1 week apart, should be drawn. The first specimen should be drawn as soon as possible after the onset of symptoms and then frozen. The second specimen should be drawn at least 1 week later, and then both specimens should be assayed at the same time.
   B. Draw a 10-mL blood sample.
4. Postprocedure care:
   A. None.
5. Client and family teaching:
   A. Fast for 8 hours before testing.
   B. Return in 1 week for follow-up testing.
6. Factors that affect results:
   A. Reject hemolyzed or grossly lipemic specimens.
   B. False-negative results may be caused by immunosuppression or antibiotic therapy.
7. Other data:
   A. A single positive antibody is insufficient to support a diagnosis because low persistent levels are common.

BAEP

(see Brainstem auditory evoked potential, Diagnostic)

BANDING IN GENETIC DISORDERS, DIAGNOSTIC

Norm. Cytogenic techniques with numerical designations map each chromosome for abnormalities.
Female   44 autosomes +
              2X chromosomes
          Karyotype: 46,XX
Male   44 autosomes + 1X and
              1Y chromosomes
          Karyotype: 46,XY

Usage. Assists in the diagnosis of genetic and neoplastic disorders.

Description. Banding techniques are used for chromosome identification. Human chromosomes are numbered in 23 pairs. Each chromosome pair has a unique pattern with intricate detail produced by different distributions of DNA in the chromosomes. Banding helps detect different regions of the same chromosome for use in identification of both the chromosome and chromosomal abnormalities. R banding uses a reverse Giemsa stain called acridine orange, which produces reverse contrast to the light Q bands detected by quinacrine mustard and dark and light crossband G bands detected with trypsin and Giemsa stain. R dark bands are useful for observing the very dark ends of chromosomes. The chromosome count per cell and banded karyotype with interpretation is included in the testing.

Professional Considerations
1. Consent form NOT required.
2. Preparation:
   A. Tube: Green topped.
3. Procedure:
   A. Draw a 4-mL blood sample.
4. Postprocedure care:
   A. None.
5. Client and family teaching:
   A. Results are normally available in 1-2 weeks.
   B. Refer the client with abnormal results for genetic counseling.
6. Factors that affect results:
   A. Heparin in the specimen collection tube must be sodium heparin.

7. Other data:
   A. This method is used widely in European countries, especially France.

BANDS, BLOOD
(see Differential leukocyte count, Peripheral blood)

BARBITURATES, QUANTITATIVE, BLOOD

Norm. Negative.

LEVELS DURING BARBITURATE THERAPY		SI UNITS
Amobarbital	**Trough**	
Therapeutic	1-5 µg/mL	4.4-22.1 µmol/L
Toxic	>10 µg/mL	>44.2 µmol/L
Panic	>70 µg/mL	>309.4 µmol/L
Butabarbital		
Therapeutic	1-2 µg/mL	4.4-8.4 µmol/L
Toxic	10-40 µg/mL	44.2-176.8 µmol/L
Pentobarbital		
Therapeutic	1-5 µg/mL	4.4-22.1 µmol/L
Therapeutic coma	20-50 µg/mL	88.4-221 µmol/L
Toxic	>10 µg/mL	>44.2 µmol/L
Panic	>60 µg/mL	>265.2 µmol/L
Phenobarbital		
Therapeutic	15-40 µg/mL	66.3-176.8 µmol/L
Toxic	35-80 µg/mL	154.7-353.6 µmol/L
Panic	>100 µg/mL	>442 µmol/L
Secobarbital		
Therapeutic	1-2 µg/mL	4.2-8.4 µmol/L
Toxic	3-40 µg/mL	13.3-176.8 µmol/L
Panic	>50 µg/mL	>221 µmol/L

Panic Level Symptoms and Treatment

Symptoms. Central nervous system depression (ataxia, confusion, drowsiness) progressing to respiratory depression, hypotension, and coma. Death may occur with ingestion of 1 g of pentobarbital or with 1.5 g of phenobarbital or 2 g of secobarbital.

Treatment:
Note: Treatment choice(s) depend on client history and condition and episode history.

Protect airway and provide oxygen.
Gastric lavage with tap water or saline up to 24 hours after ingestion.
Do NOT induce emesis.
Administer activated charcoal.
Diurese with urea if hemodynamically stable and adequate renal function is present.
Alkalinize urine.
Delay absorption by subcutaneous or intramuscular routes by packing sites with ice or using tourniquets.

	REMOVED BY HEMODIALYSIS	REMOVED BY HEMOPERFUSION	REMOVED BY PERITONEAL DIALYSIS
Amobarbital	Yes	Yes	No
Pentobarbital	No	Yes	
Phenobarbital	Yes	Yes	Yes
Secobarbital	No		No

Usage. Drug abuse, overdose, suicide attempt, and monitoring blood levels during barbiturate therapy, for example, in the treatment of catatonia.

Description. Barbiturates are a group of central nervous system depressants used as hypnotics, anticonvulsants, and sedatives and preoperatively. They are believed to act at the level of the reticular activating system. Barbiturates are metabolized in the liver and excreted by the kidneys. Overdose may lead to coma and death from respiratory arrest.

Professional Considerations
1. Consent form NOT required unless the specimen may be used as legal evidence.
2. **Preparation:**
   A. Tube: Red topped, red/gray topped, gold topped, lavender topped, or black topped.
   B. Do NOT draw the sample for amobarbital or phenobarbital level during hemodialysis.
   C. Sample for pentobarbital MAY be drawn during hemodialysis.
   D. Screen client for the use of herbal preparations or natural remedies such as *Valeriana officinalis* and kavakava (*Piper methysticum*).
3. **Procedure:**
   A. Collection should be witnessed if the specimen may be used as legal evidence.
   B. Draw a 2-mL TROUGH blood sample.
   C. Obtain serial measurements at the same time each day.
4. **Postprocedure care:**
   A. If the specimen may be used as legal evidence, write the client's name, the exact time of the blood draw, and the contents of the tube on the tube label and the laboratory requisition. Sign and have the witness sign the laboratory requisition. Transport the specimen to the laboratory in a sealed plastic bag labeled as legal evidence.
   B. Refrigerate the specimen if not tested immediately.
5. **Client and family teaching:**
   A. For intentional overdose, refer the client and family for crisis intervention.
   B. Client with panic level symptoms will require intensive care for at least 24 hours.
   C. Physical and psychologic addiction occur in clients taking barbiturates over a long period of time. Serious withdrawal symptoms that may occur include severe headache, body pains, numbness or burning in the arms and legs, seizures, hallucinations, chest pain, sweating, and breathing difficulties. Seek medical treatment if any of these symptoms occur.
   D. If activated charcoal was given for elevated levels, the client should drink 4-6 glasses of water each day for 2 days to prevent constipation. Activated charcoal will also cause stools to be black for a few days.
6. **Factors that affect results:**
   A. Reject hemolyzed specimens to avoid falsely decreased results.
   B. Drugs that may cause falsely elevated results include atropine sulfate, dexchlorpheniramine maleate, ethotoin, glutethimide, meperidine hydrochloride, phenytoin, salicylamide, and theophylline.
   C. Amobarbital cross-reactivity may occur with any of the other barbiturates. Pentobarbital cross-reactivity may occur with secobarbital or phenobarbital.
   D. Barbiturates can decompose after embalming and analysis then may lead to false negatives.
7. **Other data:**
   A. Panic level symptoms may occur with smaller doses if alcohol is also ingested.
   B. Use of barbiturates increases the risk of nasopharyngeal carcinoma, congenital heart defects, and cleft palate.

C. Herbal or natural remedies that may cause excessive sedation when used with barbiturates include valerian and kavakava (*Piper methysticum*). However, *Valeriana officinalis* (allheal, setwall, garden heliotrope, vandalroot) may reduce symptoms of benzodiazepine withdrawal.

D. Kyushin ("save-heart," a patented natural cardiotonic, dried toad venom), licorice, plantain leaves (found in Nature Cleanse Tablets, Botanical Cleanse, or Blessed Herb brands), uzara (*Dicoma anomala*) root, hawthorn, and ginseng may interfere with either digoxin pharmacodynamically or with digoxin monitoring.

BARIUM ENEMA (BE), DIAGNOSTIC

Norm. Requires interpretation. Characteristics examined include filling, passage pattern of barium, and the contour, patency, position, and mucosal pattern of the colon.

Usage. Part of the diagnostic work-up for bowel obstruction, celiac sprue, colorectal cancer, diverticulitis, diverticulosis, gastroenteritis, Hirschsprung's disease, intestinal cancer, intestinal polyps, intussusception, irritable bowel syndrome, rectal stenosis, stercoral appendicular fistula and ulcerative colitis.

Description. A fluoroscopic and radiographic examination of the large intestine after rectal instillation of barium sulfate with or without air for the purpose of identifying structural abnormalities or slowing of normal intestinal activity. The American Cancer Society recommends a screening double contrast barium enema every 5 years beginning at age 50. Positive results should be followed with a colonoscopy.

Professional Considerations
1. Consent form NOT required.

Risks
Constipation, dizziness, infection, intestinal impaction, rectal or bowel perforation, rectovaginal perforation, and vasovagal reaction.

Contraindications
Severe active ulcerative colitis accompanied by toxicity and megacolon, perforated intestine, toxic megacolon, tachycardia.

Precautions
During pregnancy, risks of cumulative radiation exposure to the fetus from this and other previous or future imaging studies must be weighed against the benefits of the procedure. Although formal limits for client exposure are relative to this risk-benefit comparison, the United States Nuclear Regulatory Commission requires that the cumulative dose equivalent to an embryo/fetus from *occupational* exposure not exceed 0.5 rem (5 mSv). Risk of exposure to the uterus from a barium enema is 2-4 rad. Radiation dose to the fetus is proportional to the distance of the anatomy studied from the abdomen and decreases as pregnancy progresses.

2. Preparation:
   A. Laxatives or cathartic suppositories or both are usually indicated the day before and on the morning of the test to facilitate complete emptying of the intestines. However, they may be contraindicated for certain clients with conditions such as ulcerative colitis or intestinal obstruction. There is no difference between using Picolax or Fleet Phospho-Soda as laxatives except Picolax tastes better and provokes less nausea.
   B. If the client is pregnant, notify the physician before exam preparation.
   C. See *Client and family teaching.*
3. Procedure:
   A. After baseline abdominal radiographs are taken, the client lies in a Sims position on a tilt table and receives a slow administration of barium sulfate or barium sulfate with air insufflation through a rectal tube.
   B. As the client assumes different positions, the filling is monitored by fluoroscopy.
   C. Spot films are taken during and after the filling.
   D. The rectal tube is withdrawn, and the barium expelled, after which another film is taken to examine the pattern of the intestinal

B

mucosa and to determine how well emptying has occurred.

4. **Postprocedure care:**
   A. Where not contraindicated, the client should increase fluid intake for 24-48 hours.
   B. Where not contraindicated, a mild cathartic may be prescribed to facilitate emptying of the barium from the intestine.
   C. Stools should be inspected by the client or the health care professional for passage of barium for 48 hours. Barium stools will look chalky white in color.
   D. Failure to have a bowel movement within 2 days after the test should be reported to the physician.

5. **Client and family teaching:**
   A. It is important to have the bowel emptied of stool before the procedure. A low-residue diet may be prescribed for 1-3 days before the test, although it does not offer any advantage over a normal diet in preparation for the test if purgatives are used.
   B. A clear liquid diet is usually prescribed for 1 day before and on the morning of the test. A normal diet may be resumed after the procedure.
   C. A laxative may be prescribed before and after the procedure.
   D. The procedure takes about 60 minutes. It is important to hold your breath when you are asked to do so during the procedure.
   E. Make sure all the barium empties from the intestinal tract after the procedure. Drinking fluids and taking laxatives or enemas after the procedure may be prescribed for this purpose.
   F. See *Postprocedure care.*
   G. Call the physician if stomach or lower abdominal pain is experienced or if stools are much smaller than the normal diameter.

6. **Factors that affect results:**
   A. Failure to achieve complete emptying of the intestinal tract before the test may necessitate a repeated barium enema.

7. **Other data:**
   A. The barium enema should be performed before a barium swallow.
   B. There is evidence that occult stool testing reduces mortality from colon cancer. There is no similar current evidence regarding BE for screening of colon cancer.
   C. Absorbed dose is 20-80 mGy to the embryo and 10-20 mGy to the fetus.

BARIUM SWALLOW, DIAGNOSTIC

Norm. Requires interpretation. Characteristics examined include filling of the pharynx and esophagus, mucosal patterns, and esophageal size, contour, and peristaltic motion.

Usage. Part of the diagnostic work-up for achalasia, bronchoesophageal fistula, duodenal ulcer, dysphagia, esophageal diverticula, esophageal varices, head and neck cancer, hiatal hernia, hypertrophic pyloric stenosis, pharyngeal muscle disorders, piriform sinus fistula, polyps, strictures, Plummer-Vinson syndrome, stomach cancer, tracheoesophageal compression, and ulcers.

Description. A fluoroscopic and radiographic examination of the pharynx and esophagus as mixtures of barium sulfate are swallowed. The test takes 20-30 minutes.

Professional Considerations
1. Consent form NOT required.

Risks
Constipation, dizziness, intestinal impaction, vasovagal reaction.

Contraindications
During pregnancy; clients with upper tract dysphagia; those with a risk of barium aspiration; and clients with intestinal obstruction.

Precautions
During pregnancy, risks of cumulative radiation exposure to the fetus from this and other previous or future imaging studies must be weighed against the benefits of the procedure. Although formal limits for client exposure are relative to this risk-benefit comparison, the United States Nuclear Regulatory Commission requires that the cumulative dose equivalent to an embryo/fetus from *occupational* exposure not exceed 0.5 rem (5 mSv). Radiation dose to the fetus is proportional

to the distance of the anatomy studied from the abdomen and decreases as pregnancy progresses. For pregnant clients, consult the Radiologist/Radiology Department to obtain estimated fetal radiation exposure from this procedure.

2. **Preparation:**
   A. See *Client and family teaching.*
3. **Procedure:**
   A. The client is positioned on a tilt table.
   B. After baseline fluoroscopic examinations of the heart, lungs, and abdomen, the client takes one swallow of a thick barium mixture while cineradiographic films are taken.
   C. The client then takes several swallows of a thin barium mixture while its passage is recorded by fluoroscopy and radiography.
   D. The process is repeated with the table tilted to various positions.
   E. About 350-450 mL of barium is swallowed during the entire procedure.
4. **Postprocedure care:**
   A. Where not contraindicated, the client should increase fluid intake for 24-48 hours after the test.

B. Where not contraindicated, a mild cathartic may be prescribed to facilitate emptying of barium from the gastrointestinal tract.
C. Failure to have a bowel movement within 2 days should be reported to the physician.
5. **Client and family teaching:**
   A. Fast for 8 hours before the procedure.
   B. This procedure lasts approximately 15 minutes.
   C. Make sure all of the barium empties from the intestinal tract after the procedure. Drinking fluids and taking laxatives or enemas after the procedure may be prescribed for this purpose.
   D. See *Postprocedure care.*
   E. Call the physician if stomach or lower abdominal pain is experienced or if stools are much smaller than the normal diameter.
6. **Factors that affect results:**
   A. None.
7. **Other data:**
   A. Barium swallow is not very sensitive as an aid in the diagnosis of proximal reflux in asthmatic children.

BARR BODY ANALYSIS BUCCAL SMEAR FOR STAINING SEX CHROMATIN MASS, DIAGNOSTIC

Norm:

	NUMBER OF BARR BODIES
Normal female (XX)	1
Normal male (XY)	0
Turner syndrome (female) (XO)	0
Klinefelter syndrome (male) (XXY)	1
Klinefelter syndrome (male) (48,XXXY)	2
Klinefelter syndrome (male) (49,XXXYY)	2
Klinefelter syndrome (male) (49,XXXXY)	3

Usage. Screening for sex chromosome abnormalities.

Description. A Barr body, or sex chromatin body, is a tightly coiled, X-chromosome lying against the nuclear membrane of female cells or any cell with more than one X chromosome. It shows up as a dark-staining body in the shape of a half-moon and is absent in male cells. Barr bodies are believed to function in early embryonic development and later become inactivated to maintain gene balance of Xs to autosomes. The number of Barr bodies in a client is one less than the number of Xs.

Professional Considerations
1. Consent form NOT required.
2. **Preparation:**
   A. Rinse the mouth with mouthwash.
   B. Obtain a metal spatula, saline, two slides, and preservative.
3. **Procedure:**
   A. Gently scrape the buccal mucosa with the metal spatula dipped in saline.

B. Clean the spatula and repeat the procedure gently but firmly.
C. Smear the material on the two slides and place them in the preservative.
4. **Postprocedure care:**
A. Label the container of the slides with the client's name, the date, and the contents.
5. **Client and family teaching:**
A. Refer the client with abnormal results for genetic counseling.
6. **Factors that affect results:**
A. None known.
7. **Other data:**
A. Barr bodies do not give any information about Y chromosomes.
B. Human chromosome analysis, rather than buccal smears, should be used for evaluations of newborns with ambiguous genitalia.

BASAL GASTRIC SECRETION TEST
(see Hollander test, Diagnostic)

BASIC METABOLIC PANEL (BMP), BLOOD

Norm. See individual test listings: *Calcium, Chloride, CO_2, Creatinine, Glucose, Potassium, Sodium,* and *Urea nitrogen.*

Usage. See individual test listings.

Description. The *basic metabolic panel* (BMP) is a term defined by The Centers for Medicare and Medicaid Services (CMS) in the United States to indicate a group of tests for which a bundled reimbursement is available. The panel is one of several that replace the multichannel tests, such as SMA-7. The panel is disease oriented, meaning that payment through Medicare is available only when the test is used to diagnose and monitor a disease and payment is not available when the test is used for screening purposes in clients who have no signs and symptoms that qualify for the test. All the tests in the panel must be carried out when a BMP is ordered.

Professional Considerations
1. Consent form NOT required.
2. **Preparation:**
A. Tube: Red topped, red/gray topped, or gold topped.

B. Do NOT draw specimens during hemodialysis.
3. **Procedure:**
A. Draw a 5-mL blood sample.
4. **Postprocedure care:**
A. None.
5. **Client and family teaching:**
A. See individual test listings.
6. **Factors that affect results:**
A. See individual test listings.
7. **Other data:**
A. The selection of tests approved for inclusion in this panel is updated periodically.
B. See individual test listings.

BASOPHILS
(see Differential leukocyte count, Peripheral blood)

BASOS
(see Differential leukocyte count, Peripheral blood)

BE
(see Barium enema, Diagnostic)

BENCE JONES PROTEIN, URINE

Norm. Negative.

Positive. Amyloidosis (primary), benign monoclonal gammopathy, cryoglobulinemia, Fanconi syndrome (adult), hyperparathyroidism, multiple myeloma (high levels indicate poor prognosis), osteomalacia, and Waldenström's macroglobulinemia.

Description. A low-molecular weight, light-chain immunoglobulin synthesized by malignant plasma cells in the bone marrow and initially broken down and reabsorbed by the kidneys. In multiple myeloma, such a large amount of these proteins are produced that they exceed the kidneys' capacity to metabolize them. This causes them to spill into the urine. Prolonged production of Bence Jones protein eventually causes degeneration of the renal tubular cells, and the protein accumulates in the tubules, causing inclusions that may lead to renal failure. Subsequently, increasing amounts of the protein spill into the urine and can be detected by thermal coagulation and acid tests and confirmed by immunoelectrophoresis.

Professional Considerations
1. Consent form NOT required.
2. Preparation:
   A. Obtain a clean specimen container without preservatives.
3. Procedure:
   A. Obtain a 25-mL first morning-voided, random urine specimen in a clean container. A fresh specimen may be taken from a urinary drainage bag.
4. Postprocedure care:
   A. Send the specimen to the laboratory and refrigerate.
5. Client and family teaching:
   A. Results are normally available within 24 hours.
6. Factors that affect results:
   A. Failure to refrigerate the specimen may result in false-negative results.

B. False-positive results may be caused by chronic renal insufficiency, connective tissue diseases (such as rheumatoid arthritis, systemic lupus erythematosus (SLE), scleroderma, polymyositis, or Wegener's granulomatosis), and other malignancies (lymphoma; leukemia; and metastatic cancer of the lung or of the gastrointestinal or genitourinary tracts).
C. Drugs that may cause false-positive results include aminosalicylic acid, cephaloridine, chlorpromazine, penicillin (high doses), promazine hydrochloride, sulfisoxazole, and tolbutamide.
D. False-negative results may be caused by very alkaline urine and severe urinary tract infections in which urea splitting occurs.
7. Other data:
   A. In light-chain disease, pancytopenia is absent.

BENEDICT'S TEST, DIAGNOSTIC

Norm. Blue or negative.

Usage. Screening for disorders of glucose or amino acid metabolism.

Positive. Congenital deficiency of homogentisic acid, hyperglycemia, and melituria. Osmotic diarrhea in infants and children.

COLOR	GLUCOSE QUANTITATIVE	GLUCOSE QUALITATIVE
Blue	0 mmol/L	Negative
Green	14 mmol/L	Trace
Greenish yellow precipitate	28 mmol/L	1+
Yellow-green	56 mmol/L	2+
Brown	83 mmol/L	3+
Orange-red	>110 mmol/L	4+

Description. A copper-reduction test that detects sugars, reducing substances, and homogentisic acid in the urine. Clients with a hereditary absence of homogentisic acid oxidase are unable to metabolize homogentisic acid, a by-product of phenylalanine and tyrosine metabolism. Some of the unmetabolized homogentisic acid is excreted in the urine, and the remainder causes ochronosis, a condition characterized by joint deposition of homogentisic acid that eventually causes joint degeneration. Benedict's solution is made of quantitative and qualitative reagent, each containing cupric sulfate dissolved in sodium sulfate but in different concentrations. When Benedict's solution is heated in the presence of sugar, homogentisic acid, or other reducing substances, the cupric sulfate is reduced and a yellow-to-red precipitate forms.

Professional Considerations
1. Consent form NOT required.
2. Preparation:
   A. Obtain a clean container, two Pyrex test tubes, a wooden test-tube holder, a beaker, a Bunsen burner, a pipette, a dropper, and Benedict's solution.

3. **Procedure:**
   A. Obtain a 10-mL random urine specimen in a clean container without preservative. A fresh specimen may be taken from a urinary drainage bag.
   B. Pipette 5 mL of Benedict's solution into a Pyrex test tube.
   C. Add 8 drops of urine.
   D. Mix the test tube gently.
   E. Using the wooden test-tube holder, boil the mixture over a Bunsen burner for 2 minutes and then cool to room temperature.
   F. Observe the color of the test-tube mixture and interpret the results as noted in the table below.
4. **Postprocedure care:**
   A. Refrigerate the specimen if the test is not performed immediately.
5. **Client and family teaching:**
   A. The specimen must be free of stool and toilet tissue.
   B. Results are normally available within 24 hours.
6. **Factors that affect results:**
   A. Results are most accurate on a freshly voided specimen.
   B. Glycosuria will cause a false-positive result when Benedict's solution is used for detection of homogentisic acid.
   C. Drugs and reducing substances that may cause false-positive results include ampicillin, ampicillin sodium, aminosalicylic acid, ascorbic acid, camphor, car-

bamazepine, cefaclor, cefadroxil monohydrate, cefamandole nafate, cefazolin sodium, cefonicid sodium, cefoperazone sodium, ceforanide, cefotaxime sodium, cefotetan disodium, cefoxitin sodium, ceftazidime, ceftizoxime sodium, ceftriaxone, cefuroxime axetil, cephalexin, cephaloridine, cephalothin sodium, cephradine, cephapirin sodium, chloral hydrate, chloramphenicol, chloroform, cimetidine, formaldehyde, fructose, galactose, glucosamine, glucuronic acid, homogentisic acid, levodopa, metaxalone, moxalactam disodium, nalidixic acid, nitrofurantoin, nitrofurantoin sodium, paraldehyde, penicillin G benzathine, penicillin G potassium, penicillin G procaine, phenol, probenecid, salicylates, streptomycin sulfate, sulfonamides, tetracyclines, turpentine, and uric acid.
7. **Other data:**
   A. Any reducing substance found in the urine may cause false-positive results.
   B. Use other methods of glucose measurement to help differentiate glucosuria from urine containing homogentisic acid.

BENTIROMIDE TEST
(see Chymex test for pancreatic function, Diagnostic)

BENZODIAZEPINES, PLASMA AND URINE

Norm. Blood and urine: negative.

Urine panic level. >200 ng/mL

	THERAPEUTIC PLASMA VALUES	SI UNITS
Alprazolam	5-25 ng/mL	
High-dose therapy	25-55 ng/mL	
Panic level	>60 ng/mL	
Chlordiazepoxide	700-1000 ng/mL	2.34-3.34 μmol/L
Panic level	>5000 ng/mL	>16.70 μmol/L
Clonazepam	15-60 ng/mL	48-190 nmol/L
Panic level	>80 ng/mL	>254 nmol/L
Diazepam	100-1000 ng/mL	0.35-3.51 μmol/L
Panic level	>5000 ng/mL	>17.55 μmol/L
Flurazepam	Information not available	
Panic level	>0.2 μg/mL	>0.5 μmol/L
Lorazepam	50-240 ng/mL	156-746 nmol/L
Midazolam	Information not available	
Oxazepam	Information not available	

	THERAPEUTIC PLASMA VALUES	SI UNITS
Prazepam	0.12-1.0 µg/mL	0.4-3.1 µmol/L
Temazepam	Information not available	
Triazolam	Information not available	

Panic Level Symptoms and Treatment

Symptoms. Somnolence, confusion, ataxia, diminished reflexes, vertigo, slurred speech, respiratory depression, and coma.

Treatment:

Note: Treatment choice(s) depend on client history and condition and episode history.

Administer activated charcoal if within 4 hours of ingestion or if symptoms are present. Repeat as necessary, as benzodiazepines undergo hepatic recirculation.

Gastric lavage is not recommended, but should be considered if within 1 hour of ingestion and if ingestion of additional lethal substance is suspected. Use warm tap water or 0.9% saline.

Monitor for central nervous system depression.

Protect airway. Support breathing with oxygen and mechanical ventilation if necessary.

Flumazenil is not recommended for routine use in benzodiazepine overdose. Flumazenil has been used as a competitive antagonist to reverse the profound effects of benzodiazepine overdose. Use of flumazenil is contraindicated if concomitant tricyclic antidepressants were taken or in dependence states because of the risk of causing seizures from lowering of the seizure threshold and because it may precipitate symptoms of bezodiazepine withdrawal. Flumazenil may not completely reverse benzodiazepine effects. Close monitoring for re-sedation is required and repeated doses may be needed. Do NOT use barbiturates.

Do NOT induce emesis.

Forced diuresis or hemodialysis will NOT remove benzodiazepines. No information was found on whether peritoneal dialysis will remove these drugs.

Positive. Hepatic encephalopathy. Drugs include clorazepate dipotassium, chlordiazepoxide, clonazepam, diazepam, fluoxetine, flurazepam hydrochloride, lorazepam, midazolam, oxazepam, prazepam, sertraline, temazepam, and triazolam.

Usage. Suspected drug overdose and drug-use screening.

Description. Benzodiazepines are non-barbiturate, sedative-hypnotic, and anti-convulsant schedule-IV drugs used to treat anxiety and insomnia. They are strongly protein bound, metabolized in the liver, and excreted in urine and feces. Benzodiazepines have long half-lives of 30-200 hours. Overdose may lead to coma and death from respiratory arrest. Serum levels are used to determine therapeutic and toxic levels and the full range of benzodiazepines but are not generally helpful in gauging the effects of overdose. Detection of the presence but not the levels of only those benzodi-

azepines that are excreted as oxazepam (above) is performed by urine assay.

Professional Considerations
1. Consent form NOT required.
2. Preparation:
   A. Blood test: Tube: Lavender topped. MAY be drawn during hemodialysis. Preserve with sodium fluoride.
   B. Urine test: Obtain a clean specimen container.
   C. Screen client for the use of herbal preparations or natural remedies such as kavakava (*Piper methysticum*).
3. Procedure:
   A. Blood test: Draw a 3-mL blood sample.
   B. Urine test: Collect a 30-mL, clean, voided urine sample. A fresh specimen may be taken from a urinary drainage bag.
4. Postprocedure care:
   A. Refrigerate the urine specimen until tested.

B. Preserve blood with sodium fluoride, store at −20° C and assay within a week.

5. **Client and family teaching:**
   A. Offer substance abuse or crisis intervention counseling if applicable.
   B. Referrals to appropriate rehabilitation centers and therapeutic community programs should be offered to all addicted clients who may be interested.
   C. Results are normally available within 24 hours.
   D. If activated charcoal was given for elevated levels, the client should drink 4-6 glasses of water each day for 2 days to prevent constipation. Activated charcoal will also cause stools to be black for a few days.

6. **Factors that affect results:**
   A. False-positive urine test results are seen with oxaprozin.
   B. Nitrobenzodiazepines are stable in blood stored for up to 24 months at −20° C
   C. Their 7-amino metabolites lose 29% stability at −20° C after 2 months.
   D. Benzodiazepine levels are not affected by the administration of flumazenil. The clinical effects of flumazenil occur because of selective displacement of benzodiazepines at receptor sites.

7. **Other data:**
   A. The positive predictive value for detecting benzodiazepines in urine using the triage visual panel was 77%.
   B. Withdrawal symptoms may occur after even a single large dose of benzodiazepines.
   C. Urinalysis fails to identify 10% of coabuse of benzodiazepines in opiate addicts.
   D. Kavakava (*Piper methysticum*), a natural herbal remedy anxiolytic potentiates the effects of benzodiazepines.

BERNSTEIN TEST
(see *Acid perfusion test, Diagnostic*)

BETA-AMYLOID PROTEIN 40/42 (ABETA), CSF

Norm. Investigational findings (Tapiola, 2001):

>340 pg/mL (sensitivity 69%-78%, specificity 85% to differentiate Alzheimer's disease from controls and 59% to differentiate Alzheimer's disease from other dementias. When used in combination with the *Tau Test, CSF*, the above specificities increased to 95% and 85%, respectively.).

Usage. Monitoring progression of Alzheimer's disease.

Description. Alzheimer's disease, the most common form of dementia, is characterized by the presence of senile plaques and neurofibrillary tangles. The senile plaques contain 40/42-residue beta-amyloid protein (Abeta), a proteolytic fragment of beta- amyloid precursor protein (APP). APP is present from a very young age and functions in the development of neural stem cells. The abnormal fragment Abeta is thought to be a primary cause of Alzheimer's disease. Cerebrospinal fluid (CSF) levels generally drop the more the disease progresses because the fragments are being deposited from the CSF into the tissues of the brain. Levels in plasma are normally 100 times less than that of CSF and also decrease with disease progression.

Professional Considerations
1. Consent form IS required for the procedure used to obtain the specimen.

Risks
See *Lumbar puncture, Diagnostic*

Contraindications
See *Lumbar puncture, Diagnostic*

2. **Preparation:**
   A. See *Lumbar puncture, Diagnostic*.
   B. Obtain a sterile container for CSF Fluid.
3. **Procedure:**
   A. Collect a 1-mL sample of CSF during the lumbar puncture procedure.
4. **Postprocedure care:**
   A. See *Lumbar puncture, Diagnostic*
5. **Client and family teaching:**
   A. See *Lumbar puncture, Diagnostic*
6. **Factors that affect results:**
   A. Levels increase as the number of neurofibrillary tangles increase.
7. **Other data:**
   A. The ELISA based test for amyloid beta protein is available from Athena Neurosciences.
   B. This test is sometimes done in conjunction with hTau Antigen testing. See *Tau Test, CSF*.

BETA-1C, SERUM
(see C3 complement, Serum)

BETA-GLUCOSIDASE, DIAGNOSTIC

Norm. Positive.

Usage. Screening for Gaucher's disease, a sphingolipid storage disease.

Description. Beta-glucosidase deficiency is an autosomal recessive disease resulting in a gangliosidosis called "Gaucher's disease," which is quickly fatal in infants but progresses more slowly in older children. Beta-glucosidase is an enzyme found in peripheral blood leukocytes that normally metabolizes the glycolipid glucocerebroside. In Gaucher's disease, glucocerebroside accumulates and causes splenomegaly, hepatomegaly, anemia, thrombocytopenia, erosion of long bones and pelvic bones, and mental retardation (in infantile form).

Professional Considerations
1. Consent form NOT required.
2. Preparation:
    A. Tube: Green topped and container of ice.
    B. If the specimen must be sent to an outside laboratory for processing, notify the in-house laboratory that a specimen will be drawn.
3. Procedure:
    A. Draw a 7-mL blood sample.
    B. Place the specimen on ice.
4. Postprocedure care:
    A. Transport the specimen to the laboratory immediately.
    B. For transport to an outside laboratory, the specimen must be transported in an ice bath the same day.
5. Client and family teaching:
    A. Results are normally available within 72 hours.
6. Factors that affect results:
    A. Results are invalid for specimens not placed on ice.

7. Other data:
    A. Anemia can be severe enough to cause respiratory difficulty.
    B. Enzyme infusion therapy is recommended treatment in type 3 Gaucher's disease.

BETA-HYDROXYBUTYRATE (BHB, BHY, BOHB), BLOOD

Norm:

Plasma	<1.2 mmol/L
Serum	<3 mg/dL or <0.3 mEq/L

Usage. Helps differentiate cause of metabolic acidosis with increased anion gap; monitoring effectiveness of therapy for acute diabetic ketoacidosis.

Description. Beta-hydroxybutyrate (BHB) is one of three types of ketone bodies occurring in diabetic ketoacidosis (DKA) and is responsible for the nausea and vomiting that occurs in this condition. When DKA occurs, BHB predominates and contributes significantly to the presence of an increased anion gap. BHB is also the predominant ketone that responds to treatment for acute DKA; thus this test is more useful than the ketone bodies test for assessing the effectiveness of treatment.

Professional Considerations
1. Consent form NOT required.
2. Preparation:
    A. Tube: red-topped, green-topped or gold-topped; tube must be precooled in ice.
3. Procedure:
    A. Collect a 2-mL blood sample.
4. Postprocedure care:
    A. Place specimen on ice and deliver to the laboratory immediately.
5. Client and family teaching:
    A. If elevated because of diabetic ketoacidosis, levels will decrease with treatment.
6. Factors that affect results:
    A. None found.
7. Other data:
    A. None.

BETA₂-MICROGLOBULIN, BLOOD AND 24-HOUR URINE

Norm:

		SI UNITS
Blood	<2 µg/mL	<170 nmol/L
Urine	<120 µg/24 hours	<10 mmol/day

Increased. AIDS, aminoglycoside toxicity, Burkitt's lymphoma Daudi, Crohn's disease, hepatitis, leukemia (chronic lymphocytic), malignancies (some), mercury exposure, multiple myeloma, osteitis fibrosa cystica, preeclampsia, renal disease (glomerular, end stage), sarcoidosis, vasculitis and Waldenström's microglobulinemia.

Description. An amino acid peptide component of lymphocytes that increases in inflammatory conditions and when lymphocyte turnover increases, as in lymphocytic leukemia, or when T-lymphocyte helper (OKT4) cells are attacked by human immunodeficiency virus. Beta$_2$-microglobulin is metabolized by the renal tubules, with over 99% being reabsorbed. Blood beta$_2$-microglobulin becomes elevated with malfunctioning glomeruli but drops with malfunctioning tubules. The test (both blood and urine) is most often used for evaluation of renal disease, chronic lymphocytic leukemia, and AIDS. Although beta$_2$-microglobulin levels rise with HIV infection, the levels do not always correlate with the stages of the infection.

Professional Considerations
1. Consent form NOT required.
2. Preparation:
   A. Tube: Lavender topped or 3-L urine collection container and toluene preservative.
   B. Follow protective isolation precautions for clients with AIDS.
   C. Write the exact beginning time of the 24-hour urine collection on the laboratory requisition.
3. Procedure:
   A. Draw a 2-mL blood sample.
   B. For 24-hour urine, discard the first morning-urine specimen. Save all urine voided for 24 hours in a refrigerated, clean, 3-L container to which toluene preservative has been added. Document the quantity of urine output during the specimen collection period. Include voiding at the end of the 24-hour period. For catheterized clients, keep the drainage bag on ice and empty the urine into the collection container hourly.
4. Postprocedure care:
   A. Compare the quantity of urine in the specimen container with uri-

nary output records. If the specimen contains less urine than was recorded as output, some of the sample may have been discarded, thus invalidating the results.
   B. Document the quantity of urine output and the ending time for the 24-hour collection period on the laboratory requisition.
5. Client and family teaching:
   A. Offer support and referrals for AIDS, cancer, or Crohn's disease as appropriate. The national AIDS Hotline is (800) 342-AIDS; AIDS Clinical Trials Information Services, National Institutes of Health, is (301) 496-8210.
   B. Save all urine voided in the 24-hour period. Urinate before defecating to avoid loss of urine. If any urine is accidentally discarded, discard the entire specimen and restart the collection the next day.
   C. Results are normally available within 24 hours.
6. Factors that affect results:
   A. Results are invalidated if the client has received radioactive dyes within 1 week before the test.
7. Other data:
   A. Results can be normal in HIV infection.
   B. See also *Acquired immunodeficiency syndrome (AIDS) evaluation battery, Diagnostic.*

BETKE-KLEIHAUER STAIN (FETAL HEMOGLOBIN STAIN, KLEIHAUER-BETKE STAIN, K-B), DIAGNOSTIC

Norm:

	HBF CELLS
Adults	<2%
Children	
Newborn	60%-90%
6 months	<5%
1 year	<2%

Usage. Assessment of fetal-maternal hemorrhage in the newborn for determination of the amount of Rh immune globulin (RhoGAM) needed. Routinely performed on RhD-negative women after the birth of an RhD-positive child.

Increased. Anemia (aplastic, congenital hemolytic, myeloblastic, myelophthisic, untreated pernicious, refractory, sickle cell, sideroblastic, spherocytic), diabetes, erythroleukemia, Fanconi's anemia, hereditary persistence of fetal hemoglobin (HPFH), hyperthyroidism, hypothyroidism, infants (small-for-gestational-age, with chronic intrauterine anoxia, with developmental abnormalities), leakage of fetal hemoglobin into maternal bloodstream, leukemia (all types, acute, chronic), myelofibrosis, paroxysmal nocturnal hemoglobinuria, pregnancy, thalassemia, thyrotoxicosis, and trisomy D syndrome. Drugs include anticonvulsants.

Description. This test measures the amount of hemoglobin present in the fetal form (HbF) compared to the adult form (HbA). When blood is present in the stool, emesis, or mucus of a newborn, this test differentiates "swallowed blood syndrome" as a result of maternal bleeding from infant gastrointestinal hemorrhage.

Professional Considerations
1. Consent form NOT required.
2. Preparation:
    A. Tube: Lavender topped, or obtain a clean container for the mucus specimen.
3. Procedure:
    A. Draw a 2-mL blood sample.
    B. For gastrointestinal or mucus specimens from an infant, use a clean glass or plastic container to collect a small amount of emesis, stool, or mucus.
4. Postprocedure care:
    A. None.
5. Client and family teaching:
    A. Cord blood may be sent as a positive control.
    B. Results are normally available within 24 hours.
6. Factors that affect results:
    A. Reject hemolyzed specimens or specimens received more than 6 hours after collection.
    B. Smears must be fixed within 1 hour after preparation.
7. Other data:
    A. A newborn cord blood specimen is recommended as a source of fetal blood to be used as a positive control.
    B. Flow cytometry is more precise than Kleihauer-Betke manual technique.

BGP
(*see Osteocalcin, Plasma or serum*)

BHB
(*see Beta-hydroxybutyrate, Blood*)

BHY
(*see Beta-hydroxybutyrate, Blood*)

BICARBONATE (HCO$_3^-$), PLASMA

Norm:

		SI UNITS
Adult		
Normal venous range	22-29 mEq/L	22-29 mmol/L
Normal arterial range	21-28 mEq/L	21-28 mmol/L
Newborn		
Normal venous range	16-24 mEq/L	16-24 mmol/L
Panic venous range	≤15 mEq/L	≤15 mmol/L
	or >35 mEq/L	or >35 mmol/L

Increased. Anoxia, burns (extensive), compensated respiratory acidosis, gastric lavage, fat embolism, gastric suction, hypokalemia, metabolic alkalosis, and vomiting. Drugs include barbiturates (causing respiratory depression), corticosteroids (chronic use), diuretics, laxative (abuse), opiates (causing respiratory depression), oral glutamine, and alkaline salts.

Decreased. Compensated respiratory alkalosis, diabetes mellitus, diarrhea, ethylene glycol poisoning, metabolic acidosis, and renal failure. Drugs include acid salts, ammonium chloride, acetazolamide, cholestyramine, cyclosporin A, methanol, and salicylate toxicity. Herbal or natural remedies include products containing aristolochic acids (*Akebia* spp., *Aristolochia* spp., *Asarum* spp., birthwort, *Bragantia* spp., *Clematis* spp., *Cocculus* spp., *Diploclisia* spp., Dutchman's pipe, Fang chi, Fang ji, Fang chi, Guang fang ji, Kan-Mokutsu, *Menispernum* spp., Mokutsu, Mu tong, *Sinomenium* spp., and *Stephania* spp.)

Description. Bicarbonate is part of the bicarbonate–carbonic acid buffering system and is mainly responsible for regulating the pH of body fluids. It also facilitates the transport of carbon dioxide from the body tissues to the lungs. In the digestive tract, bicarbonate is secreted by the pancreas and liver into the duodenum to neutralize the acid chyme entering from the stomach. Serum bicarbonate levels are approximated from the serum carbon dioxide level minus 1.2 mmol (the average concentration of carbonic acid). More accurate diagnoses regarding the buffering system can be determined by obtainment of an arterial blood sample for blood gas analysis.

Professional Considerations
1. Consent form NOT required.
2. Preparation:
   A. Tube: Green topped.
3. Procedure:
   A. Draw a 1-mL blood sample anaerobically.
   B. Do NOT draw specimen during dialysis.
4. Postprocedure care:
   A. None.
5. Client and family teaching:
   A. Results are normally available within 2 hours.
6. Factors that affect results:
   A. Ingestion of acidic or alkaline solutions may cause increased or decreased results, respectively.
   B. Underfilling Vacutainer tube lowers serum bicarbonate values.
   C. Prolonged tourniquet application before phlebotomy increases serum bicarbonate.
7. Other data:
   A. Bicarbonate does not improve the hemodynamic condition when lactic acidosis is present.
   B. Not reliable in assessing fluid deficit in children.

BILE, URINE

Norm. Reagent screening test: Negative.

Quantitative. <0.2 mg/dL.

Increased or Positive. Biliary tract obstruction, cirrhosis, hepatitis (acute, alcoholic, chronic, drug induced), hyperthyroidism, infectious mononucleosis, septicemia, and tumor (biliary tract, liver).

Description. This is a routine test used to detect unsuspected liver disease where jaundice is absent. The test is also used in the differential diagnosis of jaundice because plasma bilirubin present as a result of hemolytic disorders exists in a water-soluble form that cannot be filtered by the kidneys. Bilirubinuria is detected by a yellow foam that forms in a shaken specimen or by a yellow-orange to brown urine color. Serial levels can guide clinical management of liver and biliary disorders.

Professional Considerations
1. Consent form NOT required.
2. Preparation:
   A. Obtain a clean container and a paper bag.
3. Procedure:
   A. Obtain a 50-mL random urine specimen in a clean glass or plastic container. A fresh specimen may be taken from a urinary drainage bag.
4. Postprocedure care:
   A. Write the collection time on the laboratory requisition.
   B. Place the specimen in the paper bag and transport it to the laboratory immediately.
   C. Refrigerate the specimen if the test will not be performed within 1 hour of collection.
5. Client and family teaching:
   A. Inform the nurse immediately after the specimen has been obtained.
   B. Do not contaminate the urine specimen with stool.
   C. Results are normally available within 24 hours.
6. Factors that affect results:
   A. Reject specimens received more than 1 hour after collection.
   B. Drugs that may cause false-positive results include chlorpromazine, mefenamic acid, phenothiazines, and salicylates.

C. Drugs that may cause false-negative results include ascorbic acid, ethoxazene hydrochloride, and phenazopyridine.
D. False-positive results may be caused by contamination of the specimen with stool.
E. False-negative results may be caused by prolonged exposure of the specimen to room temperature or to light.
7. Other data:
A. Bilirubinuria is an insensitive indicator of liver disease.
B. Urinary bile acids are higher in formula-fed infants compared to breastfed infants.

C. Doxorubicin HCl (Adriamycin) chemotherapy and its metabolites are found in urine and bile.

BILIRUBIN, DIRECT (CONJUGATED), SERUM
(see Bilirubin, Serum)

BILIRUBIN, INDIRECT (UNCONJUGATED, FREE), SERUM
(see Bilirubin, Serum)

BILIRUBIN (TOTAL, DIRECT [CONJUGATED] AND INDIRECT [UNCONJUGATED]), SERUM

Norm:

		SI UNITS
Total Bilirubin		
1 Month–Adult	<1.5 mg/dL	1.7- 20.5 µmol/L
Premature Infant		
Cord	<2.8 mg/dL	<48 µmol/L
24 hours	1-6 mg/dL	17-103 µmol/L
48 hours	6-8 mg/dL	103-137 µmol/L
3-5 days	10-12 mg/dL	171-205 µmol/L
Full-Term Infant		
Cord	<2.8 mg/dL	<48 µmol/L
24 hours	2-6 mg/dL	34-103 µmol/L
48 hours	6-7 mg/dL	103-120 µmol/L
3-5 days	4-6 mg/dL	68-103 µmol/L
Direct Bilirubin	0.0-0.3 mg/dL	1.7-5.1 µmol/L
Indirect Bilirubin	0.1-1.0 mg/dL	1.7-17.1 µmol/L

Increased Total Bilirubin. Alcoholism, anemia (pernicious), biliary calculi, biliary obstruction, biliary scar tissue, carcinoma of pancreas head, cholangitis, cirrhosis, Crigler-Najjar syndrome, Dubin-Johnson syndrome, erythroblastosis fetalis, fasting (prolonged), Gilbert's disease, graft-versus-host disease (GVHD), hemolysis (autoimmune), hemorrhage, hepatic cryosurgery, hepatitis (alcoholic, infectious, toxic, viral, obstructive), hereditary spherocytosis, impaired liver function, malaria, mononucleosis (infectious), myocardial infarction, pancreatitis (biliary tract origin), pulmonary embolism, sickle cell anemia, toxic shock syndrome, transfusion reactions, and tumor. Drugs include acetazolamide, aminophenol, androgens, antimalarials, ascorbic acid, asparaginase, aspirin, barbiturates, carmustine, cholinergics, chlordiazepoxide, chloroquine hydrochloride, chloroquine phosphate, chlorothiazide sodium, chlorpromazine hydrochloride, cholinergics, clindamycin, dextran, diazoxide, dicumarol (dicoumarin), epinephrine bitartrate, epinephrine borate, epinephrine hydrochloride, erythromycin, ethyl alcohol (ethanol), ethoxazene hydrochloride, floxuridine, flurazepam, fosinopril, histidine, hydroxychloroquine sulfate, imipramine, indican, indomethacin, iproniazid, iron, isoniazid, isoproterenol hydrochloride, levodopa, lincomycin, meclofamate, methanol, methyldopa, methyltestosterone, morphine sulfate, niacin, novobiocin, novobiocin sodium, oral contraceptives, penicillin, phenazopyridine, phenelzine sulfate, phenothiazines, phenprocoumon, phenylbutazone, primaquine phosphate, procainamide hydrochloride, protein, pyrazinamide, pyrimethamine, quinacrine hydrochloride, quinidine gluconate, quinidine polygalacturonate, quinidine sulfate, radiographic dyes, rifampin, streptomycin sulfate, tetracyclines, theophylline, thiazide diuretics, tyrosine, vitamin A, and warfarin sodium. Herbs and natural remedies that have the potential to cause hepatotoxicity and elevate values include akee fruit (ackee, *Blighia sapida*), *Atractylis gummifera*, Azadirachta indica (see margosa), *Berberis vulgaris* (barberry), *Callilepsis laureola* (blazing star, *Liatris spicata*), chaparral tea (*Larrea tridentata*), cocaine, comfree ("knitbone," *Symphytum*), *Crotalaria* (bush tea), cycasin (a toxin from a Cycas species of sago palm of Guam), germander (genera *Teucrium* and *Veronica;* do not confuse with safe skullcap, a name often falsely used in selling germander), *Heliotropium* (germander, valerian), $jin^1bu^2huan^4$ ("gold-in-convertible", Jin Bu Huan Anodyne Tablets, patent medicine with misidentified constituents: essence of *t'ienchi [tianqi]* flowers, "Noto-ginseng"; also *kombucha;* also *Lycopodium serratum,* or club moss; but with plant alkaloid levo-tetrahydropalmatine, a potent neuroactive substance), ma^2huang^2 (*Ephedra*), margosa (*Melia azadirachta,* Azadirachta indica), maté tea (*Ilex paraguayensis*), mistletoe, pennyroyal, sassafras, skullcap (*Scutellaria;* do not confuse with unsafe germander), $syo\text{-}saiko\text{-}to$ ($xiao^3$ $chai^2$ hu^2 $tang^1$, "minor *Bupleurum* combination"), *Teucrium polium* (golden germander), and valerian (*Valeriana officinalis,* garden heliotrope).

Increased Direct Bilirubin. Biliary obstruction, carcinoma of head of the pancreas, cirrhosis, Dubin-Johnson syndrome, hepatitis (acute, alcoholic, infectious, viral, toxic), and rotor syndrome. Also drugs that increase total bilirubin levels: vinho abafado ("augmented Port wine," Brazil), $chuan^1lian^2$ ($huang^2lian^2$, Cantonese *ch'uen lin, Coptis chinensis/japonicum,* goldenthread) tonic, yin^1chen^2 (*Artemisia scoparia, A. capillaris,* mugwort, wormwood).

Increased Indirect Bilirubin. Anemia (pernicious), autoimmune hemolysis, Bartter syndrome, cirrhosis (acute, alcoholic, nonalcoholic), Crigler-Najjar syndrome, erythroblastosis fetalis, Gilbert's disease, hepatitis (all types), hereditary spherocytosis, intracavitary and soft-tissue hemorrhage, malaria, myocardial infarction, septicemia, sickle cell disease, and transfusion reaction (hemolytic). Also, drugs that increase total bilirubin levels.

Decreased Total, Direct, and Indirect Bilirubin. Phototherapy. Drugs include barbiturates, caffeine, chlorine, citrate, corticosteroids, dicophane, ethyl alcohol (ethanol), penicillin, protein, salicylates, sulfonamides, thioridazine, and urea.

Description. Bilirubin is produced in the liver, spleen, and bone marrow and is also a by-product of hemoglobin breakdown. Total bilirubin levels can be broken down into direct (conjugated) bilirubin, which is primarily excreted through the intestinal tract, and indirect (free) bilirubin, which circulates primarily in the bloodstream. Total bilirubin levels rise with any type of jaundice, whereas direct and indirect levels rise depending on the cause of the jaundice. Direct (conjugated) bilirubin is that portion of bilirubin that is normally excreted primarily by the gastrointestinal tract, with only small amounts entering the bloodstream. When obstructive or hepatic jaundice occurs, increasing amounts of conjugated bilirubin enter the bloodstream, rather than the gastrointestinal tract, and they are filtered and excreted by the kidneys. Indirect bilirubin (free or unconjugated bilirubin) is the portion of bilirubin that normally circulates in the bloodstream. When hemolytic jaundice occurs, increasing amounts of free bilirubin accumulate in the bloodstream as a result of increased hemoglobin breakdown. There is no direct laboratory test for indirect bilirubin; rather, it is a calculation of total bilirubin minus direct bilirubin.

Professional Considerations
1. Consent form NOT required.
2. **Preparation:**
   A. See *Client and family teaching.*
   B. Tube: Red topped, red/gray topped, or gold topped or a lancet

and capillary tube for heelstick specimens. Also obtain foil.

C. Do NOT draw blood during hemodialysis.

3. **Procedure:**
   A. Draw a 1-mL blood sample.
   B. For babies, collect heelstick blood in a capillary tube. Prewarming the heel is not necessary. Cleanse the lateral curvature of the heel with an alcohol wipe and allow it to dry. Puncture the lateral curvature of the heel with a lancet and collect blood in a capillary tube. Avoid puncturing the posterior curvature of the heel.

4. **Postprocedure care:**
   A. Leave the heelstick site open to air.
   B. Protect the sample from light. Wrap it in foil or place it in a darkened refrigerator if the test will not be run immediately.

5. **Client and family teaching:**
   A. Eat a diet low in yellow foods (such as carrots, yams, yellow beans, pumpkin) for 3-4 days before sampling.
   B. Fast for 4 hours before sampling.
   C. Serum levels will be elevated with the use of alcohol, morphine, theophylline, ascorbic acid, and aspirin.
   D. Results are normally available within 24 hours.

6. **Factors that affect results:**
   A. Reject hemolyzed or grossly lipemic specimens.
   B. Results are invalidated if the client received a radioactive scan within 24 hours before the test.
   C. Cord blood values may be elevated.
   D. Drugs that may cause falsely elevated values include acetazolamide, androgens, chlordiazepoxide, chlordiazepoxide hydrochloride, chlorpromazine, erythromycin, erythromycin ethylsuccinate, indomethacin, isoniazid, methanol, nitrofurantoin, nitrofurantoin sodium, oxacillin sodium, oxyphenbutazone, phenothiazines, phenylbutazone, salicylates, sulfinpyrazone, sulfonylureas, sulfonamides, and vitamin A.

7. **Other data:**
   A. Indirect bilirubin levels may increase in hemolytic disease in the newborn to >20 mg/dL.
   B. Neonate treatment for serum bilirubin >15 mg/dL may include

exchange transfusion or phototherapy. Phototherapy converts bilirubin into a colorless compound that has no effects on the neonate.

C. Biliary atresia can be differentiated from infantile hepatitis using bilirubin conjugates with Micronex chromatography.

BILIRUBIN, TOTAL, SERUM
(see Bilirubin, Serum)

BILIRUBIN, URINE

Norm. Negative ≤0.02 mg/dL (≤0.34 μmol/L, SI units).

Positive or Increased. Arsenic ingestion, cirrhosis, hepatitis (alcoholic, chronic, acute, drug induced), hyperthyroidism, malignancy (hepatic or biliary tract), mononucleosis (infectious), and septicemia. Herbal or natural remedies that have the potential to cause hepatotoxicity and elevate values include akee fruit (ackee, *Blighia sapida*), *Atractylis gummifera*, Azadirachta indica (see margosa), *Berberis vulgaris* (barberry), *Callilepsis laureola* (blazing star, *Liatris spicata*), chaparral tea (*Larrea tridentata*), cocaine, comfree ("knitbone," *Symphytum*), *Crotalaria* (bush tea), cycasin (a toxin from a *Cycas* species of sago palm of Guam), germander (genera *Teucrium* and *Veronica;* do not confuse with safe skullcap, a name often falsely used in selling germander), *Heliotropium* (germander, valerian), jin[1]bu[2]huan[4] ("gold-inconvertible," Jin Bu Huan Anodyne Tablets, patent medicine with misidentified constituents: essence of *t'ienchi [tianqi]* flowers, "Noto-ginseng"; also *kombucha;* also *Lycopodium serratum,* or club moss; but with plant alkaloid levo-tetrahydropalmatine, a potent neuroactive substance), ma[2]huang[2] (*Ephedra*), margosa (*Melia azadirachta,* Azadirachta indica), maté tea (*Ilex paraguayensis*), mistletoe, pennyroyal, sassafras, skullcap (*Scutellaria;* do not confuse with unsafe germander), Syo-saiko-to (xiao[3] chai[2]hu[2] tang[1], "minor *Bupleurum* combination"), *Teucrium polium* (golden germander), and valerian (*Valeriana officinalis,* garden heliotrope).

Description. Screens for the presence of conjugated bilirubin in the urine. Bilirubin is a by-product of hemoglobin breakdown that is normally excreted by the gastrointestinal tract. When obstructive or hepatic jaundice occurs, conjugated bilirubin enters the bloodstream, rather than the gastrointestinal tract, and is filtered and excreted by the kidneys.

Professional Considerations
1. Consent form NOT required.
2. Preparation:
   A. Obtain Icotest tablets, N-Multistix, or Chemstrips for urine samples, and a clean container.
3. Procedure:
   A. Collect a 20-mL fresh random urine sample in a clean container.
   B. Follow package directions exactly for either Icotest tablets, NMultistix, or Chemstrips for urine samples.
4. Postprocedure care:
   A. None.
5. Client and family teaching:
   A. Phenothiazines and ascorbic acid may affect results.
   B. Results are normally available within 24 hours.
6. Factors that affect results:
   A. Drugs that may cause false-positive results with Icotest tablets include salicylates.
   B. Drugs that may cause falsenegative results with Icotest tablets include ascorbic acid.
   C. Drugs that may cause false-positive N-Multistix or Chemstrip bilirubin results include phenazopyridine, phenothiazines and etodolac (nonsteroidal anti-inflammatory).
   D. A delay in performing the test may result in false-negative results.
7. Other data:
   A. Even trace amounts of bilirubin in the urine require further diagnostic investigation.
   B. Pruritus associated with hepatic cholestasis can be improved with the use of phototherapy.
   C. There is good agreement between the use of Multistix and Clinitek 200+ analyzer.

BIOGRAPH IMAGING, DIAGNOSTIC
(see Dual modality imaging, Diagnostic)

BIOPSY, ANAEROBIC, CULTURE

Norm. No growth.

Positive. Cellulitis, decubiti, gingivitis, gangrenous or inflamed tissues and wounds caused by *Actinomyces, Arachnia, Bacteroides fragilis, Bacteroides melaninogenicus, Bifidobacterium, Clostridium, Eubacterium, Fusobacterium, Lactobacillus, Peptostreptococcus, Propionibacterium, Veillonella*, and others.

Description. Many anaerobic bacteria are present as part of the normal flora in humans. They obtain energy for growth and metabolism from fermentation reactions, rather than from oxygen. When displaced from their location into other body tissues or spaces, they become pathogenic. Anaerobes of clinical importance in humans most commonly cause infections in the skin, intestinal tract, vagina, brain, upper respiratory tract, lungs, and peritoneum. Special collection methods are necessary for the isolation of anaerobes. Anaerobic cultures are grown on complex media, and identification is made using colony morphology, pigmentation, fluorescence, and gas-liquid chromatography.

Professional Considerations
1. Consent form IS required for the biopsy.

Risks
See *Biopsy, Site-specific, Specimen.*

Contraindications
See *Biopsy, Site-specific, Specimen.*

2. Preparation:
   A. Obtain the baseline PT and PTT values.
   B. Alert laboratory personnel that an anaerobic specimen will be arriving shortly.
   C. Obtain povidone-iodine solution, sterile drapes, a biopsy tray, and a sterile specimen container or Petri dish.
3. Procedure:
   A. The site is prepared with povidone-iodine, allowed to dry, and then draped.
   B. Ultrasound may be helpful for needle guidance in obtaining internal organ needle biopsy specimens.

C. A biopsy of the tissue is obtained by the physician, with care being taken to avoid contamination of the specimen with other area organisms and to minimize exposure of the specimen to air.
D. After it is obtained, the biopsied material is quickly placed on premoistened sterile gauze in a sterile, 100-mm Petri dish or in a sterile container with the cap loosened.
E. An anaerobic transport container such as the Bio-Bag type A Anaerobic Culture Set (Marion) may be used. It consists of a gas-impermeable plastic bag and two ampules: one that generates hydrogen and the other that releases resazurin indicator.
F. Place the container or Petri dish inside the plastic bag with both ampules and seal the bag with a heat sealer.
G. Crush the gas-generator ampule. Hydrogen from the gas-generator ampule should combine with oxygen in the presence of a catalyst to produce water vapor condensation inside the bag. (See *Anaerobic culture* for instructions for liquid specimens.)
4. Postprocedure care:
   A. Write the collection time on the laboratory requisition.
   B. Transport the sample to the laboratory immediately.
   C. Apply a dry, sterile dressing to the biopsy site.
   D. Observe the site for drainage, redness, edema, or pain until it is healed.
5. Client and family teaching:
   A. Report signs of infection at the operative site to the physician: increasing pain, redness, swelling, purulent drainage, or fever >101° F (≥38.3° C).
   B. Results are normally available within 4 days.
6. Factors that affect results:
   A. Overexposure to air may cause the anaerobe to die.
   B. Do not refrigerate the specimen.
7. Other data:
   A. The use of swabs to obtain anaerobic cultures is not recommended. When necessary, commercial anaerobic swab sets consisting of two containers must be used.

B. Cultures of an unwashed small intestinal mucosal biopsy specimen are as useful as a culture of small intestinal aspirate for bacterial overgrowth analysis.
C. Bacterial growth is more frequent in COPD clients with exacerbation and in those with bronchial inflammation than in stable COPD clients.

BIOPSY, FUNGUS, CULTURE

Norm. No growth.

Positive. *Blastomyces dermatitidis, Coccidioides immitis, Cryptococcus neoformans, Histoplasma capsulatum, Sporothrix schenckii, Candida albicans, Candida tropicalis, Aspergillus fumigatus, Aspergillus flavus,* and others.

Description. Fungi are slow growing, eukaryotic organisms that can grow on living and nonliving organic materials and are subdivided into yeasts and molds. Only a few fungi species infect humans. Normal host defense mechanisms limit the damage they cause superficially. Factors that predispose persons to fungal infections by lowering the normal host defense mechanisms include administration of broad-spectrum antibiotics or cancer chemotherapy, invasive lines, poor nutritional status, parenteral nutrition, surgery, trauma, and long-term use of steroids. Some fungi can be inhaled or introduced by traumatic inoculation into deep tissue spaces and cause serious infections. Although tentative identification of fungi can be made quickly with staining techniques, culture of the organism on special fungal culture media is required to confirm a diagnosis of a fungal infection.

Professional Considerations
1. Consent form IS required.

Risks
See *Biopsy, Site-specific, Specimen.*

Contraindications
See *Biopsy, Site-specific, Specimen.*

2. Preparation:
   A. Obtain the baseline PT/PTT or ACT.

B. Obtain a sterile container, a culture dish, or an appropriate tube. See procedure on next page for other site-specific supplies needed.

3. **Procedure:**
A. *Hair:* Examine the scalp with a Wood's lamp and remove fluorescent, fractured, or distorted hairs, and place them in a dry, sterile culture dish.
B. *Skin:* Cleanse the skin with an alcohol wipe. Remove any scales at the circumference of the lesion with a sterile scalpel. Obtain a scalpel or punch biopsy and place the tissue in a dry, sterile culture dish.
C. *Nails:* Cleanse the nails with an alcohol wipe. Scrape off the outermost layer or scrapings from beneath the edge of the nails with a scalpel and place them in a dry, sterile culture dish.
D. *Bone marrow:* Cleanse the skin over the aspiration site with povidone-iodine solution and allow it to dry completely. A physician performs an aspiration of enough bone marrow for two inoculations of media and either leaves it in the sterile syringe or injects it into a green-topped tube containing heparin. The specimen can be refrigerated no longer than 12 hours before being cultured.
E. *Tissues:* Biopsied material obtained during surgery should be placed in a sterile cup containing a small amount of saline without preservatives. For abscess drainage, a portion of the abscess wall should be submitted. The specimen can be refrigerated no longer than 10 hours before being cultured.

4. **Postprocedure care:**
A. Write the exact time of the specimen collection on the laboratory requisition.
B. Write any current antifungal therapy on the laboratory requisition.
C. Transport the specimen to the laboratory immediately.
D. Apply a dry, sterile dressing to the bone marrow aspiration or biopsy site. Observe the site for redness, tenderness, edema, or drainage until healed.

5. **Client and family teaching:**
A. Preliminary results are normally available within 5 days, the final results in 6 weeks.
B. If fungus is suspected, treatment is started as a life-saving measure before the final results are obtained.
C. Report signs of infection at the operative site to the physician: increasing pain, redness, swelling, purulent drainage, or fever >101° F (≥38.3° C).

6. **Factors that affect results:**
A. Do not refrigerate hair, skin, or nail specimens.
B. Best results are obtained if cultures are inoculated immediately. Other than noted above, the maximum time allowed between specimen collection and inoculation is 3 hours.

7. **Other data:**
A. No growth for 4-6 weeks is required for fungal culture results to be confirmed as negative.
B. Open-lung biopsy provides a better yield than bronchoalveolar lavage in immunocompromised clients.
C. Ultrasound-guided, fine-needle aspiration is recommended in clients with pulmonary or pleural aspergillosis.
D. Green onion is one spice that grows *Aspergillus.*
E. LY 303,366 is a promising antifungal agent against *Aspergillus.*
F. Fungus is more frequent in fingernails than toenails and females more than males, and the highest prevalence of fungi is 50-70 years of age.

BIOPSY, MYCOBACTERIA, CULTURE

Norm. No growth.

Positive. *Mycobacterium ulcerans, M. tuberculosis, M. bovis, M. marinum, M. kansasii, M. simiae, M. asiaticum, M. scrofulaceum, M. szulgai, M. gordonae, M. flavescens, M. xenopi, M. avium, M. intracellulare, M. gastri, M. leprae, M. malmoense, M. haemophilum, M. nonchromogenicum, M. terrae, M. triviale, M. fortuitum, M. chelonei, M. phlei, M. smegmatis,* and *M. vaccae.*

Description. Mycobacteria are rod-shaped, aerobic bacteria that resist decolorizing chemicals after staining, properties termed acid-fastness and alcohol-fastness. Nineteen *Mycobacterium* species are capable of producing human disease characterized by destructive granulomas that can necrose, ulcerate, and cavitate. *Mycobacterium tuberculosis* is transmitted by the airborne route most commonly to the lungs, where it survives well, causes areas of granulomatous inflammation, and, if not dormant, causes cough, fever, and hemoptysis. Mycobacterial infections can also occur in superficial body parts and internal organs.

Professional Considerations
1. Consent form IS required for the biopsy.

Risks
See *Biopsy, Site-specific, Specimen.*

Contraindications
See *Biopsy, Site-specific, Specimen.*

2. Preparation:
   A. Obtain the baseline PT/PTT or ACT.
   B. Obtain a sterile container large enough to hold the tissue biopsy specimen.
3. Procedure:
   A. Place a large (pea-sized) amount of biopsied material in a sterile container and transport it to the laboratory immediately.
4. Postprocedure care:
   A. Specific to site and surgery.
   B. Write the exact time of the specimen collection on the laboratory requisition.
5. Client and family teaching:
   A. If tuberculosis is suspected, wear a mask until no longer infectious, and cough only into the mask. Do not cough into the air outside the mask because this can spread the disease.
   B. Results may take up to 2 months, but treatment is started before results if tuberculosis is suspected.
   C. Report signs of infection at the operative site to the physician: increasing pain, redness, swelling, purulent drainage, or fever >101° F (≥38.3° C).
6. Factors that affect results:
   A. Do not refrigerate the specimen.

B. The maximum time allowed between specimen collection and inoculation is 3 hours.
C. Antituberculous drug therapy may cause negative results because of the inhibition of the growth of *M. tuberculosis.*
D. A high–carbon dioxide atmosphere for growth may increase the number of positive cultures.
E. A culture medium containing glycerin accelerates growth.
7. **Other data:**
   A. Cultures for *M. tuberculosis* may take 3-8 weeks to grow.
   B. Bone marrow biopsy for *Mycobacterium* should be performed only on severely immunocompromised clients.
   C. Liver biopsy can be performed to diagnose infection in HIV-infected clients who have unexplained fever and abnormal liver function test results.
   D. Rifampin + ofloxacin + minocycline is the best bactericidal combination for *M. leprae.*
   E. Clarithromycin is used for the treatment of early lesions of *M. ulcerans* and in combination with rifabutin for multidrug-resistant tuberculosis.
   F. *M. avium* has increased dramatically with AIDS. Clarithromycin + ethambutol is standard treatment with alternatives being azithromycin, rifabutin, ciprofloxin, clofazamine, and amikacin.

BIOPSY, ROUTINE, CULTURE

Norm. No growth.

Usage. Cellulitis, decubiti, inflamed tissues and wounds, and internal organs.

Description. An excision or a needle-punch sample of tissue suspected to be infected is taken and inoculated on bacterial culture media.

Professional Considerations
1. Consent form IS required for the biopsy.

Risks
See *Biopsy, Site-specific, Specimen.*

B

Contraindications
See *Biopsy, Site-specific, Specimen.*

2. Preparation:
   A. Obtain the baseline PT/PTT or ACT.
   B. Obtain a sterile container large enough to hold the tissue biopsy.
3. Procedure:
   A. Decubiti should be debrided before the biopsy.
   B. Surface wounds, skin, nails, and mucosal surfaces should be cleansed with an alcohol wipe and allowed to dry just before the biopsy.
   C. Obtain 20-500 mg of tissue by excision with a scalpel or with a needle punch using an aseptic technique. Take care not to contaminate the specimen with surrounding tissue.
   D. Place the biopsied material in a sterile container and transport it to the laboratory immediately.
4. Postprocedure care:
   A. Specific to site and surgery.
   B. Write the collection time on the laboratory requisition.
5. Client and family teaching:
   A. Final results may take up to a week, but treatment may occur after biopsy culture.
   B. Report signs of infection at the operative site to the physician: increasing pain, redness, swelling, purulent drainage, or fever >101° F (≥38.3° C).
6. Factors that affect results:
   A. Do not refrigerate the specimen.
   B. The maximum amount of time allowed between specimen collection and inoculation is 3 hours.
7. Other data:
   A. Final results may take up to 7 days.
   B. Cultures of the prostate are to be interpreted with pathologic characterization of locations contiguous to the tissue of the cultures.

BIOPSY, SITE-SPECIFIC, SPECIMEN

Norm. Interpreted by pathologist.

Usage. Abscess (abscess wall), acute interstitial nephritis (kidney), adrenal feminization (testis), alcoholic myopathy (muscle), alveolar proteinosis (lung), amebiasis (rectum), amyloidosis (tissue), amyotrophic lateral sclerosis (muscle), arthritis (joint), bronchogenic carcinoma (lung, lymph node, pleura), brucellosis (spleen, tissue), carcinoma of pancreas head (pancreas), cardiac transplant rejection, cat-scratch disease (lymph node), Chagas' disease (lung, lymph node), chancroid (lymph node), celiac disease (small intestine), cholesterol ester storage disease (liver), chromoblastomycosis (tissue), chronic inflammatory splenomegaly (spleen), cirrhosis (liver), coccidioidomycosis (joint), coccidiosis (small intestine), colon cancer (colon), de Quervain's thyroiditis (thyroid), Dubin-Johnson syndrome (liver), farmer's lung (lung), fatty liver (liver), female infertility, filariasis (lymph node), galactosemia (liver), Gaucher's disease (skin), germinal aplasia (testis), glucuronyltransferase deficiency (liver), goiter (thyroid), Goodpasture syndrome (kidney), glycogenesis (liver), gonorrhea (rectum), Hamman-Rich syndrome (lung), Hashimoto's thyroiditis (thyroid), hemochromatosis (liver), hepatitis (liver), Hirschsprung's disease (rectum), histiocytosis (spleen), Hurler syndrome (skin), Hodgkin's disease (lymph node, spleen), hypophosphatemia (bone), hyperthyroidism (muscle), hypertension (endomyocardium), immunodeficiency (lymph node), infectious mononucleosis (lymph node), jaundice (liver), kidney transplant rejection (kidney), Kimmelstiel-Wilson syndrome (kidney), Klinefelter syndrome (testis), Legionnaire's disease (lung), leprosy (nasal scrapings, lepromatous lesion), leukemia (spleen), lymphangitis (lymph node), lymphatic leukemia (lymph node), lymphogranuloma venereum (lymph node), lymphoma (lymph node), malabsorption (small intestine), male infertility (testicle), McArdle syndrome (muscle), menstrual irregularities (endometrium), metabolic diseases (muscle, skin), metachromatic leukodystrophy (nerve), metastasis (liver, lymph node), mitochondrial myopathy (muscle), muscular dystrophy (muscle), myasthenia gravis (muscle), myotonia congenita (muscle), myotubular myopathy (muscle), narcotic addiction (liver), nemaline myopathy (muscle), Niemann-Pick disease (rectum, skin), osteomalacia (bone), osteopenia (bone), parasitic infections (spleen), pelvic inflammatory disease (endometrium), pleural tumor (pleura), pneumoconiosis (lung, lymph node), *Pneumocystis* pneumonia (lung), polyarteritis nodosa (tissue), polymyalgia rheumatica (muscle, temporal artery), polymyositis (muscle), poststreptococcal glomerulonephritis (kidney), proctitis (rectum), rat-bite fever (joint fluid), renal disease (kidney tissue), Reye syndrome (liver), rheumatoid pleurisy (pleura), Riedel's thyroiditis (thyroid), Rocky Mountain spotted fever (skin), sarcoidosis (lung, lymph node, tissue), schistosomiasis (bladder, rectum), scleroderma (tissue), septic pyelophlebitis (liver), Sjögren syndrome (kidney), Stein-Leventhal syndrome (ovary), stiff-man syndrome (muscle), stomach carcinoma (bone marrow, liver, lymph node), systemic lupus erythematosus (full-thickness skin, tissue), temporal arteritis (temporal artery), toxemia of pregnancy (kidney), trichinosis (muscle), tuberculosis (bone marrow, lung, lymph node, spleen), tularemia (lymph node), Turner syndrome (ovary, testis), ulcerative colitis (liver, rectum), villous adenoma (rectum), visceral larva migrans (liver), Wegener's granulomatosis (kidney), Whipple's disease (lymph node, small intestine), Wilson's disease (liver), and yellow fever (liver).

Description. Excisional biopsy (remove entire lump), incisional (remove part of lump), or needle punch or fine needle aspiration (FNA) (where you withdraw a small sample through a 22-25 gauge needle) done under sterile technique and examined for cell morphology and tissue abnormalities. The procedure takes 15-30 minutes. Each specimen is evaluated by gross examination (looking at it), microscopically (under a microscope), and through tissue processing (staining and preserving).

Professional Considerations

1. Consent form IS required for most specimens and is specific to the institution.

Risks

Allergic reaction to local anesthetic (itching, hives, rash, tight feeling in the throat, shortness of breath, bron-

chospasm, anaphylaxis, death). Infection, hematoma, mild to severe bleeding, organ damage, and hemorrhage. Vasovagal reaction. Death is possible from biopsies of internal organs.

Contraindications

Previous allergy to local anesthetic. Biopsy may be contraindicated in clients with coagulation defects.

2. **Preparation:**
   A. Obtain the baseline PT/PTT or ACT.
   B. Type and crossmatch may be prescribed 24 hours before the biopsy.
   C. Obtain sterile containers, one with 10% formaldehyde, the other with sterile saline.

3. **Procedure:**
   A. Decubiti should be debrided before the biopsy.
   B. Surface wounds, skin, and mucosal surfaces should be cleansed with an alcohol wipe and allowed to dry just before the biopsy.
   C. Obtain 20-500 mg of tissue by needle aspiration, excision, or needle-punch using an aseptic technique. Do not contaminate the specimen with other tissue in the area.
   D. Place the biopsied material in a sterile container of 10% formaldehyde and in another with sterile saline. Transport the specimens to the laboratory immediately.

4. **Postprocedure care:**
   A. Specific to site and surgery. A dry, sterile dressing or a Band-Aid dressing is required.
   B. Write the collection time on the laboratory requisition.
   C. Assess vital signs and the site for bleeding or hematoma formation every 15 minutes × 4 and then every 30 minutes × 2.
   D. Observe for signs of infection (fever, chills, hypotension, tachycardia) every 24-48 hours.

5. **Client and family teaching:**
   A. Fast from food, and drink only clear liquids after midnight and before the biopsy.
   B. Report signs of infection at the operative site to the physician: increasing pain, redness, swelling, purulent drainage, or fever >101° F (≥38.3° C).

C. Check temperature every 6 hours for 24 hours, and notify the physician if fever, chills, faintness, weakness, or dizziness occurs. Place pressure over the site for 10 minutes if bleeding is noted.

D. Results are normally available within 72 hours.

6. **Factors that affect results:**
   A. Do not refrigerate the specimen.

7. **Other data:**
   A. The full report may take up to 5 days.
   B. Sentinel node biopsy (Specific for breast cancer).

BLADDER TUMOR–ASSOCIATED ANTIGEN

(*See BTP test for bladder cancer, diagnostic*)

BLASTOMYCOSIS (GILCHRIST'S) SKIN TEST, DIAGNOSTIC

Norm. Negative.

Usage. Diagnosis of Blastomyces dermatitidis.

Description. Blastomycosis, a chronic granulomatous and suppurative fungal disease of the lungs and skin, occurs primarily in 20- to 40-year-old males in rural areas throughout the world. There is no evidence of transmission from one client to another, and there is usually no epidemic. The mode of transmission is believed to be inhalation of spores from soil. The spores then disseminate by invading the blood and lymphatic systems. Blastomycosis skin lesions may be erythematous nodes or papular lesions, which can break down, ulcerate, drain, and spread. ARDS can develop from pulmonary blastomycosis and has a mortality rate of 89%.

Professional Considerations
1. Consent form NOT required.
2. **Preparation:**
   A. Obtain a sterile container for the biopsy specimen.
3. **Procedure:**
   A. Using a sterile technique, a biopsy specimen is taken from the periphery of a skin lesion where pus and yeast cells are found. A wet mount of the specimen shows broadly attached buds on thick-walled cells.

4. **Postprocedure care:**
   A. Apply a dry, sterile dressing to the site if bleeding occurs.
5. **Client and family teaching:**
   A. Report signs of infection at the biopsy site to the physician: increasing pain, redness, swelling, purulent drainage, or fever >101° F (≥38.3° C).
   B. Results are normally available within 72 hours.
6. **Factors that affect results:**
   A. Treatment with amphotericin B may cause false-negative results.
7. **Other data:**
   A. Blastomycosis is a general term used in parts of the world to refer to any infection caused by budding yeasts in the tissue.
   B. Endemic areas in the United States include northeast Tennessee, Vilas County (Wisconsin), Mississippi, and the Ohio River valley.

BLEEDING TIME, DUKE, BLOOD

Norm. 1-5 minutes.

Increased. Anemia (aplastic, pernicious), collagen diseases, congenital heart disease, disseminated intravascular coagulopathy, drug sensitivity, ethyl alcohol ingestion along with aspirin ingestion, factor deficiency (I, II, V, VII, VIII, IX, XI), fibrinolytic activity, Glanzmann's disease, hemorrhagic disease of the newborn, Hodgkin's disease, hypothyroidism, idiopathic thrombocytopenic purpura, infections (measles, mumps, streptococcal), leukemia (acute), liver disease (severe), mononucleosis (infectious), multiple myeloma, purpura hemorrhagica, scurvy, thrombasthenia, thrombocytopathy, thrombocytopenia purpura (secondary caused by allergy), von Willebrand's disease, and uremia. Drugs include anticoagulants (oral), aspirin, indomethacin, and phenylbutazone. Herbs or natural remedies that may inhibit platelet activity include feverfew (*Tanacetum parthenium*), *Ginkgo biloba*, garlic, ginger, and ginseng.

Decreased. Not clinically significant.

Description. The duration of active bleeding from a standardized superficial puncture wound of the skin is measured.

It is most helpful as an indicator of platelet abnormality, either in their number or function.

Professional Considerations

1. Consent form NOT required.

Risks

Bleeding, hematoma, infection, ecchymoses.

Contraindications

This test is contraindicated in clients with a platelet count <50,000/mm³, in clients with severe bleeding disorders, or in clients who have taken medications containing aspirin within 7 days before the test.

2. **Preparation:**
   A. Obtain alcohol wipes, a lancet, a stopwatch, and filter paper.
   B. Screen client for the use of herbal preparations or natural remedies such as feverfew (*Tanacetum parthenium*), *Ginkgo biloba*, garlic, ginger, ginseng.
3. **Procedure:**
   A. Cleanse the site for puncture with an alcohol wipe and allow it to dry completely.
   B. Make a small lancet puncture in the fingertip or ear lobe and simultaneously start the stopwatch.
   C. Remove blood from the wound by gently blotting with filter paper, without exerting pressure on the wound, every 30 seconds.
   D. When blood flow ceases, stop timing with the stopwatch. If bleeding continues for more than 20 minutes, discontinue the test and apply pressure to the site.
4. **Postprocedure care:**
   A. Apply a dry, sterile dressing to the site after bleeding stops.
5. **Client and family teaching:**
   A. Do not take aspirin for 7 days before the test.
   B. Call the physician if there are signs of infection at the test site: increasing pain, bleeding, redness, swelling, purulent drainage, or fever >101° F (≥38.3° C).
   C. Results are normally available within 24 hours.
6. **Factors that affect results:**
   A. A uniform incision is difficult to make without considerable skill.
   B. Pressing too hard on the blood with the filter paper disturbs the platelet plug and prolongs bleeding time.
7. **Other data:**
   A. The depth of the puncture with the lancet is difficult to standardize and results in difficulty reproducing bleeding times.
   B. Daily administration of 75 mg of aspirin for 2 weeks in healthy pregnant women yielded results of Duke's bleeding time within normal limits.

BLEEDING TIME, IVY, BLOOD

Norm. 1-9 minutes. Panic range: >15 minutes. Shorter in men than in women, and shorter in clients over 50 years of age.

Increased. Anemia (aplastic, pernicious), collagen diseases, congenital heart disease, disseminated intravascular coagulopathy, drug sensitivity, ethyl alcohol ingestion along with aspirin ingestion, factor deficiency (I, II, V, VII, VIII, IX, XI), fibrinolytic activity, Glanzmann's disease, hemorrhagic disease of the newborn, Hodgkin's disease, hypothyroidism, idiopathic thrombocytopenic purpura, infections (measles, mumps, streptococcal), leukemia (acute), liver disease (severe), mononucleosis (infectious), multiple myeloma, purpura hemorrhagica, scurvy, thrombasthenia, thrombocytopathy, thrombocytopenia purpura (secondary because of allergy), von Willebrand's disease, and uremia. Drugs include anticoagulants (oral), aspirin, indomethacin, ketorolac, and phenylbutazone. Herbs or natural remedies that may inhibit platelet activity include feverfew (*Tanacetum parthenium*), *Ginkgo biloba*, garlic, ginger, and ginseng.

Decreased. Not clinically significant.

Description. The duration of active bleeding from superficial incisions of the skin is measured. It is most helpful as an indicator of platelet abnormality, either in their number or function. This method is more sensitive than the Duke bleeding time because a blood pressure cuff is used to increase venous pressure and ensure capillary filling without interfering with venous return.

Professional Considerations

1. Consent form NOT required for most labs.

Risks

Bleeding, hematoma, infection, ecchymoses, scar, or keloid formation.

Contraindications

This test is contraindicated in clients who require upper- extremity restraints, have edematous or very cold arms, or are prone to keloid formation. It should not be performed if there are contraindications to placing or inflating a blood pressure cuff on the arm (casts, rash, dressings, arteriovenous fistula). Other contraindications include platelet count <50,000/mm^3, severe bleeding disorders, skin infectious diseases, and senile skin changes or if the client has taken medications containing acetyl groups within 7 days before the test.

2. Preparation:
   A. See *Client and family teaching.*
   B. Obtain a blood pressure cuff, a manometer, alcohol wipes, a stopwatch, a lancet, and filter paper.
   C. Screen client for the use of herbal preparations or natural remedies such as feverfew (*Tanacetum parthenium*), *Ginkgo biloba,* garlic, ginger, and ginseng.
3. Procedure:
   A. Cleanse the volar aspect of the forearm with an alcohol wipe and allow it to dry completely. Choose a site with no superficial veins.
   B. Place the blood pressure cuff on the upper arm and inflate it to 40 mm Hg.
   C. Make two small incisions or puncture wounds 2-3 mm deep with the lancet on the site that was cleansed with alcohol. Start timing with the stopwatch.
   D. Remove blood from the wounds by gently blotting with filter paper, without exerting pressure on the wound, every 30 seconds.
   E. When the blood flow ceases, stop timing with the stopwatch. If bleeding continues for more than 20 minutes, discontinue the test and apply pressure to the site.
   F. Calculate the bleeding time by averaging the bleeding time of both incisions.

4. Postprocedure care:
   A. If the bleeding time is normal, apply a dry dressing to the site. If the bleeding time is prolonged, apply a pressure bandage to the site.
5. Client and family teaching:
   A. Do not take aspirin for 7 days before the test.
   B. Call the physician if there are signs of infection at the test site: increasing pain, bleeding, redness, swelling, purulent drainage, or fever >101° F (≥38.3° C).
   C. Results are normally available within 24 hours.
6. Factors that affect results:
   A. A uniform incision is difficult to make without considerable skill.
   B. Pressing too hard on the blood with the filter paper disturbs the platelet plug and prolongs bleeding time.
7. Other data:
   A. The depth of the puncture with the lancet is difficult to standardize and results in difficulty reproducing bleeding times.
   B. Healthy pregnant women given 75 mg of aspirin for 2 weeks have an increased bleeding time by Ivy tests.
   C. Nitric oxide does not affect IV bleeding time.

BLEEDING TIME, MIELKE, BLOOD

Norm. 2.5-8 minutes.

Increased. Anemia (aplastic, pernicious), collagen diseases, congenital heart disease, disseminated intravascular coagulopathy, drug sensitivity, ethyl alcohol ingestion along with aspirin, factor deficiency (I, II, V, VII, VIII, IX, XI), fibrinolytic activity, Glanzmann's disease, hemorrhagic disease of the newborn, Hodgkin's disease, hypothyroidism, idiopathic thrombocytopenic purpura, infections (measles, mumps, streptococcal), leukemia (acute), liver disease (severe), mononucleosis (infectious), multiple myeloma, purpura hemorrhagica, scurvy, thrombasthenia, thrombocytopathy, thrombocytopenia purpura (secondary because of allergy), von Willebrand's disease, and uremia. Drugs include anticoagulants (oral), aspirin, indomethacin, and phenylbutazone. Herbs or natural remedies that may inhibit platelet activity include feverfew (*Tanacetum parthenium*), Ginkgo biloba, garlic, ginger, and ginseng.

Decreased. Not clinically significant.

Description. The duration of active bleeding from a standardized superficial incision of the skin is measured. It is particularly helpful as an indicator of platelet abnormality, either in the number or function of the platelets. This method is more sensitive than the Duke bleeding time because a blood pressure cuff is used to increase venous pressure and ensure capillary filling without interfering with venous return. Because the template standardizes the length and depth of the incision, this is the most accurate manual method for measuring bleeding time. An automated Surgicutt instrument is available to further standardize the incision.

Professional Considerations
1. Consent form NOT usually required.

Risks
Bleeding, hematoma, infection, ecchymoses, scar, or keloid formation.

Contraindications
In clients who require upper-extremity restraints, have edematous or very cold arms, or are prone to keloid formation. The test should not be performed if there are contraindications to placing or inflating a blood pressure cuff on the arm (casts, rash, dressings, arteriovenous fistula). Other contraindications include platelet count <50,000/mm^3, severe bleeding disorders, skin infectious diseases, and senile skin changes, or if the client has taken medications containing acetyl groups within 7 days before the test.

2. **Preparation:**
   A. See *Client and family teaching.*
   B. Obtain a blood pressure cuff and a manometer, alcohol wipes, a stopwatch, a template, and filter paper.
   C. Screen client for the use of herbal preparations or natural remedies such as feverfew (*Tanacetum parthenium*), Ginkgo biloba, garlic, ginger, and ginseng.
3. **Procedure:**
   A. Cleanse the volar aspect of the forearm with an alcohol wipe and

allow it to dry completely. Choose a site with no superficial veins.
   B. Place the blood pressure cuff on the upper arm and inflate to 40 mm Hg.
   C. *Manual incision:* Using a specially calibrated template to pass the blade through, make two incisions 9 mm long and 1 mm deep on the site that was cleansed with alcohol. Start timing with the stopwatch.
   D. *Automated incision:* Place the Surgicutt instrument on the site that was cleansed with alcohol and start the stopwatch at the same time as the device is triggered. The device will make a standardized puncture incision 5 mm long by 1 mm deep. Repeat at a second site.
   E. Remove the blood from the wound by gently blotting with the filter paper, without exerting pressure on the wound, every 30 seconds.
   F. When the blood flow ceases, stop timing with the stopwatch. If bleeding continues for more than 20 minutes, discontinue the test and apply pressure to the site.
   G. Calculate the bleeding time by averaging the bleeding time of both incisions.
4. **Postprocedure care:**
   A. If the bleeding time is normal, apply the dressing to the site. If the bleeding time is prolonged, apply a pressure bandage to the site.
   B. A butterfly closure may be required for 24 hours.
5. **Client and family teaching:**
   A. Do not take aspirin for 7 days before the test.
   B. Call the physician if there are signs of infection at the test site: increasing pain, bleeding, redness, swelling, purulent drainage, or fever >101° F (≥38.3° C).
   C. Results are normally available within 24 hours.
6. **Factors that affect results:**
   A. With standardized incisions, one incision yields as much information as two non-standardized incisions.
   B. Pressing too hard on the blood with the filter paper disturbs the platelet plug and prolongs the bleeding time.
7. **Other data:**
   A. None

BLEEDING TIME ASPIRIN TOLERANCE TEST

(see Aspirin tolerance test, Diagnostic)

BLOOD BIOPSY

(see Circulating cancer cell test, Blood)

BLOOD CULTURE, BLOOD

Norm. Negative or no growth.

Positive. Anthrax, bacteremia and septicemia (common in low-birth-weight infants).

Description. Blood is inoculated in aerobic and anaerobic laboratory culture media and observed for growth of pathogenic organisms. Blood cultures may be positive in either bacteremia or septicemia. Bacteremia is a localized infection, as in a particular organ or area of tissue, in which a small portion of the infectious bacteria escapes into the bloodstream. It may occur transiently, without infection after tooth brushing or specialized procedures such as dental surgery, bronchoscopy, tonsillectomy, endoscopy, cystoscopy, and transurethral resection. Septicemia occurs when a large amount of pathogenic microorganisms are dispersed throughout the bloodstream and is usually accompanied by systemic shock symptoms. Blood cultures are generally drawn as the fever is spiking, from two different sites at the same time (one immediately after the other) and again 3 hours later. The number and frequency may vary by institution and practitioner, although more than 2 or 3 is neither helpful nor cost-effective in assessment of persons with endocarditis. For clients in whom antimicrobial therapy has preceded blood cultures, the number of times cultured may be doubled (that is, double cultures drawn four different times). Results are reported as the amount of growth after a specific number of days.

Professional Considerations

1. Consent form NOT required.
2. **Preparation:**
   A. Obtain alcohol, a sterile gauze, povidone- iodine, two needles, two 30-mL syringes, and two anaerobic and two aerobic culture bottles.
   B. MAY be drawn during hemodialysis.
3. **Procedure:**
   A. Palpate the vein to determine location. Do not touch the site after cleansing.
   B. Cleanse the site for culture with an alcohol wipe and allow it to dry.
   C. Cleanse the site with povidone-iodine and allow it to dry completely or for at least 1 minute.
   D. Draw 10-20 mL of blood into a syringe. Avoid aspirating air into the syringe. If bacteremia is suspected, increase the volume of blood drawn to 30 mL.
   E. Place a fresh needle on the syringe.
   F. Remove the caps from the vacuum culture bottles and inject 5-10 mL into a vacuum bottle containing an anaerobic culture medium and 5-10 mL into a vacuum bottle containing an aerobic culture medium. If bacteremia is suspected, inject at least 15 mL into each bottle. Depending on the size of the bottle, more blood may be required to obtain at least a 1:10 dilution. Mix both bottles gently.
   G. Immediately repeat the above procedure at a different site.
4. **Postprocedure care:**
   A. Cleanse the puncture site with antiseptic and apply pressure.
   B. Write the collection time on the laboratory requisition.
   C. Write the presumptive diagnosis and the recent antimicrobial therapy on the laboratory requisition.
   D. Transport the specimens to the laboratory for incubation within 1 hour.
5. **Client and family teaching:**
   A. Call the physician if there are signs of infection at the culture site: increasing pain, redness, swelling, purulent drainage, or fever >101° F (≥38.3° C).
   B. Antibiotic or antifungal treatment will begin after the cultures are taken and before the final results.
   C. The first results are normally available in 24 hours and continue for up to 2 weeks.
6. **Factors that affect results:**
   A. Reject specimens received more than 1 hour after collection.
   B. Increasing the volume of blood cultured in suspected bacteremia may yield more positive cultures.

C. False-negative results or delayed growth may be obtained when blood cultures are drawn after antimicrobial therapy has begun.
D. Some common skin flora that may contaminate blood cultures include *Staphylococcus epidermidis*, diphtheroids, and *Propionibacterium*.
E. There is a higher incidence of positive blood cultures in clients receiving hyperalimentation.

7. **Other data:**
A. Pathogenic species most often cultured include *Actinobacter, Bacteroides, Brucella, Citrobacter, Clostridium, Enterobacter, Escherichia coli, Francisella, Haemophilus, Klebsiella, Leptospira, Listeria, Mycobacterium, Neisseria, Nocardia, Pseudomonas, Salmonella, Serratia, Staphylococcus, Streptococcus,* and *Vibrio*.
B. The contamination rate for blood cultures collected using an iodophor (povidone-iodine) is greater than when iodine tincture is used.
C. Clients on antimicrobial therapy have an enhanced yield for staphylococci using a FAN bottle compared to the standard aerobic BacT/Alert bottle.
D. Eleven percent of blood cultures are negative in infective endocarditis.
E. Instillation of 1.5 mL of taurolidine 2% into central line daily decreases catheter-related bloodstream infections.

BLOOD, FUNGUS, CULTURE

Norm. Negative or no growth.

Usage. Definitive diagnosis of systemic fungal infections.

Description. Fungi are slow-growing, eukaryotic organisms that can grow on living and nonliving organic materials and are subdivided into yeasts and molds. Factors that predispose clients to fungal infections by lowering the normal host defense mechanisms include administration of broad-spectrum antibiotics or chemotherapy, history of severe trauma or burns, invasive lines, poor nutritional status, parenteral nutrition, surgery, trauma, and long-term use of steroids. Some fungi may be inhaled or introduced by traumatic inoculation into deep tissue spaces and cause serious infections. Although tentative identification of fungi can be made quickly with staining techniques, culture of the organism in special fungal culture media is required to confirm a diagnosis of a fungal infection. Fungal cultures are generally inoculated on at least three media to facilitate recovery of all etiologic agents.

Professional Considerations
1. Consent form NOT required.
2. **Preparation:**
A. Obtain alcohol wipes, sterile gauze, povidone-iodine, two needles, two 20-mL syringes, and two fungal culture bottles.
3. **Procedure:**
A. Palpate the vein to determine the location. Do not touch the site after cleansing.
B. Cleanse the site for culture with an alcohol wipe and allow it to dry.
C. Cleanse the site with povidone-iodine and allow it to dry completely or for at least 1 minute.
D. Remove the caps from two fungal culture vacuum bottles, cleanse the rubber stoppers with an alcohol wipe and 2% iodine, and allow them to dry.
E. Draw a 10-mL blood sample into a syringe.
F. Place a fresh needle on the syringe and inject the 10 mL of blood into a vacuum bottle containing a blood culture medium specific for fungi. Mix the bottle gently.
G. Immediately repeat the above procedure at a different site.
4. **Postprocedure care:**
A. Wipe the venipuncture site with an antimicrobial agent.
B. Write the collection time on the laboratory requisition.
C. Write the presumptive diagnosis and recent antifungal therapy on the laboratory requisition.
D. Incubate the culture bottles at 25°-30° C in the laboratory.
5. **Client and family teaching:**
A. Preliminary results will be available within 72 hours and final results in 30 days.
B. Treatment for potential infection will begin before results are obtained and may include macrophage colony-stimulating

factor, amphotericin B, itraconazole, or fluconazole.

6. **Factors that affect results:**
   A. Some common skin floras that may contaminate blood cultures include *Staphylococcus epidermidis*, diphtheroids, and *Propionibacterium*.
7. **Other data:**
   A. Fungal cultures of blood must be incubated at least 30 days before being reported as negative.
   B. Fungi most often cultured from blood include *Blastomyces dermatitidis, Coccidioides immitis, Cryptococcus neoformans, Histoplasma capsulatum, Histoplasma duboisii,* *Paracoccidioides brasiliensis, Candida albicans, Aspergillus fumigatus,* and *Pseudallescheria boydii*.
   C. The BacT/Alert system may miss some fungi growth. This problem can be overcome by prolonged incubation and terminal subculture when fungal infection is considered to be likely.
   D. Detection of amphotericin B resistance of yeast isolates (*Candida* species, *Torulopsis glabrata, Saccharomyces cerevisiae, Cryptococcus neoformans*) within 12-14 hours after inoculation of the test medium is possible.

BLOOD GASES, ARTERIAL (ABG), BLOOD

Norm. Must be corrected for body temperature.

		SI UNITS
pH		
Adults	7.35-7.45	7.35-7.45
Panic values	≤7.2 and >7.6	≤7.2 and >7.6
Children		
Birth-2 months	7.32-7.49	7.32-7.49
2 months-2 years	7.34-7.46	7.34-7.46
Over 2 years	7.35-7.45	7.35-7.45

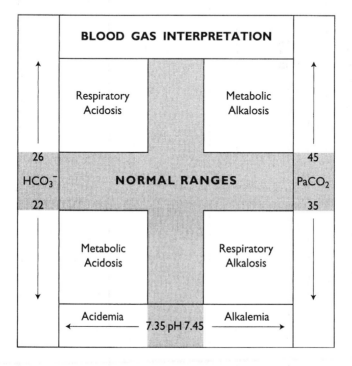

		SI UNITS
PaCO$_2$	35-45 mm Hg	4.7-6.0 kPa
Panic values	≤20 mm Hg	<2.7 kPa
	>70 mm Hg	>9.4 kPa
PaO$_2$	75-100 mm Hg	10.0-13.3 kPa
Panic values	≤40 mm Hg	<5.3 kPa
HCO$_3^-$	22-26 mEq/L	22-26 mmol/L
Panic values	≤10 mEq/L	<10 mmol/L
	>40 mEq/L	>40 mmol/L
O$_2$ Saturation	96%-100%	0.96-1.00
Panic value	≤60%	<0.60
Oxyhemoglobin Dissociation Curve	No shift	

Increased pH. Alkali ingestion, Cushing's disease, diarrhea, fever, high altitude, hyperventilation, hysteria, intestinal obstruction (pyloric, duodenal), metabolic alkalosis, peptic ulcer therapy, renal disease, respiratory alkalosis, salicylate intoxication, and vomiting (excessive). Drugs include sodium bicarbonate.

Increased PaCO$_2$. Acute intermittent porphyria, aminoglycoside toxicity, asthma (late stage), brain death, coarctation of the aorta, congestive heart failure, electrolyte disturbance (severe), emphysema, empyema, hyaline membrane disease, hyperemesis, hypothyroidism (severe), hypoventilation (alveolar), metabolic alkalosis, near drowning, pleural effusion, pleurisy, pneumonia, pneumothorax, poisoning, pulmonary edema, pulmonary infection, renal disorders, respiratory acidosis, respiratory failure, shock, tetralogy of Fallot, transposition of the great vessels, and vomiting. Drugs include aldosterone, ethacrynic acid, metolazone, prednisone, sodium bicarbonate, and thiazides.

Increased PaO$_2$. Hyperbaric oxygenation and hyperventilation.

Increased HCO$_3^-$. Anoxia, metabolic alkalosis, and respiratory acidosis.

Increased O$_2$ Saturation. High altitudes, hypocapnia, hypothermia, increased cardiac output, hyperbaric oxygenation, increased oxygen affinity for hemoglobin, oxygen therapy, positive end-expiratory pressure (PEEP) added to mechanical ventilation, respiratory alkalosis.

Decreased pH. Addison's disease, asthma, cardiac disease, diabetic ketoacidosis, diarrhea, emphysema, dysrhythmias, hepatic disease, hypercapnia, hypoventilation, malignant hyperthermia, metabolic acidosis, myocardial infarction, nephritis, nephrosis, pneumonia, pulmonary edema, pulmonary embolism, pulmonary infection, pulmonary malignancy, pulmonary obstructive disease, renal disease, respiratory acidosis (also caused by large volumes of lactated Ringer's), respiratory failure, sepsis, and shock.

Decreased PaCO$_2$. Dysrhythmias, asthma (early stage), diabetic ketoacidosis, diabetes mellitus, fever, high altitude, hyperventilation, metabolic acidosis, respiratory alkalosis, and salicylate intoxication. Drugs include acetazolamide, dimercaprol, methicillin sodium, nitrofurantoin, nitrofurantoin sodium, tetracycline, and triamterene.

Decreased PaO$_2$. Acute respiratory distress syndrome, anoxia, anesthesia, aortic valve stenosis, arteriovenous shunt, asthma, atelectasis, atrial septal defect, berylliosis, carbon monoxide poisoning, cerebrovascular accident, coarctation of the aorta, emphysema, flail chest, Hamman-Rich syndrome, head injury, hyaline membrane disease, hypercapnia, hypoventilation, lung resection, lymphangitic carcinomatosis, near drowning, phrenic nerve paralysis, pickwickian syndrome, pain causing restricted diaphragmatic breathing, pleural effusion, pneumonia, pneumothorax, poisoning, poliomyelitis (acute), pulmonary adenomatosis, pulmonary embolism, pulmonary infection, pulmonary hemangioma, pulmonic stenosis, respiratory failure, sar-coidosis, shock, smoke inhalation, sta-tus epilepticus, tetanus, transposition of the great vessels, tricuspid atresia, and ventricular septal defect.

Decreased HCO_3^-. Hypocapnia, me-tabolic acidosis, and respiratory alkalo-sis.

Decreased O_2 Saturation. Acute res-piratory distress syndrome, anesthesia, anoxia, anorexia, aortic valve stenosis, arteriovenous shunt, asthma, atelectasis, atrial septal defect, berylliosis, carbon monoxide poisoning, cerebrovascular accident, coarctation of the aorta, con-genital heart defects, decreased cardiac output, decreased oxygen affinity for hemoglobin, emphysema, fever, flail chest, Hamman-Rich syndrome, head injury, hyaline membrane disease, hypercapnia, hypoventilation, hypoxia, lung resection, lymphangitic carcino-matosis, near drowning, phrenic nerve paralysis, pickwickian syndrome, pain causing restricted diaphragmatic breath-ing, pleural effusion, pneumonia, pneu-mothorax, poisoning, poliomyelitis (acute), pulmonary adenomatosis, pul-monary embolism, pulmonary infection, pulmonary hemangioma, pulmonic stenosis, respiratory acidosis, respira-tory failure, sarcoidosis, shock, smoke

inhalation, status epilepticus, tetanus, transposition of the great vessels, tricus-pid atresia, and ventricular septal defect.

Oxyhemoglobin Dissociation Curve. See diagram below.

Shift to Left. 2,3,-DPG deficiency, high altitude, hypocapnia, hypother-mia, and respiratory alkalosis.

Shift to Right. Cluster headaches, emphysema, fever, hypercapnia, increased production of 2,3-DPG, and respiratory acidosis.

Description. The arterial blood gas test measures the dissolved oxygen and carbon dioxide in the arterial blood and reveals the acid-base state and how well the oxygen is being carried to the body. The *pH* is the measurement of free H^+ ion concentration in circulating blood. Intracellular metabolism results in the continuous production of hydrogen ions, which are buffered as either an acid (HCO_3^-) or a base (H_2CO_3). The body demands that pH remain constant. The kidneys and lungs regulate pH by preserving the ratio of acid to base. Any alteration in the ratio between *bicarbonate* and carbonic acid will cause a reciprocal change in release or uptake

NORMAL OXYHEMOGLOBIN DISSOCIATION CURVE

of free H^+, thereby altering pH value. Significant deviations in pH can be life threatening. Both *bicarbonate* (HCO_3^-) and *carbonic acid* (H_2CO_3) are components of the body's acid-base system that influence pH. The *partial pressure of carbon dioxide* (pCO_2, $PaCO_2$) is the amount of carbon dioxide in the blood based on the pressure it exerts in the bloodstream and represents the degree of alveolar ventilation occurring. When pH decreases, more CO_2 dissociates from carbonic acid and is exhaled through the lungs, counteracting the pH reduction and increasing the breathing rate. The *partial pressure of oxygen* (pO_2, PaO_2) is the amount of oxygen dissolved in plasma and represents the status of alveolar gas exchange with inspired air. *Oxygen saturation* (O_2 Sat) is the amount of oxygen actually bound to hemoglobin (as a percentage of the maximum amount that could be bound) and available for transport throughout the body. SaO_2 applies to arterial hemoglobin saturation:

Oxygen saturation = Oxygen content ×
(100/Oxygen capacity)

The *oxyhemoglobin dissociation curve* represents the affinity of hemoglobin for oxygen by demonstrating the normal levels of arterial oxygen saturation (O_2 Sat, SaO_2) of hemoglobin at varying partial pressures of oxygen. *P-50* is the partial pressure of oxygen at which the given hemoglobin sample is 50% saturated. The Hem-O-Scan machine analyzes and plots the hemoglobin-oxygen dissociation on a curve. When the curve is shifted to the left, more oxygen is delivered to the tissues for a given partial pressure of oxygen; when the shift is to the right, less oxygen is delivered to the tissues. Generally, decreased oxygen saturation to <90%-92% must be addressed by thorough assessment of the client and clinical status.

Professional Considerations
1. Consent form NOT required.

Risks
Two percent overall complication rate with brachial artery puncture. Prolonged bleeding, hematoma, infection, or nerve damage near puncture site. Arterial occlusion.

Contraindications and Precautions
In clients with bleeding disorders or anticoagulated states, repeated sampling from an invasive arterial catheter is preferred over arterial punctures.

2. **Preparation:**
   A. A modified Allen's test should be performed on both wrists before radial artery specimens are drawn. This test is performed to ensure adequate ulnar artery blood flow to the hand, in the event that the radial artery becomes occluded as a procedural complication. Occlude both the ulnar and radial arteries with two fingers for 10 seconds. Then release the pressure over the ulnar artery and observe the hand. If the pink coloring does not return to the hand within 15 seconds, this extremity should NOT be used for arterial puncture.
   B. Obtain a blood gas syringe, a 23-gauge needle, a povidone-iodine swab, alcohol wipes, sterile gloves, sterile gauze, and a container of ice.
   C. The client should rest for 30 minutes before specimen collection.
3. **Procedure:**
   A. The site for arterial puncture may be anesthetized with 1%-2% lidocaine.
   B. Attach a 1-inch long, 23-gauge needle to a plastic or glass blood gas syringe containing 0.5 mL of lithium heparin (1000 U/mL). Rotate the syringe to coat the inside surface with heparin (1000 U/mL) and eject the heparin through the needle into the sterile gauze.
   C. Cleanse the site for puncture with povidone-iodine solution and then with alcohol and allow it to dry.
   D. While wearing a sterile glove, palpate the artery and puncture the skin at a 30-45-degree angle (for radial artery), a 45-60-degree angle (for brachial artery), or a 45-90-degree angle (for femoral artery) with the bevel of the needle turned up.

E. Advance the needle until the artery is punctured, and allow the syringe to self-fill with at least 0.6 mL of arterial blood.

F. Remove the syringe and needle and apply pressure to the sterile gauze over the site while discarding the needle, expelling the air from the syringe, and quickly capping the syringe with a rubber stopper and gently mixing the specimen.

G. Immediately place the specimen in an ice bath.

4. **Postprocedure care:**

A. Record the client's body temperature and the mode and amount of oxygen delivery on the laboratory requisition.

B. Transport the specimen to the laboratory for processing within 15 minutes.

C. If the specimen was obtained by means of direct arterial puncture, hold pressure over the site for 5-10 minutes.

5. **Client and family teaching:**

A. Results are normally available within 30 minutes.

B. The client's temperature is necessary for calculation and interpretation of the results.

C. Results are interpreted according to the disease or condition and compared to previous blood gas results.

6. **Factors that affect results:**

A. Reject clotted specimens.

B. If the client is receiving endotracheal suctioning or respiratory therapy treatments, the specimen should be drawn at least 20 minutes after either procedure.

C. Failure to expel all air from the blood gas syringe will result in a falsely elevated PaO_2 and a falsely decreased $PaCO_2$.

D. Failure to place the specimen in an ice bath may result in a decreased pH, PaO_2, and oxygen saturation.

E. Failure to expel the heparin from the syringe before specimen collection may result in decreased pH, $PaCO_2$, and PaO_2.

F. Specimen storage at room temperature accelerates the fall in pH.

G. Elevated body temperature decreases the oxygen saturation result.

H. Clients with a history of cigarette smoking can have decreased arterial oxygen saturation after anesthesia.

I. Elevated WBC causes a rapid pH drop.

J. Sodium fluoride can cause either an increase or a decrease in pH.

K. A prolonged time lapse between collection and testing may result in a decreased pH.

L. Herbs or natural remedy effects: In one study, people who received 20 mg of ginseng twice each day for 3 months demonstrated improved arterial blood oxygen and walking distance, as well as pulmonary function test measurements (FVC, FEV_1, and PEFR).

7. **Other data:**

A. If arterial blood is not practical to obtain, venous blood may be obtained by venipuncture, but accuracy is evident only for monitoring pH, $PaCO_2$, and base excess.

B. Evaluation of pH should take into consideration alterations in electrolyte, carbon dioxide, oxygen, and bicarbonate levels.

C. Samples of cord blood stored in heparinized syringes for >30 minutes result in significant changes in pH and pCO_2.

D. Earlobe gas analysis is an accurate substitute for arterial sampling.

E. In anemia, oxygen saturation may be normal, but hypoxia may still be present because of decreased oxygen-carrying capacity.

F. Continuous oxygen saturation monitoring by pulse oximetry is useful during cardiac catheterization in conjunction with intracardiac pressure measurement in the detection of intracardiac abnormalities.

G. A base deficit of less than or equal to −6 indicates a high mortality in trauma.

H. See also *Pulse oximetry, Diagnostic*.

BLOOD GASES, CAPILLARY, BLOOD

Norm. Must be corrected for body temperature.

		SI UNITS
pH		
Adults	7.35-7.45	7.35-7.45
Panic values	<7.2 or >7.6	<7.2 or >7.6
Children (arterialized capillary sample)		
Birth-2 months	7.32-7.49	7.32-7.49
2 months-2 years	7.34-7.46	7.34-7.46
Over 2 years	7.35-7.45	7.35-7.45
pCO$_2$	26.4-41.2 mm Hg	3.5-5.4 kPa
Panic values	<20 mm Hg	<2.7 kPa
	>70 mm Hg	>9.4 kPa
pO$_2$	75-100 mm Hg	10.0-13.3 kPa
Panic values	<40 mm Hg	<5.3 kPa
HCO$_3^-$	22-26 mEq/L	22-26 mmol/L
Panic values	<10 mEq/L	<10 mmol/L
	>40 mEq/L	>40 mmol/L
O$_2$ Saturation	96%-100%	0.96-1.00
Panic value	<60%	<0.60

Increased pH. See *Blood gases, Arterial, Blood.*

Increased pCO$_2$. See *Blood gases, Arterial, Blood.*

Increased pO$_2$. See *Blood gases, Arterial, Blood.*

Increased HCO$_3^-$. See *Blood gases, Arterial, Blood.*

Increased O$_2$ Saturation. See *Blood gases, Arterial, Blood.*

Decreased pH. See *Blood gases, Arterial, Blood.*

Decreased pCO$_2$. See *Blood gases, Arterial, Blood.*

Decreased pO$_2$. Capillary pO$_2$ interpretation is limited to assessment for hypoxia.

Decreased HCO$_3^-$. See *Blood gases, Arterial, Blood.*

Decreased O$_2$ Saturation. See *Blood gases, Arterial, Blood.*

Description. A method for determining acid-base status from a heelstick for capillary blood. Used mostly in infants to assess pH and pCO$_2$. (See *Blood gases, Arterial,* for complete description of the test components.)

Professional Considerations
1. Consent form NOT required.
2. Preparation:
   A. Warmth may be applied to the heel for 15 minutes before collection but is not necessary.
   B. Obtain alcohol wipes, a lancet, sterile gauze, two capillary tubes with a metal stirrer, and a magnet.
3. Procedure:
   A. Cleanse an area on the medial or lateral plantar surface of the heel with an alcohol wipe and allow it to dry.
   B. Using a 2.5-mm lancet, puncture the heel until a free flow of blood is obtained.
   C. Wipe away the first drop of blood.
   D. Completely fill two heparinized, 250-mL capillary tubes without air bubbles and add a heparinized metal stirrer. Quickly seal them and mix well by maneuvering a magnet around the tubes.
4. Postprocedure care:
   A. Place the capillary tubes in an ice bath.

B. Write the client's temperature, mode and amount of oxygen delivery, and the type and site of the specimen collection on the laboratory requisition.
C. Place pressure on the heel for 5-10 minutes and leave the site open to air to heal.
D. Transport the specimens to the laboratory within 15 minutes.
5. **Client and family teaching:**
   A. The client's temperature is important in evaluating results.
   B. Results are normally available within 30 minutes.
   C. Results are interpreted according to disease or condition and compared to previous gases.
6. **Factors that affect results:**
   A. Avoid milking the heel.
   B. Reject hemolyzed or clotted specimens.
   C. Storage at room temperature accelerates the fall in pH.
   D. Elevated white blood counts cause a rapid pH drop.

E. Sodium fluoride can cause either an increase or a decrease in pH.
F. A prolonged time lapse between collection and testing may result in decreased pH.
G. Capillary blood gas specimens are contraindicated in low cardiac output, vasoconstriction, shock, and hypotension because the results will not be valid.
7. **Other data:**
   A. Avoid puncturing over previous puncture sites.
   B. Avoid puncturing the posterior curvature of the heel.
   C. Specimens may also be taken from the earlobe in adults.
   D. Evaluation of pH should take into consideration alterations in electrolyte, carbon dioxide, oxygen, and bicarbonate levels.
   E. Capillary blood gases accurately reflect arterial pH and pCO_2 in pediatric clients.

BLOOD GASES, UMBILICAL CORD ANALYSIS, BLOOD

Norm:

	UMBILICAL VEIN	UMBILICAL ARTERY
pH	7.26-7.49	7.15-7.43
pO_2	15.4-48.2 mm Hg	10-33.8 mm Hg
pCO_2	23.2-61.7 mm Hg	31.1-74.3 mm Hg
HCO_3^-	16.3-24.9 mEq/L	13.3-27.5 mEq/L
Base excess	−5.1 to 0.1 mEq/L	−6.1 to −3.9 mEq/L

Usage. Evaluation of fetal oxygen status at birth and to examine the acid-base balance of the neonate. See also *Blood gases, Arterial, Blood.*

Description. The analysis of umbilical blood gases measures and records the pH, pO_2, pCO_2, bicarbonate, and base excess of the neonate after delivery. These assessments of both arterial and venous blood provide immediate feedback of the adequacy of fetal oxygenation for energy production. This method may be used to correlate diagnosis of respiratory acidosis, metabolic acidosis, or mixed respiratory-metabolic acidosis. The value of base excess helps differentiate between respiratory and metabolic acidosis, providing an indication as to whether the fetus has sufficient buffer reserves to neutralize

hydrogen ions and acids. (See *Blood gases, Arterial, Blood,* for a complete description of each test component.)

Professional Considerations
1. Consent form NOT required.
2. **Preparation:**
   A. Obtain two prepackaged, heparinized blood gas syringes, or aspirate 0.2 mL of a 100 U/mL heparin solution into two 3-mL syringes.
   B. Obtain two 18- or 20-gauge needles and two caps for the syringes.
   C. Obtain a 10-20 cm (4- to 8-inch) segment of umbilical cord.
3. **Procedure:**
   A. Connect needles to syringes.
   B. Using a 45-degree angle, insert the needle, bevel down, into the

umbilical artery and withdraw 1-3 mL of blood into the syringe. Repeat this technique on the umbilical vein.

C. Discard needles. Aspirate air from syringes and cap the syringes. Label them with the mother's name, date and time of collection, and source of blood, specifying whether the sample is arterial or venous cord blood.

4. **Postprocedure care:**
   A. Place samples on ice and transport to the lab immediately.
   B. Discard samples if not tested within 1 hour.

5. **Client and family teaching:**
   A. Results should be available within 1 hour.

B. Results are interpreted according to maternal history, intrapartum management, delivery information, and neonate status.

6. **Factors that affect results:**
   A. Hemolysis affects results.
   B. Improper capping or prolonged exposure of the specimen to air invalidates results.

7. **Other data:**
   A. Umbilical blood gas testing does not provide definitive diagnosis. Alterations in maternal and neonate status must be assessed and taken into consideration to confirm any medical diagnosis.

BLOOD GASES, VENOUS, BLOOD

Norm. Must be corrected for body temperature.

		SI UNITS
pH	7.32-7.43	7.32-7.43
Panic value	<7.2 or >7.6	<7.2 or >7.6
pCO$_2$	38-50 mm Hg	5.0-6.7 kPa
pO$_2$	20-49 mm Hg	2.6-6.5 kPa
HCO$_3^-$	22-26 mEq/L	22-26 mmol/L
Panic value	<10 mEq/L	<10 mmol/L
	>40 mEq/L	>40 mEq/L
O$_2$ Saturation	60%-80%	0.60-0.80

Increased pH. See *Blood gases, Arterial, Blood.*

Increased pCO$_2$. See *Blood gases, Arterial, Blood.*

Increased pO$_2$. Interpretation of oxygen levels is not appropriate on venous blood specimens.

Increased HCO$_3^-$. See *Blood gases, Arterial, Blood.*

Increased O$_2$ Saturation. Interpretation of oxygen saturation is not appropriate on venous blood specimens.

Decreased pH. See *Blood gases, Arterial, Blood.*

Decreased pCO$_2$. See *Blood gases, Arterial, Blood.*

Decreased pO$_2$. Interpretation of oxygen levels is not appropriate on venous blood specimens.

Decreased HCO$_3^-$. See *Blood gases, Arterial, Blood.*

Decreased O$_2$ Saturation. Interpretation of oxygen saturation is not appropriate on venous blood specimens.

Description. A method for assessing acid-base status and for cellular hypoxia without performing an arterial puncture. Venous blood gases may be used in situations where assessment of oxygenation is unnecessary. (See *Blood gases, Arterial, Blood* for complete descriptions of the test components.)

Professional Considerations

1. Consent form NOT required.
2. Preparation:
   A. The client should rest quietly for 30 minutes before specimen collection.
   B. Obtain alcohol wipes, a tourniquet, a needle, a syringe or Vacutainer, heparin, and a green-topped tube.
3. Procedure:
   A. Draw 1 mL of heparin (1000 U/mL) into a 3-mL syringe and coat the inside of the syringe with heparin. Eject the heparin.
   B. Draw a 2-mL venous blood sample into the syringe, taking care to avoid getting air bubbles mixed with the blood.
   C. Inject blood from the syringe into the tube.
   D. Alternatively, perform a Vacutainer collection directly into a heparinized, green-topped tube and remove the tube from the Vacutainer before removing the needle from the vein.
   E. The specimen may be obtained from cord blood.
4. Postprocedure care:
   A. Place the specimen on ice.
   B. Write the client's temperature and the type of specimen on the laboratory requisition.
   C. Write the mode and amount of oxygen delivery on the laboratory requisition.
5. Client and family teaching:
   A. Do not pump your fist during collection.
   B. The client's temperature is needed to interpret results.
   C. Results are normally available within 30 minutes.
   D. Results require interpretation depending on disease or condition and compared to previous gases.
6. Factors that affect results:
   A. Avoid using a tourniquet, if possible. If one is used, it should be left in place while the sample is being drawn.
   B. Reject clotted specimens or specimens not received on ice.

C. Storage at room temperature accelerates the fall in pH.
D. Elevated white blood counts cause a rapid pH drop.
E. Sodium fluoride can cause either an increase or a decrease in pH.
F. A prolonged time lapse between collection and testing may result in decreased pH.

7. Other data:
   A. For data on oxygenation, arterial blood is required.
   B. Evaluation of pH should take into consideration alterations in electrolyte, carbon dioxide, oxygen (i.e., COPD), and bicarbonate levels.

BLOOD GROUP ANTIGEN OF SEMEN, VAGINAL SWAB

Norm. Blood group antigens may be identified in 80% of the population. Blood group matches the victim's where coitus has not occurred or where the perpetrator's blood group matches the blood group of the victim. Blood group differs from the victim's where coitus has occurred with a perpetrator of a different ABO blood group.

Usage. Rape trauma investigation.

Description. Approximately 80% of the population (both males and females) is classified as having a dominant secretor gene that causes them to secrete their ABO blood group antigen in their body fluids. Samples of vaginal fluid are analyzed for soluble A, B, and H blood group substances for the purpose of identifying the blood group of the perpetrator of a sexual assault. Although the results can be compared with the blood group antigen obtained from body fluid of the suspected assailant, this test cannot confirm this client as the perpetrator. However, it can rule out a suspect if the blood group antigens are different.

Professional Considerations

1. Consent form NOT required unless results may be used for legal evidence.
2. Preparation:
   A. Obtain a speculum, a cotton wool swab supplied in a sexual offense

kit, glass slides, and a Coplin jar of 95% ethyl alcohol (ethanol).

3. **Procedure:**
   A. If the specimen may be used as legal evidence, have the specimen collection witnessed.
   B. Position the woman in a lithotomy position and drape her for privacy and comfort.
   C. Gently scrape the walls of the vagina with a plain cotton wool swab until it is saturated.
   D. Roll the swab onto two glass slides and place the slides in a Coplin jar of 95% ethyl alcohol (ethanol).

4. **Postprocedure care:**
   A. Write the client's name, the date, the exact time of collection, and the specimen source on the laboratory requisition. Sign and have the witness sign the laboratory requisition.
   B. Transport the specimen to the laboratory immediately in a sealed plastic bag marked as legal evidence. All persons handling the specimen should sign and mark the time of receipt on the laboratory requisition.

5. **Client and family teaching:**
   A. Offer the client and family immediate counseling or crisis intervention and support. Survivors of sexual assault should be referred to appropriate crisis-counseling agencies as well as gynecologic follow-up study. Facilitate the connection if desired by the client.

   B. Referral for HIV testing should be reviewed and offered to all sexual assault victims.
   C. Preventive treatment for chlamydiosis, gonorrhea, and syphilis should be provided to all survivors of sexual assault.
   D. The option of postcoital contraceptive should be reviewed with all survivors of sexual assault.
   E. Results will be available within 5 days.
   F. The National Coalition Against Sexual Assault phone number is (202) 483-7165.

6. **Factors that affect results:**
   A. Results are inconclusive if the blood groups of the victim and the suspect are the same.
   B. Vaginal swabs for blood group antigen detection should be collected as soon as possible after the rape. Semen is rarely detected in the vagina more than 72 hours after coitus.
   C. Negative results may be obtained if the assailant was sexually dysfunctional or has had a vasectomy or if the woman bathed, douched, or defecated after the rape.

7. **Other data:**
   A. Vaginal swabs can be examined by use of an MHS-5-ELISA (SEMA kit), which is sensitive to cases of azoospermia or aspermia.
   B. See also *Acid phosphatase, Vaginal swab; Precipitin test against human sperm and blood, Vaginal swab.*

BLOOD INDICES, BLOOD

Norm:

MEAN CORPUSCULAR HEMOGLOBIN (MCH)		SI UNITS
Adults	26-34 pg	1.61-2.11 fmol
Children		
Newborn		
1 day old	1-38 pg	2.36 fmol
2-3 days	37 pg	2.30 fmol
4-8 days	36 pg	2.23 fmol
9-13 days	33 pg	2.05 fmol
2-8 weeks	30 pg	1.86 fmol
3 months	28 pg	1.73 fmol
4-5 months	27 pg	1.67 fmol
6-11 months	26 pg	1.61 fmol
1-2 years	25 pg	1.55 fmol

MEAN CORPUSCULAR HEMOGLOBIN (MCH)		SI UNITS
3 years	26 pg	1.61 fmol
4-10 years	27 pg	1.67 fmol
11-15 years	28 pg	1.73 fmol

B

MEAN CORPUSCULAR HEMOGLOBIN CONCENTRATION (MCHC)		
Adults	31%-38%	19.2-23.58 mmol/L
Children		
Newborn		
1-3 days	36%	22.34 mmol/L
2-8 days	35%	21.72 mmol/L
9-13 days	34%	21.10 mmol/L
2-8 weeks	33%	20.48 mmol/L
3-5 months	34%	21.10 mmol/L
6-11 months	33%	20.48 mmol/L
1-2 years	32%	19.86 mmol/L
3 years	35%	21.72 mmol/L
4-15 years	34%	21.10 mmol/L

MEAN CORPUSCULAR VOLUME, MEAN CELL VOLUME (MCV)		
Adults	82-98 μm^3	82-98 fL
Children		
Newborn		
1 day	106 μm^3	106 fL
2-3 days	105 μm^3	105 fL
4-8 days	103 μm^3	103 fL
9-13 days	98 μm^3	98 fL
2-8 weeks	90 μm^3	90 fL
3 months	82 μm^3	82 fL
4-5 months	80 μm^3	80 fL
6-11 months	77 μm^3	77 fL
1 year	78 μm^3	78 fL
2 years	77 μm^3	77 fL
3 years	79 μm^3	79 fL
4-10 years	80 μm^3	80 fL
11-15 years	82 μm^3	82 fL

Increased MCV. Alcoholism (chronic), anemia (acquired hemolytic, aplastic, immune hemolytic, macrocytic induced by megaloblastic anemias, pernicious [early]), benzene exposure, cigarette smokers, cirrhosis, chronic lymphocytic leukemia, cytomegalovirus, diabetic ketoacidosis, diabetes mellitus, DNA synthesis disorders (inherited), folate deficiency, hepatic disease, infants, leukocytosis (pronounced), methanol poisoning, newborns, obese, pancreatitis, peripheral arterial disease, preleukemia, reticulocytosis, sprue, and vitamin B_{12} deficiency. Drugs include blood stored at room temperature more than 2 days, hydroxyurea, zidovudine (AZT).

Increased MCH. Anemia (macrocytic, pernicious), cold agglutinin conditions, cigarette smokers, dysproteinemia, infants, newborns, and presence of monoclonal blood proteins. Drugs include heparin calcium and heparin sodium.

Increased MCHC. High titer of cold agglutinins, dehydrated hereditary stomatocytosis, hereditary spherocytosis, infants, intravascular hemolysis, lipemia, newborns, obese. Drugs include heparin calcium, heparin sodium, and chemical components from smoking.

Decreased MCV. Anemia (chronic, dyserythropoietic, hypochromic, iron deficiency, microcytic, pyridoxine responsive, sickle cell), alpha- or beta-thalassemia, Brunner's gland hartoma, chlorosis, chronic disease, colorectal cancer, diverticulitis, diverticulosis, endocarditis, G6PD deficiency, gangrene, hemoglobin E, hemoglobin H, leukocytosis (pronounced), malaria, myocarditis, nephropathy (nonimmune), pruritus, radiation therapy, red blood cell fragmentation, subacute bacterial endocarditis, and warm autoantibodies. Drugs include stavudine.

Decreased MCH. Anemia (iron deficiency, microcytic, normocytic), cyanotic congenital heart disease. Drugs include blood stored at room temperature more than 2 days, enalaprilat (Vasotec).

Decreased MCHC. Aluminum intoxication, anemia (iron deficiency, chronic, hypochromic, megaloblastic, microcytic, sideroblastic), benzene exposure, colorectal cancer.

Description. Blood indices encompasses a group of six different blood tests, the MCH, MCHC, MCV, RBC, Hct, and Hb, that are used to establish the characteristics and hemoglobin content of the red blood cells. (See *Red blood cell; Hematocrit; Hemoglobin.*) They assist in the diagnosis and differentiation of compensated and uncompensated anemias. A stained blood smear is prepared to study the shape and size of the red blood cell. Combined with staining, the indices assist in determinations of red blood cell morphology. This visual or electronic counting of erythrocytes is regarded as the most reliable index for distinguishing and differentiating erythrocyte morphology. MCH is the average weight of the hemoglobin of each red blood cell, expressed in picograms. MCHC is a calculated value of the amount of hemoglobin present in the red blood cell compared to its size. A ratio of weight to volume is expressed as a percentage. MCV is a calculated value, expressed in cubic micrometers, of the average volume of an erythrocyte.

Professional Considerations
1. Consent form NOT required.
2. Preparation:
   A. Tube: Lavender topped.

3. Procedure:
   A. Draw a 7-mL blood sample. A stained blood smear is prepared.
4. Postprocedure care:
   A. The collection tube should be filled completely, inverted, and gently rotated to thoroughly mix the anticoagulant.
   B. The serum sample is stable at room temperature for 10 hours, may be refrigerated for up to 18 hours, and should not be frozen.
5. Client and family teaching:
   A. Results are normally available within 24 hours.
   B. All results must be available to make an accurate interpretation associated with the diagnosis or condition.
6. Factors that affect results:
   A. Reject hemolyzed specimens.
   B. High altitude affects MCV (standard deviation [SD] = .810 fL), MCH (SD = .583 pg), and MCHC (SD = .630 g/dL)
7. Other data:
   A. Bone marrow suppression in the chronically ill can be a frequent cause of anemia.
   B. Production of macroreticulocytes is an early sign of engraftment after bone marrow transplantation.
   C. Hemoglobin E trait is common in Bengali, Burmese, Khmer, Malay, Thai and Vietnamese groups.
   D. See also *Red blood cell morphology, Blood.*

BLOOD SUGAR, FASTING
(see Glucose, Blood)

BLOOD TYPE
(see ABO group and Rh type, Blood)

BLOOD UREA NITROGEN
(see Urea nitrogen, Plasma or Serum)

BLOOD UREA NITROGEN/ CREATININE RATIO, BLOOD

Norm:

Normal	10:1-15:1
Diminished urea concentration:	<10:1
Inadequate renal function:	>15:1

Increased. Azotemia, burns, cachexia, catabolic states, Cushing's disease, dehydration, delirium, excessive protein intake, fever, gastrointestinal bleeding, glomerular disease, heart failure, hemorrhage, hypercalcemia, hypertension, impaired renal blood flow, ileal conduit, infection, muscle or tissue destruction, prerenal azotemia, shock, surgery, swallowing of food into the upper airway, thyrotoxicosis, urinary reabsorption (ureterocolostomy), and urinary tract obstruction (rare). Drugs include tetracyclines and steroids.

Decreased. Diarrhea, diet (inadequate protein intake), hemodialysis, hepatic insufficiency, hyperammonemias (genetic), intravenous therapy (prolonged), ketosis, marasmus, malnutrition, pregnancy, renal failure (muscular people, chronic), rhabdomyolysis, syndrome of inappropriate antidiuretic hormone secretion (SIADHS), and vomiting. Drugs include phenacemide. Drugs that increase only the creatinine and not the blood urea nitrogen (BUN) include cephalosporins, cimetidine, tetracyclines, and trimethoprim.

Description. The BUN/creatinine ratio assists in the interpretation of laboratory values in assessing renal failure and in the evaluation of an elevated BUN level. This test is a more sensitive indicator of the relationship between BUN and creatinine than each separate test because BUN rises at a greater rate than creatinine in renal disease.

Professional Considerations
1. Consent form NOT required.
2. Preparation:
   A. Tube: Red topped, red/gray topped, or gold topped.
   B. Do NOT draw specimen during hemodialysis.
3. Procedure:
   A. Draw a 5-mL blood sample.
4. Postprocedure care:
   A. None.
5. Client and family teaching:
   A. Assess knowledge and provide information about adequate dietary protein.
6. Factors that affect results:
   A. Low-protein diet lowers BUN value.
7. Other data:
   A. Before a change in BUN is significant, there exists approximately 60% renal impairment.

BLOOD VOLUME, BLOOD

Norm:

Blood Volume	8.5%-9% of body weight
Adult female	54.01-63.89 mL/kg
Adult male	52.95-70.13 mL/kg

Erythrocyte Volume	
Adult female	21.65-26.83 mL/kg
Adult male	24.16-32.38 mL/kg

Plasma Volume	
Adult female	31.53-38.01 mL/kg
Adult male	28.27-38.63 mL/kg

Usage. Anemia, differentiation of relative polycythemia from absolute polycythemia, preoperative or postoperative evaluation to estimate need for replacement blood, and unexplained hypotension. Decreased in preeclampsia but normal in gestational hypertension.

Description. Blood volume comprises plasma and cellular components and varies with body weight, muscle mass, height, age, sex, environment, and physical activity. This nuclear medicine test uses a dilution technique that measures blood volume after radiolabeled albumin and radiolabeled red blood cells are injected intravenously. A tagged sample of the client's blood is then measured for blood volume, erythrocyte volume, and plasma volume with a scintillation well counter. This test is based on the principle of adding a known quantity of tracer substance to an unknown quantity of diluent (blood). The final tracer concentration should be inversely proportional to the volume of blood. Radiolabeled albumin is used to measure plasma volume, and the radiolabeled red blood cells are used to measure volume of the cellular component of blood. This test is helpful in differentiating between fluid shifts or other causes of decreased plasma volume (relative polycythemia) and increased red blood cell mass (absolute polycythemia).

Professional Considerations
1. Consent form NOT required.

Risks
Allergic reaction to radiolabeled albumin (itching, hives, rash, tight feeling in the throat, shortness of breath, bronchospasm, anaphylaxis, death), hematoma or infection at injection site.

Contraindications
Previous allergy to radioactive dyes, iodine, or shellfish; during pregnancy; while breast-feeding; hypersensitivity to iodine; extended clotting times; in edematous or hemorrhaging clients.

2. **Preparation:**
    A. Have emergency equipment readily available.
    B. Obtain alcohol wipes, a tourniquet, a 19-gauge needle, five syringes, one glass green-topped tube, two plastic green-topped tubes, a centrifuge bag, a sterile glass beaker of 3 mL Strumia formula solution, chilled sterile 0.9% saline solution, and centrifuge.
    C. Draw a 25-mL blood sample and inject into a sterile centrifuge bag to which 3-mL of Strumia formula solution has been added. Add 50-100 mCi of ^{51}Cr (sodium chromate) to the container and gently agitate it for 3 minutes. Then fill the bag with sterile, chilled 0.9% saline and centrifuge it at a 45-degree angle for 7 minutes. Remove the supernatant fluid and resuspend the cells in 10 mL of sterile 0.9% saline solution.
    D. Obtain a mixture of 5 mL of ^{125}I-albumin in 20 mL of sterile normal saline solution for plasma volume measurement.
    E. Lugol's solution may be used to prevent uptake of ^{125}I-albumin by the thyroid gland.

3. **Procedure:**
    A. Draw an 8-mL blood sample in a heparinized green-topped tube and label it as the baseline sample.
    B. *Injection for red blood cell volume measurement:* Draw 2-3 mL of the ^{51}Cr-labeled red blood cell solution into a syringe with a 19-gauge needle. Note the exact amount in the syringe. Inject the mixture directly into a vein in the right arm of the client.
    C. *Injection for plasma volume measurement:* Draw 2-3 mL of the ^{125}I-albumin at 2 mCi/mL into a syringe. Note the exact amount in the syringe. Inject the mixture directly into a vein in the right arm of the client.
    D. *Recovery of tagged blood for blood volume determination:* At 10 and 20 minutes after the two tracer injections, draw an 8-mL blood sample from the left arm in a heparinized plastic, rather than glass, green-topped tube. Label each sample with the time drawn.
    E. Using the multi dose vials from which the ^{51}Cr-tagged red blood cells and ^{125}I-albumin were drawn as controls, measure blood volume, red blood cell volume, and plasma volume of the samples with a scintillation well counter.

4. **Postprocedure care:**
    A. None.

5. **Client and family teaching:**
    A. This test involves injection of a nuclear medicine tracer, followed by two timed blood sample collections. Total test time is less than 1 hour.
    B. Results are normally available within 24 hours.

6. **Factors that affect results:**
    A. Blood volume is usually highest in the morning.
    B. Glass tubes used for the tagged sample may cause falsely low plasma volume results because glass absorbs energy from ^{125}I-albumin.
    C. The ^{51}Cr rate of tagging red blood cells varies with pH, type of anticoagulant, and body temperature. In general, tagging should be complete by 5 minutes after injection.
    D. If the client has recently taken polyvitamins or antibiotics, ^{51}Cr

may not label the client's own red blood cells. Blood bank ^{51}Cr-labeled group O-Rh-negative blood should be substituted.
  E. Injection through intravenous tubing or tissue extravasation of tracer will cause falsely decreased results.
  F. Two post–tracer injection blood samples are required both to establish that mixing of ^{51}Cr-labeled red blood cells is complete and to determine the rate of loss of the ^{125}I-albumin tracer.
  G. If the 10- and 20-minute sample results vary by more than 3%, a third sample should be drawn 60-90 minutes after the initial injection.
7. **Other data:**
  A. No isolation of the client is necessary.
  B. Furosemide (Lasix) has no effect on blood volume, shape, or viscosity.
  C. Ringer's solution expands blood volume by 20%-25% in awake individuals and by 60% during general anesthesia.

BLOOD VOLUME DETERMINATION STUDIES, DIAGNOSTIC

Norm. Requires interpretation.

Usage. Differential diagnosis of pericardial effusion from pericardial cysts or tumors, diagnosis of peripheral vascular disease, and thrombophlebitis.

Description. A nuclear medicine study of circulation dynamics in which a tracer is circulated in the blood for a period of time. Measures of diluted radioactivity are used to calculate the volume distribution of compartments and regions of the circulation. Pericardial effusions are detected by examination of the blood volumes in and around the heart. Peripheral vascular disease and thrombophlebitis are detected by examination of the rates at which the venous pools of the legs change in volume with exercise and posture changes.

Professional Considerations
1. Consent form IS required.

Risks
Allergic reaction to radiolabeled albumin (itching, hives, rash, tight feeling in the throat, shortness of breath, bronchospasm, anaphylaxis, death), hematoma, or infection at injection site.

Contraindications
Previous allergy to iodine, radiographic dye, seafood, or a nuclear medicine radiolabeled-albumin tracer.

Precautions
During pregnancy, risks of cumulative radiation exposure to the fetus from this and other previous or future imaging studies must be weighed against the benefits of the procedure. Although formal limits for client exposure are relative to this risk-benefit comparison, the United States Nuclear Regulatory Commission requires that the cumulative dose equivalent to an embryo/fetus from *occupational* exposure not exceed 0.5 rem (5 mSv). Radiation dose to the fetus is proportional to the distance of the anatomy studied from the abdomen and decreases as pregnancy progresses. For pregnant clients, consult the Radiologist/Radiology Department to obtain estimated fetal radiation exposure from this procedure.

2. **Preparation:**
  A. Have emergency equipment readily available.
  B. Establish intravenous access in an arm vein.
3. **Procedure:**
  A. A tracer of labeled albumin, red blood cells, or substances bound by plasma proteins is injected intravenously and allowed to circulate. The circulatory compartment to be studied is scanned, and a scintillation well counter is used to compare the diluted radioactivity of the compartment with a standard. This is followed by calculation of the volume distribution of the compartment.
4. **Postprocedure care:**
  A. Encourage the oral intake of fluids.
5. **Client and family teaching:**
  A. The risk of radioactivity from this test is less than that of a regular radiograph.

6. **Factors that affect results:**
   A. Blood volume is highest in the morning.
7. **Other data:**
   A. No isolation of the client is necessary.
   B. Health care professionals working in a nuclear medicine area must follow federal standards set by the Nuclear Regulatory Commission. These standards include precautions for handling the radioactive material and monitoring of potential radiation exposure.

BLUE LIGHT TEST
(see Tonometry test for glaucoma, Diagnostic)

B-LYMPHOCYTES, BLOOD

Norm:

		SI UNITS
Adults	270-640/mm^3 or 270-640/μL	270-640 cells × 10^6 /L
	5%-15% of circulating lymphocytes	0.05-0.15
	or 25%-35% of total lymphocytes	0.25-0.35
Children		
Newborn	61% of total lymphocytes	0.61
Infants	60% of total lymphocytes	0.60
6 years	42% of total lymphocytes	0.42
12 years	38% of total lymphocytes	0.38

Increased. Active antibody formation in young children, agranulocytosis, bacterial infections (acute, chronic), brucellosis, Burkitt's lymphoma, carcinoma, chickenpox, cytomegalovirus, DiGeorge syndrome, hepatitis (viral), hyperthyroidism, influenza, leukemia (lymphocytic), leukosarcoma, lymphocytosis (infectious), lymphoma (non-Hodgkin's), measles, malnutrition, mononucleosis (infectious), multiple myeloma, multiple sclerosis, mumps, parathyroid fever, pertussis, pneumonia (viral), polyneuropathy, scurvy, syphilis, thyrotoxicosis, tuberculosis, tularemia, typhoid fever, typhus, and Waldenström's macroglobulinemia.

Decreased. Anemia (aplastic), burns, cardiac failure, Cushing's disease, Hodgkin's disease, immunoglobulin deficiency, leukemia (chronic granulocytic, monocytic), lymphatic irradiation, stress reactions, systemic lupus erythematosus (SLE), terminal carcinoma, thymic hypoplasia (children), trauma, uremia, and X-linked agammaglobulinemia. Drugs include corticotropin, cortisone acetate, epinephrine bitartrate, epinephrine borate, epinephrine hydrochloride, intravenous immunoglobulin, and nitrogen mustard.

Description. B-lymphocytes are white blood cells with a short life span that are produced by bone marrow and are responsible for humoral immunity and production of immunoglobulin and specific antibodies. They are found in the lymph nodes, spleen, bone marrow, and blood and are a primary defense against virulent, encapsulated, bacterial pathogens. When stimulated by an antigen, they transform themselves into plasma cells that rapidly secrete antibodies. These antibodies neutralize viruses, interfere with the absorption of foreign proteins, and detoxify other proteins. They loose their ability to respond to antigenic or mutogenic stimulation with age.

Professional Considerations
1. Consent form NOT required.
2. **Preparation:**
   A. Tube: Green topped.
3. **Procedure:**
   A. Draw a 5-mL blood sample.
4. **Postprocedure care:**
   A. None.
5. **Client and family teaching:**
   A. Inform the physician of past (6-month) history of colds and infections.
6. **Factors that affect results:**
   A. Medications containing epinephrine cause unreliable results.

B

7. **Other data:**
   A. Plasma cells seldom appear in the blood, but they may appear in increased numbers in severe infections, especially in children, to reinforce immunity when sufficient antibodies are not available.

BMD
(see Bone densitometry, Diagnostic)

BMP
(see Basic metabolic panel, Blood)

BMR
(see Basal metabolic rate, Diagnostic)

BNP, PLASMA
(see Natriuretic peptides, Plasma)

BODY FLUID, AMYLASE, SPECIMEN

Norm. Negative.

Positive. Benign ovarian cyst fluid, esophageal rupture, necrotic bowel, pancreatic ascites, pancreatic duct trauma, pancreatitis (with or without pseudocyst), perforated peptic ulcer, and malignant pleural effusions in the presence of cancer of the lung, breast, gastrointestinal tract, ovary, and lymphoma. Small cell lung carcinoma metastasis to the liver resulting in necrosis.

Description. Amylase is produced in large quantities by the pancreas, salivary glands, and certain malignant tumors. It is produced in lesser quantities by the fallopian tubes and lungs. Amylase from the pancreas and salivary glands is normally contained in the gastrointestinal tract. The presence of a significant amount of amylase in a body fluid specimen indicates a pathologic process.

Professional Considerations
1. Consent form NOT required. See individual procedures for procedure-specific risks and contraindications.
2. **Preparation:**
   A. Obtain a pleural or peritoneal aspiration tray and a clean con-

tainer or red-topped tube. Sterile 0.9% saline is needed for peritoneal lavage.
3. **Procedure:**
   A. Obtain a body fluid specimen by needle aspiration of pleural or peritoneal fluid, or by catheter irrigation and aspiration of the peritoneum, and inject it into a clean container or red-topped tube.
4. **Postprocedure care:**
   A. Apply a dry, sterile dressing to the site.
5. **Client and family teaching:**
   A. Results are normally available within 72 hours.
6. **Factors that affect results:**
   A. When ascitic fluid is being collected, the location of the collection site or of the catheter tip will likely affect the level of amylase that may be present. For example, a catheter directed to the left upper quadrant may produce a false-negative specimen.
7. **Other data:**
   A. A common finding of lung carcinoma with pleural effusion.
   B. Amylase levels indicative of saliva can be obtained on penile swabs, vaginal swabs, and breast swabs in sexual assault cases.

BODY FLUID, ANAEROBIC CULTURE

Norm. Negative. No growth.

Positive. Aspiration pneumonia, biliary tract infections, bite wounds, bronchiectasis, chronic osteomyelitis, chronic sinus infection, dental and mouth infections, deep tissue infection or necrosis, gastrointestinal infections (especially of the colon), gynecologic intraabdominal or extraabdominal infections, immunodeficiency states, immunosuppressive therapy, infections caused by *Actinomyces, Arachnia, Bacteroides fragilis, Bacteroides melaninogenicus, Bifidobacterium, Clostridium, Coccidioides, Eubacterium, Fusobacterium, Lactobacillus, Peptostreptococcus, Propionibacterium, Veillonella,* and others, malignancy, and trauma (accidental, surgical). Drugs include aminoglycosides.

Description. The test identifies anaerobic bacterial infections in body fluids, including ascitic fluid, bile, cerebrospinal fluid, pleural fluid, and synovial fluid, and from wounds and abscesses. Anaerobes live and grow where there is no free oxygen and obtain energy for growth and metabolism from fermentation reactions rather than from oxygen. Anaerobes are part of the normal flora of the skin, oral cavity, lower gastrointestinal tract, urethra, and the female external genital tract. When displaced from their location into other body tissues or spaces, they become pathogenic, causing localized abscesses in oxygen-poor body cavities and specific body organs. Untreated anaerobic infections may lead to bacteremia. Special collection methods are necessary for isolation of anaerobes. Anaerobic cultures are grown on complex media, and identification is made by means of colony morphology, pigmentation, fluorescence, and gas-liquid chromatography.

Professional Considerations

1. Consent form IS required for some of the procedures used to obtain the specimen. See specific procedures for risks and contraindications.
2. **Preparation:**
   A. Notify laboratory personnel that an anaerobic specimen will be arriving.
   B. For the needle and syringe method, obtain a needle, a syringe, a sterile "gassed-out" tube (a tube flushed with oxygen-free carbon dioxide or nitrogen gas), and a double stopper.
   C. For the two-tube swab method, obtain several sterile swabs prepared and stored in oxygen-free carbon dioxide tubes and tubes containing pre reduced transport media with a methylene blue indicator as needed.
3. **Procedure:**
   A. *Needle and syringe method:* Expel all air from the syringe. Aspirate the specimen directly into the syringe. Carefully expel any air from the syringe. Immediately inject the specimen into a sterile "gassed-out" tube, preferably with a double stopper to prevent the introduction of air when the specimen is injected. If this anaerobic transport tube is not available, the needle can be tightly capped or embedded in a sterile rubber stopper. Since the

specimen must be centrifuged, the volume should be over 2 mL. In the presence of extensive wounds involving large amounts of tissue or multiple lesions, several samples should be taken.
   B. *Two-tube swab method:* Collect the specimen on at least two sterile swabs that have been prepared and stored in oxygen-free tubes. Expose the swabs to air as briefly as possible. Keeping the methylene blue transport tube upright, quickly place the swabs in the tubes and close them tightly. Never let the swab samples dry out.
   C. Alternatively, an anaerobic transport container may be used.
4. **Postprocedure care:**
   A. Apply a sterile dressing over the aspiration site.
   B. Keep the specimen at room temperature and transport it to the laboratory within 30 minutes for immediate processing. Some anaerobes survive for only a short time after collection.
   C. Write the specimen source, any recent antibiotic therapy, and the client's diagnosis and symptoms on the laboratory requisition.
5. **Client and family teaching:**
   A. Results are normally available within 72 hours.
   B. Report signs of infection at the aspiration site to the physician: increasing pain, redness, swelling, purulent drainage, or fever >101° F (≥38.3° C).
   C. Treatment of the condition may begin before the results are obtained.
6. **Factors that affect results:**
   A. Reject small specimens (a few drops) in a syringe received more than 10 minutes after collection.
   B. Reject larger specimens (>1 mL) in a syringe received more than 1 hour after collection.
   C. Reject specimens in anaerobic oxygen-free vials or tubes received more than 3 hours after collection.
   D. Exposure of the specimen to air may cause false-negative results.
   E. Failure to use anaerobic transport specimen containers may cause false-negative results.
   F. Do not use methylene blue indicator tubes if the ring of blue extends beyond the top surface of the tube.

B

G. Letting the specimens dry out invalidates the results.

H. The client's symptoms, condition, and type of organism suspected determine the specific type of anaerobic culture medium selected.

7. Other data:

A. Malignancy, immunosuppressive deficiency states, immunosuppressive therapy, and some types of antibiotic therapy favor the multiplication of endogenous anaerobes.

B. The use of swabs to obtain anaerobic cultures is not recommended. When necessary, commercial anaerobic swab sets consisting of two containers must be used.

BODY FLUID, FUNGUS, CULTURE

Norm. Negative. No growth.

Positive. *Blastomyces dermatitidis, Coccidioides immitis, Cryptococcus neoformans, Histoplasma capsulatum, Sporothrix schenckii, Candida albicans, Candida tropicalis, Aspergillus fumigatus, Aspergillus flavus,* and others.

Description. Fungi are slow-growing, eukaryotic organisms that can grow on living and nonliving organic materials and are subdivided into yeasts and molds. Normal human host defense mechanisms limit the damage they cause superficially. Some fungi can be inhaled or introduced by traumatic inoculation into deep tissue spaces and cause serious infections. Factors that predispose a client to a fungal infection include immunosuppression, treatment with corticosteroids or broad-spectrum antibiotics, or debilitated states. Although tentative identification of fungi can be made quickly with staining techniques, culture of the organism on special fungal culture media is required to confirm a diagnosis of a fungal infection.

Professional Considerations

1. Consent form NOT required for the culture but may be required for the procedure used to obtain the specimen.

2. Preparation:

A. Obtain a sterile specimen container, sterile gloves, a needle, a syringe, and any necessary aspiration trays, depending on the site to be cultured.

B. For urine collection, obtain a sterile container and povidone-iodine wipes. If the client will be collecting the specimen independently, instructions should include a demonstration.

C. Obtain the specimen early in the day so that it may be processed promptly.

3. Procedure:

A. Use an aseptic technique to collect a specimen of the body fluid to be cultured.

B. The specimen should be examined for yeast cells at the bedside whenever possible or placed in a sterile container and transported promptly to the laboratory.

C. Urine collection:

i. Instruct the client to void and discard the urine.

ii. Thirty minutes later, while holding the labia open or foreskin back, cleanse the urethral meatus in an outward circular motion with each of three povidone-iodine wipes. Allow the iodine to dry while protecting the urethral meatus from contamination.

iii. Instruct the client to void a small amount and then stop the stream of urine.

iv. Place the sterile specimen container under the urethral meatus and have the client void into it, filling it no more than halfway before again stopping the stream of urine. Cap the specimen container.

4. Postprocedure care:

A. Apply an appropriate dressing as needed.

B. Write the collection date and time, specimen source, suspected disease, and any recent antibiotic or antifungal therapy on the laboratory requisition.

C. Transport the specimen to the laboratory immediately.

D. Do not refrigerate.

5. Client and family teaching:

A. Preliminary results are normally available within 72 hours, final results in about 30 days.

B. Treatment is usually begun before final results.

6. Factors that affect results:

A. Best results are obtained if cultures are inoculated immediately.

Other than noted above, the maximum time allowed between specimen collection and inoculation is 3 hours.

7. **Other data:**
   A. Four to 6 weeks are required for fungal culture results.

B. More yeast is acquired using Fan bottles.
C. *Sporothrix schenckii* infection is on the increase in HIV-positive clients.
D. Coccidioidomycosis can be associated with hypercalcemia.

BODY FLUID, GLUCOSE, SPECIMEN

Norm:

		SI UNITS

Cerebrospinal Fluid. Lags behind blood glucose levels by 2-4 hours. Fasting to 4 hours postprandially 50%-80% of serum glucose:

Adult	40-80 mg/dL	2.2-4.4 mmol/L
Premature infant	24-63 mg/dL	1.3-3.5 mmol/L
Full-term infant	34-119 mg/dL	1.9-6.6 mmol/L
Child	35-75 mg/dL	1.9-4.1 mmol/L
Peritoneal fluid	70-100 mg/dL	3.8-5.5 mmol/L
Pleural fluid	Same as blood glucose level, with a time lag of 2-4 hours or no less than 40 mg/dL (2.2 mmol/L) below blood glucose	
Fasting	60-110 mg/dL	3.3-6.1 mmol/L
Synovial fluid	No more than 10 mg/dL (0.6 mmol/L, SI units) lower than blood glucose level	

Increased CSF Glucose. Brain tumor, cerebral hemorrhage, cerebral trauma, diabetic coma, hyperglycemia, hypothalamic lesions, increased intracranial pressure, and uremia.

Increased Peritoneal, Pleural, or Synovial Fluid Glucose. Hyperglycemia and primary and symptomatic diabetes.

Decreased CSF Glucose. Brain abscess, brain tumor, cancer, central nervous system sarcoidosis, choroid plexus tumor, coccidioidomycosis, increased intracranial pressure, encephalitis (mumps or herpes simplex origin), hypoglycemia, leukemic infiltration, lupus myelopathy, lymphocytic choriomeningitis, lymphoma, melanomatosis, meningeal carcinomatosis, meningitis (acute pyogenic, aseptic, chemical, cryptococcal, fungal, granulomatous, pyogenic, rheumatoid, tuberculous, viral), neurosyphilis, rheumatoid arthritis, subarachnoid hemorrhage, toxoplasmosis, and tuberculoma of brain.

Decreased Peritoneal Fluid Glucose. Peritoneal carcinomatosis, peritonitis (tuberculous), and hypoglycemia.

Decreased Pleural Fluid Glucose. Infection (bacterial), effusion (malignant, neoplastic, rheumatoid, septic, tuberculous), and hypoglycemia.

Decreased Synovial Fluid Glucose. Arthritis (inflammatory, noninflammatory, rheumatoid, septic, tuberculous) and hypoglycemia.

Description. Body fluid glucose content is similar to blood serum glucose content. Most abnormalities result in a decreased body fluid glucose caused by increased utilization of glucose by the pathogenic process. This test is interpreted when a blood glucose level is compared to the body fluid glucose level.

Professional Considerations
1. Consent form IS required for the procedure used to obtain the specimen. See specific procedures for risks and contraindications.

Risks
See appropriate procedure being performed.

Contraindications
See appropriate procedure being performed.

2. **Preparation:**
   A. Tube: Red topped, red/gray topped, or gold topped for blood glucose specimen.
   B. Obtain a sterile specimen container, a tube, or an evacuated glass bottle, and a sterile tray (arthrocentesis, lumbar puncture, paracentesis, thoracentesis) depending on the procedure being performed.
3. **Procedure:**
   A. Draw a 5-mL blood sample for glucose in a red-topped tube.
   B. Collect the appropriate specimen as follows:
      i. *Cerebrospinal fluid (CSF):* Collect 3-5 mL of cerebrospinal fluid in a sterile glass tube by means of a spinal tap no more than 4 hours postprandially.
      ii. *Peritoneal fluid:* Collect 5 mL of peritoneal fluid in a sterile glass tube by a paracentesis immediately after blood glucose specimen collection.
      iii. *Pleural fluid:* Collect 5 mL of pleural fluid in a sterile glass tube by thoracentesis 2-4 hours after blood glucose specimen collection.
      iv. *Synovial fluid:* Collect 3-5 mL of synovial fluid in a sterile gray-topped tube containing sodium fluoride by arthrocentesis immediately after blood glucose specimen collection.
4. **Postprocedure care:**
   A. Apply a sterile dressing to the sites.
   B. Write the specimen source and collection time on the laboratory requisition.
   C. Transport the specimens to the laboratory immediately. Analysis must be performed promptly on freshly collected specimens to avoid erroneous results caused by glycolysis.
   D. For CSF collection, see *Lumbar puncture, Diagnostic.*

5. **Client and family teaching:**
   A. Report to the physician if there are signs of infection at the collection site: increasing pain, redness, swelling, purulent drainage, or fever >101° F (≥38.3° C).
   B. Results are normally available within 24 hours.
6. **Factors that affect results:**
   A. This method provides the least reliable diagnosis of bacterial peritonitis.
7. **Other data:**
   A. None.

BODY FLUID, MYCOBACTERIA, CULTURE

Norm. No growth after 8 weeks.

Usage. Diagnose the presence of *Mycobacterium* in body fluid.

Description. Mycobacteria are non-motile, non-sporeforming, straight, or slightly curved rods that resist staining by Gram's method or by acid solutions because of their high-lipid-containing cell walls. They grow slowly, with colonies developing after 2 days to 8 weeks of incubation. Some species are found in soil and water. Others are obligate parasites. The most common mycobacteria causing human disease are *Mycobacterium asiaticum, M. avium-scrofulaceum* complex, *M. fortuitum, M. haemophilum, M. kansasii, M. leprae, M. malmoense, M. marinum, M. simiae, M. szulgai, M. tuberculosis complex, M. ulcerans,* and *M. xenopi.* These organisms may attack any organ, but the primary site of infection is usually the lungs. Tubercle bacillus is the most common *Mycobacterium* infection in the United States, except in clients with AIDS. The bacilli are usually inhaled and are small enough to be carried into the alveoli without being expelled.

Professional Considerations
1. Consent form NOT required for the culture but may be required for the procedure used to obtain the specimen.

Risks
Complications of nasogastric tube insertion include bleeding, dysrhythmias, esophageal perforation, laryngospasm, and decreased mean pO_2.

Contraindications

For nasogastric tube insertion: esophageal varices.

2. **Preparation:**
   A. Obtain a sterile specimen container.
   B. For gastric lavage, obtain a nasogastric tube, lubricant, sterile water, a sterile 50-mL syringe, and a sterile specimen container.
   C. For paracentesis, thoracentesis, pericardiocentesis, or arthrocentesis obtain the appropriate sterile procedure tray.
3. **Procedure:**
   A. *Sputum specimen:* Collect an early-morning sputum specimen of 5-10 mL on three separate days. Label the specimens sequentially.
   B. *Gastric lavage:* Used for clients who cannot produce sputum. The specimen should be obtained in the early morning after an 8-hour fast from food and fluids. Insert a nasogastric tube into the stomach. Instill 20-50 mL of sterile water into the stomach through the nasogastric tube with a sterile syringe and then aspirate the fluid out of the stomach with the syringe. Remove the nasogastric tube.
   C. *Peritoneal fluid:* Collect 5-10 mL of peritoneal fluid in a sterile syringe by paracentesis using an aseptic technique.
   D. *Pleural fluid:* Collect 5-10 mL of pleural fluid in a sterile syringe by thoracentesis using an aseptic technique.
   E. *Pericardial fluid:* Collect 5-10 mL of pericardial fluid in a sterile syringe by pericardiocentesis using an aseptic technique.
   F. *Synovial fluid:* Collect 5-10 mL of synovial fluid in a sterile syringe by arthrocentesis using an aseptic technique.
   G. *Urine:* Collect first morning-voided specimens by the clean-catch technique or by aspiration from an indwelling urinary catheter or suprapubic puncture on 3 separate days. Label the specimens sequentially. See clean-catch collection instructions in the test *Body fluid, Routine, Culture.*
4. **Postprocedure care:**
   A. Apply a dry sterile dressing to the aspiration site. Observe the

site for drainage or bleeding hourly × 4.
   B. For specimens obtained by pericardiocentesis or thoracentesis, assess vital signs every 15 minutes × 4, then every 30 minutes × 2, and then hourly × 4. Observe for dysrhythmias for 24 hours.
   C. Write the specimen source, collection time, current antibiotic or antifungal therapy, and clinical diagnosis on the laboratory requisition. The request to culture the specimen for *Mycobacterium* must be specified on the laboratory requisition.
   D. Transport the specimen to the laboratory promptly. Refrigerate urine specimens if not cultured immediately.
5. **Client and family teaching:**
   A. *Needle aspiration:* Call the physician if there are signs of infection at the procedure site: increasing pain, redness, swelling, purulent drainage, or fever >101° F (≥38.3° C).
   B. *Sputum:* Deep coughs are necessary to produce sputum rather than saliva. To produce the proper specimen, take in several breaths without fully exhaling each and then expel sputum with a "cascade cough."
   C. Results are normally available within 72 hours.
6. **Factors that affect results:**
   A. Specimens are best if collected in the early morning upon arising and before eating or drinking.
7. **Other data:**
   A. Sputum induction by respiratory therapy may be required.
   B. Povidone-iodine solution at 0.02% inactivates *Mycobacterium tuberculosis, M. avium,* and *M. kansasii* within 30 seconds.

BODY FLUID, ROUTINE, CULTURE

Norm. No growth.

Usage. Identification and isolation of aerobic infectious organisms.

Positive Urine Culture. Titers >100,000/mL indicate urinary tract infection (viral [cytomegalovirus] or bacterial [frequently *Escherichia coli, Klebsiella, Proteus, Staphylococcus,* or *Streptococcus*]).

Negative Urine Culture. Titers <1000/mL are not considered clinically significant but more likely result from contamination caused by poor collection technique.

Description. Routine body fluid culture is an aseptic collection of an aerobic culture that may be performed on ascitic, pericardial, pleural, or synovial fluids and on bone marrow or urine. For urine specimens collected by suprapubic puncture, anaerobic culture may be performed.

Professional Considerations
1. Consent form NOT required for the culture but may be required for the procedure used to obtain the specimen.
2. Preparation:
   A. Obtain povidone-iodine solution, sterile towels, and an appropriate sterile tray (paracentesis, thoracentesis, arthrocentesis, bone marrow aspiration).
   B. For the clean-catch urine culture, obtain povidone-iodine wipes and a sterile specimen container.
   C. For the urine culture for indwelling urinary catheter, obtain alcohol wipes, a needle, and a 10-mL syringe.
   D. For the urine culture from suprapubic puncture, force fluids (200 mL/hour for 6 hours), and instruct the client not to void. The bladder must be full and distended for puncture. Obtain a sterile red-topped tube (or an anaerobic culture container for recovery of anaerobic organisms), povidone-iodine, and an aspiration tray.
   E. Cultures should be obtained before antibiotic or antifungal therapy is started whenever possible.
3. Procedure:
   A. *Ascitic, pericardial, pleural, or synovial fluid:*
      i. Cleanse the collection site with povidone-iodine and allow it to dry.
      ii. The physician uses an aseptic technique to collect a minimum of 2 mL of fluid by paracentesis, pericardiocentesis, thoracentesis, or arthrocentesis and transfers it into a

closed, sterile container or Petri dish that is free of preservative.
   B. *Bone marrow:*
      i. The physician uses an aseptic technique to collect a small amount of bone marrow via bone marrow aspiration and transfers it into a Petri dish that is free of any preservative.
      ii. See *Bone marrow aspiration analysis, Specimen,* for procedural details.
   C. *Urine culture from clean-catch specimen* (also known as *Urine culture, Routine, Specimen*): The clean-catch urine technique must be used to decrease the risk of specimen contamination.
      i. Have the client void to empty the bladder of long-standing urine. Thirty minutes later, obtain a 10-mL clean-catch urine specimen or sample from a straight or indwelling catheter in a sterile container.
      ii. *Female:* While holding the labia minora apart, cleanse the mucous membranes surrounding the periphery of the urethral meatus by using antiseptic-moistened cotton balls. Use the first cotton ball to wipe from front to back on one side, followed by the same procedure with the second cotton ball on the opposite side; then cleanse directly over the meatus with the third cotton ball. Discard each cotton ball after one use.
      Male: Retract the foreskin and cleanse the glans of the penis with soap and water. Then cleanse the glans with antiseptic-moistened cotton balls, using a circular motion from the urethral meatus outward and discarding each cotton ball after one use.
      iii. Have the client void a small amount of urine and discard. Then stop the stream and place the specimen container in the urine path and void 30-90 mL (1-3 ounces) of urine into the container. Avoid contaminating the container by touching the inside of the container to the body.

D. *Urine culture from indwelling catheter:*
  i. Clamp the tubing for 15 minutes to allow the urine to accumulate in the upper portion of the tubing.
  ii. Cleanse the needle port of the rubber catheter with an alcohol wipe and allow it to dry.
  iii. Insert a sterile needle attached to a syringe through the port and withdraw 10 mL of urine. Collect only fresh urine as it drains. Do not collect urine that has already passed the collection point.
  iv. Remove the syringe and discard the needle. Expel the syringe contents into a sterile specimen cup and cap tightly. Remove the clamp from the tubing.
E. *Urine culture from suprapubic puncture:*
  i. Cleanse the skin around the aspiration site with povidone-iodine and allow it to dry.
  ii. Drape the aspiration site with sterile towels.
  iii. The physician performs the suprapubic puncture into the bladder and withdraws at least 10 mL of urine.
  iv. For aerobic culture, the needle is removed from the syringe after withdrawal, and the urine is expelled into a sterile container.
  v. For anaerobic culture, a fresh needle is placed on the syringe, and the urine is quickly injected into an anaerobic culture container.
F. Body fluids and bone marrow aspirates may be inoculated into blood culture media.

4. **Postprocedure care:**
A. Apply a dry, sterile dressing to the aspiration site. Observe the site for drainage or bleeding hourly × 4.
B. For specimens obtained by pericardiocentesis or thoracentesis, assess vital signs every 15 minutes × 4, then every 30 minutes × 2, and then hourly × 4. Observe for dysrhythmias for 24 hours.
C. Write the specific collection site, date, time, client's age, diagnosis, and recent antibiotic or antifun-

gal therapy on the laboratory requisition. Requests for anaerobic culture must be specified on the requisition.
D. Send the specimen to the laboratory immediately. Urine specimens should be refrigerated if not cultured immediately. Specimens from other sites should not be refrigerated.

5. **Client and family teaching:**
A. Call the physician if signs of infection appear at the procedure site: increasing pain, redness, swelling, purulent drainage, or fever >101° F (≥38.3°C).
B. Results are usually available within 5 to 30 days.
C. Treatment may begin before culture results.

6. **Factors that affect results:**
A. Reject specimens not tightly sealed.
B. Refrigeration decreases the accuracy of results for all except urine specimens.
C. Antibiotic or antifungal therapy initiated before specimen collection may produce false-negative results.
D. The most frequent interference with urine culture results is improper collection technique, which results in specimen contamination.
E. An early-morning urine specimen yields the highest concentration of microorganisms.

7. **Other data:**
A. Preliminary results are reported in 24 hours. At least 48 hours is required for the isolation of organisms in the presence of pathogens. Fungi and mycobacteria may take several weeks. Gram stains should be available within 1 hour.
B. *Mycobacterium* and *Chlamydia* infections of the urinary tract are not diagnosed by this test.
C. If cytomegalovirus is suspected, several urine specimens are recommended because the virus is shed intermittently.
D. Urine for culture should be sent on infants suspected of UTI because 4%-6% would otherwise be misdiagnosed.

BODY FLUID ANALYSIS, SPECIMEN

Norm:

PERICARDIAL FLUID

Appearance	Clear to pale yellow
Glucose	
Transudate	Approximates whole blood levels (whole blood adult norm, 60-89 mg/dL; whole blood child norm, 51-85 mg/dL)
Exudate	Lower than whole blood levels
Lactate dehydrogenase	
Transudate	≤Client's serum LD (serum adult norm, 45-90 U/L; serum child norm, 60-170 U/L)

Other
Interleukin-1beta > 45 pg/ml indicates ischemic heart disease.

PERITONEAL FLUID		SI UNITS
Appearance	Clear or pale yellow	
Albumin	Negative	
Alkaline Phosphatase		
Adult female	76-250 U/L	
Adult male	90-239 U/L	
Ammonia	<50 g/L	
Cholesterol		
Transudate	<46 mg/dL	<1.19 mmol/L
Exudate	≥46 mg/dL	≥1.19 mmol/L
Glucose		
Transudate	60-110 mg/dL	3.3-6.1 mmol/L
Exudate	Lower than whole blood levels (whole blood adult norm, 60-89 mg/dL; child norm, 51-85 mg/dL)	
Lactic Acid	10-20 mg/dL	1.1-2.3 mmol/L
Lactate Dehydrogenase		
Transudate	≤Client's serum LD serum (adult norm, 45-90 U/L; child norm, 60-170 U/L)	
Exudate	>Client's serum LD	
pH	7.4	7.4
Specific Gravity		
Transudate	<1.016	<1.016
Exudate	≥1.016	≥1.016
Total Protein		
Transudate	<2.5 g/dL	<25 g/L
Exudate	>3 g/dL	>30 g/L

PERITONEAL FLUID—cont'd		SI UNITS
Volume	<100 mL	
White Blood Cells		
Transudate	<100/mm³	<100 × 10⁹ /L
Exudate	>1000/mm³	>1000 × 10⁹ /L
Other		

Interleukin-8 and macrophage migration inhibitory factor (MIF) are elevated in women with endometriosis.

Matrix metalloproteinases (MMP)-2 and MMP-9 are overexpressed in ovarian cancer in peritoneal fluid.

Dendritic cells in peritoneal fluid are significantly higher than in peripheral blood in infertile women.

PLEURAL FLUID		SI UNITS
Appearance	Clear, slightly amber	
Cholesterol		
Transudate	<60 mg/dL	<1.55 mmol/L
Exudate	≥60 mg/dL	≥1.55 mmol/L
Glucose		
Transudate	Approximates whole blood levels (whole blood adult norm, 60-89 mg/dL; child norm, 51-85 mg/dL)	
Exudate	Lower than whole blood levels	
Lactate Dehydrogenase		
Transudate	≤Client's serum LD (serum adult norm, 45-90 U/L; child norm, 60-170 U/L)	
Exudate	>Client's serum LD	

Pleural fluid LD > 7500IU/L may indicate *Streptococcus pneumoniae.*

pH	7.4	
Specific Gravity		
Transudate	<1.016	<1.016
Exudate	≥1.016	≥1.016
Total Protein		
Transudate	<2.5 g/dL	<25 g/L
Exudate	>3 g/dL	>30 g/L
Volume	<25 mL	
White Blood Cells		
Transudate	<100/mm³	<100 × 10⁹ /L
Exudate	>1000/mm³	>1000 × 10⁹ /L
Other		

Amylase rich pleural effusion (ARPE) common in lung cancer, adenocarcinoma, and mesothelioma.

SYNOVIAL FLUID		SI UNITS
Appearance	Clear or colorless to pale yellow	
Crystals	Absent	
Glucose		
Transudate	≤10 mg/dL lower than blood glucose (whole blood adult norm, 60-89 mg/dL; child norm, 51-85 mg/dL)	
Exudate	Lower than whole blood levels	
Lactate Dehydrogenase		
Transudate	≤Client's serum LD (serum adult norm, 45-90 U/L; child norm, 60-170 U/L)	
Exudate	>Client's serum LD	
pH	7.4	
Specific Gravity		
Transudate	<1.016	<1.016
Exudate	>1.016	>1.016
Total Protein		
Transudate	1-3 g/dL	10-30 g/dL
Exudate	>3 g/dL	>30 g/dL
Volume	<4 mL	
Viscosity	High	
White Blood Cells		
Transudate	<100/mm^3	<100 × 10^9 /L
Exudate	>1000/mm^3	>1000 × 10^9 /L

Increased Volume

PERICARDIAL FLUID	PERITONEAL FLUID
Cardiac tamponade	Abscess
Constrictive pericarditis	Ascites
Central venous catheter insertion	Hepatic disease
Pericardial effusion	Peritonitis
	Portal hypertension

PLEURAL FLUID	SYNOVIAL FLUID
Bacterial pneumonia	Amyloidosis
Bronchogenic carcinoma	Aseptic necrosis
Chronic hepatic disease	Bacterial infection
Congestive heart failure	Charcot's joint
Constrictive pericarditis	Connective tissue disease
Hypertrophic pulmonary	Crystal-induced arthritis
osteoarthropathy	Epiphyseal dysplasia
Hypoproteinemia	Gout
Lymphoma	Hemochromatosis
Metastatic carcinoma	Osteoarthritis
Neoplasm	Osteochondritis dissecans

Increased Volume—cont'd

PLEURAL FLUID	SYNOVIAL FLUID
Nephrotic syndrome	Paget's disease
Pulmonary infarct	Polymyositis
Rheumatoid disease	Psoriasis
Systemic lupus erythematosus	Regional enteritis
Trauma	Reiter's disease
Tuberculosis	Rheumatic arthritis
Viral pneumonia	Sarcoidosis
	Scleroderma
	Sickle cell disease
	Subacute bacterial endocarditis
	Systemic lupus erythematosus
	Traumatic arthritis
	Ulcerative colitis
	Villonodular synovitis

Causes of Turbidity

PERICARDIAL FLUID	PERITONEAL FLUID
Abscess	Abscess

PLEURAL FLUID	SYNOVIAL FLUID
Abscess	Abscess
Bacterial infection	Floating cartilage fragments
Rheumatic fever	Inflammation
Rheumatoid disease	Leukocytes
Tuberculosis	Pseudogout
	Rheumatoid arthritis
	Septic arthritis
	Systemic lupus erythematosus
	Tuberculous arthritis

Causes of Milky Color

SYNOVIAL FLUID
Gouty arthritis
Lymphatic drainage
Rheumatoid arthritis
Systemic lupus erythematosus
Tuberculous arthritis

Pink or Red Color

PERICARDIAL FLUID	PERITONEAL FLUID
Hemorrhage	Hemorrhage
Trauma	Trauma
Traumatic tap	Traumatic tap

PLEURAL FLUID	SYNOVIAL FLUID
Congestive heart failure	Hemophilic arthritis
Hemorrhage	Hemorrhage
Pancreatitis	Joint fracture
Pneumonia	Neurogenic arthropathy
Postmyocardial infarction syndrome	Osteoarthritis
Pulmonary infarction	Pigmented villinodular synovitis

Pink or Red Color—cont'd

PLEURAL FLUID	SYNOVIAL FLUID
Trauma	Recent hemarthrosis
Traumatic tap	Rheumatoid arthritis
Tumor	Septic arthritis
	Trauma
	Traumatic arthritis
	Traumatic tap
	Tumor

Increased Lactic Acid. Infection (pleural, peritoneal) and malignancy

Decreased Glucose

PERICARDIAL FLUID	PERITONEAL FLUID
(Not applicable)	Rheumatoid effusion

PLEURAL FLUID	SYNOVIAL FLUID
Bacterial infection	Inflammatory arthritis
Malignancy	Noninflammatory arthritis
Neoplastic effusion	Rheumatoid arthritis
Septic effusion	Rheumatoid effusion
Tuberculous effusion	Septic arthritis
	Tuberculous arthritis

Decreased pH

PLEURAL FLUID	PERITONEAL FLUID
Empyema	Peritoneal effusion
Esophageal rupture	
Loculated effusion	
Parapneumonic effusion	
Tuberculous effusion	

Decreased Synovial Fluid Viscosity. Gout, inflammatory joint disease, rheumatic fever, rheumatoid arthritis, sepsis, septic arthritis, and trauma.

Increased Synovial Fluid Viscosity. Hashimoto's thyroiditis, hypothyroidism.

Description. A sample of body fluid is obtained for analysis of its various components and for detection of the presence of abnormal constituents that may be caused by pathogenic processes. Some conditions that may cause abnormalities include neoplasm, infection, inflammation, leakage of gastrointestinal tract contents or secretions, trauma, and hemorrhage.

Professional Considerations
1. Consent form IS required for the procedure used to obtain the specimen. See specific procedures for risks and contraindications.
2. **Preparation:**
   A. Obtain sterile tubes or evacuated glass bottles for the specimens.
   B. Obtain a sterile specimen container, a tube, or an evacuated glass bottle, and a sterile tray (arthrocentesis, pericardiocentesis, paracentesis, thoracentesis) depending on the procedure being performed.
   C. Obtain alcohol wipes, a tourniquet, a needle, a syringe, and a gray-topped tube for blood glucose, and a red-topped tube for lactate dehydrogenase comparisons to body fluid levels.
3. **Procedure:**
   A. A sample of body fluid is obtained by needle aspiration under sterile conditions.

B. The amount collected varies based on the purpose of the procedure and type of specimen.

C. Draw a 7-mL blood sample in the gray-topped tube for whole blood glucose and a 7-mL blood sample in the red-topped tube for lactate dehydrogenase levels.

4. **Postprocedure care:**
   A. Apply a sterile dressing to site.

5. **Client and family teaching:**
   A. Report signs of infection at the collection site to the physician: increasing pain, redness, swelling, purulent drainage, or fever >101° F (≥38.3° C).
   B. Results are normally available within 72 hours.

6. **Factors that affect results:**
   A. None.

7. **Other data:**
   A. Ascitic fluid collection versus fluid from an over distended bladder can be differentiated with a urea nitrogen analysis. Urine urea nitrogen should be greater than 12 g/dL, whereas ascitic fluid should be less.
   B. A pleural fluid pH >7.30 and glucose >60 mg/dL predicts decreased survival from neoplastic metastasis to the lung.
   C. See also *Body fluid, Glucose, Specimen; Body fluid analysis, Cell count, Specimen; Body fluid, Amylase, Specimen.*

BODY FLUID ANALYSIS, CELL COUNT, SPECIMEN

Norm:

PERICARDIAL FLUID		SI UNITS
Red blood cells	None	
White blood cells	<500/mm³	
Polymorphonuclear leukocytes	0%-25%	0-0.25

PERITONEAL FLUID		
Cell count	<500/mm³	
Red blood cells	None	
Transudate	Few	
Exudate	Variable	
White blood cells	<300/μL	0-0.30 × 10⁹ /L
Polymorphonuclear leukocytes	0%-25%	0-0.25

PLEURAL FLUID		
Cell count	<1000/mm³	
White blood cells		
Transudate	Few	
Exudate	Many	
Eosinophils	0%-10%	0-0.10
Lymphocytes	0%-50%	0-0.50
Neutrophils	0%-50%	0-0.50
Polymorphonuclear leukocytes	0%-25%	0-0.25

SYNOVIAL FLUID		
Red blood cells	None	
White blood cells	0-200/μL	0-0.20 × 10⁹/L
Neutrophils	0%-25%	0-0.25
Lymphocytes	0%-78%	0-0.78
Monocytes	0%-71%	0-0.71
Macrophages (clasmatocytes)	0%-26%	0-0.26
Polymorphonuclear leukocytes	0%-25%	0-0.25
Synovial cells	0%-12%	0-0.12
Unclassified	0%-21%	0-0.21

Increased Leukocytes. Acute gouty arthritis, carcinoma (pleural fluid), chylothorax (pleural fluid), congestive heart failure (pleural fluid), empyema (pleural fluid), gonorrheal arthritis, inflammation (pleural fluid), lymphatic leukemia, lymphocytic leukemia (pleural fluid), lymphomas (pleural fluid), parapneumonic effusion (pleural fluid), postpneumonic effusion (pleural fluid), rheumatic fever, rheumatoid arthritis, septic arthritis, tuberculosis (pleural fluid), tumors, and uremia (pleural fluid).

Increased Polymorphonuclear Cells. Bacterial inflammation, bacterial peritonitis, and infectious processes (acute).

Increased Eosinophils. Infarcts, parasites, pneumothorax, postpneumonic effusions, rheumatic fever, rheumatoid arthritis, and tumors.

Increased Plasma Cells. Chronic inflammation, Hodgkin's disease, and lymphoma. Atypical plasma cells may be associated with multiple myeloma.

Decreased Glucose. Rheumatoid effusion (synovial fluid).

Description. The specific body fluid is tested for white blood count and differential, total red blood cell count, protein, lactate dehydrogenase, and other tests. The various cell counts of body fluids assist in the differentiation of exudate from transudate. Body fluid analysis may be performed on the following body fluids: ascitic, cyst, joint, pericardial, peritoneal, pleural, and synovial.

Professional Considerations
1. Consent form IS required for the procedure used to obtain the specimen. See specific procedures for risks and contraindications.
2. **Preparation:**
   A. The client should be properly positioned and the specimen site cleaned and prepped.
   B. Obtain heparin 1000 U/mL concentration.
   C. Obtain a sterile specimen container, a tube or an evacuated glass bottle, and a sterile tray

(arthrocentesis, pericardiocentesis, paracentesis, thoracentesis) depending on the procedure being performed.
3. **Procedure:**
   A. A sample of body fluid is obtained by needle aspiration under sterile conditions.
   B. The amount collected varies based on the purpose of the procedure and the type of specimen.
4. **Postprocedure care:**
   A. Apply a small dressing to the aspiration site.
   B. To each 100 mL of body fluid add 1 mL of heparin 1000 Units/mL concentration. Additional heparin will not alter results.
   C. Write the specimen source on the laboratory requisition.
   D. Transport the specimen to the laboratory immediately.
5. **Client and family teaching:**
   A. Report signs of infection at the operative site to the physician: increasing pain, redness, swelling, purulent drainage, or fever >101°F (>38.3°C).
   B. See individual procedure listings for procedure-specific teaching.
   C. Results are normally available within 72 hours.
6. **Factors that affect results:**
   A. Reject contaminated or hemolyzed specimens.
7. **Other data:**
   A. Ascitic fluid collection versus fluid from an over distended bladder can be differentiated with a urea nitrogen analysis. Urine urea nitrogen should be greater than 12 g/dL, whereas ascitic fluid should be less.

BODY FLUID CYTOLOGY, SPECIMEN
(see Brushing cytology, Specimen; Bronchial washing, Specimen, Diagnostic; Cerebrospinal fluid, Cytology, Specimen; Cytologic study of breast cyst, of effusions, of nipple discharge, Respiratory tract or urine, Diagnostic; Oral cavity cytology, Specimen)

BOHB
(see Beta-hydroxybutyrate, Blood)

BONE DENSITOMETRY (DUAL ENERGY X-RAY ABSORPTIOMETRY, DEXA), DIAGNOSTIC

Norm:

Bone mineral density (BMD)	Percentage within range of standard deviations from the norm provided by manufacturer of device used for the test. Each manufacturer provides a database of BMDs from many persons for comparison to those with similar age, race, sex, and ethnicity. Low BMD indicates androgen deprivation in prostate cancer, cystic fibrosis or osteoporosis.
Z-score	(% young adult) within range of manufacturer's norms.
T-score	(age-matched) within range of manufacturer's norms.

Usage. Measurement of bone mass or density, evaluation for predicting risk of fracture, skeletal morphometry, and body-composition analysis (less common). Bone densitometry is one of the diagnostic criteria for osteoporosis established by the World Health Organization.

Description. Considered the standard of comparison often used for diagnosis of osteoporosis, bone densitometry, approved by the FDA in 1988, is also known as dual-energy x-ray absorptiometry (DEXA). The procedure is carried out using an x-ray device that scans the heel, finger, lumbar spine, non dominant proximal femur or forearm and determines bone mineral density (BMD). The site selected for scanning is determined by the purpose of the test. The BMD measurement at one site can allow prediction of the risk of fracture at another site of the body. For assessment of general fracture risk, either the spine or the neck of the femur is measured. This test is not indicated if treatment decisions will not be affected by the results. In addition to the BMD, results are also often reported as a "Z-score" and a "T-score." The Z-score rep-

resents a comparison to the peak bone mass scores in other persons and helps one to predict the risk of future fracture. The T-score represents a comparison to the person's bone density to that of others of the same age.

Professional Considerations
1. Consent form NOT required.

Precautions
During pregnancy, risks of cumulative radiation exposure to the fetus from this and other previous or future imaging studies must be weighed against the benefits of the procedure. Although formal limits for client exposure are relative to this risk-benefit comparison, the United States Nuclear Regulatory Commission requires that the cumulative dose equivalent to an embryo/fetus from *occupational* exposure not exceed 0.5 rem (5 mSv). Radiation dose to the fetus is proportional to the distance of the anatomy studied from the abdomen and decreases as pregnancy progresses. For pregnant clients, consult the Radiologist/Radiology Department to obtain estimated fetal radiation exposure from this procedure.

2. **Preparation:**
   A. Notify radiologist if client is pregnant.
   B. Remove any metal items, such as buckles, jewelry, or buttons, from the area to be scanned.
3. **Procedure:**
   A. The client is positioned for the radiograph. For spinal or femoral densitometry, the client lies on a radiograph table. For peripheral densitometry, the client may sit upright in a chair and place the foot, finger, or forearm on a smaller device designed for peripheral densitometry.
   B. The scan is taken.
4. **Postprocedure care:**
   A. None.
5. **Client and family teaching:**
   A. The procedure is painless and uses minimal radiation.
   B. The scan takes only a few minutes.
   C. It is important to lie as still as possible during the scan.
6. **Factors that affect results:**
   A. The trabecular area of the spine is the preferred site for repeated

testing because it has a high rate of bone turnover and thus will show the greatest magnitude of change with treatment for osteoporosis.

B. Spinal abnormalities such as scoliosis can impair accuracy of results. An additional method of evaluation of bone density should be used in these persons.

7. **Other data:**

A. Other techniques used to measure bone density include: single x-ray absorptiometry (SXA), quantitative computed tomography (QCT), and quantitative ultrasonography (QUS).

B. See also *Bone ultrasonometry, Diagnostic.*

BONE GLA PROTEIN
(see Osteocalcin, Plasma or serum)

BONE MARROW ASPIRATION ANALYSIS, SPECIMEN (BONE MARROW BIOPSY, BONE MARROW IRON STAIN, IRON STAIN, BONE MARROW)

Norm. Red marrow contains connective tissue, fat cells, and hematopoietic cells. Yellow marrow contains connective tissue and fat cells. Interpretation of cell count and histopathology by a hematologist, pathologist, or oncologist is required.

Response to Staining. Iron stain for hemosiderin: 2+.

Periodic Acid–Schiff (PAS) Glycogen Reactions. Negative.

Sudan Black B (SBB) Granulocyte. Negative.

Differential Cell Count

	ADULT (%)	CHILD (%)	INFANT (%)
Basophils	0.1	0.06	0.07
Eosinophils	3.1	3.6	2.6
Hemocytoblasts	0.1-1.0		
Lymphocytes (all stages)	2.7-24	16	49
Megakaryocytes	0.03-0.5	0.1	0.05
Plasmacytes	0.1-1.5	0.4	0.02
Promyelocytes	0.5-8.0	1.4	0.76
Reticulum cells	0.1-2.0		
Undifferentiated cells	0.0-0.1		
Neutrophils, total	56.5	57.1	32.4
Metamyelocytes	9.6-24.6	23.3	11.3
Neutrophilic	10-32		
Eosinophilic	0.3-3.7		
Basophilic	0-0.3		
Monocytes (all stages)	0-2.7		
Myeloblasts	0.1-5.0	1.2	0.62
Myelocytes	4.2-15	18.4	2.5
Neutrophilic	5.0-20		
Eosinophilic	0.1-3.0		
Basophilic	0-0.5		
Segmented granulocytes	6.0-12.0	12.9	3.6
Neutrophilic	7.0-30		
Eosinophilic	0.2-4.0		
Basophilic	0-0.7		
Band cells	9.5-15.3	0	14.1
Neutrophilic	10-35		
Eosinophilic	0.2-2.0		
Basophilic	0-0.3		

Continued

Differential Cell Count—cont'd

	ADULT (%)	CHILD (%)	INFANT (%)
Erythroid series			
Normoblasts, total	25.6	23.1	8.0
Pronormoblasts	0.2-4.0	0.5	0.1
Basophilic normoblasts	1.5-5.8	1.7	0.34
Polychromatophilic normoblasts	5.0-26.4	18.2	6.9
Orthochromic normoblasts	3.6-21	2.7	0.54
Promegaloblasts	0		
Basophilic megaloblasts	0		
Polychromatic megaloblasts	0		
Orthochromic megaloblasts	0		

M:E Ratio. (The myeloid:erythroid ratio is the ratio of white blood cells to nucleated red blood cells.)

Adult	6:1-2:1
Birth	1.85:1
2 weeks	11:1
1-2 months	5.5:1
1-20 years	2.95:1

Usage. Helps to distinguish primary and metastatic tumors. Assists in the identification, classification, and staging of neoplasias. Aids evaluation of the progress or response to the treatment of neoplasias. Assists in the definitive diagnosis of blood disorders. Culture of an aspirated sample can aid in the identification of infections such as histoplasmosis or tuberculosis. Histologic examination aids in the diagnosis of carcinoma, granulomas, lymphoma, or myelofibrosis. Iron stain showing decreased hemosiderin levels may indicate iron deficiency or malnutrition from anorexia nervosa and SBB stain differentiates acute granulocytic leukemia from acute lymphocytic leukemia.

Increased Eosinophils. Bone marrow carcinoma, eosinophilic leukemia, hypereosinophilic syndrome, lymphadenoma, myeloid leukemia, and pernicious anemia (relapse).

Increased Lymphocytes. Aplastic anemia, hypoplasia of the bone marrow, infectious lymphocytosis or mononucleosis, lymphatic leukemoid reactions, lymphocytic leukemia (B-cell and T-cell), lymphoma, macroglobulinemia, myelofibrosis, and viral infections.

Increased Megakaryocytes. Acute hemorrhage, aging, chronic myeloid leukemia, hypersplenism, idiopathic thrombocytopenia, infection, megakaryocytic myelosis, myelofibrosis, pneumonia, polycythemia vera, and thrombocytopenia.

Increased Plasma Cells. Agranulocytosis, amyloidosis, aplastic anemia, carcinomatosis, collagen disease, hepatic cirrhosis, Hodgkin's disease, hypersensitivity reactions, infection, irradiation, macroglobulinemia, malignant tumor, multiple myeloma, rheumatic fever (acute), rheumatoid arthritis, serum sickness, syphilis, and ulcerative colitis.

Increased Granulocyte. Hypoplasia of the bone marrow, infections, myelocytic leukemia, myelocytic leukemoid reaction, and myeloproliferative syndrome.

Increased Normoblasts. Anemia (iron deficiency, hemolytic, megaloblastic), blood loss (chronic), erythema, erythroid-type myeloproliferative disorders, hypoplasia of the bone marrow, and polycythemia vera.

Increased M:E Ratio above 7:1. Decreased hematopoiesis, erythroid hypoplasia, infection, leukemoid reactions, and myeloid leukemia.

Increased Diffuse Bone Marrow Hyperplasia. Myeloproliferative syndromes and pancytopenia reactions.

Decreased Megakaryocytes. Anemia (aplastic, pernicious), bone marrow hyperplasia (with carcinomatous or leukemic deposits), cirrhosis, irradiation (excessive), and thrombocytopenia purpura. Drugs include benzene, chlorothiazides, and cytotoxic drugs.

Decreased Granulocyte. Agranulocytosis, barbiturate coma, hyperplasia of the bone marrow, and ionizing radiation.

Decreased Normoblasts. Anemia (aplastic, hypoplastic), folic acid or vitamin B_{12} (cyanocobalamin) deficiency.

Decreased M:E Ratio below 2:1. Agranulocytosis, anemia (iron deficiency, normoblastic, pernicious, posthemolytic, posthemorrhagic), erythroid activity (increased), hepatic disease, myeloid formation (decreased), polycythemia vera, sprue, and steatorrhea.

Decreased Diffuse Bone Marrow Hypoplasia. Aging, cellular infiltrations, dengue fever, hepatitis C virus, myelofibrosis, myelosclerosis, myelotoxic agents, osteoporosis, rubella, and viral infections.

Description. Bone marrow is the soft, organic, spongelike material contained in the medullary cavities, long bones, and some haversian canals and within the spaces between trabeculae of cancellous bone. It is composed of red and yellow marrow, with the chief function being production of erythrocytes, leukocytes, and platelets. Only the rusty, red marrow produces blood cells. The yellow marrow is formed of connective tissue and fat cells, which are inactive. During infancy and childhood, bone marrow is primarily red marrow, but, in the adult, 50% is red marrow. The bone marrow aspiration procedure is a way to obtain a sample of bone marrow by needle. A stained blood smear of the sample is evaluated for bone marrow morphology and examination of blood cell erythropoiesis, cellularity, differential cell count, bone marrow iron stores, and M:E ratios. This test is used mainly in the diagnosis and management of anemia, fever, leukemia, lymphoma, pancytopenia, and thrombocytopenia.

Professional Considerations
1. Consent form IS required.

Risks
Bleeding, heart damage (with sternal biopsy), hemorrhage, infection, and meningitis.

Contraindications
Bone marrow aspiration is contraindicated in hemophilia, hemostasis, and coagulation defects.

2. **Preparation:**
   A. Obtain a bone marrow aspiration tray, laboratory slides and stains, and a lavender-topped or green-topped tube.
   B. Obtain a sterile container of Zenker's acetic acid solution if a bone marrow biopsy is to be performed.
   C. Pain medication may be given to lessen procedure discomfort.
3. **Procedure:**
   A. The most common sites for bone marrow aspiration include the sternum (preferred for bone marrow biopsy), the posterior superior iliac spine (for needle biopsy), and the anterior iliac crest and vertebral spinous process in the adult. For infants under 18 months, the anterior tibia site is used, and for children, the iliac crest is preferred.
   B. The designated site is prepped, shaved, and draped. After a local anesthetic is injected and under sterile technique, a $\frac{1}{8}$-inch stab wound is made. A Jamshidi needle with the stylet in place is inserted until the outer surface of the bone is impinged. The needle guard is engaged, and the outer needle is inserted with a boring motion, about 3 mm deep, into the bone marrow cavity.
   C. *For bone marrow aspiration:* The stylet is removed, and a 10-mL syringe is attached to the needle. When aspiration of 0.2 to 0.5 mL of bone marrow has entered the syringe, it is removed and given to a technician for preparation of a stained blood smear. A second syringe may be attached and a 2-mL sample of bone marrow withdrawn and placed into a lavender-topped tube containing EDTA or a heparinized green-topped tube.
   D. *For bone marrow biopsy:* The stylet is removed, and a biopsy or inner needle with a trephine tip is inserted. A tissue plug is removed and placed into a container of Zenker's acetic acid solution.
   E. The needle is withdrawn.
4. **Postprocedure care:**
   A. Apply a pressure dressing to the bone marrow aspiration site.

B. Observe the aspiration site for bleeding.
5. **Client and family teaching:**
  A. Bone marrow aspiration is painful but only for a few moments. Pre-procedure pain medicine may be used to lessen the discomfort. It is also normal to experience a deep pressure feeling as the bone marrow is withdrawn.
  B. It is important to lie very still during the procedure.
  C. Results are normally available within 24-72 hours.
  D. Call the physician if there are signs of infection at the procedure site: increasing pain, redness, swelling, or purulent drainage, or for fever >101°F (>38.3° C).
6. **Factors that affect results:**
  A. Cytotoxic drugs, folic acid, iron, liver or vitamin B_{12} agents, and recent blood transfusions should be noted before the biopsy.
  B. Chloramphenicol causes higher frequency (90%) of marrow hypocellularity.
  C. Send the specimen to the laboratory immediately.
7. **Other data:**
  A. The presence of normal bone marrow at one site does not eliminate the possibility of disease elsewhere in the bone marrow.
  B. Normal M:E ratio may be associated with aplastic anemia, myeloma, and myelosclerosis.

BONE MARROW BIOPSY, DIAGNOSTIC
(*see Bone marrow aspiration analysis, Specimen*)

BONE MARROW IRON STAIN
(*see Bone marrow aspiration analysis, Specimen*)

BONE MARROW SCAN, DIAGNOSTIC

Norm. Even concentration of the radionuclide throughout the reticuloendothelial system, red blood cells, and bone marrow.

Usage. Assists in the diagnosis of defects in bone marrow or bone marrow depression after chemotherapy or radiation, in the differential determinations of myeloproliferative disorders and with increased pulmonary uptake consideration of pneumocystis carinii pneumonia. Differentiates acute from chronic hemolysis and bone infarction from osteomyelitis in sickle cell disease. Aids in the selection of bone marrow biopsy sites and in the staging of Hodgkin's disease, lymphomas, and metastatic diseases of the bone marrow. Assists in evaluation of hyperplasia of the bone marrow associated with chronic hemolytic anemia and polycythemia vera.

Description. The bone marrow scan is a nuclear medicine study in which the radionuclide indium chloride is administered intravenously and followed by radiographic imaging of the entire body. This scan can be nonspecific in conditions of diffuse disease such as osteomyelitis and tumor. However, areas of increased vascularity and hyperproliferation of bone marrow can be demonstrated much earlier with a bone marrow scan than by conventional radiography.

Professional Considerations
1. Consent form IS required.

Risks
Hematoma at injection site.

Precautions
During pregnancy, risks of cumulative radiation exposure to the fetus from this and other previous or future imaging studies must be weighed against the benefits of the procedure. Although formal limits for client exposure are relative to this risk-benefit comparison, the United States Nuclear Regulatory Commission requires that the cumulative dose equivalent to an embryo/fetus from *occupational* exposure not exceed 0.5 rem (5 mSv). Radiation dose to the fetus is proportional to the distance of the anatomy studied from the abdomen and decreases as pregnancy progresses. For pregnant clients, consult the Radiologist/Radiology Department to obtain estimated fetal radiation exposure from this procedure.

Contraindications
Pregnancy or during breast-feeding.

B

2. **Preparation:**
   A. The client should void before the procedure.
   B. Have emergency equipment readily available.
3. **Procedure:**
   A. The radionuclide indium chloride is administered intravenously.
   B. Whole-body imaging is planned for 48 hours after intravenous injection.
   C. If the radioisotope ^{99m}Tc-sulfur colloid is given, the scan can be completed 1 hour after the intravenous injection.
4. **Postprocedure care:**
   A. None.
5. **Client and family teaching:**
   A. Notify the physician for previous reaction to radionuclide.
   B. An IV tube may be inserted for the scan and removed after the scan is complete. Some technicians may use direct venipuncture for the injection.
   C. Results are normally available within 24 hours.
   D. In women who are breast-feeding, formula should be substituted for breast milk for 1 or more days after the procedure.
6. **Factors that affect results:**
   A. None found.
7. **Other data:**
   A. Health care professionals working in a nuclear medicine area must follow federal standards set by the Nuclear Regulatory Commission. These standards include precautions for handling the radioactive material and monitoring of potential radiation exposure.
   B. Indium scan is positive in 20-30% of clients after other imaging methods failed to detect metastasis.

BONE SCAN (BONE SCINTIGRAPHY), DIAGNOSTIC

Norm. Even concentration of radioactive isotope throughout the osseous tissues.

Usage. Detection, staging, and evaluation of osseous metastatic disease. Detection of pathologic conditions that cause increased uptake, including acute haematogenous osteomyelitis (AHOM), aseptic necrosis, bone fractures, bone infarction, bone infection, bone metastasis, bone necrosis, bone tumors, bone trauma, osseous metastatic disease, osteoarthritis, osteoid osteoma, osteomyelitis, Paget's disease, renal osteodystrophy, temporomandibular joint disease, transient osteoporosis, tuberculosis, and soft-tissue calcification. Differentiation of cellulitis from osteomyelitis. Monitoring of degenerative bone disorders, bone grafts, and prosthetic joint replacements. Aids in the selection of a biopsy site in the abnormal bone, in the evaluation of the effectiveness of arthritides, and in suspected abuse of a child.

Description. A nuclear medicine radioactive isotope study that will show bone changes from a few weeks up to 6 months before conventional radiographs will show such changes. Diagnostic sensitivity is 95.2% and accuracy 78.7%. The radioactive isotope ^{99m}Tc-diphosphonate (technetium diphosphate) is administered intravenously. As the entire body is scanned, images from the low-level radioactive isotope in the bony tissues are recorded on paper or film, creating two-dimensional images of the skeletal outlines. The epiphyses of growing bones or new bone formation shows up as areas of high metabolism, or concentration, and are called "hot spots," whereas areas of low concentration, associated with ischemia or tumor displacement, are referred to as "cold spots." Increased uptake of the isotope by bone tissue indicates an abnormality in that area. There is a phenomenon called bone scan flare, which shows an increase in bone lesions with improvement while the client is receiving chemotherapy for either breast or small-cell lung or non-small-cell lung cancers. Bone scintigraphy is especially important in detecting metastatic tumors and fractures not immediately seen on radiograph, especially in the spine, ribs, face, and small bones of the hands and feet. This test is invaluable in evaluating clients with osteomyelitis. Its disadvantage is that when it shows an abnormality, it is nonspecific as to the pathologic process present.

Professional Considerations
1. Consent form NOT required.

Risks
Hematoma at injection site.

Contraindications
Clients who cannot lie still for an extended period of time.

Precautions
During pregnancy, risks of cumulative radiation exposure to the fetus from this and other previous or future imaging studies must be weighed against the benefits of the procedure. Although formal limits for client exposure are relative to this risk-benefit comparison, the United States Nuclear Regulatory Commission requires that the cumulative dose equivalent to an embryo/fetus from *occupational* exposure not exceed 0.5 rem (5 mSv). Radiation dose to the fetus is proportional to the distance of the anatomy studied from the abdomen and decreases as pregnancy progresses. For pregnant clients, consult the Radiologist/Radiology Department to obtain estimated fetal radiation exposure from this procedure.

2. **Preparation:**
   A. The client should not drink unnecessary fluids for 2-4 hours.
   B. Obtain an alcohol wipe, a tourniquet, a needle, a syringe, and a radioactive isotope.
   C. Remove all jewelry and metal objects.
   D. Sedatives are used only if the client is unable to lie still for the scan.
   E. The client should void before the intravenous radioisotope is administered.
3. **Procedure:**
   A. ^{99m}Tc-diphosphonate (technetium diphosphate) is administered intravenously into a vein of the arm.
   B. During the next 2-3 hours, the client must drink 32 ounces of water to promote renal filtering of excess tracer.
   C. The client should void just before the scan to remove any tracer not picked up by bone that was filtered by the kidney.
   D. 1-3 hours after the injection, the client is placed in a supine position on the scanning table and instructed to lie still while the entire body is scanned and two-dimensional images of the skeleton are recorded.

4. **Postprocedure care:**
   A. If deep sedation was used, follow institutional protocol for postsedation monitoring. Typical monitoring includes continuous ECG monitoring and pulse oximetry, with continual assessments (every 5-15 minutes) of airway, vital signs, and neurologic status until the client is lying quietly awake, is breathing independently, and responds appropriately to commands spoken in a normal tone. The client should not operate a motor vehicle for 24 hours after receiving sedation.
   B. Check the injection site for redness or swelling. If a hematoma is present, apply warm soaks.
   C. Encourage oral fluid intake.
5. **Client and family teaching:**
   A. The radioisotope delivers less radiation than a regular radiograph, and the scanning machine is detecting the injected isotope, rather than exposing him or her to radiation.
   B. Do not drink fluids for 4 hours before the scan.
   C. The radioisotope will be injected intravenously before the scan.
   D. Most of the radioactive material will be excreted from the body through urine and stool within 48 hours and is not harmful to other people nearby.
   E. Results are normally available within 24 hours.
   F. In women who are breast-feeding, formula should be substituted for breast milk for 1 or more days after the procedure.
6. **Factors that affect results:**
   A. Failure to void before the test may cause an over distended urinary bladder, which can interfere with pelvic imaging.
7. **Other data:**
   A. Health care professionals working in a nuclear medicine area must follow federal standards set by the Nuclear Regulatory Commission. These standards include precautions for handling the radioactive material and monitoring of potential radiation exposure.
   B. 32% of bone scans give false-positive results for persons with T1 or T2 breast cancer.

C. Routine bone scans are not warranted in clients with squamous cell carcinoma of the head and neck.

BONE RADIOGRAPHY, DIAGNOSTIC

Norm. Negative.

Usage. Identification of abnormal growth patterns by serial radiography. Detection of ankylosing spondylitis, congenital abnormalities, fractures, healing fractures, hyperparathyroidism, infection, joint destruction, osteomalacia, osteomyelitis, osteoporosis, the presence of joint fluid, rickets, and tumors.

Description. Specific bones are radiographed in several positions for visualization of the bone from all angles. Sensitivity is 56% in bone stress injuries, specificity 94% and accuracy 67% (Kiuru MJ et al, 2002).

Professional Considerations
1. Consent form NOT required.

Precautions
During pregnancy, risks of cumulative radiation exposure to the fetus from this and other previous or future imaging studies must be weighed against the benefits of the procedure. Although formal limits for client exposure are relative to this risk-benefit comparison, the United States Nuclear Regulatory Commission requires that the cumulative dose equivalent to an embryo/fetus from *occupational* exposure not exceed 0.5 rem (5 mSv). Radiation dose to the fetus is proportional to the distance of the anatomy studied from the abdomen and decreases as pregnancy progresses. For pregnant clients, consult the Radiologist/Radiology Department to obtain estimated fetal radiation exposure from this procedure.

2. Preparation:
   A. Handle injured parts carefully.
   B. Shield the client's testes, ovaries, or pregnant abdomen.
3. Procedure:
   A. The client is placed on the radiography table in several positions, with a radiograph taken in each position.

B. The client must lie still for the radiograph.
4. Postprocedure care:
   A. The client remains in the radiology department until it is determined that the films are satisfactory.
5. Client and family teaching:
   A. The amount of exposure to radiation is minimal and not dangerous.
   B. It is important to stay still during the radiograph.
   C. Results are normally available within 24 hours.
6. Factors that affect results:
   A. Movement results in an unsatisfactory radiograph.
   B. Too little or too much exposure results in a radiograph that is too light or too dark and may need to be repeated for interpretation.
7. Other data:
   A. Wear a lead apron if remaining in the room with the client during radiography.

BONE SCINTIGRAPHY, DIAGNOSTIC
(*see Bone scan, Diagnostic*)

BONE ULTRASONOMETRY, DIAGNOSTIC

Norm. The lower the T-score, the greater the risk for fracture.
T-score ≤1.0 = Low bone mass, at increased risk for fracture.

Usage. This test is used to determine a qualitative ultrasound measurement of the calcaneus. This along with clinical factors is used to assist in determining osteoporosis, primary hyperparathyroidism, risk for fracture, and type I Gaucher's disease.

Description. This procedure uses a ultrasonometer to measure bone density of the heel and identify bone fragility and risk for osteoporosis. The ultrasonometer is an ultrasound device that measures the speed of sound and broadband ultrasonic attenuation of an ultrasound beam passed through the heel. The process determines a quantitative ultrasound index (QUI), expressed as a T-score and an estimate of the bone mineral density (BMD in g/cm^2) of the heel. Ultrasonographic bone densitometry of the heel is most useful as a screening tool. It is not recommended for frequent monitoring of response to osteoporosis treatment because the heel does not respond quickly to treatment. A 3-year interval is recommended by the manufacturer as necessary to identify improvement. Other methods of bone density testing should be used if more frequent monitoring is needed. (Test below is based on information available for the Sahara Clinical Bone Sonometer approved by the FDA in 1998. At least 15 commercial systems are available.)

Professional Considerations
1. Consent form NOT required.

Risks
None.

Contraindications
The Sahara should not be used in clients whose skin is abraded or have an open sore in an area that comes in contact with the system.

2. Preparation:
   A. The client must remove shoes and socks or stockings.
3. Procedure:
   A. If the test has been performed in the past, select the same foot for testing.
   B. The client's heel is covered with Sahara Coupling Gel and then rested against the ultrasonometer.
4. Postprocedure care:
   A. Remove gel from heel.
5. Client and family teaching:
   A. The test takes only a few seconds, and results are available during the same visit.
   B. No x rays or radiation is involved.
   C. *T-Score (−2.5 to −4.0)*
      i. Treatment is usually indicated in this range.
      ii. Treatment is almost always indicated if there has been an osteoporotic fracture.
   D. *T-Score (−0.5 to −2.5)*
      Treatment may be indicated in this range if:
      i. A family history of osteoporosis.
      ii. History of smoking.
      iii. Underweight or have experienced a weight loss.

      iv. The range is close to a −2.5 T score.
      v. There is a likelihood of bone loss.
   E. *T-Score (+1.0 and above)*
      i. Values in this range are good. Continue to maintain a healthy life-style, exercise and eat a good diet.
   F. With extra risk factors consider a baseline DEXA scan.
6. Factors that affect results:
   A. Sahara Coupling Gel should be used as directed, and no other gels should be substituted because water-based gels have been associated with coupling delays.
   B. Avoid measuring bone density on a foot or limb that has had a recent reduction in use because of immobilization, fracture, etc.
7. Other data:
   A. Although ultrasound bone sonometry allows one to predict the risk of hip fracture in elderly females almost as well as dual-energy x-ray absorptiometry (DXA) does, the latter is considered the standard of comparison often used for measuring bone density.
   B. Testing can be done in a physician's office. Medicare reimbursement is not available for this test because of its designation as a screening test.

BORDETELLA PERTUSSIS, CULTURE

Norm. No growth.

Usage. Diagnosis of pertussis (whooping cough).

Description. Pertussis is a highly communicable, acute bacterial infection of the tracheobronchial tree caused by *Bordetella pertussis,* a gram-negative coccobacillus. The disease occurs commonly in children throughout the world and can be prevented in 99.8% of cases by vaccination of 3 doses of DTaP (diphtheria, tetanus and acellular pertussis) vaccine. Mode of transmission is believed to be either direct contact with the respiratory discharges of infected clients or by inhalation of airborne droplets. It is most communicable in the early stages, before the paroxysmal cough appears. Pertussis is characterized by an explosive cough, followed by a "whooping" sound on inspiration and may include respiratory distress and apnea as symptoms. Pertussis can lead to CNS encephalopathy and pulmonary hypertension, and there are known cases of reinfection up to 12 years after initial diagnosis.

Professional Considerations
1. Consent form NOT required.
2. **Preparation:**
   A. Wear mask and gloves when collecting the specimen.
   B. Obtain a culture tube, flexible wire swab, penlight, and tongue blade or "cough plate."
3. **Procedure:**
   A. Obtain a sterile swab of the nasopharynx or have the client cough onto a cough plate held in front of his or her mouth.
   B. To obtain nasopharyngeal swab:
      i. With the client's head tilted back, use a penlight and tongue depressor to visualize the nasopharynx.
      ii. Gently pass the swab through the nostril and into the nasopharynx, keeping the swab near the septum and floor of the nose.
      iii. Rotate the swab quickly and remove it carefully, making sure it does not touch the tongue or the sides of the nostril.
4. **Postprocedure care:**
   A. Hand-deliver the specimen to the laboratory immediately.
   B. Inform laboratory personnel if pertussis is suspected because a special growth medium is required.
5. **Client and family teaching:**
   A. Observe for signs of pertussis in other children who were in contact with the infected child and who were not immunized.
   B. Therapy may begin before culture results are supplied.
   C. In the absence of antibiotic therapy, the period of communicability is considered to be from 7 days after exposure to 3 weeks after the paroxysmal cough appears. With erythromycin treatment, the period of communicability extends 7 days after the treatment is initiated.
   D. Results are normally available within 72 hours.

6. **Factors that affect results:**
   A. An insufficient specimen or current antibiotic therapy may cause false-negative results.
7. **Other data:**
   A. Immunization is available for pertussis prevention. Oral administration of rotavirus vaccine can be given with DTP and oral administration of polio vaccine without interference to children at 2, 4, and 6 months of age.
   B. Resistance to erythromycin can occur and alternatives for treatment include clarithromycin, azithromycin, trimethoprimsulfamethoxazole or the newer fluoroquinolones, such as gatifloxacin.
   C. A preliminary report should be available in 24 hours.

BORRELIA BURGDORFERI C6 PEPTIDE ANTIBODY, SERUM

Norm.

Usage. Definitive testing for active Lyme disease; Should be used in place of Lyme disease IgG and IgM antibody testing for those who are suspected of recurrent Lyme disease, or who have been vaccinated for Lyme disease in the past. Differentiation of symptoms of Lyme disease from *B. burgdorferi* vaccine-related side-effects.

Description. See *Lyme disease antibody, Blood for a description of Lyme disease.* This blood test identifies the C6 glycoprotein, a newly discovered peptide, which is part of the variable antigen VlsE[1,2]. C6 is important because it can definitively confirm active infection with *Borrelia burgdorferi*, the causative agent of Lyme disease, even in those who have previously had the disease or been vaccinated for it. In this group of people, the active disease could be present, but traditional IgG and IgM antibody testing could indicate immunity. This is because the antibodies can remain present for up to 20 years after the acute disease resolves in those who previously had Lyme disease, yet the person can become reinfected. In addition, 25% of people vaccinated for Lyme disease fail to develop enough OpsA antibodies for active immunity. It is the OpsA antibodies that cause the false-positive results on traditional tests. Because the C6 peptide does not target OpsA antibodies for measurement, it is ideal for definitive testing.

Professional Considerations
1. Consent form IS required.
2. **Preparation:**
   A. Tube: Red topped, red/gray topped, or gold topped.
3. **Procedure:**
   A. Draw a 3-mL blood sample.
4. **Postprocedure care:**
   A. Separate serum and freeze until testing.
5. **Client and family teaching:**
   A. No fasting or special preparation is required.
6. **Factors that affect results:**
   A. None.
7. **Other data:**
   A. The trade name for this test is the *Borrelia burgdorferi* C6 Peptide Antibody DetectR™.

BOTULISM, DIAGNOSTIC PROCEDURES, STOOL

Norm. Negative culture.

Usage. To diagnose the presence of *Clostridium botulinum or baratti* (Harvey et al, 2002) in the culture of feces.

Botulism Symptoms and Emergency Treatment

Symptoms. Afebrile, diarrhea, dizziness, double or blurred vision, dysarthria, dysphagia, fatigue, gastrointestinal pain, headache, hypotonia, nausea, weakness, vomiting. Cardiac and respiratory paralysis is possible.

Treatment:
Note: Treatment choice(s) depend on client history and condition and episode history.
1. Establish IV access.
2. Administer trivalent botulism antitoxin (Connaught Laboratories, Ltd.) (*Note:* Anaphylaxis is possible if the antitoxin is given to clients with asthma, hay fever, horse or horse serum allergies, or past exposure to horse serum.)
3. Follow package insert instructions for sensitivity testing before antitoxin administration.
4. Induce vomiting (with extreme caution) with syrup of ipecac, if the syrup can be given soon after the ingestion of the contaminated food. (Induction of emesis is contraindicated in clients with no gag reflex or with central nervous system depression or excitation.)
5. Use gastric lavage if emesis does not produce the contaminated food.
6. Give activated charcoal slurry.
7. Give saline cathartic solution if no ileus is present.
8. Monitor for respiratory decompensation, which may occur suddenly in clients with botulism. Elective intubation is advisable for large ingestions.
9. Notify the state health department and the Centers for Disease Control and Prevention (CDC) 404-639-2206. The after-hours medical emergency number is 404-639-2888.

Description. Botulism is a severe food poisoning resulting from the ingestion of the bacterial endotoxins of *Clostridium botulinum* or *Clostridium baratti*. The exotoxin from *C. botulinum* exerts central nervous system actions and may lead quickly to death if an antidote is not administered before the onset of neurologic symptoms. Botulism most frequently occurs in home-canned food that has not been sufficiently heated during the canning process or food left at room temperature for days such as foil-wrapped baked potatoes. It is often acquired in infants from ingestion of soil or honey.

Professional Considerations
1. Consent form NOT required.
2. **Preparation:**
   A. Obtain a sterile specimen container.
3. **Procedure:**
   A. Collect a stool specimen directly into a sterile, wide-mouthed, waxed container with a tight-fitting lid. Be sure there is no urine or paper in the specimen.
   B. If a stool specimen is not readily available, a rectal swab may be substituted. Insert a sterile microbio-

logic swab into the rectum and leave in place for 10 seconds. Remove the swab and send it to the laboratory in a culture container.

4. Postprocedure care:
   A. Properly seal the container to avoid leakage and contamination of others.
   B. Refrigerate the specimen if it cannot be sent immediately to the laboratory.
5. Client and family teaching:
   A. Avoid contaminating the stool with urine or toilet paper.
   B. Botulism may be prevented by cooking foods sufficiently to inactivate the toxins.
   C. An antitoxin is available for botulism.
   D. If activated charcoal was given for elevated levels, the client should drink 4-6 glasses of water each day for 2 days to prevent constipation. The activated charcoal will also cause stools to be black for a few days.
   E. Results are normally available within 72 hours.
6. Factors that affect results:
   A. Specimens not refrigerated invalidate the results.
7. Other data:
   A. In infant botulism, the organism and the toxin can be found in the bowel contents but not in serum. The presence of the toxin can be demonstrated by injection of mice with 0.4 mL of the suspected food, the client's fecal extract, and his or her serum. The presence of toxin results in flaccid paralysis within 24 hours and death within 3 days.
   B. The treatment for botulism is to give an antitoxin. However, the antitoxin inactivates only unbound toxins.
   C. See also *Clostridial toxin, Serum*.

BRAIN BIOPSY, DIAGNOSTIC

Norm. Normal tissue.

Usage. Confirmation of Alzheimer's disease, cerebral amyloid angiopathy, cerebral blastomycosis, cerebral Whipple's disease, Creutzfeldt-Jakob disease, encephalitis, granulomatous angiitis, HIV complications, identification and classification of tumors of the brain or metastasis to the brain, neuronal ceroid lipofuscinosis.

Description. Specimens of brain tissue are obtained during a craniotomy and sent to the pathology laboratory. The electron microscope is used to identify and classify tumors for more accurate diagnosis, on which proper therapy and prognosis depend. The pathologist may also examine the specimen for antigen localization, which identifies the cell of origin of the antigen. This identifies the origin of metastatic carcinoma.

Professional Considerations
1. Consent form IS required.

Risks
Blindness, cerebrovascular accident, headache, hemorrhage (silent after stereotactic brain biopsy), infection, meningitis, paralysis.

Contraindications
Anticoagulant therapy, bleeding disorders, increased intracranial pressure.

2. Preparation:
   A. Obtain a specimen container.
   B. Arrange for immediate handling of the specimen in pathology department.
3. Procedure:
   A. A fresh specimen of brain tissue is placed into a plastic container with saline-moistened, sterile gauze and given to the pathologist who is in the operating room or waiting in the laboratory for the immediate delivery of the specimen.
   B. If immediate preparation of the specimen by the pathologist is not possible, the specimen is immediately cut into 1-mm cubes and placed into a vial of 2%-4% phosphate, cacodylate-buffered glutaraldehyde, paraformaldehyde, or other fixative, according to the policy of the institution.
4. Postprocedure care:
   A. Tailor care to the procedure used to gain access to the brain tissue.
5. Client and family teaching:
   A. Results are normally available within 24 hours.
6. Factors that affect results:
   A. The specimen must be fresh.
   B. Placing the specimen in formalin, in the wrong fixative, or taking more than 2-3 minutes to place it in the fixative after collection invalidates the results.

C. If antigen localization is done, the antisera must be available.

7. **Other data:**
   A. Brain scans are usually performed before surgery to assist in specific localization of the tumor for biopsy.

BRAIN ECHOGRAM
(see Brain ultrasonography, Diagnostic)

BRAIN NATRIURETIC PEPTIDE, PLASMA
(see Natriuretic peptides, Plasma)

BRAIN SCAN, CEREBRAL FLOW AND PATHOLOGY, DIAGNOSTIC

Norm. Negative.

Usage. Abscess of the brain, brain ischemia, brain tumors, contusions, cerebral vascular accidents, hematomas, and causes of seizures. Posttraumatic stress disorder.

Description. A nuclear medicine scan of the brain after the intravenous injection of a radioactive isotope. An immediate scan after the injection will show changes in the cerebral blood flow from one side of the brain compared to the other side. A later scan will show pathogenic tissue, which has a greater concentration of the isotope present than normal tissue has. This method of brain scanning has largely been replaced by newer, faster, and better quality SPECT scanning.

Professional Considerations
1. Consent form IS required.

Risks
Infection.

Contraindications
Pregnancy and in clients who cannot lie still for an extended length of time.

2. **Preparation:**
   A. Potassium chloride capsules are given 2 hours before the isotope injection to prevent an inordinate amount of the isotope uptake in the choroid plexus. Too much uptake in the choroid plexus would simulate a pathologic condition in the cerebrum.

3. **Procedure:**
   A. The client is placed in a supine position on the scanning table with the isotope scanner in position over the head.
   B. The radioactive isotope is injected into a vein in the arm, and the scan is started immediately for the study of cervical flow.
   C. The scan is repeated 1 hour later to detect the presence of pathogenic tissue.

4. **Postprocedure care:**
   A. Encourage the oral intake of fluids.

5. **Client and family teaching:**
   A. Most of the radioactive material will be excreted from the body through urine and stool within 48 hours and is not harmful to other persons nearby.
   B. Venous access will be necessary.
   C. Results are normally available within 24 hours.

6. **Factors that affect results:**
   A. None found.

7. **Other data:**
   A. Health care professionals working in a nuclear medicine area must follow federal standards set by the Nuclear Regulatory Commission. These standards include precautions for handling the radioactive material and monitoring of potential radiation exposure.
   B. See also *Single-photon emission computed tomography (SPECT scan), Brain, Diagnostic.*

BRAIN ULTRASONOGRAPHY (BRAIN ECHOGRAM, BRAIN ULTRASOUND, ECHOENCEPHALOGRAM), DIAGNOSTIC

Norm. Normal position of the brain's midline structures and normal blood-flow velocity.

Usage. Diagnosis of brain deformities in newborns and infants, Leigh syndrome, space-occupying lesions, structural shifts caused by cerebral edema, subdural hematoma, or extradural hematoma. Determination of viability of brain tissue based on the sequential measurement of blood flow velocity. Brain ultrasonograms can also be used for early detection of cerebral ischemia during a carotid endarterectomy while cerebral blood flow is interrupted. Ventriculomegaly.

Description. An ultrasound beam is transmitted through the skull. The time required for the beam to be reflected back to the transducer is converted to an electrical impulse displayed on an oscilloscope screen and measured to determine the structure, position, and blood flow of the brain. A shift in the third ventricle of more than 3 mm from midline is abnormal. An enlargement of the third ventricle of more than 10 mm in the adult or of more than 7 mm in the child is abnormal.

Professional Considerations
1. Consent form NOT required.
2. Preparation:
    A. Remove jewelry and metal objects from the client's head and neck.
    B. Obtain ultrasonic gel or paste.
3. Procedure:
    A. The client is placed in a supine position.
    B. A small transducer, with water-soluble paste applied to it, is placed on the side of the head over the temporoparietal region.
    C. Ultrasonic beams are sent into the head, and their reflection is recorded on the oscilloscope and photographed.
4. Postprocedure care:
    A. Cleanse the paste from the scalp.
5. Client and family teaching:
    A. Do not drink hot or cold caffeine-containing beverages on the morning of the test.
    B. It is normal to hear an echo that sounds like repetitious humming or a musical note as the brain structures reflect the ultrasonic beam.
    C. This procedure takes approximately 1 hour.
    D. Results are normally available within 24 hours.
6. Factors that affect results:
    A. Failure to remove jewelry and metal objects from the head and neck will interfere with the clarity of the oscilloscope pictures.
7. Other data:
    A. Follow-up studies using computed tomographic scan or radionucleotides may be indicated.
    B. Enlarged fourth ventricle is a physiologic variant in early fetal life of 14-16 weeks.

BRAIN ULTRASOUND
(*see Brain ultrasonography, Diagnostic*)

BRAINSTEM AUDITORY-EVOKED POTENTIAL (BAEP), DIAGNOSTIC

Norm. Morphologically normal waveform activity generated by electrical response to auditory stimulation.

Usage. Employed as an adjunct in the diagnosis of neurologic hearing deficits or children with language impairments, in the diagnosis and treatment of migraines, acoustic neuromas, chronic renal failure and tuberculous meningitis, and in the determination of brain death versus reversible coma.

Adults. May be prescribed to test the time required for nerve signals to travel from the ear to the brainstem.

Description. A series of rapid clicks is delivered through earphones applied to the client. The brainstem response (electrical potential activity) is recorded through electrodes applied to the client's head. This recording (a series of waveform activities) is then interpreted by a physician skilled in electroencephalography.

Professional Considerations
1. Consent form NOT required.
2. Preparation:
    A. The test is generally performed in a neurology clinic or neurology diagnostic area though portable test equipment is available and the test can be performed at the bedside.
    B. No pretest medication or preparation is required. The rationale behind the test should be explained to the client or family before the procedure.
3. Procedure:
    A. An electrode is placed on the scalp at the vertex, and a reference electrode is placed on the ear lobe.
    B. Headphones, which mask the auditory responses of the outer ear, are applied.
    C. Auditory stimulation occurs, and the brainstem response is recorded as waveform activity.
4. Postprocedure care:
    A. Electrodes and headset are removed. The client may require transport from the test area back to the nursing unit.

B. The test results are interpreted by the appropriate physician.

C. No other special postprocedure care is required.

5. **Client and family teaching:**

A. Occasionally this test is used to determine brain death or the possible reversibility of coma. In this situation close contact with the family by all members of the health care delivery team and the provision of emotional and educational support is essential.

B. Parental teaching is important when the test is used to determine the presence of neural hearing loss in infants and children.

6. **Factors that affect results:**

A. Experience of the physician interpreting the results.

B. Proper function of the acoustic and recording equipment.

7. **Other data:**

A. There has been developed a variation of this technique in which direct application of the recording electrodes to the brainstem is accomplished during neurosurgery to direct certain neurosurgical procedures.

BRAZELTON NEONATAL BEHAVIORAL ASSESSMENT SCALE, DIAGNOSTIC

Norm. Normal reflexes and responses to stimulation in the newborn. Girls show higher levels of functioning when compared to boys in newborn infants of optimal health.

Usage. Evaluation of the newborn-caretaker unit to assess infant's behavior and responses to the environment and to provide recommendations for care giving and interactions. This test has been primarily used in the research arena, though it has been applied clinically to assess neurobehavioral functioning in full-term infants who were exposed to cocaine, is assessing tactile-kinesthetic stimulation in preterm infants.

Description. The newborn is administered the Neonatal Behavioral Assessment Scale (NBAS) multiple times in the first 10 days of life to study four levels of function of the neonate: physiologic, motor, state, and attentional/interac-tional. Function is determined by assessment of the response to 28 behavioral items with 7 supplementary items, all scored on a 9-point scale, and 18 reflex items, scored on a 4-point scale. The hypothesis is that a newborn's behavior is dependent on not only genetics but also intrauterine nutrition, infection, drug abuse, and perinatal events. All these factors contribute to a child's temperament and may explain why different babies respond to touch, sound, or visual stimuli in different ways. Once the child has been assessed, Brazelton believes that recommendations can be made how best to interact with that child by describing the behavioral strengths and weaknesses.

Professional Considerations

1. Consent form NOT required.

2. **Preparation:**

A. If the scale is to be used for research, training is required. Training takes up to several months, with renewal each 3 years. This is necessary for reliability of the test.

B. Obtain a manual, training handbook, examination video, and testing kit, which are available from the Brazelton Institute, 1295 Boylston St., Suite 320, Boston, MA 02215.

C. Obtain needed equipment: light, rattle, and bell.

D. Provide a quiet environment and dim lighting.

3. **Procedure:**

A. Using the scoring manual, the baby and caregiver are evaluated, and a score is given.

4. **Postprocedure care:**

A. None.

5. **Client and family teaching:**

A. The test is more accurate if a caretaker is available to interact with the neonate during the test.

B. The test takes about 30 minutes to perform.

C. Repetition improves the reliability of the test.

6. **Factors that affect results:**

A. The tester must be appropriately trained.

B. If neonate is crying, hungry, or sleepy, assessment may not be accurate.

7. **Other data:**

A. None.

BRCA TUMOR SUPPRESSOR GENES I AND 2, BLOOD

Norm. Negative

Usage. BRCA testing is completed to determine a client's genetic risk for breast or ovarian cancer.

Positive. Presence of BRCA1 or BRCA2 gene mutation(s).

Negative. Absence of BRCA1 or BRCA2 gene mutation(s).

Description. BRCA1 and BRCA2 are inherited breast cancer tumor suppressor genes, which can be recognized on the human genome. BRCA1 and BRCA2 are found on chromosomes 17 and 13, respectively. Inherited mutations of these genes have been found to be associated with an increased risk of familial breast and ovarian cancer occurrences. Carriers of BRCA1 mutations have an increased risk of ovarian cancer (epithelial or transitional cell) and microglandular adenosis and carriers of BRCA 2 are at increased risk for Fanconi's anemia and pancreatic cancer. Persons with BRCA1 and BRCA2 mutations have an increased risk of breast cancer. Manual direct sequencing or automated fluorescent sequencing of DNA can detect mutations of these genes.

Professional Considerations
1. Consent form IS required.
2. **Preparation:**
   A. Tube: Lavender topped
3. **Procedure:**
   A. Draw 10 mL blood sample.
   B. Send sample immediately to the laboratory.
4. **Postprocedure:**
   A. None
5. **Client and family teaching:**
   A. A complete family history, including first- and second-degree relatives before the test, should be taken.
   B. Genetic counseling is to be completed before and after testing.
   C. Affected relative(s) should be tested first to determine whether the mutation exists.
   D. Clients should be informed of any test limitations, possibilities for discovery of unrelated DNA findings including nonpaternity, treatment options, cost, and other emotional, legal, or insurance consequences of testing.
   E. Clients with a positive familial history of breast or ovarian cancer should be provided with education for prevention and early detection of breast or ovarian cancer regardless of their decision to undergo genetic testing for BRCA1 and BRCA2 gene mutation.
6. **Factors that affect results:**
   A. Clients receiving chemotherapy or radiation treatment should not be concurrently tested for BRCA1 or BRCA2. (Chemotherapy and radiation may alter DNA transcription.) The recommended waiting period for testing is 3-4 weeks after discontinuation of these treatment modalities or immediately before the next chemotherapy or radiation treatment course.
   B. In clients with a history of blood transfusion, a waiting period of 3 months after transfusion is suggested before testing.
7. **Other data:**
   A. Screening cost for BRCA1 and BRCA2 mutation is $2100 to $2600.

BREAST ULTRASONOGRAPHY (BREAST ECHOGRAM, BREAST ULTRASOUND), DIAGNOSTIC

Norm. Normal breast tissue boundaries demonstrate bright echo reflections. The nipple and skin reflections are higher than the areola echo reflection. Fat demonstrates low reflectivity, with a mixture of low and strong echoes, whereas connective tissue and ligaments are bright. Tumors and cysts are absent. the breasts of young women have less fatty tissue than the breasts of the women.

Usage. Detection of tiny breast tumors, differentiation of breast cysts from breast tumors less than $^{1}/_{4}$ inch in diameter; screening for breast abnormalities in low-risk clients or where mammography is not readily available; helpful for clients with radiographically dense breasts or breast prostheses or with extensive nodal involvement; and evaluation of symptomatic clients with breast inflammation or who are pregnant or lactating.

Description. A noninvasive test, with a sensitivity of 98.3% and specificity of 91.7%, in which a picture of breast tissue is produced on a screen by the beaming of high-frequency sound waves into the breast and the computer processing of the signals received back through a transducer. The time required for the ultrasonic beam to be reflected back to the transducer from differing densities of tissue is converted by a computer to an electrical impulse displayed on an oscilloscopic screen to create a three-dimensional picture of the breast. An advantage of this test is that it can display all breast tissue, whereas radiography cannot. In clients with fibrocystic breast disease, the water path method of ultrasonography may be used.

Professional Considerations
1. Consent form NOT required.
2. **Preparation:**
   A. Obtain ultrasonic gel or paste.
3. **Procedure:**
   A. The client is positioned supine and obliquely and rolled 35 degrees toward the side of the breast that will be examined. A sponge, blanket roll, or folded towel may be used to support the shoulders and hips. The client's arm on the same side to be examined should be placed behind the head.
   B. A greasy, conductive paste is applied to the 5.0- or 7.5-MHz, small-diameter, high frequency transducer.
   C. The transducer is passed methodically over all the skin of the breast. Any known breast mass is identified, and the surrounding area in a 3-cm square is marked on the breast. The breast and marked area are scanned transversely from the inferior margin toward the head in small intervals, followed by sagittal scans moving medially to laterally. Scanning is performed with light pressure.
   D. Photographs are taken of the oscilloscopic display.
   E. Dedicated water-path breast instrumentation:
      i. The client is positioned either prone on a special bed, with the breast suspended over and into water, or supine with a bag of water overlying the breast.
      ii. Scanning is performed in 1- to 2-mm intervals through the water path with a transducer.

Any lesions are identified in two axes.
4. **Postprocedure care:**
   A. Cleanse the skin of the ultrasonic paste.
5. **Client and family teaching:**
   A. Wear a two-piece outfit to facilitate breast exposure for exam (if the test is performed on an outpatient basis).
   B. Some facilities request that no deodorants, powders, or perfumes be worn the day of the test.
   C. The procedure will take approximately 30 minutes.
   D. A breast ultrasonogram may improve the accuracy of the diagnosis when used as an adjunct to mammography.
   E. Results are normally available in 1-2 days.
6. **Factors that affect results:**
   A. Compression of the breast may be used to eliminate nipple shadows, enable the use of high-frequency transducers, and improve delineation of the tissue. However, compression causes a misrepresentation of the breast anatomy.
7. **Other data:**
   A. Negative ultrasonographic results should not be used to conclude a lesion is benign.
   B. Ultrasonography of the breast should not be used as a screening method for breast cancer because of its high rates of false-positive and false-negative outcomes.

BREATH HYDROGEN ANALYSIS, DIAGNOSTIC

Norm. <20 ppm elevation over fasting level.

Usage. Assessment of orocecal transit time; determination of bronchiectasis, irritable bowel syndrome, lactose intolerance, hypolactasia; screening for early diagnosis of necrotizing enterocolitis; and evaluation of peptic ulcer disease before and during treatment with ranitidine.

Description. This test measures the hydrogen exhaled at specific intervals during the first 3 hours after ingestion of the carbohydrate (such as lactose, lactulose, fructose, or sucrose) being studied. In the normal client, hydrogen is produced exclusively by the bacterial metabolism of carbohydrates. Clients who are unable to digest or absorb carbohydrates in the small intestine have an increased volume of carbohydrates reaching the colon. These carbohydrates are metabolized in the colon, producing hydrogen, which is absorbed in the colon and exhaled by the lungs. The hydrogen breath test detects higher than normal levels and abnormal timing of peak releases of exhaled hydrogen. Ranitidine inhibits the action of histamine on the H_2-receptors of the parietal cells of the stomach, thus reducing hydrochloric acid production. The breath test can be used to evaluate hydrogen release after administration of the ranitidine.

Professional Considerations
1. Consent form NOT required.
2. Preparation:
   A. See *Client and family teaching.*
   B. Obtain a syringe or balloon.
3. Procedure:
   A. After measurement of a basal breath hydrogen level, an oral dose of lactose, 1 g/kg of body weight, is given.
   B. End-alveolar air is expired into a 30-mL glass syringe or a special plastic balloon.
   C. The breath sample is injected into an analyzer to determine H_2 and CO_2 concentration.
   D. A rise of 720 ppm in exhaled hydrogen is diagnostic for lactose malabsorption.
   E. Clients with bacterial overgrowth of the small intestine will have an increased production of hydrogen, with an early peak (within 3 hours) of hydrogen release after carbohydrate ingestion.
   F. Clients with disease of the small intestine and carbohydrate malabsorption have a later peak of hydrogen release.
4. Postprocedure care:
   A. Resume normal diet.
5. Client and family teaching:
   A. Fast from midnight before the test. A carbohydrate-controlled diet the day before the test affects the fasting breath hydrogen levels and may improve the test accuracy.
   B. Do not use laxatives or enemas for 3 days before being tested.
   C. Do not smoke for at least 15 minutes before being tested.
6. Factors that affect results:
   A. Diarrhea within 3 days before the test invalidates the results.
   B. Storage of the samples allows for leakage of the gases. A glass syringe stored on its side with the barrel lubricated with mineral oil will have negligible leakage over a 2-week period. Upright storage may result in leakage of mineral oil and loss of the barrel seal.
   C. High-fiber diet increases results.
7. Other data:
   A. Hydrogen content increases as carbohydrate malabsorption increases.

BREATH TEST (CARBON-13 OR CARBON-14 UREA BREATH TEST)
(see Urea breath test, Diagnostic)

BROMIDES, SERUM
Norm. Negative.

		SI UNITS
Reference range	0-11.7 mg/dL	0-11.7 mmol/L
Panic levels		
Bromide ion	>120 mg/dL	
Sodium bromide	>150 mg/dL	
	>15 mEq/L	>15 mmol/L

Panic Levels Symptoms and Treatment

Symptoms. Abdominal pain, ataxia, central nervous system depression (coma), cyanosis, eye irritation (if inhaled), gastrointestinal tract corrosion (if swallowed), increased cerebrospinal fluid pressure, mental disturbance (confusion, hallucinations, irritability, mania), rash, tachycardia, respiratory irritation (if inhaled), shock, vertigo, vomiting.

Treatment:

Note: Treatment choice(s) depend on client history and condition and episode history.

For bromide poisoning caused by inhalation:

Give oxygen.

Maintain patent airway and support breathing.

Monitor for and treat pulmonary edema.

For bromide poisoning from ingestion:

Induce vomiting with syrup of ipecac. (Induction of vomiting is contraindicated in clients with no gag reflex or with central nervous system depression or excitation.)

Perform gastric lavage.

General intervention:

Administer 1 g of NaCl in water orally every hour until serum bromide level is less than 50 mg/dL.

Monitor for and treat shock symptoms.

Monitor liver and kidney function.

Hydrate and provide mild diuresis.

Both hemodialysis and peritoneal dialysis WILL remove bromides.

Usage. Screening for bromide toxicity.

Increased. Exposure to vapors in photography and chemical industries, exposure to bromides in pesticides, and ingestion of over-the-counter medications such as Bromo-Seltzer or nonsteroidal antiinflammatory drugs (NSAIDS).

Description. The element bromine is a reddish brown, nonvolatile liquid that gives off suffocating vapors that are highly toxic and severely irritating to the skin. Bromine replaces chlorine in the body tissues, resulting in sedation and depression of the central nervous system. For this reason, it was used in the past as a medication to sedate clients until more effective, less toxic medications became available.

Professional Considerations

1. Consent form NOT required.
2. Preparation:
   A. Tube: Red topped, red/gray topped, gold topped, or green topped.
   B. Do NOT draw during hemodialysis.
3. Procedure:
   A. Draw a 5-mL blood sample.
4. Postprocedure care:
   A. Monitor closely for signs of bromide toxicity.

5. Client and family teaching:
   A. Bromide poisoning rarely causes death.
6. Factors that affect results:
   A. Falsely elevated levels may occur in clients receiving iodine therapy.
   B. Age over 45 years and female sex indicates high normal levels.
7. Other data:
   A. Alcoholics are especially susceptible to bromide intoxication.

BRONCHIAL ASPIRATE, FUNGUS, CULTURE

Norm. Negative. No growth.

Usage. Diagnosis of the presence and type of potentially pathogenic fungi in the bronchi.

Positive. *Aspergillus fumigatus, Aspergillus flavus, Blastomyces dermatitides, Candida albicans, Candida tropicalis, Coccidioides immitis, Cryptococcus neoformans, Histoplasma capsulatum,* and *Sporothrix schenckii.*

Description. Fungi are slow-growing, eukaryotic organisms that can grow on living and nonliving organic materials and are subdivided into yeasts and molds. Normal human host defense mechanisms limit the damage they cause superficially. Some fungi can be inhaled or introduced by traumatic inoculation into deep tissue spaces and cause serious infections. Although tentative identification of fungi can be made quickly with staining techniques, culture of the organism on special fungal culture media is required to confirm a diagnosis of a fungal infection.

Professional Considerations

1. Consent form is NOT required unless a bronchoscopy is used to obtain the specimen.
2. Preparation:
   A. Obtain a sterile container or suction trap, suction tubing, sterile suction catheter, and gloves.
   B. Prepare a suction machine or a wall suction.
   C. See *Bronchoscopy, Diagnostic (Preparation),* if this method is used.
3. Procedure:
   A. A specimen trap is inserted into the suctioning line of a flexible, fiberoptic bronchoscope or between the suctioning catheter and a regular suctioning line.

B

When the bronchoscope is in place or the suction catheter is completely inserted into a bronchus, suction is applied, and a specimen is obtained while the suction trap is held upright.

B. Specimens obtained by expectoration should be collected early in the morning after the client has removed any dentures and gargled and rinsed the mouth with water. A deep cough is required to deliver a good specimen, and the specimen should be expectorated directly into a sterile cup.

4. **Postprocedure care:**
   A. Write the collection time on the laboratory requisition.
   B. Write any current antibiotic or antifungal therapy on the laboratory requisition.
   C. Transport the specimen to the laboratory immediately.
   D. See *Bronchoscopy, Diagnostic,* if this method is used.

5. **Client and family teaching:**
   A. See *Bronchoscopy, Diagnostic,* if this method is used.
   B. To produce a specimen by coughing, take several breaths in without fully exhaling in between. When you feel you cannot breathe any more air in, cough out forcefully and catch the sputum in a specimen cup.
   C. 4-6 weeks are required for a final fungal culture report.

6. **Factors that affect results:**
   A. The specimen should be obtained with the first suctioning.
   B. A break in the sterile technique invalidates the results.
   C. The best results are obtained if the cultures are inoculated immediately. The maximum time allowed between specimen collection and inoculation is 3 hours.

7. **Other data:**
   A. None.

BRONCHIAL ASPIRATE, ROUTINE, CULTURE

Norm. No growth or growth of only normal upper respiratory flora.

Usage. Diagnosis of infections of the tracheobronchial tree.

Description. Sputum obtained by bronchoscopy, routine tracheal suctioning, or coughing is cultured and Gram stained. Suctioned samples may be obtained nasotracheally, endotracheally, or through a tracheostomy.

Professional Considerations
1. Consent form NOT required.
2. **Preparation:**
   A. Obtain a sterile container or suction trap, suction tubing, a sterile suction catheter, and gloves.
   B. Prepare the suction machine or wall suction.
   C. See *Bronchoscopy, Diagnostic (Preparation),* if this method is used.
3. **Procedure:**
   A. A specimen trap is inserted into the suctioning line of a flexible, fiberoptic bronchoscope or between the suctioning catheter and a regular suctioning line. When the bronchoscope is in place or the suction catheter is completely inserted into the bronchi, suction is applied, and a specimen is obtained while the suction trap is held upright.
   B. Specimens obtained by expectoration should be collected early in the morning after the client has removed any dentures and gargled and rinsed the mouth with water. A deep cough is required to deliver a good specimen, and the specimen should be expectorated directly into a sterile cup.
4. **Postprocedure care:**
   A. Write the collection time on the laboratory requisition.
   B. Write any current antibiotic or antifungal therapy for the client on laboratory requisition.
   C. See *Bronchoscopy, Diagnostic,* if this method is used.
5. **Client and family teaching:**
   A. To produce a specimen by coughing, take several breaths in, without fully exhaling in between. When you feel you cannot breathe any more air in, cough out forcefully and catch sputum into a specimen cup.
   B. See *Bronchoscopy, Diagnostic,* if this method is used.
   C. Cultures with no growth can be reported in 48 hours. Results take up to 10 days.

6. Factors that affect results:
   A. The specimen should be obtained with the first suctioning.
   B. Reject specimens more than 4 hours old.
7. Other data:
   A. Pulmonary nocardiosis is best treated with a combination of imipenem and amikacin.

BRONCHIAL CHALLENGE TEST
(see Methacholine challenge test, Diagnostic)

BRONCHIAL WASHING (BRONCHOALVEOLAR LAVAGE) SPECIMEN, DIAGNOSTIC

Norm. Negative for culture and cytologic testing.

Usage. Diagnosis of infections, for example *Mycobacterium szulgai* and *Bipolaris hawaiiensis*, and pathologic processes in the lungs.

Description. Procedure useful to obtain respiratory tract specimens for culture and cytologic testing when very few secretions are present. Specimens are obtained from a normal saline wash, which is instilled into the bronchi and then suctioned out. Saline may be instilled through a bronchoscope, an endotracheal tube, or a tracheal tube. A bronchoalveolar wash will provide a specimen from the alveoli and is done by insertion of the flexible fiberoptic bronchoscope as far into the bronchiole as possible and instillation of the saline at that point. This procedure is used when adequate deep sputum specimens cannot be obtained and is often helpful in the diagnosis of *Pneumocystis* pneumonia.

Professional Considerations
1. Consent form is NOT required unless the washing is done by bronchoscopy. See *Bronchoscopy, Diagnostic*, for risks and contraindications if bronchoscopy is used to obtain the specimen.
2. Preparation:
   A. Obtain a specimen trap, suction tubing, a sterile suction catheter, and sterile gloves.
   B. Prepare a wall suction or a suction machine.
   C. If the washing is performed during bronchoscopy, obtain sterile specimen containers for the bronchoscope.
   D. See *Bronchoscopy, Diagnostic*, if this procedure is used.
3. Procedure:
   A. A specimen trap is inserted into the suctioning line from the bronchoscope, or between the suctioning catheter and the suctioning line.
   B. Up to 20 mL of normal saline is instilled into the respiratory tract through the bronchoscope, the endotracheal tube, or the tracheal tube, and the specimen is obtained when suction is applied to the bronchoscope catheter or suction catheter.
4. Postprocedure care:
   A. Write the time of specimen collection and any current antibiotic or antifungal therapy on the laboratory requisition.
   B. See *Bronchoscopy, Diagnostic*, if this procedure is used.
5. Client and family teaching:
   A. See *Bronchoscopy, Diagnostic*, if this procedure is used.
   B. Results are normally available within 1-2 days.
6. Factors that affect results:
   A. Bronchial washing specimens must be collected using a sterile technique.
7. Other data:
   A. May be used to diagnose *Pneumocystis carinii* in client with AIDS.
   B. High number of neutrophils found in bronchial washing fluid of COPD clients.

BRONCHOALVEOLAR LAVAGE, SPECIMEN
(see Bronchial washing, Specimen, Diagnostic)

BRONCHOSCOPY, DIAGNOSTIC

Norm. Normal larynx, trachea, and bronchi.

Usage. Used to examine the bronchi for abscesses, aspiration pneumonia, hemoptysis, and unresolved pneumonias, strictures, tumors, and removal of foreign objects and to obtain deep sputum specimens and tissue biopsy specimens.

Description. Direct visual examination of the larynx, trachea, and bronchi with a rigid bronchoscope or a flexible fiberoptic bronchoscope.

Professional Considerations
1. Consent form IS required.

Risks
Bleeding, bronchospasm, cardiopulmonary arrest, dysrhythmias, hypotension, hypoxia, pneumothorax.

Contraindications
Pregnancy; clients with severe shortness of breath who cannot tolerate interruption of high-flow oxygen. Such clients may be intubated for the procedure to ensure optimal oxygenation. Sedatives are contraindicated in clients with central nervous system depression.

2. **Preparation:**
   A. Obtain vital signs, activated partial thromboplastin time, platelet count, and prothrombin time.
   B. Remove any dentures or eyeglasses.
   C. Sedation may be prescribed. Sedation includes benzodiazepines in 63% of cases, opioid in 14%, and both in 12% (Smyth & Stead, 2002).
   D. Prepare suctioning equipment.
   E. Have emergency resuscitation equipment readily available.
3. **Procedure:**
   A. The nasopharynx and oropharynx are anesthetized with a local anesthetic.
   B. The client is placed in a sitting or supine position.
   C. After the tube is passed through the mouth or nose into the larynx, more local anesthetic is sprayed into the trachea to inhibit the cough reflex.
   D. If the client has a large endotracheal tube in place, the flexible bronchoscope can be inserted through it.
   E. The trachea and bronchi are visually examined for abnormal color, structure, or lesions.
   F. Mucus is then suctioned until clear, bronchial washings are performed and the specimens are collected, and biopsy specimens are obtained if the flexible tube is used.
   G. The rigid bronchoscope is used to retrieve foreign bodies and excise lesions.

   H. The client is observed for impaired respirations or laryngospasms throughout the procedure.
4. **Postprocedure care:**
   A. No food or fluids are given until the gag reflex has returned, about 2 hours after the procedure.
   B. The client should not attempt to swallow saliva until the gag reflex has returned. Saliva should be expectorated into an emesis basin. Observe the client's sputum for blood if a biopsy was performed. If a tumor is suspected, collect post bronchoscopy sputum specimens for cytologic examination.
   C. Observe postanesthesia precautions if a sedative was given. If deep sedation was used, follow institutional protocol for postsedation monitoring. Typical monitoring includes continuous ECG monitoring and pulse oximetry, with continual assessments (every 5-15 minutes) of airway, vital signs, and neurologic status until the client is lying quietly awake, is breathing independently, and responds appropriately to commands spoken in a normal tone.
   D. Observe closely for postprocedure complications, including bronchospasm, bacteremia, bronchial perforation (indicated by facial or neck crepitus), cardiac dysrhythmias, fever, hemorrhage from the biopsy site, hypoxemia, laryngospasm, pneumonia, and pneumothorax.
5. **Client and family teaching:**
   A. Fast from the midnight before the procedure. Your diet will be restarted a few hours after the procedure.
   B. Arrange for transportation home after the procedure because you will not be permitted to drive for 24 hours after receiving sedation.
   C. Notify the physician if you are experiencing fever or difficulty in breathing during the next 48-72 hours.
   D. You can begin drinking or eating approximately 2 hours after the procedure.
6. **Factors that affect results:**
   A. The procedure should be stopped if the client becomes uncooperative or if impaired respiratory function is noted.

7. Other data:
   A. Intermittent negative-pressure ventilation is safe during interventional rigid bronchoscopy.
   B. Virtual bronchoscopy (use of computed tomography) has shown promise for assessing complications of lung transplantation.

BRUCELLOSIS AGGLUTININS, BLOOD

Norm. Negative. Titers of 1:20–1:80 are normal in farmers with cattle, swine, goats, or sheep, or in endemic areas without clinical manifestations.

Positive. Brucellosis caused by *Brucella abortus, B. canis, or B. melitensis.* Titers >1:160 indicate past or present infection. A fourfold increase in the titer within 2 weeks indicates an acute infection.

Description. Brucellosis (Bang's disease, Malta fever, Mediterranean fever, undulant fever) is a systemic disease acquired from animals that lasts days to years. It is found with greatest frequency in Europe, North Africa, Asia, Mexico, and South America. *Brucella* is an obligate parasite on animals. The mode of transmission to humans is through direct body tissue contact with fluids, milk, and dairy products of infected animals or by transmission to infants by breast-feeding. Onset may be acute or insidious, and symptoms may include arthralgia, body aches, chills, diaphoresis, depression, fever(s), headache, weakness, pneumonitis, and nonpurulent meningitis. In this test, *Brucella* antigens are mixed with a client's serum and observed for an agglutination reaction. A positive reaction is followed by serial dilutions of serum and retesting. The results are expressed as the highest titer showing agglutination. Agglutination indicates the presence of antibodies generated by any of three closely related *Brucella* species and is used in the indirect diagnosis of human brucellosis.

Professional Considerations
1. Consent form NOT required.
2. Preparation:
   A. Tube: Red topped, red/gray topped, or gold topped.
3. Procedure:
   A. Draw a 5-mL venous blood sample.

4. Postprocedure care:
   A. Send the specimen to the laboratory for immediate testing.
5. Client and family teaching:
   A. Serial testing is recommended for clients with positive titers. Titers usually begin rising 5-30 days after exposure and peak in 1-2 months.
6. Factors that affect results:
   A. Reject hemolyzed specimens.
   B. Falsely elevated titers may occur in clients who have received Brucella skin testing.
   C. Falsely elevated titers may occur with cross-reactions of the *Brucella* test antigens with agglutinins produced by clients with tularemia, cholera, and *Proteus vulgaris* Ox-19 infections, and in clients recently vaccinated against cholera.
   D. Falsely depressed titers may occur in immunosuppressed clients or clients receiving antibiotic therapy.
7. Other data:
   A. Isolation of the organism is necessary to confirm the diagnosis.
   B. Brucellosis is a reportable disease in most areas.
   C. Serum calcium levels are >2.35 mmol/L, in persons with brucellosis.

BRUSHING CYTOLOGY, SPECIMEN, DIAGNOSTIC

Norm. Negative. Requires interpretation.

Positive. Allergic reaction, asbestosis, Barrett's esophagus, cryptosporidiosis, echinococcosis, Goodpasture syndrome, infection (herpes virus, cytomegalovirus, measles virus, fungus), Legionnaires' disease, neoplasm (primary or metastatic), paragonimiasis, pneumonia (lipoid, *Pneumocystis carinii*), pulmonary infection (anaerobic), and strongyloidiasis.

Description. A brushing is taken (usually by means of endoscopy, bronchoscopy, cystoscopy, or gastroscopy) from a particular body site, smeared onto a slide, stained, examined microscopically, and possibly cultured. The specimens may be examined for bacterial and tumor antigens. Possible sites may be the bronchus, colon, esophagus, stomach, oropharynx, small bowel, trachea, or urethra.

Professional Considerations
1. Consent form NOT required.
2. Preparation:
   A. Obtain a brush, a glass slide, and fixative container.
   B. Label the slide with the client's name.
3. Procedure:
   A. Obtain a brushing from a body site or a lesion.
   B. Gently roll the brush over the slide and immediately fix in 95% ethyl alcohol (ethanol).
   C. For bronchial brushings, omit the slide and transport the disposable brush immediately to the laboratory.
   D. The specimens for the culture require a double-sheathed brush sealed with the sheath after specimen collection.
4. Postprocedure care:
   A. Write on the laboratory requisition the date, the site brushed, and the client's diagnosis, age, and history pertinent to this test.
   B. Transport the fixative container or brush to the laboratory.
5. Client and family teaching:
   A. The test is painless.
   B. Results are normally available within 24 hours.
6. Factors that affect results:
   A. Do NOT allow the slide to dry before fixing in alcohol.
7. Other data:
   A. May be used to diagnose *Pneumocystis carinii* in clients with AIDS.

BTA TEST FOR BLADDER CANCER, DIAGNOSTIC

Norm. Bladder tumor–associated antigen negative.

Usage. Used in the diagnosis of superficial transitional cell carcinoma of the urinary bladder. Has a 61% sensitivity, 74% specificity, 64% accuracy, 88% positive predictive value, and 38% negative predictive value for bladder carcinoma (Lokeshwar et al, 2002).

Positive. Presence of bladder tumor–associated antigen in urine sample.

Negative. Absence of bladder tumor–associated antigen in urine sample.

Description. BTA test is a noninvasive tumor-marker quantitative enzyme immunoassay. The tumor marker is an antigen named "human complement factor H–related protein" (hCFHrp). hCFHrp is not detectable in healthy epithelial cells but has been identified in bladder cancer cells. hCFHrp is similar to human complement factor (hCFH), which plays a role in the prevention of cell lysis through interruption of a complement pathway. hCFH causes lysis of foreign cells in a host by inhibiting the development of a membrane attack complex. Cancer cells are believed to be protected from lysis by hCFHrp, which also interrupts a complement pathway, thereby facilitating invasion to the host.

Professional Considerations
1. Consent form NOT required.
2. Preparation:
   A. Urine specimen suggested amount is 35 mL (minimum of 2 mL).
3. Procedure:
   A. Collect voided or catheterized urine sample in clean urine specimen container without additives. Urine specimens cannot be collected in foam or paper cups.
   B. Transport to lab on ice.
4. Postprocedure care:
   A. None
5. Client and family teaching:
   A. Obtain complete current and past medical history.
   B. Dipstick urine to verify absence of hematuria before test.
   C. Inform client that a positive bladder tumor antigen test will be confirmed by biopsy of bladder tissue.
6. Factors that affect results:
   A. False-positive tests occur 9% of cases (Friedrich et al, 2002) including any condition that causes hCFHrp to be present in the bladder. These conditions are renal lithiasis, nephritis, renal neoplasm, urinary tract infections, cystitis, history or presence of urinary stents or nephrostomy tubes, genitourinary cancer, bowel interposition segment, and trauma to the urinary system. A false negative test occurs in 2% of those tested and is associated with tumor recurrence.
   B. Hematuria may yield false-positive tests, and therefore urine samples should be first tested for presence of blood.
   C. If blood is detected in urine sample, urine cytologic testing is suggested.

7. Other data:
   A. None

BUCCAL SMEAR FOR SEX CHROMATIN EVALUATION, DIAGNOSTIC

(see Barr body analysis, Buccal smear for staining sex chromatin mass, Diagnostic)

BUN

(see Urea nitrogen, Plasma or Serum)

BUN/CREATININE RATIO, BLOOD

(see Blood urea nitrogen/creatinine ratio, Blood)

C1q IMMUNE COMPLEX DETECTION, SERUM

Norm. None detected.

Increased or Positive. Arthritis, glomerulonephritis (acute), hepatitis (serum), IgA nephropathy, infectious disease, inflammatory bowel disease, neoplasms, primary biliary cirrhosis, rheumatic disease, subacute bacterial endocarditis, systemic lupus erythematosus, thrombotic thrombocytopenic purpura, and vasculitis.

Description. *Complement* is a term describing 20 specific serum globulin proteins that, in combination with antigen-antibody complexes, cause lysis of erythrocytes sensitized to the antibody contained in the complex. The nine major complement components are labeled C1 to C9. C1q immune complex is a component of C1 complement that is bound into a circulating immune complex (CIC) when foreign antigens

react with IgG or IgM antibodies in the body. It is very important because immune complex reactions involving the C1q component activate the classic pathway of the complement cascade. Many tests for circulating immune complexes are based on C1q-binding properties. Exacerbations of immune complex disease cause elevated CICs because the lymphoreticular system is unable to clear the immune complex effectively. This test is used in serial monitoring of the progress of immune complex disease that activates the classic pathway of the complement cascade.

Professional Considerations
1. Consent form NOT required.
2. Preparation:
   A. Tube: Red topped, red/gray topped, or gold topped.
3. Procedure:
   A. Draw a 3-mL venous blood sample.
4. Postprocedure care:
   A. Send the specimen to the laboratory immediately because complement is very unstable.
5. Client and family teaching:
   A. Serial measurements are recommended.
   B. Results are normally available within 24 hours.
6. Factors that affect results:
   A. The presence of serum cryoglobulins may cause false-positive results.
   B. Recent heparin therapy may interfere with accurate results.
   C. Reject hemolyzed specimens.
7. Other data:
   A. False-negative results occur about 10% of the time; therefore a negative result does not rule out disease.
   B. See also *Complement components, Serum; Complement fixation, Serum; and Complement total, Serum.*

C3 ACTIVATOR, SERUM
(see C3 proactivator, Serum)

C3 COMPLEMENT (BETA-1C GLOBULIN), SERUM

Norm:

		SI UNITS
Adult	83-177 mg/dL	0.83-1.77 g/L
Cord blood	65-111.8 mg/dL	0.65-1.12 g/L
Child	86.6-135.8 mg/dL	0.87-1.36 g/L

Increased. Acute-phase plasma protein response such as infection, dermatomyositis, inflammation, keratoconus, malignancy with metastasis, necrotizing disorders, rheumatic fever, and rheumatoid arthritis.

Decreased. Anemia (pernicious, folic acid deficiency), anorexia nervosa, arthralgias, celiac disease, cirrhosis, congenital C3 deficiency, disseminated intravascular coagulation, glomerulonephritis (acute), membranoproliferative, poststreptococcal hepatitis (chronic active), hypocomplementeric nephritis, immune complex disease, infection (recurrent pyogenic), liver disease (chronic), malnutrition (protein), multiple myeloma, multiple sclerosis, real transplant rejection, septicemia (gram negative), serum sickness, subacute bacterial endocarditis, systemic lupus erythematosus (active, with renal involvement), and uremia.

Description. *Complement* is a term describing 20 specific serum globulin proteins that, in combination with antigen-antibody complexes, cause lysis of erythrocytes sensitized to the antibody contained in the complex. The nine major complement components are labeled C1 to C9. C3 complement is one of the nine major components of total complement protein and is involved in both the classic and alternative pathways of the complement cascade that function in humoral immunologic responses. Activation of the complement cascade functions in phagocytic activity, destruction of foreign bacteria, and the inflammatory response. This test evaluates the integrity of the cascade and is increased during acute-phase responses and inflammatory processes. Serial C3 levels may reflect the progress of such conditions based on the return of values to normal levels.

Professional Considerations
1. Consent form NOT required.
2. Preparation:
   A. Tube: Red topped, red/gray topped, or gold topped.
3. Procedure:
   A. Draw a 3-mL venous blood sample.
4. Postprocedure care:
   A. None.
5. Client and family teaching:
   A. Serial measurements are recommended.

B. Results are normally available within 24 hours.
6. Factors that affect results:
   A. Complement is heat sensitive and deteriorates rapidly. Send the specimen to the laboratory immediately.
   B. Reject hemolyzed specimens or specimens received more than 1-2 hours after collection.
   C. Freeze serum if not tested within 2 hours.
7. Other data:
   A. See also *C3 proactivator, Serum; Complement components, Serum; Complement fixation, Serum; Complement total, Serum.*

C3 PROACTIVATOR (ALTERNATE PATHWAY FACTOR B, C3 ACTIVATOR), SERUM

Norm. 20-42 mg/dL, or 0.20-0.42 g/L (2.16-4.54 mmol/L, SI units).

Increased. Burns, childhood nephrotic syndrome, diffuse intravascular coagulation, inflammation, subacute bacterial endocarditis, bacteremia (with shock symptoms), paroxysmal nocturnal hemoglobinuria, rheumatoid arthritis, and sickle cell disease.

Decreased. Chronic liver disease, glomerulonephritis (acute), and systemic lupus erythematosus.

Description. Used in serial monitoring of the progress of immune complex diseases. A factor involved in the alternate pathway of the complement cascade, which is involved in the humoral immune response. Polysaccharides, bacterial endotoxins, or aggregated IgA or IgG immunoglobulins reacting with factor B produce an enzyme that activates the C3 component of complement and initiation of the alternative pathway of the complement cascade.

Professional Considerations
1. Consent form NOT required.
2. Preparation:
   A. Tube: Red topped, red/gray topped, or gold topped.
3. Procedure:
   A. Draw a 3-mL venous blood sample.

B. Allow the specimen to clot at room temperature for 30 minutes.
C. Refrigerate the specimen at 4° C for 1 hour.
D. Remove the specimen from the refrigerator.
4. Postprocedure care:
   A. Send the specimen to the laboratory after refrigerating, as described above.
5. Client and family teaching:
   A. Serial measurements are recommended.

6. Factors that affect results:
   A. Reject hemolyzed specimens or specimens received more than 2 hours after collection.
   B. Freeze the serum if the test cannot be performed within 2 hours after collection.
7. Other data:
   A. See also *C3 complement, Serum; Complement components, Serum; Complement fixation, Serum; Complement total, Serum.*

C4 COMPLEMENT, SERUM

Norm:

		SI UNITS
Female	15-52 mg/dL	0.73-2.53 µmol/L
Male	15-60 mg/dL	0.73-2.91 µmol/L

Increased. Cancer, chronic urticaria, dermatomyositis, juvenile rheumatoid arthritis, keratoconus, and rheumatoid spondylitis.

Decreased. Chronic bronchitis, cigarette smoking, congenital C4 complement deficiency, cryoglobulinemia, glomerulonephritis, Henoch-Schönlein purpura, hepatitis (chronic active), hereditary angioedema, hypergammaglobulinemic state, immune complex disease, lupus nephritis, pesticide workers exposed to pyrethroids, renal transplant rejection, serum sickness, subacute bacterial endocarditis, systemic lupus erythematosus (active), and tubulointerstitial nephritis and uveitis (TINU syndrome).

Description. *Complement* is a term describing 20 specific serum globulin proteins that, in combination with antigen-antibody complexes, cause lysis of erythrocytes sensitized to the antibody contained in the complex. The nine major complement components are labeled C1 to C9. C4 complement is one of the nine components of total complement protein and is involved in only the classical pathway of the complement cascade that functions in humoral immunologic responses and is normally present in human colostrum. C4 complement deficiency is an inherited autosomal recessive trait and results in decreased resistance to infection. Activation of the complement cascade functions in phagocytic activity, destruction of foreign bacteria, and the inflammatory response. C3 and C4 levels are helpful in distinguishing the cause of glomerulonephritis, as C3 is decreased, but C4 is usually normal when the cause is poststreptococcal.

Professional Considerations
1. Consent form NOT required.
2. **Preparation:**
   A. Tube: Red topped, red/gray topped, or gold topped.
3. **Procedure:**
   A. Draw a 3-mL blood sample.
4. **Postprocedure care:**
   A. Allow the specimen to clot for 15-30 minutes at room temperature and then refrigerate.
   B. Freeze the serum if not processed immediately.
5. **Client and family teaching:**
   A. Serial measurements are recommended.
6. **Factors that affect results:**
   A. Complement is heat sensitive and deteriorates rapidly. Send the specimen to the laboratory immediately.
   B. Reject hemolyzed specimens or specimens received more than 1-2 hours after collection.

C

7. Other data:
A. See also *C3 complement, Serum; Complement components, Serum; Complement fixation, Serum; Complement total, Serum.*

C6 PEPTIDE
(*see Borrelia burgdorferi C6 peptide antibody, Serum*)

¹⁴C-CHOLATE BREATH TEST
(*see Bile salt absorption test, Diagnostic*)

CA 15-3 (CARBOHYDRATE ANTIGEN 15-3, CANCER ANTIGEN 15-3), SERUM

Norm. <31 U/mL.

Increased. Breast cancer (prebiopsy increases associated with 14% 5-year survival rate), liver cancer, lung cancer, ovarian cancer, prostate cancer, pregnancy (higher in third trimester), during lactation, systemic lupus erythematosus, hepatitis, benign gynecologic tumors, chronic pelvic inflammatory disease, cirrhosis, tuberculosis, sarcoidosis.

Usage. Used to monitor response to treatment in breast cancer clients. A prognostic marker in node-negative breast cancer with risk of relapse increasing from 10 U/mL.

Decreased. Positive response to therapy.

Description. The MUC1 gene is a high-molecular-weight glycoprotein found in specific tissues throughout the body. (See *Mucin-like carcinoma associated antigen, Blood.*) The MUC1 gene has many varieties of carbohydrate chains that are termed *mucin-like* antigens, and one of these is the carbohydrate antigen15-3 (CA 15-3) that circulates in the bloodstream when cancer is present. Approximately 80% of clients with metastatic breast cancer have elevated CA 15-3 levels and 36% of cases show elevations in relapse. Approximately 50% of clients with ovarian carcinoma have increased values (95% specificity and 92% predictive value), although CA 15-3 is not routinely used to monitor ovarian cancer clients. CA

125 levels are used preferentially to monitor ovarian cancer clients. Clients with high concentrations of CA 15-3 have a significantly worse prognosis than clients with low CA 15-3 concentrations. Preoperative concentrations of CA 15-3 may have a role in the selection of clients for adjuvant treatment and may serve as independent prognostic indicators in breast cancer. Preoperative levels >40 U/mL correlate well with large tumor size, metastasis, and higher grade. Postoperative levels >86 U/mL are indicative of metastatic disease, but normal levels do not exclude metastasis. Transient elevations of CA 15-3 often occur in the first weeks of therapy and should not be confused with treatment failure. Although individual levels may not be useful in monitoring disease status, trends are useful, and a change of 25%, whether a decrease or an increase, is good evidence for either response to therapy or recurrence, respectively. Because of its low detection rate in early disease and in micrometastatic disease, CA 15-3 is not a useful screening test and is also not likely to detect early recurrent disease. CA 15-3 levels are measured via monoclonal antibody immunoassay.

Professional Considerations
1. Consent form NOT required.
2. Preparation:
   A. Tube: Red topped or serum separator (red/gray or gold topped).
3. Procedure:
   A. Collect a 3-mL blood sample.
   B. Refrigerate specimen.
4. Postprocedure care:
   A. None.
5. Client and family teaching:
   A. CA 15-3 is not a useful screening test for early carcinoma.
   B. Results are normally available within 3 working days.
6. Factors that affect results:
   A. Persons with benign breast or ovarian disease may have elevated levels.
   B. Results are invalidated if the client has received radioisotopes within the prior 30 days.
7. Other data:
   A. Results >25 U/mL are found in women with metastatic breast carcinoma.
   B. CA 15-3 when used with CA 125 can improve the management of women presenting with a pelvic mass.

CA 19-9 (CARBOHYDRATE ANTIGEN 19-9, GICA, GASTROINTESTINAL CANCER ANTIGEN), BLOOD

Norm:

		SI UNITS
Norm	<37 AU/mL	<37 kU/L
Metastasis	>1000 AU/mL	>1000 kU/L

Usage. Used to monitor gastrointestinal, pancreatic, and colorectal malignancies. CA 19-9 with carcinoembryonic antigen is useful when clients are being monitored for possible recurrence of gastric carcinoma.

Increased. Gastrointestinal, pancreatic, hepatobiliary, lung, testicular and colorectal malignancies, acute pancreatitis, cholangitis, cirrhosis, echinococcus infection, hydronephrosis, and hypothyroidism.

Description. The MUC1 gene is a high molecular weight glycoprotein found in specific tissues throughout the body. (See *Mucin-like carcinoma associated antigen, Blood.*) The MUC1 gene has many varieties of carbohydrate chains that are termed *mucinlike* antigens, and one of these is the carbohydrate antigen 19-9 (CA 19-9) that circulates in the bloodstream when cancer is present. CA 19-9 is a glycoprotein present on a wide variety of adenocarcinomas of the gastrointestinal and hepatobiliary systems. The CA 19-9 is produced in excess by the adenocarcinomas and released into the blood, enabling measurement. CA 19-9 is considered the standard of comparison often used marker for pancreatic cancer, along with CT, to differentiate from benign pancreatic disease. A total of 70-80% of pancreatic cancers, 60% of hepatobiliary cancers, and 50-60% of gastric carcinomas have elevated CA 19-9 levels. In pancreatic adenocarcinoma, 96% of tumors with CA 19-9 levels >1000 U/mL are considered unresectable. Serial elevated postoperative CA 19-9 levels often predict relapse of pancreatic carcinoma before clinical or radiographic findings, but the CA 19-9 levels are not often monitored because of the paucity of effective treatment for relapsed pancreatic carcinoma. Because of the lack of both sensitivity and specificity of CA 19-9, it is not considered useful as a screening test for early pancreatic cancer. Of note, the CA 19-9 glycoprotein is not expressed in Lewis (a–b–) individuals (nonsecretors) who account for approximately 7% of the US population and approximately 20% of the population of Japan, leading to the possibility of false-negative results when CA 19-9 levels are being obtained. CA 19-9 is measured using a double monoclonal immunoassay.

Professional Considerations
1. Consent form NOT required.
2. Preparation:
   A. Tube: Red topped, serum-separator (red/gray or gold topped) for serum samples, lavender topped for plasma samples.
3. Procedure:
   A. Blood sample is collected in the appropriate tube and refrigerated.
   B. Specimen should be refrigerated or frozen immediately.
4. Postprocedure care:
   A. None.
5. Client and family teaching:
   A. CA 19-9 is not useful as a screening test.
   B. Results are usually available within 3 working days.
6. Factors that may affect results:
   A. Reject hemolyzed specimen or specimen left at room temperature.
   B. Nonsecretor client. Individuals who are Lewis (a–b) phenotype (6% of the population) cannot synthesize CA 19-9, CA 50, and CA 195, and this inability may account for the lesser diagnostic value of these markers.
   C. Specimen left at room temperature.
   D. Results are invalidated if the client has received radioisotopes within the prior 30 days.
7. Other data:
   A. Elevated levels are found in cystic fibrosis and in human seminal fluid.

C

CA 50 (CARBOHYDRATE ANTIGEN 50, CANCER ANTIGEN 50), BLOOD

Norm. <17 U/mL.

Increased. Gastrointestinal (GI) tract tumors, biliary tract tumors, cholangiocarcinoma, oral cancer, pancreatic cancer, transitional cell carcinoma, non–small-cell lung cancer, benign extrahepatic jaundice, cirrhosis, cystic fibrosis.

Usage. Used with other tumor markers to determine prognosis, monitor response to therapy, and monitor for relapse.

Decreased. Positive response to therapy.

Description. The MUC1 gene is a high-molecular-weight glycoprotein found in specific tissues throughout the body. (See *Mucinlike carcinoma associated antigen, Blood.*) The MUC1 gene has many varieties of carbohydrate chains that are termed *mucinlike* antigens, and one of these is the carbohydrate antigen 50 (CA 50) that circulates in the bloodstream when cancer is present. CA 50 is found in the blood of clients with GI tumors and biliary tract tumors and appears to be a more sensitive marker for disease progression than that for regression. Although studies have shown relatively high specificity and sensitivity when CA 50 levels are used to aid in diagnosing pancreatic cancer, the specificity is high only when combined with specific signs and symptoms of pancreatic cancer. The CA 50 is not a widely used marker in the evaluation of clients with GI tumors because other markers are more reliable and more readily available.

Professional Considerations
1. Consent form NOT required.
2. Preparation:
   A. Tube: Red topped, red/gray or gold topped.
3. Procedure:
   A. Collect a 7-mL blood sample in appropriate tube.
4. Postprocedure care:
   A. Evaluate other antigen tests and the liver function studies.
5. Client and family teaching:
   A. This test is not used as a screening test for early carcinoma.

B. Results are normally available within 7 working days.
6. Factors that affect results:
   A. False-positive results occur in benign liver disease.
   B. Results are invalidated if the client has received radioisotopes within the prior 30 days.
7. Other data:
   A. CA 50 is higher for more undifferentiated and advanced-stage bladder tumors.
   B. CA 50 cannot be used as a tumor marker in cirrhotic clients because cytolysis increases this test result.

CA 72-4 (CARBOHYDRATE ANTIGEN 72-4, CANCER ANTIGEN 72-4, TUMOR-ASSOCIATED GLYCOPROTEIN 72, TAG 72), BLOOD

Norm. Negative.

Usage. Can be used in combination with carcinoembryonic antigen (CEA) and CA 19-9 for detection of gastric cancer. CA 72-4 is specific (100%) for esophageal, gastric, and colorectal cancer, but not very sensitive (18%, 32%, 56%) when tested alone. When used in combination with the CEA and CA 19-9 test, sensitivities increased to 46%, 50%, and 89%, respectively (Lopez et al, 1999). The test is more sensitive than CA 125 for ovarian cancer and has been found to be most elevated in mucinous type of ovarian cancer; it is less sensitive than CA-19 for pancreatic cancer.

Description. The MUC1 gene is a high-molecular-weight glycoprotein found in specific tissues throughout the body. (See *Mucinlike carcinoma associated antigen, Blood.*) The MUC1 gene has many varieties of carbohydrate chains that are termed *mucin-like* antigens, and one of these is the carbohydrate antigen 72-4 (CA72-4) that circulates in the bloodstream when cancer is present. CA 72-4 is elevated in several types of gastrointestinal cancer and in ovarian cancer and levels are most useful when evaluated in combination with other carbohydrate antigens. CA 72-4 is not helpful in detecting micrometastasis of colorectal cancer, but is positive in advanced metastatic tumors. It is being investigated for its usefulness as a prognostic indicator of survival in gastric cancer. CA 72-4 levels are determined using a monoclonal antibody immunoassay.

Professional Considerations
1. Consent form NOT required.
2. Preparation:
   A. Tube: Red topped, serum-separator (red/gray or gold topped) for serum samples, lavender topped for plasma samples.
3. Procedure:
   A. Blood sample is collected in the appropriate tube and refrigerated.
   B. Specimen should be refrigerated or frozen immediately.
4. Postprocedure care:
   A. None.
5. Client and family teaching:
   A. CA 72-4 is not useful as a screening test.
   B. Results are usually available within 3 working days.
6. Factors that may affect results:
   A. Reject hemolyzed specimen or specimen left at room temperature.
   B. Results are invalidated if the client has received radioisotopes within the prior 30 days.
   C. Positive tests may occur in 85% of invasive ductal breast carcinomas, more than 85% of gastrointestinal adenocarcinomas (gastric, colon, pancreatic, and esophageal), and in ovarian and endometrial adenocarcinomas. Specificity can be improved with concurrent testing for other tumor markers.
7. Other data:
   A. None.

CA 125 (CARBOHYDRATE ANTIGEN 125, CANCER ANTIGEN 125), BLOOD

Norm. <35 U/mL (<35 kU/L, SI units).

Usage. Used to aid in the management of clients with malignancies that produce the CA 125 glycoprotein; especially useful in monitoring ovarian carcinoma and breast cancer.

Increased. Abdominal inflammation, cirrhosis, endometriosis, luteal phase of menstrual cycle, menses, neoplasms (breast, cervix, colon, endometrium, fallopian tube, gastrointestinal tract, liver, lung, lymphoma, non-Hodgkin lymphoma, ovary, pancreas), nonmucinous ovarian epithelial neoplasms, ovarian abscess, pancreatitis (acute), pelvic inflammatory disease, pelvic or peritoneal tuberculosis, peritonitis (acute), polyarteritis nodosa, pregnancy (higher in first and third trimester with median 23 U/ml), serosal (pericardial, pleural, peritoneal) inflammation, Sjögren syndrome, and systemic lupus erythematosus.

Description. The MUC1 gene is a high molecular weight glycoprotein found in specific tissues throughout the body. (See *Mucin-like carcinoma associated antigen, Blood.*) The MUC1 gene has many varieties of carbohydrate chains that are termed *mucin-like* antigens, and one of these is the carbohydrate antigen 125 (CA125) that circulates in the bloodstream when cancer is present. The CA 125 epitope is present on most adult tissues derived from the coelomic epithelium. The CA 125 level is used to aid in the management of clients with malignancies that produce the glycoprotein in amounts large enough to be measured in the blood. It is rarely found in normal ovarian tissue but is found in 80% of epithelial ovarian cancers. Twenty-six percent of women with benign ovarian tumors also have an elevated CA 125 level. Although CA 125 cannot distinguish benign from malignant tumors, levels >65 U/mL are associated with malignancy in 90% of pelvic masses. Clients with very high CA 125 levels (>450 U/mL) have poor median survival, whereas clients with levels less than 55 U/mL tend to do somewhat better. CA 125 is used to monitor response to chemotherapy and to monitor for recurrence. Because a normal CA 125 level does not exclude the presence of disease, serial CA 125 levels, in combination with second-look surgery, are recommended for monitoring clients for disease recurrence. It is preferable not to perform the assay until 3 weeks after primary chemotherapy and at least 2 months after abdominal surgery. In endometrial carcinoma, an elevated CA 125 correlates well with higher grade, higher stage, increased myometrial invasion, and reduced survival. CA 125 levels are obtained by means of a CA 125 II immunoassay, which uses monoclonal antibodies.

Professional Considerations
1. Consent NOT required.
2. Preparation:
   A. Tube: Red topped, red/gray or gold topped.
3. Procedure:
   A. Draw a 1-mL blood sample.
   B. Specimen may remain at room temperature for up to 7 days but must be refrigerated if assay not performed within 7 days.
4. Postprocedure care:
   A. None.
5. Client and family teaching:
   A. This test is not used as a screening test for early carcinoma.
   B. Results should be available within 3 working days.
6. Factors that affect results:
   A. Antineoplastic therapy may lower results.
   B. Results are invalidated if the client has received radioisotopes within the prior 30 days.
7. Other data:
   A. Sensitivity of this test to ovarian cancer is 75-80%.
   B. See also *Prostasin, Serum*. Combining serum prostasin levels and CA125 levels as a marker for ovarian cancer reveals a sensitivity of 94% (compared with a sensitivity of 64.9% for CA125 and of 51.4% for prostasin).

CA 549 (CARBOHYDRATE ANTIGEN 549, CANCER ANTIGEN 549), BLOOD

Norm. <10-15.5 U/mL (No definitive cutoff yet agreed upon).

Usage. Monitoring for breast cancer disease response to treatment; Monitoring for early detection of breast cancer recurrence.

Increased. Breast cancer (low sensitivity [0.51] early in the disease, but high specificity [0.93]). In advanced breast cancer, sensitivity is about 0.70 alone, and 0.79 in combination with other markers, such as carcinoembryonic antigen (CEA) or CA 15-5.

Decreased. Positive response to therapy.

Description. The MUC1 gene is a high-molecular-weight glycoprotein found in specific tissues throughout the body. (See *Mucin-like carcinoma associated antigen, Blood*.) The MUC1 gene has many varieties of carbohydrate chains that are termed *mucin-like* antigens, and one of these is the carbohydrate antigen 549 (CA549) that circulates in the bloodstream when cancer is present. One of the newest serum markers, CA 549, is present in the serum of clients with moderate–to advanced breast cancer. Levels increase as the disease progresses, and decrease as the disease goes into remission. CA 549 is also increased when breast cancer metastasizes. It can be used as a marker alone or in combination with other tests such as CA 15-5 or CEA. However, because CEA is elevated in a variety of other conditions and types of cancer, it is less sensitive than CA 549 for breast cancer. Because of its low detection rate in early disease, CA 549 is not a useful screening test and is also not likely to detect early recurrent disease. CA 549 levels are determined using a monoclonal antibody immunoassay.

Professional Considerations
1. Consent form NOT required.
2. Preparation:
   A. Tube: Red topped or serum separator (red/gray or gold topped)
3. Procedure:
   A. Collect a 3-ml blood sample.
   B. Refrigerate specimen.
4. Postprocedure care:
   A. None.
5. Client and family teaching:
   A. Results are normally available within 3 working days.
6. Factors that affect results:
   A. CA 549 is normal in clients with benign breast disease.
   B. CA 549 can be normal in early breast cancer.
   C. False-positive results are possible, but infrequent in other types of cancer, such as liver, colon, lung and prostate cancer, and in healthy persons.
   D. Results are invalidated if the client has received radioisotopes within the prior 30 days.
7. Other data:
   A. Because CA 549 is commonly found on immunohistochemical staining of biopsies of a variety of

carcinomas, the immunohisto-chemical method of CA 549 detection is not useful for differentiating breast cancer. Sensitivity can be improved if other cancer markers are also tested.

CAC, BLOOD
(see Circulating anticoagulant, Blood)

CADMIUM, SERUM AND 24-HOUR URINE

Norm:

		SI UNITS
Serum		
Nonsmoker	0.1-0.50 µg/dL	0.89-4.45 nmol/L
Excess exposure	>10 µg/dL	>89 nmol/L
Panic level	>41 µg/dL	>365 nmol/L
Urine		
Nonsmoker	0.5-4.7 µg/L	4.4-41.8 nmol/L
Excess exposure	>10 µg/L	>88.97 nmol/L

Panic Level Symptoms and Treatment

Symptoms. Abdominal cramps, acute renal failure, diarrhea, exhaustion, headache, nausea, pulmonary edema (when cadmium dust or fumes are inhaled), shock, vertigo, vomiting.

Treatment:
Note: Treatment choice(s) is/are dependent upon client history and condition and episode history.
Give demulcents.
Use gastric lavage with milk or water.
Induce vomiting with a saline cathartic or a syrup of ipecac if within $\frac{1}{2}$ hour of exposure. (Induction of vomiting is contraindicated in clients with no gag reflex or with central nervous system depression or excitation.)
Give saline or sorbitol cathartic.
Closely monitor and support respiratory and hemodynamic status.
Activated charcoal is NOT helpful.
Monitor for liver and kidney damage.
$CaNa_2$-EDTA will enhance cadmium removal for acute exposure only.

Increased. Bladder cancer, early delivery due to maternal exposure, industrial exposure to cadmium dust and fumes such as in torch cutters, ingestion of contaminated water or food stored in cadmium-plated containers, lung cancer. Drugs include traditional Indian or Croatian remedies, herbal remedies from Lublin's drugstores (Poland).

Decreased. Not clinically significant.

Description. Cadmium is a heavy metal with a half-life of 15-20 years in humans that is obtained from zinc ores and is used in the manufacture of alloys, in storage batteries, and in electroplating. The general population is exposed to small amounts daily through fertilizers, food, water, air, and cigarette smoke. Cadmium is a respiratory tract irritant that can produce fatal pulmonary edema, proliferative interstitial pneumonia, and cardiovascular collapse if inhaled as dust or fumes. Cadmium ingestion poisoning produces a sudden onset of severe gastrointestinal symptoms within 30 minutes. Chronic exposure can produce osteomalacia and renal, lung, and hepatic disorders and can also cause severe gastroenteritis. Cadmium is not metabolized in the body. It accumulates in tissue, concentrating primarily in the kidneys and the liver. More than 95% of the blood cadmium is contained in the erythrocytes. Serum levels are used for diagnosis of acute cadmium intoxication. Urine cadmium levels are measured to detect chronic exposure. It is believed that urine cadmium levels >10 mg/L (>88.97 nmol/L, SI units) are indicative of renal tubular damage.

Professional Considerations
1. Consent form NOT required.
2. **Preparation:**
   A. *Serum:* Tube: Green topped or black topped.
   B. *Urine:* Obtain a 3-L, metal-free container without a preservative.
3. **Procedure:**
   A. *Serum:* Draw a 5-mL blood specimen in a metal-free tube.
   B. *Urine:*
      i. Discard the first morning urine specimen.
      ii. Save all the urine voided for 24 hours in a refrigerated, clean, metal-free, 3-L container without preservatives. Include the urine voided at the end of the 24-hour period. For catheterized clients, keep the drainage bag on ice and empty urine into the collection container hourly.
4. **Postprocedure care:**
   A. Send the serum specimen to the laboratory immediately.
   B. *Urine:*
      i. Compare urine quantity in the specimen container with the urinary output record for the test. If the specimen contains less urine than was recorded as output, some urine may

have been discarded, thus invalidating the test.
      ii. Document the quantity of urine output for the collection period on the laboratory requisition.
      iii. It is best to send the entire specimen to the laboratory so that it can be measured and mixed well before being tested.
5. **Client and family teaching:**
   A. *Urine:* Save all the urine voided in the 24-hour period and urinate before defecating to avoid loss of urine. If any urine is accidentally discarded, discard the entire specimen and restart the collection the next day.
   B. A client with elevated levels should identify and reduce sources of cadmium exposure and see the physician regularly for monitoring of the effects of chronic cadmium exposure.
6. **Factors that affect results:**
   A. Reject hemolyzed specimens.
   B. Urine levels increase with aging.
   C. Cadmium levels normally increase with aging.
7. **Other data:**
   A. Death may occur if pulmonary edema, shock, or renal failure is caused by cadmium poisoning.

CALCITONIN (THYROCALCITONIN), PLASMA OR SERUM

Norm:

		SI UNITS
Serum		
Adult female	<25 pg/mL	<25 ng/L
Adult male	<40 pg/mL	<40 ng/L
Term newborn, cord blood	30-240 pg/mL	30-240 ng/L
Neonate, 2 days old	91-580 pg/mL	91-580 ng/L
Neonate, 7 days old	77-293 pg/mL	77-293 ng/L
Plasma		
Basal		
Female	≤0.105 ng/mL	
Male	≤0.155 ng/mL	

Increased. Anemia (pernicious), cancer (breast, lung, thyroid), chronic renal failure, Cushing's disease (type II), ectopic calcitonin production, hypercalcemia, islet cell tumors, medullary cancer of the thyroid, parathyroid adenoma or hyperplasia, pheochromocytoma, renal failure (chronic), sepsis, thyroiditis, uremia, and Zollinger-Ellison syndrome.

Decreased. Chronic autoimmune thyroiditis.

Description. Calcitonin (thyrocalcitonin) is a thyroid gland polypeptide hormone that helps maintain normal serum calcium and phosphorus levels. It is secreted in response to hypercalcemia. Its functions include inhibition of calcium absorption from the gastrointestinal tract, inhibition of calcium resorption from the bone and soft tissues by osteoclasts and osteocytes, and increasing the amount of renal calcium excretion. Calcitonin functions in calcium homeostasis by antagonizing parathyroid hormone and vitamin D to lower serum calcium levels.

Professional Considerations
1. Consent form NOT required.
2. **Preparation:**
   A. See *Client and family teaching.*
   B. Tube: Green-topped tube, or chilled red-topped or chilled red/gray-topped, or gold-topped tube.
   C. Notify laboratory personnel that a specimen for calcitonin measurement will be delivered.
3. **Procedure:**
   A. Draw a 3-mL venous blood sample.
4. **Postprocedure care:**
   A. Send the specimen to the laboratory immediately for immediate serum separation into a plastic tube, followed by freezing.
5. **Client and family teaching:**
   A. Fast (except for sips of water) for 8 hours before sampling.
   B. A few days are required for completion of this test in the laboratory.
6. **Factors that affect results:**
   A. Reject hemolyzed specimens.
7. **Other data:**
   A. Calcitonin levels do not differ significantly by race.

CALCIUM, CALCULATED IONIZED, SERUM

Norm. 46-50% of total calcium.

Increased. See *Calcium, Ionized, Blood.*

Decreased. See *Calcium, Ionized, Blood.*

Description. Calcium is a cation that is absorbed into the bloodstream from dietary sources. Calcium functions in bone formation, nerve impulse transmission, contraction of myocardial and skeletal muscles, and in blood clotting by converting prothrombin to thrombin. Calcium is stored in the teeth and bones, and circulating calcium is filtered by the kidneys, with most being reabsorbed when serum calcium levels are normal. Calculated ionized calcium is an indirect method for calculating the amount of ionized (biologically active) calcium based on serum protein levels. Normally, 46-50% of total calcium is ionized, and most of the remainder (40%) is bound to proteins. The remaining 8%-10% is complexed with anions such as bicarbonate and lactate and is biologically inactive. Of the portion bound to proteins, 80% is bound to albumin, and 20% is bound to globulin. Calculated ionized calcium is also called protein-corrected total calcium and is used as a formula to calculate the amount of protein-bound calcium and to deduct that from the total calcium level to derive an estimate of the biologically active ionized calcium. This method is often imprecise and unreliable, especially in clients with low or high protein levels, and is being replaced by newer laboratory methods for ionized calcium measurement.

Professional Considerations
1. Consent form NOT required.
2. **Preparation:**
   A. See *Calcium, Total, Serum; Albumin Serum, Urine and 24-Hour urine;* and *Protein, Serum,* for instructions on drawing the blood for the results needed for the calculation.
3. **Procedure:**
   A. Obtain total calcium, albumin, and globulin levels and calculate the amount of ionized calcium with the following formulas:
   Step 1. % of protein-bound Ca^{++} = 8(Albumin g/dL) + 2(Globulin g/dL) + 3
   Step 2. % of ionized Ca^{++} = Total calcium mg/dL − % of protein-bound Ca^{++}
4. **Postprocedure care:**
   A. Not applicable.
5. **Client and family teaching:**
   A. None.
6. **Factors that affect results:**
   A. Results are unreliable for hypoproteinemic or hyperproteinemic states. The ion-selective

electrode procedure should be used for these clients.
B. Serum ionized-calcium concentration is significantly decreased in the elderly.
7. **Other data:**
A. Other formulas exist for calculation of ionized calcium. Many of these formulas have been dis-

puted, which makes the reliability of this calculation questionable.
B. There is a negative correlation between serum calcium and triglycerides in young and elderly hypertensives.
C. See also *Calcium, Ionized, Blood, and Calcium, Total, Serum.*

CALCIUM, IONIZED (FREE CALCIUM, DIALYZABLE CALCIUM), BLOOD

Norm. 46-56% of total serum calcium.

		SI UNITS
Serum		
Adults	4.64-5.28 mg/dL	1.16-1.32 mmol/L
Newborn	2.24-2.46 mEq/L	
Cord blood	5.2-6.40 mg/dL	1.30-1.60 mmol/L
2 hours old	4.84-5.84 mg/dL	1.21-1.46 mmol/L
1 day old	4.40-5.44 mg/dL	1.10-1.36 mmol/L
3 days old	4.60-5.68 mg/dL	1.15-1.42 mmol/L
5 days old	4.88-5.92 mg/dL	1.22-1.48 mmol/L
Children, teens	4.80-5.52 mg/dL	1.20-1.38 mmol/L
Capillary Blood		
6-36 hours old	4.20-5.48 mg/dL	1.05-1.37 mmol/L
60-84 hours old	4.40-5.68 mg/dL	1.10-1.42 mmol/L
108-132 hours old	4.80-5.92 mg/dL	1.20-1.48 mmol/L
Whole Blood		
Adults		
18-60 years	4.60-5.08 mg/dL	1.15-1.27 mmol/L
60-90 years	4.64-5.16 mg/dL	1.16-1.29 mmol/L
>90 years	4.48-5.28 mg/dL	1.12-1.32 mmol/L
Plasma		
Adults	4.12-4.92 mg/dL	1.03-1.23 mmol/L

Increased. Acidemia, hypervitaminosis D, malignancy, hyperparathyroidism (primary), tumors that produce or elevate parathyroid hormone, varicose veins. Drugs include hydrochlorothiazide (chronic use), lithium compounds, and rilmenidine.

Decreased. Alkalemia; burns; after citrate-containing blood transfusions; hyperosmolar states; hypoparathyroidism (primary); magnesium deficiency; multiple organ failure; pancreatitis; postoperatively; pseudohypoparathyroidism; sepsis; trauma; and vitamin D deficiency. Drugs include anticonvulsants, danazol, foscarnet, furosemide, and hyperosmolar solutions.

Description. Calcium is a cation that is absorbed into the bloodstream from dietary sources. Calcium functions in bone formation, nerve impulse transmission, contraction of myocardial and skeletal muscles, and in blood clotting by converting prothrombin to thrombin. Calcium is stored in the teeth and bones, and circulating calcium is filtered by the kidneys, with most being reabsorbed when serum calcium levels are normal. Ionized calcium is a cation that circulates freely in the bloodstream and constitutes 46%-50% of all circulating calcium. Levels increase and decrease directly with increases and decreases in blood pH. For every 0.1 pH unit decrease, ionized calcium increases 1.5%-2.5%. Ionized calcium is sometimes considered a more sensitive and reliable indicator of primary hyperparathyroidism for clients with low levels of albumin than total serum calcium is because ionized calcium is not affected by changes in serum albumin concentrations. Total serum calcium values increase and decrease directly with serum albumin levels, but ionized calcium levels do not. See *Calcium, Total, Serum.*

Professional Considerations
1. Consent form NOT required.
2. Preparation:
   A. The client should lie supine for 30 minutes.
   B. Tube: Red-topped, red/gray-topped, gold-topped, or green-topped tube that does not contain zinc heparin. Also obtain ice.
   C. Do NOT draw during hemodialysis.
3. Procedure:
   A. Completely fill the tube with blood without using a tourniquet. Use a Vacutainer to collect the specimen directly into the tube without removing the tube stopper.
   B. Capillary tubes from heelstick specimens are also acceptable.
   C. Place the specimen immediately on ice.
4. Postprocedure care:
   A. Deliver the specimen to the laboratory immediately and refrigerate.

5. Client and family teaching:
   A. Results are normally available within 4 hours.
   B. For chronic hypocalcemia, food sources high in calcium include milk, egg yolks, cheese, beans, cauliflower, chard, kale, and rhubarb.
6. Factors that affect results:
   A. Prolonged exposure of the serum to air causes an increase in pH that in turn causes an increased ionized calcium level. Collect the specimens anaerobically.
   B. The test must be performed within 48 hours of specimen collection.
   C. A diurnal variation exists, with the lowest values occurring in the early morning hours (0200-0400) and the highest values occurring at midevening.
   D. Levels may decrease from baseline in women taking oral contraceptives, and may increase from baseline in women taking injectable contraceptives.
7. Other data:
   A. This is the most reliable test for diagnosing hyperparathyroidism in clients with low albumin.
   B. See also *Calcium, Total, Serum,* and *Calcium, Calculated ionized, Serum.*

CALCIUM, TOTAL, SERUM

Norm:

		SI UNITS
Adults		
18-60 years	8.6-10.0 mg/dL	2.15-2.50 mmol/L
60-90 years	8.8-10.2 mg/dL	2.20-2.55 mmol/L
>90 years	8.2-9.6 mg/dL	2.05-2.40 mmol/L
Children		
Cord blood	8.2-11.2 mg/dL	2.05-2.80 mmol/L
Premature infant	6.2-11.0 mg/dL	1.55-2.75 mmol/L
≤10 days	7.6-10.4 mg/dL	1.90-2.60 mmol/L
10 days–2 years	9.0-11.0 mg/dL	2.25-2.75 mmol/L
2-12 years	8.8-10.8 mg/dL	2.20-2.70 mmol/L
12-18 years	8.4-10.2 mg/dL	2.10-2.55 mmol/L
Panic Levels		
Tetany	<7 mg/dL	<1.75 mmol/L
Coma	>12 mg/dL	>2.99 mmol/L
Possible death	≤6 mg/dL	≤1.50 mmol/L
	≥14 mg/dL	≥3.49 mmol/L

Panic Level Symptoms and Treatment

Note: Treatment choice(s) depend on client history and condition and episode history.

Symptoms of hypercalcemia. Constipation, ECG changes (shortened ST-segment), lethargy, muscle weakness, nausea, neurologic depression (headache, apathy, reduced level of consciousness) progressing to coma, vomiting.

Treatment of hypercalcemia panic levels

Correct the cause.
Give normal saline and diuretics to speed renal calcium excretion.
Give calcitonin or steroids to move calcium intracellularly.
Hemodialysis WILL remove calcium.

Symptoms of hypocalcemia. Convulsions, carpopedal spasm (positive Trousseau's sign), dysrhythmias, ECG changes (prolonged ST-segment and QT interval), facial spasm (positive Chvostek's sign), muscle cramps, numbness, tetany, tingling, and muscle twitching, spasms of the larynx.

Treatment of hypocalcemia panic levels

Implement seizure precautions.
Maintain continuous ECG monitoring.
Correct the cause.
Give calcium, magnesium, and vitamin D replacement.
IV calcium chloride or calcium gluconate 100 mg of elemental calcium or 4-7 mL of 10% calcium chloride mixed in 50-100 mL of solution over 20 minutes. Follow with calcium infusion at 1-2 mg/kg/hour.

Increased. Acidosis (respiratory), acromegaly, acute tubular necrosis (recovery phase), Addison's disease, berylliosis, bacteremia, coccidioidomycosis, diet (high calcium), ectopic neoplasms that produce parathyroid hormone, familial hypocalciuric hypercalcemia, hepatic disease (chronic advanced), histoplasmosis, hyperparathyroidism (primary, tertiary renal), hyperthyroidism, hypervitaminosis (vitamin D or A intoxication), immobility (prolonged), infants (idiopathic), leukemia, lymphoma, malignancy (bladder, breast, kidney, lung), metastatic bone cancer, milk-alkali (Burnett) syndrome, multiple endocrine neoplasia, multiple myeloma, mycoses, osteoporosis, Paget's disease, peptic ulcer diet, pheochromocytoma, polycythemia vera, porphyria, renal calculi, renal osteomalacia (induced by aluminum), renal transplantation, respiratory disease, rhabdomyolysis, sarcoidosis, and tuberculosis. Drugs include anabolic steroids, androgens, antacids (alkaline), calcium gluconate, calciferol, calcium salts, calusterone, chlorothiazide sodium, chlorthalidone, danazol, diethylstilbestrol, dihydrotachysterol, diuretics, ergocalciferol, estrogens, indomethacin, isotretinoin, lithium carbonate, parathyroid hormone, progesterone, secretin, tamoxifen, testolactone, theophylline (toxicity), thiazide diuretics, thyroid hormones, vitamin A, and vitamin D.

Decreased. Alkalosis, bacteremia, blood transfusions (excessive without replacement of calcium), burns, cachexia, celiac disease, chronic renal disease, cystic fibrosis of pancreas, diarrhea, Fanconi syndrome (with renal tubular acidosis), hypomagnesemia, hypoparathyroidism, hypoproteinemia, infection (severe), malabsorption, malaria (uncomplicated), Milkman syndrome, nephritis, nephrosis, nephrotic syndrome, obstructive jaundice, osteomalacia, pancreatitis (acute), parathyroidectomy, pregnancy (late), pseudohypoparathyroidism, renal failure, renal insufficiency, renal tubular acidosis, rickets, sprue, starvation, toxic shock syndrome, thyroidectomy with accidental removal of parathyroid gland, and vitamin D deficiency. Drugs include acetazolamide, albuterol, alprostadil, aminoglycosides, antacids, anticonvulsants, asparaginase, aspirin, barbiturates (in elderly), calcitonin, carbamazepine, carbenoxolone, carboplatin, corticosteroids, cholestyramine resin, fluorides, furosemide, gastrin, gentamicin, glucagon, glucose, heparin, hydrocortisone, indapamide, insulin, iron, isoniazid, laxatives (excessive), magnesium salts, mercurial diuretics, mestranol, mithramycin, methicillin, phenobarbital, phenytoin, phosphates, plicamycin, and saline (in hypercalcemic state) tetracycline (during pregnancy).

Description. Calcium is a cation that is absorbed into the bloodstream from dietary sources and functions in bone formation, nerve impulse transmission, contraction of myocardial and skeletal muscles, and in blood clotting by converting prothrombin to thrombin. Calcium is stored in the teeth and bones, and circulating calcium is filtered by the kidneys, with most being reabsorbed when serum calcium levels are normal. To maintain a normal calcium balance and counteract any excreted calcium, at least 1 g of calcium must be ingested daily. Normally, 46%-50% of total calcium is ionized and most of the remainder (40%) is bound to proteins. Only ionized calcium can be used by the body. The remaining 8%-10% is complexed with anions such as bicarbonate and lactate and is biologically inactive. Total serum calcium values increase and decrease directly with serum albumin levels, but ionized calcium levels do not. For every 1 g/dL decrease in albumin, total serum calcium decreases by 0.8 mg/dL. When acidosis is present, more calcium is ionized. In alkalosis, most is bound to protein and cannot be used by the body.

Professional Considerations
1. Consent form NOT required.
2. Preparation:
   A. Tube: Red topped, red/gray topped, or gold topped.
   B. Do NOT draw during hemodialysis.
3. Procedure:
   A. Leaving the tourniquet in place less than 1 minute, draw a 1-mL venous blood sample.
4. Postprocedure care:
   A. Send the specimen to the laboratory for spinning within 1 hour.
5. Client and family teaching:
   A. Eat a diet with normal calcium levels, 800 mg/day (15-20 mmol/day, SI units), for 3 days before sampling.
   B. Fast, except for water, for 8 hours (only for multichannel tests).
   C. For elevated levels, avoid foods high in calcium, ambulate when possible, and increase fluid intake unless contraindicated.
6. Factors that affect results:
   A. Reject hemolyzed specimens.
   B. Falsely elevated values may be caused by hemolysis, dehydration, or hyperproteinemia.
   C. Falsely decreased values may be caused by dilutional hypervolemia, administration of intravenous sodium chloride or by the administration of sulfobromo-sulphalein sodium (Bromsulphalein) dye within 2 days before specimen collection.
   D. Serum calcium should be corrected for the serum albumin. For every gram below 4 mg/dL, add 0.8 to the calcium level.
7. Other data:
   A. Hypercalcemia can induce digoxin toxicity and decreased neuronal permeability.
   B. High intakes of calcium reduced the risk of rectal cancer by 45%.
   C. See also *Calcium, Calculated ionized, Serum,* and *Calcium, Ionized, Blood.*

CALCIUM, URINE

Norm. Semiquantitative Sulkowitch test: 1+ to 2+.

QUANTITATIVE TESTS		SI UNITS
Random specimen	<40 mg/dL	<1.0 mmol/L
24-hour specimen		
Low-calcium diet	<150 mg/day	<3.7 mmol/day
Normal-calcium diet	100-250 mg/day	2.5-6.2 mmol/day
High-calcium diet	250-300 mg/day	6.2-7.5 mmol/day

Increased. Acromegaly, amyotrophic lateral sclerosis, bone metastasis, cancer (primary) of the breast or lung, Crohn's disease, diabetes mellitus, diet (high calcium or high sodium chloride), ectopic hyperparathyroidism, Fanconi syndrome (with renal tubular acidosis), glucocorticoid excess, hypercalcemia, hyperparathyroidism, hyperthyroidism, hypervitaminosis D, hypocitraturia, idiopathic hypercalciuria, immobility (long term), leukemia, lymphoma, metastasis, medullary sponge kidney, multiple myeloma, nephrolithiasis, osteoporosis, Paget's disease, renal tubular acidosis, sarcoidosis, ulcerative colitis, and Wilson's disease. Drugs include ammonium chloride, androgens, anabolic steroids, antacids, calcipotriol, cholestyramine, EB 1089 (vitamin D analog), furosemide, mercurial diuretics, parathyroid hormone, potassium citrate, and vitamin D.

Decreased. Chronic renal failure, familial hypocalciuric hypercalcemia, hypocalcemia, hypoparathyroidism, malabsorption, milk-alkali syndrome, metastatic carcinoma of the prostate, nephrosis, osteomalacia, preeclampsia, pseudohypoparathyroidism, renal insufficiency, renal osteodystrophy, rickets (vitamin D resistant), steatorrhea, and vitamin D deficiency. Drugs include aspirin, indomethacin, oral contraceptives, sodium phytate, thiazide diuretics, and viomycin.

Description. A cation that is absorbed into the bloodstream from dietary sources and that functions in bone formation, nerve impulse transmission, contractility of muscles, and blood clotting. Calcium is stored in the bones and circulating calcium is filtered by the kidneys, with most being reabsorbed when serum calcium levels are normal. When serum calcium levels rise above normal, the kidneys reabsorb less calcium, and elevated levels of calcium appear in the urine. Whereas quantitative tests must be performed by a laboratory, the Sulkowitch test is a semiquantitative test suitable for home use.

Professional Considerations
1. Consent form NOT required.
2. **Preparation:**
   A. Note daily dietary level of calcium intake for the previous 3 days on the laboratory requisition.
   B. Obtain a 3-L container with hydrochloric acid (HCl) additive or an acid-washed glass bottle for 24-hour collection. Write the

starting date and the time on the container.
   C. Obtain a small container to collect a random sample.
3. **Procedure:**
   A. *24-hour collection (quantitative):*
      i. Discard the first morning-urine specimen.
      ii. Begin to time a 24-hour urine collection.
      iii. Save all the urine voided for 24 hours in a clean, plastic, 3-L container to which 10 mL of 6N HCl has been added or in an acid-washed glass bottle. Include the urine voided at the end of the 24-hour period.
   B. *Random specimen collection (quantitative):*
      i. When evaluating for hypocalciuria, collect a postprandial specimen. When evaluating for hypercalciuria, collect an early-morning specimen before breakfast. Obtain a 100-mL random urine specimen in a clean container. A fresh specimen may be taken from a urinary drainage bag.
   C. *Sulkowitch test (semiquantitative):*
      i. Obtain a 20-mL random urine specimen.
      ii. Follow the package instructions.
4. **Postprocedure care:**
   A. Compare the urine quantity in the specimen container with the urinary output record for the test. If the specimen contains less urine than what was recorded as output, some urine may have been discarded, thus invalidating the test.
   B. Document the quantity of urine output for the collection period on the laboratory requisition.
   C. Send the specimen to the laboratory within 1 hour.
5. **Client and family teaching:**
   A. The client should consume a diet with normal calcium levels, 600-800 mg/day (15-20 mmol/day, SI units), for 3 days.
   B. Save all the urine voided in the 24-hour period and urinate before defecating to avoid loss of urine. If any urine is accidentally discarded, discard the entire

specimen and restart the collection the next day.

C. Clients with elevated levels should be told to notify the physician for symptoms of renal calculi (flank or abdominal pain, severe dysuria).

6. Factors that affect results:
   A. Failure to add HCl to the collection container before the collection is started will result in falsely decreased results.
   B. All the urine voided for the 24-hour period must be included to avoid a falsely low result.
   C. For a random specimen, a delay in processing may cause falsely decreased results.
   D. Elevated urine phosphate may caused decreased results.

7. Other data:
   A. 20-25% of clients who form calcium stones have hyperuricosuria.
   B. See also *Calcium, Total, Serum*.

CALCIUM DISODIUM EDTA MOBILIZATION TEST, 24-HOUR, URINE

(see Lead mobilization test, 24-Hour urine)

CALIFORNIA ENCEPHALITIS VIRUS TITER (LA CROSSE VIRUS TITER), SERUM

Norm. Less than a fourfold increase in titer in paired sera (acute and convalescent sera).

Usage. Supports the diagnosis of viral encephalitis.

Description. The California encephalitis virus commonly produces aseptic meningitis, which occurs in the summer and is clinically indistinguishable from enteroviral disease. Encephalitis is an inflammation of the brain caused by an arbovirus infection transmitted by infected mosquitoes and tics. It causes an abrupt onset of severe frontal headache, fever of 38-40° C, stiff neck, sore throat, and sometimes lethargy, bronchitis, pneumonia, meningitis, convulsions, and coma. Incidence is highest in children and in the inhabitants of tundra, taiga, and leafy forest and the north central states of the United States including Indi-

ana, Tennessee, North Carolina, and West Virginia. Risk increases with number of hours spent outdoors and living residence with one or more tree holes within 100 meters.

Professional Considerations
1. Consent form NOT required.
2. Preparation:
   A. Tube: Red topped, red/gray topped, or gold topped.
   B. MAY be drawn during hemodialysis.
3. Procedure:
   A. Draw a 15-mL venous blood sample.
   B. Repeat the test for a convalescent serum specimen in 10-14 days.
4. Postprocedure care:
   A. Send the specimen to the laboratory within 2 hours.
5. Client and family teaching:
   A. Return in 10 days to 2 weeks for repeat testing.
6. Factors that affect results:
   A. Reject hemolyzed specimens.
   B. The serum should be separated from the clot within 2-3 hours.
7. Other data:
   A. The virus can rarely be isolated from blood or spinal fluid in the acute phase.
   B. Serologic diagnosis can be made by demonstration of rising antibody titers between the acute and convalescent specimens.
   C. Specific serologic diagnosis may be complicated by cross-reactions in clients with prior exposure to dengue or other flaviviruses.

cAMP

(see Cyclic adenosine monophosphate, Serum and Urine)

CAMPYLOBACTER-LIKE-ORGANISM (CLO) TEST (RAPID UREASE TEST), SPECIMEN

Norm. Negative (CLO test gel turns yellow 24 hours after specimen insertion).

Positive. Presence of *Helicobacter pylori* (amount present is decided by deepening in color of the specimen).

Description. This is a simple test used to determine the presence of *H. pylori* in

C

gastric mucosal biopsy specimens. *H. pylori* has been implicated as a primary etiologic factor in duodenal ulcer disease, gastric ulcer, and nonulcer dyspepsia. By causing chronic inflammation, *H. pylori* may weaken mucosal defenses and allow acid and pepsin to disrupt the epithelium. *H. pylori* produces large amounts of urease enzyme which can be found in 83% of dental plaque scrapings and 59% of tongue scrapings. Although urease primarily allows *H. pylori* to utilize urea as a nitrogen source, the breakdown of urea also produces high local concentrations of ammonia, which enable the organism to tolerate a low pH. Simple tests such as the CLO test enable a rapid diagnosis. The CLO test is a sealed plastic slide holding an agar gel that contains urea, a pH indicator, phenol red, buffers, and bacteriostatic agents that help prevent false color changes that could lead to false-positive readings. If the urease enzyme of *H. pylori* is present in an inserted tissue sample, the resulting degradation of urea causes the pH to rise, and the color of the gel turns from yellow to a bright magenta color.

Professional Considerations

1. Consent form NOT required but IS required for the endoscopy procedure used to obtain the specimen. See *Gastroesophagoduodenoscopy, Diagnostic,* for risks and contraindications.
2. **Preparation:**
   A. See *Client and family teaching.*
   B. Inspect the CLO test slide to make sure that the well is full and is a yellow color. If a CLO test slide has an orange color, it should be used with caution because it may give a false-positive result.
   C. See also *Esophagogastroduodenoscopy, Diagnostic.*
3. **Procedure:**
   A. Immediately before endoscopy, place the CLO test on a warming plate at 30°-40° C. Warming helps to speed the chemical reaction.
   B. Obtain a tissue sample from the gastric mucosa by endoscopy. Place the sample immediately in the well of the CLO test slide.
4. **Postprocedure care:**
   A. Be certain that the tissue specimen is completely immersed so that it will have maximum contact with the urea and bacteriostat in the gel.
   B. Reseal the CLO test container.
   C. Keep the CLO test in a warm place for the next 3 hours.
   D. See also *Esophagogastroduodenoscopy, Diagnostic.*
5. **Client and family teaching:**
   A. Do not take antibiotics or bismuth salts for at least 3 weeks before the test.
   B. This test will help identify whether the *H. pylori* bacteria is present in your stomach. The bacterium is believed to be a cause of ulcers and gastritis.
   C. Since *H. pylori* therapy is only 50%-75% effective, it is important that you return for retesting 28 days after completing therapy to confirm complete eradication of *H. pylori.*
   D. See also *Esophagogastroduodenoscopy, Diagnostic.*
6. **Factors that affect results:**
   A. False-negative results may occur when very low numbers of *H. pylori* are present or when the bacterium has a patchy distribution.
   B. The CLO test will be less sensitive if the client has recently been taking antibiotics or bismuth.
7. **Other data:**
   A. The CLO test has proved to be an accurate test with few false-negative results.

CAMPYLOBACTER PYLORI

(see Helicobacter pylori, Quick office serology, Serum and titer, Blood or Campylobacter-like organism test, Specimen)

C-ANCA

(see Anti-neutrophil cytoplasmic antibody screen, Serum)

CANNABINOIDS, QUALITATIVE, BLOOD OR URINE

Norm. None present. Negative.

Usage. Testing for use of marijuana.

Description. Marijuana is derived from an Asiatic herb, *Cannabis sativa,* and contains many biologically active chemicals, with most of the pharmacologic effects resulting from 9-tetrahydrocannabinol (THC). THC has an unusually high lipid solubility, and so it is widely distributed in the body, with a high affinity for brain tissue. THC affects mood, memory, motor coordination, cognitive ability, sensorium, time sense, and self-perception. THC also significantly increases cortical and cerebellar blood flow and suppresses immunologic function of macrophages. The effects are dose related and are three to four times more potent when smoked than when ingested or injected. THC is metabolized to numerous active and inactive metabolites called cannabinoids. Seventy percent of the dose from smoking THC is excreted within 72 hours in the urine and feces. Because of slow release of THC from tissue storage sites, urine may test positive for 2-5 days after marijuana use by infrequent smokers. The primary psychoactive metabolite, which is also the most abundant and inactive, is 11-hydroxy-THC. Most immunoassay tests use antibodies directed at 11-hydroxy-THC. Immunoassays are also available to measure the drug THC, which can be used in the treatment of persistent nausea and vomiting associated with cancer chemotherapy or to decrease the pain of glaucoma.

Professional Considerations
1. Consent form NOT required but is usually obtained for preemployment testing or for medicolegal specimens.
2. Preparation:
   A. Tube: Red topped, red/gray topped, or gold topped. Also obtain a sterile plastic urine collection container.
   B. Do NOT draw during hemodialysis.
3. Procedure:
   A. If specimens are being obtained for medicolegal purposes, the collection, transportation, and processing should be performed in the presence of a witness.
   B. Draw a 5-mL venous blood sample.
   C. Obtain a random 50-mL urine specimen in a sterile plastic container.
4. Postprocedure care:
   A. Write the exact time of the specimen collection and the source, date, and client's name on the laboratory requisition.

B. If the specimen may be used as legal evidence, sign and have the witness sign the laboratory requisition. Transport the specimen to the laboratory in a sealed plastic bag labeled as legal evidence. Each client handling the specimen should sign and write the time of specimen receipt on the laboratory requisition.
5. Client and family teaching:
   A. The long-term effects of marijuana use include impaired lung structure, chromosomal mutation, higher incidence of birth defects, mononucleic white blood cells, memory impairment, flashbacks, and impairment of fertility.
   B. Offer substance abuse counseling referral to all clients using cannabinoids without a medical prescription.
6. Factors that affect results:
   A. Serum levels of THC peak within 10-30 minutes of inhalation and within 3 hours of ingestion depending on the dosage.
   B. Urine levels peak from 2 to 6 hours after THC has entered the system.
   C. Urine levels are detectable for 4-6 days in acute users and for 20-77 days in chronic users.
   D. Urine loss is 23% if stored at room temperature for 10 days and 8%-20% if frozen for up to 3 years.
   E. The use of Stealth adulterant in the urine sample will cause negative results in a positive sample.
7. Other data:
   A. Because of the cardiac stimulant effects, cannabinoids may pose a threat to clients with cardiovascular disease.
   B. Marijuana is the most widely used illicit drug in the United States.
   C. The signs and symptoms of *Cannabis* intoxication are tachycardia; conjunctival infection; hypotension; muscle weakness; tremors; unsteadiness; increased deep tendon reflexes; psychologic and cognitive impairments; hallucinations; loss of consciousness; and, rarely, death.
   D. Common street names for marijuana include Acapulco gold, bhand, blunts, chronic (or "the chronic"), Colombian, ganja, grass, hash, hash oil, hay, herb, J,

jay, jive stick, joint, loco weed, Mary Jane, Panama red, pot, reefer, rope, smoke, stick, tea, and weed.

CAPILLARY FRAGILITY TEST (RUMPEL-LEEDE TOURNIQUET TEST), DIAGNOSTIC

Norm. Negative or 1+.
Within a radius of 2.5 cm:

    Females = 10 or less petechiae
    Males = 5 or less petechiae

Increased. Aplastic anemia, acute leukemia, chronic nephritis, decreased estrogen level in postmenopausal female, disseminated intravascular coagulation, dysproteinemia, factor VII deficiency, fibrinogen deficiency, Glanzmann's disease, hereditary telangiectasia, influenza, idiopathic thrombocytopenia purpura, liver disease, measles, polycythemia vera, prothrombin deficiency, scarlet fever, *Stachybotrys chartarum* fungus, thrombocytopenia, scurvy, vascular purpura, vitamin K deficiency, and von Willebrand's disease. Drugs include long-term steroid use, and selective serotonin reputake inhibitor antidepressants. Herbal or natural remedies include *ruscus aculeatus* (butcher's broom).

Decreased. Drugs include glucocorticoids.

Description. This test, also known as the tourniquet test, is a nonspecific evaluation to measure capillary wall weakness and deficiencies in platelet number and function. An inflated blood pressure cuff at a specific pressure for a fixed period of time produces increased pressure and hypoxia in the capillaries distal to the cuff. Decreased capillary resistance causes the capillaries to rupture, which leads to bleeding and the formation of petechiae.

Professional Considerations
1. Consent form NOT required.

Risks
Bleeding, infection, hematoma, ecchymosis.

Contraindications
The test is contraindicated if routine tourniquet use for drawing blood specimens produces petechiae. This test is contraindicated in clients who have edematous or very cold arms or if there are contraindications to placing or inflating a blood pressure cuff on the arm (such as casts, rash, dressings, arteriovenous fistula). Other contraindications include platelet count <50,000/mm³, severe bleeding disorders, anticoagulant therapy, or senile skin changes, or if the client has taken medications containing aspirin within 7 days before the test.

2. **Preparation:**
   A. Obtain a blood pressure cuff, manometer, and watch.
   B. Inspect the arm carefully for the presence of preexisting petechiae.
3. **Procedure:**
   A. Apply a blood pressure cuff to the arm and inflate to a level midway between the client's systolic and diastolic pressures but not higher than 100 mm Hg.
   B. Leave the cuff inflated for 5 minutes and observe the arm at least 1 inch distal to the cuff for the formation of petechiae.
   C. The test results are reported in a range from negative to +4, depending on the number of petechiae appearing in a 5-cm diameter circle:

       Negative = No petechiae
       +1 = 1-10 petechiae
       +2 = 11-20 petechiae
       +3 = 21-50 petechiae
       +4 = >50 petechiae

   If preexisting petechiae are present, count the number of additional petechiae formed during the test.
4. **Postprocedure care:**
   A. Deflate and remove the blood pressure cuff.
   B. Client should open and close the hand to hasten blood return to the distal extremity.
5. **Client and family teaching:**
   A. A good explanation of the test procedure is essential because the test may cause discomfort to the client.
6. **Factors that affect results:**
   A. Failure to keep the cuff inflated for 5 minutes.
7. **Other data:**
   A. A positive test in women over 40 years old may not be pathogenic.

B. A variation of this positive-pressure test is the negative-pressure test, in which a small suction cup is applied for 1 minute to the skin and the number of resulting petechiae are counted.

C. The test should not be repeated on the same extremity for at least 1 week.

CAPTOPRIL RENOGRAPHY
(*see Renocystogram, Diagnostic*)

CARBAMAZEPINE, BLOOD

Norm. Negative.

	TROUGH	SI UNITS
Therapeutic value	4-12 µg/mL	17-51 µmol/L
Value for persons taking concurrent antiepileptic medications	4-8 µg/mL	17-34 µmol/L
Panic level	>20 µg/mL	>84 µmol/L

Panic Level Symptoms and Treatment

Symptoms

Stage I (Levels >25 µg/mL)—stupor, coma up to 24 hours, seizures, respiratory depression.

Stage II (Levels 15-25 µg/mL)—adventitial choreiform movements, combativeness, hallucinations, moderate stupor.

Stage III (Levels 11-15 µg/mL)—mild drowsiness

Stage IV (Levels <11 µg/mL)—ataxia and nystagmus with otherwise normal neurologic status. Relapse to earlier stages may recur unexpectedly. Ataxia, blurred vision, CNS depression, coma, diplopia, dizziness, drowsiness, dysrhythmias (conduction defects, right bundle branch block, sinus tachycardia), dystonic reaction, hallucination, hypotension, nystagmus, reduced myocardial contractility, pulmonary edema, respiratory depression, seizures (when levels exceed 20 g/mL), vomiting.

Treatment:
Note: Treatment choice(s) depend on client history and condition and episode history.
Do NOT induce emesis.
Perform gastric lavage if the drug has been recently ingested (most effective mechanism to reduce absorption).
Maintain and protect airway.
Give activated charcoal unless ileus is present.
Treat hypotension with fluids and vasopressors.
Treat seizures with diazepam, phenobarbital, or phenytoin.
Monitor for cardiovascular toxicity (ECG, vital signs, renal function, electrolytes, CBC).
Carbamazepine CANNOT be hemodialyzed out of the body.
Hemoperfusion for at least 4 hours WILL remove 50 mg to 2.4 grams of carbamazepine in most clients.

Increased. Drug abuse, glossopharyngeal neuralgia, renal failure (increases metabolite 10,11-epoxide), tic douloureux, and trigeminal neuralgia. Drugs include calcium-channel blockers, cimetidine, erythromycin, fluoxetine, influenza vaccine, isoniazid, propoxyphene, verapamil, and vigabatrin.

Decreased. Convulsions, epilepsy, and seizures. Drugs include phenobarbital, primidone, and phenytoin.

Description. Carbamazepine (CBZ) is an anticonvulsant, anticholinergic sedative, antidepressant, and muscle relaxant that is used alone or with other anticonvulsants to treat seizures. This drug is metabolized in the liver, with a half-life of 10-30 hours in adults and 8-19 hours in children. Steady-state levels occur in 2-6 days. This drug is affected by circadian rhythm and therefore should be ingested at a consistent time of day. CBZ crosses the placenta and appears in breast milk. For rapid detection, the fluorescence polarization assay method can be used.

Professional Considerations
1. Consent form NOT required.
2. Preparation:
   A. Serum should be drawn before the morning dose is given.
   B. Tube: Green topped, red topped, red/gray topped, or gold topped.
   C. MAY be drawn during hemodialysis.
3. Procedure:
   A. Draw a 7-mL TROUGH venous blood sample.
   B. Obtain serial measurements at the same time each day.
4. Postprocedure care:
   A. Reject hemolyzed specimens.
5. Client and family teaching:
   A. Early toxic signs include fever, sore throat, oral ulcers, easy bruising, unusual bleeding, and joint pain.
   B. Levels should be checked weekly × 12 during initiation of therapy and then monthly for 2-3 years.
   C. If activated charcoal was given for elevated levels, the client should drink 4-6 glasses of water each day for 2 days to prevent constipation. Activated charcoal will also cause stools to be black for a few days.

6. Factors that affect results:
   A. Absorption of the drug is enhanced with the eating of food.
   B. Therapeutic values should be toward the lower norms when both CBZ and other anticonvulsants are taken.
   C. Peak levels occur 2-4 hours after oral dosage.
7. Other data:
   A. Side effects include bone marrow depression, eosinophilia, hepatic dysfunction, and urticaria.
   B. CBZ can be responsible for testing positive on a tricyclic antidepressant immunoassay.
   C. Serum levels of breast-fed infants are 20% of maternal CBZ values.
   D. Antemortem serum concentration of CBZ is not significantly different from whole blood concentrations 72 hours after death.
   E. The trade name for CBZ is Tegretol.

CARBOHYDRATE ANTIGEN 19-9, BLOOD
(see CA 19-9, Blood)

CARBOHYDRATE ANTIGEN 50, BLOOD
(see CA 50, Blood)

CARBOHYDRATE ANTIGEN 72-4, BLOOD
(see 72-4, Blood)

CARBOHYDRATE ANTIGEN 125, BLOOD
(see CA 125, Blood)

CARBOHYDRATE ANTIGEN 549, BLOOD
(see CA 549, Blood)

CARBON-13 OR CARBON-14 UREA BREATH TEST
(see Urea breath test, Diagnostic)

CARBON DIOXIDE, PARTIAL PRESSURE (pCO$_2$), BLOOD

Norm:

		SI UNITS
Arterial sample	35-45 mm Hg	4.7-6.0 kPa
Panic level	<20 mm Hg	<2.6 kPa
	>70 mm Hg	>9.2 kPa
Arterialized capillary sample (<2 years of age)	26.4-41.2 mm Hg	3.5-5.4 kPa
Venous sample	38-50 mm Hg	5.0-6.7 kPa

Increased. Acute intermittent porphyria, aminoglycoside toxicity, asthma (late stage), brain death, coarctation of the aorta, congestive heart failure, cystic fibrosis, electrolyte disturbance (severe), emphysema, empyema, extubation after coronary artery bypass graft, hyaline membrane disease, hyperemesis, hypothyroidism (severe), hypoventilation (alveolar), metabolic alkalosis, near drowning, pleural effusion, pleurisy, pneumonia, pneumothorax, poisoning, pulmonary edema, pulmonary infection, renal disorders, respiratory acidosis, respiratory failure, shock, tetralogy of Fallot, transposition of the great vessels, and vomiting. Drugs include aldosterone, bicarbonate (HCO$_3$$^-$), ethacrynic acid, glucose-insulin-kalium mixture, hydrocortisone, laxatives, metolazone, morphine, prednisone, thiazides, tromethamine, and viomycin.

Decreased. Dysrhythmias, asthma (early stage), diabetic ketoacidosis, diabetes mellitus, epileptic spike waves, fever, high altitude, hyperventilation, metabolic acidosis, respiratory alkalosis, and salicylate intoxication. Drugs include acetazolamide, dimercaprol, dimethadione, methicillin sodium, nitrofurantoin, nitrofurantoin sodium, phenformin, tetracycline, and triamterene.

Description. Carbon dioxide gas present in air and also occurring as a nutritional metabolite is essential to the body's regulation of acid-base buffer system. This test measures the partial pressure exerted by carbon dioxide (pCO$_2$) dissolved in the blood and reflects the body's ability to produce carbonic acid and the efficiency of lung alveoli to excrete carbon dioxide. Laboratory measurement of pCO$_2$ assists in differentiating respiratory from metabolic causes of acidosis and alkalosis.

Professional Considerations
1. Consent form NOT required.
2. **Preparation:**
   A. The client should rest for 30 minutes before specimen collection.
   B. Obtain a 22-gauge needle, a green-topped tube, a glass syringe, heparin, 2% lidocaine, sterile gauze, and ice.
   C. Do NOT draw during hemodialysis.
3. **Procedure:**
   A. Brachial, femoral, and radial arteries are choice sites for obtaining blood specimens. If an arterial site is selected, anesthetize surrounding tissue.
   B. Draw a 5-mL anaerobic arterial or mixed venous blood sample into a heparinized, green-topped tube or glass syringe.
   C. To maintain the blood specimen anaerobically, completely fill syringe or green-topped tube with blood. If using a syringe, place the needle in a rubber stopper or apply a rubber cap immediately. Avoid pulling back on the syringe plunger. When using a green-topped vacuum tube, remove it from the adapter before removing the needle from the artery or vein and do not remove the stopper from the tube.
   D. Place the specimen immediately in an ice bath and send the specimen to the laboratory while maintaining anaerobic integrity.
4. **Postprocedure care:**
   A. Hold direct pressure over the site for 3-5 minutes.

B. Write the time of collection on the requisition.
5. **Client and family teaching:**
   A. Results are normally available within 4 hours.
6. **Factors that affect results:**
   A. Reject specimens containing air bubbles, not packed in ice, or received more than 15 minutes after collection. Test results are more accurate if performed within 15-20 minutes after specimen collection.
7. **Other data:**
   A. The pCO_2 level must be analyzed with consideration given to electrolyte and pH levels.
   B. See also *Carbon dioxide, Total content, Blood,* because pCO_2 is only a measure of the pressure exerted by carbon dioxide present in the blood.

CARBON DIOXIDE (CO_2) TOTAL CONTENT, BLOOD

Norm:

		SI UNITS
Adult	22-30 mEq/L	22-30 mmol/L
	38-50 mm Hg	
Panic level	<15 mEq/L	<15 mmol/L
	>50 mEq/L	>50 mmol/L
Neonates–2 years	32-44 mm Hg	
Child >2 years	22-26 mEq/L	22-26 mmol/L

Increased. Adrenal cortex hormone imbalance, airway obstruction, alcoholism, aldosteronism, bradycardia, cardiac disorders, emphysema, fat embolism, hypoventilation, metabolic alkalosis, pneumonia, pulmonary dysfunction, prolonged nasogastric tube drainage, pyloric obstruction, renal disorders, respiratory acidosis, respiratory disease, and vomiting (severe). Drugs include antacids, corticotropin, cortisone acetate, mercurial diuretics, sodium bicarbonate, and thiazide diuretics.

Decreased. Alcoholic ketosis, dehydration, diabetic ketoacidosis, diarrhea (severe), drainage of intestinal fluid (gastric suction), head trauma, high fever, hepatic disorders, hyperventilation, lactic acidosis, malabsorption syndrome, metabolic acidosis, renal disorders, renal failure (acute), respiratory alkalosis (compensated), salicylate intoxication, starvation, and uremia. Drugs include acetazolamide, ammonium chloride, aspirin, chlorothiazide diuretics, dimercaprol, methicillin, nitrofurantoin, paraldehyde, and tetracycline.

Description. Carbon dioxide (CO_2) gas is present in air and also occurs as a nutritional metabolite. Total carbon dioxide level reflects the total amount of carbon dioxide in the body (that is, in solution bound to proteins and bound as bicarbonate, carbonate, and carbonic acid) and is a general guide to the body's buffering capacity. Total CO_2 content is a bicarbonate and base solution that is regulated by the kidneys. CO_2 gas is acidic and is regulated by the lungs. Since over 80% of CO_2 is present in the form of bicarbonate, this test is a good reflection of bicarbonate level. Elevated or decreased levels indicate an acid-base imbalance and are related to hyperventilation or hypoventilation from a variety of causes as well as a metabolic cause. Total CO_2 is generally measured with electrolytes in the SMA-6 test but may be measured alone.

Professional Considerations
1. Consent form NOT required.
2. **Preparation:**
   A. Tube: Green topped. Obtain a container of ice for the arterial samples.
   B. Do not allow the client to clench-unclench the hand before blood drawing.
   C. Do NOT draw during hemodialysis.
3. **Procedure:**
   A. Collect the specimen without a tourniquet or quickly after tourniquet application, to prevent stasis.
   B. Completely fill a heparinized green-topped tube with venous blood to prevent diffusion of CO_2

into the tube. Collect the specimen directly into the tube without exposing to the air.

C. In the newborn, blood may be drawn from the heel, fingertips, or toes.

D. Write the body temperature on the laboratory requisition.

4. **Postprocedure care:**
   A. Place the arterial sample on ice immediately.
   B. Transport the specimen to the laboratory within 15 minutes.

5. **Client and family teaching:**
   A. Results are normally available within 4 hours.

6. **Factors that affect results:**
   A. Pumping the fist before venipuncture may cause falsely elevated results.
   B. High altitudes require a decrease in values of 5 mm Hg/mile (3 mm Hg/km).
   C. A clotted sample or air bubbles in the sample invalidate the results.
   D. Hyperthermia causes an increased CO_2 level. Values must be corrected for temperature abnormalities.

7. **Other data:**
   A. See also *Carbon dioxide, Partial pressure, Blood.*

CARBON MONOXIDE (CO), BLOOD

Norm:

	% OF TOTAL HEMOGLOBIN
Rural environment, nonsmoker	0.05-2.5
Heavy smoker	5-10
Acute toxicity	>25
Newborn	10-12

Panic Level Symptoms and Treatment

Symptoms. Symptoms correlate poorly with blood levels. Levels over 10% cause dizziness, headache, dyspnea on exertion, and impaired judgment. Levels over 30% additionally cause nausea, syncope, tachycardia, tachypnea, and vomiting. Deep coma, convulsions, respiratory failure, and death may occur at levels over 50%.

Treatment:

Note: Treatment choice(s) depend on client history and condition and episode history.

100% oxygen by high-flow mask until CO level is less than 10%.

Continuous ECG monitoring.

Laboratory work: arterial blood gas, electrolytes, creatine kinase, and urinalysis. Repeat blood carbon monoxide measurements every 2-4 hours until results are <15%.

Treat metabolic acidosis only if pH is <7.15. Acidosis increases availability of oxygen to the tissues from a right shift in the oxyhemoglobin dissociation curve. Acidosis will resolve as the CO levels normalize.

Cerebral edema is possible. Observe for and treat seizures with diazepam, phenobarbital, or phenytoin. Perform frequent neurologic checks.

Hyperbaric oxygen for severely elevated levels (e.g., >40% or when symptoms continue after 4 hours of treatment) and in all clients who are pregnant.

Both hemodialysis and peritoneal dialysis WILL remove carbon monoxide.

Increased. Accidental or intentional inhalation of fumes from combustion of carbon-containing fuels (caused by smoking or exposure to passive smoke, automobile exhaust fumes, or gas-burning appliances).

Decreased. Not clinically significant.

Description. Carbon monoxide (CO) is a chemical asphyxiant found in the fumes of automobile exhaust, improperly functioning furnaces, and defective gas-burning appliances. When inhaled, it combines with the hemoglobin in the red blood cells with an affinity 200 times greater than oxygen. This produces a hemoglobin derivative, carboxyhemoglobin, which is unable to transport or release oxygen throughout the body, resulting in hypoxia. CO induces toxicity according to level and duration of exposure.

Professional Considerations
1. Consent form NOT required.
2. Preparation:
   A. Tube: Lavender topped or green topped.
   B. Do NOT draw during hemodialysis.
3. Procedure:
   A. If specimen will be tested immediately, draw a 5- to 10-mL blood sample as soon as possible after exposure. Prevent contamination of the specimen with room air.
   B. If specimen will not be tested immediately, draw a specimen as above but completely fill a heparinized, green-topped tube.
4. Postprocedure care:
   A. Deliver the specimen to the blood gas laboratory immediately.
5. Client and family teaching:
   A. For accidental inhalation, refer the client or family for crisis intervention.

B. CO cannot be seen, tasted, or smelled. It can be emitted by gas fireplaces; poorly vented gas clothes dryers; charcoal, wood, gas or coal stoves; cars; and kerosene heaters. An in-home CO detector is an inexpensive safety essential that can provide early warning of rising levels.
6. Factors that affect results:
   A. Draw a sample before administering oxygen, if possible.
   B. Newborn levels are higher than adult levels because fetal hemoglobin has a higher affinity for CO than does adult hemoglobin.
7. Other data:
   A. The results are most accurate if tested immediately, but the specimen may be stored in the refrigerator for several hours if the tube is completely filled and tightly stoppered.
   B. Expired breath carbon monoxide (COHbe) is correlated with clinical severity in carbon monoxide poisoning.

CARBOXYHEMOGLOBIN, BLOOD
(see Carbon monoxide, Blood)

CARCINOEMBRYONIC ANTIGEN (CEA), SERUM

Norm:

		SI UNITS
Nonsmoker	<3.0 ng/mL	<3.0 mg/L
Smoker	<5.0 ng/mL	<5.0 mg/L

Usage. CEA is a helpful marker in establishing prognosis, determining effectiveness of therapy, and recognizing recurrent disease in clients with adenocarcinoma, especially those arising in the colon or stomach (elevated in 25% of cases). CEA is the marker of choice for monitoring colorectal carcinoma, and levels above 15 ng/ml indicate high-risk clients and the need for adjuvant or neoadjuvant chemotherapy.

Increased. Adenocarcinoma of the colon, rectum, breast, lung, pancreas, and stomach; hepatocellular carcinoma;

medullary carcinoma of the thyroid; inflammatory bowel disease; COPD; cirrhosis; cholelithiasis; chronic hepatitis; obstructive jaundice; cholangitis; liver abscess; emphysema; bronchitis.

Decreased. Not clinically significant.

Description. CEA is a glycoprotein that functions as a homotypic intercellular adhesion molecule that promotes aggregation of human colorectal carcinoma cells. It is likely that CEA facilitates metastasis of colorectal carcinoma cells to the liver and lung. Moderately differentiated tumors usually secrete more CEA than either poorly or well-differentiated tumors. Measurement of the CEA level is useful in establishing prognosis, monitoring effectiveness of therapy, and recognizing recurrent disease. CEA is the marker of choice for monitoring colorectal cancer. High preoperative levels are associated with metastatic disease and poorer prognosis. CEA levels should return to normal 4-6 weeks after surgery, and elevated postoperative levels signal early recurrence or incomplete resection. CEA is measured preoperatively and every 2 months for at least 2 years. Progressive elevations of CEA are often the first evidence of recurrent tumor, many times present 3 to 36 months before clinical symptoms and often before CT-evident lesions. Transient elevations of CEA may be noticed after chemotherapy or radiation therapy secondary to tumor cell necrosis or membrane damage, permitting the escape of CEA into the circulation. CEA is the most frequently used tumor marker in pleural fluid where an elevated CEA level is highly suggestive of malignancy but may be elevated in complicated parapneumonic effusions and empyema. An elevated CSF/serum CEA ratio is found in 90% of leptomeningeal cancers. Because the liver is the major site of clearance of CEA, single measurements of CEA may not be useful in clients with liver disease, but progressively rising CEA levels are highly suggestive of disease. CEA levels are obtained by means of an immunoreactive assay using double monoclonal antibodies.

Professional Considerations
1. Consent form NOT required.
2. **Preparation:**
   A. Tube: Red topped or serum separator for serum. Lavender topped for plasma.

B. May be drawn during hemodialysis.
3. **Procedure:**
   A. Draw a 1-mL venous blood sample without hemolysis.
   B. Specimen may be kept at room temperature or refrigerated for 24 hours but should be frozen if assay not performed within 24 hours after collection.
4. **Postprocedure care:**
   A. None.
5. **Client and family teaching:**
   A. Results are usually available in 1-3 working days.
6. **Factors that affect results:**
   A. Hemolysis of specimen.
   B. Thawing of frozen specimen.
   C. Recently administered isotopes.
   D. Specimen not separated within 6 hours of collection.
   E. CEA results obtained with a different assay method and different specimen typed cannot be used interchangeably. It is recommended that only one assay method and specimen type be used consistently.
7. **Other data:**
   A. Cells must be separated from the serum or plasma within 6 hours. The specimen is then stable at room temperature for 3 days or in a refrigerator for 1 week.
   B. Levels may exceed 10 ng/mL (10 mg/L, SI units) in acute inflammatory disorders and 12 ng/mL (12 mg/L, SI units) in the presence of neoplasm.

CARCINOGENIC ANTIGEN 15-3
(see CA 15-3, Serum)

CARDIAC CATHETERIZATION (ANGIOCARDIOGRAPHY, CARDIOANGIOGRAPHY, AND CORONARY ANGIOGRAPHY), DIAGNOSTIC

Norm. Normal heart anatomy with normal chamber volumes and pressures, normal wall and valve motion, and patent coronary arteries. Normal cardiac output and chamber pressures are listed below:

	NORMAL PRESSURES
Cardiac output (CO):	4-8 L/min

	NORMAL PRESSURES
Right-sided Heart Catheterization	
Right atrial (RA)	3-11 mm Hg
Right atrial mean	6 mm Hg
Right ventricular systolic	20-30 mm Hg
Right ventricular end-diastolic	<5 mm Hg
Pulmonary artery systolic (PAS)	20-30 mm Hg
Pulmonary artery end-diastolic pressure (PAEDP)	8-15 mm Hg
Pulmonary artery mean (PAM)	<20 mm Hg
Pulmonary artery wedge pressure (PAWP) or pulmonary capillary wedge pressure (PCWP)	4-12 mm Hg
Left-sided Heart Catheterization	
Ascending aorta systolic	140 mm Hg
Ascending aorta diastolic	90 mm Hg
Ascending aorta mean	105 mm Hg
Left ventricle (LV) systolic	140 mm Hg
Left ventricular end-diastolic pressure (LVEDP)	8-12 mm Hg
Left atrium mean (LAM)	12 mm Hg

C

Usage. Identification, documentation, and quantitation of congenital disorders of the heart and diseases and disorders of the greater vessels of the heart; evaluation of cardiac muscle function; evaluation of coronary artery patency; identification of ventricular aneurysms; and identification and quantitation of the severity of acquired or congenital cardiac valve disease. This procedure is safe in morbidly obese clients.

Description. Cardiac catheterization involves passing a catheter through the brachial or femoral artery or antecubital or femoral vein into the left or right side of the heart through the aorta or vena cava, respectively. Angiographic films can be taken after radiopaque dye is injected from the catheter tip. The dye makes it possible to visualize chamber function, valve function, and chamber size. Measurements of oxygen content and pressure and flow rate of blood can be obtained in each chamber, along with the cardiac output and perfusion of the coronary arteries.

Professional Considerations
1. Consent form IS required.

Risks
Air embolism, allergic reaction to dye (itching, hives, rash, tight feeling in the throat, shortness of breath, bronchospasm, anaphylaxis, death), asystole,

cardiac tamponade, cerebrovascular accident (left-sided heart catheterization), congestive heart failure, cerebrovascular accident, dysrhythmias, embolus (left-sided heart catheterization), endocarditis, hematoma, hemorrhage, hemothorax, hypovolemia, infection, myocardial infarction, pneumothorax, pulmonary edema, pulmonary embolism (right-sided heart catheterization), renal toxicity, retroperitoneal bleed, thrombophlebitis (right-sided heart catheterization with antecubital site), thrombus (left-sided heart catheterization), and vagal response (right-sided heart catheterization). This invasive procedure poses a 2% risk of complications.

Contraindications and Precautions
Pregnancy, (because of radioactive iodine crossing the blood-placental barrier), severe cardiomyopathy, severe dysrhythmias, uncontrolled congestive heart failure. This procedure should be performed with extreme caution on clients allergic to local anesthetics, iodine, shellfish, or radiopaque contrast material. Steroids and diphenhydramine should be given before the procedure to these clients.

2. Preparation:
   A. See *Client and family teaching.*
   B. Routine cardiac medications may be given with a small sip of water.

C. Record the baseline height and weight for the calculation of dye dosage.

D. Sedation is usually prescribed for relaxation, but the client remains awake.

E. Assess peripheral pulses and mark them for easy location.

F. Assess baseline ECG and arterial blood pressure and monitor continuously because of the potential for occurrence of cardiac dysrhythmias during the procedure.

G. Have emergency cardiac medications and emergency equipment readily available.

3. **Procedure:**

A. *Left-sided heart catheterization:* In a cardiac catheterization laboratory under fluoroscopy, a long catheter is inserted through a percutaneously inserted sheath into the brachial or femoral artery retrograde through the aorta into the left ventricle or to the beginning of the coronary arteries. Radiopaque dye is then injected from the catheter tip, and the patency of the coronary arteries (coronary angiography, coronary arteriography, cineangiography, or angiocardiography), left ventricular function (contrast ventriculography), and bicuspid and aortic valve function are assessed and recorded radiographically.

B. *Right-sided heart catheterization:* In a cardiac catheterization laboratory under fluoroscopy, a long catheter is inserted through a percutaneously inserted sheath into an antecubital or femoral vein through the vena cava, right atrium, and right ventricle and into the pulmonary artery. Heart chamber and pulmonary artery pressures may be measured as well as cardiac output, tricuspid and pulmonary valve function, and right ventricular function. Radiographic films of the procedure are made.

4. **Postprocedure care:**

A. Maintain bed rest for 4-6 hours.

B. Apply a pressure dressing to the arterial catheter insertion site and immobilize the extremity for 4-6 hours. A sandbag may be placed over an arterial site. Check the dressing and site for bleeding and hematoma formation along with vital sign and pulse checks. Bed rest and extremity immobilization may be extended in clients receiving heparin.

C. Check vital signs and peripheral pulses, color, skin temperature, and sensation of the procedural extremity every 15 minutes × 4, then every 30 minutes × 2, and then hourly for 8-12 hours. Also check for low back or flank pain, which may indicate a retroperitoneal bleed.

D. Assess for dysrhythmias, chest pain, or symptoms of cardiac tamponade.

E. An analgesic may be prescribed for catheterization site discomfort.

F. Encourage the oral intake of fluids if not contraindicated.

G. Resume diet.

5. **Client and family teaching:**

A. Fast from food for 8 hours and from fluids for 3 hours before the procedure.

B. The procedure lasts 1-3 hours.

C. A momentary warm flush and metallic taste or racing pulse may be experienced when the dye is injected. It is also normal to feel a few skipped beats when the catheter is in the ventricle.

D. If coronary angiography will be performed, you might experience momentary chest pain while the dye is injected into the arteries, but no damage will result.

E. It is important to lie motionless throughout the procedure. Symptoms of more than momentary chest pain should be verbalized immediately.

F. Vital signs, pulse checks, and assessments for pain will be taken after the procedure at frequent intervals.

G. Report any difficulty breathing during and after the procedure.

6. **Factors that affect results:**

A. Atherosclerosis of peripheral vessels prohibits easy passage of the catheter.

7. **Other data:**

A. The procedure should be stopped for severe chest pain, neurologic symptoms of a cerebrovascular accident, cardiac dysrhythmias, or hemodynamic changes.

B. Because of the risk of complete coronary artery occlusion from plaque disruption or coronary artery perforation, it is advisable (and legally required in many states) to have backup cardiothoracic surgery availability whenever a cardiac catheterization is performed.

C. African Americans and females are less likely to be referred for cardiac catheterization (Shire, 2002).

CARDIAC ENZYMES/ISOENZYMES (CK, LD, ALT, AST), BLOOD

Norm. Results are method dependent and should be compared with the reference values of the laboratory performing the test.

		SI UNITS
Creatine Kinase (CK)		
Adult female	<80 U/L	<1.33 mkat/L
Adult male	<90 U/L	<1.50 mkat/L
Newborn	<200 U/L	<3.33 mkat/L

	% OF TOTAL CK	FRACTION OF TOTAL CK
CK Isoenzymes		
CK_1BB (brain)	0-3	0-0.03
CK_2MB (heart)	0-6	0-0.06
CK_3MM (muscle)	90-97	0.90-0.97

		SI UNITS
Lactate Dehydrogenase (LD)		
Wróblewski method 30° C	150-450 U	72-217 IU/L
Adult		
≤60 years	45-90 U/L	45-90 U/L
>60 years	55-102 U/L	55-102 U/L
Child		
Newborn	160-500 U/L	160-500 U/L
Neonate	300-1500 U/L	300-1500 U/L
Infant	100-250 U/L	100-250 U/L
Child	60-170 U/L	60-170 U/L

	% OF TOTAL LD	FRACTION OF TOTAL CK
Lactate Dehydrogenase Isoenzymes (Agarose, Electrophoresis)		
Fraction LD_1	14-26	0.14-0.26
Fraction LD_2	29-39	0.29-0.39
Fraction LD_3	20-26	0.20-0.26
Fraction LD_4	8-16	0.08-0.16
Fraction LD_5	6-16	0.06-0.16

		SI UNITS
Aspartate Aminotransferase (AST, SGOT)		
Adult female		
≤60 years	8-20 U/L	8-20 U/L
>60 years	10-20 U/L	10-20 U/L

Continued

		SI UNITS
Aspartate Aminotransferase (AST, SGOT)—cont'd		
Adult male		
≤60 years	8-20 U/L	8-20 U/L
>60 years	11-26 U/L	11-26 U/L
Children		
Newborn	16-72 U/L	16-72 U/L
Infant	15-60 U/L	15-60 U/L
1 year	16-35 U/L	16-35 U/L
5 years	19-28 U/L	19-28 U/L

		SI UNITS
Alanine Aminotransferase (ALT, SGPT)		
Adult female		
≤60 years	8-20 U/L	8-20 U/L
>60 years	7-16 U/L	7-16 U/L
Adult male		
≤60 years	8-20 U/L	8-20 U/L
>60 years	6-24 U/L	6-24 U/L
Children		
Newborn	5-28 U/L	5-28 U/L
Infant	5-28 U/L	5-28 U/L

Increased. Patterns in myocardial infarction are generally as follows:

CK. Total CK levels may be normal in acute myocardial infarction, even when the CK-MB isoenzyme is elevated. CK levels begin rising before LD and AST levels. In general, CK begins rising at 4-8 hours, peaks at 12-24 hours, and returns to baseline level by 3-4 days after the onset of myocardial damage.

CK Isoenzymes. CK_2MB begins rising at 6 hours, peak at 18 hours, and returns to baseline level by 72 hours after the onset of myocardial damage. CK-MB subforms are a new test in which results are available within 1 hour.

LD. Total LD levels begin rising at 24 hours, peak at 3-4 days, and return to baseline level in 8-12 days.

LD Isoenzymes. LD_1 peaks with an LD_1:LD_2 ratio inversion 48 hours after onset of damage.

AST. AST initially rises at 6-10 hours, peaks at 12-48 hours, and returns to baseline by 4-6 days after the onset of myocardial damage.

AST/ALT Ratio. ≥3.1, or double that of the baseline level after myocardial damage.

Increases in Selected Other Conditions. Cardiomyopathy (total CK, CK_1BB, CK_2MB, total LD), congestive heart failure (CK_2MB [rare], total LD, AST, ALT), myocardial infarction (total CK, CK_2MB, CK_3MM, total LD, LD_1, LD_2, LD_1:LD_2 inversion, AST [pronounced], ALT [slight], AST/ALT ratio), myocarditis (total CK, CK_2MB), pericarditis (AST), pulmonary infarction (total CK, AST, total LD, LD_2, LD_3), and severe angina (total CK [rare], CK_2MB).

Decreased. See individual test listings. Decreases not applicable for myocardial infarction.

Description. Cardiac enzymes are a group of enzymes released by the heart as a result of myocardial injury. They aid in the differential diagnosis of myocardial infarction from congestive heart failure, pericarditis, pulmonary infarction, angina, and other conditions. CK is an enzyme found in specific body tissues, and lactate dehydrogenase is an enzyme present in many tissues. Both are composed of subcomponent isoenzymes that are released in fairly consistent patterns when myocardial injury occurs. Isoenzyme CK_2MB (found mainly in the heart) is normally absent in the serum but becomes present and increases in a specific pattern when released from damaged myocardial cells. Isoenzymes LD_1 and LD_2 (found mainly in the heart and red blood cells) are normally present in a fairly constant ratio of about 1:2 in the serum but begin rising after myocardial damage until the ratio reverses. Serial levels of CK and LD and isoenzymes of both are evaluated for demonstration of characteristic patterns of rise and fall when differentiating suspected acute myocardial infarction from other disorders that may cause similar symptoms. Serum AST is an enzyme found in several body organs, including large amounts in the heart, but is nonspecific for myocardial injury. It is sometimes compared to serum ALT levels, which are found mainly in the liver, with only small amounts in the heart and other organs. An AST level that rises much more than an ALT level can help identify whether the cause is cardiac injury. See also *Creatine kinase, Serum; Lactate dehydrogenase, Blood; Alanine aminotransferase, Serum;* and *Aspartate aminotransferase, Serum,* for discussion of abnormalities from causes other than cardiac.

Professional Considerations
1. Consent form NOT required.
2. Preparation:
   A. Tube: Red topped, red/gray topped, or gold topped.
   B. MAY be drawn during hemodialysis.
3. Procedure:
   A. Draw a 5-mL venous blood sample without hemolysis.
   B. Samples are drawn immediately with suspected myocardial infarction and serially at 12, 24, and 48 hours or every 8 hours for three samples.
4. Postprocedure care:
   A. The serum should be separated and left at room temperature for LD and ALT measurement; the CK serum should be frozen if not tested within 24 hours of specimen collection.
5. Client and family teaching:
   A. Samples will be drawn in a set sequence to evaluate changes in laboratory results to facilitate the plan of care.
6. Factors that affect results:
   A. Reject hemolyzed specimens, which invalidate several values.
   B. Drugs that may cause falsely elevated LD, AST, and ALT levels include heparin (porcine, bovine). See individual tests for a more

detailed listing of drugs that affect the results.
   C. Alcohol ingestion within 24 hours of specimen collection causes increased values.
   D. If intramuscular injections must be given, they should be given after or at least 1 hour before this test.
7. Other data:
   A. Previous terminology used for aspartate aminotransferase includes serum glutamic oxaloacetic transaminase (SGOT). Previous terminology for alanine aminotransferase includes serum glutamic pyruvic transaminase (SGPT) and glutamic pyruvate transaminase (GPT). Previous terminology used for lactate dehydrogenase includes lactic acid dehydrogenase (LDH).
   B. Echocardiography can diagnose ischemic heart disease before a rise in cardiac enzymes is detected.
   C. CK-MB subform results are available within the hour and are very reliable for telling if a person has had an MI. This should replace CK-MB in emergency departments.

CARDIAC NATRIURETIC HORMONES
(see Natriuretic peptides, Atrial, Brain, C-type, Plasma)

CARDIAC OUTPUT, THERMODILUTION, DIAGNOSTIC

Norm. 4-8 L/minute.

Usage. Evaluation of hemodynamic instability (heart failure, pulmonary hypertension), shock states, determination of optimal myocardial function preoperatively by Starling curve, evaluation of response to fluid administration and inotropic drugs. Cardiac output is performed to determine the amount of blood being propelled forward by the heart.

Description. Cardiac output is the product of heart rate and stroke volume. It is the volume of blood ejected from the heart over a period of 1 minute. The determinants of cardiac output are preload, afterload, and heart rate in beats per minute and stroke volume in milliliters per beat (CO = HR × SV). Stroke volume is the volume of blood ejected with each ventricular contraction and is the difference between the volume of the left ventricle at end diastole and the volume remaining in the ventricle at end systole. In an average-sized adult at rest, cardiac output is approximately 4-8 L/min. In diseased states, cardiac output is usually found to be less than normal and may be so low that an adequate blood supply to the body's tissues cannot be delivered. A low cardiac output may be the result of poor filling of the ventricle (reduced preload) or poor forward emptying of the ventricle (increased afterload). Some causes of low resting cardiac output are diminished myocardial function resulting from myocardial infarction, aortic stenosis, arterial hypertension, and cardiomyopathy. The thermodilution method of cardiac output determination measures the change in core temperature in the pulmonary artery before and after injection of a specific quantity of injectate of a known temperature. The change in temperature reflects the cardiac output in an inverse manner and is used to plot a cardiac-output thermodilution curve. A low cardiac output produces a greater change in temperature for a longer period of time than does a high cardiac output.

Professional Considerations
1. Consent form IS required for insertion of pulmonary artery catheter.

Risks
Pulmonary embolus from dislodgement of clot on catheter. See *Pulmonary artery catheterization, Diagnostic,* for catheter-specific risks and contraindications.

Contraindications
None. Injections should be kept to the minimum volume needed for clients who are fluid overloaded.

2. **Preparation:**
   A. Client must have a pulmonary artery catheter in place.
   B. Obtain a cardiac output tubing, a 10-mL syringe, and injectate. Also obtain ice if injectate is less than 10° C cooler than the client's core temperature. Iced injectate should also be used for hemodynamically unstable clients and hypothermic clients.
3. **Procedure:**
   A. The client may be positioned up to 60 degrees of head-of-bed elevation but should be positioned

similarly for each cardiac output measurement. Hemodynamically unstable clients should be positioned supine.
B. Cardiac output is performed through a 2- or 3-lumen pulmonary artery catheter. A 3-lumen catheter contains two lumens that exit in the right atrium for measurements of central venous pressure, cardiac output injection, and fluid infusions and one lumen that exits in the pulmonary artery, plus a thermistor at the distal catheter tip in the pulmonary artery for measurement of core blood temperature.
C. A computation constant is selected for the specific injectate temperature and quantity, and the catheter in use is entered into the computer that will calculate cardiac output. The injectate used must be at least 10° C cooler than the client's core temperature for the most accurate thermodilution curve.
D. After the catheter placement has been verified, a bolus of 5 or 10 mL of iced or room-temperature intravenous fluid (D_5W or NS) is injected into the external catheter port that exits into the right atrium. The injection should begin as the client begins exhalation and should be completed within 4 seconds.
E. As the fluid exits into the right atrium, it cools the blood that is in the right atrium. This volume of cooled blood moves into the right ventricle and then into the pulmonary artery.
F. In the pulmonary artery, the catheter thermistor senses the temperature change as the cooled blood passes over it. The thermistor will record a decrease in temperature followed by a gradual return to body temperature as the cold solution flows distally. The resulting temperature change is plotted on a temperature-time curve by the cardiac output computer.
G. Generally, three (3) cardiac output readings are obtained and averaged to calculate cardiac output. However, the procedure may be stopped and the cardiac output calculated if the second measurement is within 10% of the first measurement.

C

4. Postprocedure care:
   A. Resume slow flush infusion to maintain patency of the cardiac-output lumen, if used before injection.
5. Client and family teaching:
   A. The client will not feel injections.
6. Factors that affect results:
   A. Too much or too little of injectate solution injected will produce erroneous values.
   B. Injection not completed within 4 seconds will produce a falsely high value.
   C. If the catheter is kinked, the cardiac output value will be falsely high.
   D. If the catheter is not inserted far enough for the cardiac output port to be distal to the tip of the introducer (sheath, Cordis) retrograde injection into the cordis will produce a falsely high cardiac output.
   E. Changes in stroke volume resulting from dysrhythmias or changing heart rates can produce wide variations in serial cardiac output readings.
   F. An incorrect catheter computation constant entered into the cardiac output calculation will produce an erroneous value.
7. Other data:
   A. One single duration-controlled injection thermodilution measurement is as accurate as the mean of four phase-controlled measurements.

CARDIAC RADIOGRAPHY, DIAGNOSTIC

Norm. Normal size, shape, and appearance of the heart and lungs. Posteroanterior and lateral views should demonstrate no enlargement or bulging of the right ventricle, right ventricular outflow tract, left ventricle, or pulmonary veins, and no aortic abnormalities. The left cardiac border should be convex, rather than straight.

Usage. Congestive heart failure, abnormalities of the aortic arch (calcifications); some aneurysms; transposition; evaluation of the appearance, size, and shape of the heart and lungs; and verification of invasive line placement and position.

Description. A radiograph of the thoracic area and subsequent examination of the film for abnormalities. The procedure of choice is that carried out in the radiology department with the client in a standing or erect sitting position for posteroanterior and left-lateral views of the chest. The posteroanterior position provides the most realistic view of cardiac size and shape. In this position, the heart is closer to the film than in an anteroposterior view, resulting in less distortion of cardiac size and shape as a result of shadows created by distance.

Professional Considerations
1. Consent form NOT required.

Risk
Hypotension while holding breath; fetal damage during first trimester of pregnancy.

Contraindications
Assess for contraindications to performing the Valsalva maneuver (recent myocardial infarction, bradycardia). If these conditions are present, teach the client how to hold the breath without bearing down.

Precautions
During pregnancy, risks of cumulative radiation exposure to the fetus from this and other previous or future imaging studies must be weighed against the benefits of the procedure. Although formal limits for client exposure are relative to this risk:benefit comparison, the United States Nuclear Regulatory Commission requires that the cumulative dose equivalent to an embryo/fetus from occupational exposure not exceed 0.5 rem (5 mSv). Radiation dosage to the fetus is proportional to the distance of the anatomy studied from the abdomen and decreases as pregnancy progresses. For pregnant clients, consult the Radiologist/Radiology Department to obtain estimated fetal radiation exposure from this procedure.

2. Preparation:
   A. Remove radiopaque objects above the waist such as jewelry and clothing with snaps. Also remove electrocardiographic patches with snaps when not contraindicated.
   B. The abdomen and pelvis should be shielded by lead during pregnancy.

3. **Procedure:**
   A. For the posteroanterior view, position the client standing or sitting erect with arms held slightly out from the sides, chest expanded, and shoulders pressed forward. The radiographic film is placed against the anterior chest.
   B. For left lateral views, the client stands with his or her arms elevated from the shoulders and forearms resting on the arm of the radiographic equipment if necessary. The radiographic film is placed against the left side of the chest.
   C. The client must take a deep breath and hold it while the radiograph is taken.
   D. For clients unable to stand or sit erect, an anteroposterior view is taken with the client sitting in as high a Fowler's position as possible and the radiographic plate positioned behind the back and chest.
4. **Postprocedure care:**
   A. Replace the electrocardiographic monitoring patches and leads, if removed.

5. **Client and family teaching:**
   A. You must breathe in and hold your breath and lie very still during the procedure.
6. **Factors that affect results:**
   A. Radiopaque objects such as jewelry and wires create shadows on the film.
   B. The cardiac size and shape appear larger in an anteroposterior radiograph than in a posteroanterior radiograph.
   C. Cardiopulmonary congestion requires an increase in exposure.
   D. Inadequate films result when the client is unable to hold a deep inspiration during exposure.
   E. Movement obscures the clarity of the picture.
   F. Thoracic deformity such as scoliosis affects radiographic interpretation.
7. **Other data:**
   A. Although contraindicated during the first trimester, this is the procedure of choice when necessitated during pregnancy because the amount of radiation delivered is up to 20 times less than that of the nuclear medicine cardiac series.

CARDIOANGIOGRAPHY, DIAGNOSTIC
(see Cardiac catheterization, Diagnostic)

CARDIOPULMONARY SLEEP STUDY
(see Polysomnography, Diagnostic)

CAROTENE, SERUM

Norm:

		SI UNITS
Adult	50-200 µg/dL	0.74-3.72 µmol/L
	50-300 IU/L	
Child	40-130 µg/dL	0.3-2.3 µmol/L
Infant	0-40 µg/dL	0.0-0.7 µmol/L

Increased. Amenorrhea, anorexia nervosa, diarrhea, diabetes mellitus, excessive dietary carotene intake, hypercholesterolemia, hyperlipidemia, hypervitaminosis A, hypothyroidism, myxedema, nephritis (chronic), nephrotic syndrome, and pancreatitis.

Decreased. Celiac disease, cystic fibrosis, fever, HIV, infectious hepatitis, jaundice (obstructive), kwashiorkor, liver disease, low-fat diet, malabsorption, pancreatic insufficiency, poor dietary intake, pregnancy, and steatorrhea.

Description. Carotene is a fat-soluble precursor of vitamin A that exists in green and yellow vegetables. A small portion of carotene is absorbed from the intestines and contributes to the yellow serum color. With the aid of fats and bile salts, however, the majority of carotene

C

is normally converted to retinol in the intestines and then absorbed into the bloodstream and stored in the liver. Since low values indicate poor dietary intake or malabsorption, this test is most commonly used as a screening test for malabsorption syndrome. Carotenemia, or elevated carotene levels, is characterized by yellow skin pigmentation with no scleral color change. The client may also have malaise, itching, or weight loss. The condition is usually benign and treated with changes in diet.

Professional Considerations
1. Consent form NOT required.
2. **Preparation:**
   A. Tube: Red topped, red/gray topped, or gold topped; and a paper bag.
   B. See *Client and family teaching.*
3. **Procedure:**
   A. Draw a 6-mL venous blood sample.
   B. Place the specimen in a paper bag or otherwise protect it from light.
4. **Postprocedure care:**
   A. Transport the specimen to the laboratory for immediate spinning and freezing in a plastic vial until carotene can be measured.
   B. If results are low because of poor dietary intake, institute diet teaching.
5. **Client and family teaching:**
   A. You may have to eliminate carotene-rich foods for 2-3 days. A high-carotene diet may be prescribed for several days if the test purpose is to evaluate ability to absorb carotene.
   B. Fast for 8 hours before sampling.

6. **Factors that affect results:**
   A. Reject hemolyzed specimens.
   B. Women have higher levels than men.
7. **Other data:**
   A. This is a nonspecific test. There may be an overlap between carotene levels of normal clients and those with malabsorption syndromes. Dietary intake must be considered when one is interpreting results.
   B. Increased intake of beta-carotene by lactating mothers increases the supply of milk beta-carotene to breast-fed infants.
   C. High-dose beta-carotene may enhance lung tumorigenesis thus lowering the risk of lung cancer.

CAROTID DOPPLER (CAROTID ARTERY ECHOGRAM, CAROTID ARTERY ULTRASOUND), DIAGNOSTIC
(see Transcranial Doppler ultrasonography, Diagnostic)

CAROTID PHONOANGIOGRAPHY (CPA), DIAGNOSTIC
(see Color Duplex Ultrasonography)

CAT SCAN
(see Cerebral computed tomography, Diagnostic; Chest tomography, Diagnostic; Computed tomography of the body, Diagnostic; Tomography paranasal sinuses, Diagnostic)

CATECHOLAMINES, FRACTIONATION, PLASMA
(see Catecholamines, Plasma)

CATECHOLAMINES, FRACTIONATION FREE, PLASMA
(see Catecholamines, Plasma)

CATECHOLAMINES, PLASMA

Norm. Values vary by laboratory.

		SI UNITS
Fractionation		
Standing		
Epinephrine	0-140 pg/mL	0-762 pmol/L
Norepinephrine	200-1700 pg/mL	1088-9256 pmol/L
Dopamine	0-30 pg/mL	0-163 pmol/L

Continued

336 CATECHOLAMINES, PLASMA

		SI UNITS
Supine		
Epinephrine	0-110 pg/mL	0-599 pmol/L
Norepinephrine	70-750 pg/mL	381-4083 pmol/L
Dopamine	0-30 pg/mL	0-163 pmol/L
Fractionation Free		
Total	150-650 pg/mL	886-3843 pmol/L

Increased Epinephrine. Anger, electroconvulsive therapy, exercise (extreme), fear, ganglioblastoma (slight increase), ganglioneuroma (slight increase), hypoglycemia, hypotension, hypothyroidism, ketoacidosis (diabetic), kidney disease, myocardial infarction (acute), neuroblastoma (slight increase), paragangliomas (slight increase), pheochromocytoma (continuous or intermittent increase), postoperatively, prolonged exposure to cold, shock, stress, thyrotoxicosis, and volume depletion. Drugs include epinephrine bitartrate, epinephrine borate, epinephrine hydrochloride, and ethyl alcohol (ethanol) (in large amounts).

Increased Norepinephrine. Anxiety, burns, exercise (extreme), ganglioblastoma (large increase), ganglioneuroma (large increase), hypoglycemia, hypotension, hypothyroidism, ketoacidosis (diabetic), kidney disease, myasthenia gravis, myocardial infarction (acute), neuroblastoma (large increase), paragangliomas (large increase), pheochromocytoma (slight increase), postoperatively, progressive muscular dystrophy, shock, thyroid disease, thyrotoxicosis, and volume depletion. Drugs include ethyl alcohol (ethanol) (in large amounts) and norepinephrine bitartrate.

Increased Dopamine. Ganglioneuroma and neuroblastoma. Drugs include dopamine hydrochloride.

Increased Catecholamines (Any). Drugs include aspirin, decongestants, sympathomimetics, and tricyclic antidepressants.

Decreased Epinephrine. Alzheimer's disease.

Decreased Norepinephrine. Anorexia nervosa, autonomic nervous system dysfunction, and orthostatic hypotension.

Decreased Dopamine. Parkinson's disease.

Decreased Catecholamines (Any). High altitude exposure. Drugs include barbiturates, clonidine, and reserpine.

Description. The catecholamines (epinephrine, norepinephrine, and dopamine) are found in the adrenal medulla, neurons, and the brain. This test is used to help rule out the presence of catecholamine-secreting tumors such as pheochromocytoma.

Epinephrine is a hormone and neurotransmitter synthesized from tyrosine and secreted after the splanchnic nerve is stimulated because of hypoglycemia, stress, fear, or anger. Epinephrine acts during the body's fight-or-flight response to dilate the bronchioles, increase the heart rate, increase glycogenolysis to provide more glucose for body fuel, and decrease peripheral resistance and blood flow to the skin and kidneys.

Norepinephrine is the predominant catecholamine hormone and neurotransmitter secreted by the adrenal medulla in response to splanchnic nerve stimulation and is also secreted by certain neurons in the peripheral nervous system. Synthesized from dopamine and in the presence of tyramine, norepinephrine acts to increase blood pressure through constriction of the peripheral vasculature, dilate the pupils, and relax the gastrointestinal system. It also functions as an intermediary in epinephrine synthesis.

Dopamine is a neurotransmitter found in the brain, sympathetic ganglia, liver, lungs, intestines, and retina. A product of dopa decarboxylation, dopamine acts to dilate renal arteries, increase the heart rate, and constrict the peripheral vasculature.

In a fractionated test, total catecholamines are differentiated into the portions comprising epinephrine, norepinephrine, and dopamine. Plasma levels reveal the balance between synthesis, release, uptake, catabolism, and excretion of catecholamines. In pheochromocytoma, the tumor secretes increased amounts of catecholamines, causing paroxysmal or persistent hypertension. Therefore, catecholamine levels are most helpful when drawn during or just after a hypertensive episode. Total catecholamine levels exceeding 1000 pg/mL are suggestive of pheochromocytoma, and levels over 2000 pg/mL are presumptive of this condition. In normal clients, epinephrine and norepinephrine results should be higher when the clients are standing than when they are supine. Absence of this difference may indicate autonomic nervous system dysfunction.

Professional Considerations

1. Consent form NOT required.
2. **Preparation:**
   A. See *Client and family teaching.*
   B. Insert heparin lock 24 hours before the test.
   C. Tubes: Two chilled lavender topped or green topped.
   D. Notify laboratory personnel that a specimen for plasma catecholamine levels will be drawn and must be spun and frozen immediately upon arrival in the laboratory.
3. **Procedure:** Baseline-level specimens should be collected between 0600 (6 AM) and 0800 (8 AM) as follows:
   A. The client should relax in a recumbent position before the procedure for 40-60 minutes.
   B. Withdraw and discard 3 mL of heparin and blood from the heparin lock. Draw a 10-mL venous blood sample from the heparin lock and inject it into a chilled, green-topped or lavender-topped tube, depending on laboratory requirements. Once the specimen is collected, relock the site according to institutional protocol.
   C. Follow postprocedure care instructions and have the specimen transported to the laboratory immediately.
   D. Have the client stand for 10 minutes and draw a second specimen as in step 3B. Remove or flush the

heparin lock according to institutional protocol.
4. **Postprocedure care:**
   A. Mix the specimen well by gently inverting several times, but avoid agitation. Place the specimen in an ice bath and transport it to the laboratory immediately. Write the body position (supine or standing) and the collection time on the laboratory requisition.
5. **Client and family teaching:**
   A. Explain test and guidelines thoroughly, since without the client's compliance, the results are unreliable.
   B. Do not eat foods high in amines within 48 hours before the test. These foods include avocados, bananas, beer, cheese, chocolate, cocoa, fava beans, grains, tea, vanilla, walnuts, and wine.
   C. Do not consume the herb coffee (*Coffea*) within 48 hours before the test.
   D. Medications that increase catecholamines may be prescribed to be withheld for 48 hours. Diuretics, antihypertensives, and sympathomimetics (including nonprescriptive cold and allergy medications) must be withheld for 5-14 days.
   E. Follow a normal-sodium diet for 3 days and fast from food and fluids for 10-12 hours before sampling.
   F. Avoid strenuous exercise and tobacco smoking immediately before testing.
   G. Evaluate the client's understanding of the importance of following pretest instructions to ensure accuracy of the results.
   H. Results may not be available for at least 1 week.
6. **Factors that affect results:**
   A. Reject specimens received in the laboratory more than 5 minutes after collection. Plasma catecholamine levels drop quickly if the red blood cells are not separated within 5 minutes of specimen collection. The specimen should be spun in a refrigerated centrifuge or chilled carrier. Plasma should be separated from the red blood cells and frozen upright in a plastic vial at −70° C.
   B. The trauma of direct venipuncture may increase the amount of catecholamines in the specimen.

C. Stressors such as a cold or hypoglycemia may cause elevated results.
D. The results may be invalid if the client has undergone a radioactive scan within 1 month before specimen collection.
E. The results of this test are unreliable in clients taking ascorbic acid, chloral hydrate, chlorpromazine, decongestants, hydralazine, isuprel, levodopa, methenamine mandelate, methyldopa, phenothiazines, quinine, quinidine, theophylline, or tricyclic antidepressants.
F. Drugs that may cause falsely elevated results include amphetamines, bronchodilators, isopro-terenol hydrochloride, and vasodilators.
G. Drugs that may cause falsely decreased results include anticonvulsants, antidysrhythmics, and barbiturates.
H. A diet high in amines may elevate the results.

7. **Other data:**
A. Because plasma catecholamine levels are difficult to measure, urine catecholamine measurements are more often used.
B. This test is often used in conjunction with urinary levels and VMA determinations to diagnose pheochromocytoma or neuroblastoma.
C. The complete analysis may take up to 1 week.

CATECHOLAMINES, URINE

Norm:

		SI UNITS
Random Urine		
Total Catecholamines	0-18 µg/dL	0-103 nmol/dL
Daytime Specimen		
Total Catecholamines	1.4-7.3 µg/hr	8-43 nmol/hr
24-Hour Urine		
Total Catecholamines	0-135 µg/24 hours	0-796 nmol/24 hours
Panic level	>200 µg/24 hours	>1180 nmol/24 hours
Epinephrine		
Adult	0-15 µg	0-82 nmol/D
Children		
1-4 years	0-6 µg/D	0-33 nmol/D
4-10 years	0-10 µg/D	0-55 nmol/D
10-15 years	0.5-20 µg/D	2.7-110 nmol/D
Epinephrine panic level	>50 µg/D	>295 nmol/D
Norepinephrine		
Adult	0-100 µg/D	0-590 nmol/D
Children		
1-4 years	0-29 µg/D	0-170 nmol/D
4-10 years	8-65 µg/D	47-380 nmol/D
10-15 years	15-80 µg/D	89-470 nmol/D
Dopamine		
4 years to adult	65-400 µg/D	384-2364 nmol/D
4 years or less	40-260 µg/D	236-1535 nmol/D

Increased. Adrenocortical adenoma, burns, exercise (strenuous), ganglioneuroma, neuroblastoma, pheochromocytoma, seizures (tonic-clonic epileptic) and other catecholamine-secreting tumors and stress (severe anger, anxiety). Drugs include caffeine, ethyl alcohol (ethanol) (large amounts), reserpine (short-term use), and sympathomimetics.

Decreased. Anorexia nervosa, familial dystonia, and idiopathic orthostatic hypotension. Drugs include guanethidine sulfate, phenothiazines, and reserpine (chronic use).

Description. Catecholamines are a group of hormones that are secreted from the adrenal medulla (epinephrine and norepinephrine) and are also released from nerve endings (epinephrine, norepinephrine, and dopamine). These hormones function in the fight-or-flight response, sympathetic nervous system functioning, blood pressure and hemodynamic controls, and response to stressors. Catecholamines are degraded and excreted by the kidneys and can be measured in random urine samples. In pheochromocytoma, the tumor secretes increased amounts of catecholamines, causing paroxysmal or persistent hypertension. Therefore, 24-hour urine catecholamine levels are helpful in detecting paroxysmal secretion that occurs throughout the day and may be missed by random plasma levels.

Professional Considerations
1. Consent form NOT required.
2. **Preparation:**
   A. Obtain a clean container for random urine.
   B. For 24-hour collections, obtain a clean, 3-L container to which hydrochloric acid (HCl) preservative has been added.
3. **Procedure:** Random or 24-hour urine:
   A. *Random collection:* Collect a 50-mL random urine specimen in a clean container.
   B. *24-hour collections:*
      i. Discard the first morning-urine specimen.
      ii. Begin to time a 24-hour urine collection.
      iii. Save all the urine voided for 24 hours in a refrigerated, 3-L container to which HCl preservative has been added. Include the urine voided at the end of the 24-hour period.
      iv. For catheterized clients, keep the drainage bag on ice and empty the urine into the acidified collection container hourly.
4. **Postprocedure care:**
   A. Compare the urine quantity in the specimen container with the urinary output record for the test. If the specimen contains less urine than was recorded as output, some of the sample may have been discarded, invalidating the test.
   B. Document the 24-hour urine quantity on the laboratory requisition.

C. Keep the specimen chilled until testing.
5. **Client and family teaching:**
   A. Save all the urine voided in the 24-hour period, and urinate before defecating to avoid loss of urine.
6. **Factors that affect results:**
   A. All the urine voided for the 24-hour period must be included to avoid a falsely low result.
   B. The client should have a quiet environment and avoid strenuous exercise throughout the specimen collection period.
   C. Foods that may cause falsely elevated levels include bananas, beer, Chianti wines, cheese, and walnuts.
   D. An herb that may cause falsely elevated levels is coffee (*Coffea*).
   E. Hypoglycemia may cause falsely elevated levels.
   F. Drugs that may cause unreliable results as a result of interference with the laboratory fluorescence testing method include ascorbic acid, ampicillin, ampicillin sodium, chloral hydrate, epinephrine bitartrate, epinephrine borate, epinephrine hydrochloride, erythromycin, erythromycin ethylsuccinate, hydralazine hydrochloride, methenamine mandelate, methyldopa, methyldopate hydrochloride, niacin, quinidine gluconate, quinidine polygalacturonate, quinidine sulfate, riboflavin, salicylates, tetracyclines, and vitamin B complex.
7. **Other data:**
   A. A random urine sample may be prescribed just after a hypertensive episode for pheochromocytoma diagnosis.
   B. Urine samples are easier to study than plasma catecholamines and so are more frequently used for diagnosis.
   C. Urine levels of vanillylmandelic acid (VMA) (urinary metabolite of epinephrine), metanephrine (urinary metabolite of epinephrine and norepinephrine), and homovanillic acid (urinary metabolite of dopamine) are often prescribed with this test.
   D. 24-hour urine catecholamines are more reliable than plasma catecholamines.

CATHEPSIN-D, SPECIMEN

Norm:

Normal reference range	<30 pmol/mg CP
Borderline positive	30-70 pmol/mg CP
Positive (high-risk)	>70 pmol/mg CP

Increased. Increased total antigen amounts of cathepsin D in breast tissue have been associated with increased disease recurrence, more frequent metastasis, and increased mortality in breast cancer clients and is increased in squamous cell carcinoma of the head and neck including laryngeal squamous carcinoma. Presence of cathepsin D in aortic aneurysm walls increases mechanical resistance of arteries.

Decreased. Not clinically significant.

Description. Cathepsin D is an independent prognostic factor associated with high risk for metastasis in breast cancer. It is an estrogen-inducible lysosomal protease that is believed to have a role in tumor invasion and metastasis. The overexpression of cathepsin D is associated with visceral and increased soft-tissue metastases and decreased overall survival. Current thought is that cathepsin D is more of a marker of increased metabolism rather than a specific marker for cancer.

Professional Considerations

1. Consent NOT required but IS required for the procedure used to obtain the specimen. See the specific procedure for risks and contraindications.
2. Preparation:
   A. Obtain biopsy equipment.
3. Procedure:
   A. Specimen requirement: 0.5-1.0 g of solid tumor, trimmed of excess fat.
   B. The tissue is cut into small pieces and then quick-frozen on dry ice in a cryostat or in liquid nitrogen within 20 minutes of excision.
   C. The specimen is placed in a 60-mL biopsy bottle without formalin, with the cap secured.
   D. Label the specimen bottle with the client's name, the date collected, and the client's identification number.
   E. The tissue must remain frozen.
4. Postprocedure care:
   A. Apply a dry, sterile dressing to the biopsy site.
   B. Use a mild analgesic for site tenderness.
5. Client and family teaching:
   A. Use a mild analgesic for site tenderness.
   B. Notify the physician for increased or purulent drainage, redness, or increasing tenderness at the site.
   C. This test is investigational.
6. Factors that affect results:
   A. None found.
7. Other data:
   A. Cathepsin D may be prescribed in combination with other prognostic tests. The test has been recommended for investigative use only and should not be used as a diagnostic procedure without confirmation of the diagnosis by another medically established diagnostic product or procedure.

CBC
(see Complete blood count, Blood)

CBL
(see Vitamin B$_{12}$, Serum)

CCCT
(see Circulating cancer cell test, Blood)

CD4
(see Acquired immunodeficiency syndrome evaluation battery, Diagnostic)

CDT
(see Transferrin, Carbohydrate deficient, Serum)

CEA
(see Carcinoembryonic antigen, Serum)

C-erb-2
(see HER-2/neu oncogene, Specimen)

CEREBRAL ANGIOGRAPHY (CEREBRAL ANGIOGRAM), DIAGNOSTIC

Norm. Symmetric pattern of vascular circulation to the brain with no areas of absent vessels. The vessels are smooth, and there are no areas of pooling of the contrast dye (which would indicate bleeding from the vessels or aneurysm).

Usage. Suspected cerebral aneurysm or other cerebral vascular disease such as carotid occlusion in Behçet's disease, Churg-Strauss syndrome, Parry-Romberg syndrome, fistulas, spasms, atherosclerosis, or arteriovenous malformations; tumors of the brain; and work-up for transient ischemic attack or other neurologic signs and symptoms. The need for angiography may be suggested by brain scan findings.

Description. Cerebral angiography is a procedure performed in the radiology department using a special radiographic machine with a rapid biplane cassette changer. It involves a series of radiographic views of the cerebral circulation obtained after intra-arterial injection of a contrast medium showing the patterns of circulation, any interruptions to circulation, or changes in vessel wall appearance.

Professional Considerations
1. Consent form IS required.

Risks
Allergy to contrast medium, aphasia, embolus, hematoma, hemiplegia, hemorrhage, infection, loss of consciousness, renal toxicity, transient ischemic attack.

Contraindications
Atherosclerosis; coagulopathy, dehydration; previous allergy to iodine, shellfish, or contrast medium; renal disease; hepatic disease; thyroid disease; or allergy to contrast medium; during breast-feeding.

Precautions
During pregnancy, risks of cumulative radiation exposure to the fetus from this and other previous of future imaging studies must be weighed against the benefits of the procedure. risk of exposure to the uterus from cerebral angiopraphy is <10 mrad. Radiation dosage to the fetus decreases as pregnancy progresses.

2. **Preparation:**
   A. See *Client and family teaching.*
   B. Have emergency equipment readily available.
   C. Remove all jewelry and metal objects such as hairpins from the client's head area.
   D. Obtain sterile gauze, tape, alcohol, or other skin-cleansing agent, arterial catheter, razor, contrast medium, normal saline or heparinized normal saline, syringes, and automatic contrast injector.
   E. For clients who are unable to cooperate and especially for children, a general anesthetic may be administered by an anesthesia professional.

3. **Procedure:**
   A. The client is placed supine on a special radiographic table.
   B. A site for intra-arterial injection is selected and prepared by cleansing of the skin with 70% alcohol or povidone-iodine solution and injection of a local anesthetic.
      i. Carotid artery: The client's neck must be hyperextended by placement of a rolled towel under the shoulders, and his or her head must be immobilized with tape.
      ii. Femoral artery: The area must be shaved before cleansing. A long catheter is threaded through the femoral artery to the aortic arch.
      iii. Brachial artery: The area may require shaving before cleansing. The brachial artery is the least common injection site. A blood pressure cuff is applied distal to the injection site and inflated before the injection to prevent contrast medium flow to the lower arm.
   C. Needle and catheter placement appropriate to the site is performed by the physician and verified by fluoroscopy.
   D. Contrast medium is injected, and the client is carefully observed for signs of an allergic reaction such as hives, flushing, or stridor.
   E. A series of radiographs of the head, both of the anterior and lateral views, are taken during the 5-15 seconds after the injection. Approximately another 6 seconds

after the arteries appear, capillary and venous blood flow may be studied by radiographs.

F. The contrast injection may be repeated, and the views varied to complete the study, as indicated by the suspected abnormalities.

G. The artery catheter is kept open with continuous or intermittent flushing or with heparinized normal saline.

4. Postprocedure care:
    A. The catheter is withdrawn and pressure is applied to the artery for at least 15 minutes.
    B. Apply a dry, sterile or pressure dressing to the site and observe for bleeding or hematoma formation at the catheter insertion site.
    C. Maintain bedrest for 12-24 hours.
    D. Assess neurologic status and vital signs hourly for 4 hours and then every 4 hours for 20 hours.
    E. For femoral or brachial approaches, immobilize the leg or arm straight for 12 hours. Check color, motion, temperature, sensation, and distal pulses of the immobilized extremity every 15 minutes for 4 hours, then every 30 minutes for 2 hours, then every 1 hour for 4 hours, and then every 4 hours for 12 hours.
    F. For the carotid approach, observe for respiratory distress, dysphagia, or hoarseness, which may indicate extravasation of the dye.
    G. If general anesthesia was used, continue the assessment of respiratory status and follow institutional protocol for postsedation monitoring. Typical monitoring includes continuous ECG monitoring and pulse oximetry, with continual assessments (every 5-15 minutes) of the airway, vital signs, and neurologic status until the client is lying quietly awake, is breathing independently, and responds appropriately to commands spoken in a normal tone.

5. Client and family teaching:
    A. Fast from food and fluids for 4-8 hours before the procedure.
    B. It is important to lie still for this test. A sensation of burning may be felt because of the injection of the contrast medium, but this feeling lasts for only a few moments.

6. Factors that affect results:
    A. Head movement during the study obscures the clarity of the radiographs.
    B. Radiopaque objects such as earrings obstruct the view of the internal vasculature.

7. Other data:
    A. The femoral artery approach has the advantage of providing visualization of both carotid arteries and both vertebral arteries, extending the study to the supply vessels.

CEREBRAL COMPUTED TOMOGRAPHY, DIAGNOSTIC

Norm. Normal-appearing skull and symmetry and size of cerebral or other brain tissue. Cerebrum appears with black-gray shadings, and bone or other very dense tissues appear white. There is normally no evidence of tumor, high-density to whitish hematoma, edema, or congenital abnormalities such as hydrocephalus.

Usage. Brain tumor (astrocytoma, meningioma, metastatic, or primary lesions); cerebral atrophy or infarction; cerebral edema; cerebrovascular accident (CVA); evaluation of neurologic symptoms; evaluation of effects of surgery, radiation, or chemotherapeutic treatment of intracranial tumors; head injury; hematoma (epidural, subdural); hydrocephalus; subarachnoid hemorrhage and other acute hemorrhage.

Description. Computed tomography (CT) uses special radiographic equipment and computers to produce a series of images (or tomographs) of cross sections of the brain tissues. Images may be "slices" taken of the skull and brain across anteroposterior, horizontal, sagittal, or coronal planes. Although contrast medium may be used, the test is often noninvasive and therefore provides a safe, effective diagnostic tool for the study of tumors of the brain, evaluation of neurologic clinical changes, evaluation of CVA or intracranial bleeds, and assessment of clients with possible head injury for hematoma before symptoms are evident. For evaluation of vascular malformations, high-resolution CT (HRCT) is preferred. HRCT improves upon traditional CT technology by providing optimized spatial resolution of body structures and better differentiation of normal from abnormal blood vessels. For rapid evaluation after stroke symptoms appear, Spiral (Helical) CT is the preferred method. (See also *Computed tomography of the body, Diagnostic* for further description of the different types of CT technology available.)

Professional Considerations
1. Consent form IS required when contrast medium is injected as part of the study.

Risks
Allergic reaction to contrast media (itching, hives, rash, tight feeling in the throat, shortness of breath, bronchospasm, anaphylaxis, death), dehydration, renal toxicity, vomiting.

Contraindications
Claustrophobia; dehydration; severe liver or kidney disease; previous allergy to contrast medium, iodine, or shellfish; pregnancy (relative contraindication); and renal insufficiency if CT with contrast will be performed. Weight >136 kg, or >300 pounds, may exceed the capabilities of some scanners.

Precautions
During pregnancy, risks of cumulative radiation exposure to the fetus from this and other previous of future imaging studies must be weighed against the benefits of the procedure. although formal limits for client exposure are relative to this risk:benefit comparison, the United States Nuclear Regulatory Commission requires that the cumulative dose equivalent to an embryo/fetus from occupational exposure not exceed 0.5 rem (5 mSv). risk of exposure to the uterus from cerebral CT is <10 mrad. Radiation dosage to the fetus decreases as pregnancy progresses.

2. **Preparation:**
   A. Remove all jewelry, hairpins, wigs, or dentures.
   B. Establish intravenous access if contrast medium will be used.
   C. Have emergency equipment readily available for CT with contrast medium if necessary.
3. **Procedure:**
   A. The client is placed on a movable radiographic table in a supine position. The table has a special-ized headrest with straps that are positioned to immobilize the head.
   B. The table head is moved into a circular CT scanner, which moves around the client's head, taking an extensive series of radiographs at each degree of a 180-degree arch.
   C. The automated computer then produces a reconstruction of the images, which shows slices through the skull and the brain.
   D. The study may then continue to include intravenous administration of contrast material. A second series of views is completed. The client is observed for rash or respiratory difficulty, which may indicate reaction to the contrast medium. Reactions develop within 30 minutes.
4. **Postprocedure care:**
   A. None for CT without contrast.
   B. For CT with contrast, observe for side effects such as headache, nausea, and vomiting and delayed hypersensitivity reaction.
   C. Resume previous diet.
5. **Client and family teaching:**
   A. You must lie very still for this test.
   B. If a contrast medium will be used, fast from midnight before the test.
   C. Results are normally available the same day.
   D. Inform CT personnel if you feel claustrophobic in enclosed spaces.
6. **Factors that affect results:**
   A. Movement of the client's head interferes with the quality of the films.
   B. Metal objects such as jewelry or hairpins interfere with complete visualization.
7. **Other data:**
   A. Intracerebral hemorrhage is higher among Hispanics as a result of chronic hypertension; therefore cerebral CT should be considered.

CEREBROSPINAL FLUID, CYTOLOGY, SPECIMEN
(see *Cerebrospinal fluid, Routine, Culture and cytology*)

CEREBROSPINAL FLUID, FUNGUS, CULTURE
(see *Cerebrospinal fluid, Routine, Culture and cytology*)

CEREBROSPINAL FLUID, GLUCOSE, SPECIMEN

Norm. (Fasting) 50-80% of serum glucose.

		SI UNITS
Adult	40-80 mg/dL	2.2-4.4 mmol/L
Premature infant	24-63 mg/dL	1.3-3.5 mmol/L
Full-term infant	34-119 mg/dL	1.9-6.6 mmol/L
Child	35-75 mg/dL	1.9-4.1 mmol/L

Increased. Brain tumor, cerebral hemorrhage, cerebral trauma, diabetic coma, hyperglycemia, hypothalamic lesions, increased intracranial pressure, and uremia.

Decreased. Brain abscess, brain tumor, cancer, central nervous system sarcoidosis, choroid plexus tumor, coccidioidomycosis, glut-1 deficiency, encephalitis (mumps or herpes simplex origin), hypoglycemia, increased intracranial pressure, leukemic infiltration, lupus myelopathy, lymphocytic choriomeningitis, lymphoma, melanomatosis, meningeal carcinomatosis, meningitis (acute pyogenic, aseptic, chemical, cryptococcal, fungal, granulomatous, *Haemophilus influenzae*, pyogenic, rheumatoid, tuberculous, viral), neurosyphilis, rheumatoid arthritis, subarachnoid hemorrhage, toxoplasmosis, and tuberculoma of brain.

Description. Cerebrospinal fluid (CSF) glucose content is related to the blood serum glucose content of 1-4 hours earlier. Most abnormalities result in a decreased CSF glucose because of increased utilization of glucose by the pathogenic process. This test is interpreted by comparison of a blood glucose level to a CSF glucose level.

Professional Considerations
1. Consent form IS required for the lumbar puncture, which is necessary to obtain the specimen. See *Lumbar Puncture, Diagnostic,* for procedure risks and contraindications.
2. Preparation:
   A. Obtain a lumbar puncture tray, sterile drapes, and 1-2% lidocaine.
   B. Tube: Red topped, red/gray topped, or gold topped.
3. Procedure:
   A. Draw a 1-mL blood sample.
   B. 3-10 mL of CSF is collected by a physician in sequentially numbered sterile glass tubes through a spinal tap between L3-4 or L4-5 or from the ventricles of the brain during special procedures.
4. Postprocedure care:
   A. Transport the specimens to the laboratory immediately. Analysis must be performed on a freshly collected specimen to avoid erroneous results from glycolysis.
   B. Refrigerate the CSF if it is not analyzed promptly.
5. Client and family teaching:
   A. See *Lumbar puncture, Diagnostic.*
6. Factors that affect results:
   A. Falsely decreased levels may be caused by cellular and bacterial utilization if the test is not performed immediately.
   B. See *Lumbar puncture, Diagnostic.*
7. Other data:
   A. See *Lumbar puncture, Diagnostic.*

CEREBROSPINAL FLUID, IMMUNOGLOBULIN G (IgG), IMMUNOGLOBULIN G RATIOS AND IMMUNOGLOBULIN G INDEX, IMMUNOGLOBULIN G SYNTHESIS RATE, SPECIMEN

Norm:

IgG:	0.5-5 mg/dL (5-50 mg/L, SI units), or <12% of CSF total protein
IgG/albumin ratio:	22-28% of serum IgG/albumin ratio
IgG index:	0.3-0.7
Immunoglobulin G synthesis rate:	− 9.9 to +3.3 mg/day or 0.0 to 0.8 mg/day

Increased. Brain tissue destruction, Claude syndrome, CNS infection (chronic), CNS lupus erythematosus, CNS vasculitis, Guillain-Barré syndrome, Landau-Kleffner syndrome, Miller Fischer syndrome, multiple sclerosis, neurosyphilis, and Sjögren syndrome (primary with CNS involvement).

Decreased Immunoglobulin G. Not applicable.

Decreased Immunoglobulin G Index. Contamination of cerebrospinal fluid (CSF) with blood from spinal tap, intracerebral hemorrhage, or disturbance of the blood-brain barrier.

Decreased Immunoglobulin G Synthesis Rate. Not applicable.

Description. *IgG antibodies* constitute a portion of immunoglobulin proteins secreted by beta-lymphocytes. They act as antibacterial and antiviral neutralizers of toxins produced by bacteria and viruses by activating phagocytic cells. Although slow to develop, they remain present in CSF long after the bacteria and viruses have disappeared and reappear rapidly on subsequent exposure to the antigens. IgG antibodies are identified by electrophoretic testing of the CSF that separates the protein into its component factors.

The *IgG ratio* and *IgG index* help rule out the possibility that blood has entered the CSF, bringing with it increased amounts of IgG antibodies. If this is the case, IgG and albumin will be present in about the same proportion in which they are present in the bloodstream, as evidenced by the IgG/albumin ratio of CSF compared to the IgG/albumin ratio of serum.

The *IgG index* measures CSF production of IgG by the following formula:

(CSF IgG/CSF albumin) ÷
      (serum IgG/serum albumin)

The elevation of either measure indicates the presence of CNS disease.

The *IgG synthesis rate* helps rule out the possibility that blood has entered the CSF, bringing with it increased amounts of IgG antibodies. If this is the case, IgG synthesis will be greater in CSF than in serum, indicating the presence of CNS disease. The rate is calculated according to the "formula of Tourtellote":

$$IgG \text{ synthesis (mg/day)} = \\ [(IgG_{CSF} - IgG_{SERUM}/369) - \\ (Alb_{CSF} - Alb_{SERUM}/230) \times \\ (IgG_{SERUM}/Alb_{SERUM}) \, 0.43] \times 5$$

Professional Considerations

1. Consent form IS required for the lumbar puncture, which is necessary to obtain CSF. See *Lumbar puncture, Diagnostic,* for procedure risks and contraindications.

2. **Preparation:**
   A. A CT scan is typically performed to rule out increased intracranial pressure before lumbar puncture in critically ill clients or those with changed mental status.
   B. Obtain a lumbar puncture tray, sterile drapes, and 1-2% lidocaine.
   C. Tube: Red topped, red/gray topped, or gold topped.

3. **Procedure:**
   A. 3-10 mL of CSF is collected by a physician in sequentially numbered sterile glass tubes through a spinal tap between L3-4 or L4-5 or from the ventricles of the brain during special procedures.
   B. Draw a 2-mL blood sample for IgG/albumin ratio (also known as IgG/albumin index) and comparison of the serum and CSF IgG.

4. **Postprocedure care:**
   A. See also *Lumbar puncture, Diagnostic.*
   B. Transport the specimens to the laboratory immediately.
   C. Refrigerate the CSF if it is not analyzed promptly.

5. **Client and family teaching:**
   A. See *Lumbar puncture, Diagnostic.*

6. **Factors that affect results:**
   A. This test should be performed on tube 2 or higher to lessen the chance of contamination of the specimen with blood from a traumatic spinal tap.
   B. The results are invalidated if the client has recently undergone a myelogram.
   C. Immunoglobulin G synthesis rate norms vary by laboratory.
   D. Protein >100 mg/dL results in yellow-tinged CSF.

7. **Other data:**
   A. The possibility exists that CSF IgG may be elevated because of leakage of serum into the spinal canal during disruption of the blood-brain barrier. The CSF IgG

ratios and IgG index test should be performed to rule out this possibility.

B. The IgG synthesis rate sensitivity is 70-96%, which is slightly less sensitive and reproducible than the IgG index.

C. In one study, 55% of clients with multiple sclerosis had an elevated IgG synthesis rate.

D. See also *Lumbar puncture, Diagnostic.*

CEREBROSPINAL FLUID, LACTIC ACID, SPECIMEN

Norm:

	SI UNITS
9-26 mg/dL	1.13-3.23 mmol/L

Increased. Brain abscess, central nervous system carcinoma, cerebral infarct, cerebral ischemia, cerebral trauma, hydrocephalus, hypotension, increased cerebrospinal fluid (CSF), white blood cells, intracranial hemorrhage, low CSF glucose, meningitis (bacterial, fungal, tuberculous), multiple sclerosis, respiratory alkalosis, and seizures.

Decreased. Not clinically significant.

Description. Elevated CSF lactic acid levels indicate increased glucose utilization and anaerobic metabolism associated with decreased oxygenation of the brain or increased intracranial pressure. This test aids in the differentiation of meningitis and in identification of central nervous system disease processes.

Professional Considerations
1. Consent form IS required for the lumbar puncture, which is necessary to obtain CSF. See *Lumbar puncture, Diagnostic,* for procedure risks and contraindications.

2. **Preparation:**
   A. A CT scan is typically performed to rule out increased intracranial pressure before the lumbar puncture in critically ill clients or those with changed mental status.
   B. See also *Lumbar puncture, Diagnostic.*
   C. Obtain a lumbar puncture tray, sterile drapes, and 1-2% lidocaine.

3. **Procedure:**
   A. 3-10 mL of CSF is collected by a physician in sequentially numbered sterile glass tubes through a spinal tap between L3-4 or L4-5 or from the ventricles of the brain during special procedures.

4. **Postprocedure care:**
   A. See *Lumbar puncture, Diagnostic.*

5. **Client and family teaching:**
   A. See *Lumbar puncture, Diagnostic.*

6. **Factors that affect results:**
   A. Discard the first specimen because it is most likely to be contaminated with blood.
   B. Lactic acid determination should be performed on tube 2 or higher to lessen the chance of blood contamination.
   C. Refrigerate the CSF if it is not analyzed promptly.

7. **Other data:**
   A. Cell counts and other chemical and serologic studies may also be performed on this sample.
   B. See also *Lumbar puncture, Diagnostic.*

CEREBROSPINAL FLUID, MYCOBACTERIA, CULTURE
(*see Cerebrospinal fluid, Routine, Culture and cytology, Specimen*)

CEREBROSPINAL FLUID, MYELIN BASIC PROTEIN, OLIGOCLONAL BANDS, PROTEIN, AND PROTEIN ELECTROPHORESIS, SPECIMEN

Norm:

		SI UNITS
Myelin Basic Protein		
Negative	<4 ng/mL	<4 mg/L
Active demyelination	>6 ng/mL	>6 mg/L

		SI UNITS
Oligoclonal Bands	Absent	
Total Protein		
Adults		
20-40 years		
Lumbar	15-45 mg/dL	150-450 mg/L
Cisternal	15-25 mg/dL	150-250 mg/L
Ventricular	5-15 mg/dL	50-150 mg/L
40-50 years	20-50 mg/dL	200-500 mg/L
50-60 years	20-55 mg/dL	200-550 mg/L
>60 years	30-60 mg/dL	300-600 mg/L
Children		
Premature infant	400 mg/dL	4000 mg/L
Full-term newborn	20-170 mg/dL	200-1700 mg/L
1-4 weeks	30-150 mg/dL	300-1500 mg/L
4-12 weeks	20-100 mg/dL	200-1000 mg/L
3-6 months	15-50 mg/dL	150-500 mg/L
6 months–10 years	10-30 mg/dL	100-300 mg/L
10-20 years	15-45 mg/dL	150-450 mg/L

		FRACTION OF TOTAL CSF PROTEIN
Protein Electrophoresis		
Prealbumin	2-7%	0.02-0.07
Albumin	45-76%	0.45-0.76
Alpha$_1$ globulin	1.1-7%	0.01-0.07
Alpha$_2$ globulin	3-12%	0.03-0.12
Beta globulin	7.5-18%	0.07-0.18
Gamma globulin	3-13%	0.03-0.13

Increased Myelin Basic Protein. Cerebral infarcts, demyelinating diseases, and multiple sclerosis (acute).

Increased Oligoclonal Bands. CNS lesions (destructive), CNS lupus erythematosus, CNS vasculitis, diabetes mellitus, Guillain-Barré syndrome, multiple sclerosis, neurosyphilis, panencephalitis (progressive rubella, subacute sclerosing), polyneuropathy, Sjögren syndrome (primary involving the CNS) and spinal arteriovenous malformation.

Increased Protein. Anesthetics (spinal), arteriosclerosis (cerebral), aseptic meningeal reaction, brain abscess, brain tumor, cerebral aneurysm (ruptured), coccidioidomycosis, cord tumor, diabetic neuropathy, encephalitis (postinfectious), Froin syndrome, Guillain-Barré syndrome, head trauma (bloody), heavy metal poisoning, hemorrhage (intracerebral, subarachnoid), herpes zoster, hyperproteinemia, infections (acute, coxsackievirus, echovirus), lead encephalopathy, measles, meningitis (acute pyogenic, bacterial, cryptococcal, fungal, tuberculous, viral), meningoencephalitis (bacterial, mycotic), multiple sclerosis, mumps, myxedema, neuropathy (retrobulbar), poliomyelitis (acute anterior), polyneuritis (ascending), sarcoidosis, syphilis (tabes dorsalis, general paresis, meningovascular), systemic lupus erythematosus, thrombosis (cerebral), and toxoplasmosis (congenital). Drugs that increase cerebrospinal fluid (CSF) protein at toxic levels include ethyl alcohol (ethanol), isopropanol, phenytoin, and phenytoin sodium.

Protein Electrophoresis

Increased beta globulin. Cerebrovascular disease, meningitis (acute), neoplasms.

Increased gamma globulin. Multiple sclerosis, neurosyphilis, and subacute sclerosing leukoencephalitis.

Increased IgG. Guillain-Barré syndrome, meningoencephalitis (viral), multiple sclerosis, neurosyphilis, subacute sclerosing panencephalitis, and systemic lupus erythematosus of the CNS.

Decreased myelin basic protein. Not applicable.

Decreased oligoclonal bands. Multiple sclerosis.

Decreased protein. Not applicable.

Description. *Myelin basic protein* is a part of the myelin protein that composes the sheath surrounding myelinated nerves. The myelin sheath surrounds and insulates nerve axons and functions to speed nerve impulse conduction. In demyelinating diseases, the myelin sheath is broken down, resulting in the release of myelin basic protein into the CSF. The detection of myelin basic protein in CSF aids in the diagnosis and staging of demyelinating diseases.

Oligoclonal bands are identified by means of protein electrophoresis, which separates CSF protein into its component factors. They are present only in certain CNS diseases that cause the normally homogeneous gamma globulin to break up into specific bands called "oligoclonal bands." This signifies the presence of antibodies produced in the CNS. Oligoclonal bands help differentiate CNS diseases that produce similar signs and symptoms.

Elevated CSF *protein* levels provide a nonspecific indicator of serious disease. Protein levels normally remain constant and are elevated in CSF only during increased tissue catabolism or by a disturbance in the normal capillary impermeability to plasma proteins.

Electrophoretic testing of CSF separates the protein into its component factors. Synthesis of the immunocompetent cells contained in the CNS and small amounts of protein that diffuse from the bloodstream account for the protein content of the CSF. Under normal circumstances, CSF contains minute amounts of protein. Inflammation and infection increase the permeability of blood vessels, allowing all proteins to more easily cross the blood-brain barrier. Certain disease states produce characteristic changes in specific types of CSF protein, such as albumin,

alpha globulin, beta globulin, and gamma globulin. Electrophoresis is a measurement of proteins, which under the influence of an electrical field, at a pH of 8.6, separate by charge, size, and shape. This separation produces homogeneous bands that are plotted on specially treated paper. IgG immunoglobulin is the principal immunoglobulin represented with protein electrophoresis.

Professional Considerations
1. Consent form IS required for the lumbar puncture, which is necessary to obtain CSF. See *Lumbar puncture, Diagnostic,* for procedure risks and contraindications.
2. Preparation:
   A. A CT scan is typically performed to rule out increased intracranial pressure before the lumbar puncture in critically ill clients or those with changed mental status.
   B. See *Lumbar puncture, Diagnostic.*
3. Procedure:
   A. 3-10 mL of CSF is collected by a physician in sequentially numbered sterile glass tubes through a spinal tap between L3-4 or L4-5 or from the ventricles of the brain during special procedures.
4. Postprocedure care:
   A. Apply a Band-Aid over the spinal tap site.
   B. See also *Lumbar puncture, Diagnostic.*
   C. Refrigerate the CSF if it is not analyzed promptly.
   D. Monitor for headaches, dizziness, or change in level of consciousness.
5. **Client and family teaching:**
   A. See also *Lumbar puncture, Diagnostic.*
6. **Factors that affect results:**
   A. Discard the first specimen.
   B. Myelin basic protein determination should be performed on tube 2.
   C. Cell counts and other chemical and serologic studies may also be performed on this specimen.
   D. Transport the specimens to the laboratory immediately. Analysis must be performed promptly on freshly collected specimens to avoid erroneous results from cell lysis and disintegration.
   E. Falsely elevated protein levels may result from a traumatic spinal puncture.

F. Drugs that may cause falsely elevated CSF protein results include aspirin, chlorpromazine, phenacetin, salicylates, streptomycin sulfate, and sulfonamides.

7. **Other data:**
A. Serum electrophoresis should be performed if oligoclonal bands are found in the CSF. Oligoclonal bands would be considered abnormal only if they are absent in the serum.
B. Protein >100 mg/dL results in yellow-tinged CSF.
C. See also *Lumbar puncture, Diagnostic.*

CEREBROSPINAL FLUID, OLIGOCLONAL BANDS, SPECIMEN
(see Cerebrospinal fluid, Myelin basic protein, oligoclonal bands, protein and protein electrophoresis, Specimen)

CEREBROSPINAL FLUID, PROTEIN, SPECIMEN
(see Cerebrospinal fluid, Myelin basic protein, oligoclonal bands, protein and protein electrophoresis, Specimen)

CEREBROSPINAL FLUID, PROTEIN ELECTROPHORESIS, SPECIMEN
(see Cerebrospinal fluid, Myelin basic protein, oligoclonal bands, protein and protein electrophoresis, Specimen)

C

CEREBROSPINAL FLUID, ROUTINE, CULTURE AND CYTOLOGY

Norm:

Routine culture. No growth.

Fungus culture. No growth after several weeks.

Mycobacteria culture. No growth after 8 weeks.

Cytology. Cerebrospinal fluid free of abnormal cells.

		SI UNITS
Adults and children	0-5 cells/μL	$0\text{-}5 \times 10^6/L$
Newborn	0-30 cells/μL	$0\text{-}30 \times 10^6/L$
Adults		
Neoplastic cells	Negative	Negative
Erythrocytes	0-10/μL	$0\text{-}10 \times 10^6/L$
Leukocytes	0-10/μL	$0\text{-}10 \times 10^6/L$
Differential lymphocytes	63-99%	
Beta-lymphocytes	0-4%	
T-lymphocytes	89-97%	
Monocytes	3-37%	
Neutrophils	Absent	
Eosinophils	0-5%	
Children		
Neoplastic Cells	Negative	Negative
Erythrocytes		
Newborn	0-675/μL	$0\text{-}675 \times 10^6/L$
Leukocytes		
Infants	0-30/μL	$0\text{-}30 \times 10^6/L$
1-4 years	0-20/μL	$0\text{-}20 \times 10^6/L$
5-20 years	0-10/μL	$0\text{-}20 \times 10^6/L$

Cytology Usage. Establish the presence of primary or metastatic neoplasm; diagnosis of cryptococcal meningitis, bacterial meningitis, or cerebral hemorrhage, brain abscess, encephalitis (postinfection, tick borne), lead encephalopathy, medulloblastoma, neurosyphilis, sarcoidosis (meningeal), and study of CNS changes related to acquired immunodeficiency syndrome.

Positive Routine Culture. CNS infections, encephalitis, meningitis, and sepsis neonatorum.

Negative Routine Culture. Normal finding.

Positive Fungus Culture. Brain abscess, meningitis, and systemic fungal infections.

Negative Fungus Culture. Normal finding.

Positive Mycobacteria Culture. Mycobacterial meningitis. The most common mycobacteria causing human disease are *Mycobacterium asiaticum, M. avium-scrofulaceum complex, M. fortuitum, M. haemophilum, M. kansasii, M. leprae, M. malmoense, M. marinum, M. simiae, M. szulgai, M. tuberculosis complex, M. ulcerans,* and *M. xenopi.*

Negative Mycobacteria Culture. Normal finding.

Description. This test includes cultures for anaerobic, aerobic, and acid-fast organisms, bacteria, protozoa, fungi, or viruses. A culture of cerebrospinal fluid (CSF) for fungus is performed to detect systemic fungal infections and normally harmless fungi that become pathogenic in the presence of immunosuppressive conditions. Although tentative identification of fungi can be made quickly with staining techniques, a culture of the organism on a special fungal culture medium is required to confirm a diagnosis of a fungal infection. Cell count and cytologic examination (the number and character of cells) is performed to identify the presence of abnormal cells, infective organisms, or variations in the usually low numbers of red and white blood cells. Abnormalities include increases in the numbers of normal cells or the presence of neoplastic cells.

Professional Considerations

1. Consent form IS required for the lumbar puncture, which is necessary to obtain CSF. See *Lumbar puncture, Diagnostic,* for procedure risks and contraindications.
2. Preparation:
   A. A CT scan is typically performed to rule out increased intracranial pressure before the lumbar puncture in critically ill clients or those with changed mental status.
   B. Hand washing significantly decreases false-positive coagulase negative staphylococcal culture rates.
   C. See also *Lumbar puncture, Diagnostic.*
3. Procedure:
   A. 3-10 mL of CSF is collected by a physician in sequentially numbered sterile glass tubes through a spinal tap between L3-4 or L4-5 or from the ventricles of the brain during special procedures.
4. Postprocedure care:
   A. Write the specimen source, collection time, current antibiotic or antifungal therapy, and clinical diagnosis on the laboratory requisition.
   B. Monitor for headaches, dizziness, or change in level of consciousness.
   C. Transport the specimens to microbiology immediately. Analysis must be performed promptly on freshly collected specimens.
   D. See also *Lumbar puncture, Diagnostic.*
5. Client and family teaching:
   A. See *Lumbar puncture, Diagnostic.*
   B. Growth of fungi may take several weeks.
6. Factors that affect results:
   A. The results are invalid when the specimen stands over 1 hour at room temperature.
   B. Previous radiation, intrathecal therapy, myelogram, or pneumoencephalogram may cause cytologic changes that produce false results.
   C. Microbiologic studies should be performed on tube 3 or higher to lessen the chance of skin contamination.
   D. At least 5 mL is necessary to detect fungal and mycobacterial infections.

7. **Other data:**
   A. Glucose and protein determinations may also be performed on this specimen.
   B. If CNS infection is strongly suspected but initial cell counts are normal, the test should be repeated a few hours later to detect rising white cell counts.
   C. Store CSF for culture in a bacteriologic incubator when not tested promptly.
   D. A portion of the sample should be frozen at −20° C when viral meningitis is suspected.
   E. For positive CSF cultures, sensitivity = 92%, specificity = 95%, false-positive = 5%, and false-negative = 8%. The results are most accurate when samples are obtained before the initiation of antibiotic therapy.
   F. CSF specimens: most common organism for adults is *Cryptococcus* and most common diagnosis for children was medulloblastoma.
   G. See also *Lumbar puncture, Diagnostic*.

CEREBROSPINAL FLUID, ROUTINE ANALYSIS, SPECIMEN

Norm:

		SI UNITS
Appearance	Clear, colorless	
Specific gravity	1.006-1.008	1.006-1.008
Pressure	50-175 mm H_2O	50-175 mm H_2O
pH	7.30-7.40	
AST	0-19 U	
Bicarbonate	22.9 mEq/L	
Calcium	2.1-2.7 mEq/L	1.05-1.35 mmol/L
	4.2-5.4 mg/dL	1.05-1.35 mmol/L
Chloride	118-132 mEq/L	118-132 mmol/L
Cholesterol	0.2-0.6 mg/dL	
pCO_2	42-52 mmHg	
Creatinine	0.4-1.5 mg/dL	
Glucose (fasting)	40-80 mg/dL	2.2-4.4 mmol/L
Glutamine	6-16 mg/dL	
Iron	1-2 mg/dL	
Lactate	10-18 mg/dL	
LD	1/10 of serum level	
Magnesium	2.0-3.1 mEq/L	
Phosphorus	1.2-2.1 mEq/L	
Potassium	2.7-3.9 mEq/L	0.15-0.45 g/L
Protein	15-45 mg/dL	150-450 mg/L
Sodium	138-154 mEq/L	
Urea	6-28 mg/dL	
Uric acid	0.5-4.5 mg/dL	
WBC	0-10 mg/L	

Increased. Acute anterior poliomyelitis (*protein, WBC*), alcoholism (*pressure [possibly]*), aseptic meningeal reaction (*protein, WBC*), brain abscess (*protein, neutrophils*), brain tumor (*pressure, protein, glucose*), cerebellitis (*protein*), cerebral hemorrhage (*RBC, pressure, protein*), cerebral thrombosis (*protein, lymphocytes*), cerebral trauma (*pressure, glucose*), coccidioidomycosis (*pressure, protein, WBC*), coma (diabetic) (*glucose*), cord tumor (*protein, WBC*), diabetes mellitus (*protein*), encephalitis (postinfectious) (*pressure, protein, lymphocytes*), Guillain Barré (*protein*), head trauma (*pressure, protein*), herpes zoster (*protein, WBC*), infections (*protein*), hyperglycemia (*glucose*), hypothalamic lesions (*glucose*), lead encephalopathy (*pressure, protein, WBC*), leptomeningeal carcinomatosis (*malignant cells*), meningitis (acute pyogenic) (*pressure,* protein, neutrophils), meningitis (aseptic) (pressure, protein, WBC), meningitis (cryptococcal, fungal, tuberculous, viral) (pressure, protein, lymphocytes), meningoencephalitis (primary amebic) (pressure, protein, WBC), measles (pressure [possibly], protein, WBC), multiple sclerosis (protein, lymphocytes), mumps (pressure [possibly], protein, WBC), polyneuritis (protein, lymphocytes), pseudotumor cerebri (pressure), subarachnoid hemorrhage (endothelin, pressure, protein), subdural hematoma (pressure, protein, lymphocytes), syphilis (protein, lymphocytes), uremia (pressure, protein, glucose), and viral infections (coxsackievirus and echovirus) (neutrophils).

Decreased. Only decreased glucose is significant. See *Cerebrospinal Fluid, Glucose, Specimen.*

Description. Analysis of cerebrospinal fluid (CSF) components is performed to aid diagnosis of a wide variety of CNS diseases, including infectious and malignant diseases.

Professional Considerations
1. Consent form IS required for the lumbar puncture, which is necessary to obtain CSF. See *Lumbar puncture, Diagnostic,* for procedure risks and contraindications.
2. Preparation:
   A. A CT scan is typically performed to rule out increased intracranial pressure before the lumbar puncture in critically ill clients or those with changed mental status.
   B. See *Lumbar puncture, Diagnostic.*
3. Procedure:
   A. 3-10 mL of CSF is collected by a physician in sequentially numbered sterile glass tubes through a spinal tap between L3-4 or L4-5 or from the ventricles of the brain during special procedures.

4. Postprocedure care:
   A. Apply a Band-Aid over the spinal tap site.
   B. See also *Lumbar puncture, Diagnostic.*
   C. Transport specimens to the laboratory immediately.
   D. Monitor for headaches, dizziness, or change in level of consciousness.
5. Client and family teaching:
   A. See *Lumbar Puncture, Diagnostic.*
6. Factors that affect results:
   A. Discard the first specimen.
   B. Cell counts, chemistry, and serology should be performed on tube 2.
   C. Microbiologic studies should be performed on tube 3 or higher to lessen the chance of skin contamination.
   D. The analysis must be performed promptly on freshly collected specimens to avoid erroneous results from cell lysis, disintegration, and continued glycolysis.
   E. Colored or very cloudy spinal fluid requires additional mixing with 0.5 mL of sterile sodium citrate per 5 mL of CSF to prevent clotting. This item is not applicable if tuberculous meningitis is suspected.
   F. Withdraw at least 10.5 mL of CSF to avoid false-negative results for leptomeningeal carcinomatosis.
7. Other data:
   A. Handle specimens cautiously to prevent self-contamination.
   B. Refrigerate the CSF if it is not analyzed promptly.
   C. Cloudy specimens may be caused by elevated white blood cells. Yellow specimens may be caused by elevated protein. Pink or red specimens may be caused by red blood cells.
   D. See also *Lumbar puncture, Diagnostic.*

CERULOPLASMIN (CP), SERUM

Norm:

		SI UNITS
Adult	14-40 mg/dL	0.93-2.65 µmol/L
Newborn	1-30 mg/dL	0.06-1.99 µmol/L
6-12 months	15-50 mg/dL	0.99-3.31 µmol/L
1-12 years	30-65 mg/dL	1.99-4.30 µmol/L

Increased. Cancer (breast), cardiovascular disease, cirrhosis, diabetes mellitus, epilepsy, infection, pregnancy, primary sclerosing cholangitis, rheumatoid arthritis, hepatitis, myocardial infarction, and thyrotoxicosis. Drugs include oral contraceptives, estrogens, phenytoin (Dilantin), and methadone.

Decreased. Aceruloplasminemia, hepatic disease, Klippel-Trenaunay syndrome, kwashiorkor, malabsorption (such as sprue), meningococcal sepsis, nephrosis, nephrotic syndrome, in early infancy, and Wilson's disease (<23 mg/dL).

Description. Ceruloplasmin is an alpha$_2$-globulin transport protein that transports copper and aids in mobilizing iron stores. It is an acute-phase reactant that becomes elevated during stress, pregnancy, and infection. This test is most often used to aid diagnosis of Wilson's disease, in which subnormal quantities of ceruloplasmin are manufactured by the liver. The resulting tissue deposition of copper causes brain and liver damage.

Professional Considerations
1. Consent form NOT required.
2. Preparation:
   A. Tube: Red topped, red/gray topped, or gold topped.
3. Procedure:
   A. Draw a 1-mL blood sample.
4. Postprocedure care:
   A. None.
5. Client and family teaching:
   A. Results may not be available for several days.
6. Factors that affect results:
   A. Hemolysis invalidates the results.
   B. The results are unreliable in infants under 3 months old.
7. Other data:
   A. The serum level of ceruloplasmin is determined by electrophoresis.

CERVICAL CULTURE

Norm. Negative for pathogenic vaginal microorganisms.

Positive. The most common organisms recovered in positive cervical cultures include *Actinomyces, Candida, Chlamydia, Mobiluncus, Gardenella,* herpes simplex, *Mycoplasma hominis, Neisseria gonorrhoeae, Trichomonas,* and *Ureaplasma urealyticum.*

Description. A cervical culture is included in routine gynecologic examinations or in cases of cervicitis, endometritis, leukorrhea, vaginitis, suspected infection, or rape. A smear is usually included as well. The specimen is obtained by means of a vaginal examination. Although cultures are considered the standard for diagnosis of cervical infections, because of their specificity they are difficult to collect. Newer nucleic acid and antigen/antibody detection methods are becoming available that can detect the organisms in a urine specimen.

Professional Considerations
1. Consent form NOT required.
2. Preparation:
   A. The client must disrobe below the waist.
   B. Obtain a speculum, a sterile Culturette, glass slides, two spatuli, potassium hydroxide, and a sterile 0.9% saline.
3. Procedure:
   A. Position the client in the dorsal lithotomy position and drape for privacy and comfort.
   B. Insert a speculum into the vagina and expose the cervix and vaginal walls.
   C. Collect exudate from the cervix or vagina or both on a sterile Culturette. The exudate may be expressed from the cervix by being gently pressed between two spatuli. Smear exudate onto two glass slides. Place one slide in the potassium hydroxide fixative and the other in the sterile 0.9% saline.
4. Postprocedure care:
   A. Write the clinical data, specimen source, and any recent antibiotic therapy on the laboratory requisition.
   B. Send the specimen to the laboratory within 2 hours. Do not refrigerate the specimen.
5. Client and family teaching:
   A. Do not douche for 24 hours before the test.
   B. Several days may be required for growth in the culture. Empiric therapy is often begun while the client awaits culture results.

C. Instruct the client with a positive culture on the preventive measures appropriate to the grown organism, where applicable.

D. The client with a positive test for a sexually transmitted organism should inform all sexual partners of the infection, return for a follow-up culture 7-10 days after finishing the medication prescribed for the infection, and refrain from sexual activity with another person until negative follow-low-up cultures are received.

6. **Factors that affect results:**
   A. The test must be repeated if the Culturette is contaminated by touching the speculum or walls of the labia or if other contamination occurs during the procedure.
   B. If *Actinomyces* is suspected, a special anaerobic culture container with a theocolate broth must be obtained.
   C. *Chlamydia* is difficult to culture with this method.

7. **Other data:**
   A. A fish odor from a fresh slide treated with potassium hydroxide is a positive indication for *Gardenella.*
   B. Yeast vaginal infections, especially *Candida*, are easily noted microscopically when spores are stained by potassium hydroxide.
   C. On saline-treated culture slides, the *Trichomonas* organism has a typical pear shape and flagella.
   D. Wet vaginal swab PCR detects more chlamydia and more gonorrhea than routine cervical culture.

CERVICAL CULTURE FOR *NEISSERIA GONORRHOEAE,* CULTURE

Norm. No *Neisseria gonorrhoeae* is isolated.

Positive. Gonorrheal infection of the female genitalia.

Negative. No infection is detected.

Description. *N. gonorrhoeae* is a pyogenic, gram-negative, oxidase-positive coccus that is an obligate parasite of humans. It is the causative organism of the sexually transmitted infection called "gonorrhea." *N. gonorrhoeae* inhabits the mucous membranes of the genital tract and may also be found in the oral mucosa of clients who engage in oral sex. The symptoms include dysuria, purulent urethral discharge, proctitis, and pharyngitis. Females are often asymptomatic. Left untreated, gonorrhea leads to skin lesions, arthritis, meningitis, and reproductive problems. The cervix is the best site for obtaining accurate culture specimens in females.

Professional Considerations
1. Consent form NOT required.
2. **Preparation:**
   A. The client should disrobe below the waist.
   B. Obtain a special packaged culture swab with culture medium, a speculum, and warm water.
3. **Procedure:**
   A. Place the client in the dorsal lithotomy position.
   B. Lubricate the speculum with warm water and insert it into the vagina to expose the cervix.
   C. Clean off any mucus with a dry cotton swab.
   D. Insert a sterile cotton-tipped swab into the endocervical canal and move the swab from side to side.
   E. Hold the swab in place for several seconds and then withdraw it and place it in a special culture medium (Jembec or Mager-Martin).
   F. Alternatively, gently compress the cervix between the speculum blades to express exudate onto the swab.
   G. Cultures of the throat and the anus may also be taken to test for *N. gonorrhoeae.*
4. **Postprocedure care:**
   A. Send the specimen to the laboratory immediately. Do not refrigerate the specimen.
5. **Client and family teaching:**
   A. Do not douche for 24 hours before the test.
   B. Gonorrhea is a reportable disease.
   C. If your test is positive, you should inform all your sexual partners of the infection, return for follow-up culture 7-10 days after finishing antibiotics, and refrain from sexual activity with another person until negative follow-up cultures are received.
   D. Instruct the client with a positive culture on the preventive measures appropriate to a grown organism, where applicable.

6. **Factors that affect results:**
   A. A lubricant gel should not be used.
   B. Care must be taken not to contaminate the culture tip by touching the sides of the vagina during the procedure.
7. **Other data:**
   A. This test is often included in a rape-trauma work-up.

B. Women with cervical *N. gonorrhoeae* or cervical *Chlamydia trachomatis* are at high risk for endometriosis.
C. For positive results, the client should also be serologically tested for syphilis.
D. See also *Neisseria gonorrhoeae smear, Specimen.*

CERVICAL/VAGINAL CYTOLOGY, SPECIMEN
(*see Pap smear, Diagnostic*)

CHAGAS'S DISEASE SEROLOGIC TEST
(*see Trypanosomiasis serologic test, Blood*)

CHEM-6, -7, -12, -20
(*see SMA-6, -7, -12, -20, Blood*)

CHEMISTRY PROFILE, BLOOD

Norm:

		SI UNITS
Albumin (Nephelometric, Colorimetric)		
Adults	3.5-5.5 g/dL	35-55 g/L
>60 years	3.4-4.8 g/dL	34-48 g/L
Average at rest	0.3 g/dL	3 g/L
Alkaline Phosphatase		
Adults		
20-60 years		
Bodansky	2-4 U/dL	10.7-21.5 IU/L
King-Armstrong	4-13 U/dL	28.4-92.3 IU/L
Bessey-Lowrey-Brock	0.8-2.3 U/dL	13.3-38.3 IU/L
Elderly	Slightly higher	
Newborn	1-4 times adult values	
Children: Values remain high until epiphyses close.		
Females		
2-10 years	100-350 U/L	
10-13 years	110-400 U/L	
Males		
2-13 years	100-350 U/L	
13-15 years	125-500 U/L	
Aspartate Aminotransferase		
Adult females		
<60 years	8-20 U/L	8-20 U/L
≥60 years	10-20 U/L	10-20 U/L
Adult males		
<60 years	8-20 U/L	8-20 U/L
≥60 years	11-26 U/L	11-26 U/L

Continued

		SI UNITS
Aspartate Aminotransferase—cont'd		
Children		
Newborn	16-72 U/L	16-72 U/L
Infant	15-60 U/L	15-60 U/L
1 year	16-35 U/L	16-35 U/L
5 years	19-28 U/L	19-28 U/L
Bilirubin		
1 month–adult	<1.5 mg/dL	1.7-20.5 µmol/L
Premature infant		
Cord	<2.8 mg/dL	<48 µmol/L
24 hours	1-6 mg/dL	17-103 µmol/L
48 hours	6-8 mg/dL	103-137 µmol/L
3-5 days	10-12 mg/dL	171-205 µmol/L
Full-term infant		
Cord	<2.8 mg/dL	<48 µmol/L
24 hours	2-6 mg/dL	34-103 µmol/L
48 hours	6-7 mg/dL	103-120 µmol/L
3-5 days	4-6 mg/dL	68-103 µmol/L
Calcium		
Adult	4.5-5.5 mEq/L	
	8.2-10.2 mg/dL	2.05-2.54 mmol/L
Child	4.5-5.8 mEq/L	
	9.0-11.5 mg/dL	2.24-2.86 mmol/L
Infant	5.0-6.0 mEq/L	
	8.6-11.2 mg/dL	2.15-2.79 mmol/L
Newborn	3.7-7.0 mEq/L	
	7.0-11.5 mg/dL	1.75-2.87 mmol/L
Panic levels	≤10 mEq/L	
	≥13 mEq/L	
Tetany	<7 mg/dL	<1.75 mmol/L
Coma	>12 mg/dL	>2.99 mmol/L
Possible death	≤6 mg/dL	≥1.50 mmol/L
	≥14 mg/dL	≥3.49 mmol/L
Creatinine		
Jaffe, manual method	0.8-1.5 mg/dL	70-133 µmol/day
Jaffe, kinetic or enzymatic method		
Adults		
Female	0.5-1.1 mg/dL	44-97 µmol/L
Male	0.6-1.2 mg/dL	53-106 µmol/L
Elderly	May be lower	May be lower
Children		
Cord blood	0.6-1.2 mg/dL	53-106 µmol/L
Newborn	0.8-1.4 mg/dL	71-124 µmol/L
Infant	0.7-1.7 mg/dL	62-150 µmol/L
1 year of age, female	≤0.5 mg/dL	≤44 µmol/L
1 year of age, male	≤0.6 mg/dL	≤53 µmol/L
2-3 years, female	≤0.6 mg/dL	≤53 µmol/L
2-3 years, male	≤0.7 mg/dL	≤62 µmol/L
4-7 years, female	≤0.7 mg/dL	≤62 µmol/L
4-7 years, male	≤0.8 mg/dL	≤71 µmol/L
8-10 years, female	≤0.8 mg/dL	≤71 µmol/L
8-10 years, male	≤0.9 mg/dL	≤80 µmol/L
11-12 years, female	≤0.9 mg/dL	≤80 µmol/L
11-12 years, male	≤1.0 mg/dL	≤88 µmol/L
13-17 years, female	≤1.1 mg/dL	≤97 µmol/L

		SI UNITS
Creatinine—cont'd		
Children—cont'd		
13-17 years, male	≤1.2 mg/dL	≤106 μmol/L
18-20 years, female	≤1.2 mg/dL	≤106 μmol/L
18-20 years, male	≤1.3 mg/dL	≤115 μmol/L
Lactate Dehydrogenase		
Wróblewski method	150-450 U	72-217 IU/L
30° C		
Adult		
<60 years	45-90 U/L	45-90 U/L
≥60 years	55-102 U/L	55-102 U/L
Newborn	160-500 U/L	160-500 U/L
Neonate	300-1500 U/L	300-1500 U/L
Infant	100-250 U/L	100-250 U/L
Child	60-170 U/L	60-170 U/L
Phosphorus		
Adults <60 years	3.0-4.5 mg/dL	0.97-1.45 mmol/L
Females ≥60 years	2.8-4.1 mg/dL	0.90-1.30 mmol/L
Males ≥60 years	2.3-3.7 mg/dL	0.74-1.20 mmol/L
Children		
Cord blood	3.7-8.1 mg/dL	1.19-2.62 mmol/L
Premature infant	5.4-10.9 mg/dL	1.74-3.52 mmol/L
Newborn	3.5-8.6 mg/dL	1.13-2.78 mmol/L
Infant	4.5-6.7 mg/dL	1.45-2.16 mmol/L
Child	4.5-5.5 mg/dL	1.45-1.78 mmol/L
Protein, Total		
Adults	6.0-8.0 g/dL	60-80 g/L
Children		
Premature infant	4.3-7.6 g/dL	43-76 g/L
Newborn	4.6-7.4 g/dL	46-74 g/L
Infant	6.0-6.7 g/dL	60-67 g/L
Child	6.2-8.0 g/dL	62-80 g/L
Urea Nitrogen		
Young Adults (<40 Years)	5-18 mg/dL	1.8-6.5 mmol/L
Adults	5-20 mg/dL	1.8-7.1 mmol/L
Elderly (>60 Years)	8-21 mg/dL	2.9-7.5 mmol/L
Children		
Cord blood	21-40 mg/dL	7.5-14.3 mmol/L
Premature infant, first 7 days	3-25 mg/dL	0.1-0.9 mmol/L
Full-term newborn	4-18 mg/dL	1.4-6.4 mmol/L
Infant	5-18 mg/dL	1.8-6.4 mmol/L
Child	5-18 mg/dL	1.8-6.4 mmol/L
Mild Azotemia	20-50 mg/dL	7.1-17.7 mmol/L
Panic Level	>100 mg/dL	>35.7 mmol/L
Uric Acid		
Adult females	2.4-6.0 mg/dL	143-357 μmol/L
		0.17-0.45 mmol/L
Adult males	3.4-7.0 mg/dL	202-416 μmol/L
		0.21-0.51 mmol/L
Children	2.5-5.5 mg/dL	119-327 μmol/L
		0.15-0.33 mmol/L
Elderly	3.5-8.5 mg/dL	204-550 μmol/L
		0.21-0.51 mmol/L
Panic level	>12 mg/dL	>714 μmol/L

Increased. See individual test listings.

Decreased. See individual test listings.

Description. A chemistry profile is a group of several laboratory tests performed on one blood sample and measured on an automated instrument. It can be performed for routine screening on healthy populations or for the purpose of detecting specific changes for a client. This profile generally includes the following tests: *Albumin, Serum; Alkaline phosphatase, Serum; Aspartate aminotransferase, Serum; Bilirubin, Serum; Calcium, Serum; Creatinine, Serum; Lactate dehydrogenase, Blood; Phosphorus, Serum; Protein, Total, Serum; Urea nitrogen, Plasma or Serum;* and *Uric acid, Serum.* See individual test listings for individual test descriptions.

Professional Considerations
1. Consent form NOT required.
2. **Preparation:**
   A. Tube: Red topped, red/gray topped, or gold topped.
   B. Do NOT draw during hemodialysis.
3. **Procedure:**
   A. Draw a 5-mL blood sample.
4. **Postprocedure care:**
   A. None.
5. **Client and family teaching:**
   A. See individual test listings.
   B. Results are normally available within 24 hours.
6. **Factors that affect results:**
   A. Anabolic steroids increase AST, ALT and CK levels.
   B. See individual test listings.
7. **Other data:**
   A. See individual test listings.

CHEST TOMOGRAPHY, DIAGNOSTIC

Norm. Normal structures and organ content of the chest, including the chest wall, the lungs, the heart, and the diaphragm; absence of neoplasm, infective process, or structural changes.

Usage. Asbestosis, asthma, COPD, pulmonary embolism, metastatic tumor of lung or thoracic skeleton; primary tumors of the thoracic skeleton; chondrosarcoma, myeloma, or Ewing's sarcoma in children; osteomyelitis of the spine, sternum, or ribs; work-up after chest trauma for dislocations of the sternoclavicular joint; diagnosis and evaluation of the extent and involvement of soft-tissue sarcomas or lymphomas, hemangiomas, and nerve sheath tumors; examination of mediastinal injury, infection, and sternal involvement; axillary space study of lymph node abnormalities for evidence of metastatic processes, infection, or axillary vein thrombosis. Although the mammogram is more widely used, cancer of the breast with other breast abnormalities may be seen by chest tomography to diagnose or aid in the diagnosis of breast tissue diseases. Pleura are examined for lung effusions, cause of hemoptysis, extent and location of infection, empyemas, plaques typical of asbestos disease, bulbous emphysema, and fibrotic pleural disease. The diaphragm is examined for hernias or tumors. The heart may be examined for cardiomyopathy, pericardial effusion, location and extent of congenital anomalies, tumor, or calcifications. Also, great vessel abnormalities and aortic aneurysms can be noted.

Description. Tomographic scanning is special radiographic scanning using scintillation detectors that can produce transverse sectional views of the chest area, providing a two-dimensional image. With computed tomography (CT or CAT scan) of the lung, the specialized computers produce a series of cross-sectional or transverse views of the whole thoracic area. The test aids diagnostic study of the chest wall, breast tissue, axillary space, lungs, pleural space, diaphragm, spinal cord and spine at the thoracic level rib structure, sternum, and mediastinal space. (See also *Computed tomography of the body, Diagnostic* for further description of the different types of CT technology available.)

Professional Considerations
1. Consent form IS required if procedure will be performed with IV contrast.

Risks
None.

Contraindications
Screen client for contraindications to performing the Valsalva maneuver (recent myocardial infarction, bradycardia). If conditions are present, teach the client how to hold breath without bearing down.

Precautions

During pregnancy, risks of cumulative radiation exposure to the fetus from this and other previous or future imaging studies must be weighed against the benefits of the procedure. Although formal limits for client exposure are relative to this risk:benefit comparison, the United States Nuclear Regulatory Commission requires that the cumulative dose equivalent to an embryo/fetus from occupational exposure not exceed 0.5 rem (5 mSv). Radiation dosage to the fetus is proportional to the distance of the anatomy studied from the abdomen and decreases as pregnancy progresses. For pregnant clients, consult the Radiologist/Radiology Department to obtain estimated fetal radiation exposure from this procedure.

2. **Preparation:**
   A. The client must disrobe above the waist and remove all jewelry and metal objects.
   B. Shield the uterus if the client is a pregnant female.
3. **Procedure:**
   A. The test is performed with a specialized x-ray scintillator and computer in a radiology laboratory with specialized personnel.
   B. The client is placed in a supine position on the CT radiographic table, which moves into the x-ray scintillography machine for a series of views. The client will be asked to take a deep breath and hold it for some views. The automated computer then produces reconstructed images that show "slices" of the chest.
   C. The test takes approximately 15 minutes for all views, transverse and oblique.
4. **Postprocedure care:**
   A. None.
5. **Client and family teaching:**
   A. The procedure may be frightening for the client, who must cooperate for the best results. Fear usually stems from fear of enclosed spaces. Good explanations and preparation are necessary.
   B. This test is noninvasive and carries no risk.
6. **Factors that affect results:**
   A. Movement of the client interferes with the accuracy of the films.
   B. Jewelry and metal objects obstruct the views.

7. **Other data:**
   A. None.

CHEST RADIOGRAPHY (CHEST X-RAY, CXR), DIAGNOSTIC

Norm. Normal anatomy and no pathologic changes evident.

Usage. Chest radiography may be used as a general screening tool preoperatively or for general physical examinations or may be prescribed for a specific diagnostic purpose. Provides information regarding the anatomic location and abnormalities of the heart, great vessels, lungs, soft tissue of the chest and mediastinum, and the bones. Many types of pulmonary, cardiac, and orthopedic abnormalities may be seen on a chest radiograph, particularly if serial films are available for study. Pulmonary uses include abscess, acute respiratory distress syndrome (ARDS), atelectasis, Bethlem myopathy, bronchitis, cystic fibrosis, emphysema, fibrosis bullae, hemothorax, malignancies of the lung, pleural effusion, pneumonia, pneumothorax, pulmonary edema, and tuberculosis calcific changes. Cardiac uses include congestive heart failure and determination of heart size. Uses in the great vessels include abnormalities of aortic arch (calcification), some aneurysms, and transposition. Orthopedic uses include bone tumors, fracture of clavicles, kyphosis, rib fractures, scoliosis, and spinal fractures. General uses include placement of central lines, endotracheal tubes, tracheostomy tubes, chest tubes, nasogastric tubes, pacemaker wires and intra-aortic balloon pumps, foreign bodies, lymph node enlargement, mediastinal changes, and pulmonary artery catheter placement.

Description. X-rays are passed through the chest and react on a special photographic plate. Normally the lungs are radiolucent. Bones and fluid-containing bodies such as the heart, the aorta, and any tumor or infiltrate are denser than the lungs and can be easily visualized. Chest radiographs can be performed with the client standing or sitting upright, during inhalation, and in anteroposterior, posteroanterior, and lateral views. Portable, in-bed, anteroposterior chest radiographs can be performed for clients too ill to transport to the radiology department.

Professional Considerations
1. Consent form NOT required.

Risks
Fetal teratogenicity, vasovagal response (hypotension, bradycardia) to breath-holding.

Contraindications
Screen the client for contraindications to performing the Valsalva maneuver (recent myocardial infarction, bradycardia). If these conditions are present, teach the client how to hold breath without bearing down.

Precautions
During pregnancy, risks of cumulative radiation exposure to the fetus from this and other previous or future imaging studies must be weighed against the benefits of the procedure. Although formal limits for client exposure are relative to this risk:benefit comparison, the United States Nuclear Regulatory Commission requires that the cumulative dose equivalent to an embryo/fetus from occupational exposure not exceed 0.5 rem (5 mSv). Radiation dosage to the fetus is proportional to the distance of the anatomy studied from the abdomen and decreases as pregnancy progresses. For pregnant clients, consult the Radiologist/Radiology Department to obtain estimated fetal radiation exposure from this procedure.

2. **Preparation:**
   A. Remove from the chest area all jewelry, clothing with snaps, electrocardiographic patches (if not contraindicated), and other metal objects that may interfere with the interpretation of the results.
   B. Females should be asked if they are pregnant or if there is any possibility that they may be pregnant.
3. **Procedure:**
   A. The client is positioned sitting or standing upright in front of the x-ray machine, with arms held slightly out from the sides, chest expanded, and shoulders pressed forward. The radiographic film is placed against the anterior chest.
   B. For lateral views, the client stands with his or her arms elevated from the shoulders and with the fore-arms resting on the arm of the radiographic equipment, if necessary. The radiographic film is placed flush against the right or left side of the chest.
   C. As the client holds very still and takes in a deep breath and holds it, one or more radiographs are taken.
   D. For portable radiographs, the client is positioned sitting in a high Fowler's position, and the portable x-ray machine is moved into place in front of the chest for the radiographic exposure onto the plate positioned behind the back and chest.
4. **Postprocedure care:**
   A. Replace the electrocardiographic patches and wires if they have been removed.
   B. Return personal belongings to the client and help him or her dress.
   C. In the event of usage of a portable x-ray machine, help the client return to a comfortable position.
5. **Client and family teaching:**
   A. It is important to breathe in deeply, hold your breath, and remain motionless while the radiograph is taken.
   B. A radiograph takes approximately 15 minutes to complete and verify that the images are properly exposed.
   C. No restrictions are necessary on food or fluid intake.
   D. No sedation is used for this procedure.
   E. Views are taken in various positions on the table or chair.
6. **Factors that affect results:**
   A. "Vascular structures that can simulate neoplasms include normal structures such as the subclavian artery and left brachiocephalic, azygos, and pulmonary veins and abnormal structures such as congenital and acquired anomalies of the thoracic aorta and its branches, pulmonary arteries and veins, superior and inferior venae cavae, and azygos and hemizygous veins. Other entities such as postoperative changes, massive pulmonary embolism, false ventricular aneurysm, and esophageal varices can also be misinterpreted. Important radiographic features that help distinguish these vascu-

lar structures from true neoplasms include proximity to known vascular structures, smooth margination, mural calcification, round or oval configuration, poor or nonvisualization in one of two orthogonal views, and absence or altered position of normal vascular structures. Knowledge of client history and a detailed understanding of normal mediastinal anatomic structures and common variants help in making the correct diagnosis. Familiarity with these entities will result in the proper, most cost-efficient evaluation" [Cole et al, 1995].

B. Clothing, jewelry, and metal objects cause shadows on the film.

C. Movement obscures the clarity of the picture.

D. Improper positioning makes radiographs difficult to interpret.

E. Portable radiographs are not so reliable as those performed in radiology departments. The anteroposterior position may cause the heart to appear larger than it is.

F. Overexposure or underexposure results in inadequate visualization.

G. The experience of the physician interpreting the films affects the accuracy of the findings.

7. **Other data:**

A. Chest radiography is not suggested as a first-line screening tool for tuberculosis or cancer because of possible dangers from frequent radiographic exposure.

B. Health care workers in areas near frequent usage of x-rays should wear an x-ray badge to track exposure level. They should wear a lead apron when remaining in the room with the client during exposure. For portable radiographs, health care workers should stand at least 5 feet from the x-ray source during exposure.

CHLAMYDIA CULTURE AND GROUP TITER, SPECIMEN (CULTURE)

Norm:

<table>
<tr><td><1:16</td><td>= Normal titer</td></tr>
<tr><td>>1:16</td><td>= Previous exposure to Chlamydia</td></tr>
<tr><td>1:32 in babies</td><td>= Positive for Chlamydia trachomatis</td></tr>
</table>

1:16 in adults = Positive for *Chlamydia psittaci*

Usage. Suspected *Chlamydia psittaci* or *C. trachomatis* infections, including lymphogranuloma venereum or trachoma eye infection.

Description. *Chlamydia* are intracellular parasites with the characteristics of bacteria and of viruses that cause psittacosis, pneumonia, eye infections, and lymphogranuloma venereum. The mode of transmission for *C. psittaci* is thought to be inhalation of the organism from the droppings of, or direct contact with, infected birds. The mode of transmission for *C. trachomatis* is direct contact of the infant with the mother's cervix during birth or direct contact through sexual activity. The culture method is more widely used for diagnosis of *C. trachomatis* and the Group Titer is more often used for diagnosis of *C. psittaci* (because of danger to laboratory workers of inhalation transmission of the disease). *C. trachomatis* diseases include (1) lymphogranuloma venereum venereal disease characterized by edema and infection of the lymph nodes of the inguinal, perirectal, and intra-abdominal areas; (2) a less serious, often asymptomatic genital infection; (3) trachoma (a serious eye infection); and (4) neonatal infections (usually conjunctivitis and pneumonia in babies of infected mothers). *Chlamydia* group titer uses complement fixation or microimmunofluorescence to measure the amount of IgG antibodies to *Chlamydia*. It is a nonspecific, in vitro, antigen-antibody study that detects previous exposure to *Chlamydia* organisms. *Chlamydia* infection is confirmed by a fourfold increase in serial titers.

Professional Considerations

1. Consent form NOT required.

2. **Preparation:**

A. Culture: Obtain sterile cotton-tipped culture swabs, a cytobrush, and a culture medium. Where *Chlamydia psittaci* is suspected, health care workers should wear a mask when obtaining a specimen to avoid inhalalation of the microorganism.

B. Group Titer Test: Tube: Red topped, red/gray topped, gold topped, or SST.

3. **Procedure:**

A. Culture: The specimens for culture are obtained by vigorous scraping or swabbing of suspected sites. A cytobrush may be used. Purulent drainage does not provide accurate or adequate results. Obtaining two specimens is recommended, as *Chlamydia* lives inside normal cells and thus is difficult to diagnose. See *Culture, Routine Specimen* for collection instructions.

B. Draw a 5-mL blood sample.

4. Postprocedure care:
   A. Transport the specimen to the laboratory immediately.

5. Client and family teaching:
   A. Several days may be required for titer results. Empiric therapy is often started while you await the results. Chlamydia is curable with medication.
   B. For elevated titer, your sexual partner(s) should subsequently be tested.

C. Chlamydia infection may cause difficulties with conception in the future and, in pregnancy, may cause premature labor.

6. Factors that affect results:
   A. Reject hemolyzed specimens.
   B. Serious illness, immune disorders, and immunosuppressive therapy may interfere with antigen-antibody reaction and show false-negative results.
   C. Antibiotic therapy may cause false-negative results.

7. Other data:
   A. *Chlamydia* titer is not used in neonatal infection diagnosis because the mother's autoantibodies to *Chlamydia* are present in the neonate for up to 9 months.
   B. Transmission of *Chlamydia trachomatis* from infected men to female sexual partners is 65%.

CHLORAMPHENICOL, BLOOD

Norm. Negative.

		SI UNITS
Therapeutic level	10-25 μg/mL	31-77 μmol/L
Trough level	<5 μg/mL	<15 μmol/L
Gray baby syndrome	40-100 μg/mL	124-309 μmol/L
Panic level	>50 μg/mL	>154 μmol/L

Panic Level Symptoms and Treatment

Symptoms. Hematopoietic toxicity, including reversible bone-marrow suppression and irreversible aplasia, may occur; hemolysis; allergic reaction; and peripheral neuritis.

Treatment:
Note: Treatment choice(s) depend on client history and condition and episode history.
Monitor closely.
Maintain peak serum levels below 25 μg/mL by dose adjustments.
Hemodialysis WILL remove the drug.
Peritoneal dialysis will NOT remove chloramphenicol.

Usage. Evaluation for appropriate dosing when chloramphenicol is used for treatment of *Chlamydia* or vancomycin-resistant *Enterococcus*, infants with severe anaerobic infections, *Haemophilus*

influenzae, meningitis, *Mycoplasma*, rickettsias, *Salmonella*, or typhoid fever.

Description. Chloramphenicol is a potent, broad-spectrum, synthetic antibiotic used for gram-negative, gram-positive, and anaerobic microorganisms when other antibiotics cannot be used or are ineffective. It is metabolized by the liver and excreted by the kidneys, with a half-life of 2.5-3.0 hours in clients with normal hepatic and renal function. Chloramphenicol levels, complete blood counts, and reticulocyte levels must be closely monitored during therapy because of the risk of bone marrow depression side effects.

Professional Considerations
1. Consent form NOT required.
2. Preparation:
   A. Tube: Red topped, red/gray topped, gold topped, or green topped or lavender topped.
   B. Do NOT draw during hemodialysis.
3. Procedure:
   A. Draw a 1-mL blood sample. For a trough level, draw the specimen

just before the next dose. For a peak level, draw the specimen 15 minutes after completion of the dose.

4. **Postprocedure care:**
   A. Send the specimen to the laboratory for immediate separation of test sample. Freeze the sample after separation if not tested immediately.
5. **Client and family teaching:**
   A. Results are normally available within 24 hours.
6. **Factors that affect results:**
   A. Concurrent use of phenobarbital may reduce chloramphenicol levels.
   B. Toxic levels are more likely to occur in clients with impaired renal or hepatic function.
   C. Therapeutic levels may last for up to 8 hours after administration.
7. **Other data:**
   A. Bone marrow suppression is most commonly dose related but may

occur up to 2 months after completion of any dose of therapy and be irreversible.
B. Can cause gray baby syndrome in premature infants with impaired hepatic function and in newborns less than 3 weeks old, resulting in cardiovascular collapse and death.
C. Chloramphenicol-resistant bacterial isolates are also resistant to tetracycline.
D. *Streptococcus pneumoniae* and *Streptococcus pyogenes* are resistant to chloramphenicol in 3.9% and 2.2% of clients, respectively, and 26.1% are resistant to enterocci. *Salmonella typhi* and *Salmonella worthington* are also resistant to chloramphenicol.

CHLORAZEPATE DIPOTASSIUM
(see Benzodiazepines, Plasma and Urine)

CHLORDIAZEPOXIDE (LIBRIUM), BLOOD

Norm. Negative.

		SI UNITS
Therapeutic levels	700-1000 ng/mL	2.34-3.34 μmol/L
Panic level	>5000 ng/mL	>16.7 μmol/L

Panic Level Symptoms and Treatment

Symptoms. Drowsiness, dysarthria, ataxia, and confusion.

Treatment:
Note: Treatment choice(s) depend on client history and condition and episode history.
Gastric lavage not recommended, but should be considered if within 1 hour of ingestion and if ingestion of additional lethal substance is suspected. Use warm tap water or 0.9% saline.
Administer activated charcoal if within 4 hours of ingestion or if symptoms are present. Repeat as necessary, because benzodiazepines undergo hepatic recirculation.
Monitor for central nervous system depression.
Protect airway. Support breathing with oxygen and mechanical ventilation, if necessary.

Flumazenil is not recommended for routine use in benzodiazepine overdose. Flumazenil has been used as a competitive antagonist to reverse the profound effects of benzodiazepine overdose. Use of flumazenil is contraindicated if concomitant tricyclic antidepressants were taken or in dependence states because of the risk of causing seizures from lowering of the seizure threshold and because it may precipitate symptoms of benzodiazepine withdrawal. Flumazenil may not completely reverse benzodiazepine effects. Close monitoring for re-sedation is required and repeated doses may be needed.
Do NOT use barbiturates.
Do NOT induce emesis.
Forced diuresis or hemodialysis will NOT remove benzodiazepines to any significant extent. No information was found on whether peritoneal dialysis will remove these drugs.

Usage. Drug abuse, ongoing monitoring for therapeutic dosage, and overdose. Also used in conjunction with clidinium for treatment of acute thrombocytopenic purpura.

Description. Chlordiazepoxide is a mild benzodiazepine used for relief of mild to severe anxiety and tension; withdrawal symptoms of acute alcoholism, preoperative apprehension, and anxiety. It is also used for the short-term treatment of insomnia, acute treatment for seizures, and management of alcohol withdrawal symptoms. Chlordiazepoxide is metabolized by the liver and excreted by the kidneys, with a half-life of 5-30 hours. Overdose may lead to respiratory depression and coma. Levels chronically over the therapeutic range may cause renal dysfunction. Use is safe during pregnancy and lactation.

Professional Considerations
1. Consent form NOT required.
2. **Preparation:**
   A. Tube: Red topped, red/gray topped, or gold topped.
   B. Do NOT draw during hemodialysis.
3. **Procedure:**
   A. Collect a 3-mL blood sample.
4. **Postprocedure care:**
   A. None.

5. **Client and family teaching:**
   A. For the client who takes chlordiazepoxide regularly, watch for, and call the physician in the event of, early signs of overdose: drowsiness, unsteady gait, or confusion.
   B. For an intentional overdose, refer the client and his or her family for crisis intervention.
   C. Referrals to appropriate rehabilitation centers and therapeutic community programs should be offered to all addicted clients who may be interested.
   D. If activated charcoal was given for elevated levels, the client should drink 4-6 glasses of water each day for 2 days to prevent constipation. The activated charcoal will also cause stools to be black for a few days.
6. **Factors that affect results:**
   A. Kidney disease elevates blood levels.
7. **Other data:**
   A. The drug should be tapered off rather than abruptly withdrawn.
   B. The drug is one of the most frequent inappropriately prescribed drugs for the elderly.
   C. See also *Benzodiazepines, Plasma and Urine.*

CHLORIDE, SERUM

Norm:

		SI UNITS
Children and adults	97-107 mEq/L	97-107 mmol/L
Premature infants	95-110 mEq/L	95-110 mmol/L
Full-term infants	96-106 mEq/L	96-106 mmol/L
Panic levels	<80 mEq/L	<80 mmol/L
	>115 mEq/L	>115 mmol/L

Panic Level Symptoms and Treatment

Symptoms. Impaired mentation, hypotension, and cardiac dysrhythmias.

Treatment. Correct the underlying disorder.

Increased. Acidosis (hyperchloremic, nephrotic), alcoholism, alkalosis (respiratory), hyperaldosteronism (primary), anemia, bromism, congestive heart failure, Cushing's disease, dehydration, diabetes insipidus, diarrhea (sodium loss > chloride loss), eclampsia, fever, head trauma, hypercorticoadrenalism, hypernatremia, hyperparathyroidism, hyperventilation, hypoproteinemia, intestinal fistula (sodium loss > chloride loss), nephritis (acute), nephrosis, neurogenic hyperventilation, ostomies, prostatic obstruction, renal failure (acute), salicylate intoxication, seawater aspiration (severe), serum sickness, uremia, ureterosigmoidostomy, and urinary obstruction. Drugs include acetazolamide, ammonium chloride, boracic acid, boric acid, chlorothiazide, cholestyramine, cyclosporin A, glucocorticoids, guanethidine sulfate, imipenem-cilastin sodium, oxyphenbutazone, phenylbutazone, sodium bromide, sodium chloride, and spironolactone. Herbal or natural remedies include products containing aristolochic acids (*Akebia* spp., *Aristolochia* spp., *Asarum* spp., birthwort, *Bragantia* spp., *Clematis* spp., *Cocculus* spp., *Diploclisia* spp., Dutchman's pipe, Fang chi, Fang ji, Fang chi, Guang fang ji, Kan-Mokutsu, *Menispernum* spp., Mokutsu, Mu tong, *Sinomenium* spp., and *Stephania* spp.)

Decreased. Acidosis (diabetic, diarrheal, lactic, metabolic, tubular, respiratory), Addison's disease, amyotrophic lateral sclerosis (indication of shorter survival), anesthesia, burns, CNS disorders, cholera, congestive heart failure, diabetic ketoacidosis, diaphoresis, diarrhea (severe), edema, emphysema, fasting, fever, freshwater aspiration, heat exhaustion, heavy-metal poisoning, hypertrophic pyloric stenosis, hypokalemia, hyponatremia, hypoventilation, infections (acute), intestinal obstruction, nephritis, paralytic ileus, pneumonia, pyelonephritis (chronic), pyloric obstruction, pyloric stenosis (infants), renal failure (chronic), rickettsial diseases, suction (gastric), syndrome of inappropriate antidiuretic hormone secretion, typhus fever, ulcerative colitis, uremia, vomiting, Waterhouse-Friderichsen syndrome, and water intoxication. Drugs include aldosterone, amiloride hydrochloride, bumetanide, corticotropin, dextrose infusions (prolonged), ethacrynic acid, furosemide, mercurial diuretics, prednisolone, prednisolone acetate, prednisolone sodium phosphate, prednisolone tebutate, sodium bicarbonate, spironolactone, triamterene, and thiazide diuretics.

Description. Chloride, a hydrochloric acid salt, is the most abundant body anion in the extracellular fluid. It functions in counter-balancing cations such as sodium and also acts as a buffer during oxygen/carbon dioxide exchange in red blood cells. Chloride also aids in digestion, osmotic pressure, and water balance. It is measured in serum, along with other electrolytes to evaluate electrolyte acid-base balance.

Professional Considerations
1. Consent form NOT required.
2. Preparation:
   A. Tube: Red topped, red/gray topped, or gold topped.
   B. Do NOT draw during hemodialysis.
3. Procedure:
   A. Draw the specimen from an extremity that does not have saline infusing into it. Draw a 3-mL blood sample without a tourniquet if possible.
   B. The sample may be taken from infants from a capillary heelstick.
   C. Do NOT allow the client to clench-unclench the hand before blood drawing.
4. Postprocedure care:
   A. None.
5. Client and family teaching:
   A. Results are normally available in ≤4 hours.
6. Factors that affect results:
   A. Reject hemolyzed specimens.
   B. Any condition accompanied by prolonged vomiting or diarrhea will alter levels.
   C. Potassium chloride, ammonium chloride, acetazolamide, methyldopa, diazoxide, and bromides may cause falsely elevated results.
   D. Drugs such as ethacrynic acid, furosemide, thiazide diuretics, and bicarbonate may lead to decreased levels.
7. Other data:
   A. In respiratory acidosis, chloride excretion is a necessary component of renal compensation.
   B. Useful interpretation of the results requires clinical knowledge of the client.

CHLORIDE, SWEAT, SPECIMEN

Norm:

		SI UNITS
Adults	10-70 mEq/L	10-70 mmol/L
Children	5-45 mEq/L	5-45 mmol/L

Increased. Cystic fibrosis (levels >60 mEq/L are indicative of cystic fibrosis in children <20 years). Also Addison's disease, adrenal insufficiency, diabetes insipidus (hereditary nephrogenic), ectodermal dysplasia, fucosidosis, glucose-6-phosphate dehydrogenase deficiency, hypothyroidism, malnutrition, mucopolysaccharidosis, pseudohypoaldosteronism type 1, and renal failure.

Decreased. Hypoaldosteronism and sodium depletion. Drugs include mineralocorticoids.

Description. Chloride is an electrolyte normally excreted in sweat and urine combined chemically with sodium or other cations. It functions in the maintenance of acid-base balance and electrical neutrality of the body. Sweat chloride levels are found to be especially high in children with cystic fibrosis, a genetic disease that affects exocrine gland functioning, including the sweat glands of the skin, which secrete abnormally high levels of sodium, potassium, and chloride electrolytes. Sweat chloride levels are often high in genetic carriers of the cystic fibrosis genome as well. Genetic carriers have one recessive defective gene and one dominant normal gene and have no other manifestations of the disease. This test involves the stimulation of sweat production by iontophoresis, the painless delivery of a small amount of electric current to the skin.

Professional Considerations
1. Consent form NOT required.

Risks
None.

Contraindications
In clients with dermatitis.

2. **Preparation:**
   A. Obtain equipment for the iontophoresis and preweighed gauze or filter paper, sterile water, normal saline, forceps, weighing bottle, tape, plastic, and pilocarpine.
3. **Procedure: Gibson-Cooke technique:**
   A. Wash and dry the right forearm or right thigh with distilled water.
   B. Place a small amount of the pilocarpine-soaked gauze on the skin of the area to be studied and attach it to the positive electrode. Place a

small amount of the saline-soaked gauze on the skin and attach it to the negative electrode.
   C. Deliver 4 mA of current in 15- to 20-second intervals for 5 minutes.
   D. Remove and discard the electrodes.
   E. Place the preweighed, dry, sterile gauze or filter paper over the pilocarpine gauze site. Cover it with plastic and seal it with waterproof tape.
   F. After 30-40 minutes, droplets visible beneath the plastic indicate an adequate accumulation of sweat.
   G. Remove and discard the tape and plastic.
   H. Remove the gauze or filter paper with forceps and place it directly into a weighing bottle, seal it tightly, and send it to the laboratory.
4. **Postprocedure care:**
   A. It is normal for the studied area to remain reddened for several hours.
5. **Client and family teaching:**
   A. The test is not painful but does cause a minor tingling sensation.
   B. Parents are able to stay with the child during the test to help provide distraction.
   C. Skin erythema will fade within 24 hours.
6. **Factors that affect results:**
   A. Improper cleansing of the test area may cause unreliable results.
   B. The hands have a higher sweat chloride content than arms or legs and thus should be avoided as a study site.
   C. Hot weather could deplete sodium chloride stores and affect the results.
   D. Poor or incomplete sealing of the test site could result in falsely increased chloride levels by allowing evaporation of sweat.
   E. Falsely low values may occur in clients with edema or hypoproteinemia.
   F. Increased levels may be caused by skin rashes or lesions over the testing site.
7. **Other data:**
   A. A positive sweat test in itself is not diagnostic of cystic fibrosis. The clinical picture and family history are important considerations.
   B. Repetition of both borderline and positive tests is recommended.

CHLORIDE, URINE

Norm:

		SI UNITS
24-Hour Urine		
Adult	110-250 mEq/24 h	110-250 mmol/day
>60 years	95-195 mEq/24 h	95-195 mmol/day
Spot Urine		
	15-115 mEq/L	15-115 mmol/L
Child		
Infant	2-10 mEq/L	2-10 mmol/L
12 months–6 years	15-40 mEq/L	15-40 mmol/L
6-10 years		
Female	18-74 mEq/L	18-74 mmol/L
Male	36-110 mEq/L	36-110 mmol/L
10-14 years		
Female	36-173 mEq/L	36-173 mmol/L
Male	64-176 mEq/L	64-176 mmol/L

Increased. Cushing syndrome, dehydration, hypernatremia, salicylate toxicity, syndrome of inappropriate antidiuretic hormone secretion (SIADHS), and starvation. Drugs include chlorothiazide diuretics and mercurial diuretics.

Decreased. Addison's disease, congestive heart failure (prolonged), diarrhea, diaphoresis, emphysema, low-salt diet, malabsorption syndrome, nasogastric suction (prolonged), pyloric obstruction, and renal damage.

Description. Chloride is the most abundant extracellular anion. It is normally excreted by the kidney to help maintain the normal fluid and electrolyte and acid-base balance of the body. The amount of chloride excreted in the urine is an indication of the state of electrolyte balance.

Professional Considerations
1. Consent form NOT required.
2. **Preparation:**
   A. Obtain a clean, 3-L specimen container without preservatives.
   B. Write the beginning time of collection on the laboratory requisition and specimen container.
3. **Procedure:**
   A. Discard the first morning urine specimen.
   B. Begin to time a 24-hour urine collection.
   C. Save all the urine voided for 24 hours in a clean, 3-L container without preservatives. Refrigera-

tion is unnecessary. Include the urine voided at the end of the 24-hour period.
4. **Postprocedure care:**
   A. Compare the urine quantity in the specimen container with the urinary output record for the test. If the specimen contains less urine than what was recorded as output, some of the sample may have been discarded, invalidating the test.
   B. Document the quantity of the urine output for the 24-hour collection period on the laboratory requisition.
   C. Send the specimen to the laboratory for refrigeration.
5. **Client and family teaching:**
   A. Save all the urine voided in the 24-hour period and urinate before defecating to avoid loss of urine. If any urine is accidentally discarded, discard the entire specimen and restart the collection the next day.
6. **Factors that affect results:**
   A. All the urine voided for the 24-hour period must be included to avoid a falsely low result.
   B. Bromides may cause falsely elevated results.
7. **Other data:**
   A. Dietary intake should be considered when results are being evaluated. This is a useful test for monitoring the effects of a low-salt diet.
   B. Urine chloride levels are more precise than urine sodium levels for differentiating between saline

responsiveness and saline-resistant conditions associated with metabolic alkalosis.

CHLORPHENTERMINE
(*see Amphetamines, Blood*)

CHLORPROMAZINE
(*see Phenothiazines, Blood*)

CHOLANGIOGRAM
(*see Endoscopic retrograde cholangiopancreatography, Diagnostic; Intravenous cholangiography, Diagnostic; Percutaneous transhepatic cholangiography, Diagnostic; or T-tube cholangiography, Postoperative, Diagnostic*)

CHOLECYSTOGRAPHY RADIOGRAPHY, DIAGNOSTIC

Norm. Good visualization of the gallbladder; no stones and no filling defects.

Usage. Diagnosis of gallbladder disorder such as calculus, stones, polyps, tumors (cancer gallbladder or non-Hodgkin's lymphoma), or duct defects. Usually complaints of right upper quadrant, right epigastric pain, or both, of unknown cause.

Description. Oral cholecystography is used to study the dye-filled gallbladder by radiographic film. Stones or calculi can be seen as darker shadows, and filling defects indicate polyps or tumors after opacification of the gallbladder by radiopaque contrast medium. The gallbladder and the contour and patency of the cystic duct and hepatic ducts are also studied.

Professional Considerations
1. Consent form IS required.

Risks
Respiratory failure, shock, allergic reaction to dye (itching, hives, rash, tight feeling in the throat, shortness of breath, bronchospasm, anaphylaxis, death); renal toxicity.

Contraindications
Known abdominal infection or inflammation; vomiting; previous allergy to iodine, iopanoic acid, radiographic dye, or shellfish; renal or hepatic failure; pregnancy, unless the benefits outweigh the risks; jaundice with bilirubin >2 mg/dL; or severe vomiting or diarrhea.

2. **Preparation:**
   A. See *Client and family teaching.*
   B. Have emergency equipment readily available.
   C. If diarrhea or vomiting occurs before the test, consult the radiologist to see if the test should be rescheduled.
3. **Procedure:**
   A. A series of radiographic films are taken of the right upper quadrant of the client's abdomen with the client in several positions.
4. **Postprocedure care:**
   A. The dye is excreted in the urine. Mild dysuria is common.
   B. A fatty meal may enhance dye excretion. The client may resume a normal diet.
   C. Observe for allergic reaction to radiographic dye (listed above) for 24 hours.
5. **Client and family teaching:**
   A. On the evening before the test, eat a low-fat meal and then fast beginning at midnight before the test or after step B, whichever is earlier.
   B. Take six 0.5-g iopanoic acid tablets by mouth 12 hours before the test. The tablets should be taken with a large amount of water at 5-minute intervals. Then fast from food and fluids until the test is completed.
   C. If preparing for the test at home, go to the nearest emergency room if experiencing rash, itching, or hives, or difficulty in breathing after taking iopanoic acid tablets.
   D. The procedure will take approximately 1 hour.
6. **Factors that affect results:**
   A. Hepatic failure with bilirubin >1.8 mg/dL will interfere with gallbladder visualization. The dye must be processed in the liver before it passes into the gallbladder. The test will be canceled for a high bilirubin level.
   B. Vomiting or diarrhea will inhibit dye uptake and result in inadequate visualization of the gallbladder. If either occurs, the test should be postponed and the dye are administered. Alternatively, other visualization methods may be used.
   C. A fatty diet will cause the dye to pass through the system too rap-

idly for gallbladder visualization to be performed 12 hours after the dye tablets are taken.

7. **Other data:**

A. Occasionally, after the above procedure, the client is given a fatty meal or Bilevac (fatty synthetic) to test gallbladder contractility. Further radiographs are then taken in 1-2 hours.

B. Contractility studies may also be accomplished 15 minutes after the first set of radiographs by intravenous injection of fatty sincalide.

C. Cholecystography is being replaced by ultrasonography, which is now the diagnostic test of choice, or by MRI/CT in selected situations.

CHOLESTEROL, BLOOD

Norm. There is variation in recommended norms in the literature.
(*Note:* Range given applies to a healthy population consuming a typical North American diet.)

AGE	MALE mg/dL	SI UNITS mmol/L	FEMALE mg/dL	SI UNITS mmol/L
Total Cholesterol				
Adult (10% higher levels for African Americans)				
20-24 years	124-218	3.21-5.64	122-216	3.16-5.59
25-29 years	133-244	3.44-6.32	128-222	3.32-5.75
30-34 years	138-254	3.57-6.58	130-230	3.37-5.96
35-39 years	146-270	3.78-6.99	140-242	3.63-6.27
40-44 years	151-268	3.91-6.94	147-252	3.81-6.53
45-49 years	158-276	4.09-7.15	152-265	3.94-6.86
50-54 years	158-277	4.09-7.17	162-285	4.20-7.38
55-59 years	156-276	4.04-7.15	172-300	4.45-7.77
60-64 years	159-276	4.12-7.15	172-297	4.45-7.69
65-69 years	158-274	4.09-7.10	171-303	4.43-7.85
≥70 years	144-265	3.73-6.86	173-280	4.48-7.25
Child				
Cord blood	44-103	1.14-2.66	50-108	1.29-2.79
≤4 years	114-203	2.95-5.25	112-200	2.90-5.18
5-9 years	121-203	3.13-5.25	126-205	3.26-5.30
10-14 years	119-202	3.08-5.23	124-201	3.21-5.20
15-19 years	113-197	2.93-5.10	119-200	3.08-5.18
High-Density Lipoprotein Cholesterol (HDL)				
Adult (African-American levels approximately 10 mg/dL higher)				
20-24 years	30-63	0.78-1.63	33-79	0.85-2.04
25-29 years	31-63	0.80-1.63	37-83	0.96-2.15
30-34 years	28-63	0.72-1.63	36-77	0.93-1.99
35-39 years	29-62	0.75-1.60	34-82	0.88-2.12
40-44 years	27-67	0.70-1.73	34-88	0.88-2.28
45-49 years	30-64	0.78-1.66	34-87	0.88-2.25
50-54 years	28-63	0.72-1.63	37-92	0.96-2.38
55-59 years	28-71	0.72-1.84	37-91	0.96-2.35
60-64 years	30-74	0.78-1.91	38-92	0.98-2.38
65-69 years	30-75	0.78-1.94	35-96	0.91-2.48
≥70 years	31-75	0.80-1.94	33-92	0.85-2.38
Child				
Cord blood	6-53	0.16-1.37	13-56	0.34-1.45
5-9 years	38-75	0.98-1.94	36-73	0.93-1.89
10-14 years	37-74	0.96-1.91	37-70	0.96-1.81
15-19 years	30-63	0.78-1.63	35-74	0.91-1.91

Continued

| | MALE | | FEMALE | |
AGE	mg/dL	SI UNITS mmol/L	mg/dL	SI UNITS mmol/L
Low-Density Lipoprotein Cholesterol (LDL)				
Adult				
20-24 years	66-147	1.71-3.81	57-159	1.48-4.12
25-29 years	70-165	1.81-4.27	71-164	1.84-4.25
30-34 years	78-185	2.02-4.79	70-156	1.81-4.04
35-39 years	81-189	2.10-4.90	75-172	1.94-4.45
40-44 years	87-186	2.25-4.82	74-174	1.92-4.51
45-49 years	97-202	2.51-5.23	79-186	2.05-4.82
50-54 years	89-197	2.31-5.10	88-201	2.28-5.21
55-59 years	88-203	2.28-5.26	89-210	2.31-5.44
60-64 years	83-210	2.15-5.44	100-224	2.59-5.80
65-69 years	98-210	2.54-5.44	92-221	2.38-5.72
≥70 years	88-186	2.28-4.82	96-206	2.49-5.34
Child				
Cord blood	20-56	0.52-1.45	21-58	0.54-1.50
5-9 years	63-129	1.63-3.34	68-140	1.76-3.63
10-14 years	64-133	1.66-3.44	68-136	1.76-3.52
15-19 years	62-130	1.61-3.37	59-137	1.53-3.55

		SI UNITS
Cholesterol Esters	60-75% of total or <210 mg/dL	0.60-0.75 <5.43 mmol/L
Free Cholesterol	<50 mg/dL	<1.29 mmol/L
LDL:HDL Ratio	<3	<3

Increased Total Cholesterol. Anemia (aplastic), anorexia nervosa, atherosclerosis, bile duct blockage, carbon disulfide occupational exposure as in viscose rayon workers, coronary heart disease, celiac disease, cholestasis, cirrhosis (biliary), congestive heart failure, Cushing's disease, debrancher deficiency, diabetes mellitus (poorly controlled), eclampsia, Forbes' disease, glomerulonephritis, *Helicobacter pylori*, hepatic cholesterol ester storage disease, hepatic phosphorylase deficiency, hypercholesterolemia (idiopathic), hyperlipoproteinemia, hypothyroidism, jaundice (obstructive, cholestatic), leukemia, limit dextrinosis, lipid disorders, lipoidosis, nephrosis, nephrotic syndrome, Niemann-Pick C disease, obesity, pancreatectomy, pancreatitis (chronic), periodontal pockets, pregnancy, starvation (early), stress, type III glycogen deposition disease, type VI glycogen storage disease, and von Gierke's disease. Drugs include amiodarone, anabolic steroids, androgens, catecholamines, chenodeoxycholic acid, cinchophen, chlorpropamide, corticosteroids (glucogenic), cyclosporin A, diuretics, epinephrine, epinephrine bitartrate, epinephrine borate, epinephrine hydrochloride, epinephrine (racemic), ergocalciferol, isotretinoin, levodopa, miconazole, oral contraceptives, phenytoin, phenytoin sodium, sulfonamides, thiazides.

Decreased Total Cholesterol. Abetalipoproteinemia, acanthocytosis, amylopectinosis, Andersen's disease, anemia (pernicious, hemolytic, hypochromic), Bassen-Kornzweig syndrome, brancher deficiency, cancer, chromium enriched diet, cirrhosis (Laënnec's, portal), depression, epilepsy, familial lecithin-cholesterol acyltransferase deficiency (absent cholesterol esters), gastric bypass surgery, Gaucher's disease, Hansen's disease, hepatic disease, hepatitis (toxic, viral), hyperthyroidism, hypobetalipoproteinemia, infections (severe), intestinal obstruction, jaundice (hepatocellular), leprosy, liver cellular necrosis, malnutrition, pancreatic carcinoma, porphyria (acute, intermittent), premenstrual time phase, steatorrhea, suicidal behavior, Tangier disease, tuberculosis, type IV glycogen deposition disease, and uremia.

Drugs include allopurinol, aminosalicylic acid, androgens, asparaginase, azathioprine, carbutamide, cholestyramine, chlorpropamide, chlortetracycline, clofibrate, clomiphene, colchicine, colestipol, cyproterone acetate, dextrothyroxine, doxazosin, erythromycin, estrogens, fenfluramine, gemfibrozil, glucagon, haloperidol, heparin sodium, hydralazine, interferon, isoniazid, kanamycin, ketoconazole, levothyroxine sodium, lovastatin, MAO inhibitors, neomycin, niacin, neomycin, orlistat, phenformin, pravastatin, prazosin, probucol, simvastatin, tamoxifen, tetracyclines, thiazides, thyroxine, trimethadione, and vitamin A. Herbs or natural remedies include guar gum, *meshasringi* (*Gymnema sylvestre, mesha shringi,* Indian milkweed vine), *methi* (fenugreek leaves), *tundika* (*Coccinia indica*).

Description. Cholesterol is a sterol compound synthesized exogenously in the liver from dietary fats and endogenously within cells. It is present in all body tissues and is a major component of low-density lipoproteins (LDL), brain and nerve cells, cell membranes, and some gallstones. Hypercholesterolemia, combined with low levels of high-density lipoprotein (HDL), increases the risk for developing arteriosclerosis. Levels under 200 mg/dL (5.17 mmol/L, SI units) are *desirable.* Levels from 200 to 239 mg/dL (5.17 to 6.18 mmol/L, SI units) are classified as *borderline high,* and levels over 239 mg/dL (>6.18 mmol/L, SI units) are classified as *high.* Cholesterol levels tend to decrease temporarily with major illness or surgery.

Professional Considerations
1. Consent form NOT required.
2. Preparation:
   A. See *Client and family teaching.*
   B. Tube: Red topped, red/gray topped, or gold topped.
   C. Screen the client for the use of herbal preparations or natural remedies such as *dai-saiko-to* (Chinese: *da⁴-chai²hu²-tang¹,* 'major *Bupleurum* preparation': mixture of *Pinellia, Scutellaria, Zizyphus,* ginseng, licorice, and ginger) and *saiko-ka-ryukotsuboreito* (Chinese: *chai²hu²-jia¹-long²gu³- mu³li⁴-tang¹,* '*Bupleurum* with added-dragon bone-oyster-preparation', composed of *Bupleurum, Pinellia,* ginger, *Scutellaria,*

Zizyphus, cinnamon, China root fungus [*fu²ling², hoelen, Poria cocos, P. sclerotium*], *Codonopsis,* Chinese rhubarb, ginseng, oyster shell, and fossil bone for calcium).
3. Procedure:
   A. Leave the tourniquet on for as short a time as possible and no more than 2 minutes.
   B. *Total cholesterol and cholesterol esters:* Draw a 1-mL blood sample.
   C. *HDL cholesterol:* Draw a 1-mL blood sample.
4. Postprocedure care:
   A. Transport the specimen to the laboratory immediately.
5. Client and family teaching:
   A. Consume a diet containing consistent levels of cholesterol for 3 weeks before this test.
   B. If more than total cholesterol will be measured, fast from food and liquids, except for water, for 12-14 hours and from alcohol for 24 hours before the test.
   C. The evening meal before the test should be free of high-cholesterol foods and have less than 30% total fat content.
   D. Drugs affecting the results should be withheld for 24 hours, whenever possible.
   E. Desirable cholesterol levels and risk for coronary heart disease are listed in this section in the *Lipid Profile, Blood Test.* These may be used to identify and teach desirable levels to clients.
   F. Screen the client for the use of herbal preparations or natural remedies such as dai-saiko-to and saiko-ka-ryukotsuboreito (see above).
6. Factors that affect results:
   A. Reject hemolyzed specimens.
   B. Levels may be lower when collected with the client recumbent for 20 minutes or more than in those samples collected when the client is standing erect.
   C. Cholesterol levels should always be drawn at the same time of day after the same type of diet the day before, with the client in the same position.
   D. Drugs that may cause falsely elevated results include ascorbic acid, bromides, chlorpromazine, corticosteroids, iodides, viomycin, and vitamin A.

E. Drugs that may cause falsely decreased levels include nitrates, nitrites, and propylthiouracil.
7. **Other data:**
   A. Total cholesterol specimen is stable for 7 days at room temperature when nonhemolyzed.
   B. Cholesterol esters convert to free cholesterol when left at room temperature.
   C. Estrogen therapy benefits the vasculature of hypercholesterolemic postmenopausal women.
   D. Follow-up physician office visits do not benefit further CHD risk factor modification for work-site employees.
   E. Chinese herbs or natural remedies *dai-saiko-to* and *saiko-ka-ryukotsuboreito* increase high-density lipoproteins.
   F. See also *Low-density lipoprotein cholesterol, Blood; High-density lipoprotein cholesterol, Blood.*

CHOLINESTERASE II
(*see Pseudocholinesterase, Plasma*)

CHOLINESTERASE (PSEUDO), PLASMA
(*see Pseudocholinesterase, Plasma*)

CHORIONIC VILLI SAMPLING, DIAGNOSTIC

Norm. No detection of chromosome or genetic defects.

Usage. Detection of genetic defects, chromosomal abnormalities, and acquired disorders in fetuses in women who are at high risk. Disorders such as beta-glucuronidase deficiency, hemophilia (factor VIII or IX), cystic fibrosis, mental retardation, Down syndrome, chromosome abnormalities, fragile X syndrome, beta-thalassemia, and Duchenne muscular dystrophy. Infections.

Description. Chorionic villi sampling (CVS) consists in extracting a small amount of villous tissue directly from the chorion. This procedure can be performed at about 10 weeks of gestation and does not require in vitro culturing of cells because sufficient numbers are directly available in the extracted tissue. The procedure allows prenatal diagnosis at about 2 months of gestation rather than at nearly 5 months of gestation. This procedure is the method of choice for prenatal diagnosis in the first trimester of pregnancy.

Professional Considerations
1. Consent form IS required.

Risks
Bleeding, hematoma, infection, intrauterine death, spontaneous abortion. Limb reduction defects may occur, possibly caused by vascular accident from decreased perfusion in distal portions of limbs or from thrombosis at the sampling site or from inadvertent amnion puncture resulting in either amniotic bands or loss of amniotic fluid, with subsequent compression and deformity (Gruber et al. 1994). See also *Amniocentesis and amniotic fluid analysis, Diagnostic.* CVS involves slightly higher fetal loss rate than amniocentesis does, with most estimates ranging from 1-2%.

Contraindications
Morbid obesity, retroverted uterus with intervening bowel.

2. **Preparation:**
   A. Arrange for a laboratory technician to be present to evaluate the sample on location.
   B. Must have complete family history.
   C. Provide continuous fetal heart tone monitoring.
   D. See *Amniocentesis and amniotic fluid analysis, Diagnostic.*
   E. See *Obstetric ultrasonography, Diagnostic.*
3. **Procedure:**
   A. Transabdominal CVS:
      i. The client is positioned supine.
      ii. Under ultrasonic guidance, a long 20-gauge needle is inserted percutaneously through the abdomen into villous tissue.
   B. Transcervical CVS:
      i. The client is placed in dorsal lithotomy position.
      ii. Under ultrasonic guidance, a malleable catheter is inserted through the cervix into villous tissue.
      iii. The perineum, vagina, and cervix are prepared with antiseptic solution.
      iv. A sterile speculum is placed into the vagina to allow visualization of the cervix.

v. The catheter is advanced through the cervix into the chorion frondosum under ultrasonic guidance.

4. Postprocedure care:
   A. Suggest maternal serum alpha-fetoprotein (MSAFP) screening at 15-20 weeks of gestation.
   B. See *Amniocentesis and amniotic fluid analysis, Diagnostic.*
   C. See *Obstetric ultrasonography, Diagnostic.*

5. Client and family teaching:
   A. The advantage of CVS, as opposed to amniocentesis, is earlier diagnosis of genetic defects.
   B. Explore the couple's expectations and review the risks and limitations of the test.
   C. Refer the client with abnormal results for genetic counseling.

6. Factors that affect results:
   A. Specimens not large enough invalidate the results.
   B. Specimens not labeled invalidate the results.

7. Other data:
   A. CVS is not indicated if neural tube defect is suspected.
   B. See also *Amniocentesis and amniotic fluid analysis, Diagnostic.*

CHRISTMAS FACTOR, BLOOD
(see Factor IX, Blood)

CHROMIUM, SERUM

Norm. 0.18-0.47 ng/mL (35-90 nmol/L, SI units) or <0.5 mg/L.

Increased. Chromium toxicity, hypocholesterolemia, clients with metal or ultrahigh molecular weight polyethylene cementless total hip arthroplasty, tannery workers.

Decreased. Aging, diabetes mellitus, total parenteral nutrition.

Description. Chromium is a trace element normally found in the body. It may aid amino acid transport, especially to the liver and heart. Chromium may also enhance insulin activity and proper glucose utilization. Industrial exposure to chromium in tanning, electroplating, steel and metal industries, photography, and the paint, dye, and explosives industries

may cause toxicity, resulting in liver and kidney impairment, dermatitis, convulsions, and coma. Respiratory tract cancers have been linked to chromium exposure.

Professional Considerations
1. Consent form NOT required.
2. Preparation:
   A. Tube: Blue topped, metal free.
3. Procedure:
   A. Draw a 5-mL blood sample.
4. Postprocedure care:
   A. None.
5. Client and family teaching:
   A. Results are normally available within 24-48 hours.
6. Factors that affect results:
   A. Reject hemolyzed specimens.
   B. Results are invalidated if the client has undergone a recent diagnostic test involving the injection of radioactive chromium.
   C. Laboratory equipment used to measure chromium must be free of metal and stainless steel. Measurement must be performed under laminar air-flow conditions.
7. Other data:
   A. Occupational exposure causes dermatitis, skin ulcerations, perforations of the nasal septum, asthma, and cancer of the nasal mucosa or lungs.
   B. There is a loss of chromium in breast milk despite adequate dietary intake.
   C. See also *51Cr, Blood; Chromium, Urine.*

CHROMIUM, URINE

Norm:

	SI UNITS
0.1-2.0 µg/L	1.9-38.4 nmol/L

Increased. Aging, chromium toxicity, total hip replacement clients, tannery workers.

Decreased. Diabetes (children), pregnancy, total parenteral nutrition.

Description. Chromium is a trace element required by the body for its participation in the action of insulin on cell surfaces. Chromium is therefore important in glucose utilization. Deficiencies in chromium are being studied related to glucose intolerance and malnutrition. Chromium is mainly excreted by the kidneys, but it is currently difficult to measure chromium in small amounts in the urine. Chromium toxicity occurs from high exposure in the tanning, electroplating, steel and other metal industries, photography, and the paint, dye, and explosives industries and may also occur in clients with chronic renal disease. Toxicity may result in liver and kidney impairment, dermatitis, convulsions, and coma. Respiratory tract cancers have been linked to chromium exposure. This test is used to detect chromium toxicity.

Professional Considerations
1. Consent form NOT required.
2. **Preparation:**
   A. Prepare a 3-L container for chromium collection by leeching it for 48 hours in 10% nitric acid and then washing it with metal-free, distilled water.
   B. Write the exact starting time of the urine collection on the laboratory requisition.
3. **Procedure:**
   A. Collect a 24-hour urine specimen in an airtight, specially prepared 3-L container free of preservatives and metals.
   B. Avoid contamination of the urine with stool.
4. **Postprocedure care:**
   A. Compare urine quantity in the specimen container with the urinary output record for the test. If the specimen contains less urine than what was recorded as output, some of the sample may have been discarded, invalidating the test.
   B. Document quantity of urine output for the collection period on the laboratory requisition.
5. **Client and family teaching:**
   A. Save all the urine voided in the 24-hour period and urinate before defecating to avoid loss of urine. If any of the urine is accidentally discarded, discard the entire specimen and restart the collection the next day.
   B. Results are normally available within 24 hours.
6. **Factors that affect results:**
   A. Falsely elevated values may result from urine exposed to metal (as in collections from a metal urinal or bedpan) or contaminated with stool.

B. Laboratory equipment used to measure chromium must be free of metal and stainless steel. Measurement must be performed under laminar air-flow conditions.
   C. All the urine voided for the 24-hour period must be included to avoid a falsely low result.
7. **Other data:**
   A. Most laboratories currently use urine as a gross screening for toxicity. Because of the difficulty detecting small amounts of chromium in urine, serum levels are more accurate for determination of the level of toxicity.

CHROMOSOME ANALYSIS, BLOOD

Norm. A total of 46 chromosomes with 22 matched pairs plus XX for females and XY for males.

Usage. Diagnosis of chromosome abnormalities leading to Down syndrome, ring 20 syndrome (epilepsy), microphthalmia, other physical or mental retardation, and sex chromosome disorders such as Turner syndrome or Klinefelter syndrome; establishes sex in hypogonadism or unclear genitalia; part of the work-up for amenorrhea, infertility (male and female), frequent miscarriages, and other chromosome-related disorders and some leukemias and transitional-cell carcinoma of the bladder; used in genetic counseling for prospective parents and those with a family history of genetic disease.

Description. Chromosome analysis involves karyotyping human chromosomes from a culture of leukocytes from peripheral blood. Cell replication of the cultured leukocytes is chemically halted in metaphase, and microscopic photographs are taken of the chromosomes within the cell nucleus. The chromosome pictures are enlarged, and the chromosomes are paired, sorted, and studied for symmetry of pairs, number of chromosomes, identification of sex chromosomes, and staining patterns.

Professional Considerations
1. Consent form NOT required.
2. **Preparation:**
   A. See *Client and family teaching.*
   B. Preschedule this test with the laboratory.

C. Tube: Green topped.
3. **Procedure:**
   A. Draw a 7-mL blood sample.
4. **Postprocedure care:**
   A. Write the date and time of specimen collection on the laboratory requisition.
   B. Send the specimen to the laboratory immediately.
5. **Client and family teaching:**
   A. Fast for 3 hours and do not eat fatty foods for 12 hours before specimen collection.
6. **Factors that affect results:**
   A. Reject hemolyzed specimens or specimens received more than 24 hours after collection.
7. **Other data:**
   A. Karyotyping may be completed on other tissues including tumor cells, bone marrow, amniocentesis, or buccal smear.
   B. Some forms of leukemia, especially chronic myelogenous, are noted by chromosome assay of blood.
   C. Chromosomal anomalies account for up to 15.7% of male infertility.

CHS
(see Pseudocholinesterase, Plasma)

CHYMEX TEST FOR PANCREATIC FUNCTION (BENTIROMIDE TEST, CHYMOTRYPSIN), DIAGNOSTIC

Norm. Greater than 70% the administered dose of *para*-aminobenzoic acid (PABA) appears in the urine of the client within 6 hours of administration.

Usage. This is a test used to evaluate pancreatic exocrine (digestive) function. It is frequently employed in the management of clients with chronic pancreatitis and may be used to determine if clients with this illness will require chronic pancreatic enzyme therapy.

Description. N-Benzoyl-L-tyrosyl-*para*-aminobenzoic acid (BT-PABA, bentiromide) is administered orally. The pancreatic digestive enzyme chymotrypsin cleaves this material to PABA, which is then readily absorbed across the intestinal mucosa into the systemic circulation. The PABA subsequently appears in the urine. Failure of significant amounts of PABA to appear in the urine implies reduced amounts of chymotrypsin in the intestinal tract, and the diagnosis of pancreatic insufficiency is consequently established.

Professional Considerations
1. Consent form NOT required.

Risks
Infection.

Contraindications
Previous history of allergic reaction to BT-PABA or PABA.
Previous BT-PABA testing within 7 days of the test.
The safety of this test has not been established during pregnancy.

Adverse Reactions
Central nervous system: Headache
Respiratory: Stridor
Gastrointestinal: Diarrhea, nausea, vomiting

2. **Preparation:**
   A. There are several medications and foods that interfere with the results of this test and should be discontinued before testing (see under *Factors that affect results*).
   B. Pancreatic enzyme therapy can interfere with the test (creating a "false-negative" result) and should be discontinued at the discretion of the client's physician before the test.
3. **Procedure:**
   A. 500 mg of BT-PABA (bentiromide) is given to the client orally after an overnight fast.
   B. The bentiromide is usually administered with 250 mL of water, and oral water intake is encouraged for several hours after the agent is administered.
   C. All urine is collected for 6 hours after the bentiromide is given.
   D. Urine volume is measured, and a sample of urine is submitted to the laboratory for PABA determination. In this manner the total amount of PABA excreted in the urine can be calculated.
   E. The results of the test are determined as a percentage when the amount of PABA excreted in the urine (in milligrams) is divided by the amount of BT-PABA

administered (500 mg) and this number is multiplied by 100.
4. **Postprocedure care:**
   A. Complete urine output needs to be collected for 6 hours after the administration of the BT-PABA.
   B. Encourage oral fluid intake.
5. **Client and family teaching:**
   A. The rationale behind the test should be discussed before the administration of the BT-PABA.
   B. The client should be informed of the necessity of collecting all urine passed during the 6 hours after the administration of the BT-PABA.
6. **Factors that affect results:**
   A. Foods that interfere with urine PABA determination: prunes, cranberries (these should be eliminated from the diet for 72 hours before the test).
   B. Medications that interfere with urine PABA determination: acetaminophen, chloramphenicol certain sunscreens, local anesthetic agents, thiazide diuretics, sulfonamides.
   C. Renal or hepatic insufficiency.
   D. Ongoing therapy with pancreatic enzymes.
7. **Other data:**
   A. An empiric trial of pancreatic enzyme therapy is occasionally done in clients with presumed pancreatic insufficiency in place of a formal BT-PABA test.
   B. Other tests utilized to confirm the diagnosis of pancreatic exocrine insufficiency include the secretin test and the CCK-pancreozymin tests.

CHYMOTRYPSIN TEST
(*see Chymex test for pancreatic function, Diagnostic*)

CIRCULATING ANTICOAGULANT (CAC, LUPUS ANTICOAGULANT), BLOOD

Norm. Negative. No CAC identified.

Positive. Indicates the presence of an inhibitor (CAC). There are two types of CAC: one is a specific factor inhibitor—an immunoglobulin that interferes with the function of any one clotting factor—and the other is a lupus anticoagulant—an immunoglobulin that interferes with phospholipid in coagulation tests.

Description. Circulating anticoagulants (CACs) and lupus anticoagulants develop spontaneously or are acquired in association with autoimmune diseases or certain medication exposure. Clients with systemic lupus erythematosus, malignancies such as multiple myeloma, or chronic inflammatory diseases such as ulcerative colitis and rheumatoid arthritis as well as renal transplant recipients are known to develop these antibodies. CACs may also develop during complications post partum or in clients taking chlorpromazine or similar drugs. In the laboratory they prolong the PT (prothrombin time), PTT (partial thromboplastin time), APTT (activated partial thromboplastin time) or all of them. CACs are detected by a test called a "mixing study," in which normal plasma is added to client plasma and the PT, PTT, or APTT is repeated. Failure to correct the clotting to normal is a positive test. Additional tests are used to determine whether the CAC is a specific factor inhibitor or a lupus anticoagulant.

Professional Considerations
1. Consent form NOT required.
2. **Preparation:**
   A. Tube: Blue topped.
3. **Procedure:**
   A. Draw this specimen last or discard 1-2 mL of blood into a syringe or tube, leaving the needle in place.
   B. Attach a second syringe or tube and draw a 5-mL blood sample into a blue-topped tube.
   C. Mix the specimen well by gently inverting the tube several times and transport it within 1 hour of collection.
4. **Postprocedure care:**
   A. Write the collection time on the laboratory requisition.
5. **Client and family teaching:**
   A. The client must not take IV heparin for 4-8 hours, or subcutaneous heparin for 24 hours. Some other anticoagulant drugs may interfere with the test. Warfarin (Coumadin) does not interfere.
6. **Factors that affect results:**
   A. Drugs that may cause false-positive results include heparin, hirudin, and argatroban.
   B. Contact of the specimen with the tissue thromboplastin may cause false-negative results. This is the

reason for the double-draw procedure.
C. Reject hemolyzed, diluted, iced, or clotted specimens and specimens received more than 1 hour after collection.
D. Separate and refrigerate plasma if the test cannot be performed within 2 hours of collection.
7. **Other data:**
A. Specific factor inhibitors cause severe bleeding. Severe clinical bleeding is rare with the lupus anticoagulant unless there are other clotting abnormalities such as thrombocytopenia.

CIRCULATING CANCER CELL TEST (CCCT^SM, BLOOD BIOPSY), BLOOD

Norm. Negative.

Usage. Has potential for use as a general screening for the presence of various types of tumors that shed endothelial cells into the bloodstream; Early detection of tumor recurrence.

Description. A newly-developed test that screens for a higher than normal amount of epithelial cells in the bloodstream, targets and removes normal cells from the sample, and then uses histologic and DNA examination on the remaining sample to pinpoint cells with cancerous morphology. The principle of this test is that many common malignancies cause epithelial cell shedding into the bloodstream, often long before clinical symptoms are present and possibly even before more sensitive tumor marker tests become positive. The DNA examination portion of this test can identify cell division and DNA cell fragments, both characteristics apt to be more abundant when cancer is present. Because cancer metastasizes via the bloodstream, this test holds promise to detect spreading or recurrent cancer before further organ damage occurs.

Professional Considerations
1. Consent form IS required.
2. **Preparation:**
A. Obtain a 20-mL syringe and CCCT test kit.
3. **Procedure:**
A. Obtain a 20-mL blood sample.

4. **Postprocedure care:**
A. Package and store according to test kit instructions and send to laboratory.
5. **Client and family teaching:**
A. There is no fasting required for this test.
B. Test results may take 2-3 weeks.
6. **Factors that affect results:**
A. None.
7. **Other data:**
A. This test is available through Cell Works, Inc.

CISTERNOGRAPHY, CSF FLOW SCAN
(*see Cisternography, Radionuclide, Diagnostic*)

CISTERNOGRAPHY, RADIONUCLIDE (CSF FLOW STUDIES, CSF FLOW SCAN), DIAGNOSTIC

Norm. Normal cerebrospinal fluid (CSF) flow patterns at specific times after intrathecal injection of radiographic material into the lumbar area of the spinal cord.

1 hour:	Basal cisterns.
3-4 hours:	Radioactivity has reached the cerebral area and begun to spread to the ventricles and subarachnoid area.
24 hours:	The flow of radioactivity should be complete to convexities or subarachnoid areas, without leakage or obstruction that would interfere with bilateral symmetry of flow.
48 hours:	Radioactivity is primarily diffuse over the vertex but not in the brainstem area because it has been absorbed into the blood circulation. Symmetry is normal.

Usage. Brain atrophy; communicating hydrocephalus; suspected hydrocephalus related to CSF flow blockage (that is, tumor, cyst, subdural hematoma); CSF leakage (rhinorrhea); cerebrospinal fistulas; CSF leaks after spontaneous intracranial hypotension, trauma or neurosurgery; identification of dural tear site with basal skull fracture; evaluation of the patency of a CSF shunt; and work-up of central nervous system symptoms such as personality changes, behavioral changes, and other neurologic changes.

Description. A nuclear medicine study of the brain and cerebral blood flow. Injection of a radioisotope into the subarachnoid space through a cisternal or lumbar puncture. The head is scanned at regular intervals to determine the amount of time it takes for the radioisotope to clear from the circulating CSF. Several views are taken at specific times over 24-48 hours.

Professional Considerations

1. Consent form IS required for the lumbar puncture, the radioactive injection, or the injection by cisternal puncture.

Risks

Same as for *Lumbar puncture, Diagnostic.*

Contraindications

In elevated cerebrospinal fluid pressure; skin infection in lumbar or cisternal area.

Precautions

During pregnancy, risks of cumulative radiation exposure to the fetus from this and other previous or future imaging studies must be weighed against the benefits of the procedure. Although formal limits for client exposure are relative to this risk:benefit comparison, the United States Nuclear Regulatory Commission requires that the cumulative dose equivalent to an embryo/fetus from occupational exposure not exceed 0.5 rem (5 mSv). Radiation dosage to the fetus is proportional to the distance of the anatomy studied from the abdomen and decreases as pregnancy progresses. For pregnant clients, consult the Radiologist/Radiology Department to obtain estimated fetal radiation exposure from this procedure.

2. **Preparation:**
   A. Inspect the lumbar and cisternal areas for skin infection.
   B. Obtain povidone-iodine solution, 1-2% lidocaine, a needle, a syringe, radionuclide, and a sterile lumbar puncture tray including a spinal needle.
   C. Elevated CSF pressure should be ruled out before this procedure.

3. **Procedure:**
   A. Lumbar injection:
      i. The client is placed in a lateral position with knees drawn up and chin placed on the chest. A lumbar puncture is performed, and CSF pressure is measured. A radionuclide (indium 111, ytterbium 169, iodine 131 bound to RISA) is injected into the lumbar spine space.
      ii. The client is then returned to a hospital room and usually must lie flat between studies, especially for the first series.
      iii. Cisternograms or radiographic scans are completed at 4, 24, and 48 hours.
      iv. The progress and flow pattern of the radiographic material is then studied for diagnostic purposes.
   B. Cisternal injection:
      i. Using the lumbar puncture set, a puncture is made directly into the cisterna magna at the base of the skull. A radionuclide (indium 111, ytterbium 169, iodine 131 bound to RISA) is injected into the cisterna magna.
      ii. Cisternograms are obtained in minutes, and subsequent studies are performed in 24 and 48 hours.

4. **Postprocedure care:**
   A. The client should lie flat for 1-4 hours after the injection.
   B. Observe for headache or neurologic changes.
   C. Return the client, when scheduled, to the nuclear medicine department.

5. **Client and family teaching:**
   A. Notify the nurse or physician of any complaints of headache, dizziness, or nausea.

6. **Factors that affect results:**
   A. Movement during the scan obscures the views.
   B. Improper injection may cause inadequate visualization.

7. **Other data:**
   A. Cisternography is an expensive, invasive test.
   B. If improper injection (rather than leak) is suspected, the study should be repeated after at least 1 week. A radiograph of the spine

may be used to study a suspected leak in that area.

C. Health care professionals working in a nuclear medicine area must follow federal standards set by the Nuclear Regulatory Commission. These standards include precautions for handling the radioactive material and monitoring of potential radiation exposure.

CK
(see Creatine kinase, Serum)

CLINISTIX TEST, DIAGNOSTIC
(see Glucose qualitative, Semiquantitative, Urine)

CLINITEST, DIAGNOSTIC
(see Glucose qualitative, Semiquantitative, Urine)

CLONAZEPAM, BLOOD

Norm. Negative.

		SI UNITS
Therapeutic level	10-80 µg/L	32-254 nmol/L
Panic level	≥100 µg/L	≥254 nmol/L

Panic Level Symptoms and Treatment

Symptoms. Deteriorating level of consciousness, coma.

Treatment:
Note: Treatment choice(s) depend on client history and condition and episode history.
Gastric lavage is not recommended, but should be considered if within 1 hour of ingestion and if ingestion of additional lethal substance is suspected. Use warm tap water or 0.9% saline.
Administer activated charcoal if within 4 hours of ingestion or if symptoms are present. Repeat as necessary, as benzodiazepines undergo hepatic recirculation.
Monitor for central nervous system depression.
Protect airway. Support breathing with oxygen and mechanical ventilation, if necessary.
Flumazenil is not recommended for routine use in benzodiazepine overdose. Flumazenil has been used as a competitive antagonist to reverse the profound effects of benzodiazepine overdose. Use of flumazenil is contraindicated if concomitant tricyclic antidepressants were taken or in dependence states because of risk of causing seizures from lowering of the seizure threshold and because it may precipitate symptoms of benzodiazepine withdrawal. Flumazenil may not completely reverse benzodiazepine effects. Close monitoring for re-sedation is required and repeated doses may be needed.
Do NOT use barbiturates.
Do NOT induce emesis.
Forced diuresis or hemodialysis will NOT remove benzodiazepines to any significant extent. No information was found on whether peritoneal dialysis will remove these drugs.

Usage. Monitoring for drug abuse; monitoring for therapeutic levels with long-term use and overdose. Treatment of convulsions or myoclonus, sedation, anxiety, hallucinogen persisting perception disorder (HPPD), labile arterial hypertension, panic disorders, unipolar depression, pedophilia, and drop episodes in Coffin-Lowry syndrome. Reduce spasticity of cerebral palsy.

Description. Clonazepam is a schedule-IV benzodiazepine used for the treatment of convulsions and myoclonus. Peak levels occur within 2 hours after oral administration. The drug is metabolized in the liver and excreted by the kidneys, with a half-life of 20-40 hours. Burning mouth syndrome may occur after taking the drug. Use does not directly relate to obstetric complications.

Professional Considerations
1. Consent form NOT required.
2. **Preparation:**
   A. Tube: Red topped, red/gray topped, or gold topped.
   B. MAY be drawn during hemodialysis.
3. **Procedure:**
   A. Collect a 5-mL blood sample.
4. **Postprocedure care:**
   A. If storing, separate and freeze the serum.
5. **Client and family teaching:**
   A. If an accidental overdose occurs in clients on chronic clonazepam therapy, teach the early signs of overdose (drowsiness, ataxia, slurred speech) for which emergency room treatment must be sought in the future.
   B. Refer clients with intentional overdose, for crisis intervention.
   C. Referrals to appropriate rehabilitation centers and therapeutic community programs should be offered to all addicted clients who may be interested.
6. **Factors that affect results:**
   A. Concomitant administration of carbamazepine, phenobarbital, phenytoin or valproic acid may result in subtherapeutic clonazepam values.
7. **Other data:**
   A. For seizures, dose adjustments are necessary after 90 days because of the development of tolerance.
   B. Physical dependence can occur. Discontinuation must be accomplished by tapering off to avoid status epilepticus.
   C. For the first 3 weeks of treating major depression clonazepam with fluoxetine is superior.
   D. See also *Benzodiazepines, Plasma and Urine.*

CLOSTRIDIAL TOXIN, SERUM

Norm. Negative.

Positive. Botulism (foods that are undercooked or left out such as baked potatoes). Wound botulism from use of injected black tar heroin.

Negative. Absence of spore-forming bacterium microorganism *Clostridium botulinum.*

Botulism Symptoms and Emergency Treatment

Symptoms. Diarrhea, dizziness, double-vision, fatigue, gastrointestinal pain, headache, nausea, weakness, vomiting. Cardiac and respiratory paralysis is possible.

Treatment:
Note: Treatment choice(s) depend on client history and condition and episode history.
1. Establish IV access.
2. Administer trivalent botulism antitoxin (Connaught Laboratories, Ltd). (Note: Anaphylaxis is possible if the antitoxin is given to clients with asthma, hay fever, horse or horse serum allergies, or past exposure to horse serum.) Follow the package insert instructions for sensitivity testing before antitoxin administration.
3. Induce vomiting with syrup of ipecac if the syrup can be given soon after ingestion of the contaminated food. (Induction of emesis is contraindicated in clients with no gag reflex or with central nervous system depression or excitation.)
4. Perform gastric lavage if emesis does not produce the contaminated food.
5. Give activated charcoal slurry.
6. Administer saline cathartic if no ileus is present.
7. Monitor for respiratory decompensation, which may occur suddenly in clients with botulism. Elective intubation is advisable for large ingestions.
8. Notify the state health department and the Centers for Disease Control and Prevention at 404-639-2206. (The after-hours medical emergency number is 404-639-2888.)

Description. Clostridia are gram-positive anaerobes of the family Bacillaceae characterized by production of exothermic spores, enzymes, and potent endotoxins. *Clostridium* species are found in soil, freshwater, and marine sediments, and some species are part of the human lower gastrointestinal tract. *C. botulinum* causes botulism, a neuroparalytic disease transmitted by the clostridial spores that survive improper cooking of food. Botulism causes acute flaccid paralysis and may lead to death if not treated with antitoxin before the onset of neurologic symptoms. Infant botulism is represented by hypotonia, feeding disruption, and a weak cry. Because of the severity of the disease and the potential for an epidemic among other clients ingesting the affected food, cases of suspected botulism must be immediately reported to the state department of health and the Centers for Disease Control and Prevention. Serum samples are used to confirm the diagnosis by identification of the toxin of *C. botulinum*.

Professional Considerations
1. Consent form NOT required.
2. Preparation:
   A. Vials: aerobic and anaerobic culture vials.
   B. It may be necessary for this test to be performed by an outside laboratory.
3. Procedure:
   A. Collect a 15- to 20-mL blood sample from each of two sites aseptically in the two culture vials, one for the aerobic and one for the anaerobic culture.
   B. Double the amount of cultures collected for clients on whom antibiotic therapy has been instituted.
4. Postprocedure care:
   A. Note antibiotic therapy on the laboratory requisition.
5. Client and family teaching:
   A. Results may not be available for several days. Empiric therapy is typically started while results are being awaited.
6. Factors that affect results:
   A. Antibiotic therapy may interfere with organism identification.
7. Other data:
   A. 20-50 g of stool and the food suspected of causing botulism should also be collected and sent for testing with the serum sample. See *Botulism, Diagnostic procedures, Stool*.

CLOSTRIDIUM DIFFICILE TOXIN ASSAY, STOOL

Norm. Negative. No *C. difficile* toxin detected.

Positive. Antibiotic-related pseudomembranous enterocolitis.

Usage. Determine the presence or absence of *C. difficile* toxin A.

Description. *C. difficile* is a large, gram-positive, rod-shaped bacteria that releases two necrotizing toxins (toxin A [enterotoxin] and toxin B [cytotoxin]) causing a potentially fatal (1.5%) pseudomembranous colitis, especially in clients receiving antibiotics. *C. difficile* enterocolitis is the most common cause of diarrheal disease in hospitalized clients. Although it is part of the normal flora of the intestine, antibiotics to which it is resistant may increase the amount of *C. difficile* in the intestine. *C. difficile* enterocolitis is associated most commonly with clindamycin, ampicillin, and cephalosporin therapy but is possible with any antibiotic therapy. The test includes detection of toxin produced by the organism in the stool of a client.

Professional Considerations
1. Consent form NOT required.
2. Preparation:
   A. Obtain a sealed plastic feces specimen container, no preservative; a sealed sterile or nonsterile container with lid.
3. Procedure:
   A. Obtain a freshly passed fecal specimen of 25 g of solid stool or 25-50 mL of liquid stool in a sterile, tightly sealed plastic container. Normally, three sequential specimens are collected.
4. Postprocedure care:
   A. Send the specimen to the laboratory for processing within 3-4 hours.
   B. The specimen may be refrigerated for up to 24 hours before being tested.
   C. Freeze the specimen if the test will not be performed within 24 hours. Transportation to an outside laboratory should be performed with the specimen stored in dry ice.
5. Client and family teaching:
   A. For outpatients, cohabitants should also be tested.

6. **Factors that affect results:**
   A. Exposure of the specimen to carbon dioxide may deactivate the toxins.
7. **Other data:**
   A. Results generally take up to 2 days.
   B. Culture is sometimes also prescribed but often recovers organisms that do not produce toxin.
   C. Many normal infants and up to 21% of adults may have *C. difficile* as a transient or permanent part of their normal flora. Therefore cultures of *C. difficile* are not diagnostic.
   D. *C. difficile* has been isolated in hospitals in 18% of patients (Miller MA et al, 2002) and from curtains, bookshelves, bedpans, and linens and accounts for 73% of pathogenic disease.
   E. Infection control programs have been shown to decrease the incidence of *C. difficile* by 60%.
   F. Treatment includes 10 days of oral metronidazole with vancomycin as second-line therapy (intravenous or intracolonic).

CLOT RETRACTION, BLOOD

Norm. 30-60 minutes for beginning of retraction; 1-2 hours for partial clot retraction; 6-24 hours for complete clot retraction.

Increased. Not applicable.

Decreased. Anemia (aplastic), disseminated intravascular coagulation (DIC), factor XIII deficiency, fibrinogen deficiency, fibrinolytic activity (increased), Glanzmann's thrombasthenia, Hodgkin's disease, hyperfibrinogenemia, hypofibrinogenemia, idiopathic thrombocytopenia purpura, leukemia (acute), multiple myeloma, platelet deficiency, platelet dysfunction, polycythemia vera, and thrombocytopenia purpura (secondary).

Description. A test performed on whole blood that determines the length of time required for firm clot formation by platelets and fibrinogen. Clot retraction decreases clot size during formation of the hemostatic plug. Test results indicate platelet and fibrinogen quantity and function. This test is rarely used.

Professional Considerations
1. Consent form NOT required.
2. **Preparation:**
   A. Tube: Red topped, red/gray topped, or gold topped.
3. **Procedure:**
   A. Collect and discard 3 mL of blood, leaving the needle in place in the vein.
   B. Attach a fresh syringe and collect 4-10 mL of blood.
   C. Observe the tube for clotting. When a clot has formed, observe after 2, 6, 12, and 24 hours for retraction from the walls of the test tubes and record the findings as no retraction, partial retraction, or complete retraction; time taken for beginning retraction; and complete retraction; clot consistency; amount of serum surrounding clot; and serum cell volume.
4. **Postprocedure care:**
   A. Observe for bleeding from the venipuncture site for 15 minutes if the client has a known coagulopathy.
5. **Client and family teaching:**
   A. Results are normally available within 24-48 hours.
6. **Factors that affect results:**
   A. Hemolysis invalidates results. Reject hemolyzed specimens.
   B. Plastic test tubes prolong the test results.
   C. Low platelet count, aspirin therapy, increased fibrinolysis, and hypofibrinogenemia will result in abnormal clot retraction. Drugs that interfere include c7E3\Fab and recombinant activated factor VII (rFVIIa).
   D. In DIC, afibrinogenemia, and severe hemophilic state, clot formation may not occur.
7. **Other data:**
   A. This test is only a measure of platelet function and is now considered useful mainly in the diagnosis of Glanzmann's thrombasthenia.

CLOT UREA SOLUBILITY, BLOOD
(see Factor XIII)

CMP
(see Comprehensive metabolic panel, Blood)

CNH
(see Natriuretic peptides, Plasma)

CO, BLOOD
(see Carbon monoxide, Blood)

CO₂, BLOOD
(see Carbon dioxide, Partial pressure, Blood; Carbon dioxide, Total content, Blood)

COAGULATION FACTOR ASSAY, BLOOD

Norm. Factors VIII, IX, and XII are present and normal.

Usage. Detection of the type of hemophilia or other coagulation abnormalities.

HEMOPHILIA TYPE	PT	PTT	ADSORBED PLASMA	AGED NORMAL SERUM
Factor III	Normal	Increase	Corrects	No change
Factor IX	Normal	Increase	No change	Corrects
Factor XI	Normal	Increase	Partial	Partial
Factor II	Normal	Increase	Corrects	Corrects

Description. A blood assay completed by special coagulation laboratories to determine the presence of a congenital or acquired blood clotting factor deficiency that may cause hemophilia or other blood coagulation disorders. The client's blood is mixed with normal serum or specially prepared plasma or serum with a known specific deficiency. The results are studied for prothrombin time (PT), partial thromboplastin time (PTT), and activated partial thromboplastin time (APTT) as well as clot solubility to urea. The pattern (see table above) of clotting, PT, PTT, and any change when cross-mixed with the special agent plasma gives results that can determine the specific factor deficiency. For example, in hemophilia:

1. Test plasma adsorbed contains only factors XI and XII and so would specifically correct a client's plasma deficiency in these factors and therefore identify the problem.
2. Test plasma aged contains VII, IX, and XI and is known to lack I, V, and VIII.

Professional Considerations
1. Consent form NOT required.
2. **Preparation:**
   A. Preschedule the study with the special coagulation laboratory.
   B. Tube: 2.7-mL blue topped or 4.5-mL blue topped, a control tube, and a waste tube or syringe. Also obtain a container of ice.
3. **Procedure:**
   A. Perform a venipuncture and withdraw 2 mL of blood into a syringe or vacuum tube. Remove the syringe or tube, leaving the needle in place. Attach a second syringe, and draw two blood samples, one in a citrated blue-topped tube and the other in a control tube. The sample quantity should be 2.4 mL for a 2.7 mL tube and 4.0 mL for a 4.5-mL tube. Mix the sample gently by inverting the tube several times. Place the specimens immediately in the container of ice.
4. **Postprocedure care:**
   A. Write the collection time on the laboratory requisition.
   B. Refrigerate the specimen during transport, and transport it to the laboratory immediately. The test should be completed within 2 hours.
   C. Observe the venipuncture site closely for any client with known coagulopathy.
5. **Client and family teaching:**
   A. The client should not have warfarin (Coumadin) therapy for 2 weeks or heparin therapy for 2 days.
6. **Factors that affect results:**
   A. Reject clotted or nonrefrigerated specimens.

B. The double-draw procedure is required to avoid contact of the blood with tissue thromboplastin, which may cause false-negative results.

C. Drugs that may cause false-negative results include bishydroxycoumarin, heparin calcium, heparin sodium, and warfarin sodium.

D. Oral contraceptives may cause abnormally high levels of factors II, VII, IX, and X.

7. **Other data:**
A. It is normal for healthy premature infants to have low (50% of normal) levels of factors II, III, IX, X, XI, and XII, even though a normal premature infant does not bleed spontaneously.

COCAINE, BLOOD

Norm. None detected.

		SI UNITS
Therapeutic range	100-500 ng/mL	330-1650 μmol/L
Panic (fatal) level	>1000 ng/mL	>3300 μmol/L

Panic Level Symptoms and Treatment

Symptoms. Short-lived CNS and sympathetic stimulation, hypertension, tachypnea, tachycardia, and mydriasis.

Treatment:
Note: Treatment choice(s) depend on client history and condition and episode history.
Provide airway and cardiac support. Prolonged resuscitation is indicated if cardiac arrest occurs secondary to cocaine intoxication.
Induce emesis if oral ingestion. (Note: Induction of emesis is contraindicated in clients with no gag reflex or with central nervous system depression or excitation).
Perform gastric lavage if oral ingestion.
Perform whole-bowel irrigation for ingested packs of cocaine. Administer activated charcoal into the body cavity where ingested packs are found.
Administer benzodiazepines for convulsions or other sympathomimetic symptoms, such as arrhythmias.
Do NOT use beta blockers.
Provide cool environment or hypothermia if the client is febrile.
Monitor renal function for damage from rhabdomyolysis.
Monitor for hypoglycemia.

Consider need for continuous ECG monitoring.

Usage. Determination of therapeutic cocaine levels or diagnosis of drug abuse or drug overdose.

Description. Cocaine is a schedule-II, central nervous system stimulant and a local anesthetic used clinically for its bronchodilator and vasoconstrictor effects, which result in increased blood pressure, respiratory rate, and heart rate. It is readily absorbed through mucous membranes, detoxified in the liver, and excreted by the kidneys and acts for 2 hours or less. Cocaine is also a drug of abuse, and street names for it include C, coke, crack, girl, lady, happy dust, gold dust, and stardust. Cocaine administration compromises the heart's antioxidant defense system, and an overdose may lead to cardiopulmonary failure.

Professional Considerations
1. Consent form NOT required unless the specimen may be used for legal evidence.
2. **Preparation:**
A. Tube: Green topped or lavender topped. Also obtain ice. Use of gray-top Vacutainer tube containing cholinesterase inhibitor sodium fluoride will prevent enzymatic degradation of the blood sample.
3. **Procedure:**
A. If the specimen will be used as legal evidence, have the specimen collection witnessed.

B. Draw a 5- to 10-mL blood sample and place the tube immediately on ice.

4. **Postprocedure care:**
   A. If the specimen will be used as legal evidence, seal the bag and label it as legal evidence. Label the specimen with the exact time drawn, the client's name, and the specimen source. Sign the laboratory requisition and have the witness sign it also. Laboratory personnel in receipt of the specimen must also sign the requisition and record the time of receipt on it.
   B. Transport the specimen to the laboratory immediately.

5. **Client and family teaching:**
   A. For overdose, refer the client and the family for crisis intervention and psychologic support.
   B. Referrals to appropriate rehabilitation centers and therapeutic community programs should be offered to all addicted clients who may be interested.
   C. Cocaine can cause lung and kidney problems, heart attacks, strokes, aortic dissection, intestinal ischemia, hallucinations, feelings of suicide, and death. It is an addictive drug. When you stop using cocaine, withdrawal symptoms may include depression, lack of energy, sleep disturbances, chills, muscle aches, fast heartbeat, sweating, and chest pain.

6. **Factors that affect results:**
   A. Reject specimens not received on ice. Cocaine is rapidly hydrolyzed in blood, and iced specimens must be processed by gas chromatography within 1 hour.

7. **Other data:**
   A. Because cocaine is so rapidly hydrolyzed, the blood specimen would have to be drawn just after use to show that it was positive for abuse. Therefore levels of urinary cocaine or its metabolite, benzoylecgonine, are more accurate screening methods for drug abuse.
   B. The use of cocaine, even one time, can cause rhabdomyolysis, a disease that causes muscle tissue destruction.
   C. Cocaine and tobacco use are associated with significant risk for spontaneous abortion.

D. Cocaine has adverse effects on fetuses (with motor development deficiencies still detectable at 2 years of age), but it has no adverse effect on the placenta.

COCCIDIOIDES SEROLOGY, BLOOD OR CSF

Norm. Negative.

Usage. Detection of *Coccidioides* infection. Occurs primarily in desert southwest United States and can result in pericarditis or acute respiratory distress syndrome. Found in persons with HIV, occupational archeological dinosaur site workers and donor transfer in lung transplantation.

Description. See *Coccidioidomycosis skin test, Diagnostic*. The *Coccidioides* serologic tests are three tests on blood or cerebrospinal fluid that help diagnose coccidioidomycosis. The tube precipitin test is positive 7-21 days after the start of the infection and becomes negative about 6 months later. The latex agglutination (LA) test is more sensitive than the precipitin test but produces more false-positive results than the precipitin test does. CF test of spinal fluid is highly sensitive and specific during active infection.

Professional Considerations
1. Consent form NOT required.
2. **Preparation:**
   A. Tube: Red topped, red/gray topped, or gold topped.
3. **Procedure:**
   A. Draw a 3-mL blood sample.
   B. An acute sample should be drawn as soon as possible after symptoms appear.
   C. The convalescent sample should be drawn at least 7-14 days after the acute sample and preferably 14-21 days after the onset of symptoms.
4. **Postprocedure care:**
   A. None.
5. **Client and family teaching:**
   A. Results usually take several days because the sample is normally sent to a reference laboratory.
   B. Return at specified date for serial specimen collection.
6. **Factors that affect results:**
   A. Up to 10% false-positive results occur in the LA test.

7. **Other data:**
   A. See also *Coccidioidomycosis skin test, Diagnostic.*

COCCIDIOIDOMYCOSIS SKIN TEST, DIAGNOSTIC

Norm. Negative or no skin reaction.

Positive. Skin induration >5 mm diameter indicates exposure to *Coccidioides* but gives no indication of duration. Associated with hypercalcemia.

Usage. Determine the exposure to fungal infections affecting the pulmonary system.

Description. *Coccidioides immitis* is a fungus found in the soil of dry climates of the southwest United States and Latin America. Spores in the dust are inhaled, causing respiratory infection that is mild and asymptomatic or may cause acute to chronic pulmonary cavities and septic shock. A rare 1% of infected individuals develop disseminated disease or infection that is fatal. The course of the disease includes fever, malaise, and respiratory complaints, which become self-limiting as the client develops antibodies. In the disseminated form, the skin, bones, internal organs, and meninges are infected. This test is performed by injection of a *Coccidioides* antigen sample and observation for signs of an antibody reaction.

Professional Considerations
1. Consent form NOT required.

2. **Preparation:**
   A. Obtain an alcohol wipe, a syringe, a subcutaneous needle, and a *Coccidioides* antigen sample.
3. **Procedure:**
   A. Cleanse the volar aspect of the lower arm with an alcohol wipe and allow it to dry.
   B. Inject 0.1 mL of 1:100 dilution of coccidioidin or spherulin (which is more sensitive) subcutaneously.
   C. Circle the injection site with a pen or marker.
4. **Postprocedure care:**
   A. Read the skin test 24 and 48 hours after the injection.
5. **Client and family teaching:**
   A. The injection causes a stinging sensation.
   B. Do not wash off the marking until the test is read. Return in 24-48 hours to have the test site read.
6. **Factors that affect results:**
   A. Low dilution of the antigen preparation (that is, 1:10) may produce a cross-reaction, indicating other fungal diseases.
   B. The skin test may be negative in the severe, disseminated form of the disease.
7. **Other data:**
   A. Cross-reactions occur in clients with histoplasmosis.
   B. The advantage of skin testing is that results are available in approximately 24-48 hours.
   C. The main disadvantage is the time needed to develop antibodies.
   D. Clients with facial lesions are more likely to have meningitis.

CODEINE, SERUM AND URINE

Norm. Negative.

		SI UNITS
Serum		
Therapeutic level	10-100 ng/mL	33-334 nmol/L
Panic level	>200 ng/mL	>668 nmol/L
Urine		
Therapeutic level	5-30 mg/L	
Panic level	31-250 mg/L	

Panic Level Symptoms and Treatment

Symptoms. CNS depression (including somnolence, convulsions, stupor, coma), ataxia, vomiting, rash and itching of the skin, respiratory depression, miosis, hypotension, and skeletal muscle flaccidity.

Treatment:
Note: Treatment choice(s) depend on client history and condition and episode history.
Maintain patent airway and support breathing.
Administer vasopressors to support blood pressure.
Administer naloxone in repeated doses as needed.
Administer activated charcoal.
Administer gastric lavage.
Administer laxative.
Monitor fluid status. Administer IV fluids as needed.
Perform neurologic checks every hour.
Hemodialysis will NOT remove codeine.

Usage. Codeine therapy and codeine overdose.

Description. Codeine is a schedule-II narcotic analgesic used for relief of mild-to-moderate pain and as an antitussive. Codeine is also found in combination with other analgesics in schedule III and IV medications. Drug effects of codeine are dose related. It is metabolized by the liver and excreted as norcodeine and conjugated morphine by the kidneys, with a half-life of 2.5-4.0 hours. Codeine can induce pancreatitis and manic psychotic episodes.

Professional Considerations
1. Consent form NOT required unless the specimen may be used as legal evidence.
2. Preparation:
   A. Obtain a clean urine container.
   B. Tube: Red topped, red/gray topped, or gold topped.
   C. The specimen MAY be drawn during hemodialysis.
3. Procedure:
   A. If the specimen may be used as legal evidence, have the specimen collection witnessed.
   B. *Serum:* Draw a 5-ml blood specimen.
   C. *Urine:* Collect 50 mL of urine in a clean container without preservatives. A fresh specimen may be taken from a urinary drainage bag.
4. Postprocedure care:
   A. If the specimen is being collected for legal purposes, sign and have the witness sign the laboratory requisition. Also write the date, time and specimen source on the requisition. Transport the specimen to the laboratory in a sealed plastic bag labeled as legal evidence. Each person handling the specimen should write the date and time he or she received the specimen on the requisition.
5. Client and family teaching:
   A. In the event of accidental overdose, the early sings of overdose for which to seek emergency treatment include drowsiness, ataxia, or slurred speech, or all three.
   B. Refer clients with intentional overdose, for crisis intervention.
   C. Referrals to appropriate rehabilitation centers and therapeutic community programs should the offered to all addicted clients who may be interested.
6. Factors that affect results:
   A. Some metabolites may affect urine codeine levels; thus confirmatory serum codeine measurement must also be drawn.
   B. Lengthened codeine half-life is associated with end-stage renal disease.
7. Other data:
   A. Accidental overdose with codeine-containing cough medications occurs in children.
   B. Endogenous plasma codeine is elevated in clients with anorexia nervosa and bulimia nervosa.

COGNITIVE TESTS, EVENT-RELATED POTENTIALS, DIAGNOSTIC

Norm. Normal recognition and reaction time.

Usage. Alzheimer's disease, dementia, depression, Huntington's disease, multiple sclerosis, myoclonic dystrophy, postcoma unawareness, psychiatric illnesses, and other clinical or experimental situations in which cognitive function disorders are suspected.

Description. A test devised to measure perceptomotor skills, sensory acuity, and ability to discriminate. Attention span is also tested because the client is asked to indicate it by pressing a button quickly after recognizing certain auditory or visual clues. When combined with evoked potential recordings, the test can give information about possible areas of error (such as a psychiatric disorder in which a hysterical loss of hearing shows positive brain response to sound but the client is unable to respond). Lack of expected response may be found to result from physical hearing loss rather than from psychiatric causes.

Professional Considerations
1. Consent form NOT required.
2. Preparation:
   A. Obtain earphones, a multichannel recorder with response button, and stimulus equipment.
3. Procedure:
   A. This test is carried out in a specialized psychophysiology laboratory.
   B. The client is seated in a quiet environment in a comfortable chair.
   C. After headphones are placed over the client's ears, a pattern or patterns of auditory cues are given.
   D. The client must respond to the cues by pushing a button as quickly as possible to signify his or her recognition of the proper cue.
   E. Visual cues consisting of patterns of light flashes are also utilized. A multichannel recorder notes the stimulus and response so that the time lapse as well as correctness of response can be determined.
   F. In some tests, an evoked potential is also recorded and determined. One electrode (active) is placed between the vertex and the auditory meatus. Neutral electrodes are attached to the earlobes, and an evoked potential recording of the hearing test is obtained along with the above recordings.
4. Postprocedure care:
   A. Remove the headphones.
5. Client and family teaching:
   A. You must cooperate if the results are to be of value. You will be asked to recognize certain demonstrated tones through earphones and respond by pressing the button provided.
6. Factors that affect results:
   A. Hearing loss or visual disorders impair the client's ability to respond to the auditory and visual cues.
   B. The test is not helpful in clients who are unable to cooperate or comprehend the instructions.
   C. Noise or other distractions in the testing environment may interfere with the client's comprehension of the testing cues.
7. Other data:
   A. See also *Brainstem auditory evoked potential, Diagnostic.*

COLD AGGLUTININ SCREEN, BLOOD

Norm. Negative or <1:32. Titers >1:40 are positive.

Usage. This test is indicated when an antibody screen or panel is suggestive of cold autoagglutination because the cold agglutinins are interfering with the examination for irregular antibodies. It also may be performed for hemolytic anemia or as part of the work-up of painful extremities in cold weather (Raynaud's) or other suspected cold reactions as in surgery. It is found in autoimmune hemolytic anemia, B-cell non-Hodgkin's lymphoma, chickenpox, lymphocytic leukemia, myelodysplastic syndrome, systemic lupus erythematosus, T-cell lymphoma and uterine sarcoma.

Description. Cold agglutinins are antibodies that are able to agglutinate

C

(clump) type O human blood cells at cold (<20° C) temperatures but not at room or higher temperatures. Cold agglutinins are present in small amounts in the circulation of many people and react at severely cold temperatures (4° C). Increased levels may follow infections. Their presence and reactivity at temperatures of 20° C or below are termed "wide amplitude" cold agglutination. Positive cold agglutinins can cause agglutination or clumping of antigens, which leads to thrombosis, pain in the extremities, and hemolysis.

Professional Considerations
1. Consent form NOT required.
2. **Preparation:**
   A. Tube: Red topped, red/gray topped, or gold topped.
3. **Procedure:**
   A. Draw a 4-mL blood sample.
4. **Postprocedure care:**
   A. The specimen is separated and then stored at 4° C for 2 hours or overnight.
5. **Client and family teaching:**
   A. Results are normally available within 48 hours.
6. **Factors that affect results:**
   A. Reject hemolyzed specimens.
7. **Other data:**
   A. Autoagglutination can occur in clients with positive results when exposed to cold and occurs especially in the extremities where body temperatures are normally lowest. It may also occur during surgery, especially during open-heart surgery, where the perfusate for bypass is 15-32° C.
   B. Cold agglutinins are not found in normal (room-temperature) blood cross-match methods.
   C. This is not to be confused with *Cold agglutinin titer,* which is a specific test for *Mycoplasma* pneumonia. The only connection is that among other infections, *Mycoplasma* infection may cause the presence of these cold agglutinins.

COLD AGGLUTININ TITER, SERUM

Norm. Negative or titer <32 or <1:32.

Positive. Titer >40 or >1:40 in combination with acute respiratory symptoms usually indicates *Mycoplasma pneumoniae* infection, usually *Mycoplasma* pneumonia, viral pneumonia, or primary atypical pneumonia. An agglutination reaction present even at very high titers is suggestive of *M. pneumoniae,* especially if the test is specific for anti-I antigens. Positive titers as a result of *M. pneumoniae* infection rise after about 10 days, peak at 12-25 days, and then diminish by 30 days with an acute infection. Positive titers may also indicate cirrhosis (hypertrophic, syphilitic), hemolytic anemia, Hodgkin's disease, lymphoma, mononucleosis infection, pleuropneumonia-like organism (PPLO), PNH, trypanosomiasis, and tuberculosis (febrile).

Negative. Titer <1:32 is negative for *M. pneumoniae* or related infection.

Description. Cold agglutinins are antibodies that cause clumping or agglutination of type O red blood cells at cold temperatures. The cold agglutinin titer tests for cold agglutinins at 2-8° C—those antibodies that result from *M. pneumoniae* infection. A titer is the highest dilution of a serum that will demonstrate a specific antigen-antibody reaction. *M. pneumoniae* is a nonbacterial infective agent that causes a pneumonia characterized by fever and a nonproductive or nonpurulent cough.

Professional Considerations
1. Consent form NOT required.
2. **Preparation:**
   A. Tube: Red topped, red/gray topped, gold topped, or lavender topped.
3. **Procedure:**
   A. Draw a 4-mL blood sample.
   B. Usually at least two serial samples are taken. The first is taken 1 week after the onset of illness. The second is taken 12-25 days after the onset of illness, and a third may be taken 30 days after the onset.
4. **Postprocedure care:**
   A. Transport the specimen to the laboratory immediately. The blood is allowed to clot at 37° C and the serum is then separated from the cells and cooled for testing.
5. **Client and family teaching:**
   A. Results are normally available within 48 hours.

6. **Factors that affect results:**
   A. Reject hemolyzed specimens or refrigerated specimens. Refrigeration before separation of serum may cause false-negative results.
   B. Antibiotic therapy may decrease antibody production.
   C. False-positive results may occur in clients with malaria, congenital syphilis, peripheral vascular disease, hepatic cirrhosis, anemia, and respiratory diseases. In such cases, the titer pattern is more constant, without peaks.
   D. The sample must not be allowed to clot at room temperature.
7. **Other data:**
   A. Culture methods for *M. pneumoniae* are available, but the cold agglutinin titer is more reliable for diagnosis.
   B. Serial titers are most helpful because the *M. pneumoniae* titers follow a specific pattern that peaks during the third to fourth week after infection.
   C. Newer cold agglutinin methods that test agglutination reactions specific to major antigen types make this test much more specific. *M. pneumoniae* is related to the I-I antigen system. Anti-M or anti-P are associated with other cold agglutinin activity and diseases.

COLONOSCOPY, DIAGNOSTIC

Norm. The intima of the large intestine is normally orange-pink in color, with folds and smooth indentations covered with mucus. Blood vessels may be visible below the epithelial surface.

Usage. Visualization of the mucosa of the entire colon and terminal ileum. Screening for intestinal abnormalities, including diverticula, polyps, tumors, ulcerative areas, infection, inflammation, irritation, bleeding sites, or strictures. Also used to study and biopsy or remove tumors, polyps, ulcerative colitis, parasitic disease, or other causes of diarrhea.

Description. A fiberoptic endoscopy study in which the lining of the large intestine is visually examined for inflammation or other changes of the mucosal surface and for bleeding sites or strictures. The test is indicated after a positive test for fecal occult blood or after a positive screening sigmoidoscopy or double-contrast barium enema, after bleeding of the lower GI tract, and when a client experiences a changing patterns bowel function. The American Cancer society recommends a screening colonoscopy every 10 years in adults over age 50. See also *Sigmoidoscopy, Diagnostic.*

Professional Considerations
1. Consent form IS required.

Risks
Dysrhythmias, hemorrhage, myocardial infarction, perforation of colon, peritonitis, respiratory depression.

Contraindications
Recent myocardial infarction or pulmonary embolus; retained barium from an earlier study; second or third trimester pregnancy. Sedatives are contraindicated in clients with central nervous system depression.

2. **Preparation:**
   A. See *Client and family teaching.*
   B. A tap-water enema may be prescribed to be given just before the test and/or person may ingest 28 tablets (42 g) of sodium phosphate or drink magnesium citrate the day before to cleanse the bowel.
   C. Sedation may be prescribed such as 2-3 mg midazolam and 80 mg propofol IV just before procedure.
   D. Prepare suction equipment, emergency equipment, naloxone, lubricant, cytology brush, and containers of fixative for cytology specimens.
   E. Record baseline vital signs.
3. **Procedure:**
   A. The client is positioned lying on the left side with knees flexed and draped for privacy and comfort.
   B. The flexible fiberoptic endoscope is inserted through the anus, and the rectum and colon are visualized. Insufflation occurs to aid in visualization. However, insufflation of CO_2 rather than air

reduces abdominal pain and bowel distention after colonoscopy.

C. Specimens may be obtained for cytologic testing.

D. Photographs are taken of anomalies present.

E. Polyps may be removed with colonoscopy biopsy forceps or an electrocautery snare.

4. **Postprocedure care:**

A. Place the tissue specimens in fixative of 10% formalin. Place the cytology specimens in 95% ethyl alcohol (ethanol). Label the specimens and send them to the laboratory immediately.

B. Observe the client and check vital signs every 15-30 minutes until fully recovered. If sedation was used, follow institutional protocol for postsedation monitoring. Typical monitoring includes continuous ECG monitoring and pulse oximetry, with continual assessments (every 5-15 minutes) of airway, vital signs, and neurologic status until the client is lying quietly awake, breathing independently, and responding appropriately to commands spoken in a normal tone.

C. After the client has fully recovered, he or she may resume a normal diet.

D. Observe for signs of colon perforation, which include abdominal pain or distention, malaise, fever, purulent rectal drainage, or lower gastrointestinal bleeding.

5. **Client and family teaching:**

A. Follow a clear liquid diet for 48 hours before the test and resume normal diet after the test.

B. Bowel preparation is very important. A laxative is usually prescribed the evening before the test, unless contraindicated. Examples are 10 ounces of magnesium citrate or 3 tablespoons of castor oil.

C. Make arrangements for transportation home after the procedure because driving is not permitted for 24 hours after receiving sedation.

D. Take deep, slow breaths during the procedure. The urge to defecate is normal and can be relieved with this type of breathing.

E. An increase in flatus is normal, and minor amounts of blood in the stool are expected after polyp removal.

6. **Factors that affect results:**

A. Soap-suds enemas irritate the mucosa, increase mucus production, and hinder visibility.

B. Barium from any previous gastrointestinal work-up makes colon visualization impossible.

C. Failure to clean the lower intestine makes colon visualization impossible.

D. Strictures or other abnormalities from previous surgery, radiation, or severe, chronic inflammatory disease may interfere with passage of the colonoscope.

7. **Other data:**

A. The findings from this procedure may be useful to the surgeon during laparotomy to exclude other lesions.

B. Virtual endoscopic magnetic resonance colonography which uses 3-D imaging does not identify polyps smaller than 5 mm.

C. Music therapy has been shown to reduce anxiety and the need for sedation in persons undergoing colonoscopy.

COLOR DUPLEX ULTRASONOGRAPHY, DIAGNOSTIC

Norm. Description of normal tissues, structure, and blood flow.

Usage. Noninvasive study that is performed to assess characteristics of blood flow including alterations of normal flow (i.e., sexual dysfunction), direction of flow, and presence of flow (i.e., thrombosis of upper extremity, vertebrobasilar ischemic disease). Tissue perfusion and tumor vascularization (i.e., acute pancreatitis) can also be assessed.

Description. Color duplex refers to the fact that this test presents on the screen a simultaneous display of Doppler information and the ultrasonographic image. High-frequency sound waves are passed over the structure, and a computer analyzes the time required for the impulse to be reflected back to a transducer. The computer converts this impulse to an electrical impulse that is viewed on the screen to create a three-dimensional picture of the structure, using color as a guide. The "Doppler" effect refers to a change in frequency that occurs when the sound wave is reflected from a moving object. The computer can display this change in frequency as sound or as color changes in the pictures or both ways. Different colors are used to represent flow, one color toward the transducer, and one away from the transducer. Speed of flow can be indicated by changes in the color shade.

Professional Considerations
1. Consent form NOT required.
2. **Preparation:**
   A. Obtain ultrasonic gel or paste.
3. **Procedure:**
   A. The patient is positioned on the bed or on an examination table so as to allow access to the structure that is to be studied.
   B. The area that is to studied is covered with the ultrasonic gel or paste, and the transducer is slowly passed over the area. The technician may use a longitudinal or a transverse approach in an attempt to obtain the best visualization of the structure.
   C. Video is obtained of the display for later review.
   D. The procedure should last less than 45 minutes depending on what structures are being visualized.
4. **Postprocedure care:**
   A. Remove gel or paste from the skin.
   B. Place client back to a comfortable position.
5. **Client and family teaching:**
   A. You will not be allowed to eat or drink during the test.
   B. The test is painless and the ultrasonic waves cannot be felt.
   C. You must lie as still as possible during the test.
   D. The area that is being studied will be uncovered, but you will otherwise be covered.
6. **Factors that affect results:**
   A. Abdominal fat can alter the intensity of a beam "looking" at abdominal structures.

B. If the beams pass through substances such barium, gas, or food particles, the clarity of the image can be diminished.
C. Client movement can affect the image clarity.

COLOR VISION TESTS, DIAGNOSTIC

Norm. The client is able to identify all the colors, symbols, and patterns presented.

Usage. Screening for retinal disease or color vision deficiency (such as red-green or blue-yellow deficiency).

Description. A test using pseudo-isochromatic plates with numbers or letters buried in a matrix of colored dots. Deficits can be genetic and result from one or more of the three-color cone systems, or acquired.

Professional Considerations
1. Consent form NOT required.
2. **Preparation:**
   A. Obtain an eye patch or hand-held occluder, test kit, and pointer.
3. **Procedure:**
   A. One eye is occluded, and the test booklet is held approximately 14 inches (35 cm) in front of the unoccluded eye.
   B. Sample plates of different patterns of primary colors with a background of a variety of colors are shown to the client, one at a time.
   C. The client is asked to identify the patterns of the primary colors and to trace the patterns with a pointer.
4. **Postprocedure care:**
   A. None.
5. **Client and family teaching:**
   A. Bring corrective glasses or lenses to the test.
   B. There are no food or fluid restrictions.
   C. The test is painless.
6. **Factors that affect results:**
   A. Conduct the test in a well-lighted area.
   B. Abnormalities of the ocular media, the retina, or the optic nerve can affect results and should be ruled out if color blindness is discovered.

C. The client may be unable to cooperate and participate in the test.
7. **Other data:**
   A. Color blindness may include more than one kind of spectral color.
   B. Color vision is not affected by laser in situ keratomileusis (LASIX) surgery.

COLORECTAL CANCER ALLELOTYPING FOR CHROMOSOME 17P AND 18Q (P53 OR DCC GENE), SPECIMEN AND BLOOD

Norm. Normal gene sequence.

Usage. Detection of mutations in tumor-suppressor genes, which are associated with approximately half of human cancers, including colorectal, breast, bladder, esophageal, liver, lung, ovarian, brain (p53) and colorectal, breast, brain, pancreas, leukemias, and male germ cell cancers (DCC).

Description. The progression of colon adenoma to invasive cancer frequently involves mutations in the p53 and DCC (deleted in colorectal cancer) genes, which are tumor-suppressor genes located on chromosome 17p and 18q, respectively. Most attention is given to the p53 gene because it is the most common mutational event in the progression of cancer, involved in nearly half of all human cancers. p53 produces a protein that induces apoptosis in response to DNA damage, maintaining genetic stability and preventing tumor formation. Both of the alleles must be damaged in order for the mutation to be apparent. The DCC gene encodes a protein similar to an immunoglobulin and mutations of this gene are found in several cancers. The role of both p53 and DCC in determining prognosis and treatment remains unclear though breast cancers with p53 mutations appear to be relatively resistant to ionized radiation and seem to benefit significantly from CMF chemotherapy. The techniques used for analysis of the genes are immunohistochemical, to detect the gene product, and DNA analysis to detect specific mutations. Analysis may be conducted on fresh, frozen, or paraffin-embedded tissue.

Professional Consideration
1. Consent is required for biopsy. See *Biopsy, Site-specific, Specimen*, for risks and contraindications.
2. **Preparation:**
   A. Tissue specimen: Obtain solid-tissue biopsy bottle.
   B. Blood: Obtain yellow-topped or lavender-topped tube.
3. **Procedure:**
   A. Obtain tissue specimen by desired procedure or draw blood and place in appropriate container. Tissue is to be frozen quickly.
4. **Postprocedure care:**
   A. Apply clean, sterile dressing to biopsy site.
5. **Client and family teaching:**
   A. Results may not be available for several days.
6. **Factors that affect results:**
   A. Small specimens decrease the reliability of the results.
   B. Tissue specimens must not be frozen, and blood specimens must not be clotted.
7. **Other data:**
   A. The specimen must be >40% tumor.
   B. Penclomedine is in clinical trials to assess its antitumor activity in colorectal carcinoma.
   C. Increased risk of colorectal carcinoma is associated with variant alleles of the DNA repair gene XRCC1 and GSTM3*B gene variant. Reduced risk of colorectal cancer is associated with phenol sulphotransferase SULT1A1*1 genotype.

COLPOSCOPY, DIAGNOSTIC

Norm. Normal appearance of vagina and cervix. Vagina and cervix are free of lesions, and no abnormal cells or tissue are present.

Usage. Evaluation, by physician or certified nurse, of suspicious lesions or suspected cervical or vaginal cancer, evaluation of abnormal cytologic characteristics of the vagina and cervix, testing for vulvar dystrophy, and screening for cervical abnormalities in women whose mothers were treated with diethylstilbestrol (DES) when pregnant with them. Collection of cervical specimen for definitive testing after abnormal Pap smear result has been obtained.

Description. The visual examination of the vagina and cervix using a lighted colposcope that magnifies the mucosal surfaces. Colposcopy helps diagnose benign and preclinical cancerous lesions of the cervix and vagina. Attachments to the colposcope include a green filter (aids in detecting abnormalities of blood vessels in the cervix), teaching arm, or video camera. If an abnormal Pap smear has been previously obtained, the colposcopy may be performed with a loop electrosurgical excision procedure (LEEP), in which a thin wire loop electrode is used to excise cervical tissue in the area of the abnormality for lesion removal and further examination.

Professional Considerations
1. Consent form IS required.

Risks
Bleeding, infection, mild discomfort.

Contraindications
Biopsy during colposcopy is contraindicated in the presence of anticoagulant therapy, bleeding disorders, thrombocytopenia, or heavy menses.

2. Preparation:
  A. The client should disrobe below the waist and the room should be a warm temperature.
  B. Obtain a speculum, a 3% acetic acid solution, sterile cotton-tipped swabs, a colposcope, biopsy forceps, a cauterizer, a specimen cup with preservative, and sterile cotton.
  C. Obtain supplies for a PAP smear, if one will be collected during the colposcopy examination.
3. Procedure:
  A. The client is placed in the lithotomy position and draped for comfort and privacy.
  B. The vagina and cervix are exposed with a speculum.
  C. Saline may be applied to the cervix, then cervical mucus is removed with acetic acid being applied, then Lugol's iodine can be applied to outline cervix abnormalities (abnormal epithelium does not contain glycogen and therefore will not stain).

  D. The colposcope is inserted, and the walls of the vagina and cervix are visually examined for color, keratinization, lesions, blood vessel structure, inflammation, atrophy, and erosion. Suspicious areas may be biopsied, and cautery or pressure is used to control bleeding.
  E. For clients with low-grade changes on a previous PAP smear, a repeat PAP smear may be taken during colposcopy.
4. Postprocedure care:
  A. Vaginal bleeding is not abnormal. Provide a sanitary pad.
5. Client and family teaching:
  A. The procedure lasts about 15 to 20 minutes and may cause slight discomfort from the vaginal speculum.
  B. A small amount of bleeding may occur because of the sampling of tissue.
  C. Immediate complications include pain and hemorrhage and secondary hemorrhage can occur up to 14 days after.
  D. Results may not be available for several days.
  E. Refrain from sexual intercourse until receiving confirmation on a follow-up visit that the biopsy site has healed.
6. Factors that affect results:
  A. Heavy menstrual flow may interfere with adequate visualization of the cervix.
7. Other data:
  A. Colposcopy is helpful in adding information about tumor extension.
  B. Annual colposcopy provides no additional benefit compared to Papanicolaou smear for detection of cervical cancer in HIV-infected females.
  C. Colposcopically directed brush cytologic testing is a safe substitute for directed biopsy in pregnant patients.

COMPANION, DIAGNOSTIC
(*see Glucose monitoring machines, Diagnostic*)

COMPLEMENT, TOTAL, SERUM (CH$_{50}$)

Norm. 75-160 U/mL (75-160 kU/L, SI units), >33% of plasma CH$_{50}$ (fraction of plasma CH$_{50}$: >0.33, SI units).

Increased. Atopic dermatitis, diabetes mellitus, jaundice (obstructive), mixed connective tissue disease, myocardial infarction (acute), rheumatoid arthritis (adult, severe), thyroiditis, ulcerative colitis, and Wegener's granulomatosis.

Decreased. Allograft rejection, cirrhosis (advanced), glomerulonephritis (poststreptococcal acute, chronic), hemolytic anemia (autoimmune), hepatitis (chronic, active), hypogammaglobulinemia, kwashiorkor, lupus nephritis, malaria, multiple myeloma, rheumatic fever, serum sickness (acute), sinusitis (*Streptococcus pneumoniae, Neisseria*), subacute bacterial endocarditis (SBE), and systemic lupus erythematosus (SLE).

Usage. Evaluate and follow up SLE client's response to therapy; screen for complement component deficiency; evaluate cases of immune complex disease, glomerulonephritis, arthritis, SBE, and cryoglobulinemia. Hypocomplementemia that accompanies some forms of renal disease may indicate immune utilization. Identification and monitoring of immune-related diseases.

Description. The complement system comprises a series of proteins that when activated serve to amplify an immune response. Activation of the complement system lends to the elaboration of potent inflammatory mediators, facilitates particle opsonization and clearance, and may result in the direct lysis of altered mammalian cells and certain bacteria. The complement system may be activated by a number of immunologic and nonimmunologic stimuli. Complement activation proceeds by either the classical or alternative pathway. (See *Complement components, Serum.*) The test for total serum complement evaluates the integrity of the complement cascade. Total complement is depressed during the active phases of

immune diseases when various individual components are significantly depressed.

Professional Considerations
1. Consent form NOT required.
2. **Preparation:**
   A. Tube: Red topped, red/gray topped, or gold topped.
3. **Procedure:**
   A. Draw a 3-mL blood sample.
   B. Leave the specimen at room temperature to clot. Then refrigerate it at 4° C for 30 minutes to 1 hour.
4. **Postprocedure care:**
   A. Send the specimen to the laboratory for immediate testing.
5. **Client and family teaching:**
   A. Results are normally available within 48 hours.
6. **Factors that affect results:**
   A. Complement is heat sensitive and deteriorates rapidly. Send the specimen to the laboratory immediately.
   B. Freeze the specimen at −70° C if it cannot be processed immediately after 1 hour of refrigeration.
7. **Other data:**
   A. Various individual components (C1-C9) may be depressed only slightly in immune disease and may not have a significant effect on the total complement level.
   B. Low CH_{50} levels tend to correlate with active phases of immune complex diseases such as SLE (especially if associated with nephritis and cases of glomerulonephritis.
   C. Decreased complement in synovial fluid may be seen with acute arthritis. Low serum complement levels occur in some clients with severe active rheumatoid factor positive arthritis and may indicate the development of vasculitis.
   D. See *C1q immune complex detection, Serum; C3 complement, Serum; C3 proactivator, Serum; C4 complement, Serum; Complement components, Serum; Complement fixation, Serum.*

COMPLEMENT COMPONENTS, SERUM

Norm:

		SI UNITS
Classical Pathway Components		
C1	70,000-200,000 U/mL	70-200 MU/L

Continued

		SI UNITS
Classical Pathway Components—cont'd		
C1q		
Adult	14.9-22.1 mg/dL	149-221 mg/L
Maternal	9-24.8 mg/dL	90-248 mg/L
Newborn	9-20 mg/dL	90-200 mg/L
C1r		
Adult	0.025-0.10 mg/mL	0.025-0.010 g/L
C1s	0.05-0.10 mg/mL	0.05-0.10 g/L
C2	1.6-3.6 mg/dL	16-36 mg/L
C4		
Adult	10-67.5 mg/dL	100-675 mg/L
Alternative Pathway Components		
Factor D	1-5 μg/dL	1-5 mg/L
C3-Proactivator		
Adult	127-278 μg/mL	127-278 mg/L
Properdin		
Adult	10-36.5 μg/mL	10-36.5 mg/L
Cord serum	8.1-23.4 μg/mL	8.1-23.4 mg/L
Regulatory Components		
C1-INH	8-24.0 mg/dL	80-240 mg/L
C4-binding protein	18-32 mg/dL	180-320 mg/L
Factor H	40.5-71.7 mg/dL	405-717 mg/L
Factor I	0.025-0.05 mg/mL	25-50 mg/L
Anaphylatoxin inactivator	30-40 μg/mL	300-400 mg/L
S-protein	(mean) 500 μg/mL	(mean) 500 mg/L
C-3 nephritic factor	Negative	Negative
Split Products		
$C3_{desArg}$	<940 ng/mL	<940 μg/L
$C4_{desArg}$	<2.8 μg/mL	<2.8 mg/L
$C5_{desArg}$	<12 ng/mL	<12 μg/L
Bb, Ba	Negative	Negative
C4d	Trace	Trace
SC5b-9	<390 μg/mL	<390 mg/L
Terminal Pathway Components		
C3		
Adult	83-177 mg/dL	0.83-1.77 g/L
Cord serum	57-116 mg/dL	0.57-1.16 g/L
6 months	74-177 mg/dL	0.74-1.77 g/L
C5		
Adult	4.8-18.5 mg/dL	48-185 mg/L
Cord serum	3.4-6.2 mg/dL	34-62 mg/L
6 months	2.4-6.4 mg/dL	24-64 g/L
C6		
Adult	28-60 μg/mL	28-60 mg/L
Cord serum	6.9-12.7 mg/dL	69-127 mg/L
C7		
Adult	27-80 μg/mL	27-80 mg/L
C8		
Adult	40-106 μg/mL	40-106 mg/L
C9		
Adult	33-250 μg/mL	33-250 mg/L

Usage. Helps diagnose immune-mediated disease and genetic complement deficiency. C1q is higher in Alzheimer's disease and C4 complement is increased in styrene occupational exposure.

Useful in acute vascular rejection, cerebral palsy, chronic renal failure, hereditary angioedema, hyperactive xenograft rejection, paroxysmal nocturnal hemoglobinuria, pemphigus vulgaris.

Description. The complement system comprises a series of proteins that, when activated, serve to amplify an immune response. Complement accounts for 10% of serum globulins. Activation of the complement system leads to the elaboration of potent inflammatory mediators, facilitates particle opsonization and clearance, and may result in the direct lysis of altered mammalian cells and foreign bacteria. The complement system may be activated by numerous immunologic and nonimmunologic stimuli. Complement activation proceeds by classical and alternative mechanisms. The components C1-C1q, C1r, C1s, C2, and C4 are activated in the classical pathway, which is stimulated when an antigen-antibody reaction occurs. Alternative pathway components, C3 proactivator, properdin, and factor D, are stimulated possibly by mechanisms other than antigen-antibody reactions. C3 and C4 levels are most often used to evaluate the integrity of the classical and alternative pathways. Levels of other individual components may be used to monitor autoimmune activity and identify a genetic deficiency of the individual component(s).

Professional Considerations
1. Consent form NOT required.
2. **Preparation:**
   A. Tube: Red topped, red/gray topped, or gold topped.
3. **Procedure:**
   A. Draw a 7-mL blood sample.
   B. Leave the specimen at room temperature to clot. Then refrigerate at 4° C for 30 minutes to 1 hour.
4. **Postprocedure care:**
   A. Write the exact specimen collection time on the laboratory requisition.
   B. Send the specimen to the laboratory, where testing should be performed immediately.

5. **Client and family teaching:**
   A. Results are normally available within 12 hours.
6. **Factors that affect results:**
   A. Complement is heat sensitive and deteriorates rapidly.
   B. Reject hemolyzed specimens or specimens received more than 2 hours after collection.
   C. Freeze the specimen at −70° C if it cannot be processed immediately after 1 hour of refrigeration.
7. **Other data:**
   A. Complement abnormalities in disease are commonly deficiencies rather than increases.
   B. Serial measurements are recommended.
   C. See *C1q immune complex detection, Serum; C3 complement, Serum; C3 proactivator, Serum; C4 complement, Serum, Complement fixation, Serum; Complement, Total, Serum.*

COMPLEMENT FIXATION (CF), SERUM

Norm. Negative test—red cell hemolysis occurs; positive test—absence of red cell hemolysis.

Positive. In the presence of antigen-antibody reactions, hepatic psittacosis, Japanese encephalitis, *Chlamydia* pneumoniae, *Mycoplasma pneumoniae*, Q fever infection, sheep or dairy farmers.

Usage. Detection of antigens, antibodies, or both, during reactions. Clinically, complement fixation is used to detect the presence of anti-DNA, immunoglobulins, and antiplatelet antibodies.

Description. CF is a two-step process based on the principle that one or more of the complement components can be fixed (used) in an antigen-antibody reaction. The test is initiated when a known amount of complement is added to the client's serum. The added complement is then fixed. The second step detects the amount of complement fixed and the proportion of antibody or antigen in the client's serum. The second step is performed when antigenic sheep red blood cells are added to the serum. The remaining unfixed complement will lyse the sheep red blood cells. Therefore lysis occurs when the complement is unfixed, an indication that the serum is deficient in either antigen or antibody. Lysis does not occur if all the complement is fixed, an indication of the presence of antigen and antibody in the serum.

Professional Considerations
1. Consent form NOT required.
2. **Preparation:**
   A. Tube: Red topped, red/gray topped, or gold topped.
3. **Procedure:**
   A. Draw a 3-mL blood sample.
4. **Postprocedure care:**
   A. None.
5. **Client and family teaching:**
   A. Two days are required for this test because the second incubation must occur overnight.

6. **Factors that affect results:**
   A. A contaminated tube may give anticomplementary results.
   B. Gonococcal vaccine may cause a false-positive gonococcal complement fixation test.
   C. Tuberculosis may cause a false-positive leishmaniasis complement fixation test.
   D. Brucellosis and Q fever may cause a false-positive psittacosis complement fixation test.
7. **Other data:**
   A. See *C1q immune complex detection, Serum; C3 complement, Serum; C3 proactivator, Serum; C4 complement, Serum; Complement components, Serum; Complement total, Serum.*

COMPLETE BLOOD COUNT (CBC), BLOOD

Norm:

		SI UNITS
Hematocrit (HCT) (Whole Blood)		
Adult Females		
18-44 years	35-45%	0.35-0.45
45-64 years	35-47%	0.35-0.47
65-74 years	35-47%	0.35-0.47
Pregnant		
Trimester 1	35-46%	0.35-0.46
Trimester 2	30-42%	0.30-0.42
Trimester 3	34-44%	0.34-0.44
Post partum	30-44%	0.30-0.44
Adult Males		
18-44 years	39-49%	0.39-0.49
45-64 years	39-50%	0.39-0.50
65-74 years	37-51%	0.37-0.51
Children		
At birth	42-68%	0.42-0.68
Cord blood	42-60%	0.42-0.60
2 weeks	41-65%	0.41-0.65
1 month	33-55%	0.33-0.55
2 months	28-42%	0.28-0.42
4 months	32-44%	0.32-0.44
6 months	31-41%	0.31-0.41
9 months	32-40%	0.32-0.40
1 year	33-41%	0.33-0.41
4 years	31-44%	0.31-0.44
6-8 years	33-41%	0.33-0.41
9-11 years	34-43%	0.34-0.43
12-14 years (male)	35-45%	0.35-0.45
12-14 years (female)	34-44%	0.34-0.44
15-17 years (male)	37-48%	0.37-0.48
15-17 years (female)	34-44%	0.34-0.44

		SI UNITS
Hemoglobin (HGB)		
Adult Females	12-16 g/dL	7.4-9.9 mmol/L
Pregnant		
Trimester 1	11.4-15.0 g/dL	7.1-9.3 mmol/L
Trimester 2	10.0-14.3 g/dL	6.2-8.9 mmol/L
Trimester 3	10.2-14.4 g/dL	6.3-8.9 mmol/L
Post partum	10.4-18.0 g/dL	6.4-9.3 mmol/L
Adult Males	14.0-18.0 g/dL	8.7-11.2 mmol/L
Panic low level	<5 g/dL	<3.1 mmol/L
Panic high level	>18 g/dL	>11.2 mmol/L
Children		
At birth	15.5-24.5 g/dL	9.6-15.2 mmol/L
12-24 hours	19.0 g/dL	11.8 mmol/L
1 week	14.3-22.3 g/dL	8.9-13.8 mmol/L
2 weeks	10.7-17.3 g/dL	6.6-10.7 mmol/L
1 month to 1 year	9.9-15.5 g/dL	6.1-9.6 mmol/L
2 years	9.0-14.6 g/dL	5.6-9.0 mmol/L
4 years	9.4-15.5 g/dL	5.8-9.6 mmol/L
8-20 years	13.4 g/dL	8.3 mmol/L
Panic levels	<5 g/dL	<3.1 mmol/L
	>18 g/dL	>11.2 mmol/L
Red Blood Cells (RBC)		
Adult Females	4.0-6.2 million/μL	$4.0\text{-}6.2 \times 10^{12}/L$
Pregnant		
Trimester 1	4.0-5.0 million/μL	$4.0\text{-}5.0 \times 10^{12}/L$
Trimester 2	3.2-4.5 million/μL	$3.2\text{-}4.5 \times 10^{12}/L$
Trimester 3	3.0-4.9 million/μL	$3.0\text{-}4.9 \times 10^{12}/L$
Post partum	3.2-5.0 million/μL	$3.2\text{-}5.0 \times 10^{12}/L$
Adult Males	4.0-6.2 million/μL	$4.0\text{-}6.2 \times 10^{12}/L$
Children		
At birth	4.1-6.1 million/μL	$4.1\text{-}6.1 \times 10^{12}/L$
1 week	5.1 million/μL	$5.1 \times 10^{12}/L$
2 weeks	3.8-5.6 million/μL	$3.8\text{-}5.6 \times 10^{12}/L$
1 month to 1 year	3.8-5.2 million/μL	$3.8\text{-}5.2 \times 10^{12}/L$
2 years	3.6-5.5 million/μL	$3.6\text{-}5.5 \times 10^{12}/L$
4 years	4.0-5.2 million/μL	$4.0\text{-}5.2 \times 10^{12}/L$
6 years	4.7 million/μL	$4.7 \times 10^{12}/L$
8-20 years	4.8 million/μL	$4.8 \times 10^{12}/L$
Mean Cell Volume (MCV)		
Adults	82-93 μm³	82-93 fL
Children		
At birth	106 μm³	106 fL
12-24 hours	105 μm³	105 fL
1 week	103 μm³	103 fL
2 weeks	90 μm³	90 fL
1 month to 1 year	82-88 μm³	82-88 fL
2 years	77 μm³	77 fL
4 years	80 μm³	80 fL
11-15 years	82 μm³	82 fL

Continued

		SI UNITS
Mean Cell Hemoglobin (MCH)		
Adults	26-34 pg	1.61-2.11 fmol
Children		
At birth	38 pg	2.36 fmol
12-24 hours	38 pg	2.36 fmol
1 week	36 pg	2.23 fmol
2 weeks	33 pg	2.05 fmol
1 month to 1 year	26 pg	1.61 fmol
2 years	25 pg	1.55 fmol
4 years	26 pg	1.61 fmol
6 years	27 pg	1.67 fmol
8-20 years	28 pg	1.73 fmol
Mean Cell Hemoglobin Concentration (MCHC)		
Adults	31-38%	19.2-23.58 mmol/L
Children		
At birth	36%	22.34 mmol/L
1 week	34%	21.10 mmol/L
2 weeks	33%	20.48 mmol/L
1 month to 1 year	33-34%	20.48-21.10 mmol/L
2 years	32%	19.86 mmol/L
4 years	35%	21.72 mmol/L
6 years	34%	21.10 mmol/L
8-20 years	34%	21.10 mmol/L
White Blood Cells (WBC)		
Adult Females	4500-11,000/µL	$4.5\text{-}11.0 \times 10^9$L
Pregnant		
Trimester 1	6600-14,100/µL	$6.6\text{-}14.1 \times 10^9$L
Trimester 2	6900-17,100/µL	$6.9\text{-}17.1 \times 10^9$L
Trimester 3	5900-14,700/µL	$5.9\text{-}14.7 \times 10^9$L
Postpartum	9700-25,700/µL	$9.7\text{-}25.7 \times 10^9$L
Adult Males	4500-11,000/µL	$4.5\text{-}11.0 \times 10^9$L
Children		
At birth	9000-30,000/µL	$9.0\text{-}30.0 \times 10^9$L
1 month to 1 year	6000-17,500/µL	$6.0\text{-}17.5 \times 10^9$L
4 years	5700-16,300/µL	$5.7\text{-}16.3 \times 10^9$L
8-20 years	4500-13,500/µL	$4.5\text{-}13.5 \times 10^9$L
Differential White Blood Cells—Granulocytes:		
Segmented Neutrophils (Segs)	54-62%	0.54-0.62
Adults	3800/µL or mm^3	3800×10^6/L
Children		
At birth	8400/µL or mm^3	8400×10^6/L
12-24 hours	8870-12,100/µL or mm^3	$8870\text{-}12,100 \times 10^6$/L
1 week	4100/µL or mm^3	4100×10^6/L
2 weeks	3320/µL or mm^3	3320×10^6/L
1 month to 1 year	2680-2750/µL or mm^3	$2680\text{-}2750 \times 10^6$/L
2 years	2660/µL or mm^3	2660×10^6/L
4 years	3040/µL or mm^3	3040×10^6/L
6 years	3600/µL or mm^3	3600×10^6/L
8-20 years	3700-3800/µL or mm^3	$3700\text{-}3800 \times 10^6$/L
Band Neutrophils (Bands)	3-5%	0.03-0.05
Adults	620/µL or mm^3	620×10^6/L

		SI UNITS

Differential White Blood Cells—Granulocytes—cont'd

Band Neutrophils (Bands)—cont'd

Children

At birth	2540/µL or mm^3	2540 × 10^6/L
12-24 hours	2680-3460/µL or mm^3	2680-3460 × 10^6/L
1 week	1420/µL or mm^3	1420 × 10^6/L
2 weeks	1200/µL or mm^3	1200 × 10^6/L
1 month to 1 year	990-1150/µL or mm^3	990-1150 × 10^6/L
2 years	850/µL or mm^3	850 × 10^6/L
4 years	710/µL or mm^3	710 × 10^6/L
6 years	670/µL or mm^3	670 × 10^6/L
8-20 years	620-660/µL or mm^3	620-660 × 10^6/L

Eosinophils (Eos) — 1-3% — 0.01-0.03

Adults	200/µL or mm^3	200 × 10^6/L
Children		
At birth	400/µL or mm^3	400 × 10^6/L
12-24 hours	450/µL or mm^3	450 × 10^6/L
1 week	500/µL or mm^3	500 × 10^6/L
2 weeks	350/µL or mm^3	350 × 10^6/L
1 month–1 year	300/µL or mm^3	300 × 10^6/L
2 years	280/µL or mm^3	280 × 10^6/L
4 years	250/µL or mm^3	250 × 10^6/L
6 years	230/µL or mm^3	230 × 10^6/L
8-20 years	200/µL or mm^3	200 × 10^6/L

Basophils (Basos) — 0-0.75% — 0-0.0075

Adults	40/µL or mm^3	40 × 10^6/L
Children		
At birth–24 hours	100/µL or mm^3	100 × 10^6/L
1 week–6 years	50/µL or mm^3	50 × 10^6/L
8-20 years	40/µL or mm^3	40 × 10^6/L

Monocytes (Monos) — 3-7% — 0.03-0.07

Adults	300/µL or mm^3	300 × 10^6/L
Children		
At birth	1050/µL or mm^3	1050 × 10^6/L
12-24 hours	1100-1200/µL or mm^3	1100-1200 × 10^6/L
1 week	1100/µL or mm^3	1100 × 10^6/L
2 weeks	1000/µL or mm^3	1000 × 10^6/L
1 month to 1 year	700/µL or mm^3	700 × 10^6/L
2 years	530/µL or mm^3	530 × 10^6/L
4 years	450/µL or mm^3	450 × 10^6/L
6 years	400/µL or mm^3	400 × 10^6/L
8-20 years	350-400/µL or mm^3	350-400 × 10^6/L

Lymphocytes (Lymphs) — 25-33% — 0.25-0.33

Adults	2500/µL or mm^3	2500 × 10^6/L
Children		
At birth	5500/µL or mm^3	5500 × 10^6/L
12-24 hours	5800/µL or mm^3	5800 × 10^6/L
1 week	5000/µL or mm^3	5000 × 10^6/L
2 weeks	5500/µL or mm^3	5500 × 10^6/L
1 month to 1 year	6000-7000/µL or mm^3	6000-7000 × 10^6/L
2 years	6300/µL or mm^3	6300 × 10^6/L
4 years	4500/µL or mm^3	4500 × 10^6/L
6 years	3500/µL or mm^3	3500 × 10^6/L
8-20 years	2500-3300/µL or mm^3	2500-3300 × 10^6/L

Continued

		SI UNITS
Platelets (Plt)		
Adults	150,000-400,000/µL or mm^3	150-400 × 10^9/L
Panic levels	<30,000/µL or mm^3	<30 × 10^9/L
	>1,000,000/µL or mm^3	>1000 × 10^9/L
Children		
At birth	100,000-300,000/µL or mm^3	100-300 × 10^9/L
1 week	260,000/µL or mm^3	260 × 10^9/L
2 years	250,000/µL or mm^3	250 × 10^9/L
Panic levels	<20,000/µL or mm^3	<20 × 10^9/L
	>1,000,000/µL or mm^3	>1000 × 10^9/L

Increased. See individual test listings.

Decreased. See individual test listings.

Description. The complete blood count (CBC) consists of several tests that allow for the evaluation of different cellular components of the blood on a broad range of clients. The items commonly evaluated include hemoglobin, hematocrit, red blood cells, red blood cell indices, white blood cells, white blood cell differential, platelets, and microscopic examination of stained blood smears. Normal levels of the different blood components vary among different age groups, depending on the body's needs and composition (see *Norms,* above). The CBC is used for physical examinations, preoperative screening, and evaluation of acute disease or symptoms of anemia or infection. Serial values are often used to track the progress of a variety of diseases and to monitor for side effects resulting from acute or chronic use of drugs that may cause blood dyscrasias. See individual test listings as follows for detailed descriptions of CBC components: *Blood indices, Blood; Differential leukocyte count, Peripheral blood; Hematocrit, Blood; Hemoglobin, Blood; Platelet count, Blood; Red blood cell, Blood.*

Professional Considerations
1. Consent form NOT required.
2. **Preparation:**
   A. Tube: Lavender topped.
   B. Do NOT draw during dialysis.
3. **Procedure:**
   A. To avoid a hemodiluted sample, draw the sample from an extremity that does not have intravenous fluids infusing into it. Leaving the tourniquet in place no longer than 60 seconds, completely fill the tube with a venous blood sample.

Invert and gently rotate the tube to thoroughly mix the anticoagulant.
4. **Postprocedure care:**
   A. Write the specimen collection time on the laboratory requisition.
5. **Client and family teaching:**
   A. See individual test listings.
   B. Results are normally available within 4 hours.
6. **Factors that affect results:**
   A. Failure to fill the tube completely with blood causes an improper blood–anticoagulant ratio, which yields unreliable values.
   B. The serum sample is stable at room temperature for 10 hours, may be refrigerated for up to 18 hours, and should not be frozen.
   C. See also individual test listings.
7. **Other data:**
   A. See individual test listings.

COMPLEXED PSA, SERUM
(*see Prostate-Specific Antigen, Serum*)

COMPREHENSIVE METABOLIC PANEL (CMP), BLOOD

Norm. See individual test listings: *Albumin, Alkaline phosphatase, Aspartate aminotransferase, Bicarbonate, Bilirubin (Total), Calcium, Chloride, Creatinine, Glucose, Potassium, Protein (Total), Sodium,* and *Urea nitrogen.*

Usage. See individual test listings.

Description. The CMP is a term defined by The Centers for Medicare and Medicaid Services (CMS) in the United States to indicate a group of tests for which a bundled reimbursement is available. The panel is one of several that replace the multichannel tests, such as SMA-20. The panel is disease oriented, meaning that payment through Medicare is available only when the test is used to diagnose and monitor a disease, and payment is not available when the test is used for screening purposes in clients who have no signs and symptoms. All the tests in the panel must be carried out when a BMP is ordered.

Professional Considerations

1. Consent form NOT required.
2. Preparation:
   A. Tube: Red topped, red/gray topped, or gold topped.
   B. Do NOT draw specimens during hemodialysis.
3. Procedure:
   A. Draw a 5-mL blood sample.
4. Postprocedure care:
   A. None.
5. Client and family teaching:
   A. See individual test listings.
6. Factors that affect results:
   A. See individual test listings.
7. Other data:
   A. See individual test listings.

COMPRESSION ULTRASOUND (CUS), DIAGNOSTIC

Norm. Negative.

Usage. Used in conjunction with rapid ELISA D-dimer testing to assess the probability of existence of venous thrombi. Monitoring for occurrence of deep vein thrombosis in high-risk populations.

Description. Compression ultrasound (CUS) is a noninvasive diagnostic tool that has largely replaced venography (phlebography), which is the criterion standard for diagnosis of venous thrombosis. In this procedure, the transducer pressure is applied to collapse the vein being scanned. A normal vessel will collapse completely, whereas a vessel with a thrombosis will not. Although CUS poses less procedural risk than venography, it is most accurate for the detection of proximal deep vein thromboses, which occur in 85% of clients with deep vein thrombosis (DVT), and which are the source of life-threatening pulmonary emboli. However, CUS often does not identify thromboses of the calf vein(s), is unreliable in determining the patency of the pelvic veins and inferior vena cava, and is not sensitive to asymptomatic postoperative DVT. To compensate for its limitations, the CUS is often followed by a color duplex ultrasound. CUS is not indicated in non-hospitalized patients with a low clinical score for risk of DVT, if a negative D-dimer test result has been obtained. For those with moderate or higher clinical risk scores and a negative D-dimer result, the CUS is recommended. Any positive CUS confirms DVT. Michiels et al (2002) found that "the combination of a negative CUS and a negative rapid ELISA D-dimer test safely excludes DVT in patients with suspected DVT irrespective of the clinical score." Frequent involvement of both limbs suggest the use of this procedure bilaterally.

Clinical Score (Outpatients)	Risk of DVT	Rapid ELISA D-Dimer Test	CUS	Implications
Low	3-10%	Negative	N/A	Negative predictive value >99.9% to exclude DVT
Low		Positive <1000 ng/mL	Negative	Negative predictive value >99% to exclude DVT
Moderate	15-30%	Negative	Negative	Negative predictive value >99.4% to exclude DVT
Moderate	15-30%	Positive	Negative	Probability of DVT of 3-5%. Repeat CUS recommended.
High	>70%	Not recommended	Negative	Probability of DVT of 20-30%. Repeat CUS recommended.

Michiels, et al (2002)

Professional Considerations

1. Consent form is NOT required.
2. Preparation:
   A. This test may be done at the bedside.
   B. Obtain a 3-7 Mhz (for adults) 5-7 Mhz (for children) linear transducer.
3. Procedure:
   A. Establish a baseline for comparison by evaluating the asymptomatic extremity.
   B. Both non-compression and compression views are taken, beginning at the groin and proceeding distally down the common femoral vein, superficial femoral vein and popliteal vein. Transverse views are taken both without and with augmentation at each of these vessels, followed by longitudinal views via spectral and color Doppler.
   C. Repeat on the affected extremity, adding visualization of the iliac veins and inferior vena cava in the pelvis.
   D. Follow with color duplex ultrasonography if further visualization of the pelvic veins and inferior vena cava is needed.
4. Postprocedure care:
   A. Cleanse ultrasound gel off of skin.
5. Client and family teaching:
   A. This test is painless and noninvasive.
   B. Test takes about 20 minutes to complete.
   C. Radionuclide imaging may follow inconclusive tests.
6. Factors that affect results:
   A. CUS results may be positive for up to 6 months after an acute DVT.
   B. The skill of the operator affects the accuracy of the results.
7. Other data:
   A. The clinical score for determination of probability for DVT is a clinical model of complaints, signs, and symptoms, which has been found to be valid for estimating low, moderate, and high probability (Wells et al, 1995).

COMPUTED TOMOGRAPHIC PERCUTANEOUS TRANSSPLENIC PORTOGRAPHY (CT-PTSP)

(see Splenoportography, Diagnostic)

COMPUTED TOMOGRAPHY OF THE BODY (SPIRAL [HELICAL], ELECTRON BEAM, [EBCT, ULTRAFAST], HIGH RESOLUTION [HRCT]), DIAGNOSTIC

Norm. Negative. No tumor, malformations, or pathologic activity.

EBCT Norm. No coronary artery stenosis, no pulmonary embolism. EBCT has the potential to replace ventilation-perfusion scanning as the primary screening diagnostic test for pulmonary emboli.

Traditional CT Usage. Determination of the extent of primary and secondary neoplasms of the neck; evaluation of bony and inflammatory abnormalities of the spine and joints, including neoplasms, fractures, dislocations, and congenital anomalies; localization of foreign bodies in the soft tissues, hypopharynx, or larynx; and assessment of airway integrity after trauma; evaluation of retropharyngeal abscesses; investigation of suspected tracheal, thymic, mediastinal, and hilar masses; evaluation of problems identified on chest radiographics; staging of bronchogenic carcinoma and gastrointestinal tumors; detection of aortic aneurysm or aortic dissection; detection, localization, and characterization of lung disease; detection of mediastinal or diaphragmatic herniation; evaluation of musculoskeletal or soft-tissue trauma or neoplasms; evaluation of suspected congenital or other abnormalities of specific body organs such as the liver, gallbladder, pancreas, kidneys, adrenal gland, and spleen; identification and localization of sites of hemorrhage; assessment of the organs and structures of the peritoneal cavity and pelvis; and sometimes used to provide imaging identification and guidance for invasive procedures such as abscess drainage or amebic liver abscess, percutaneous biopsy, or aspirate for cytologic or histologic study.

EBCT Usage. Used with contrast for imaging the coronary arteries and coronary artery bypass grafts, and for diagnosis of aortic malformations and diseases, pulmonary emboli and other lung diseases, and for quantifying ventricular mass and volume. Used primarily in asymptomatic clients who have risk factors for heart disease.

Spiral CT Usage. Procedure of choice for lung evaluations for cancer; over 90% sensitive and specific for pulmonary embolism, except when subsegmental emboli are found; superior to ultrasonography for detection of deep venous thrombosis; 100% sensitive and 98% specific for detection of aortic injury; 80-85% sensitive for detection of metastatic liver disease; Rapid evaluation for ischemic stroke; Preferred CT method for children due to reduced length of radiation exposure and reduced dose of contrast material. Spiral CT equipment often is selected as a replacement for older CT equipment; thus, usage would be as described above for traditional CT.

High Resolution CT Usage. Procedure of choice for lung evaluations for chronic infiltrative lung diseases, and for vascular evaluations, such as brain imaging for vascular malformations.

Description. *Computed tomography (CT)* is a radiographic scan that may be performed with or without contrast on virtually any portion of the body. CT is classified as a reconstructive imaging procedure because it produces a picture of the contents of a portion of the body based on the differing densities and composition of body tissues. The picture is obtained by projection of x rays along all possible lines in the plane of the body. An x-ray detector records the intensity of the x rays from multiple angles as it is transmitted through the tissue. A computer then reconstructs the differing intensities into pixels that appear in differing shades for differing tissues and represent an anterior-to-posterior "slice" across the plane of the body. CT is used to detect very minor differences in radiographic contrast, providing radiography that portrays boundaries between tissues that are normally indistinguishable to radiographic examination. The tissue-contrast differentiation of CT is superior to that of conventional radiography.

Electron Beam CT (EBCT, Ultrafast CT) was developed specifically for evaluating the heart and other structures in the chest, such as the lungs and blood vessels. This type of CT uses an electron beam magnetically directed to can take a rapid sequence of images at the speed of light, thus providing detailed information about how the heart functions throughout the cardiac cycle. Because the images can be taken so quickly, the test takes less time than a regular CT. EBCT can detect plaques, and stenosis and can also detect minute amounts of calcific deposits, which can progress to coronary artery lesions.

Spiral (also called helical) CT, first available in the early 1990s, is an improvement in the CT technology that provides much improved resolution in a much shorter time than older CT imaging methods. Spiral CT enables the collection of multiple overlapping pictures taken in a continuous spiral pattern that can be fused to give a 3-dimensional picture of the body. Because of the continuous nature of the imaging, fewer contrast material is needed, and the procedure takes only a few minutes.

High Resolution CT (HRCT) improves on traditional CT technology by providing optimized spatial resolution of body structures and better differentiation of normal from abnormal blood vessels.

The newest equipment called *"Dual Modality Imaging"* combines CT with functional imaging modalities such as PET or SPECT for improved imaging results. (See *Dual Modality Imaging, Diagnostic.*)

Professional Considerations

1. Consent form IS required if contrast material will be injected.

Risks

Allergic reaction to dye (itching, hives, rash, tight feeling in the throat, shortness of breath, bronchospasm, anaphylaxis, death); renal toxicity; hematoma or infection at the injection site for CT with contrast.

Contraindications

CT with contrast: Previous allergy to iodine, shellfish, or radiographic dye; renal insufficiency. CT is contraindicated in clients who are unable to lie motionless.

Precautions

During pregnancy, risks of cumulative radiation exposure to the fetus from these and other previous or future imaging studies must be weighed against the benefits of the procedures. Although formal limits for client exposure are relative to this risk: benefit comparison, the United States Nuclear Regulatory Commission requires that the cumulative dose equivalent to an embryo/fetus from occupational exposure not exceed 0.5 rem (5 mSv). Radiation dosage to the fetus is proportional to the distance of the anatomy studied from the abdomen and decreases as pregnancy progresses. An abdominal CT (10-slice) exposes the first trimester fetus to 2.6 rad, but the week 35 fetus to only 1.7 rad. For pregnant clients, consult the Radiologist/Radiology Department to obtain estimated fetal radiation exposure from these procedures.

2. **Preparation:**
   A. For CT with contrast, see *Client and family teaching.*
   B. Remove radiopaque objects such as jewelry, snaps, and electrocardiographic leads with snaps (if possible).
   C. Establish intravenous access for injection of the dye and prepare emergency equipment for a possible hypersensitivity reaction.
   D. Obtain radiographic contrast medium, if the procedure will be performed with contrast.
   E. Have emergency equipment readily available if the procedure will be performed with contrast.
3. **Procedure:**
   A. The client is positioned supine, with his or her head secured and resting on a headrest on a motorized handling table. For spinal studies, the lumbar spine is straightened by flexing the knees and providing a footrest.
   B. The client must lie motionless as the table slowly advances through the circular opening of the scanner. The CT scanner sends a narrow beam of x rays across the area to be imaged in a linear fashion. While a client is being scanned, the nonabsorbed x rays are detected at the same time as the beam is transmitting. This linear scan sequence is repeated at many different angles around the client's body. The data collected consist of a series of profiles that reflect the area visualized at different angles.
   C. If contrast medium is to be used, it is injected intravenously at this time, and the scan is repeated. The client is observed for rash or respiratory difficulty, which may indicate reaction to the contrast medium. Reactions usually develop within 30 minutes if the client is allergic to the dye.
   D. For Ultrafast and Spiral CT, the client may be asked to hold his/her breath for short periods of time. Operating in the multislice scan mode, the scanner takes several pictures as the table is advanced by a 2-mm step.
4. **Postprocedure care:**
   A. Replace the electrocardiographic (ECG) leads if they were removed.
   B. For CT with contrast, observe for side effects such as headache, nausea, and vomiting. Resume previous diet if no side effects have been noted.
5. **Client and family teaching:**
   A. You must lie motionless during the scan. Because this can be a frightening test, it should be described carefully to the client before he or she enters the CT room.
   B. If contrast medium will be used, fast from food and fluids for 4 hours before the CT scan.
   C. For Ultrafast and Spiral CT imaging, you will have to hold breath for several seconds.
   D. A sensation of burning may be felt from the injection of the contrast medium.
6. **Factors that affect results:**
   A. Unavoidable internal motion of body organs such as the heart and lungs or intentional movement by the client contributes to the appearance of "tuning-fork"-like streaks across the picture.
   B. Radiopaque objects such as jewelry and snaps obscure visualization.
   C. The literature contains differing opinions concerning findings of segmental emboli cloud when pulmonary embolus is suspected.
7. **Other data:**
   A. For chest examinations the average breast dose from EBCT was comparable to that of conventional CT scanners, despite differences in dose distribution.

B. EBCT has the potential to replace ventilation-perfusion scanning as the primary screening diagnostic test for pulmonary emboli.

C. See also *Cerebral computed tomography, Diagnostic; Chest tomography, Diagnostic.*

COMPUTED TOMOGRAPHY OF THE BRAIN, DIAGNOSTIC
(see Cerebral computed tomography, Diagnostic)

CONCENTRATION TEST, URINE

Norm:

		SI UNITS
Specific gravity	1.025-1.032	1.025-1.032
Osmolality	>800 mOsm/kg of water	>800 mmol/kg of water

Increased. Dehydration.

Decreased. Congestive heart failure, diabetes insipidus, Fanconi syndrome, hydronephrosis, hypercalcemia, hypokalemia, hypoproteinemia, nephrogenic diabetes insipidus, polycystic kidneys, pyelonephritis (chronic), and sickle cell trait. Drugs include diuretics.

Description. The urine concentration test is an evaluation of renal capacity to concentrate urine in response to fluid deprivation or to dilute the urine in response to fluid overload. Urine specific gravity and osmolality are measured after mild hypernatremia is induced by 12 hours of fluid restriction and deprivation. This test is used to detect renal impairment and evaluate renal tubular function. It is also used to differentiate deficiency of antidiuretic hormone (ADH) from renal insensitivity to ADH. In clients with normal renal function and diabetes insipidus (caused by ADH deficiency), administration of exogenous ADH causes urine osmolality to increase. In clients with renal insensitivity to ADH (nephrogenic diabetes insipidus), the exogenous ADH does not cause an increase in urine osmolality.

Professional Considerations
1. Consent form NOT required.

Risks
Hypotension and associated sequelae.

Contraindications
This test may be contraindicated in clients with subnormal cardiac output because of the risk of depleting plasma volume.

2. **Preparation:**
A. See *Client and family teaching.*
B. Obtain baseline weight before the evening meal before the test and every 4 hours until the test is completed. Terminate the test if weight decreases more than 5% from the baseline weight or for orthostatic hypotension.
C. Obtain three 500-mL clean containers.
D. Monitor the client closely throughout the test for symptoms of severe dehydration or for surreptitious intake of fluids.

3. **Procedure:**
A. Collect the entire voided urine specimens in separate, refrigerated, clean containers at 0600 (6 AM), 0800 (8 AM), and 1000 (10 AM). Record the exact time and amount of each specimen.
B. If the test is being performed to differentiate diabetes insipidus from nephrogenic diabetes insipidus, exogenous ADH (vasopressin) is administered intravenously as soon as a plateau in osmolality is reached. A final urine sample is collected, as above, in 1 hour.

4. **Postprocedure care:**
A. Resume diet and fluids.
B. Record the time and amount of each specimen collected on the laboratory requisition.
C. Refrigerate the specimens until testing.

5. **Client and family teaching:**
A. Eat a high-protein dinner the day before the test.
B. Fluids are restricted to 200 mL the evening before the test, including the evening meal.

C. Fast from food and fluids from midnight before the test until the test is completed.

D. It is normal to feel very thirsty during the testing period, but you should not drink anything.

6. **Factors that affect results:**
   A. Failure to follow dietary and fluid restrictions will interfere with results.
   B. Fluid intake over 200 mL caused by intravenous therapy invalidates the results.
   C. Administration of radiographic dyes within 7 days before the test may cause increased urine osmolality.
   D. Baseline glucosuria invalidates the results.

7. **Other data:**
   A. None.

4. **Postprocedure care:**
   A. Place the swab in the transport medium according to the requirements of the laboratory performing the test.
   B. Send the swab immediately to the laboratory.

5. **Client and family teaching:**
   A. Refer the client with positive results for follow-up care, which is necessary for prevention and early detection of sequelae.

6. **Factors that affect results:**
   A. Results are invalidated if the swab dries out before being inoculated onto culture medium or before preparation of a smear.

7. **Other data:**
   A. Condyloma of the toe web is an unusual manifestation of secondary syphilis.

CONDYLOMA LATUM, VULVAR OR ANAL CULTURE FOR CYTOLOGY, SPECIMEN

Norm. Negative findings.

Description. Condyloma latum is a flat, moist, papular growth that appears on the moist skin of the genital and anal areas during the secondary stages of syphilis. It is also called flat condyloma.

Professional Considerations
1. Consent form NOT required.
2. **Preparation:**
   A. Verify the collection procedure with the individual laboratory performing the test. Smears may be required to be prepared and fixed at the bedside.
   B. Obtain sterile cotton swabs or Culturette, gloves, and transport medium.
3. **Procedure:**
   A. *Vulvar sample:* Wipe the vulva with sterile cotton or gauze. Insert a sterile, cotton-tipped swab between the vulva and leave it in place for several seconds for optimum absorption of pathogens.
   B. *Anal sample:* Insert a sterile, cotton-tipped swab into the anus approximately 2 cm. Leave the swab in place several seconds for optimum absorption of pathogens. If feces are obtained, discard the swab and repeat the procedure.

CONIZATION OF CERVIX (COLD KNIFE CONIZATION), DIAGNOSTIC

Norm. Negative. No abnormal findings.

Usage. Follow-up study for abnormal Pap smear; atypical squamous cells of undetermined significance (ASCUS); carcinoma in situ; cervical cancer, cervical intraepithelial neoplasia (CIN); used when colposcopy, cervical cytology, and colposcopy biopsies yield inconclusive findings.

Description. Conization is a biopsy of the uterine cervix that is performed after cervical smears reveal the presence of intraepithelial neoplasias. It may be performed with dilatation and curettage. The advantage that conization brings to the diagnostic process is that it provides a sample of the entire lateral margins of the transformation zone of the cervix. Cold knife conization is less expensive than laser conization and produces equally satisfactory specimens for histologic examination. The cold knife method may also be superior to the loop electrosurgical excisional procedure (LEEP) because it does not produce electrocautery artifact that interferes with examination of the cervical margins.

Professional Considerations
1. Consent form IS required.

Risks
Hemorrhage, infection, sepsis.

Contraindications
Anticoagulant therapy, bleeding disorders, thrombocytopenia. Sedatives are contraindicated in clients with central nervous system depression.

2. **Preparation:**
   A. See *Client and family teaching.*
   B. Preschedule this test with the pathology laboratory. Biopsy specimens must be processed immediately.
   C. Obtain Lugol's solution, a tenaculum, vasopressin, conization knife, suture material, Gelfoam or Surgicel (or electrocautery), and a sterile container.
3. **Procedure:**
   A. This procedure can be performed under general anesthesia, though local anesthesia is less costly and has little discomfort, nausea, or vomiting.
   B. The client is placed in a lithotomy position, and the cervix is painted with Lugol's solution (Schiller's test) to detect white, pale, or unstained areas, which may indicate lesions.
   C. A suture may be sewn on each side of the cervix to control bleeding. The anterior lip of the cervix is lifted with a tenaculum, and vasopressin (Pitressin Synthetic) is injected into several areas to control bleeding.
   D. A cone of tissue is removed from the cervical os with a cold knife (Fleming knife). Tissues that did not stain with Schiller's test are included in the cone. The specimen is transferred immediately to the laboratory in a sterile container, with or without sterile saline, according to the requirements of the laboratory performing the test.
   E. Bleeding may be controlled by packing with Gelfoam or Surgicel or by cervical sutures or electrocautery.
4. **Postprocedure care:**
   A. Provide sanitary pads and observe for heavy bleeding, which is abnormal.
   B. Perform standard postanesthesia observations and assessments if

general anesthesia or deep sedation was used.
5. **Client and family teaching:**
   A. If general anesthesia will be used, fast from food and fluids for 8 hours before the procedure.
   B. A greenish-grayish discharge from the vagina caused by the presence of the Lugol's solution is normal for several days after the test.
   C. Resume previous diet after the procedure.
6. **Factors that affect results:**
   A. Electrocautery should not be used because it distorts tissues and impairs diagnosis.
7. **Other data:**
   A. Conization should be performed in a hospital, rather than in a physician's office.
   B. Conization should be performed before dilatation and curettage, which dislodges the cervical epithelium.
   C. Residual dysplasia present in cold knife conization specimens is not predictive of residual dysplasia in hysterectomy specimens.
   D. Residual carcinoma in situ can be present even with a negative conization margin.

CONJUNCTIVAE, ROUTINE, CULTURE

Norm. No abnormal growth. Normal flora includes diphtheroids, *Staphylococcus epidermidis*, Staphylococcus pyogenes, Streptococcus pneumoniae, and *Streptococcus viridans.*

Usage. Used to establish the presence of bacterial or viral pathogens causing blepharitis, chalazion, conjunctivitis, impetigo, and stye.

Description. Conjunctivitis is an inflammation of the eye conjunctiva most commonly caused by staphylococci, nonserotypable *Streptococcus pneumoniae, Chlamydia* (causing inclusion conjunctivitis), rickettsiae, viruses, or parasites. Less commonly, the conjunctiva may be infected by *Gonococcus* and may possibly lead to blindness. Conjunctivitis may also result from allergic processes or injury to the eye. Symptoms of conjunctivitis include redness, swelling, drainage, and itching.

This condition is commonly diagnosed by culture and Gram staining or Wright staining of the drainage from the lower part of the conjunctiva.

Professional Considerations
1. Consent form NOT required.
2. Preparation:
   A. Cleanse the skin around the eye.
   B. Obtain an eye swab approved for microbiologic purposes and culture tube (Culturette).
3. Procedure:
   A. Gently but firmly, wipe a sterile, cotton-tipped swab over the inflamed lower conjunctiva or inner canthus, avoiding the eyelashes.
   B. Insert the swab into a Culturette tube and squeeze the ampule of medium.
   C. If the specimen will be tested for *Gonococcus* (most commonly in newborns), place the swab in a Transgrow bottle, not a Culturette tube.
4. Postprocedure care:
   A. Write the antibiotic therapy on the laboratory requisition.
   B. Send the swab to the laboratory immediately.
5. Client and family teaching:
   A. Where inflammation is present, the swab technique may cause transient pain.
   B. Wash hands after touching conjunctival area to avoid spread of infection to others.
6. Factors that affect results:
   A. Results are invalidated if the specimen dries out before being inoculated onto culture medium or before preparation of a slide for staining.
7. Other data:
   A. The best results are obtained if the culture is taken before antibiotic therapy is started.
   B. Candidal blepharitis is often found in immunosuppressed clients.
   C. Ciprofloxacin 0.3% ophthalmic solution is effective treatment for keratitis and conjunctivitis. About 8% of conjunctivitis is resistant to ciprofloxacin.

CONJUNCTIVAL IMPRESSION CYTOLOGY, SPECIMEN
(see Ocular Cytology, Specimen)

CONNECTING PEPTIDE, SERUM
(see C-Peptide, Serum)

CONTRACTION STRESS TEST (CST), DIAGNOSTIC
(see Fetal monitoring, External, Contraction stress test [CST] and Oxytocin challenge test [OCT], Diagnostic)

CONTRAST VENOGRAPHY
(see Venography, Diagnostic)

COOMBS' TEST, DIRECT (DIRECT ANTIGLOBULIN TEST), SERUM

Norm. Negative.

Positive. Arthritis (rheumatoid), elderly clients, erythroblastosis fetalis, hemolytic anemia (autoimmune, drug induced), infection, neoplasm, renal disorders, systemic lupus erythematosus, and transfusion reaction. Drugs include (possibly as a result of IgG erythrocyte sensitization by the drugs) aminopyrine, cephalosporins, chlorpromazine, dipyrone, ethosuximide, hydralazine hydrochloride, insulin, isoniazid, levodopa, mefenamic acid, melphalan, methyldopa, methyldopate hydrochloride, oxyphenisatin, para-aminosalicylic acid, penicillins, phenacetin, phenytoin, phenytoin sodium, procainamide hydrochloride, quinidine gluconate, quinidine polygalacturonate, quinidine sulfate, rifampin, streptomycin sulfate, sulfonamides, tetracyclines and Unasyn (ampicillin sodium plus sulbactam sodium).

Negative. Hemolytic anemia (nonautoimmune, non drug induced). Normal finding.

Usage. Used to show antigen-antibody reactions, differentiation of types of hemolytic anemias, testing for suspected erythroblastosis fetalis, and investigation of erythrocyte sensitization by drugs or blood transfusions.

Description. The direct Coombs' test involves adding Coombs' antihuman globulin serum to a client's washed red blood cells and observing for agglutination, which signals the presence of previously undetected IgG antibodies, complement, or immunoglobulins on the surfaces of the client's erythrocytes. The Coombs' antiglobulin contains antibodies to IgG and several complement components. The antibodies detected by the direct Coombs' test are difficult to detect any other way because they are left over from incomplete antigen-antibody reactions and, though present on the erythrocyte surfaces, remain invisible. The Coombs' antiglobulin causes completion of the antigen-antibody reaction, thus making the antibodies identifiable as they begin clumping.

Professional Considerations
1. Consent form NOT required.
2. Preparation:
   A. Tube: Lavender topped, red topped, red/gray topped, or gold topped.
3. Procedure:
   A. Draw a 7-mL blood sample.
   B. The sample may be obtained from cord blood.
4. Postprocedure care:
   A. Write recent transfusions and drugs on the laboratory requisition.
5. Client and family teaching:
   A. For positive results, the more specific direct Coombs' IgG test is indicated.
6. Factors that affect results:
   A. Reject hemolyzed specimens.
   B. Cord blood contaminated by Wharton's jelly may yield unreliable results.
   C. Cold agglutinins may cause false-positive results.
   D. Drugs that may cause false-negative results in the presence of acquired hemolytic anemia include heparin calcium and heparin sodium.
7. Other data:
   A. This test does not delineate the nature of the antibodies identified.
   B. The test must be completed within 24 hours of specimen collection.
   C. There is a high incidence of positive results in clients with antibodies to HIV, which indicates that this test may be helpful as a prognostic indicator for the disease course.
   D. See also *Antibody identification, Red cell, Serum.*

COOMBS' TEST, DIRECT IgG, SERUM

Norm. Negative.

Positive. Anemia (hemolytic, drug induced), autoimmune hepatitis, erythroblastosis fetalis, leukemia (chronic lymphocytic), and transfusion reaction. Drugs include (possibly as a result of IgG erythrocyte sensitization by the drugs) aminopyrine, cephalosporins, chlorpromazine, dipyrone, ethosuximide, hydralazine, hydrochloride, insulin, isoniazid, levodopa, mefenamic acid, melphalan, methyldopa, methyldopate hydrochloride, oxyphenisatin, *para*-aminosalicylic acid, penicillins, phenacetin, phenytoin, phenytoin sodium, procainamide hydrochloride, quinidine gluconate, quinidine polygalacturonate, quinidine sulfate, rifampin, streptomycin sulfate, sulfonamides, and tetracyclines.

Description. See *Coombs' test, Direct, Serum.* This test is more specific than a direct Coombs' test and is performed after a positive direct Coombs' test. The direct Coombs' IgG test mixes Coombs' antiglobulin containing only anti-IgG with the client's washed red blood cells and observing for agglutination, which signals the presence of IgG on the surface of the client's erythrocytes.

Professional Considerations
1. Consent form NOT required.
2. Preparation:
   A. Tube: Lavender topped.
3. Procedure:
   A. Draw a 7-mL blood sample.
4. Postprocedure care:
   A. Write recent transfusions and drugs on the laboratory requisition.
5. Client and family teaching:
   A. Results are normally available within 24 hours.
6. Factors that affect results:
   A. Cold agglutinins may cause false-positive results.
   B. False-negative results may occur in the presence of sensitized erythrocytes with less than 100-300 IgG molecules per cell.
7. Other data:
   A. The test must be completed within 24 hours of specimen collection.

COOMBS' TEST, INDIRECT (INDIRECT ANTIGLOBULIN TEST), SERUM

Norm. Negative.

Positive. ABO-incompatible bone marrow transplant, erythroblastosis fetalis, hemolytic anemia (drug induced), hemolytic transfusion reaction (delayed), incompatible cross-match, maternal-fetal Rh incompatibility, and prior transfusion reaction. Drugs include levodopa, mefenamic acid, methyldopa, and methyldopate hydrochloride.

Description. This test detects unexpected circulating antibodies by exposing a client's serum to group O erythrocytes that are not affected by anti-A or anti-B antibodies but do contain other known antigens. It screens for reactions to RhDu, Kell, and Duffy antigens; pretransfusion blood screening; detection of leukocyte, platelet, or rare antibodies, and screening prenatally for fetomaternal blood incompatibility. In contrast to the direct Coombs' test, which detects antibodies already attached to erythrocytes, the indirect Coombs' test detects the presence of antibodies other than those of the ABO groups that are present in the serum. One performs the test by (1) mixing erythrocytes containing known antigens to a client's serum and allowing time for unknown antibodies in the client's serum to react with the antigens and (2) the addition of Coombs' antihuman globulin serum to the mixture and observing for agglutination, indicating the presence of antibodies.

Professional Considerations
1. Consent form NOT required.
2. Preparation:
   A. Tube: Red topped, red/gray topped, or gold topped.
3. Procedure:
   A. Draw a 10-mL blood sample (adult) or a 2.5-mL blood sample (pediatric).
4. Postprocedure care:
   A. Write recent transfusions and drugs on the laboratory requisition.
5. Client and family teaching:
   A. Results are normally available within 24 hours.
   B. If results are positive, an additional sample may be needed to perform antibody identification.
6. Factors that affect results:
   A. Reject hemolyzed specimens.
   B. Cold agglutinins may cause false-positive results.
7. Other data:
   A. Negative tests on pregnant women during the first 12 weeks of gestation should be repeated at 28 weeks of gestation. A positive test at 28 weeks of gestation indicates the need for antibody-identification testing.
   B. This test must be completed within 48 hours of specimen collection.

CO-OXIMETER PROFILE (HEMOGLOBIN PROFILE), ARTERIAL OR VENOUS, BLOOD

Norm:

	% HEMOGLOBIN
Carboxyhemoglobin (COHb)	Nonsmokers: <1.5%
	Smokers: <5%
	Toxic: 15-35%
Methemoglobin (MetHb)	0.4-1.5%
Oxyhemoglobin (O_2Hb, oxygen saturation)	Arterial: 94-100%
	Venous: 60-80%
Total hemoglobin (THb)	12-15%
Volume % O_2 (%O_2)	15-23%

Usage. Helps diagnose and monitor carbon monoxide poisoning. Determination of the fractional components of hemoglobin.

Description. CO-oximetry provides a breakdown of all of the components that make up the total hemoglobin values. In monitoring critically ill clients, this test can help the clinician assess the capacity for oxygenation in critically ill clients. It can provide more accurate information than noninvasive pulse oximetry, which decreases in accuracy as hypoxemia and perfusion worsens.

Professional Considerations
1. Consent form NOT required.
2. **Preparation:**
   A. Allow time for client to relax before testing.
   B. Obtain a heparinized green-topped tube or lavender-topped tube or heparinized capillary tube and ice for venous sample, or an arterial blood gas kit and ice for an arterial sample.
   C. Document oxygen delivery amount and site of specimen collection on the laboratory requisition.

3. **Procedure:**
   A. Position client supine.
   B. *Venous sample:* Draw at least a 0.5-mL blood sample by means of venous puncture or heelstick.
   C. *Arterial sample:* Obtain 1.5-mL arterial blood sample by means of arterial puncture.
4. **Postprocedure care:**
   A. Place specimen immediately on ice.
   B. Hold pressure over the site until bleeding stops. Assess for hematoma.
5. **Client and family teaching:**
   A. Any hematoma present will gradually reabsorb into the body over several days.
6. **Factors that affect results:**
   A. Results may not be accurate if client is also receiving methylene blue.
   B. Results will be erroneous if specimen contains air bubbles.
   C. Blood substitutes give less accurate or negative carboxyhemoglobin readings.
7. **Other data:**
   A. See also *Methemoglobin, Blood; Blood gases, Arterial, Blood; Blood gases, Venous, Blood.*

COPPER (Cu), SERUM

Norm:

		SI UNITS
Adult Females	80-155 µg/dL	12.56-24.34 µmol/L
Pregnant, 40 weeks	118-302 µg/dL	18.53-47.41 µmol/L
Adult Males	70-140 µg/dL	10.99-21.98 µmol/L
Children		
≤6 months	20-70 µg/dL	3.14-10.99 µmol/L
Infant	15-65 µg/dL	2.35-10.20 µmol/L
Child	30-150 µg/dL	4.71-23.55 µmol/L

Increased. Alzheimer's disease, anemia (aplastic, pernicious, megaloblastic of pregnancy; iron deficiency), cirrhosis (biliary), elevated C-reactive protein, glomerulonephritis, hemochromatosis, Hodgkin's disease, hyperestrogenemia, hypothyroidism, hypertension, hyperthyroidism, infection, leukemia, Lofgren syndrome, lymphoma, myocardial infarction, occupation as worker in copper processing plant, pellagra, pregnancy, rheumatoid arthritis, sarcoidosis, systemic lupus erythematosus, and ulcerative colitis. Drugs include carbamazepine, estrogens and oral contraceptives, heroin that is homemade, phenobarbital, and phenytoin sodium.

Decreased. Burns, Down syndrome, hypoproteinemia, kwashiorkor, malabsorption, Menkes's (kinky-hair) syndrome, nephrosis, and Wilson's disease. Drugs include nifedipine.

Description. Copper is an essential trace element that functions in hemoglobin synthesis and activation of respiratory enzymes. Abnormally low levels cause impaired erythrocyte production and survival time and lowered catabolism by copper-containing enzymes. Copper toxicity causes jaundice, hepatic injury, headache, and vomiting and may lead to hemolytic shock. This test is most frequently used to aid diagnosis of Wilson's disease, in which serum copper levels are low, urine copper levels are high, and increased amounts of copper are deposited in body tissues.

Professional Considerations
1. Consent form NOT required.
2. Preparation:
   A. Preschedule this test with the laboratory.
   B. Obtain a stainless steel needle, plastic syringe, and navy blue–topped tube.

C. Do NOT draw during hemodialysis or peritoneal dialysis.
3. Procedure:
   A. Draw a 10-mL blood sample in a plastic syringe, using a stainless steel needle.
   B. Transfer the sample into a navy blue-topped tube without a rubber-siliconized stopper.
4. Postprocedure care:
   A. None.
5. Client and family teaching:
   A. Results are normally available within 24 hours.
6. Factors that affect results:
   A. The contact of serum with rubber-siliconized stopper yields unreliable results.
7. Other data:
   A. Serum ceruloplasmin and urine copper are usually also evaluated with this test.
   B. Serial testing and copper supplementation are recommended for clients with burns.

COPPER (Cu), URINE

Norm:

		SI UNITS
All ages	0-60 μg/24 hours	0-0.96 μmol/day
Wilson's disease	>100 μg/24 hours	>1.60 μmol/day

Increased. Alzheimer's disease, aminoaciduria, cirrhosis (biliary, Indian childhood), hepatitis (chronic, active), hyperceruloplasminemia, nephrotic syndrome, pellagra, proteinuria, and Wilson's disease (500-1000 mg/dL).

Description. Copper is an essential trace element that functions in hemoglobin synthesis and activation of respiratory enzymes. Abnormally low levels cause impaired erythrocyte production and survival time and lowered catabolism by copper-containing enzymes. Copper toxicity causes jaundice, hepatic injury, headache, and vomiting and may lead to hemolytic shock. This test is most frequently used to aid diagnosis of Wilson's disease, in which serum copper levels are low, urine copper levels are high, and increased amounts of copper are deposited in body tissues.

Professional Considerations
1. Consent form NOT required.
2. Preparation:
   A. Preschedule this test with the laboratory.
   B. Obtain a clean polyethylene, acid-washed container, pH paper, hydrochloric (HCl) or nitric acid, and a 100-mL clean container for the aliquot.
3. Procedure:
   A. Discard the first morning-urine specimen.
   B. Begin to time a 24-hour urine collection.
   C. Save all the urine voided for 24 hours in a room temperature, clean, 3-L, polyethylene, acid-washed container. Document the quantity of urine output during the specimen collection period. For catheterized clients, empty the urine drainage bag into the

acidified collection container hourly. Include the urine voided at the end of the 24-hour period. Add HCl or nitric acid as needed to maintain pH at 2.
4. **Postprocedure care:**
   A. Compare the urine quantity in the specimen container with the urinary output record for the test. If the specimen contains less urine than what was recorded as output, some of the sample may have been discarded, invalidating the test.
   B. Document the urine quantity on the laboratory requisition.
   C. Send a 100-mL aliquot to the lab.
5. **Client and family teaching:**
   A. Save all the urine voided in the 24-hour period and urinate

before defecating to avoid loss of urine. If any urine is accidentally discarded, discard the entire specimen and restart the collection the next day.
6. **Factors that affect results:**
   A. All the urine voided for the 24-hour period must be included before the aliquot is taken to avoid a falsely low result.
   B. Contact of the specimen with stool or metal invalidates results.
7. **Other data:**
   A. Serum copper and serum ceruloplasmin are usually also evaluated with this test.
   B. Significantly higher copper values are seen in females 15-19 years of age when compared to males.

COPROPORPHYRIN (UCP), URINE

Norm. Norms vary by laboratory. Consult reference range reported with results. Some reported ranges are as follows:

		SI UNITS
24-Hour Urine		
All	34-234 µg/24 hours	51-351 nmol/day
Adult females	1-57 µg/24 hours	1.5-86 nmol/day
Adult males	0-96 µg/24 hours	0-144 nmol/day
First Morning Void		
All	0.5-2.3 µg/dL	0.75-3.5 nmol/L

Increased. Acute myocardial infarction, acute poliomyelitis, anemia (hemolytic, pernicious, sideroachrestic), cirrhosis (alcoholic), coproporphyria (erythropoietic), erythroid hyperplasia, exercise, fever, hemochromatosis, hepatitis C virus, HIV, Hodgkin's disease, lead poisoning, leukemia, porphyria (congenital erythropoietic), porphyria cutanea tarda, protoporphyria (erythropoietic), thyrotoxicosis, and vitamin deficiencies. Drugs include barbiturates, chloral hydrate, chlordiazepoxide, chlorpropamide, meprobamate, and sulfonamides.

Decreased. Not clinically significant.

Description. Coproporphyrin is a compound formed during the production of the heme portion of hemoglobin. After it is metabolized, small amounts

of coproporphyrin can be found in the urine of healthy individuals. Clients with one of the congenital or acquired diseases classified as the "porphyrias" secrete and excrete increased amounts of hemoglobin-precursor compounds, including coproporphyrin. This test is most frequently used with the measurement of other urine porphyrin levels to differentiate the cause and type of porphyria occurring.

Professional Considerations
1. Consent form NOT required.
2. **Preparation:**
   A. See *Client and family teaching.*
   B. Obtain a 3-L, light-protected, clean specimen container, pH paper, sodium bicarbonate, and a 100-mL light-protected container.
3. **Procedure:**
   A. *24-Hour urine:*

i. Discard the first morning-urine specimen.

ii. Begin to time a 24-hour urine collection.

iii. Collect a 24-hour urine specimen in a refrigerated dark bottle containing 5 g of sodium carbonate. Document the quantity of urine output and keep the container tightly covered during the specimen collection period. For catheterized clients, maintain the collection bag on ice in a light-protected container and empty the bag into the refrigerated collection container hourly.

iv. Maintain the pH of the specimen between 6 and 7 by adding sodium bicarbonate as needed. Include the urine voided at the end of the 24-hour period.

v. At the end of the collection period, mix the specimen gently and transfer a 50-mL aliquot to a light-protected container and cap tightly.

B. *First morning void:*

i. Collect the entire first morning voided urine specimen in a light-protected container.

4. Postprocedure care:

A. Before taking aliquot, compare the urine quantity in a specimen container with a urinary output record for the test. If the specimen contains less urine than what was recorded as output, some of the sample may have been discarded, thus invalidating the test.

B. Send the specimen to the laboratory immediately and refrigerate it until testing.

5. Client and family teaching:

A. Barbiturates, chloral hydrate, chlorpropamide, sulfonamides, meprobamate, and chlordiazepoxide will induce porphyria and should be stopped 10 days before the test.

B. Save all the urine voided in the 24-hour period and urinate before defecating to avoid loss of urine. If any urine is accidentally discarded, discard the entire specimen and restart the collection the next day.

6. Factors that affect results:

A. All the urine voided for the 24-hour period must be included before the aliquot is taken to avoid a falsely low result.

B. Porphyrins decompose when exposed to light.

C. Drugs that may cause unreliable results include phenothiazines.

7. Other data:

A. This test is not specific for lead poisoning.

B. Uroporphyrin, protoporphyrin, delta-aminolevulinic acid (ALA), and porphobilinogen levels should also be performed.

CORONARY ANGIOGRAPHY, DIAGNOSTIC
(see Cardiac catheterization, Diagnostic)

CORONARY INTRAVASCULAR ULTRASONOGRAPHY (CORONARY SONOGRAM, CORONARY ULTRASOUND), DIAGNOSTIC

Norm. Three-dimensional view of the inside of vasculature. Normal coronary vascular anatomy; absence of coronary artery narrowing or occlusion; absence of coronary artery luminal irregularities.

Usage. Provides information regarding tissue characterization, morphology, and the precise measurement of the dimensions of the coronary arteries; identification of plaque and thrombus as well as other luminal irregularities; assessment of the coronary arteries before and after coronary angioplasty; identification of the best location for the placement of arterial stents, a coil wire used to keep arteries open in clients with occluded arteries. Helps check for stent expansion after placement of intracoronary stents. Also used for the location of atherosclerotic plaque formation before removal during cardiac catheterization.

Description. An invasive ultrasound performed from a transducer within the lumen of the coronary arteries. The intravascular ultrasound uses a tiny transducer, about 1 mm in diameter, which is fed through a catheter leading to the heart from a femoral vessel. Similar to those seen in ultrasonograms and echocardiograms, ultrasound images of the inside of the arteries appear on a monitor, offering a clear picture of the inside of the vessel. The images allow visualization of tears, precise determination of the size and shape of a plaque buildup or blood clot, or evaluation of the effectiveness of an angioplasty. This procedure is extremely useful in the evaluation of left main coronary artery narrowing. It is performed with coronary catheterization and angiography. A baseline impression, depicted through tissue differentiation, can provide insight into the progression and degree of coronary artery disease. When used with other procedures, the ultrasonogram requires about 5 minutes of time to complete.

Professional Considerations
1. Consent form IS required. Consent for this procedure may be included with the consent for cardiac catheterization and angiography.

Risks
Prolonged bleeding, hemorrhage, cerebrovascular accident, hypotension, death.

Contraindications
No different from those for cardiac catheterization.

2. Preparation:
   A. See *Cardiac catheterization, Diagnostic*. No additional prepa-

ration is necessary for this procedure.
3. Procedure:
   A. An 8-French, transducer-tipped catheter is placed over a guidewire into the coronary artery. The sound beam is swept through a series of radial positions within the perimeter of a well-defined cross-sectional plane. The echo information is then converted into a "real-time" cross-sectional image of the vessel.
   B. This procedure increases the length of a cardiac catheterization procedure by approximately 15 minutes and requires a larger dose of heparin.
4. Postprocedure care:
   A. Because additional heparinization is required when this procedure is added to a cardiac catheterization, the immediate postprocedure bed rest requirements may be prolonged.
   B. See *Cardiac catheterization, Diagnostic*.
5. Client and family teaching:
   A. See *Cardiac catheterization, Diagnostic*.
6. Factors that affect results:
   A. None found.
7. Other data:
   A. Complications of this procedure include the potential for lifting plaque or thrombus from the vessel lumen because the tip of the transducer actually enters the coronary artery, as well as potential complications listed under *Cardiac catheterization, Diagnostic*.

CORTISOL, PLASMA OR SERUM

Norm:

		SI UNITS
Adult		
8-10 AM	5-28 μg/dL	138-773 nmol/L
4-6 PM	2-14 mg/dL or ½ morning level	55-386 nmol/L
8 PM	<50% of morning level	
Child		
8-10 AM	15-25 μg/dL	414-690 nmol/L
4-6 PM	5-10 μg/dL or ½ morning level	138-276 nmol/L
8 PM	<50% of morning level	

Increased. Burns, CABG (post-op), Crohn's disease, Cushing's disease, Cushing syndrome, eclampsia, exercise, hepatic disease (severe), hyperpituitarism, hypertension, hyperthyroidism, infectious disease, obesity, osteoporosis, pancreatitis (acute), pregnancy, renal disease (severe), shock, stress (severe, heat, cold, trauma, psychologic), surgery, and virilism. Drugs include corticotropin, estrogens, oral contraceptives, yohimbine and vasopressin.

Decreased. Addison's disease, adrenal insufficiency, adrenogenital syndrome, chromophobe adenoma, craniopharyngioma, hypoglycemia, hypophysectomy, hypopituitarism, hypothyroidism, liver disease, postpartum pituitary necrosis, rheumatoid arthritis, and Waterhouse-Friderichsen syndrome. Drugs include dexamethasone, dexamethasone acetate, and dexamethasone sodium phosphate.

Description. Cortisol is a steroidal hormone released from the adrenal cortex when stimulated by secretion of adrenocorticotropic hormone (ACTH) from the pituitary gland. Cortisol is normally secreted in a diurnal pattern, with peaks and troughs occurring during specific time periods. This test is most commonly used to aid diagnosis of Cushing syndrome, in which multiple results compared from am and pm reveal no diurnal variation in cortisol levels. However, plasma or serum cortisol levels are less reliable than a 24-hour urine collection for diagnosing or ruling out Cushing syndrome.

Professional Considerations
1. Consent form NOT required.
2. Preparation:
   A. See *Client and family teaching*.
   B. Tube: Red-topped, red/gray-topped, or gold-topped tube for serum level; green topped or lavender topped for plasma level.
3. Procedure:
   A. Plasma level: Draw a 1-mL blood sample.
   B. Serum level: Draw a 1-mL blood sample.

4. Postprocedure care:
   A. Write the collection time on the laboratory requisition. Also note the client status, such as "after ACTH infusion," where applicable.
   B. Send the specimen to the laboratory for immediate spinning.
5. Client and family teaching:
   A. Fast from food and fluids for 4-8 hours before the procedure.
   B. Restrict physical activity for 10-12 hours. The client should be relaxed and recumbent for 30 minutes before the test.
6. Factors that affect results:
   A. Reject hemolyzed or lipemic specimens.
   B. Cortisol is secreted in a diurnal pattern. The highest levels occur from 5 to 10 AM, with peak levels occurring at about 8 AM.
   C. Specimens collected other than in the morning should be collected before meals.
   D. Collect specimens at the same time each day. Levels increase with exposure to bright light.
   E. Hypoglycemic states suppress plasma cortisol response.
   F. Falsely increased results may occur from amphetamines, estrogens (within 6 weeks), ethyl alcohol (ethanol), methamphetamines, nicotine, oral contraceptives (within 6 weeks), quinacrine, and spironolactone.
   G. Estrogens during pregnancy and during oral contraceptive use will falsely increase levels by increasing plasma proteins that bind with cortisol.
   H. Falsely decreased results may result when there is a delay in spinning down the sample.
7. Other data:
   A. The specimen is stable at room temperature for 1 week.
   B. Extreme elevation in the morning and no variation in the evening are suggestive of carcinoma.
   C. A single sleeping midnight cortisol level above 50 nmol/L has an 100% accuracy in the diagnosis of Cushing syndrome, 2% more accurate than the dexamethasone suppression test alone.

CORTISOL, URINE

Norm:

		SI UNITS
Adult	10-100 µg/day	27-276 nmol/day
Child >12 years	5-55 µg/day	14-152 nmol/day
Child <12 years	2-27 µg/day	5.5-74 nmol/day

Increased. Amenorrhea, Cushing syndrome, hyperthyroidism, lung cancer (small cell carcinoma), pituitary tumor, pregnancy, and stress. Drugs include corticotrophin, fluticasone propionate.

Decreased. Hypothyroidism and renal glomerular dysfunction. Drugs include dexamethasone, dexamethasone acetate, dexamethasone sodium phosphate, and inhaled glucocorticoids for asthma treatment. Ingestion of grapefruit juice.

Description. Cortisol is a steroidal hormone released from the adrenal cortex when stimulated by secretion of adrenocorticotropic hormone (ACTH) from the anterior pituitary gland. Free cortisol is unconjugated cortisol filtered by the renal glomeruli into the urine. Although it comprises less than 5% of circulating cortisol, the amount filtered follows the pattern of cortisol secretion from the adrenal cortex. Because it is excreted in a diurnal pattern, a 24-hour urine sample contains the effects of both the peak and trough cortisol levels and is thus a more accurate measurement than serum levels for diagnosing or ruling out Cushing's syndrome in which continuously high levels of cortisol are secreted.

Professional Considerations
1. Consent form NOT required.
2. **Preparation:**
   A. See *Client and family teaching*.
   B. Obtain a clean, 3-L urine container to which 10 g of boric acid or 20 mL of 33% acetic acid has been added.
3. **Procedure:**
   A. Discard the first morning urine specimen.
   B. Save all the urine voided for 24 hours in a refrigerated 3-L container to which 10 g of boric acid has been added. If the specimen is over 1 L, add 10 g of boric acid for each additional liter of urine. Include the urine voided at the end of the 24-hour period. For catheterized clients, keep the drainage bag on ice and empty urine into the collection container hourly.
   C. Alternatively, obtain a room-temperature collection as above in a 3-L container to which 20 mL of 33% acetic acid has been added.
4. **Postprocedure care:**
   A. Compare the urine quantity in the specimen container with the urinary output record for the test. If the specimen contains less urine than what was recorded as output, some of the sample may have been discarded, invalidating the test.
   B. Document the quantity of urine output for the 24-hour period on the laboratory requisition.
   C. The specimen should be frozen until testing occurs.
5. **Client and family teaching:**
   A. Do not take spironolactone or quinacrine for 7 days before the test.
   B. Because exercise increases cortisol secretion, activity should be restricted 24 hours before the test until the collection is complete.
   C. Save all the urine voided in the 24-hour period and urinate before defecating to avoid loss of urine. If any urine is accidentally discarded, discard the entire specimen and restart the collection the next day.
6. **Factors that affect results:**
   A. Stress during the test increases levels.
   B. All the urine voided for the 24-hour period must be included to avoid a falsely low result.

C. Falsely increased results may occur from amphetamines, estrogens (within 6 weeks), methamphetamines, nicotine, novosporin, oral contraceptives (within 6 weeks), quinacrine, and spironolactone.

7. **Other data:**
   A. Also measure creatinine concentration.

COXSACKIE A OR B VIRUS TITER, BLOOD

Norm. Negative. Less than a fourfold increase in titer of paired (acute and convalescent) sera.

Positive Coxsackie A. Acute febrile respiratory disease, acute flaccid paralysis, conjunctivitis (epidemic hemorrhagic), enteroviral carditis, myositis, and viral carditis.

Positive Coxsackie B. Acute febrile respiratory disease, aseptic meningitis (vital), chorioretinitis, enteroviral carditis, epidemic pleurodynia, fulminant hepatitis, hand-foot-mouth-disease, herpangina, meningitis, myocarditis, pericarditis, pleurisy, and viral carditis.

Description. The coxsackievirus is divided into two antigenically different groups, A and B, and is of the enterovirus family. Enteroviruses are easily transmitted by the fecal-oral route and are associated with epidemics, especially in newborn nurseries. Although blood is rarely used for isolation of viruses, serologic testing may be performed to detect Coxsackie A virus or Coxsackie B virus antibodies. Twenty-three species of Coxsackie A exist. Types 1, 4, 9, 16, and 23 may infect the heart, causing pericarditis progressing to heart failure. Coxsackie type A is also associated with a severe form of conjunctivitis and with respiratory disease. Six species of Coxsackie B exist. Types 1 to 5 may infect the heart, causing pericarditis progressing to heart failure. These same types may cause pleurodynia, a disease of limited duration (1 week) in which the client experiences the acute onset of chest or abdominal pain along with fever and headache. Types 2 to 5 cause most cases of vital meningitis. This test involves measuring the antibody levels in both an acute and convalescent sample of blood to detect an increase in the titer. It is a neutralization test in which diluted samples (1:2, 1:8, 1:32, 1;128, 1:512) are mixed with Coxsackie A virus or Coxsackie B virus, inoculated onto a cell culture system and observed for antigen-antibody reactions for up to 7 days. Enterovirus antibodies respond very quickly to infection; thus the earlier the acute sample is collected, the better the chance of detecting a positive test.

Professional Considerations
1. Consent form NOT required.
2. **Preparation:**
   A. Preschedule the test with the laboratory.
   B. Tube: Red topped, red/gray topped, or gold topped.
3. **Procedure:**
   A. Draw a 3- to 4-mL blood sample.
   B. Collect an acute-phase sample promptly after symptoms appear and no more than 1 week after onset.
   C. Collect the convalescent sample 2-3 days after the onset of symptoms or 2-3 weeks after the acute-phase sample.
4. **Postprocedure care:**
   A. Label the specimen as either the acute sample or the convalescent sample.
   B. The test should be specified as either *Coxsackie A virus titer* or *Coxsackie B virus titer*.
   C. Transport the specimen immediately to the laboratory. The sample should be clotted at room temperature, with serum and clot then separated and saved for simultaneous testing with the convalescent sample.
5. **Client and family teaching:**
   A. Results may not be available for several days.
6. **Factors that affect results:**
   A. Transportation of the serum to an outside laboratory may result in clot disintegration and hemolysis, thus invalidating the test.
   B. After separation, samples are stable up to 6 weeks when refrigerated. Longer storage requires freezing at −20° C.

C. Paired sera should be tested at the same time in the same laboratory.
D. False-negative Coxsackie A virus results may occur when the acute-phase titer is elevated as a result of past Coxsackie A virus infection.
E. False-negative Coxsackie B virus results may occur when the acute-phase titer is elevated as a result of past Coxsackie B virus infection.

7. **Other data:**
   A. Other tests performed to detect Coxsackie A virus or Coxsackie B virus infection include swabs of feces and the throat.

CPA
(*see Carotid phonoangiography, Diagnostic*)

CPAP TITRATION STUDY
(*see Polysomnography, Diagnostic*)

C-PEPTIDE (CONNECTING PEPTIDE), SERUM

Norm:

		SI UNITS
C-Peptide		
Adult age ≤60 years	≤4.0 ng/mL	≤4.0 µg/L
Female >60 years	1.4-5.5 ng/mL	1.4-5.5 µg/L
Male >60 years	1.5-5.0 ng/mL	1.5-5.0 µg/L
Insulin/Glucose Ratio	<0.3	

Usage. Factitious (self-medication) hypoglycemia caused by exogenous insulin overdose or insulin abuse; detection of fasting hypoglycemia or insulinoma by failure to suppress C-peptide production with exogenous insulin administration; evaluation after pancreatectomy for residual islet tissue; and evaluation of insulin reserve in insulin-dependent diabetics.

Increased. Android type of obesity, cardiac dysrhythmias (prolonged QT interval), islet cell tumor, sudden death. Drugs include oral hypoglycemic agents and sulfonylureas.

Decreased. Diabetes mellitus, pancreatic disorders in alcoholics. Drugs include rosiglitazone, troglitazone.

Description. C-peptide is an inactive, amino acid residue degradation product of proinsulin. It is formed as a by-product during the endogenous conversion of proinsulin to insulin in the pancreatic beta cells and its release is unaffected by exogenous insulin administration. C-peptide levels normally correlate with insulin levels because it is released by the beta cells in amounts similar to endogenous insulin release. This test is helpful in estimating endogenous insulin levels when insulin assay is falsely elevated by insulin antibodies.

Professional Considerations
1. Consent form NOT required.
2. **Preparation:**
   A. Tube: Red topped, red/gray topped or gold topped, and gray topped, and a container of ice.
3. **Procedure:**
   A. Draw a 7-mL blood sample for insulin and C-peptide in a chilled, red-topped tube.
   B. Pack the sample for insulin in ice.
   C. Draw a 5-mL blood sample for glucose in a gray-topped tube.
4. **Postprocedure care:**
   A. Write the collection time on the laboratory requisition.
   B. Transport the specimen to the laboratory immediately.
   C. The serum should be immediately separated in a chilled centrifuge and frozen in a plastic tube.

5. Client and family teaching:
   A. A fast from food and fluids for 8 hours may be required before sampling.
6. Factors that affect results:
   A. Reject hemolyzed specimens.
   B. Recent radioactive scans invalidate the results.
   C. C-peptide levels do not always correlate with intrinsic insulin levels in obese clients and clients with islet cell tumors.
   D. Hepatic dysfunction causes elevated levels.

7. Other data:
   A. Perform the C-peptide measurement and insulin measurement on the same sample.
   B. Pancreas graft function is attainable in clients with high preoperative C-peptide.

CPK
(see Creatine kinase, Serum)

CPS
(see Polysomnography, Diagnostic)

---

^{51}Cr (CHROMIUM)-RED CELL SURVIVAL, BLOOD

Norm:

Plasma radioactivity half-life	≤2 hours
Tagged ^{51}Cr-red blood cell half-life	25-35 days
Gamma scan	Only slight spleen, liver, and bone marrow radioactivity

Increased. Thalassemia minor.

Decreased. Anemia (congenital non-spherocytic, idiopathic acquired hemolytic, megaloblastic of pregnancy, pernicious, sickle cell), distal splenorenal shunt, elliptocytosis (with hemolysis), hemoglobin C disease, hemoglobinuria (paroxysmal nocturnal), leukemia (chronic lymphatic), spherocytosis (hereditary), and uremia.

Description. Red blood cell survival time is measured by tagging a sample of the client's red blood cells (RBCs) with radioactive ^{51}Cr. Over a 4-week period, blood samples are periodically measured for radioactivity levels to determine the amount of time taken for the tagged RBCs to disappear from the circulation. Major body organs may also be scanned with a gamma camera to locate concentrations of radioactivity. The test aids in identifying the cause of anemia and sites of RBC destruction.

Professional Considerations
1. Consent form NOT required.

Risks
Bleeding, infection, hematoma.

Contraindications
Active bleeding extended clotting times, breast-feeding, and pregnancy.

2. Preparation:
   A. For procedures 3 A-C below, collect a sterile glass beaker containing sodium chromate.
   B. For procedures 3 D-F, tubes: green topped and lavender topped.
3. Procedure:
   A. Draw a 30-mL blood sample and mix it with 100 mCi of ^{51}Cr (sodium chromate).
   B. Incubate overnight.
   C. Inject the mixture intravenously into the client.
   D. 30 minutes later, draw a 6-mL blood sample in a lavender-topped tube for measurement of baseline volumes of blood and red cells.
   E. 24 hours later, draw a 6-mL blood sample in a green-topped tube. Send the specimen to the laboratory for a same-day measurement of hematocrit and of ^{51}Cr with a scintillation well counter.
   F. Repeat procedure 3-E every 1-3 days for 4 weeks.
   G. After the last sample is drawn, draw a 6-mL blood sample in a lavender-topped tube for comparison measurement of blood and red cell volumes.
4. Postprocedure care:
   A. None.
5. Client and family teaching:
   A. No isolation is necessary.

6. **Factors that affect results:**
   A. Conditions that decrease red blood cell volume or the proportion of tagged red cells to non-tagged red cells, including blood draws, blood transfusions, chronic occult extravascular blood loss, and hemorrhage, will simulate decreased survival time.
7. **Other data:**
   A. Normal tests are seen in hemoglobin C trait and sickle cell trait and elliptocytosis without hemolysis.
   B. Normal red blood cell half-life is 60 days.
   C. This test may also be used to predict the viability of donated red blood cells.
   D. Red blood cell survival can also be measured by use of enumeration of biotinylated red blood cells, which does not expose the client to radiation.

C-REACTIVE PROTEIN, SERUM

Norm:

		SI UNITS
Qualitative	Negative	
Quantitative		
Adult	68-8200 ng/mL	68-8200 µg/L
	or 20 mg/dL	
	or <8 µg/mL	
Behring BNII assay (high sensitivity CRP):		
Females	0.175 mg/dL	
Males	0.115 mg/dL	
Kamiya K-assay (high sensitivity CRP):		
Females	0.191 mg/dL	
Males	0.139 mg/dL	
Cord blood	10-350 ng/mL	10-350 µg/L

Positive (>1:2 titer). Adenovirus pneumonia, Alzheimer's disease, ankylosing spondylitis, Castleman's tumor, Crohn's disease, empyema, gout, inflammation, Graves' disease, Hodgkin's disease, Kawasaki disease, lymphoma, malignant tumor, meningitis, metabolic syndrome, myocardial infarction, myxoma (of heart left atrium), necrosis, nephritis, non-Hodgkin's lymphoma, pancreatitis (acute), peritonitis, pharyngitis (streptococcal), pneumonia (pneumococcal), postcommissurotomy syndrome, postoperatively (first week), pregnancy (after month 3), renal infarction, rheumatic fever (acute), rheumatoid arthritis (acute), sepsis, systemic lupus erythematosus, trauma (surgical), tuberculosis, and urinary tract infection.

Positive, If >0.3 mg/dL. Associated with increased risk of developing initial or recurrent myocardial infarction.

Usage. Monitoring of rheumatoid arthritis and rheumatic fever inflammatory processes, differentiation of Crohn's disease from ulcerative colitis, predictor of myocardial infarction (plasma levels >1.6 mg/L predict future coronary events) in women and coronary heart disease in middle-aged men, and detection of the presence or exacerbation of inflammatory processes (high preoperative levels indicate increased risk for postoperative infection).

Description. C-reactive protein is an abnormal serum glycoprotein produced by the liver during acute inflammation. Because it disappears rapidly when inflammation subsides, its detection signifies the presence of a current inflammatory process. It is the best indicator of the severity of pancreatitis when measured 48 hours after the onset of symptoms. C-reactive protein has been linked to metabolic syndrome, a group of signs that include abdominal obesity, hypertriglyceridemia, low HDL-C, hypertension, and high fasting blood glucose. It is now suspected that chronic inflammation as evidenced by an chronically elevated C-reactive protein level may be an additional component of the syndrome. Its contribution is hypothesized to be regulation of the adverse lipid profile seen in metabolic syndrome. C-reactive protein interacts with the complement cascade and is detected by antiserum by means of immunoassays.

Professional Considerations

1. Consent form NOT required.
2. **Preparation:**
   A. Tube: Red topped.
3. **Procedure:**
   A. Draw a 2-mL blood sample.
4. **Postprocedure care:**
   A. Transport the specimen to the laboratory for immediate testing.
   B. Do not refrigerate the specimen.
5. **Client and family teaching:**
   A. Fast from food and fluids for 4 hours before sampling.

6. **Factors that affect results:**
   A. Drugs that may cause false-positive results include oral contraceptives.
   B. Drugs that may cause false-negative results as a result of suppression of inflammation include NSAIDs, steroids, and salicylates.
   C. Drugs that lower C-reactive protein include simvastatin.
   D. Presence of an intrauterine device may cause inflammation, which produces a positive test.
   E. Overnight refrigeration of the sample may produce a false-positive result.
7. **Other data:**
   A. Useful in monitoring postoperative inflammatory complications.
   B. Daily measurements of C-reactive protein correlate with resolution of sepsis. A decrease in CRP by 25% or more from the previous day's level is a good indicator of resolution of sepsis, with a predictive value of 97%.
   C. Elevated C-reactive protein, elevated fibrinogen, elevated amyloid A, and baseline values of IL-6 have each been independently associated with future coronary occlusion.

CREATINE KINASE (CK), SERUM

Norm. Results are method-dependent and should be compared with the reference values of the laboratory performing the test.

		SI UNITS
Creatine Kinase—Total		
Adult Females	5-25 μg/mL	
	10-135 IU/L	
	5-35 mU/mL	
Ambulatory	10-70 U/L	0.17-1.16 μKat/L
≤60 years	10-55 U/L	0.17-0.92 μKat/L
>60 years	16-80 U/L	0.27-1.33 μKat/L
Adult Males	5-35 μg/mL	
	20-170 IU/L	
	5-55 mU/mL	
Ambulatory	25-90 U/L	0.42-1.50 μKat/L
<61 years	12-80 U/L	0.20-1.33 μKat/L
61-70 years	20-110 U/L	0.33-1.83 μKat/L
>70 years	22-90 U/L	0.37-1.50 μKat/L
Children		
Newborn	65-580 IU/L at 30° C	
	10-200 U/L	0.17-3.33 μKat/L
Male	0-70 IU/L at 30° C	
Female	0-50 IU/L at 30° C	

Total levels may be normal in acute myocardial infarction, even when the CK-MB isoenzyme is elevated. In general, total CK trends in acute myocardial infarction are as follows:

Initial rise:	2-6 hours after onset of damage
Peak levels:	18-36 hours after onset of damage
Return to baseline level:	3-6 days

	% of Total CK	Fraction of Total CK (SI Units)
Creatine Kinase Isoenzymes		
CK_1-BB (Brain)	0-3	0-0.03
CK_2-MB (Heart)	0-6	0-0.06
CK_3-MM (Muscle)	90-97	0.90-0.97

CK_2-MB Trends in Acute Myocardial Infarction:

Initial rise	4-8 hours after onset of damage.
Peak levels	18-24 hours after onset of damage.
Return to baseline level	3 days after onset of damage.

Increased Total CK. Amyotrophic lateral sclerosis (values greater in limb-onset versus bulbar-onset), anoxia, atresia (biliary), bowel injury, brain tumor, burns (thermal, electrical), cancer (breast, lung, oat cell, gastrointestinal, prostatic), carbon monoxide poisoning, cardiomyopathy (cobalt-beer), carbon monoxide poisoning, carrier state (for Duchenne's muscular dystrophy), cerebrovascular accident, CNS trauma, coma (hepatic), convulsions, coughing (severe), crush syndrome, delirium tremens, dermatomyositis, ectopic pregnancy, eosinophilia-myalgia syndrome, exercise, head injury, hemodialysis, hypokalemia (severe), hypothermia, hypothyroidism, hypothyroid myopathy, infarction (bowel, cerebral, myocardial, prostate), intoxication (alcohol, salicylate), intramuscular injection (recent), labor, leptospirosis, malignant hyperthermia, meningoencephalitis, muscle spasms, muscular dystrophy (Duchenne's, limb-girdle, fascioscapulohumeral), myocarditis, myoglobinuria, myopathy (from alcoholism), myotonic dystrophy, myxedema, necrosis of striated muscle, neuroleptic malignant syndrome, organ rejection (heart transplant), parturition, polymyositis, postictal state, pregnancy, prostate injury, psychosis (acute with agitation), pulmonary edema, pulmonary embolism, renal failure, renal insufficiency (chronic), Reye syndrome, rhabdomyolysis, Rocky Mountain spotted fever, shock, skeletal muscle disorders, status epilepticus, striated muscle atrophy (acute), subarachnoid hemorrhage, surgery (bowel, cardiac, CNS, prostate), tachycardia, thyrotoxicosis, toxic shock syndrome (day 7), trauma (muscular), typhoid fever, and very muscular people. Drugs include anabolic steroids, fluvastatin, isotretinoin and combination cerivastin-gemfibrozil therapy.

Increased CK_1-BB (Brain). Anoxia, atresia (biliary), brain damage, cancer (breast, gastrointestinal, oat cell, prostatic, widespread malignancies), cerebrovascular accident (hemorrhage, infarction), hemodialysis, hypothermia, intestinal necrosis, labor, malignant hyperthermia, renal failure, shock, surgery (CNS), and uremia.

Increased CK_2-MB (Heart). Anoxia, burns (electrical, thermal), cancer (lung), carbon monoxide poisoning, cardiomyopathy (cobalt-beer), collagen vascular diseases, congestive heart failure (rare), coronary angiography (rare), coronary insufficiency (rare), hypothermia, hypothyroidism, malignant hyperthermia, muscular dystrophy (Duchenne's), myocardial infarction, myocarditis, myoglobinuria (severe), polymyositis, pulmonary embolism, renal insufficiency (chronic), Reye syndrome, rhabdomyolysis, Rocky Mountain spotted fever, surgery (cardiac, valve replacement), systemic lupus erythematosus, and trauma (cardiac). Drugs include doxycycline.

Increased CK$_3$-MM (Muscle). Cardiac catheterization (with myocardial damage), cardioversion, coronary arteriography (with myocardial damage), hypothyroidism, intramuscular injections, muscle trauma, muscular dystrophy, myocardial infarction, psychosis (acute with agitation), Reye syndrome, shock, surgery, and trauma (skeletal muscle).

Decreased Total CK. Addison's disease, anterior pituitary hyposecretion, connective tissue disease, hepatic disease (alcoholic), low muscle mass, metastatic neoplasia, postinfarction left ventricular remodeling (CK flux rates are decreased), and pregnancy (first half). Drugs include steroids.

Decreased CK$_1$-BB, CK$_2$-MB, CK$_3$-MM. Not applicable.

Description. Creatine kinase is an enzyme found in muscle and brain tissue and reflects tissue catabolism as a result of cell trauma. It catalyzes creatine-creatinine metabolism. The test is performed to detect myocardial or skeletal muscle damage or central nervous system damage resulting in increased tissue catabolism from those areas. One can determine the type of tissue damage (tissue undergoing increased catabolism) occurring by performing the CK isoenzymes test that measures the three types of isoenzymes that make up total CPK: CK$_1$-BB, CK$_2$-MB, and CK$_3$-MM. CK$_1$-BB is found mainly in brain tissue but also in the smooth muscle, thyroid gland, lungs, and prostate gland. CK$_2$-MB is found mainly in cardiac muscle but also in the tongue, diaphragm, and skeletal muscle (scant amount). CK$_3$-MM is found mainly in skeletal muscle. The isoenzyme test is usually repeated at 8- to 12-hour intervals to track trends characteristic of specific types of cell damage. Most recently, test kits have been developed to allow detection of CK$_3$-MM and CK$_2$-MB isoforms earlier than the traditional methods for CK isoenzyme detection.

Professional Considerations
1. Consent form NOT required.
2. **Preparation:**
   A. See *Client and family teaching.*

B. Tube: Red topped, red/gray topped, or gold topped.
3. **Procedure:**
   A. Collect a 5-mL blood sample.
4. **Postprocedure care:**
   A. Send the specimen to the laboratory immediately.
   B. Refrigerate the specimen if measurement will be delayed more than 2 hours. Separate the serum and freeze it if the test will not be performed within 24 hours of collection.
   C. If isoenzyme measurement is desired, specify this on the laboratory requisition.
5. **Client and family teaching:**
   A. If the test is for skeletal muscle disorder evaluation, the client should avoid strenuous physical activity for 24 hours before the test.
   B. Avoid ingestion of alcohol for 24 hours before the test.
   C. Withhold drugs that would affect the test results (see below) for 24 hours before the test, when possible.
6. **Factors that affect results:**
   A. Necessary intramuscular (IM) injections should be given after or at least 1 hour before this test.
   B. Hemolysis invalidates the results.
   C. Invasive procedures and other factors that elevate CK include cardiac catheterization (with myocardial injury), cardioversion, coronary arteriography (with myocardial injury), electric shock, electrocautery, electromyography, intramuscular injections, and muscle massage (recent).
   D. Drugs that may cause falsely increased CK values include aminocaproic acid, clofibrate, codeine, dexamethasone, dexamethasone acetate, dexamethasone sodium phosphate, digoxin, epsilon-aminocaproic acid, ethyl alcohol (ethanol), furosemide, glutethimide, guanethidine, halothane, heroin, imipramine, lithium carbonate, meperidine hydrochloride, morphine sulfate, phenobarbital, and succinylcholine chloride.

7. **Other data:**
   A. CK is considered to be a marker for Duchenne's muscular dystrophy.
   B. Evaluation of myocardial infarction should also include LDH isoenzyme measurements every 24 hours.
   C. In clients suspected of acute myocardial infarction, CK-MB testing alone may reveal more information than total CK level, which may not show an elevation initially. CK-MB measurement within 9 hours of arrival provides accurate clinical assessment in 99% cases of myocardial infarction.
   D. Troponin T is superior to CK-MB for prediction of impending complications after cardiac surgical procedures.

CREATINE KINASE ISOENZYMES (CK ISOENZYMES), SERUM
(see Creatine kinase, Serum)

CREATINE PHOSPHOKINASE (CK, CPK), SERUM
(see Creatine kinase, Serum)

CREATINE, URINE

Norm:

		SI UNITS
Adults	<6% of urine creatinine	
Adult females	≤80 mg/24 hours	0-615 μmol/day
Pregnant	≤12% of urine creatinine	
Adult males	≤40 mg/24 hours	0-307 μmol/day
Infants	Equal to urine creatinine	
Children	≤30% of urine creatinine	

Increased. Acromegaly, Addison's disease, amyotonia congenita, burns, children (growth state), Cushing syndrome, diabetes mellitus, disseminated lupus erythematosus, fractures, guanidinoacetate methyltransferase (GAMT) deficiency, hyperthyroidism, hypothyroidism, infections, injuries (crushing), leukemia, male eunuchoidism, muscular dystrophy, myasthenia gravis, myoglobinuria (acute paroxysmal), myopathy (alcoholic), myotonia (congenital Thomsen's disease), myotonic dystrophy, neurogenic atrophy, poliomyelitis, polymyositis, pregnancy, puerperium, starvation, X-linked mental retardation and raw meat diet.

Decreased. Aging (fifth to ninth decade), hypothyroidism.

Description. Creatine is a compound that functions in anaerobic muscle metabolism by combining with phosphate to yield energy used in intense muscle activity for short periods of time. Normally, phosphocreatine breaks down into creatinine, which is then excreted in the urine. In some conditions, particularly muscle diseases, creatine is released in increased amounts into the bloodstream and can be measured in the urine.

Professional Considerations
1. Consent form NOT required.
2. **Preparation:**
   A. Obtain a clean, 3-L, 24-hour urine container with toluene preservative.
3. **Procedure:**
   A. Discard the first morning urine specimen.
   B. Save all the urine voided for 24 hours in a refrigerated, clean, 3-L container to which toluene preservative has been added. Include the urine voided at the end of the 24-hour period. For catheterized clients, keep the drainage bag on ice and empty urine into the refrigerated collection container hourly.

4. Postprocedure care:
   A. Compare the urine quantity in the specimen container with the urinary output record for the test. If the specimen contains less urine than what was recorded as output, some of the sample may have been discarded, invalidating the test.
   B. Document urine quantity on the laboratory requisition.
   C. Send the entire specimen to the lab.
5. Client and family teaching:
   A. Save all the urine voided in the 24-hour period and urinate before defecating to avoid loss of urine. If any urine is accidentally discarded, discard the entire specimen and restart the collection the next day.
6. Factors that affect results:
   A. All the urine voided for the 24-hour period must be included to avoid a falsely low result.
   B. Drugs that may cause falsely elevated results include caffeine, corticosteroids, corticotropin, cortisone acetate, desoxycorticosterone acetate, desoxycorticosterone pivalate, methyltestosterone, nitrofurantoin, nitrofurantoin sodium, phenolsulfonphthalein, and sodium benzoate.
   C. Drugs that may cause falsely decreased results include anabolic steroids, androgens, and thiazide diuretics.
   D. The results may be increased after 3 weeks of pregnancy.
7. Other data:
   A. This test may be useful as a marker for testicular damage.

CREATININE, SERUM

Norm:

		SI UNITS
Jaffe, Manual Method	0.8-1.5 mg/dL	70-133 μmol/day
Jaffe, Kinetic or Enzymatic Method		
Adults		
Females	0.5-1.1 mg/dL	44-97 μmol/L
Males	0.6-1.2 mg/dL	53-105 μmol/L
Elderly	May be lower	May be lower
Children		
Cord blood	0.6-1.2 mg/dL	53-105 μmol/L
Newborn	0.8-1.4 mg/dL	71-124 μmol/L
Infant	0.7-1.7 mg/dL	62-150 μmol/L
1 year, female	≤0.5 mg/dL	≤44 μmol/L
1 year, male	≤0.6 mg/dL	≤53 μmol/L
2-3 years, female	≤0.6 mg/dL	≤53 μmol/L
2-3 years, male	≤0.7 mg/dL	≤62 μmol/L
4-7 years, female	≤0.7 mg/dL	≤62 μmol/L
4-7 years, male	≤0.8 mg/dL	≤71 μmol/L
8-10 years, female	≤0.8 mg/dL	≤71 μmol/L
8-10 years, male	≤0.9 mg/dL	≤80 μmol/L
11-12 years, female	≤0.9 mg/dL	≤80 μmol/L
11-12 years, male	≤1.0 mg/dL	≤88 μmol/L
13-17 years, female	≤1.1 mg/dL	≤97 μmol/L
13-17 years, male	≤1.2 mg/dL	≤106 μmol/L
18-20 years, female	≤1.2 mg/dL	≤106 μmol/L
18-20 years, male	≤1.3 mg/dL	≤115 μmol/L

Increased. Values are 20-40% higher in the late afternoon than in the morning. Acromegaly, allergic purpura, amyloidosis, analgesic abuse, azotemia (prerenal, postrenal), congenital hypoplastic kidneys, congestive heart failure, diabetes mellitus, diet (high meat content), gigantism, glomerulonephritis (chronic), Goodpasture syndrome, gout, hemoglobinuria, high dietary intake, hypovolemic shock, hypothyroidism, infants (first 2 weeks of life), intestinal obstruction, Kimmelstiel-Wilson syndrome, microalbuminemia, metal poisoning, multiple myeloma, muscle destruction, nephritis, nephropathy (hypercalcemic, hypokalemic), nephrosclerosis, pancreatitis (necrotizing), polyarteritis nodosa, polycystic disease, preeclampsia, pyelonephritis, renal artery stenosis or thrombosis, renal cortical necrosis, renal failure, renal vein thrombosis, renal tuberculosis, rheumatoid arthritis (active), scleroderma, sickle cell anemia, subacute bacterial endocarditis, systemic lupus erythematosus, testosterone therapy, toxic shock syndrome, uremia, urinary obstruction and vomiting. Drugs include acetohexamide, ammonia (inhaled), androgens, arginine, bleomycin-induced pulmonary toxicity, Bromsulphalein, captopril, cephalosporins (Cefoxitin), cimetidine, cincophen, clofibrate, corticosteroids, diacetic acid, diuretics, disopyramide phosphate, dopamine, fenofibrate, fosinopril, fructose, gentamicin sulfate, glucose, hydralazine hydrochloride, hydroxyurea, lipomul, lithium carbonate, losartan, mannitol, meclofenamate sodium, methicillin sodium, metoprolol tartrate, minoxidil, mithramycin, nitrofurantoin, nitrogen oxide (inhaled), propranolol, protein, pyruvate, sulfobromophthalein, sulfonamides, streptokinase, testosterone, testosterone cypionate, testosterone enanthate, testosterone propionate, triamterine, and viomycin. Herbal or natural remedies include products containing aristolochic acids (*Akebia* spp., *Aristolochia* spp., *Asarum* spp., birthwort, *Bragantia* spp., *Clematis* spp., *Cocculus* spp., *Diploclisia* spp., Dutchman's pipe, *Fang chi, Fang ji, Fang chi, Guang fang ji, Kan-Mokutsu, Menispernum* spp., *Mokutsu, Mu tong, Sinomenium* spp., and *Stephania* spp.)

Decreased. Diabetic ketoacidosis (artifactual decrease) and muscular dystrophy. Drugs include cefoxitin sodium, cimetidine, chlorpromazine, chlorprothixene, marijuana, thiazide diuretics, and vancomycin. Herbal or natural remedies include *Cordyceps sinensis*.

Description. Creatinine is produced continuously as a nonprotein end prod-

uct of anaerobic energy-producing creatine-phosphate metabolism in skeletal muscle. Because it is continually and easily excreted by the renal system, increased levels indicate a slowing of the glomerular filtration rate. Creatinine is thus a very specific indicator of renal function, revealing the balance between creatinine formation and excretion. A diurnal variation in creatinine may be related to meals, with troughs occurring around 0700 (7 AM) and peaks occurring around 1900 (7 PM).

Professional Considerations
1. Consent form NOT required.
2. **Preparation:**
   A. Tube: Red topped, red/gray topped, or gold topped.
   B. Do NOT draw during hemodialysis.
3. **Procedure:**
   A. Draw a 1-mL blood sample.
4. **Postprocedure care:**
   A. Send the specimen to the laboratory promptly and refrigerate it until tested.
5. **Client and family teaching:**
   A. Avoid excessive exercise for 8 hours and avoid excessive red meat intake for 24 hours before the test.
6. **Factors that affect results:**
   A. Some clients with long-standing chronic renal failure may have normal levels.
   B. Drugs that may cause falsely elevated levels include amphotericin B, ascorbic acid, barbiturates, capreomycin sulfate, carbutamide, cefoxitin sodium, cephalothin sodium, chlorthalidone, clonidine, colistin sulfate, dextran, doxycycline hyclate, kanamycin, levodopa, methyldopa, methyldopate hydrochloride, nitromethane fuel inhalation, *para*-aminohippurate, phenolsulfonphthalein, and sulfobromophthalein.
7. **Other data:**
   A. The specimen will remain stable for 1 week when refrigerated and for 1 month when frozen.
   B. Mean creatinine values are higher for men, non-Hispanic blacks, and older persons and are lower in Mexican Americans.

CREATININE, URINE

Norm:

			SI UNITS
Adult		14-26 mg/kg/24 hours	124-230 µmol/kg/day
Female		600-1800 mg/24 hours	5.3-16 µmol/day
Male		800-2000 mg/24 hours	7-18 µmol/day
Child		8-22 mg/kg/24 hours	71-195 µmol/kg/day

Increased. Fever, hypothyroidism and tissue catabolism. Values are 20-40% higher in the late afternoon than in the morning, are higher in blacks, and increase with age.

Decreased. Decreased renal perfusion, glomerulonephritis, cystic kidney disease, polymyositis, pyelonephritis (chronic bilateral), and shock (hypovolemic).

Description. Creatinine is produced continuously as a nonprotein end product of anaerobic energy-producing creatine-phosphate metabolism in skeletal muscle. It is continually and easily excreted by the renal system by glomerulofiltration. Decreased levels of urine creatinine indicate a slowing of the glomerular filtration rate. Creatinine is thus a very specific indicator of renal function. A diurnal variation in creatinine may be related to meals, with troughs occurring around 0700 (7 AM) and peaks occurring around 1900 (7 PM). Because this test involves the collection of a 24-hour urine sample, it captures the effects of both peaks and troughs of creatinine levels.

Professional Considerations
1. Consent form NOT required.
2. Preparation:
   A. Obtain a clean, 3-L, 24-hour urine container.
3. Procedure:
   A. Discard the first morning urine specimen.
   B. Save all the urine voided for 24 hours in a refrigerated, clean, 3-L container with or without a preservative. Include the urine voided at the end of the 24-hour period. For catheterized clients, keep the drainage bag on ice and empty it into the refrigerated collection container hourly.

4. Postprocedure care:
   A. Compare the urine quantity in the specimen container with the urinary output record for the test. If the specimen contains less urine than what was recorded as output, some of the sample may have been discarded, invalidating the test.
   B. Document the quantity of urine output and the beginning and ending times of collection on the laboratory requisition.
   C. Send the specimen to the laboratory immediately and refrigerate it until tested. Only prolonged storage times of 30 days at high temperatures above 55° C could significantly decrease levels.
5. Client and family teaching:
   A. Save all the urine voided in the 24-hour period and urinate before defecating to avoid loss of urine. If any urine is accidentally discarded, discard the entire specimen and restart the collection the next day.
6. Factors that affect results:
   A. Failure to include all the urine voided for the 24-hour period yields a falsely low result.
   B. Failure to refrigerate the specimen throughout the collection period yields a falsely low result.
   C. Drugs that may cause falsely elevated results include amphotericin B, ascorbic acid, barbiturates, capreomycin sulfate, carbutamide, cefoxitin sodium, cephalothin sodium, chlorthalidone, clonidine, colistin sulfate, dextran, doxycycline hyclate, kanamycin, levodopa, methyldopa, methyldopate hydrochloride, para-aminohippurate, phenolsulfonphthalein, sulfobromophthalein.

D. Drugs that may cause falsely decreased results include anabolic steroids, androgens, and thiazides.

7. **Other data:**
   A. Urine creatinine is stable when refrigerated for 1 week and when frozen for 1 month.

CREATININE CLEARANCE, 12- OR 24-HOUR, URINE

(see Creatinine clearance, Serum, Urine)

C

CREATININE CLEARANCE, SERUM, URINE

Norm. Corrected to 1.73 m^2 of body surface area.

AGE	ADULT FEMALE mL/min	SI UNITS mL/sec	ADULT MALE mL/min	SI UNITS mL/sec
≤20 years	84	1.4	90	1.5
21-30 years	90	1.5	96	1.6
31-40 years	96	1.6	102	1.7
41-50 years	102	1.7	108	1.8
51-60 years	108	1.8	114	1.9
61-70 years	114	1.9	120	2.0
71-80 years	120	2.0	126	2.1
81-90 years	126	2.1	132	2.2
91-100 years	132	2.2	138	2.3

AGE	CHILD mL/min	Units mL/sec
<1 year	72	1.2
1 year	45	0.8
2 years	55	0.9
3 years	60	1.0
4-5 years	71-73	1.2
6-7 years	64-67	1.1
8 years	72	1.2
9 years	83	1.4
10-11 years	89-92	1.5
12 years	109	1.8
13-14 years	86	1.4

Increased. Correlates to higher mortality risk after acute stroke. Drugs include low-molecular-weight heparin enoxaparin, perindopril. Herbal or natural remedies include *Cordyceps sinensis*.

Decreased. Acute coronary syndrome acute tubular necrosis, atherosclerosis (of renal artery), congestive heart failure, dehydration, elderly clients, glomerulonephritis, malignancy (bilateral renal), nephrosclerosis, obstruction (renal artery), phenacetin, polycystic kidney disease, pyelonephritis (advanced bilateral chronic), shock (cardiogenic, hypovolemic), thrombosis (renal vein), and tuberculosis (renal). Drugs include aminoglycosides, amphotericin B, captopril, cyclosporine, indomethacin, lithium, nitrendipine and penicillins.

Description. Creatinine is produced continuously as a nonprotein end product of anaerobic energy-producing creatine metabolism in skeletal muscle. It is continually and easily excreted by the renal system by glomerular filtration. The creatinine clearance test measures both a blood sample and a urine sample to determine the rate at which creatinine is being cleared from the blood by the kidneys. Specifically, "clearance" means the amount of blood cleared of creatinine in 1 minute and is independent of urine flow rate. Decreased results occur when over 50% of renal nephrons are damaged, thus indicating impaired glomerular filtration. Creatinine clearance is thus a very specific indicator of renal function, revealing the balance between creatinine formation and excretion.

Professional Considerations
1. Consent form NOT required.
2. **Preparation:**
   A. *Urine collection:* Obtain clean, 3-L, 24-hour urine bag or bottle(s).
   B. *Serum collection:* Tube: red topped, red/gray topped, or gold topped.
   C. Do NOT draw the specimen during hemodialysis.
3. **Procedure:**
   A. *Urine collection:*
      i. Discard the first morning urine specimen.
      ii. Begin to time a 24-hour urine collection. (2-, 6-, or 12-hour urine collections can also be performed, but a 24-hour specimen is preferable although at least an 8-hour collection is recommended.)
      iii. Save all the urine voided for 24 hours in a refrigerated, clean, 3-L container with or without a preservative. Include the urine voided at the end of the 24-hour period. For catheterized clients, keep the drainage bag on ice and empty into the refrigerated collection container hourly.
   B. *Serum collection:*
      i. Because the glomerular filtration rate remains stable, the serum specimen can be drawn at any time during the urine collection period. Draw a 7-mL blood sample in a red-topped tube for serum creatinine.
4. **Postprocedure care:**
   A. Compare the urine quantity in the specimen container with the urinary output record for the test. If the specimen contains less urine than what was recorded as output, some of the sample may

have been discarded, invalidating the test.
   B. Document the quantity of the urine output as well as the beginning and ending times for the 24-hour period on the laboratory requisition.
   C. Send the 24-hour urine specimen to the laboratory immediately and refrigerate it until tested.
   D. Urine creatinine is stable for 1 week when refrigerated and for 1 month when frozen.
5. **Client and family teaching:**
   A. Avoid strenuous exercise for 8 hours before the test.
   B. For the urine test, save all the urine voided in the 24-hour period and urinate before defecating to avoid loss of urine. If any urine is accidentally discarded, discard the entire specimen and restart the collection the next day.
6. **Factors that affect results:**
   A. Failure to refrigerate the specimen throughout the collection period allows the creatinine to decompose, causing falsely low results.
   B. Drugs that may cause falsely elevated results include amphotericin B, ascorbic acid, barbiturates, capreomycin sulfate, carbutamide, cefoxitin sodium, cephalothin sodium, chlorthalidone, cifpirome, clonidine, colistin sulfate, dextran, doxycycline hyclate, kanamycin, levodopa, methyldopa, methyldopate hydrochloride, *para*-aminohippurate, phenolsulfonphthalein, and sulfobromophthalein.
   C. Drugs that may cause falsely decreased results include anabolic steroids, androgens, and thiazides.
7. **Other data:**
   A. Elderly clients can have a normal serum creatinine and still have renal impairment. Therefore, commonly prescribed drugs usually require dose adjustments in the elderly.

CRYOFIBRINOGEN, PLASMA

Norm. Negative. No cryofibrinogen noted.

Positive. Central retinal vein occlusion, collagen vascular diseases, familial Mediterranean fever (acute), hemophilia, infections (neonatal), hepatitis C viral infection, multiple myeloma, neoplasms, scleroderma, spontaneous necrosis of the skin, thromboembolic conditions, and toxemia of pregnancy. Also associated with conditions exhibiting cryoglobulins. Drugs include methimazole and oral contraceptives.

Description. Cryofibrinogen is a complex of fibrinogen and protein fragments that precipitates at 0-4° C and redissolves when warmed. Cryofibrinogenemia refers to the presence of these precipitated complexes in plasma but not in serum. It is associated with elevations in alpha$_1$-antitrypsin, haptoglobin, alpha$_2$-macroglobulin, and hyperfibrinogenemia. Symptoms include sensitivity to cold, including urticaria, bleeding, and blood vessel damage. Cryofibrinogenemia has been associated with thromboembolic conditions, inflammatory processes, and malignancies. Cryofibrinogens have also been detected secondary to purpura and gangrene from peripheral occlusion. Positive tests require a study of cold precipitable proteins in order to differentiate cryofibrinogen from cryoglobulins. Treatment includes the use of streptokinase, streptodornase, urokinase, stanozolol or plasmapheresis.

Professional Considerations
1. Consent form NOT required.
2. Preparation:
   A. Tube: Blue topped, black topped, or lavender topped, depending on the individual laboratory requirements. Also obtain a container of warm water.
   B. The client should not receive heparin therapy for 2 days.
3. Procedure:
   A. Draw a 7-mL blood sample. Place the tube in the container of warm water.
4. Postprocedure care:
   A. Write the collection time on the laboratory requisition.
   B. Transport the specimen to the laboratory immediately. The specimen should be allowed to clot at 37° C. A portion of plasma is kept at room temperature and another portion is refrigerated overnight. The samples are then compared

for gel or white particle formation. If present, the sample is incubated ½ hour at 37° C. Absence of the gel or white particles after incubation indicates a positive test.
5. Client and family teaching:
   A. Heparin therapy within 2 days before the test may cause false-negative results.
6. Factors that affect results:
   A. Reject specimens received more than 2 hours after collection.
7. Other data:
   A. Cryofibrinogen is not to be confused with cryoglobulins, which precipitate from *serum*, rather than plasma, during cold conditions.
   B. At least 24 hours is required for results.

CRYOGLOBULIN, SERUM
(see Cryoglobulin, Qualitative, Serum)

CRYOGLOBULIN, QUALITATIVE, SERUM

Norm. Negative.

Positive Type I Cryoglobulin. Leukemia (chronic lymphocytic), lymphoma, multiple myeloma, and Waldenström's macroglobulinemia.

Positive Type II Cryoglobulin. Lymphoma, mixed essential cryoglobulinemia, multiple myeloma, rheumatoid arthritis, and Sjögren syndrome.

Positive Type III Cryoglobulin. Chronic infection, cytomegalovirus infection, endocarditis (infective), glomerulonephritis (poststreptococcal), hepatitis (acute viral, chronic active), infectious mononucleosis, kala-azar, leprosy, polymyalgia rheumatica, primary biliary cirrhosis, rheumatoid arthritis, scleroderma, Sjögren syndrome, systemic lupus erythematosus, and tropical splenomegaly syndrome.

Positive Type I, II, or III. Hodgkin's disease, infection (viral), and Raynaud's disease.

Description. Cryoglobulins are abnormal serum proteins that precipitate at low laboratory temperatures and redissolve after being warmed. They cannot be identified by serum protein electrophoresis. Cryoglobulin presence in the serum causes vascular problems most commonly of the extremities and is usually associated with immunologic disease. Three types may be delineated to help differentiate the type of disease occurring. This test involves obtaining a "cryocrit" by observation for cold precipitation of cryoglobulin after at least 72 hours of storage at 4° C and confirmation of the reversibility of the reaction by rewarming of the serum sample.

Professional Considerations
1. Consent form NOT required.
2. Preparation:
   A. See *Client and family teaching.*
   B. Tube: Red topped, red/gray topped, or gold topped.
   C. The syringe and red-topped tube should be warmed to 37° C to prevent loss of cryoglobulins.
3. Procedure:
   A. Draw a 10-mL blood sample in a tube that has been prewarmed to body temperature.
4. Postprocedure care:
   A. Keep the specimen warm and send it to the laboratory immediately for warmed clotting at 37° C.
5. Client and family teaching:
   A. Fast from food and fluids for 8 hours before the test.
   B. Clients with positive tests should avoid exposure to cold temperatures.
   C. Results may not be available for several days.
6. Factors that affect results:
   A. After separation of serum from the clot and subsequent serum centrifugation, refrigerate the sample for 3-7 days. Testing the sample before the end of the precipitation period may yield incorrect results.
7. Other data:
   A. The serum should be kept under observation for 1 week to detect late-forming cryoglobulins.
   B. Cryoglobulins are not to be confused with cryofibrinogen, which precipitates from *plasma,* rather than serum, in cold conditions.

CRYPTOCOCCAL ANTIGEN TITER, CEREBROSPINAL FLUID (CSF), SPECIMEN

Norm. Negative.

Positive. Titers of 1:8 or more indicate active meningitic *Cryptococcus neoformans* infection. Titers of 1:4 are highly suggestive of meningitic *Cryptococcus neoformans* infection.

Description. *Cryptococcus* is a yeast member of the Fungi Imperfecti group found in the soil and in contaminated bird droppings. It is believed to be transmitted to humans by inhalation from the environment. Normal host defense mechanisms prevent *Cryptococcus* from causing disease. Clients with Hodgkin's disease, sarcoidosis, acquired immunodeficiency syndrome, diabetes, and those on corticosteroid therapy or undergoing bone marrow transplantation are more susceptible to cryptococcal infection. *Cryptococcus neoformans* is the genus most commonly causing pathologic conditions in humans, with chronic meningitis being the most common manifestation. Antigen detection enables earlier diagnosis than culture does. This test uses latex agglutination to detect the presence of the cryptococcal antigen in a sample of cerebrospinal fluid. The results are reported in titers, with the level of titer corresponding to the extent of infection. Serial titers may be used to monitor response to therapy.

Professional Considerations
1. Consent form IS required for the spinal tap. See *Lumbar puncture, Diagnostic,* for risks and contraindications.
2. Preparation:
   A. See *Lumbar puncture, Diagnostic.*
3. Procedure:
   A. 5-10 mL of cerebrospinal fluid is collected through a needle inserted into the spinal canal between L3-4 and L4-5 or directly from the ventricles of the brain during special procedures. See *Lumbar puncture, Diagnostic.*
4. Postprocedure care:
   A. See *Lumbar puncture, Diagnostic.*
   B. Transport the specimen to the laboratory immediately.

5. **Client and family teaching:**
   A. *Cryptococcus* is not believed to be transmitted directly from person to person. Isolation of the clients with positive results is unnecessary.
6. **Factors that affect results:**
   A. False-positive results may occur in clients with rheumatoid arthritis. This cross-reaction may be eliminated when the sample is treated with pronase or the sample is boiled with disodium EDTA.
   B. Several commercially available kits have demonstrated sensitivities of 93-100% and specificity of 93-98% for testing for cryptococcal antigen titer in cerebrospinal fluid.
7. **Other data:**
   A. Amphotericin B and 5-fluocytosine are used to treat cryptococcal infections.
   B. A positive culture is required to confirm diagnosis of cryptococcal infections.
   C. See *Lumbar puncture, Diagnostic,* for procedural contraindications.
   D. See also *Cryptococcal antigen titer, Serum,* for further information about the disease.

CRYPTOCOCCAL ANTIGEN TITER, SERUM

Norm. Negative.

Positive. Titers of 1:8 or more are indicative of active disseminated *Cryptococcus neoformans* infection; titers of 1:4 are highly suggestive of disseminated *C. neoformans* infection.

Description. *Cryptococcus* is a yeast member of the Fungi Imperfecti group found in the soil and in contaminated bird droppings. It is believed to be transmitted to humans by inhalation from the environment. Normal host defense mechanisms prevent *Cryptococcus* from causing disease. Clients with Hodgkin's disease, sarcoidosis, acquired immunodeficiency syndrome, and those on corticosteroid therapy or receiving bone marrow transplants are more susceptible to cryptococcal infection. *C. neoformans* is the genus most commonly causing pathologic conditions in humans, with chronic meningitis being the most common manifestation. Other types of cryptococcal disease involve the lungs, the cutaneous tissue, the skeletal system, and a disseminated infection. Serologic antigen detection allows earlier diagnosis than culture does. This test involves using latex agglutination to detect the presence of the cryptococcal antigen in a sample of serum. Detection of the cryptococcal antigen in serum usually indicates systemic cryptococcosis. Results are reported in titers, with the level of titer corresponding to the extent of infection. Serial titers may be used to monitor response to therapy.

Professional Considerations
1. Consent form NOT required.
2. **Preparation:**
   A. Tube: Red topped, red/gray topped, or gold topped.
3. **Procedure:**
   A. Draw a 10-mL blood sample.
4. **Postprocedure care:**
   A. Transport the specimen to the laboratory immediately.
5. **Client and family teaching:**
   A. *Cryptococcus* is not believed to be transmitted directly from person to person. Isolation of the client is unnecessary.
   B. Results may not be available for several days.
6. **Factors that affect results:**
   A. False-positive results may occur in clients with rheumatoid arthritis. This cross-reaction may be eliminated by treatment of the sample with pronase or boiling of the sample with disodium EDTA.
   B. There are significant differences in sensitivity among five commercially available kits that test for cryptococcal antigen in serum. Kits that pretreat the specimen with pronase had greater specificity (97%) than kits that do not pretreat with pronase (83%).
7. **Other data:**
   A. Amphotericin B (fluconazole) and 5-fluocytosine (flucytosine) are used to treat cryptococcal infections.
   B. A positive culture is required to confirm diagnosis of cryptococcal infections.

CRYPTOCOCCUS ANTIBODY TITER, SERUM

Norm. Negative.

Positive. Titers ≥1:2 are highly suggestive of cryptococcal infection. Positive IFA at titers of ≥1:16 are diagnostic for cryptococcosis.

Description. *Cryptococcus* is a yeast member of the Fungi Imperfecti group found in the soil and in contaminated bird droppings. It is believed to be transmitted to humans by inhalation from the environment. Normal host defense mechanisms prevent *Cryptococcus* from causing disease. Clients with Hodgkin's disease, sarcoidosis, acquired immunodeficiency syndrome, diabetes mellitus, and those on corticosteroid therapy are more susceptible to cryptococcal infection. *C. neoformans* is the genus most commonly causing pathologic conditions in humans, with chronic meningitis being the most common manifestation. Other types of cryptococcal disease involve the lungs, the cutaneous tissue, the skeletal system, and a disseminated infection. Serologic antibody detection allows earlier diagnosis than culture does. This test involves using two tests (indirect fluorescent-antibody and tube agglutination) to detect the presence of the cryptococcal antibody in a sample of serum. The results are reported as the highest dilution demonstrating agglutination when serum is combined with yeast cells.

Professional Considerations
1. Consent form NOT required.
2. **Preparation:**
   A. Tube: Red topped, red/gray topped, or gold topped.
3. **Procedure:**
   A. Obtain a 5-mL blood sample.
4. **Postprocedure care:**
   A. None.
5. **Client and family teaching:**
   A. *Cryptococcus* is not believed to be transmitted directly from person to person. Isolation of the client is unnecessary.
6. **Factors that affect results:**
   A. False-negative results may occur in the presence of increased circulating antigens as the disease progresses. Results may then become positive as drug therapy lowers antigen levels.
   B. False-positive results may occur in the presence of antibodies from past cryptococcal infections.
7. **Other data:**
   A. Amphotericin B (fluconazole) and 5-fluocytosine (flucytosine) are used to treat cryptococcal infections.
   B. A positive culture is required to confirm diagnosis of cryptococcal infections.

CRYPTOSPORIDIUM DIAGNOSTIC PROCEDURES, STOOL

Norm. Negative.

Usage. AIDS.

Description. To detect the presence of *Cryptosporidium*, a coccidian obligate parasite that inhabits the intestinal mucosa and respiratory tracts of many animals (deer, horses, geese) and can cause diarrhea in humans. In clients with intact immune systems, cryptosporidiosis is self-limited to 2 weeks or less. In immunocompromised clients, the disease causes a severe diarrhea lasting weeks to years. In this test, *Cryptosporidium* oocysts must be distinguished from yeast cells. Iodine stains are used to differentiate yeast cells, which do stain, from *Cryptosporidium* oocysts, which do not stain. An acid-fast stain is then performed on a smear of fixed or unfixed stool to confirm the presence of *Cryptosporidium*. In a positive test, *Cryptosporidium* oocysts stain bright red, but yeast cells do not stain.

Professional Considerations
1. Consent form NOT required.
2. **Preparation:**
   A. Clarify the collection procedure with the individual laboratory that will be performing the test. Preschedule this test with the laboratory because testing must be done on a freshly collected specimen.
   B. Obtain a clear container.
3. **Procedure:**
   A. Collect a 20-g sample of stool directly into a wide-mouthed, watertight, clean container.
   B. Some laboratories require that the stool specimen be preserved immediately with a 10% formalin

solution or sodium acetate–acetic acid formalin.

C. If the client is unable to defecate into the container, substitute a sheet of waxed paper and transfer the specimen into the container.

D. Repeat the collection every other day for a total of three specimens.

4. **Postprocedure care:**
A. If a fixative is used, document the consistency of the fresh sample on the laboratory requisition or include a sample of unfixed specimen in a separate container.
B. Transport the specimen to the laboratory immediately.

5. **Client and family teaching:**
A. Contamination of the stool specimen with urine or toilet water invalidates the results.

6. **Factors that affect results:**
A. Antimicrobial therapy causes false-negative results. The test should be repeated 5-10 days after discontinuation of antibiotic therapy.
B. Do not use polyvinyl alcohol (PVA) fixative.

7. **Other data:**
A. Handle the specimen cautiously to prevent self-contamination. *Cryptosporidium* is highly contagious.

CSF ANALYSIS, CSF EXAMINATION

(see Cerebrospinal fluid, Glucose, Specimen; Cerebrospinal fluid, Immunoglobulin G, Immunoglobulin G ratios, and Immunoglobulin G index; Immunoglobulin G synthesis rate, Specimen; Cerebrospinal fluid, Routine analysis, Specimen; Cerebrospinal fluid, Routine, Culture and cytology)

CSF FLOW STUDIES, DIAGNOSTIC

(see Cisternography, Radionuclide, Diagnostic)

CST (CONTRACTION STRESS TEST), DIAGNOSTIC

(see Fetal monitoring, External, Contraction stress test [CST] and Oxytocin challenge test [OCT], Diagnostic)

CT SCAN

(see Cerebral computed tomography, Diagnostic; Chest tomography, Diagnostic; Computed tomography of the body, Diagnostic; Tomography, Paranasal sinuses, Diagnostic)

CT-PTSP

(see Splenoportography, Diagnostic)

C-TYPE NATRIURETIC PEPTIDE

(see Natriuretic Peptides, Plasma)

^{13}C-UBT, ^{14}C-UBT

(see Urea breath test, Diagnostic)

CULDOSCOPY, DIAGNOSTIC

Norm. Normal structure and arrangement of the pelvic organs; absence of inflammatory processes, lesions, adhesions, or ectopic pregnancy; and patent fallopian tubes.

Usage. Aids in the diagnosis of endometriosis, pelvic adhesions, and pelvic abnormalities not diagnosable by palpation. Exploratory procedure for adhesions or tubal blockage causing sterility or for suspected salpingitis, ectopic pregnancy, pelvic pain, or pelvic inflammatory disease. Technique for tubal sterilization.

Description. The direct visualization of the pelvic organs through a culdoscope inserted through the cul-de-sac (rectovaginal septum) of the vagina into the pelvis. The culdoscope, or pelvic endoscope, is a surgical instrument (flexible type available) with a fiberoptic light source, lens, and light hood. Although visualization of the pelvic organs is more difficult with culdoscopy than with laparoscopy, the procedure poses less risk to the woman.

Professional Considerations
1. Consent form IS required.

Risks
Inadvertent amniocentesis, pain.

Contraindications

In instances of cul-de-sac mass, fixed uterine retrodisplacement, acute gynecologic infections, thickened nodular uterosacral ligaments, and in clients who are unable to maintain a knee-chest position.

2. **Preparation:**
   A. Pain medication may be prescribed.
   B. The client should void just before the procedure and disrobe below the waist or wear a gown.
   C. Obtain an antiseptic solution, a culdoscope, a cannula and a trocar, sterile water in a warmer, perineal retractor, a speculum, a tenaculum, a local anesthetic, two needles, two syringes, indigo carmine dye, a pillow, and an absorbable suture material.
   D. The culdoscope is prewarmed in a sterile solution.
   E. Insert an indwelling urinary catheter to prevent bladder distension from urine.

3. **Procedure:**
   A. The client is placed facedown in the knee-chest position with her thighs perpendicular to the examination table and her shoulders supported with shoulder rests.
   B. A perineal retractor is inserted to expose the vaginal vault, and the area is cleansed with an antiseptic solution.
   C. A speculum is inserted through the vagina to elevate the perineum, and a tenaculum is used to pull the cervix toward the symphysis pubis, thus exposing the cul-de-sac.
   D. The rectovaginal septum is injected with local anesthetic in several places.
   E. The trocar is inserted through a cannula and pushed through the vaginal wall at the cul-de-sac and then removed. Upon removal, pneumoperitoneum occurs, aided by the knee-chest position, as air rushes into the peritoneal cavity.
   F. The culdoscope is connected to the fiberoptic light cord and inserted through the cannula into the peritoneal cavity, and the angled lens system is manipu-

lated to methodically inspect the pelvic organs. Organs and structures inspected include the posterior uterine surface, fallopian tubes and ovaries, uterosacral ligaments, pelvic peritoneum, appendix, rectum, and sigmoid colon.
   G. Dye may be injected into the uterus through the cervix, and the fallopian tubes is inspected for patency.
   H. The culdoscope is removed, and the woman is assisted into a prone position with a pillow under the abdomen to force air out of the abdominal cavity. The cannula is removed, and the cul-de-sac is sutured with absorbable sutures.

4. **Postprocedure care:**
   A. Notify the physician for more than a small amount of bleeding or for fever, chills, or an increase in abdominal pain.

5. **Client and family teaching:**
   A. You may experience abdominal cramping for several days after the procedure, until the air dissipates.

6. **Factors that affect results:**
   A. The value of this procedure depends on the skill of the operator.

7. **Other data:**
   A. Microsurgical repair of adnexal structures is sometimes performed with culdoscopy.

CULTURE, BLOOD

(see Blood culture, Blood; Blood culture with antimicrobial removal device, Culture)

CULTURE, CEREBROSPINAL FLUID, SPECIMEN

(see Cerebrospinal fluid, Routine, Culture and cytology, Specimen)

CULTURE, ROUTINE, SPECIMEN

Norm. No growth, normal flora.

Usage. Abscess, auditory infestations, bites (animal, human), blepharitis, body cavity drainage or fluids, endocarditis, inflammation, otitis externa, otitis media, respiratory secretions (mostly gram-negative rods), ulcerations, and wounds (draining, surgical traumatic, mostly *Staphylococcus aureus*).

Description. Laboratory cultures of specimens taken from various body substances are performed to isolate and identify pathogenic microorganisms causing disease. This test involves the direct microscopic inspection of a Gram-stained smear of an organism after it is grown in selected media.

Professional Considerations
1. Consent form NOT required.
2. **Preparation:**
   A. Obtain the proper specimen container for the site (see the table at the bottom of the page).
   B. Label multiple collections of the same test sequentially.
   C. Wear a mask to prevent inhalation of airborne microorganisms expelled with coughing while collecting tracheal or nasopharyngeal specimens.
3. **Procedure:**
   A. A separate specimen should be obtained for each test.
   B. *Ear culture:* Insert a cotton-tipped Culturette $\frac{1}{8}$ to $\frac{1}{4}$ inch into the external auditory canal and rotate the swab. Remove the swab without touching any other parts of the ear. Insert the swab into the Culturette tube and squeeze the end of the tube to release the contents of the medium.
   C. *Eye culture:* Swab the inner canthus of the eye with a sterile cotton-tipped Culturette swab. Insert the swab into the Culturette tube and squeeze the end of the tube to release the contents of the medium.
   D. *Nasal culture:* Have the client clear the nose of excess secretions and tilt back the head. Insert the cotton-tipped Culturette into the nostril until it reaches the posterior nares and swab it in a circular motion two times. Leave the swab in place for 15 seconds. Slowly remove the swab and place it in the Culturette tube. Squeeze the swab end of the tube to release the contents of the medium. Repeat this procedure using the other nostril for nares culture.
   E. *Nasopharyngeal culture:* Have the client tilt back the head and open the mouth. While depressing the tongue with a tongue blade, gently swab the tonsillar area from left to right. Also swab any reddened or purulent areas. Remove the swab without touching any other parts of the mouth. Insert the swab into the Culturette tube and squeeze the end of the tube to release the contents of the medium.
   F. *Sputum culture:* A first-morning sputum specimen is recommended. Chest clapping, postural drainage, or aerosol therapy, or all three, may be helpful in mobilizing tenacious secretions just before sputum collection. Have the client cough deeply several times and expel the mucus contents mobilized into a wide-mouthed, sterile specimen cup. Instruct the client to avoid otherwise contaminating the cup's inside or edges. Tightly cap the cup.

CULTURE, ROUTINE, SPECIMEN

SITE	TYPE OF STERILE CONTAINER
Ear	Cotton swab Culturette
Eye	Cotton swab Culturette
Nasal	2 cotton swab Culturettes
Nasopharyngeal	Cotton swab Culturette
Site drainage	Cotton swab Culturette
Sputum	Sterile cup with lid
Sputum, tracheal	Sputum trap
Wound, superficial	Cotton swab Culturette
Wound, deep	Sterile syringe

G. *Sputum, tracheal, culture:* Ventilated clients should be hyperoxygenated before starting the procedure. Place the sputum trap in-line between the suction tubing and suction catheter. Maintain the trap in an upright position. Using a sterile technique, insert the suction catheter tip into the tracheostomy, endotracheal tube, or nares and advance it into the trachea without applying suction. In 10 seconds or less, apply suction and obtain 3-5 mL of mucus for culture in the trap and remove the suction catheter. Cap the sputum trap.

H. *Wound, superficial site drainage:* Swab the site with the cotton-tipped end of a Culturette. Avoid touching the surrounding skin with the tip. Place the swab into the Culturette tube and squeeze the swab end to release the contents of the medium. Large wounds should have several separate cultures performed from different areas of the wound.

I. *Wound, deep:* Aspirate drainage with a syringe and needle from deep inside the wound. Remove the syringe, expel the air into sterile gauze, and either cap the needle with a rubber stopper or cork, or inject the contents into anaerobic culture medium. Transport the specimen to the laboratory immediately.

4. **Postprocedure care:**
   A. Label the container with the specimen collection date and time.
   B. Place the specimen in a sealed plastic bag.
   C. Write any recent antibiotic or antifungal therapy on the laboratory requisition.
   D. Send the specimen to the laboratory immediately. Do not refrigerate it.

5. **Client and family teaching:**
   A. The specimen collection procedure is typically painless, unless pressure is placed on an area of inflammation.
   B. *Sputum collection:* Deep coughs are necessary to produce sputum, rather than saliva. To produce the proper specimen, take several breaths in, without fully exhaling

each, and then expel sputum with a "cascade cough."
   C. Clients started on empiric therapy should continue taking drugs unless and until test results are found to be negative.

6. **Factors that affect results:**
   A. Antibiotic or antifungal therapy initiated before the specimen is taken may produce false-negative results. Obtain the culture before starting this therapy for the most accurate identification of the causative bacteria and the best clinical results.

7. **Other data:**
   A. Results for most microorganisms will not be available for 48-72 hours. Fungi and mycobacteria may take several weeks. Gram stains requested should be available within 1 hour.
   B. Normal mouth flora include *Actinomyces,* anaerobic and aerobic (non–group A) streptococci, anaerobic spirochetes, Enterobacteriaceae, *Haemo philus influenzae, Lactobacillus, Pneumococcus, Branhamella catarrhalis, Bacteroides* species, *Candida* fungi, nonpathogenic *Neisseria, N. meningitides, Staphylococcus aureus, S. epidermidis, S. pyogenes,* and *Veillonella* species.
   C. Normal throat flora include alpha-hemolytic and nonhemolytic streptococci, *Bacteroides, Candida* fungi, *Corynebacterium* species, Enterobacteriaceae, *Haemophilus influenzae, N. meningitides,* nonpathogenic *Neisseria, Pneumococcus, S. aureus,* and *S. pyogenes.*
   D. Normal nasal flora in small amounts include *B. catarrhalis, C. albicans,* diphtheroids, *H. influenzae, Neisseria* species (except *N. gonorrhoeae* and *N. meningitides), S. aureus, S. epidermidis, S. pneumoniae,* and *S. pyogenes.*
   E. Normal ear flora include *S. epidermidis, Corynebacterium,* and *S. aureus.*
   F. Normal eye flora include diphtheroids, Enterobacteriaceae, *Haemophilus, Moraxella, Neisseria, Pneumococcus, Sarcina, Staphylococcus epidermidis,* and *S. pyogenes.*
   G. Nasal cultures should generally be limited to situations where

throat specimens are not easily obtained because throat cultures are usually more advantageous for diagnosing upper respiratory tract infections.

H. Time to detection closely correlates with overall response to treatment for pulmonary tuberculosis.

CULTURE, ROUTINE, STOOL
(see Stool culture, Routine)

CULTURE, SKIN, SPECIMEN

Norm. Negative.

Usage. Abscesses, ache, anthrax, athlete's foot, burn infections, candidiasis, carbuncles, erysipelas, folliculitis, herpes simplex, *Microsporum audouinii* for ringworm of the scalp, *Neisseria meningitides* for meningococcemia, neutrophilic eccrine hidradenitis, *Prototheca* algae, pruritus, psoriasis, pyoderma, scrapings to collect ova or mites for scabies, *Staphylococcus aureus* or group A beta-hemolytic streptococci for impetigo, *Streptococcus pyogenes*, tinea cruris, vitiligo, warts, yaws, and other skin infections.

Description. A sample of infected lesions of the skin is incubated, and the growth patterns, bacterial cell staining, and microscopic appearance are studied for determination of the organism causing the disease process. The most common skin pathogens are *Aspergillus, Blastomyces, Candida, Coccidioides immitis, Cryptococcus, Enterococcus, Histoplasma capsulatum, Microsporum, Penicillium, Proteus, Rhizopus, Rhodotorula, Sporothrix schenckii, Staphylococcus, Streptococcus,* and *Trichophyton* species.

Professional Considerations
1. Consent form NOT required.
2. Preparation:
   A. Obtain 70% alcohol, sterile water, a sterile scalpel or spatula, and a sterile Petri dish or anaerobic swab culture tubes, as indicated.
3. Procedure:
   A. Cleanse the lesion site with 70% alcohol and then rinse with ster-

ile water to eliminate the effect of alcohol on any bacteria. Allow the site to dry.

B. Scrape the edge of the lesion to obtain tissue samples or purulent drainage with a sterile scalpel or spatula. Place the sample in a sterile Petri dish.

C. For an anaerobic culture, obtain purulent drainage samples from deep in the wound on a swab and carefully place them in an anaerobic culture medium.

4. Postprocedure care:
   A. Apply a dry, sterile dressing as needed.
5. Client and family teaching:
   A. If started on empiric therapy, you should continue taking the prescribed drug(s) unless and until the test results are found to be negative.
6. Factors that affect results:
   A. Obtain specimens before starting antibiotics for the most accurate bacterial identification and best clinical outcome.
   B. For burned clients, viable skin rather than eschar yields the best results.
   C. Chances of inadequate sampling of the lesion can be reduced when several separate samplings of the lesion or exudate are taken.
7. Other data:
   A. Minor normal flora of the skin include *S. aureus*, fungi of the pityriasis type, and *Staphylococcus epidermidis*, which may proliferate in clients with poor immune systems and invasive wounds.

CULTURE, URINE
(see Culture, Routine, Specimen)

CUTANEOUS IMMUNOFLUORESCENCE BIOPSY, DIAGNOSTIC

Norm. A descriptive, interpretive report of histologic study findings is made.

Usage. Bulbous pemphigoid, chilblain lesions, dermatitis herpetiformis, herpes gestationis, necrolytic migratory erythema, pemphigus, and porphyria cutanea tarda in scleroderma; indicated in the investigation of cutaneous forms of chronic discoid lupus erythematosus, blistering disease, and vasculitis; also used to confirm the histopathologic characteristics of skin lesions and to follow the results of treatment.

Description. A biopsy specimen of the skin is taken for direct epidermal immunofluorescent study. Direct immunofluorescence is a histologic technique whereby the skin sample is treated with fluorescein-conjugated human immunoglobulin antisera and then incubated and examined under ultraviolet radiation. Deposition of human immunoglobulins and complement components in skin tissue and lesions (indicating a disorder) is identified and differentiated by the immunofluorescent patterns demonstrated.

Professional Considerations
1. Consent form IS required.

Risks
Bleeding, infection.

Contraindications
May be contraindicated in bleeding disorders, anticoagulated states, and immunocompromised states.

2. **Preparation:**
   A. Obtain punch forceps, an antiseptic solution, gauze, and a sterile specimen container.

3. **Procedure:**
   A. A 4-mm punch biopsy or surgically excised specimen of involved or uninvolved skin is obtained.
   B. The specimen is quick-frozen in liquid nitrogen and stored at $-94°$ F ($-70°$ C). If the specimen is to be shipped to an outside lab, it is preserved in Michel holding solution with the pH maintained between 7.0 and 7.4.

4. **Postprocedure care:**
   A. Apply a dry, sterile dressing to the biopsy site.

5. **Client and family teaching:**
   A. The test typically is transiently painful.
   B. Place pressure over the site for 5 minutes if bleeding occurs.
   C. Results may not be available for several days.

6. **Factors that affect results:**
   A. Amount of biopsy <4 mm is insufficient.
   B. The reliability of immunofluorescence technique is affected by factors such as age and site of the lesion, type of immunofluorescence, and type of immunoglobulin. For this reason, histopathologic characteristics should also be used to confirm the results.

7. **Other data:**
   A. The final report may take up to 3 days.

CXR, DIAGNOSTIC
(see Chest radiography, Diagnostic)

CYANIDE, BLOOD

Norm:

		SI UNITS
Serum		
Nonsmoker	0.004 mg/L	0.15 µmol/L
Smoker	0.006 mg/L	0.22 µmol/L
Panic (lethal) level	>0.1 mg/L	>3.7 µmol/L
Nitroprusside therapy	0.01-0.06 mg/L	0.37-2.21 µmol/L
Whole Blood		
Nonsmoker	0.016 mg/L	0.59 µmol/L
Smoker	0.041 mg/L	1.52 µmol/L
Panic (lethal) level	>1 mg/L	>37 µmol/L
Nitroprusside therapy	0.05-0.5 mg/L	1.9-19 µmol/L

Panic Level Symptoms and Treatment

Symptoms. Headache, dizziness, abdominal pain, nausea, confusion, labored breathing, syncope, tachycardia, hypertension, convulsions, and coma before respiratory failure. Loss of consciousness, metabolic acidosis, and cardiopulmonary failure are three most common signs of cyanide poisoning in clients who die from this problem.

Treatment:
Note: Treatment choice(s) depend on client history and condition and episode history.
Oxygen 15 L by mask (adult) and amyl nitrate pearl inhalants (crush onto a cloth and place in front of mouth for inhalation for 15-30 seconds, remove for 15 seconds, and repeat process every 3 minutes), hydroxocobalamin 4 g in 24 hours for adults, sodium nitrate 3% (300 mg in 10 mL of sterile water given IV over 10 minutes for adult and may repeat × 1, and 0.33 mL/kg for children; if given too fast, causes hypotension), and sodium thiosulfate (12.5 g in 50 mL of sterile water under slow IV push for adult and 1.65 mg/kg as pediatric dose).

Usage. Cyanide poisoning or suicide and monitoring of cyanide levels during nitroprusside therapy.

Description. A determination of the presence of cyanide in the blood. Cyanide is a very toxic chemical that inactivates cellular respiration enzymes (cytochrome oxidase), poisoning their functional activity and causing death from asphyxia. The major cause of death from cyanide poisoning is suicide.

Professional Considerations
1. Consent form NOT required.
2. Preparation:
   A. Tube: Lavender topped, black topped, or green topped.
3. Procedure:
   A. Completely fill the tube with blood.
4. Postprocedure care:
   A. If cyanide poisoning is suspected, monitor neurologic and respiratory status closely and have emergency intubation equipment and oral airway available.
5. Client and family teaching:
   A. Kidneys and corneas can be harvested for transplantation after the poison level falls below lethal concentrations without adverse transplantation effects.
6. Factors that affect results:
   A. An insufficient blood sample may cause falsely low results.
7. Other data:
   A. Cyanide is an end product of combustion, cigarette smoke, artificial nail remover, metal, wood, plastic refineries, Laetrile, plants, grass (sorghum), and pits of peaches and apricots. Also found in acetonitrile (methyl cyanide), a common industrial organic solvent.

CYCLIC ADENOSINE MONOPHOSPHATE (cAMP, CYCLIC AMP), SERUM AND URINE

Norm:

		SI UNITS
Serum	5.6-10.9 ng/mL	17-33 nmol/L
Urine		
Total cAMP	112-188 mg/L or 4612 pmoles	340-570 nmol/L
cAMP portion of creatinine	3-5 mmol/g of creatinine	
cAMP portion of glomerular filtrate	6.6-15.5 mg/L	20-47 mmol/L
cAMP nephrogenous portion of glomerular filtrate	<9.9 mg/L	<30 nmol/L

Increased. Hyperparathyroidism, malignant processes combined with hypercalcemia, manic-depressives with bipolar disorder (untreated), migraine headaches, and pseudohyperparathyroidism.

Decreased. Atopic dermatitis, chronic renal failure, hypoparathyroidism, and pseudohypoparathyroidism.

Description. Nephrogenous cyclic adenosine monophosphate (cAMP) is an enzyme that increases in production in the renal tubules in response to parathyroid hormone, cAMP influences the rate of cell protein synthesis and indirectly affects renal reabsorption of phosphate, gastrointestinal calcium absorption, and skeletal calcium mobilization, cAMP in urine is the result of renal tubular cAMP secretion, and glomerulus-filtered cAMP. Thus, by comparing the serum and urine levels of cAMP with the glomerular filtration rate, one can estimate the portion of cAMP secreted by the tubules. There is some evidence that it may be secreted in a diurnal pattern. In clients with hyperparathyroidism, increased levels of nephrogenous cAMP are usually found as a result of excess parathyroid hormone production. A 24-hour urine collection may reveal increased levels of cAMP as a result of excess parathyroid hormone in the system.

Professional Considerations
1. Consent form NOT required.
2. Preparation:
   A. See *Client and family teaching.*
   B. Preschedule this test with the laboratory.
   C. Tube: Red topped, red/gray topped, or gold topped for the serum sample.
   D. Obtain a 3-L container with hydrochloric acid (HCl) preservative for the urine sample.
   E. The client should lie recumbent throughout the urine collection.
   F. For 24-hour collections, discard the first morning-urine specimen and write the beginning time on the laboratory requisition.
3. Procedure:
   A. Serum collection: Draw a 5-mL blood sample.
   B. Urine collection: Collect a 2- or 24-hour urine sample for cAMP and creatinine in a refrigerated, 3-L container. For 24-hour col-

lections, include the urine voided at the end of the 24-hour period. For catheterized clients, keep the drainage bag on ice and empty urine into the acidified collection container hourly.
4. Postprocedure care:
   A. *Serum sample:*
      i. Write the specimen collection time on the laboratory requisition.
      ii. Transport the specimen to the laboratory immediately for serum separation.
      iii. Freeze the specimen if the test cannot be performed immediately.
   B. *Urine sample:*
      i. Compare the urine quantity in the specimen container with the urinary output record for the test. If the specimen contains less urine than what was recorded as output, some of the sample may have been discarded, invalidating the test.
      ii. Write the ending time of collection and the total urine volume on the laboratory requisition.
      iii. Send the specimen to the laboratory immediately and refrigerate it until testing.
5. Client and family teaching:
   A. Limit physical exertion for 4 hours before the urine test.
   B. Urinate before defecating to avoid loss of urine for the urine test. If any urine is accidentally discarded, discard the entire specimen and restart the collection the next day.
   C. Results may not be available for more than 24 hours.
6. Factors that affect results:
   A. Reject serum specimens received more than 1 hour after collection.
   B. Radioactive scans within 7 days before the test invalidate the serum and urine results.
   C. Impaired renal function precludes the value of this urine test because results cannot be relied on for diagnosis.
   D. All the urine voided for the 24-hour period must be included to avoid a falsely low result.
7. Other data:
   A. For differentiation of hypoparathyroidism from pseudohypoparathyroidism, see *Cyclic adenosine*

monophosphate provocation test, Urine.

CYCLIC ADENOSINE MONOPHOSPHATE PROVOCATION TEST, URINE

Norm. Positive: A 10- to 20-fold increase, or 3.6-4 mmol.

Negative. Type I pseudohypoparathyroidism.

Description. A test that measures cyclic adenosine monophosphate (cAMP) response to parathyroid hormone administration. cAMP is an enzyme that influences the rate of cell protein synthesis and indirectly affects renal reabsorption of phosphate, gastrointestinal calcium absorption, and skeletal calcium mobilization. In normal clients and those with idiopathic or postoperative hypoparathyroidism, parathyroid hormone administration causes increased renal tubular production of cAMP. In clients with pseudohypoparathyroidism, a genetically transmitted, autosomal dominant disease resulting in tissue resistance to the effects of parathyroid hormone, the infusion fails to increase production of cAMP in the renal tubules, resulting in a negative test.

Professional Considerations
1. Consent form NOT required.

Risks
Allergic reaction to parathyroid hormone (itching, hives, rash, tight feeling in the throat, shortness of breath, bronchospasm, anaphylaxis, death).

Contraindications
Positive parathyroid hormone skin test. This test is contraindicated in hypercalcemia.

Precaution
Use cautiously when digitalis has been administered and in renal impairment, cardiac disease, or sarcoidosis.

2. **Preparation:**
   A. Preschedule this test with the laboratory.
   B. Obtain 300 U of parathyroid hormone and reconstitute it with sterile water for injection, as directed on the container.
   C. Obtain a needle, a syringe, and a 1-L urine collection container with hydrochloric acid (HCl) preservative.
   D. Establish intravenous access with 5% dextrose in water.
   E. Have emergency equipment readily available.
3. **Procedure:**
   A. Have the client empty the bladder.
   B. Attach a new collection bag on ice for catheterized clients.
   C. Administer the prescribed dose of parathyroid hormone over 15 minutes.
   D. Save all the urine collected in a refrigerated, 1-L container with HCl preservative. For catheterized clients, empty the drainage bag into the collection container hourly.
   E. Three hours after the completion of the infusion, mix the container gently and collect a 50- to 100-mL aliquot for cAMP measurement.
4. **Postprocedure care:**
   A. Send the specimen to the laboratory immediately. Refrigerate the specimen until testing.
   B. Observe the client for lethargy, anorexia, nausea, vomiting, vertigo, or abdominal cramps, which could result from the mobilization of calcium stores by parathyroid hormone administration.
5. **Client and family teaching:**
   A. You will not be permitted to drive for 24 hours after the test and should make arrangements for someone else to drive you home.
6. **Factors that affect results:**
   A. Radioactive scans within 7 days before the test invalidate the results.
7. **Other data:**
   A. None.

CYCLIC AMP
(see Cyclic adenosine monophosphate, Serum and Urine)

CYSTINE, QUALITATIVE, URINE

Norm. Negative.

Positive. Congenital cystinuria, Fanconi syndrome, Lowe syndrome, nephrolithiasis, nephrotoxicity (caused by heavy metals), pyelonephritis (acute), renal tubular acidosis, and Wilson's disease.

Description. Cystine is an amino acid normally absent or present in only low amounts in the urine. In conditions causing cystinuria over 300 mg/day, smooth, waxy cystine stones form in the kidneys and may be passed into the urine. Positive qualitative results should be followed by a 24-hour collection for cystine measurement because random samples may demonstrate peaks of cystine excretion in the urine.

Professional Considerations
1. Consent form NOT required.
2. Preparation:
   A. Obtain a clean container.
3. Procedure:
   A. Obtain a random urine specimen of 20 mL. A fresh specimen may be taken from a urinary drainage bag.
4. Postprocedure care:
   A. Send the specimen to the laboratory immediately.
5. Client and family teaching:
   A. Results are normally available within 24 hours.
6. Factors that affect results:
   A. Drug that may cause false-negative results include penicillamine.
7. Other data:
   A. This test should be scheduled before an intravenous pyelogram.
   B. This is not a test for cystinosis, in which the urine cystine may be normal or only slightly elevated.
   C. Acalculous cystinuria does not necessarily result in urinary stone disease.

CYSTOGRAPHY, RETROGRADE, DIAGNOSTIC

Norm. Normal and intact structure of the bladder and normal location of the bladder; absence of rupture, laceration, fistula, tumor, or reflux into the ureters.

Usage. Detection of anastomotic leak after surgery, bladder diverticuli, bladder tumors, calculi, clots or other foreign bodies, fistula, hematoma, pyelonephritis, and laceration or rupture of bladder, urinary tract infections, or vesicoureteral reflux. This test will often indicate irregularity of the bladder present in neurogenic bladders.

Description. Retrograde cystography performed by filling the bladder by injection or gravity flow (by means of a syringe barrel) with opacified contrast and sometimes air through a catheter into the bladder. This is followed by radiographs of the pelvis and bladder with the client in several positions.

Professional Considerations
1. Consent form IS required.

Risks
Bleeding, infection, urinary tract obstruction. Allergic reaction to contrast (hives, itching, rash, tight feeling in the throat, shortness of breath, bronchospasm, anaphylaxis, death) is extremely rare. Contrast should not be used in clients who have a contrast allergy or clients who have suspected major trauma to the bladder with the possibility of venous uptake of contrast or intraperitoneal spill.

Contraindications
History of allergy to radiographic dye, iodine, or shellfish; in urethral obstruction or injury, inability to pass a urethral catheter; or during the acute phase of a urinary tract infection; pregnancy (if iodinated contrast material is used, because of radioactive iodine crossing the blood-placental barrier).

2. Preparation:
   A. Obtain a straight urinary catheter and a catheter insertion tray, 50-300 mL of radiographic dye, and a syringe.
   B. The client should disrobe below the waist or wear a gown.
   C. Obtain baseline vital signs.
   D. Have emergency equipment readily available.
3. Procedure:
   A. The client is positioned supine on the radiographic table.
   B. A baseline kidney-ureter-bladder (KUB) radiograph is taken.
   C. 200-300 mL (50-100 mL for infants) of radiographic dye is instilled into the bladder by a catheter inserted through the urethra. It is recommended that the contrast be instilled through gravity using the barrel of a catheter-tipped syringe.
   D. After the catheter is clamped, the client is assisted to several different positions by a tilt table; the

physical position changes for radiographic examination of the bladder and surrounding areas.

E. The catheter is unclamped, the bladder fluid allowed to drain, and final radiographs are taken.

4. Postprocedure care:
A. Monitor vital signs every 15 minutes × 4, then every 30 minutes × 2, then hourly × 4, and then every 2 hours for 24 hours after the test only if there is gross extravasation or major trauma is identified.
B. Encourage the oral intake of fluids where not contraindicated.
C. Have the client and family members observe for signs of allergic reaction to the dye (listed above) for 24 hours.
D. Observe for urinary retention or symptoms of urinary tract infection (fever; chills; tachycardia; tachypnea; abdominal, flank, or suprapubic pain; hesitancy and frequency; dysuria; and hematuria). Notify the physician for any of these signs.
E. See *Client and family teaching.*

5. Client and family teaching:
A. A clear liquid diet and a cathartic the day before the test may improve the clarity of the results by minimizing intestinal gas and the amount of stool.
B. After the procedure, save all the urine voided for the next day and report chills or painful urination. Blood in the urine that lasts more than 4-6 hours is abnormal.

6. Factors that affect results:
A. This test should not be performed within 1 week of a previous intestinal barium examination.
B. The clarity of the radiographic images may be diminished by the presence of excess gas or stool in the lower gastrointestinal tract.

7. Other data:
A. None.

CYSTOMETRY, DIAGNOSTIC

Norm. Normal filling pattern. Absence of residual urine; sensation of fullness at 300-500 mL; urge to void at 150-450 mL; filling bladder pressure constant (≤ in a change of 15 cm of water) until capacity reached with contraction at capacity. Normal thermal

sensation when hot and cold sterile fluids are introduced into the bladder.

Usage. Evaluation of detrusor muscle function and tonicity, determination of the cause of bladder dysfunction (urinary incontinence and retention), and differentiation of the type of neurogenic bladder dysfunction.

Description. Cystometry involves assessment of bladder neuromuscular function after instillation of measured quantities of fluid or air and evaluation of the client's neurologic sensations and muscular responses. It also includes assessment of the voiding flow pattern for abnormalities. Neuromuscular dysfunction of the bladder can occur when brain or spinal cord lesions (spinal cord or brain surgery or injury; stroke) interfere with the neural pathways that transmit bladder reflexes to and from the brain or with progressive diseases (such as multiple sclerosis), congenital malformations, strokes, or postoperatively. Cystometry is most often performed in a physician's office or clinic.

Professional Considerations
1. Consent form IS required.

Risks
Clients with spinal cord lesions (usually with cervical lesions or a history of higher cord lesions) may exhibit autonomic dysreflexia (bradycardia, hypertension, flushing, diaphoresis, and headache) during instillation of fluid or carbon dioxide. Intravenous or oral nifedipine or propantheline bromide may help to counteract this response.

Contraindications
This procedure is contraindicated in the acute phase of urinary tract infection and in urethral obstruction.

2. Preparation:
A. Obtain a gas cystometer, a cystometric set, a 6- or 8-French special multiple-port transducer catheter, and an irrigation solution of sterile 0.9% saline or sterile, distilled water.
B. The client should disrobe below the waist or wear a gown.

3. Procedure:
A. The client urinates into a funnel attached to a machine that plots

the amount, flow, and time of voiding on a graph.

B. Residual urine volume, if any, is then measured by means of an inserted indwelling catheter.

C. As the client lies in a supine position, thermal sensation is evaluated by the client's reported sensations in response to the instillation of 30-60 mL of room temperature 0.9% sterile saline solution, followed by 30-60 mL of 29-32° C, 0.9% sterile saline solution through the catheter into the bladder.

D. The fluid is then drained from the bladder.

E. The client is then placed on a special commode chair attached to a cystometrogram table or placed in the semi-upright position. The client's sensations to bladder filling are measured next after the catheter is connected to a cystometer and measured amounts of sterile fluid or carbon dioxide are instilled into the bladder. Sometimes another catheter is placed into the rectum for abdominal presssure measurement. This allows true bladder muscle (detrusor) pressure to be electronically determined (Bladder pressure − Abdominal pressure = Detrusor pressure). Needle or surface electrodes may be used to measure pelvic floor muscle activity.

F. The cystometer measures and graphically records bladder pressure and volume, along with the client's reported descriptions of sensations, as when he or she first feels the urge to void or feels unable to go any longer without voiding, and any reported discomfort.

G. The instillation is stopped when the client feels uncomfortably full or if it is determined that there is an absence of filling sensation.

H. The air or fluid and catheter are removed, or the client may be asked to void the fluid.

I. The test may be repeated in standing or sitting positions or after the administration of bladder-tone stimulants such as bethanechol chloride.

4. **Postprocedure care:**

A. Encourage the oral intake of fluids when not contraindicated; 125 mL/hour for 24 hours is desirable.

B. Monitor fluid intake and urine output for 24 hours.

C. Observe for urinary retention, symptoms of urinary tract infection (fever; chills; tachycardia; tachypnea; abdominal, suprapubic, or flank pain; hesitancy and frequency; dysuria; and hematuria).

D. Hematuria for more than 4-6 hours is abnormal. More postprocedure discomfort may be experienced after carbon dioxide instillation than after irrigant instillation.

E. Analgesics may be prescribed for bladder spasms.

5. **Client and family teaching:**

A. The client must lie very still during the test.

B. The client may experience bladder spasms and see blood in his or her urine after the procedure. Spasms occurring for longer than 24 hours or bloody urine for more than 4-6 hours is abnormal. Call the physician if either of these occurs.

6. **Factors that affect results:**

A. Antihistamines may interfere with bladder function by causing relaxation.

B. Movement during the test may interfere with bladder reflexes.

7. **Other data:**

A. None.

CYSTOSCOPY, DIAGNOSTIC

Norm. Normal structure and function of the bladder; absence of urethral strictures or abnormalities, tumors, or bladder calculi; and absence of inflammation or purulent secretions.

Usage. Diagnosis of bladder cancer (99% Stage Ta grade I), diagnosis of vesicoureteral efflux in children, evaluation and differentiation of urinary tract disorders, method for obtaining bladder and ureteral biopsy specimens, sometimes used for excision of small tumors, evaluation of hematuria and of suspected urinary tract malformation in children.

Description. Cystoscopy is the direct, transurethral visualization of the bladder and urethra with the use of a lighted, magnifying cystoscope with a variety of lenses. The cystoscope is a metal instrument with a solid obturator that is placed inside a sheath within the urethra. Flexible cystoscopy is becoming more widely used as an alternative to rigid cystoscopy. Cystoscopy is indicated after other tests such as cystography show abnormalities or for symptoms such as dysuria, frequency, and incontinence or for evaluation of hematuria. It is also used as surveillance for recurrent bladder lesions such as transitional cell carcinoma. The procedure may be performed in a hospital or office by a physician or specialist urology nurse (SUN).

Professional Considerations
1. Consent form IS required.

Risks
Bleeding, infection (7.8% overall and 21.7% in enterocystoplasty clients), urinary tract obstruction.

Contraindications
Acute inflammations of the urethral passage. Sedatives are contraindicated in clients with central nervous system depression.

2. **Preparation:**
   A. See *Client and family teaching*.
   B. Obtain a cystoscopy tray, disinfectant or surgical scrub solution, a genitourinary irrigant, drapes, sterile gloves, a cystoscope with appropriate lenses, obturator and light source (today video monitoring is common and the appropriate lens connector for camera and cord connection to the video unit is recommended), filiforms and followers, and two or three sterile specimen containers (for possible biopsy, urine for culture and sensitivity, and a urine sample for cytologic testing).
   C. A sedative may be prescribed.
   D. Prophylactic antibiotics do not decrease the incidence of urinary tract infection in clients with sterile urine.
   E. The client should disrobe below the waist or wear a gown.
   F. Obtain baseline vital signs.

G. Pad the lithotomy stirrups.
H. Have emergency equipment readily available.
3. **Procedure:**
   A. The client is positioned in the supine position on the cystoscopic table for possible administration of general or regional anesthesia.
   B. The client is then placed in the lithotomy position for external genitalia cleansing and draping and cystoscopic examination.
   C. After local anesthesia (if used) is instilled into the urethra and bladder and retained for 10-20 minutes, the urethra is progressively dilated (if necessary), and a cystoscope with obturator in place is inserted through the urethra into the bladder. The cystoscope is usually placed with the obturator in place in women and under direct vision with a 0- or 30-degree lens or flexible cystoscope in men. Pain can be significantly reduced by use of 20 mL of 2% lignocaine (lidocaine) gel left in the urethra for 15 minutes.
   D. Urine specimens for culture or cytologic study may be removed through the cystoscope.
   E. The bladder is filled with genitourinary irrigant solution, and the lighted cystoscope is used with magnification to directly examine the interior walls, structures, and contents of the bladder and urethra.
   F. The bladder is inspected for tumors, calculi, diverticula, obstructions, and other lesions. The urethra is inspected for strictures and other lesions.
   G. A biopsy sample of the bladder or ureters may be taken, and tiny tumors may also be excised through the cystoscope, with bleeding controlled by electrocautery.
4. **Postprocedure care:**
   A. For general anesthesia, monitor vital signs every 15 minutes × 4, then every 30 minutes × 2, and then every 2 hours × 2. Typical postanesthesia monitoring also includes continuous ECG monitoring and pulse oximetry, with continual assessments (every 5-15 minutes) of airway and neuro-

logic status until the client is lying quietly awake, is breathing independently, and responds appropriately to commands spoken in a normal tone.

B. For local anesthesia, assist the client to a chair until strength has returned to baseline value or for at least 15-30 minutes.

C. Encourage oral intake of fluids: 125 mL/hour for 24-48 hours when not contraindicated.

D. Monitor fluid intake and urine output for 24 hours.

E. Observe for urinary retention or symptoms of urinary tract infection (fever, chills, pain [abdominal, suprapubic, or flank], tachypnea, tachycardia, hesitancy and frequency, dysuria, and hematuria). Notify the physician if any of these signs occur.

F. Observe for hematuria. Pink urine is normal initially but should clear. Frank hematuria or clotting is abnormal. Dysuria lasting more than 4-6 hours is abnormal.

G. Analgesics may be prescribed for bladder spasms, and sitz or tub baths may help decrease generalized genital area discomfort.

H. Resume diet.

5. Client and family teaching:
A. Arrange for someone to drive you home if the procedure was performed under anything other than local anesthesia because you will not be permitted to drive for 24 hours after having general anesthesia. It is also suggested that someone drive you home after local anesthesia in some situations, but this is not absolutely necessary.

B. For general anesthesia, fast from food and fluids for 8 hours. For local anesthesia, consume only clear liquids for 8 hours. You may be required to take in a large amount of fluids to promote urine flow during the procedure.

C. Clients receiving local anesthesia may feel the urge to void while the cystoscope is in place.

D. After the procedure, drink 6-8 glasses of water or other fluids per day for 2 days (unless contraindicated). Watch for warning symptoms of complications (see above). Report chills, fever, dysuria, or frank blood in the urine.

E. Do not have sexual relations until the physician confirms healing.

6. Factors that affect results:
A. None.

7. Other data:
A. Urethroscopy or retrograde pyelogram may also be combined with cystoscopy.

B. Cystoscopy may also be used as a therapeutic procedure to crush and remove calculi, perform bladder irrigation, resect tumors, or perform a transurethral resection of the prostate gland.

C. The use of intraurethral lidocaine gel has not been shown to decrease client pain during rigid cystoscopy in one study (Stein et al, 1994). Anxiety has been shown to positively correlate with pain perception.

CYSTOURETHROGRAPHY, VOIDING, DIAGNOSTIC

Norm. Normal formation of bladder and urethra, normal elimination of contrast medium through the urethra, and absence of retrograde movement of contrast medium into the ureters.

Usage. Detection of urinary tract congenital anomalies, vesicoureteral reflux, neurogenic abnormalities, enlarged prostate gland, urethral strictures, and bladder diverticula or polyps.

Description. Using fluoroscopy or radiography, voiding cystourethrography demonstrates the bladder filling by contrast medium instillation through a catheter into the bladder and then shows exiting of the contrast medium during voiding after removal of the catheter.

Professional Considerations
1. Consent form IS required.

Risks
Bleeding, hematuria, and infection. Allergic reaction to contrast (itching, hives, rash, tight feeling in the throat, shortness of breath, bronchospasm, anaphylaxis, death) is a very rare possibility, since no contrast should be absorbed into the vascular tree with this procedure.

Contraindications
Previous allergy to radiographic dye, iodine, or shellfish; in the acute phase of a urinary tract infection; urinary tract obstruction; during pregnancy (if iodinated contrast material is used, because of radioactive iodine crossing the blood-placental barrier); recent bladder surgery; and urethral obstruction, evulsion, or transection. Sedatives are contraindicated in clients with central nervous system depression.

2. **Preparation:**
   A. See *Client and family teaching*.
   B. Obtain a balloon catheter, a contrast medium, and a syringe or tubing for instillation of the contrast medium.
   C. The client should disrobe below the waist.
   D. A sedative may be prescribed. Elder and Longenecker (1995) demonstrated safety of midazolam use for excessively frightened children undergoing voiding cystourethrography.
   E. Have emergency equipment readily available.

3. **Procedure:**
   A. After the client is positioned supine, a balloon catheter is inserted through the urethra into the bladder, and the balloon is inflated.
   B. The bladder is filled with contrast medium by gravity or syringe instillation, and the catheter is clamped.
   C. Radiographic or fluoroscopic films of the lower urinary tract are taken with the client in several positions.
   D. The catheter is then removed, and the client must void in a right-sided or left-sided position with the lower leg flexed at the hip. Male testes should be shielded by lead before voiding begins.
   E. Several more radiographic or fluoroscopic films of the lower urinary tract are taken during voiding.
   F. If the client is unable to void, the bladder area is gently pressed to stimulate voiding.

4. **Postprocedure care:**
   A. Encourage oral intake of fluids, 125 mL/hour for 24 hours when this is not contraindicated.
   B. Monitor fluid intake and urine output for quantity and hematuria for 24 hours. Hematuria or dysuria that lasts more than 4-6 hours is abnormal.
   C. Observe for signs of allergic reaction to the contrast (listed above) for 24 hours.
   D. Observe for urinary retention or symptoms of urinary tract infection (fever, chills, pain [abdominal, suprapubic, or flank], tachypnea, tachycardia, hesitancy and frequency, dysuria, and hematuria). Notify physician for anuria present within 8 hours or for any of the above signs.
   E. Analgesics may be prescribed for bladder spasms, and sitz or tub baths may help decrease generalized genital area discomfort.

5. **Client and family teaching:**
   A. A clear liquid diet and a cathartic may be prescribed the day before the exam.
   B. The urge to void during the procedure is normal.
   C. Drink 6-8 glasses of water or other fluids per day for 2 days (unless contraindicated). Watch for warning symptoms of complications (see above). Report chills, fever, dysuria, or frank blood in the urine.
   D. In women who are breast-feeding, formula should be substituted for breast milk for 1 or more days after the procedure.

6. **Factors that affect results:**
   A. Although the clearest films result from the recumbent position, standing films are sometimes used for clients unable to void while lying down.
   B. Intestinal barium studies within 1 week before the test or the presence of a large amount of gas in the lower bowel may inhibit the clarity of the films.

7. **Other data:**
   A. None.

CYSTS AND NIPPLE DISCHARGE, DIAGNOSTIC
(see Cytologic study of breast cyst, Diagnostic; Cytologic study of nipple discharge, Diagnostic)

CYTOCHEMICAL STAIN
(*see Leukocyte cytochemistry, Specimen*)

CYTOLOGIC STUDY, SPECIMEN
(*see Bronchial washing, Specimen, Diagnostic; Brushing cytology, Specimen, Diagnostic; Cerebrospinal fluid, Routine, Culture and cytology, Specimen; Cytologic study of breast cyst, Effusions, Gastrointestinal tract, Nipple discharge, Respiratory tract, or Urine, Diagnostic; Ocular cytology, Specimen; Oral cavity cytology, Specimen*)

CYTOLOGIC STUDY OF BREAST CYST, DIAGNOSTIC

Norm. Absence of cells indicating malignancy or infection.

Usage. Determine if the breast lesion is a mass or a cyst, and determine if malignant cells are present.

Description. Breast cyst cytology is the microscopic study of the fluid or cells obtained by fine-needle aspiration. The lesion may have been detected by breast examination or mammogram. The fluid is fixed and examined by the cytologist on a microscopic slide. Any cells in the cyst fluid are studied for diagnosis of neoplasm, infective process, and, rarely, tuberculosis of the breast.

Professional Considerations
1. Consent form NOT required. See *Needle aspiration, Diagnostic*, for procedure-specific risks and contraindications.
2. **Preparation:**
   A. Obtain a 21- or 23-gauge long needle, a 10-mL syringe, sterile 0.9% saline, a red- or marble-topped glass tube or gold-seal plastic tube, and a clean jar.
   B. The client should disrobe above the waist.
   C. Position the client for comfort and accessibility to the cyst and drape him or her for privacy.
3. **Procedure:**
   A. The aspiration site is identified. The skin is cleansed with an alcohol wipe and allowed to dry.

B. The suspect mass is immobilized by one hand while the needle is inserted with the other hand.
C. Fluid is aspirated when one draws back on the syringe.
D. A fluid drop is placed on a clean slide, and the thin edge of a second slide is used to produce a smear.
E. The slide is then fixed immediately in 95% ethyl alcohol in a clean jar.
F. If more than a minute amount of fluid has been aspirated, place the remaining fluid in a red- or marble-topped tube.
G. If the specimen is minute, rinse the needle with 10 mL of sterile 0.9% saline and place the rinsed material into the tube.
H. Label the slide and the aspirate or wash with the client's name, and indicate the specimen source, noting which breast.
4. **Postprocedure care:**
   A. Apply pressure to the aspiration site for a short time.
   B. Write the pertinent clinical information on the laboratory requisition.
   C. Send the specimens to the laboratory for immediate evaluation.
5. **Client and family teaching:**
   A. This is the diagnostic procedure of choice for breast cysts in pregnant women because there are no radiographs or anesthesia required.
   B. This is a sterile procedure that takes approximately 10 minutes, with minimal discomfort.
   C. Watch the area for the next 72 hours for redness, drainage, and swelling, and check for fever over 101° F (38.3° C); report any of these signs to the physician or nurse.
   D. Results are normally available within 48 hours.
6. **Factors that affect results:**
   A. Immediate fixation of the smear prevents drying of the sample and distortion of the findings because of contamination.
   B. Some cytologists prefer specimens that were allowed to dry before being placed in the fixative. These should be specifically labeled because they are stained differently for study.

C. An insufficient sample may result when the breast lesion is not penetrated or it contains no fluid.

7. **Other data:**
   A. Aspiration is an inexpensive screening procedure for evaluating breast lesions. It decreases the necessity of open surgical biopsy to determine a definitive diagnosis.
   B. This test is more reliable than nipple discharge cytology for ruling out neoplasms.
   C. Culture of the aspirate is usually obtained for a complete work-up.
   D. There is no difference in the cytologic yield when a 21-G needle is compared with that of a 23-G needle.
   E. Fine-needle aspiration is a sensitive test that must be used only in the context of other diagnostic modalities.

CYTOLOGIC STUDY OF EFFUSIONS, DIAGNOSTIC

Norm. No tumor cells or infection.

Usage. Gout, lymphoproliferative disease, infections of or fistulas into serous cavities, metabolic arthritis, metastatic neoplasms, myeloproliferative disease, rheumatoid arthritis, rheumatoid pleuritis, systemic lupus erythematosus, and pulmonary TB.

Description. An effusion is an abnormal collection of fluid occurring most commonly in the pericardial sac, abdomen, pleural space, and synovial cavities. Effusions may be transudate caused by hydrostatic pressure differences or exudate caused by tumors or infective processes. Effusion cytology is the microscopic study of the fluid aspirate of the particular effusion used to differentiate the cause and type of effusion and to characterize and identify the source of infection or the tumor type.

Professional Considerations

1. Consent form IS required for the procedure used to obtain the specimen. See individual procedures for procedure-specific risks and contraindications.

2. **Preparation:**
   A. Check PT and PTT or INR. This procedure may be contraindicated in clients with coagulation defects.
   B. Obtain the appropriate procedure tray, sterile gloves and drapes, povidone-iodine solution, and 1-2% lidocaine. If a large effusion is to be drained, obtain a heparinized vacuum bottle and tubing with a clamp or stopcock.
   C. Obtain baseline vital signs.
   D. For a pericardiocentesis, monitor ECG continuously throughout the procedure.
   E. For small or loculated effusions, an ultrasonograph- or CT-guided tap will increase the chance of obtaining a specimen.

3. **Procedure:**
   A. Position the client appropriately for the procedure to be performed.
   B. Cleanse the aspiration site and surrounding skin with povidone-iodine solution and allow it to dry.
   C. Overlay the aspiration site with sterile drapes.
   D. Obtain two 3- to 10-mL samples of fluid using a sterile technique by means of arthrocentesis, pericardiocentesis, paracentesis, or thoracentesis. Place one specimen in a heparinized tube and one in a nonheparinized tube for evaluation and cytologic testing.

4. **Postprocedure care:**
   A. For a thoracentesis, a postprocedure chest radiograph MUST be performed to check for a possible pneumothorax.
   B. Monitor vital signs for indications of bleeding or hemodynamic changes.
   C. Write the name, date, source of fluid, and symptoms on the laboratory requisition.
   D. Send the specimen to the laboratory immediately. Refrigerate specimens not examined immediately.

5. **Client and family teaching:**
   A. This is a sterile procedure that takes up to 1 hour and may include moderate discomfort.
   B. It is very important to stay as still as possible during the procedure to avoid injury and complications.
   C. Results are normally available within 72 hours.

6. **Factors that affect results:**
   A. Results are most accurate when the specimen is examined within 1 hour of collection.
7. **Other data:**
   A. This method is usually more sensitive than blind biopsy for diagnosis of pleural malignancies.
   B. The addition of Ki67 immunostaining appears more sensitive than cytomorphology alone in distinguishing benign from malignant effusions.

CYTOLOGIC STUDY OF GASTROINTESTINAL TRACT, DIAGNOSTIC

Norm. Normal cells of the gastrointestinal tract. No tumor cells or infection.

Usage. Cytologic examination of exfoliation of the mucosa of the gastrointestinal tract to allow diagnosis of benign, precancerous, or malignant lesions of the esophagus, stomach, and duodenum. Also for amyloidosis, microscopic colitis, Crohn's disease, granulomatous inflammation, gastritis, *Helicobacter pylori*, leiomyosarcoma, lymphoma, intestinal spirochetosis, melanosis coli, Métrier's disease, pernicious anemia, schistosomiasis, toxic drug effect on gastric mucosa, and Whipple's disease.

Description. Brushings or fine-needle aspirations of the mucosa of the upper gastrointestinal tract are performed during endoscopic examination. Washings of the mucosa for a specimen through a nasogastric tube may be performed when endoscopy is not available or is contraindicated and neoplasm is clinically suspected. Brushings of the colon or rectum can be made by proctosigmoidoscopy.

Professional Considerations
1. Consent form NOT required for nasogastric tube method. Consent form IS required for endoscopy and sigmoidoscopy.

Risks
See individual procedures for risks and contraindications.

Contraindications
Severe gastrointestinal bleeding, varices (gastric or esophageal), and clients who are unable to cooperate.

2. **Preparation:**
   A. Preschedule this test with the laboratory.
   B. If colon washing is to be performed, administer oral cathartic as prescribed and collect the last bowel movement before the test to send to the laboratory with the washing specimen.
   C. For collection of gastric washings for cytologic examination, obtain a nasogastric (NG) tube, a lubricant, 0.9% saline, a syringe, a 500-mL clean container, a 50% ethyl alcohol (ethanol) fixative, and dry ice.
   D. For collection of endoscopic brushings for cytologic examination, obtain endoscopic equipment, a brush, glass slides labeled with the client's name, a clean container of 95% ethyl alcohol or other fixative required by the specific laboratory, and dry ice or 50% ethyl alcohol.
   E. For colon washing, obtain enema tube, 0.9% saline, a large airtight plastic container, and dry ice or 50% ethyl alcohol.
   F. See *Upper gastroduodenojejunoscopy, Diagnostic; Barium enema, Diagnostic; Proctoscopy, Diagnostic;* or *Sigmoidoscopy, Diagnostic,* for other preparations, as would be appropriate for the procedure being performed.
3. **Procedure:**
   A. *Gastric washing:*
      i. Insert a nasogastric tube.
      ii. Withdraw gastric contents with a Toomey syringe and discard.
      iii. Instill 300-500 mL of 0.9% saline solution into the stomach through the NG tube.
      iv. Have the client roll 360 degrees four or five times.
      v. Aspirate all the gastric contents into a clean, sealed container.
   B. *Endoscopic brushings for cytology:*
      i. During endoscopy, a brushing is taken from specific lesions of the esophagus, the stomach, or the duodenal area.

ii. The brush should be rolled onto a slide to cover at least a 1.5-cm diameter area.

iii. The slide should be immediately placed into a container of 95% ethyl alcohol (ethanol) or other required fixative.

C. *Colon washing:* Colon washing is performed just before barium enema washing.

i. Insert the enema tubing into the colon through the rectum.

ii. Instill 100 mL of 0.9% saline solution through the tubing.

iii. Have the client roll 360 degrees several times.

iv. Drain the fluid out of the enema tubing and instill it into an airtight container.

D. *Colon or rectal brushing:*

i. Insert the proctoscope or sigmoidoscope.

ii. Take a brushing from the lesion sites.

iii. The brush should be rolled onto a slide to cover at least a 1.5-cm diameter area.

4. **Postprocedure care:**

A. Either pack the specimen in dry ice or preserve it with 50% ethyl alcohol.

B. Write the time and source of the specimen collection on the laboratory requisition. Each separate brushing sample should be labeled with the anatomic site of collection.

C. Transport the specimen to the cytotechnologist in the pathology laboratory immediately for fixing and microscopic examination.

D. Remove the nasogastric or enema tube.

E. Resume normal diet.

F. See *Upper gastroduodenojejunoscopy, Diagnostic; Barium enema, Diagnostic; Proctoscopy, Diagnostic;* or *Sigmoidoscopy, Diagnostic,* for other postprocedure care, as appropriate for the procedure being performed.

5. **Client and family teaching:**

A. Eat a soft diet for the evening meal before the test.

B. Fast from food for 8-12 hours and from water for 1 hour before the procedure.

6. **Factors that affect results:**

A. Washings may be performed twice. Discarding the first aspirate and sending the second aspirate for study may be more reliable, especially for gastric neoplasms.

B. Contamination of the specimen with food or barium invalidates the results.

C. Reject specimens not packed in dry ice or not received promptly after collection.

D. Reject slides that were allowed to dry before fixing or those received without fixative.

E. Reject unlabeled slides.

7. **Other data:**

A. This is not so effective a diagnostic tool as radiography or endoscopy with biopsy.

B. A negative report does not rule out malignancy.

C. Gastroscopy-guided brushings are preferable to gastric washings for cytologic study.

D. Proctosigmoidoscopic smears to investigate diarrhea should be performed with no preparation of the bowel because the exudate may be washed away, the mucosa distorted, trauma of the mucosa induced, or the evidence of disease obscured or altered.

CYTOLOGIC STUDY OF NIPPLE DISCHARGE, DIAGNOSTIC

Norm. Absence of tumor cells or infection.

Usage. Diagnosis of inflammatory disease, intraductal papilloma, mammary dysplasia with ectasia of the ducts, metastasis or suspected malignancy of the breast, and papillomatosis.

Description. Nipple discharge is considered abnormal except in lactating or pregnant women, though some discharge is caused by medication. Several nipple-discharge smears are fixed on glass slides and microscopically studied for the presence of abnormal cells indicating neoplasm or infection, and rarely, tuberculosis of the breast. Abnormal cytology indicates increased relative risk for breast cancer.

Professional Considerations

1. Consent form NOT required.

2. **Preparation:**
   A. Explain the procedure. The client who assists should hold the fixative bottle under the breast so that the slide can be immediately placed in the fixative.
   B. Obtain warmed sterile saline, 6-12 clean glass slides, 6-12 clean glass bottles of 95% ethyl alcohol (ethanol), labels, and cotton or gauze.
   C. The client should disrobe above the waist.
   D. Position the client so that it is convenient to obtain the specimen, and drape him or her for privacy.
3. **Procedure:**
   A. Vigorously cleanse the nipple and then soak it in warm saline on a cotton or gauze pad for 10-15 minutes and pat it dry.
   B. Gently strip the subareolar area with a thumb and forefinger, moving toward the nipple tip. Continue until a pea-sized droplet of fluid is expressed.
   C. Place the frosted side of a clean glass microscope slide on the nipple and quickly slide it across the nipple tip to obtain a smear of fluid.
   D. Immediately place the slide into a small jar of 95% ethyl alcohol (ethanol) fixative.
   E. Label the jar with the number of the smear and whether it was taken from the right or left breast. This is especially important when both breasts are studied.
   F. Repeat steps 3A-E until four to six slides from each breast are obtained if possible.
4. **Postprocedure care:**
   A. Write a description of the discharge and the client's name, age, clinical symptoms, and which breast is being studied on the laboratory requisition.
   B. Send the specimens to the laboratory immediately.
   C. Cleanse the breast and nipple as needed.
5. **Client and family teaching:**
   A. The procedure takes about 10 minutes.
   B. Results are normally available within 48 hours.
   C. About 3% of breast cancers and 10% of benign lesions of the breast are associated with nipple discharge. Negative cytologic results do not rule out a malignancy.
6. **Factors that affect results:**
   A. Immediate fixation of the smear prevents drying of the sample and distortion of the findings because of contamination.
   B. Several (rather than 1 or 2) slides improve results because later smears include more abnormal cells if present.
   C. Medications that affect hormonal balance and may cause nipple discharge include chlorpromazines, digitalis, diuretics, oral contraceptives, phenothiazines, and steroids.
7. **Other data:**
   A. Mammography and biopsy or aspiration are more reliable diagnostic procedures for breast malignancy than cytologic study.

CYTOLOGIC STUDY OF RESPIRATORY TRACT, DIAGNOSTIC

Norm. Negative.

Usage. Diagnosis of respiratory neoplasms or premalignant cell changes related to chronic inflammation, inhaled toxins, tuberculosis, or asthma; and diagnosis of respiratory bacterial, viral, or parasitic infections.

Description. Respiratory tract cytology is the microscopic study of the number and type of cells of the respiratory tract or sputum to detect the presence of cells abnormal for that specimen, including tumor or pretumor cells or evidence of an infective process. Any anomalies of cells are correlated to clinical data for diagnosis.

Professional Considerations

1. Consent form NOT required unless the sample for study is obtained by bronchoscopy.
2. **Preparation:**
   A. An aerosol treatment just before specimen collection may help to mobilize respiratory secretions.
3. **Procedure:**
   A. Three early-morning specimens are obtained.
   B. Have the client rinse the mouth with water.

C. Instruct the client to inhale deeply and then exhale with a deep, expulsive cough and expectorate sputum directly into a sterile, wide-mouthed container.

D. Alternatively, bronchial secretions may be removed directly during bronchoscopy or by nasotracheal suctioning using a specimen trap.

4. **Postprocedure care:**
A. Write the client's name, the date, the specimen source, the specimen number, the diagnosis, and the clinical symptoms on the laboratory requisition.
B. Send the specimen to the laboratory immediately.

5. **Client and family teaching:**
A. Results are normally available within 72 hours.
B. To produce a deep sputum specimen, rather than saliva, take several deep breaths, without fully exhaling between them. When you feel as though you cannot take any more breaths, cough out forcefully and catch the sputum in the sterile cup.
C. The results may have to be confirmed by culture or biopsy.

6. **Factors that affect results:**
A. The results are most accurate when examined within 1 hour of collection.
B. The results are invalid if the sample is saliva, rather than respiratory secretions.
C. Smoking and pharmacotherapy affect the results of the analysis.

7. **Other data:**
A. About 15% of results are false negatives.
B. Sputum cytologic findings are more likely to be negative in a client with small cell carcinoma than in one with non–small cell carcinoma of the lung.
C. Culture with or without biopsy is usually more reliable than cytologic examination for diagnosis of respiratory tract neoplasm or infection.
D. The detection of the codon-12 K-*ras* mutation in BALF cells aids the diagnosis of lung cancer in clients with negative cytologic findings.

CYTOLOGIC STUDY OF URINE, DIAGNOSTIC

Norm. Normal type and amount of squamous and epithelial cells of the urinary tract and little or no cellular debris; red blood cell count (RBC) ≤3; white blood cell count (WBC) ≤4; no abnormal cells such as cytomegalic inclusion bodies, malignant cells, parasites, or yeasts.

Usage. Anemia (hemolytic), cerebral metachromatic leukodystrophy, cytomegalovirus infection (cytomegalic inclusion bodies), measles (cytomegalic inclusion bodies), renal hemosiderosis, screening for premalignant cell changes, transplant rejection, urinary tract infections (herpesvirus, fungi, *Schistosoma,* others), urinary tract inflammation (epithelial cells, RBC, WBC), and urinary tract primary or metastatic cancer (malignant cells).

Description. Urine cytology is the microscopic study of cells in urine to detect the presence of abnormal cells, including tumor or pretumor cells or evidence of an infective process. Any abnormalities found are correlated to clinical data for a diagnosis of urinary tract neoplasm, infection, or other diseases that may affect the urine.

Professional Considerations
1. Consent form NOT required.
2. **Preparation:**
A. Obtain a sterile container.
B. Hydrate the client $\frac{1}{2}$ to 1 hour before specimen collection.
3. **Procedure:**
A. Urine cytology involves centrifuging and filtering the urine, or cytocentrifuging, staining, and examining the filtered sediment.
B. For a voided specimen, have the client urinate directly into a sterile container. Tightly cover the container.
C. Catheterization may be used if it is otherwise difficult to obtain the specimen or if a high urinary tract lesion is suspected.
4. **Postprocedure care:**
A. Send the specimen to the laboratory immediately.
5. **Client and family teaching:**
A. Discard the first morning void if collecting the sample in the

morning. With the next void, urinate directly into the container and then cap it tightly.

B. Results are normally available within 48 hours.

6. Factors that affect results:
   A. An early-morning specimen is unsuitable because cell death occurs in the bladder overnight.
   B. Recent instrumentation may cause cell injury or changes that give false-positive results.
   C. Hypotonic solutions used as washing during cystourethroscopy procedures may alter the results by directly affecting cell structure and appearance.
   D. Chemotherapeutic agents such as cyclophosphamide may alter the results.

7. Other data:
   A. A voided specimen is preferred except when specific study of high urinary tract areas is needed. Urine from each ureter may be studied and compared.
   B. Cytomegalovirus (CMV) can be diagnosed by urine cytologic examination. Several specimens are recommended because cytomegalovirus is not shed continuously. The presence of CMV in the urine may indicate CMV disease or an asymptomatic reactivation of CMV disease. The herbs *Geum japonicum, Syzygium aromaticum,* and *Terminalia chebula* have demonstrated anti-murine CMV activity in mice.

CYTOLOGY, SPECIMEN
(see Cytologic study, Specimen)

CYTOLOGY, URINE
(see Cytologic study of urine, Diagnostic)

CYTOMEGALIC INCLUSION DISEASE, CYTOLOGY, URINE

Norm. Negative for inclusion body cells.

Positive. Cytomegalovirus infections of a disseminated type.

Description. Cytomegalovirus is a member of the herpesvirus family and causes cytomegalic inclusion disease, a generalized infection of infants and small children caused by intrauterine, natal, or postnatal exposure to infected secretions (blood, cervical secretions, urine, saliva, breast milk, or semen). The mode of transmission to immunocompromised clients is unknown. Cytomegalic inclusion disease symptoms may range from none in healthy-appearing children to generalized symptoms of a severe infection and is characterized by the presence of intranuclear or intracellular inclusion bodies in the kidney that are excreted in the urine. The disease may also affect the salivary glands, lung, liver, pancreas, and brain, where inclusion bodies may also be found. Severe symptoms may be fatal.

Professional Considerations
1. Consent form NOT required.
2. Preparation:
   A. Obtain a clean-catch urine kit.
   B. Hydrate the client for ½ to 1 hour.
   C. The specimen should be obtained at least 3 hours after the last void but should not be the first morning void.
3. Procedure:
   A. Urine cytology involves centrifuging and filtering the urine, or cytocentrifuging, staining, and examining the filtered sediment.
   B. The clean-catch urine technique must be used to decrease the risk of specimen contamination. See clean-catch collection instructions in the test *Body fluid, Routine, Culture.*
   C. A fresh specimen may be taken from a clean urinary drainage bag.
4. Postprocedure care:
   A. Send the specimen to the laboratory immediately.
5. Client and family teaching:
   A. Provide collection instructions (above) if the client will be obtaining the specimen independently.
   B. This test is one of the most reliable and rapid methods for diagnosing cytomegalovirus infection. Several specimens are recommended because cytomegalovirus is not shed continuously.

6. **Factors that affect results:**
   A. Specimens should be tested within 6 hours.
7. **Other data:**
   A. Cytomegalic inclusion bodies are often found in clients with cancer undergoing chemotherapy and in transplant clients receiving immunosuppressive drugs.
   B. Inclusion bodies may also be found in smears and brushings from other sources, such as bronchoalveolar lavage fluid and biopsy specimens of cytomegalovirus infected tissues.
   C. Positive urine culture with the occurrence of CMV retinitis signifies CMV retinitis in the contralateral eye of clients with unilateral disease.
   D. The herbs *Geum japonicum*, *Syzygium aromaticum*, and *Terminalia chebula* have demonstrated antimurine CMV activity in mice.

CYTOMEGALOVIRUS ANTIBODY, SERUM

Norm. Negative.

IgM	<1:8
IgH	<1:8 for those exposed
IgG	<1:16 for those exposed

Positive. A fourfold increase in the antibody titer between the acute and convalescent specimens or IgM >1:8 in a single specimen indicates a primary cytomegalovirus infective process. Cytomegalovirus (CMV) infections include congenital CMV, spontaneous CMV mononucleosis (heterophil-negative mononucleosis), posttransfusion CMV mononucleosis, and CMV in immunosuppressed clients. Disseminated infections may cause CMV retinitis, esophagitis, hepatitis, and ileocolitis. Positive in aphthous stomatitis, lichen planus, Meniere's disease, pulmonary fibrosis, and scleroderma.

Description. Cytomegalovirus is a herpesvirus. The virus is present in a large segment of the population early in life without causing apparent disease. Serologic prevalence studies show that 60-90% of US adults, depending on socioeconomic level, and very old people are positive for antibodies to CMV. Since the presence of disease is unusual, host factors predisposing to the disease should be investigated when the disease is manifested. CMV mononucleosis usually occurs in older adults, compared to Epstein-Barr mononucleosis, and presents with a lower incidence of pharyngitis and lymphadenopathy. Congenital CMV may cause a variety of developmental abnormalities and neurologic deficits in the infant or young child. In the immunosuppressed client, pulmonary or systemic infections may occur. Clients receiving tissue transplants (liver, heart, lung, kidney, and bone) are also at high risk for manifested infections. CMV immune status should be performed on all organ transplant candidates before surgery. Blood for transfusion to seronegative transplant clients and all premature neonates should be from donors without CMV antibodies.

Professional Considerations
1. Consent form NOT required.
2. **Preparation:**
   A. Tube: Red topped, red/gray topped, or gold topped.
3. **Procedure:**
   A. Draw a 3-mL blood sample. Label the tube as the acute sample.
   B. 10-14 days later, repeat the test and label the tube as the convalescent sample.
4. **Postprocedure care:**
   A. Results are normally available within 72 hours.
5. **Client and family teaching:**
   A. It is important to return in 10 days to 2 weeks for follow-up sampling to see if the infection is clearing up.
   B. Acyclovir, gancyclovir, and foscarnet are used for treatment of cytomegalovirus infections.
6. **Factors that affect results:**
   A. False-positive low titer results may occur in clients exposed to the Epstein-Barr virus, but a high titer confirms CMV. May also be falsely positive in those with rheumatoid factor in their serum.
7. **Other data:**
   A. The titer is not valid for the study of infants <6 months of age because they may have maternal antibodies present in their serum.
   B. In a CMV-positive client, CMV may be cultured from urine. The presence of the virus in the urine

may indicate CMV disease or an asymptomatic reactivation of CMV. The finding of a positive CMV blood culture has a much higher correlation with the presence of CMV disease.

C. CMV antibody titers are of little value in determining the presence of CMV infection in immunocompromised clients because of the high incidence of CMV seropositive clients in the general public. Viral isolation is necessary for diagnosis.

D. The herbs *Geum japonicum, Syzygium aromaticum,* and *Terminalia chebula* have demonstrated anti-murine CMV activity in mice.

CYTOPLASMIC NEUTROPHIL ANTIBODIES, SERUM
(see Anti-neutrophil cytoplasmic antibody screen, Serum)

D & C
(see Dilatation and curettage)

D-DIMER TEST (FIBRIN DEGRADATION FRAGMENT), BLOOD

Norm. Less than 1 μg/mL or <100 μg/L.

Positive. Indicates in vivo fibrinolytic activity. Value >4 μg/mL indicates DVT. Value >120 μg/L (plus plasmin-antiplasmin complex >5.25 nmol/L) is predictive of a future MI in males and females >65 years.

Usage. Acute thrombosis (including arterial, coronary, and deep vein), defibrination therapy, disseminated intravascular coagulation, fibrinolysis (primary and secondary), malignancy (ovarian), postoperative fibrinolytic therapy, pregnancy, (especially postpartum period), preeclampsia, rheumatoid arthritis (juvenile), sickle cell anemia vaso-occlusive crisis, surgery, and unstable angina.

Description. An assay to measure the amount of clot breakdown products specific for cross-linked fragments (D-dimer) derived from fibrin. The test can be performed on whole blood without the removal or interference of fibrinogen. It does not distinguish lysis of physiologic and pathologic thrombi but distinguishes between fibrinogenolysis and fibrinolysis. Has a 93% sensitivity for large emboli and a 50% sensitivity for smaller subsegmental emboli.

Professional Considerations
1. Consent form NOT required.
2. **Preparation:**
   A. Tube: Blue topped if other coagulation tests are being drawn at the same time. Otherwise obtain a red-topped, red/gray-topped, or gold-topped tube.
3. **Procedure:**
   A. Completely fill a blue-topped tube or draw a 5-mL sample in a red-topped, red/gray-topped, or gold-topped tube.
   B. The specimen is stable for 8 hours at room temperature or for 6 months at −20° C.
4. **Postprocedure care:**
   A. Assess the client for other signs of thrombosis, emboli, or veno-occlusive disease.
5. **Client and family teaching:**
   A. Results are normally available within 48 hours.
6. **Factors that affect results:**
   A. D-Dimer levels increase with increasing levels of tumor marker CA 125 in ovarian cancer, increasing titers of rheumatoid factors, post electrical cardioversion and with letrozole therapy in advanced breast cancer.
7. **Other data:**
   A. May be of use in veno-occlusive disease associated with sequelae of bone marrow transplantation in oncology.
   B. A normal D-dimer value excludes pulmonary embolus in 30% of clients.
   C. A negative D-dimer does not rule out the possibility of a pulmonary embolism. False-negative D-dimers are not uncommon for pulmonary emboli.

DEHYDROEPIANDROSTERONE SULFATE (DHEA-S), SERUM AND URINE, 24-HOUR

Norm:

		SI UNITS
Serum		
Adult female	0.5-2.8 µg/mL	
	or 200-800 ng/dL	
Premenopausal	60-340 µg/dL	1.6-8.9 µmol/L
	or 820-3380 ng/mL	
Postmenopausal	<130 µg/dL	
	or 100-610 ng/mL	
Pregnant (term)	230-1170 ng/mL	
Adult male	130-550 µg/dL	3.4-14.4 µmol/L
	or 270-1400 ng/dL	
Prepubertal male	2000-3350 ng/mL	
Newborn	1670-3640 ng/mL	
Child	100-600 ng/dL	
Urine		
Female	0.2-1.8 mg/day	0.7-6.2 µmol/day
Male	0.2-2 mg/day	0.7-6.9 µmol/day

Increased. Addison's disease, adrenal cortex adenoma and carcinoma, Cushing's disease, ectopic ACTH-producing tumors, female acne and hirsutism, hyperthyroidism, oligomenorrhea in female athletes, polycystic ovarian syndrome, Stein-Leventhal syndrome, and virilizing congenital adrenal hyperplasia.

Decreased. Adrenal insufficiency (primary and secondary), chronic fatigue syndrome, Crohn's disease, diabetes mellitus under poor blood glucose control, low libido, ulcerative colitis. Low levels in amniotic fluid indicate anencephaly in the fetus. Drugs include carbamazepine, dexamethasone, phenytoin.

Description. Dehydroepiandrosterone sulfate (DHEA-S) is the most abundant steroid in the circulation. It arises primarily from the adrenal cortex and is converted to testosterone. Although not androgenic itself, it is a specific and stable marker of adrenal androgen production. Levels are normally elevated in neonates and then decrease considerably until 7 years of age. At puberty, increased levels of DHEA-S from the adrenals result in the axillary and pubic hair growth, preceding gonadal androgen secretion.

Professional Considerations

1. Consent form NOT required.
2. **Preparation:**
   A. *Blood test:* Tube: Red topped, red/gray topped, gold topped, or green topped.
   B. *Urine test:* Obtain a 3-L, 24-hour urine jug without preservative.
3. **Procedure:**
   A. *Blood test:* Obtain a 1-mL blood sample.
   B. *Urine test:*
      i. Discard the first morning-urine specimen.
      ii. Save all the urine voided for 24 hours. Include the urine voided at the end of the 24-hour period. For catheterized clients, keep the drainage bag on ice and empty urine into the collection container hourly.
4. **Postprocedure care:**
   A. Freeze the serum specimen if it is not tested within 1 hour.
   B. *Urine:*
      i. Compare the urine quantity in the specimen container with the urinary output record for the test. If the specimen contains less urine than what was recorded as output, some urine may have been

discarded, thus invalidating the test.

ii. Document the quantity of urine output for the collection period on the laboratory requisition.

iii. It is best to send the entire specimen to the laboratory so that it can be measured and mixed well before being tested.

5. Client and family teaching:

A. Avoid radionuclide scans for 24 hours before this test.

B. *Urine:* Save all the urine voided in the 24-hour period and urinate before defecating to avoid loss of urine. If any urine is accidentally discarded, discard the entire specimen and restart the collection the next day.

C. Results are normally available within 24 hours.

6. Factors that affect results:

A. Radionuclides administered in the last 24 hours may increase results.

B. Phenytoin and carbamazepine cause DHEA-S levels to decrease.

7. Other data:

A. For those who exercise strenuously, such as marathon runners, DHEA-S levels will be elevated at the completion of the exercise period and for up to 36 hours after.

B. Levels decline with age in men and women. Individuals differ in the amount of DHEA-S secreted and, for unknown reasons; DHEA-S levels positively correlate with longevity. Low levels also decrease the development of atherosclerosis.

C. Women with levels >70 μg/dL have successful labor inductions.

D. A significant positive correlation exists between bone mineral density and serum DHEA-S levels in postmenopausal women.

DENSITOMETRY

(*see Bone densitometry, Diagnostic*)

DENVER DEVELOPMENTAL SCREENING TEST (DDST), DENVER II, DIAGNOSTIC

Norm. Age-appropriate tasks should be demonstrated for each area tested in children between 1 month and 6 years of age.

Usage. The Denver Developmental Screening Test (DDST) tests children in the following areas: gross and fine motor development, language skills, and personal-social skills. Norms for each chronologic age are provided. Although not diagnostic by itself, this frequently used test can identify children (such as those with HIV, hypoxic-ischemic encephalopathy, or blindness) who have global problems or problems in one specific area. This test can also be used to track children over time.

Description. The DDST is a skills test that was revised in 1990 as the Denver II to include 125 items. These easily administered items were picked to prevent any bias against gender, ethnicity, maternal education, or place of residence. Most skills are objectively visualized by the tester, but caregiver verbal reports are adequate to pass some of them.

Professional Considerations

1. Consent form NOT required.

2. Preparation:

A. Provide a quiet room with all the equipment needed for the test:

i. Denver Development Screening forms available in pads of 100 sheets from Denver Development Materials.

ii. Denver Development Screening kit, which includes a ball, bell, and other objects needed to perform test.

3. Procedure:

A. Determine chronologic age of child (see manual for explanation of age adjustment for preterm birth) and draw age line on scoring sheet.

B. Begin testing child with items in approximation but to the left of the age line. This establishes confidence. See manual for directions on repeating test items and giving instructions to child.

C. Continue testing along age line and then to the right of the age line until child fails items in each of the four categories.

4. Postprocedure care:

A. Explain results to parent or caregiver. Show adult the scoring sheet.

5. **Client and family teaching:**
   A. The test usually takes less than 1 hour and helps identify potential developmental problems in the child.
   B. A parent or person familiar to the child will be asked to stay with the child during the screening.
   C. Results are completely available within 48 hours.
6. **Factors that affect results:**
   A. Environmental distractions interfere with validity of the results.
   B. Testing by untrained clients. Screening should be performed only by clients who have successfully completed a written and an observational proficiency test.
7. **Other data:**
   A. The Denver exam is less reliable for children under 30 months of age and over $4^{1}/_{2}$ years of age. For younger children, use the Revised Denver Prescreening Developmental Questionnaire (R-PDQ).

11-DEOXYCORTISOL (COMPOUND S, 11-DOC) TEST, DIAGNOSTIC

Norm. 0-2 mg/dL (0-57.72 nmol/L, SI units). Levels are normally decreased from birth to 4 years.

Usage. Basal levels aid in diagnosis of adrenal carcinoma and congenital adrenal hyperplasia; used to measure response when metyrapone is given to diagnosing adrenal insufficiency and Cushing's disease. Low levels found in amyloidosis and posttraumatic stress disorder (PTSD). High levels found in adrenocortical tumors.

Description. Blood test used to determine a specific metabolic block in the synthesis of cortisol. Cortisol is synthesized by two successive hydroxylations of 17-alpha-hydroxyprogesterone. The first results in 11-deoxycortisol, which is then catalyzed by 11-beta-hydroxylase to yield cortisol. This test is used with the metyrapone test to allow diagnosis of primary and secondary adrenal insufficiency. Metyrapone blocks the conversion of 11-deoxycortisol to cortisol, which then stimulates the adrenals to produce more 11-deoxycortisol. A blood level of 11-deoxycortisol that is not elevated after metyrapone administration indicates the presence of adrenal insufficiency.

Professional Considerations
1. Consent form NOT required.
2. **Preparation:**
   A. Tube: Green topped.
3. **Procedure:**
   A. Obtain a 7-mL blood sample.
4. **Postprocedure care:**
   A. Deliver the specimen to the laboratory immediately. Separate and freeze the plasma.
5. **Client and family teaching:**
   A. Results are normally available within 48 hours.
6. **Factors that affect results:**
   A. Results are increased if the client is taking any glucocorticoids, such as hydrocortisone, dexamethasone, or prednisone.
7. **Other data:**
   A. 11-deoxycortisol has no glucocorticoid activity.
   B. See also *Metyrapone test.*

DESIPRAMINE
(see Tricyclic antidepressants, Plasma or Serum)

DEXA
(see Bone densitometry, Diagnostic)

DEXAMETHASONE SUPPRESSION TEST, DIAGNOSTIC

Norm. 24-hour urine values should be <50% baseline values.

Plasma cortisol	<5 µg/dL
Urine-free cortisol	<25 µg/24 hours
Urine for 17-OHCS	4 µg/24 hours

Positive. High levels of serum cortisol and 17-OHCS are present after dexamethasone is administered. Occurs in adrenal hyperplasia, adrenal incidentalomas, adrenal tumors, aldosteronism (primary), bulimia nervosa, chronic fatigue syndrome, chronic renal failure, Cushing's disease, depression, oat cell cancer of the lung, and schizophrenics with suicide attempts.

Description. Screening test for Cushing's disease and for depression. The test can be performed after a low or high dose of dexamethasone or as an overnight test with a morning blood draw. Dexamethasone is a potent synthetic glucocorticoid that is used to test the integrity of the hypothalamic-pituitary-adrenal axis. When given to normal clients, it decreases the production of cortisol and other adrenal steroids through the usual feedback systems. In clients with Cushing's disease or depression there is no suppression of ACTH. The low test dose is for screening. If results are positive, a high-dose test is given to determine the cause of Cushing's disease. If there is suppression with the high-dose test, it indicates a pituitary origin of the excess cortisol. If there is no suppression, it indicates an adrenal or ectopic tumor.

Professional Considerations

1. Consent form NOT required.
2. **Preparation:**
   A. Obtain a 3-L plastic container.
   B. Tube: Green topped, red topped, red/gray topped, or gold topped.
   C. Baseline values for plasma cortisol, urine-free cortisol, and urine 17-OHCS should be known.
3. **Procedure:**
   A. Obtain a 5-mL blood sample for plasma cortisol level.
   B. Overnight test consists in administering 1 mg of dexamethasone orally at 1100 (11:00 AM) followed by venipuncture for cortisol level the next day at 0800 (8:00 AM).
   C. The low-dose test includes a baseline measurement of urine-free cortisol or 17-OHCS followed by oral dexamethasone 0.5 mg every 6 hours for 2 days followed by a 24-hour urine for free cortisol or 17-OHCS collected on day 2.
   D. The high-dose test includes a baseline measure of urine-free cortisol or 17-OHCS followed by oral dexamethasone 2 mg every 6

hours for 2 days followed by a 24-hour urine for urine-free cortisol or 17-OHCS collected on day 2.
4. **Postprocedure care:**
   A. Send the blood sample to the laboratory within 30 minutes for serum separation and freezing.
5. **Client and family teaching:**
   A. Oral dexamethasone will be given at a specific time the evening before the blood sampling. The blood and urine samples will be collected at specific times the next day.
   B. *Urine:* Save all the urine voided in the 24-hour period and urinate before defecating to avoid loss of urine. If any urine is accidentally discarded, notify the physician immediately because the test results will be invalid.
6. **Factors that affect results:**
   A. Failure to ingest oral dexamethasone or radioactive scan performed within the previous 24 hours will elevate the results. For depressed clients, methylene blue is added to the dexamethasone tablets, and urinary excretion of the dye is monitored to indicate that the drug was ingested.
   B. False-positive results occur with acute illnesses, alcoholism, anorexia nervosa, dehydration, preclinical Cushing's syndrome (PCS), severe depression, diabetes (unstable), electroconvulsive therapy after treatment day 1, fever, malnutrition, nausea, obesity, pregnancy, high stress, and temporal lobe disease. Drugs include aspirin (drug overdose), barbiturates, carbamazepine, estrogens, glutethimide, meprobamate methaqualone, methyprylon, oral contraceptives, phenytoin, reserpine, rifampin, spironolactone, stilbestrol, and tetracycline.
   C. False-negative results occur with Addison's disease, hypopituitarism, and in clients who metabolize dexamethasone at an abnormally slow rate. Drugs include benzodiazepines (high dose), corticosteroids, and cyproheptadine.
   D. Using 1 mg of dexamethasone results in lower sensitivity in Japanese and Asian people with major depressive episodes when compared to Caucasians. Low dose 0.5 mg DST is better in Japanese and Asian clients.

7. **Other data:**
   A. Levels in some clients with Cushing's disease may be suppressed by 50%, but these clients can be identified by the metyrapone test.
   B. As a screening test for depression it is 90% specific and 45% sensitive.
   C. Female survivors of sexual abuse have significantly suppressed plasma cortisol in response to dexamethasone.
   D. See also *Metyrapone test, Serum.*

DHEA, SERUM
(*see Dehydroepiandrosterone sulfate, Serum*)

DIALYZABLE CALCIUM, SERUM
(*see Calcium, Ionized, Blood*)

DIASCAN, DIAGNOSTIC
(*see Glucose monitoring machines, Diagnostic*)

DIAZEPAM, SERUM

Norm. Negative.

		SI UNITS
Therapeutic range	100-1000 ng/mL	0.35-3.51 µmol/L
Panic level	>5000 ng/mL	>17.55 µmol/L
Lethal level	720 µg/mL	

Panic Level Symptoms and Treatment

Symptoms. Ataxia, cyanosis, coma, convulsions, diminished reflexes, mental confusion, respiratory depression, somnolence, slurred speech, vertigo.

Treatment:

Note: Treatment choice(s) depend on client history and condition and episode history.

Gastric lavage is not recommended, but should be considered if within 1 hour of ingestion and if ingestion of additional lethal substance is suspected. Use warm tap water or 0.9% saline.

Administer activated charcoal if within 4 hours of ingestion or if symptoms are present. Repeat as necessary, because benzodiazepines undergo hepatic recirculation.

Monitor for central nervous system depression.

Protect airway. Support breathing with oxygen and mechanical ventilation, if necessary.

Flumazenil is not recommended for routine use in benzodiazepine overdose. Flumazenil has been used as a competitive antagonist to reverse the profound effects of benzodiazepine overdose. Use of flumazenil is contraindicated if concomitant tricyclic antidepressants were taken or in dependence states because of the risk of causing seizures from lowering of the seizure threshold and because it may precipitate symptoms of benzodiazepine withdrawal.

Flumazenil may not completely reverse benzodiazepine effects. Close monitoring for re-sedation is required and repeated doses may be needed.

Do NOT use barbiturates.

Do NOT induce emesis.

Diazepam is a benzodiazepine

Forced diuresis or hemodialysis will NOT remove benzodiazepines to any significant extent. No information was found on whether peritoneal dialysis will remove these drugs.

Increased. Drug abuse, overdose, and suicide.

Description. Diazepam is a benzodiazepine derivative that acts on the limbic and subcortical levels of the central nervous system, producing sedation, skeletal muscle relaxation, and anticonvulsant effects. Absorbed from gastrointestinal tract, metabolized by the liver, excreted in the urine and stool, peak plasma concentration is 1-2 hours, half-life is 21-46 hours, and steady-state levels occur in 5-10 days.

Professional Considerations

1. Consent form NOT required unless sample is being collected as legal evidence.
2. Preparation:
   A. Tube: Red topped, red/gray topped, or gold topped.
   B. MAY be drawn during hemodialysis.
3. Procedure:
   A. Have the specimen collection witnessed if being collected for legal evidence.
   B. Obtain a 5-mL blood sample.
   C. For a therapeutic dose evaluation, draw the sample 2 hours after oral ingestion of diazepam.
4. Postprocedure care:
   A. For specimens collected for legal evidence, write the client's name, date, exact time of collection, and specimen source on the lab requisition. Sign and have the witness sign the lab requisition.
   B. Transport the specimen to the laboratory immediately in a sealed plastic bag marked as legal evidence. All persons handling the specimen should sign and mark the time of receipt on the laboratory requisition.
   C. Observe for side effects of ataxia, drowsiness, lethargy, nystagmus, nausea, tinnitus, and vertigo, which often subside after continued therapy.
5. Client and family teaching:
   A. Discuss the need for psychologic intervention with the family and the client if panic or lethal doses have been determined. Refer for crisis intervention for intentional overdose.
   B. Referrals to appropriate rehabilitation centers and therapeutic community programs should be offered to all addicted clients who may be interested.
   C. Expect intensive care unit placement for severe overdose.
   D. Death is rare in overdose when diazepam is taken alone.
6. Factors that affect results:
   A. Naltrexone (opiate antagonist) delays the peak level of diazepam by 1 hour.
   B. Proton pump inhibitor (PPI) medications have metabolic interactions with diazepam.
7. Other data:
   A. Heavier sedation occurs in persons with liver disease.
   B. Long-term use may deplete the body of trace elements: zinc, iron, and copper.
   C. Lorazepam is the first line therapy in preference to diazepam in adults with convulsive status epilepticus.
   D. See also *Benzodiazepines, Plasma and Urine.*

DIETHYLPROPION
(see Amphetamines, Blood)

DIFFERENTIAL LEUKOCYTE COUNT (DIFF), PERIPHERAL BLOOD

Norm:

		SI UNITS
White Blood Cells (WBC)		
Adult Females	4500-11,000/μL	$4.5\text{-}11.0 \times 10^9$/L
Pregnant		
Trimester 1	6600-14,000/μL	$6.6\text{-}14.1 \times 10^9$/L
Trimester 2	6900-17,100/μL	$6.9\text{-}17.1 \times 10^9$/L
Trimester 3	5900-14,700/μL	$5.9\text{-}14.7 \times 10^9$/L
Post partum	9700-25,700/μL	$9.7\text{-}25.7 \times 10^9$/L
Adult Males	4500-11,000/μL	$4.5\text{-}11.0 \times 10^9$/L
Children		
Newborn	9000-30,000/μL	$9.0\text{-}30.0 \times 10^9$/L
3 months	5700-18,000/μL	$5.7\text{-}18.0 \times 10^9$/L
1 year	6000-17,500/μL	$6.0\text{-}17.5 \times 10^9$/L
3 years	5700-16,300/μL	$5.7\text{-}16.3 \times 10^9$/L
10 years	4500-13,500/μL	$4.5\text{-}13.5 \times 10^9$/L

		SI UNITS
Differential White Blood Cells		
GRANULOCYTES		
Segmented Feutrophils (Segs)	54-62%	0.54-0.62
Adults	3800/μL	3800 × 10^6/L
Children		
Birth	8400/μL	8400 × 10^6/L
12 hours	12,100/μL	12,100 × 10^6/L
24 hours	8870/μL	8870 × 10^6/L
1 week	4100/μL	4100 × 10^6/L
2 weeks	3320/μL	3320 × 10^6/L
1-2 months	2750/μL	2750 × 10^6/L
4 months	2730/μL	2730 × 10^6/L
6 months	2710/μL	2710 × 10^6/L
8 months	2680/μL	2680 × 10^6/L
10 months	2600/μL	2600 × 10^6/L
12 months	2680/μL	2680 × 10^6/L
2 years	2660/μL	2660 × 10^6/L
4 years	3040/μL	3040 × 10^6/L
6 years	3600/μL	3600 × 10^6/L
8-14 years	3700/μL	3700 × 10^6/L
16-20 years	3800/μL	3800 × 10^6/L
Band Neutrophils (Bands)		
Proportion	3-5%	0.03-0.05
Adults	620/μL	620 × 10^6/L
Children		
Birth	2540/ μL	2540 × 10^6/L
12 hours	3460/μL	3460 × 10^6/L
24 hours	2680/μL	2680 × 10^6/L
1 week	1420/μL	1420 × 10^6/L
2 weeks	1200/μL	1200 × 10^6/L
1 month	1150/μL	1150 × 10^6/L
2 months	1100/μL	1100 × 10^6/L
4-10 months	1000/μL	1000 × 10^6/L
12 months	990/μL	990 × 10^6/L
2 years	850/μL	850 × 10^6/L
4 years	710/μL	710 × 10^6/L
6 years	670/μL	670 × 10^6/L
8 years	660/μL	660 × 10^6/L
10 years	645/μL	645 × 10^6/L
12-14 years	640/μL	640 × 10^6/L
16-20 years	620/μL	620 × 10^6/L
Eosinophils (Eos)		
Proportion	1-3%	0.01-0.03
Adults	200/μL	200 × 10^6/L
Children		
Birth	400/ μL	400 × 10^6/L
12-24 hours	450/μL	450 × 10^6/L
1 week	500/μL	500 × 10^6/L
2 weeks	350/μL	350 × 10^6/L
1 month-1 year	300/μL	300 × 10^6/L
2 years	80/μL	280 × 10^6/L
4 years	250/μL	250 × 10^6/L
6 years	230/μL	230 × 10^6/L
8-20 years	200/μL	200 × 10^6/L

D

Continued

		SI UNITS
GRANULOCYTES—cont'd		
Basophils (Basos)		
Proportion	0-0.75%	0-0.0075
Adults	40/µL	40×10^6/L
Children		
Birth-24 hours	100/µL	100×10^6/L
1 week-8 years	50/µL	50×10^6/L
10-20 years	40/µL	40×10^6/L
MONOCYTES (MONOS)		
Proportion	3-7%	0.03-0.07%
Adults	300/µL	300×10^6/L
Children		
Birth	1050/µL	1050×10^6/L
12 hours	1200/µL	1200×10^6/L
24 hours-1 week	1100/µL	1100×10^6/L
2 weeks	1000/µL	1000×10^6/L
1 month	700/µL	700×10^6/L
2 months	650/µL	650×10^6/L
4 months	600/µL	600×10^6/L
6-8 months	580/µL	580×10^6/L
10-12 months	550/µL	550×10^6/L
2 years	530/µL	530×10^6/L
4 years	450/µL	450×10^6/L
6 years	400/µL	400×10^6/L
8-12 years	350/µL	350×10^6/L
14 years	380/µL	380×10^6/L
16-18 years	400/µL	400×10^6/L
20 years	380/µL	380×10^6/L
LYMPHOCYTES (LYMPHS)		
Proportion	25-33%	0.25-0.33
Adults	2500/µL	2500×10^6/L
Children		
Birth-12 hours	5500/µL	5500×10^6/L
24 hours	5800/µL	5800×10^6/L
1 week	5000/µL	5000×10^6/L
2 weeks	5500/µL	5500×10^6/L
1 month	6000/µL	6000×10^6/L
2 months	6300/µL	6300×10^6/L
4 months	6800/µL	6800×10^6/L
6 months	7300/µL	7300×10^6/L
8 months	7600/µL	7600×10^6/L
10 months	7500/µL	7500×10^6/L
12 months	7000/µL	7000×10^6/L
2 years	6300/µL	6300×10^6/L
4 years	4500/µL	4500×10^6/L
6 years	3500/µL	3500×10^6/L
8 years	3300/µL	3300×10^6/L
10 years	3100/µL	3100×10^6/L
12 years	3000/µL	3000×10^6/L
14 years	2900/µL	2900×10^6/L
16 years	2800/µL	2800×10^6/L
18 years	2700/µL	2700×10^6/L
20 years	2500/µL	2500×10^6/L

Increased White Blood Cell Count.
Abscess, actinomycosis, amebiasis, Andersen's disease, anemia (acquired hemolytic), anorexia, anoxia, anthrax, appendicitis, bacterial infections, blastomycosis, bronchitis, burns, chickenpox, cholecystitis (acute), choledocholithiasis, cholera, cirrhosis (with necrosis), colon cancer, convulsive seizures, Crohn's disease, croup, Cushing syndrome, cytomegalovirus, dengue fever, diphtheria, dissecting aortic aneurysm, diverticulitis, diverticulosis, dysproteinemia, eclampsia, electrical injury, emotional stress, empyema (acute subdural), endocarditis, Epstein-Barr virus, erythroblastosis fetalis, exercise, exposure to ultraviolet radiation, fascioliasis, fatty liver, fever of undetermined origin, G6PD deficiency, gangrene, glomerulonephritis (poststreptococcal), gout (acute), halothane toxicity, heart transplant rejection, hemorrhage, hepatitis (alcoholic), hepatoma, hookworm, Hodgkin's disease, idiopathic myelofibrosis, infection (bacterial, parasitic), infectious mononucleosis, intestinal obstruction, ketoacidosis, lactic acidosis, Legionnaires' disease, leukemia, leukocytosis, lymphoma, meningitis, menstruation, myocardial infarction, myocarditis, pancreatitis, peritonitis, pneumonia, pneumomediastinum, poisoning (arthropods, chemicals, metals, venom), polycythemia vera, postoperative surgical stress, pregnancy, paroxysmal tachycardia, preleukemia, pylephlebitis, rat-bite fever, red blood cell hemolysis, retroperitoneal fibrosis, rheumatic fever, rubeola, sepsis, shock, smallpox, stress, strongyloidiasis, suppurative cholangitis, systemic lupus erythematosus, tonsillitis, toxic shock syndrome, transfusion reaction, trauma, trichuriasis, tuberculosis, tularemia, tumor necrosis, ulcers, ultraviolet radiation, uremia, yellow fever, visceral larva migrans, Wegener's granulomatosis, and Weil's disease. Drugs include allopurinol, anesthetics, atropine sulfate, barbiturates, diethylcarbamazine, epinephrine bitartrate, epinephrine borate, epinephrine hydrochloride, erythromycin, steroids, streptomycin sulfate, and sulfonamides. Herbs or natural remedies that increase granulocyte colony-stimulating factor (GCSF) include Japanese *sho-saiko-to* (TJ-9, *xiao chaihu tang,* Minor *Bupleurum* Combination) and those that increase lymphocyte counts include *Viscum album* (European mistletoe; Plenosol, viscumin and viscotoxin) and *Echinacea purpurea* (purple coneflower; echinacin).

Increased Neutrophils.
Acute infections, allergies, anemia, anoxia, anxiety, appendicitis, asthma, burns, cancer, chickenpox, cholecystitis, cholera, colitis, Cushing syndrome dermatitis, diabetic acidosis, Di Guglielmo's disease, diphtheria, diverticulitis, diverticulosis, eclampsia, electroconvulsive therapy treatment, empyema, emphysema, endocarditis, fear, G6PD deficiency, gangrene, gout, hemorrhage, inflammation, ketoacidosis, labor and delivery, leukemia, leukocytosis, lymphoma, meningitis (purulent), myocardial infarction, osteomyelitis, otitis media, pancreatitis, panic, peritonitis, pernicious anemia, pneumonia, poisoning (carbon monoxide, lead, mercury, arsenic, turpentine), polycythemia vera, postoperative surgical stress, pulmonary infarction, pyelonephritis, pyemia, rheumatic fever, rheumatoid arthritis, salpingitis, scarlet fever, septicemia, smallpox, smoking, thyroiditis, tonsillitis, transfusion reaction, typhus, and uremia. Drugs include acetylcholine, benzene, blood stored for more than 2 days at room temperature, carbon monoxide, casein, chlorpropamide, corticosteroids, corticotropin, digitalis, epinephrine, ethylene glycol, histamine, heparin, insect venoms, lead, lithium, mercury, potassium chloride, and turpentine.

Increased Bands.
Pharyngitis.

Increased Segmented.
Pernicious anemia.

Increased Eosinophils.
Addison's disease, allergies, atheroembolic renal disease, asthma, brucellosis, cancer (bone, brain, ovary, testes), chorea, coccidioidomycosis, dermatitis, diverticulitis, diverticulosis, eczema, gangrene, hay fever, Hodgkin's disease, leprosy, leukemia (chronic granulocytic), leukocytosis, Löffler syndrome, malaria, metastatic carcinoma, parasitic infections, pemphigus, pernicious anemia, phlebitis, polycythemia vera, psoriasis, pruritus caused by jaundice, radiation therapy, rheumatoid arthritis, rhinitis,

sarcoidosis, scarlet fever, sickle cell anemia, splenectomy, Sjögren syndrome, thrombophlebitis, tuberculosis, and ulcerative colitis. Drugs include antibiotics (associated with allergic reactions), allopurinol, aminosalicylic acid, anticonvulsants, blood stored for more than 2 days at room temperature, cephalosporins, chlorpropamide, digitalis, heparin, imipramine, methotrexate, nitrofurantoin, penicillin, phenothiazine, procainamide, procarbazine, propranolol, quinidine, streptomycin, sulfonamides, and tetracycline.

Increased Basophils. Allergic reaction to food/drugs/inhalants, chickenpox, chronic myelogenous leukemia, erythroderma, Heinz-body anemia, Hodgkin's disease, hypothyroidism, irradiation, leukocytosis, myelofibrosis, myxedema, nephrosis, periarteritis nodosa, polycythemia vera, serum sickness, sinusitis, smallpox, splenectomy, ulcerative colitis, and urticaria. Drugs include antithyroids, desipramine, and estrogens.

Increased Lymphocytes. Brucellosis, cytomegalovirus, diverticulitis, diverticulosis, endocarditis, hepatitis, Hurler syndrome, infectious mononucleosis, leukocytosis, lymphocytic leukemia, pertussis, syphilis, toxoplasmosis, and xerostomia. Drugs include aspirin, blood stored for more than 2 days at room temperature, carbon disulfate poisoning, haloperidol, lead intoxication, levodopa, phenytoin, and tetrahydrochloride poisoning.

Increased Monocytes. Brucellosis, carbon disulfide poisoning, Epstein-Barr virus, Hodgkin's disease, leukemia (AML, CML), leukocytosis, multiple myeloma, phosphorus poisoning, rheumatoid arthritis, salmonellosis, sarcoidosis, syphilis, systemic lupus erythematosus, tetrahydrochloride poisoning, tuberculosis, and ulcerative colitis. Drugs include haloperidol and methsuximide.

Decreased White Blood Cell Count. Agranulocytosis, AIDS, alcoholism, anaphylactic shock, anemia (aplastic, pernicious), amyloidosis, anorexia nervosa, anthrax, arsenic poisoning, brucellosis, cachexia, chemical toxicity, chemotherapy, cirrhosis, Colorado tick fever, dengue fever, disseminated lupus erythematosus, Felty syndrome, Gaucher's disease, heavy chain disease, hepatitis (infectious, viral), Hodgkin's disease, hypersplenism, hypothermia, idiopathic myelofibrosis, infection (severe bacterial, viral), influenza, Legionnaires' disease, leishmaniasis, leukemia (some forms), leukopenia, lymphoma, measles, mononucleosis, myxedema, paratyphoid fever, pharyngitis, *Pneumocystis* pneumonia, preleukemia, protein therapy, psittacosis, Q fever, radiation therapy, renal trauma, rheumatic fever, rubella, sepsis neonatorum, shock, Sjögren syndrome, stiff-man syndrome, stomatitis, strongyloidiasis, toxoplasmosis, tuberculosis, tularemia, and typhoid fever. Drugs include acetaminophen, aminoglutethimide, aminopyrine, antibiotics, antineoplastics, antithyroids, arsenicals, aurothioglucose, bismuth, chloramphenicol, chloroquine phosphate, diazepam, diethylcarbamazine, ethotoin, furosemide, immunosuppressives, meprobamate, methyldopa, methyldopate hydrochloride, methsuximide, phenothiazines, phenylbutazone, phenytoin, phenytoin sodium, primidone, procainamide hydrochloride, quinacrine hydrochloride, quinine sulfate, sulfonamides, and vitamin A.

Decreased Neutrophils. Acromegaly, Addison's disease, agranulocytosis, anaphylactic shock, anorexia nervosa, aplastic anemia, brucellosis, cachexia, carcinoma, Chediak-Higashi syndrome, chemotherapy, cirrhosis, Colorado tick fever, dengue fever, Felty syndrome, folic acid deficiency, Gaucher's disease, hypersplenism, hypopituitarism, hypothyroidism, infections, infectious hepatitis, infectious mononucleosis, influenza, iron deficiency anemia, kala-azar, malaria, measles, mumps, myelofibrosis, myeloma, paratyphoid fever, paroxysmal nocturnal hemoglobinuria, pernicious anemia, pneumonia, psittacosis, radiation therapy, Rocky Mountain spotted fever, rubella, rubeola, sarcoma, septicemia, thyrotoxicosis, tularemia, typhoid fever, vitamin B_{12} deficiency, and yellow fever. Drugs include alcohol, aminophylline, antipyrine, aminopyrine, ampicillin, arsenic, aspirin, barbiturates, carbimazole, cephalothin, chemotherapeutic agents, chloramphenicol, chlorpromazine, chlorpropamide, cinchophen, DDT, diazepam, dinitrophenol, diuretics, electroconvulsive therapy treatment, gold salts, imipramine, indomethacin, isoniazid, mephenytoin, 6-mercaptopurine, methaphenolene hydrochloride, methicillin, *para*-aminobenzoic acid, penicillin, phenacetin, phenylbutazone, phenylhydrazine, phenytoin, procainamide, quinine, rauwolfia, streptomycin, sulfonamides, tolbutamide, tripelennamine hydrochloride, and urethan.

Decreased Eosinophils. Acromegaly, anemia (aplastic), coccidioidomycosis, congestive heart failure, Cushing syndrome, disseminated lupus erythematosus, eclampsia, fascioliasis, Goodpasture syndrome, hypersplenism, infections, infectious mononucleosis, schistosomiasis, and stress. Drugs include adrenocorticotropic hormone, corticotropin, epinephrine, glucocorticoids, methysergide, niacin, niacinamide, procainamide, and thyroxine.

Decreased Basophils. Acute infection, anaphylaxis, Cushing syndrome, hyperthyroidism, ovulation, pregnancy, radiation therapy, thyrotoxicosis, and stress. Drugs include chemotherapy, corticosteroids, corticotropin, procainamide, and thiotepa.

Decreased Lymphocytes. Aplastic anemia, Cushing syndrome, Hodgkin's disease, immunoglobulin deficiencies, leukemia (chronic granulocytic, monocytic), lymphosarcoma, renal failure, systemic lupus erythematosus, thymic hypoplasia in children, and uremia. Drugs include asparaginase, chlorambucil, cortisone, epinephrine, glucocorticoids, lithium compounds, mechlorethamine, niacin, nitrogen mustard, and radiation therapy to the lymphatics.

Decreased Monocytes. Aplastic anemia and hairy-cell leukemia. Drugs include blood stored for more than 2 days at room temperature.

Description. The differential white blood cell count (Diff) provides an assessment of each leukocyte distribution on two stained glass slides of peripheral blood. One hundred white blood cells are identified and then classified (differentiated) according to their morphology. A relative percentage of each type of cell is then determined and reported. White blood cells (leukocytes) function in the body's immune defense system. Three main types of white blood cells exist: granulocytes, monocytes, and lymphocytes, and are identified and counted by microscopic examination of stained blood films. *Granulocytes,* manufactured by bone marrow, are subdivided into neutrophils, eosinophils, and basophils and function in bacterial phagocytosis. Neutrophils are further subclassified as either segmented or band neutrophils. Segmented neutrophils (Segs) are more mature and have two to five lobes, which increase (shift to the right) during pathologic conditions. Band neutrophils (Bands) are less mature and increase in number (shift to the left) during conditions causing increased white blood cell (WBC) production. Eosinophils are leukocytes that contain course round granules. Eosinophils become active in the later stages of inflammation. These cells act as phagocytes and are active in allergic reactions and parasitic infections. Eosinophils are under the influence of the adrenal cortex. *Monocytes* are manufactured by bone marrow function both in antigen recognition and in phagocytosis of cellular debris. *Lymphocytes* formed by the lymphatic system function in humoral and cell-mediated immune responses to foreign antigens.

Professional Considerations
1. Consent form NOT required.
2. **Preparation:**
   A. Tube: Lavender-topped glass or lavender-sealed plastic.
   B. Screen client for the use of herbal preparations or natural remedies such as Japanese *sho-saiko-to* (TJ-9, *xiao chaihu tang,* Minor *Bupleurum* Combination) and those that increase lymphocyte counts include *Viscum album* (European mistletoe; Plenosol, viscumin and viscotoxin) and *Echinacea purpurea* (purple coneflower; echinacin).
3. **Procedure:**
   A. Draw a 3.5-mL blood sample.
   B. Do not leave tourniquet in place longer than 60 seconds.

4. **Postprocedure care:**
   A. Apply pressure at the site of the venipuncture because bleeding may occur because of disease entity.
   B. Record the collection time because counts vary according to time of day.
5. **Client and family teaching:**
   A. Results are normally available within 24 hours.
6. **Factors that affects results:**
   A. In leukemia, cryofibrinogenemia, and cryoglobulinemia, WBC results performed on an electronic cell counter are unreliable. The counts must be performed manually.
   B. The most accurate leukocyte counts are obtained from capillary punctures. For EDTA-anticoagulated blood (lavender-topped tube), the most accurate counts are obtained within 4 hours of the specimen collection.
   C. The serum sample is stable at room temperature for 10 hours and refrigerated for 18 hours and should not be frozen.
   D. Leukocyte differential relative values reported as percentages should be converted to absolute values by multiplication of the percentage by the total WBC count before interpretation.
7. **Other data:**
   A. "Shift to the left" means that there are an increased number of immature neutrophils in the peripheral blood. Neutrophils are usually illustrated from left (young cells) to right (mature cells) in the differential. A low total WBC count with a left shift indicates a recovery from bone marrow depression or an infection of such intensity that the demand for neutrophils in the tissue is greater than the capacity of the bone marrow to release them in the circulation. A high total WBC count with a left shift indicates an increased release of neutrophils by the bone marrow in response to an overwhelming infection or inflammation.
   B. "Shift to the right" means cells have more than the usual number of nuclear segments. This is found in liver disease, Down syndrome, or megaloblastic and pernicious anemia.
   C. The eosinophil count may be used with the Thorn test to evaluate adrenocortical stimulation.
   D. An automated WBC may not reveal the "shifts."
   E. Differential leukocyte counts do not differ in clients with or without chronic graft-versus-host disease after allogeneic bone marrow transplant.

DIFFUSING CAPACITY FOR CARBON MONOXIDE (DL_{CO}, TRANSFER FACTOR), DIAGNOSTIC

Norm. The predicted values are based on prediction equations calculated according to gender, age, height, weight, and hemoglobin. Results are considered abnormal if they are less than 80% of the predicted values. The average normal for resting subjects by the single-breath and steady-state methods is 25 mL/min/mm Hg.

Usage. Identify and monitor the course of parenchymal lung disease processes and pulmonary hypertension in scleroderma; Monitor for pulmonary drug toxicity; distinguish chronic bronchitis (normal DL_{CO}) from emphysema (low DL_{CO}); distinguish interstitial fibrosis from pleural fibrosis.

Increased. Asthma, alveolar hemorrhage, polycythemia. Diseases or conditions associated with increased pulmonary blood flow such as left-to-right shunts, tachycardia, and exercise. Medications include inhaled budesonide corticosteroid.

Decreased. Acute myocardial infarction, alveolar fibrosis (associated with sarcoidosis, asbestosis, berylliosis, pneumoconiosis in coal miners, idiopathic pulmonary fibrosis, O_2 toxicity, or silicosis), asbestosis, bone marrow transplant following total body irradiation, bronchiolitis obliterans with organizing pneumonia, diseases associated with anemia (such as chronic renal failure), histiocytosis X, lung resection, metal fume fever, mitral stenosis, mixed connective tissue diseases (dermatomyositis, inflammatory bowel disease, polymyositis, rheumatoid arthritis, Wegener's granulomatosis), obstructive lung diseases (emphysema, cystic fibrosis), parenchymal loss or replacement, pneumonia, posture of upright position, primary pulmonary hypertension, pulmonary edema, pulmonary emboli, restrictive lung disease, space-occupying lesions, systemic disease with pulmonary involvement (progressive systemic sclerosis, scleroderma, systemic lupus erythematosus). Drugs include amiodarone and bleomycin affecting the alveolocapillary membrane, marijuana smoking, acute and chronic ethyl alcohol ingestion, freebasing cocaine, cigarette smoking.

Description. Carbon monoxide (CO) is a gas that is readily taken from the alveolus and bound to hemoglobin (Hb) in pulmonary capillary blood. The diffusing capacity rate of the lung provides a measure of the lung's gas exchange mechanism. It assesses the amount of functioning pulmonary capillary bed in contact with functioning alveoli. Therefore it can provide useful information on gas-exchange properties of the lung. Thus transport or flow or uptake of carbon monoxide is a unique way to noninvasively determine the ability of the alveolar capillary membrane to transport oxygen into the blood. It is reported in cubic centimeters (of CO) per minute per millimeters of Hg or millimoles (of CO) per minute per kilopascals at $0°$ C, 760 mm Hg, dry (that is, STPD). There are several methods for determining the DL_{CO}. The two most commonly used in the clinical setting are the steady-state technique and the single-breath technique.

Comparison of Steady-State and Single-Breath Methods for Determination of DL_{CO}

Steady State	Single Breath
Generally easier for the subject to perform because no special breathing maneuvers are required.	Far less susceptible to development of CO back pressure and to effects of V/Q abnormalities.
Adaptable to use during exercise and other applications where breath holding is not feasible.	Tends to be more reproducible.
	Generally yields higher values (than steady-state methods do) in a given subject.

Professional Considerations
1. Consent form NOT required.
2. **Preparation:**
   A. Assess medication record for recent analgesic that may depress respiratory function.
   B. Bronchodilators and intermittent positive-pressure breathing therapy may be withheld before the tests.
   C. The client should wear loose-fitting and comfortable clothing the day of the test.
   D. Document the client's age, gender, height, and weight on the test requisition.
   E. Dentures should not be removed.
   F. See *Client and family teaching.*
3. **Procedure:**
   A. The equipment used for this test contains a sample pump and bag, a calibrated spirometer of test gas, and both a helium analyzer and a carbon monoxide analyzer.

   B. The client is positioned sitting upright with feet on the floor.
   C. A nose clip is applied to ensure consistent air flow through the mouth.
   D. *Single-breath Maneuver:*
      i. The client exhales completely, rapidly inhales from the spirometer to reach maximum capacity, and then holds his or her breath for 10 seconds.
      ii. Upon exhalation, 0.5-1.0 liter of exhaled air is collected and analyzed for helium and carbon monoxide.
      iii. The test is repeated after 4 minutes.
      iv. *Note:* Variations of this test have been published, with one method measuring DL_{CO} on inhalation, breath holding, and exhalation. A third method is designed for clients

who cannot hold their breath for 10 seconds or achieve an adequate flow rate and is based on a slow, submaximal breath and requires different equipment.

E. *Steady-state Method:*
  i. The client is instructed to breath in and out through the mouthpiece while exercise is done or other maneuvers are carried out and measurements are taken.

4. **Postprocedure care:**
  A. Resume all medications including bronchodilators and intermittent positive-pressure breathing therapy.
  B. Test results are normally available within 30 minutes.

5. **Client and family teaching:**
  A. Teach proper breathing technique for the test.
  B. The procedure takes approximately 20 minutes.
  C. Refrain from smoking or eating a heavy meal for 3-4 hours before the test.
  D. Refrain from drinking alcohol for 24 hours before the test.

6. **Factors that affect results:**
  A. Reasonable airway mechanics, lung volumes, and client cooperation are required for accurate measurements.
  B. An inadequate seal around the mouthpiece invalidates the results.
  C. A supine body position increases DL_{CO}.
  D. Exercise increases diffusing capacity.
  E. Gastric distension, hypoxia, narcotics, sedatives, and pregnancy may alter the results.
  F. Bronchodilators administered before the tests may obscure true pulmonary function.
  G. Results are adjusted for high or low Hb levels using the following equation:

  $$\text{Corrected } DL_{CO} = \text{Actual } DL_{CO} \times 10.2 + \text{Observed Hb (g/dL)} / 1.7 + \text{Observed Hb (g/dL)}$$

  H. Single-breath method results are invalidated and reported with anecdotal notation for any of the following reasons:

  i. Inspired VC <90% of highest historical VC
  ii. Client is unable to hold breath at least 9 seconds or holds longer than 11 seconds.
  iii. Inspiration that is too slow (such as longer than 2.5-4 seconds).

7. **Other data:**
  A. Diffusion capacity for carbon monoxide is routinely performed in a pulmonary function laboratory.
  B. Proper interpretation of results needs to account for inherent assumptions regarding CO distribution and timing procedures.
  C. The abbreviation for the single-breath method is $DL_{CO}{}^{SB}$.

DIFFUSION-WEIGHTED IMAGING
(see Magnetic resonance imaging, Diagnostic)

DIGITAL MAMMOGRAPHY
(see Mammography, Diagnostic)

DIGITAL SUBTRACTION ANGIOGRAPHY (DSA) AND TRANSVENOUS DIGITAL SUBTRACTION, DIAGNOSTIC

Norm. Normal carotid arteries, vertebral arteries, abdominal aorta and branches, renal arteries, and peripheral vessels.

Usage. Aneurysms, aortic valvular stenosis, arterial occlusion, bypass surgery (postoperative), carotid stenosis, dural sinus thrombosis, hepatocellular carcinoma, jugular tumors, nutcracker renal phenomenon, pheochromocytoma, pulmonary emboli, thoracic outlet syndrome, and ulcerative plaques.

Description. A noninvasive computer imaging procedure that allows examination of the arteries in the body after an IV injection of contrast medium. Images of the cardiac region are subtracted from images obtained after contrast medium injection as the dense images of soft tissue and bone are removed by the computer. There is less discomfort and risk of complications than with an arteriogram, but visualization of the arteries is less precise, and visualization of stenotic lesions in sequential branches may not occur.

Professional Considerations
1. Consent form IS required.

Risks
Allergic reaction to dye (itching, hives, rash, tight feeling in the throat, shortness of breath, bronchospasm, anaphylaxis, death), aphasia, hemiplegia, hemorrhage, paresthesia, thromboemboli, infection, renal toxicity from contrast medium.

Contraindications
Recent myocardial infarction, severe renal failure, previous allergy to dye, iodine, or shellfish; during pregnancy (because of radioactive iodine crossing the blood-placental barrier).

2. Preparation:
   A. Assess for normal renal function.
   B. Have emergency equipment readily available.
   C. Glycogen may be administered intravenously to reduce motion artifacts by stopping peristalsis.
   D. Record baseline vital signs.
3. Procedure:
   A. A local anesthetic is given over the basilic or cephalic veins in the antecubital area.
   B. Venous catheterization is performed and iodine contrast medium is injected at a rate of 14 mL/second.
   C. Radiographic images are taken of arteries made visible by the contrast medium.
4. Postprocedure care:
   A. Monitor vital signs every 15 minutes until stable.
   B. Observe the puncture site of catheterization for infection, hemorrhage, and hematoma.

C. Force fluids after the procedure to help flush the contrast medium through the kidneys. A liter of IV fluid may be given as a precautionary measure to clients having an increased risk of developing renal toxicity from the contrast medium, such as the elderly, and clients with dehydration, diabetes, or multiple myeloma.
D. Monitor renal function (BUN and creatinine) for 2 days after the procedure in all clients to be sure the levels remain normal. If the levels become abnormally elevated, indicating nephrotoxicity, continuous IV fluids should be given until the levels return to normal limits. An adverse reaction to IV contrast medium should be noted in a prominent place on the chart and the client informed that he or she should not receive a contrast medium in the future.
E. If the study is necessary in a client with renal insufficiency, a newer, less nephrotoxic agent should be used, even though it is more expensive, and the client should be well hydrated.
5. Client and family teaching:
   A. You must remain still during the procedure.
   B. The procedure takes approximately 45 minutes.
   C. In women who are breast-feeding, formula should be substituted for breast milk for 1 or more days after the procedure.
6. Factors that affect results:
   A. Small amounts of motion by the individual including swallowing and respirations obscure results.
   B. Intracardiac or intra-arterial injection of contrast medium can also obscure results.
7. Other data:
   A. The femoral vein may also be used for catheterization.

DIGITOXIN, SERUM

Norm. Negative.

	TROUGH	SI UNITS
Therapeutic values	10-32 ng/mL	13.1-41.9 nmol/L
Panic level	>35 ng/mL	>45.8 nmol/L

Panic Level Symptoms and Treatment

Symptoms (occur with concentrations >25 μg/mL). Anorexia, hyperkalemia, mental status changes, nausea, vomiting, diarrhea, and visual distortion in which objects appear yellow or green or have a halo around them. Serious toxic symptoms are bradycardia and atrioventricular (AV) nodal block.

Treatment:

Note: Treatment choice(s) depend on client history and condition and episode history.
1. Continuous ECG monitoring is necessary. Watch for prolonged PR-interval, widening QRS-interval, lengthening QTc, and AV block.
2. Transcutaneous pacing for rhythms progressing to AV block.
3. Discontinue medication.
4. For acute overdose, empty the stomach by inducing emesis (with extreme caution) with syrup of ipecac or by gastric lavage or warm 0.9% saline or tap water. Do NOT induce emesis if signs of central nervous system depression are evident or if the client has no gag reflex.
5. Give activated charcoal.
6. Treat hypokalemia with a potassium supplement.
7. Treat hyperkalemia with IV glucose and insulin.
8. For potentially life-threatening toxicity, administer digoxin-specific antibody fragments (Fab). The dose depends on the amount of digitoxin (or oleandrin) to be neutralized, usually 240 mg (six 40-mg vials reconstituted with sterile water to provide a solution of 10 mg/mL) given by IV push or as an infusion over 15-30 minutes.
9. Hemodialysis will NOT remove digitoxin but will be helpful in treating serious hyperkalemia.

Usage. Prophylactic management and treatment of heart failure and to control the ventricular rate in atrial fibrillation or atrial flutter. May also be used to treat and prevent recurrent paroxysmal atrial tachycardia. Monitoring of serum levels is performed during initial digitoxin therapy, if toxicity is suspected from symptoms, and for assessment of medication compliance. After a stable dose is established, routine monitoring is not usually necessary.

Description. Long-acting cardiac glycoside with a half-life is 5-7 days and with peak concentrations occurring in 1-3 hours; 90% is metabolized in the liver and excreted in the urine. The main property of a cardiac glycoside is its positive inotropic effect on the myocardium. It also decreases the conduction velocity through the AV node and prolongs the effective refractory period of the AV node. It reduces diastolic blood pressure and heart rate during sleep. Serum digitoxin levels are elevated in oleander plant poisoning.

Professional Considerations
1. Consent form NOT required.
2. **Preparation:**
   A. Tube: Red topped, red/gray topped, or gold topped.
   B. Specimens should be drawn 6-8 hours after the last dose of digitoxin.
   C. The specimen MAY be drawn during hemodialysis.
3. **Procedure:**
   A. Draw a 3-mL TROUGH blood sample.
   B. Obtain serial measurements at the same time each day.
4. **Postprocedure care:**
   A. If toxic levels are found, withhold the drug and notify the physician.
   B. Be sure to request the right drug level. There will be an error in results if digoxin is requested instead of digitoxin.
5. **Client and family teaching:**
   A. Results are normally available within 24 hours.
   B. If activated charcoal was given for elevated levels, the client should drink 4-6 glasses of water each day for 2 days to prevent constipation. The activated charcoal will also cause stools to be black for a few days.
   C. Refer clients with intentional overdose for crisis intervention.
6. **Factors that affect results:**
   A. Radioactive tracer within 24 hours falsely elevates results.

B. Recent administration of digoxin may increase results.

C. Serum potassium, calcium, or magnesium imbalances may falsely elevate results.

D. Drug interactions include carbamazepine, cholestyramine, heparin, kaolin-pectin, neomycin, phenobarbital, phenytoin, quinidine, rifampin, valproic acid and verapamil, which may elevate results. Herbs include Chinese medicines Chan Su and Lu-Shen-Wan that increase results.

E. Results may be elevated in hepatic or renal dysfunction.

F. A rebound of the digitoxin level may occur 2-3 days after Fab administration.

7. **Other data:**

A. Treatment of supraventricular tachycardia and atrial fibrillation may need to have drug levels in the high therapeutic range.

B. Digoxin is a metabolite of digitoxin, and so digoxin-specific antibody fragments are effective in the treatment of toxicity.

C. Use with caution in the elderly because the mean half-life is 25.2 days, which is significantly higher than that in younger clients.

D. Toxicity usually results from hepatic or renal dysfunction, hypokalemia, hypothyroidism, severe hypoxic heart or respiratory disease, or variations in the client response to the dose.

D

DIGOXIN, SERUM

Norm. Negative

	TROUGH	SI UNITS
Therapeutic level	0.5-2.0 ng/mL	0.6-2.6 nmol/L
Dysrhythmias appear	1.5-2.0 ng/mL	1.9-2.6 nmol/L
Congestive heart failure	0.8-1.5 ng/mL	1.0-1.9 nmol/L
Panic level (adult)	>2.4 ng/mL	>3.2 nmol/L
Panic level (children)	>3.0 ng/mL	>3.8 nmol/L

Panic Level Symptoms and Treatment

Symptoms. Anorexia, hyperkalemia, mental status changes, nausea, vomiting, diarrhea, and visual distortion in which objects appear yellow or green or have a halo around them. Serious toxic symptoms are bradycardia and AV nodal block. 87% of people with levels over 2 ng/mL have toxic symptoms.

Treatment:

Note: Treatment choice(s) depend on client history and condition and episode history.

1. Continuous ECG monitoring is necessary. Watch for prolonged PR-interval, widening QRS-interval, lengthening QTc, and AV block.

2. Transcutaneous pacing for rhythms progressing to AV block.

3. Discontinue medication.

4. For acute overdose soon after ingestion, empty stomach by inducing emesis with syrup of ipecac or by gastric lavage or warm 0.9% saline or tap water. Do NOT induce emesis if signs of central nervous system depression are evident or if the client has no gag reflex.

5. Give activated charcoal.

6. Treat hypokalemia with potassium supplement.

7. Treat hyperkalemia with IV glucose and insulin.

8. For potentially life-threatening toxicity, administer digoxin-specific antibody fragments (Fab). The dose depends on the amount of digoxin to be neutralized, usually 240 mg (six 40-mg vials reconstituted with sterile water to provide a solution of 10 mg/mL) given by IV push or as an infusion over 15-30 minutes. Hemodialysis and peritoneal dialysis will NOT remove digoxin but will be helpful in treating serious hyperkalemia. Hemoperfusion WILL remove digoxin.

Increased. Hepatic dysfunction, renal dysfunction. Drug interactions include amiodarone, antacids, captopril, cholestyramine, clarithromycin, erythromycin, flecainide, fluoxetine, heparin, ibuprofen, itraconazole (arrhythmias of ventricular premature contraction, AV block and ST depression so decrease dose of digoxin by 50%), kaolin-pectin, midazolam, neomycin, nitrendipine, phenobarbital, phenytoin, propafenone, quinidine, rifampin, spironolactone, and verapamil, which may increase results. Herbal or natural remedies that contain cardiac glycosides include pleurisy root. Herbs or natural remedies that may potentiate cardiac glycoside effects include *Ephedra* (*ma huang*; ephedrine). The herbal remedy sarsaparilla may increase the absorption of digoxin.

Decreased. Drugs include bisacodyl. An herb or natural remedy that decreases digoxin peak and trough concentrations is St. John's wort (*Hypericum perforatum*). Other herbal or natural remedies include Senna (*Cassia senna, Cassia angustifolia*).

Usage. Prophylactic management and treatment of heart failure and Ebstein tricuspid valve anomaly and for control of the ventricular rate in atrial fibrillation or atrial flutter. May also be used to treat and prevent recurrent paroxysmal atrial tachycardia. Monitoring of serum levels is performed during initial digoxin therapy, if toxicity is suspected from symptoms, and for assessment of medication compliance. After a stable dose is established, routine monitoring is not usually necessary.

Description. Cardiac glycoside with prompt action and less prolonged effect than digitoxin and is rapidly excreted in the urine. Half-life is 32-51 hours in adults and 11-50 hours in children, with peak concentrations reached in 1-5 hours. Steady-state levels are reached after 7-11 days in adults and after 2-10 days in children. The main property of a cardiac glycoside is its positive inotropic effect on the myocardium. It also decreases the conduction velocity through the AV node and prolongs the effective refractory period of the AV node.

Professional Considerations
1. Consent form NOT required.
2. Preparation:
   A. Tube: Red topped, red/gray topped, or gold topped.
   B. Specimens should be drawn 6-8 hours after last dose of digoxin.
   C. MAY be drawn during hemodialysis.
   D. Screen client for the use of herbal preparations or natural remedies such as St. John's wort, eleuthero (Siberian ginseng, *Eleutherococcus senticosus*), ma^{2}huang^2 (*Ephedra*), "Chomper" (by Arise and Shine, with glycoside-like compounds found in the toxic plant Digitalis lanata), plantain leaves (found in Nature Cleanse Tablets, Botanical Cleanse, or Blessed Herb brands), Kyushin ("save-heart", a patented natural cardiotonic, dried toad venom), uzara (*Dicoma anomala*) root, hawthorn, ginseng.
3. Procedure:
   A. Draw a 1-mL TROUGH blood sample.
   B. Obtain serial measurements at the same time each day.
4. Postprocedure care:
   A. Be sure to request the right drug level to be drawn. There will be an error in results if digitoxin is requested instead of digoxin.
   B. If toxic levels are found, withhold the drug and notify the physician.
5. Client and family teaching:
   A. Results are normally available within 24 hours.
   B. A rebound of the digoxin level may occur 2-3 days after Fab administration.
   C. Do not drink grapefruit juice because it can inhibit the absorption of digoxin.
   D. Refer clients with intentional overdose for crisis intervention.
6. Factors that affect results:
   A. Radioactive tracer within 24 hours may falsely elevate results.
   B. Serum potassium, calcium, or magnesium imbalances may increase results.
   C. Grapefruit juice inhibits the absorption of digoxin.
   D. Use of Digibind therapy to treat digoxin toxicity actually increases the serum level of digoxin initially, by as much as double,

and serum digoxin levels are misleading for the next 2 weeks after Digibind therapy.

E. Herbs or natural remedies that may cause falsely elevated results include eleuthero (Siberian ginseng, *Eleutherococcus senticosus*), Chomper, plantain leaves (found in Nature Cleanse Tablets, Botanical Cleanse or Blessed Herb brands), Kyushin, uzara root, hawthorn, ginseng (see all above).

F. Levels correlate poorly with clinical signs of toxicity.

7. **Other data:**
A. Treatment of supraventricular tachycardia and atrial fibrillation may need to have drug levels in the high therapeutic range.
B. Use with caution in the elderly.
C. Toxicity usually results from hepatic or renal dysfunction, hypokalemia, hypothyroidism, severe hypoxic heart or respiratory disease, or variations in the client response to the dosage. Visual disturbances can occur with therapeutic blood levels.
D. Anticonvulsants have been reported to increase hepatic clearance of digoxin.
E. Trade names include Lanoxicaps, Lanoxin, Digoxin Elixir, and Lanoxin Elixir.
F. The herbal remedy natural licorice may cause potassium loss, which increases the risk of digoxin toxicity. Artificial licorice does not cause potassium loss.
G. In obese persons the use of digoxin increases the risk of developing diabetes mellitus.

DILATATION AND CURETTAGE (D & C), DIAGNOSTIC

Norm. No abnormal cells.

Usage. Acquired and congenital cervical stenosis, cancer, diagnosis and treatment of abnormal uterine bleeding, dysmenorrhea, insertion of an IUD, insertion of a radium device for treatment of cancer, pedunculated leiomyomas, preceding a hysterography or hysteroscopy, and uterine polyps.

Description. A widening of the cervical canal with a dilator and then a scraping of the uterine canal with a curette. The test is performed for diagnostic purposes less frequently than in the past because other modalities, such as endometrial biopsy, hysteroscopy and pelvic ultrasonography, have become available for use. D & C is usually performed therapeutically after an incomplete abortion or miscarriage.

Professional Considerations
1. Consent form IS required.

Risks
The primary complication is perforation of the uterus. If a perforation occurs and the client is stable, a laparoscopy can be performed to evaluate the perforation. If a perforation is suspected during a suction curettage, a laparoscopy must be performed to continue the procedure to be sure that bowel is not aspirated into the uterus. If the client becomes unstable, emergency surgery is necessary. Arthralgias, though uncommon, can be painful side effects.

Contraindications
Clients with coagulopathies or active vaginal infections.

2. **Preparation:**
A. Ascertain any drug allergies.
B. Perineal shave may be preferred.
C. The client should void before the procedure.
D. An enema may be prescribed before the procedure.
E. An intravenous line may be initiated.
F. Obtain containers of 10% formalin solution for tissue specimens.
G. Measure and document baseline vital signs.

3. **Procedure:**
A. Regional or general anesthesia (thiopental-isoflurane most cost effective) is initiated.
B. The cervical canal is dilated with a dilator, and the uterine canal is scraped with a curette.
C. Tissue specimens are placed in containers of 10% formalin and sent to the laboratory for analysis. If an infection is suspected, part of the specimen should be placed in a sterile container without fixative and sent to the laboratory for culture and sensitivity.

4. **Postprocedure care:**
   A. Assess vital signs every 15 minutes until stable and then every hour × 4 after general anesthesia. Additional monitoring after general anesthesia typically includes continuous ECG monitoring and pulse oximetry, with continual assessments (every 5-15 minutes) of airway, vital signs, and neurologic status until the client is lying quietly awake, is breathing independently, and responds appropriately to commands spoken in a normal tone.
   B. After regional anesthesia, assess vital signs when the procedure is completed and continue to monitor if unstable.
   C. Assess the perineal pad for color and amount of drainage.
   D. Assess for postanesthesia sensation.
   E. Assess and medicate for cramping.
   F. Dexamethasone 8 mg IV is an effective antiemetic for preventing postoperative nausea and vomiting 0-24 hours after propofol-based anesthesia after D & C.
5. **Client and family teaching:**
   A. The procedure takes approximately 45 minutes.
   B. The procedure is accompanied by cramping similar to menstrual cramps. Medications will be given to keep this tolerable.
   C. Call the physician for signs of infection: fever >101° F (38.3° C), pelvic or vaginal pain, purulent vaginal drainage, or for excessive bleeding.
6. **Factors that affect results:**
   A. None found.
7. **Other data:**
   A. Hysteroscopy does not improve the sensitivity of D & C in detecting hyperplasia or endometrial carcinoma but is superior in detecting focal lesions of the uterine cavity in postmenopausal bleeding.

DINITROPHENYLHYDRAZINE (DNPH) TEST, DIAGNOSTIC

Norm. Normal amino acid screen.

Usage. Biotinidase deficiency, cystinuria, Hartnup's homocystinuria disease, maple syrup urine disease, oasthouse urine disease, PKU, tyrosinemia, tyrosinosis, lactic acidosis, fructose-1, 6-diphosphatase deficiency, ketosis, seizures, and unexplained mental retardation.

Description. Metabolic screening test to detect inherited disorders in the metabolism of branched-chain amino acids.

Professional Considerations
1. Consent form NOT required.
2. **Preparation:**
   A. Obtain a clean specimen container.
3. **Procedure:**
   A. Obtain a 15-mL random urine specimen.
4. **Postprocedure care:**
   A. Keep the urine sample refrigerated or frozen.
5. **Client and family teaching:**
   A. Results are normally available within 72 hours.
6. **Factors that affect results:**
   A. Radiopaque contrast dye may increase the results.
   B. Falsely elevated results occur if valproic acid, penicillin derivatives, or benzoic acid preservatives have been ingested within 3 days of the urine collection.
7. **Other data:**
   A. A 24-hour urine sample may also be obtained.
   B. Peritoneal dialysis may be used to clear amino acids from the body.
   C. One of the branched-chain amino acids produces a metabolite that causes the urine to smell like maple syrup.
   D. The test can also be performed on a newborn heel stick blood spot as part of the neonatal screening for metabolic disorders.

DIPYRIDAMOLE-THALLIUM SCAN
(*see Heart scan, Diagnostic*)

DIRECT ANTIGLOBULIN TEST
(*see Coombs' test, Direct, Serum*)

DISCOVERY IMAGING, DIAGNOSTIC
(*see Dual modality imaging, Diagnostic*)

DISOPYRAMIDE PHOSPHATE, SERUM

Norm:

	TROUGH
Therapeutic	2-5 µg/mL
Panic level	>7 µg/mL

Panic Level Symptoms and Treatment

Symptoms. Prolonged QT interval and ventricular tachycardia, heart failure, hypotension.

Treatment:
Note: Treatment choice(s) depend on client history and condition and episode history.
Stop medication.
Monitor ECG for R-on-T phenomenon.
Support airway, breathing, and blood pressure.
Hemodialysis WILL remove disopyramide. No information was found on peritoneal dialysis's effect on disopyramide levels.

Usage. Monitoring for therapeutic dosage during disopyramide phosphate.

Description. A quinidine-like type 1a antidysrhythmic agent used to treat atrial and ventricular dysrhythmias. It depresses myocardial responsiveness, slows automaticity, and raises the cardiac tissue threshold, prolonging the effective refractory period. It also prolongs cardiac conduction. Disopyramide is metabolized by the liver, with a half-life of 4-10 hours. Up to 80% is excreted in the urine. Steady-state levels are reached after 25-30 hours. Overdose treatment includes catecholamine infusion and gastric lavage to restore blood pressure followed by percutaneous cardiopulmonary support. Known to produce cardiac arrhythmias in clients receiving macrolide antibiotics (erythromycin, clarithromycin) simultaneously with disopyramide, hypoglycemia in clients with type 2 diabetes mellitus, neuropathy and pneumonitis.

Professional Considerations
1. Consent form NOT required.

2. Preparation:
   A. Note the time the last dose was taken.
   B. Note on the laboratory requisition if the client is taking phenytoin because this may cause decreased levels of disopyramide phosphate.
   C. Obtain a siliconized red-topped or gold-sealed tube.
   D. Do NOT draw this specimen during hemodialysis.

3. Procedure:
   A. Draw a 1-mL TROUGH blood sample.
   B. Draw a peak sample 2-3 hours after the oral dose.
   C. Draw a trough sample just before the next dose.
   D. Obtain serial measurements at the same time each day.

4. Postprocedure care:
   A. Assess the results before administration of the next dose.

5. Client and family teaching:
   A. The next dose of medication is dependent on these test results.
   B. Explain the need and timing of the peak and trough blood samples.
   C. Refer clients with intentional overdose for crisis intervention.

6. Factors that affect results:
   A. Results are elevated in renal and hepatic dysfunction and with drug use of azithromycin.
   B. Blood levels are difficult to monitor because the levels of free (unbound) disopyramide change considerably over a dosing interval.
   C. Metabolism increases with concomitant treatment with phenobarbital, phenytoin, and rifampin.
   D. Interaction of disopyramide with propranolol includes bradycardia and arrhythmia in chick embryos.

7. Other data:
   A. Other trade names include DSP, Napamide, Norpace, and Rythmodan.
   B. Metabolite has an anticholinergic effect, causing dry mouth, urinary retention, constipation, blurred vision, exacerbation of glaucoma, and dryness of bronchial secretions.
   C. Use with caution with myasthenia gravis because it may precipitate a crisis.
   D. Do not use with clients in heart failure or shock.
   E. More than 6 µg/mL may be needed to suppress ventricular dysrhythmias.

D

F. Enhances the effect of warfarin and oral antihyperglycemics. Does not affect digoxin and digitoxin levels.

G. Improves myocardial oxygen supply-demand balance in clients with hypertrophic obstructive cardiomyopathy (HOCM) and controls hypotension and bradycardia in neurocardiogenic syncope.

H. Cibenzoline has comparable efficacy to disopyramide for the prevention of recurrence of atrial tachyarrhythmia and is better tolerated.

DNA PLOIDY (STEMLINE DNA ANALYSIS), SPECIMEN

Positive. Aneuploid, polyploid.

Negative. Diploid.

Usage. Determining prognosis in bladder cancer (squamous), breast cancer, hepatocellular carcinoma (HCC), and laryngeal squamous-cell carcinoma.

Description. Malignant cells demonstrate greater proliferation than normal cells do and tend to have disordered cellular division whereby aneuploid DNA is present in individual cells. This abnormality increases with the degree of malignancy. Clinical studies indicate that the proportion of proliferating cells in a breast tumor biopsy specimen and the degree of aneuploidy have prognostic significance for breast cancer. Longer disease-free periods after treatment tend to occur in individuals whose tumor has lower degrees of proliferation and fewer aneuploid cells.

Professional Considerations

1. A consent form is required for the biopsy itself but not for the test performed.
2. Preparation:
   A. Obtain a sterile formalin specimen container.
   B. The specimen may be obtained by needle or surgical biopsy.
3. Procedure:
   A. Place the tissue specimen in a sterile formalin specimen container.
4. Postprocedure care:
   A. Send the specimen to pathology as soon as possible.
5. Client and family teaching:
   A. DNA ploidy is only one means of measuring the degree of malignancy and prognosis of breast cancer. Other prognostic factors include status of axillary nodes, presence of estrogen and progesterone receptors, tumor size and extension into chest wall or skin, and distant metastasis.
   B. Use a mild analgesic for biopsy site pain.
6. **Factors that affect results:**
   A. An inadequate sample size may yield false-negative results.
7. **Other data:**
   A. DNA ploidy analysis may offer additional prognostic information in individuals with prostatic adenocarcinoma, lymphoma, bladder carcinoma, renal cell carcinoma, malignant melanoma, and head and neck cancers.
   B. Relatively few cells are needed to perform DNA ploidy flow cytometry. Therefore, tumors and response to treatment can be monitored for changes in the DNA content of the cells by serial needle biopsy.

DNPH, DIAGNOSTIC
(see Dinitrophenylhydrazine test, Diagnostic)

DOPPLER ULTRASONOGRAPHIC, TRANSCRANIAL, DIAGNOSTIC
(see Doppler ultrasonographic flow studies, Diagnostic)

DOPPLER ULTRASONOGRAPHIC FLOW STUDIES, TRANSCRANIAL, DIAGNOSTIC
(see Doppler ultrasonographic flow studies, Diagnostic)

DOPPLER ULTRASONOGRAPHIC FLOW STUDIES (INCLUDES CAROTID DOPPLER, CAROTID ARTERY ECHOGRAPHY, CAROTID ARTERY ULTRASONOGRAPHY, TRANSCRANIAL DOPPLER ULTRASONOGRAPHY), DIAGNOSTIC

Norm. Normal intracranial arterial flow velocity. Normal carotid artery anatomy or unimpeded blood flow of that portion of the circulation evaluated.

Usage. *Transcranial Doppler ultrasonography* is used to evaluate blood flow through the cerebral arteries. Diagnostic in intracranial aneurysms, arteriovenous malformations, and Mayo-Mayo syndrome. Allows assessment of blood supply in intracranial neoplasms. Used intraoperatively to monitor velocity in the middle portion of cerebral artery during carotid endarterectomy. Used in the evaluation of collateral circulation stenosis, vasoconstriction as a result of insult, and cerebral dynamics after head injury and in establishing brain death in adults. Used to predict the risk of stroke in children with sickle cell anemia. *Carotid Doppler ultrasonography, carotid artery ultrasonography,* and *carotid artery echography* are used for detection or preoperative evaluation of atherosclerotic carotid artery disease, cerebrovascular disease, renal artery stenosis, and deep vein thrombosis; postoperatively for evaluating carotid endarterectomy and cardiac function.

Description. A noninvasive, hand-held mechanical ultrasonograph that uses a low-frequency (2-2.5 MHz) sector transducer through temporal, orbital, and suboccipital acoustic windows of the skull. Constant-frequency ultrasonic waves are transmitted into the vessel of interest by a transducer either in the form of fixed-wave or pulsed signals. Using the color and power technique of the Doppler signal instead of the frequency shift, it records the anatomy, flow direction, and mean blood flow velocity in real-time imaging. Doppler ultrasonography can display very small quantitative and qualitative volumes, allowing great morphologic detail. Interferences about the presence of obstruction to blood flow can be made with this procedure. When this technique is combined with a static image of the vessel provided by B-mode ultrasonography, the procedure is referred to as "duplex Doppler sonography." When a color image is generated by changes in blood flow, the term "color Doppler" is applied.

Professional Considerations
1. Consent form is NOT required.

2. **Preparation:**
   A. Although portable ultrasonographic equipment is available, this test is frequently performed within the radiology suite.
   B. Occasionally clients are required to fast before abdominal ultrasonographic procedures. No other pretest preparation or medication is required.
   C. Remove any restrictive clothing to allow access to the portion of the client's body to be studied.
   D. Client is usually positioned recumbent with a small pillow supporting the head.
   E. See *Client and family teaching.*
3. **Procedure:**
   A. The test is generally performed in a darkened room either by a radiology technician or a radiologist who is seated at the bedside.
   B. Acoustic jelly is applied to the skin in the area over the part of the circulatory system of interest.
   C. The ultrasound transducer is applied to the skin, and acoustic jelly and ultrasonographic recordings are made. The procedure is painless and usually brief (minutes).
   D. Ultrasonic waves are released from the transducer and reflected back to it. An image is then generated within the ultrasound apparatus where it is displayed on a viewing screen. The sound waves used during the test are not audible to the client.
   E. For transcranial Doppler ultrasonography, time-averaged mean blood-flow velocity of >200 cm/second is indicative of cerebral ischemia. Stenosis >60% diameter reduction is reported immediately.
4. **Postprocedure care:**
   A. Wipe ultrasonic gel from the client's body.
   B. Although preliminary results of the procedure may be available in the radiology suite, the client should be informed that a physician interpretation is required before the test results are available.
5. **Client and family teaching:**
   A. The test takes approximately 60 minutes, can be performed at the bedside, and is painless and safe.

B. Results are usually available in 24 hours.

C. Vascular (carotid) surgery may occur because of the test results, and this will require special educational and emotional support for the client and family.

6. **Factors that affect results:**

A. The accuracy of this test is highly dependent on the skill of the operator (technician or radiologist) and the interpreter of the results.

B. The body habitus of the client and technical condition of the equipment may affect the test results.

C. Accurate transmission and reflection of ultrasonographic signals can be affected by the presence of calcium (bone or calcification deposits) or gas overlying the vessel of interest, and condition may preclude the achievement of accurate results.

D. Intramural calcification may inhibit sound penetration, leading to false-positive results.

E. Flow velocity is age dependent and decreases continuously from early childhood to adulthood.

F. Detection of small aneurysms is limited by insonation angles and spatial resolution.

G. Transcranial procedure:

   i. ICP, blood pressure and volume, hematocrit, and subarachnoid hemorrhage affect flow velocity in transcranial Doppler scanning.

   ii. False-negative exams of vasospasm are associated with chronic high blood pressure, increased intracranial pressure, severe spasm of the carotid siphon, and distal vasospasm.

   iii. Use of tobacco and caffeine.

   iv. In clients with occlusive cerebrovascular disease, false-positive and false-negative results have been reported when one is evaluating for cross flow through the anterior and posterior communicating arteries.

7. **Other data:**

A. In previous years carotid endarterectomy was almost always preceded by carotid arteriography; however, the high diagnostic accuracy of carotid ultrasonography (when performed by experienced operators) has eliminated this requirement in many cases.

B. Most accurate for diagnosis of proximal DVT but less reliable in isolated calf vein thrombi.

C. See also *Ankle-brachial index, Diagnostic.*

DOPPLER ULTRASONOGRAPHIC FLOW STUDIES, DUPLEX
(see Doppler ultrasonographic flow studies, Diagnostic)

DOXEPIN, BLOOD
(see Tricyclic antidepressants, Plasma or Serum)

DRUG SCREEN, BLOOD
(see Toxicology, Drug screen, Blood)

DRUG SCREEN, URINE
(see Toxicology, Drug screen, Urine)

DUAL ENERGY X-RAY ABSORPTIOMETRY
(see Bone densitometry, Diagnostic)

DUAL MODALITY IMAGING (PET/CT, SPECT/CT, BIOGRAPH, DISCOVERY VH HAWKEYE, DISCOVERY VI POSITRACE, DISCOVERY LS, GEMINI) DIAGNOSTIC

Norm. Findings are interpreted by a radiologist specializing in the types of imaging used.

Usage. Cancer staging via precise localization of tumor-targeted radiopharmaceuticals; Monitoring response to radioimmunotherapy. More accurate assessment of myocardial perfusion than other single mode studies. Planning for and evaluating success of radiation therapy.

Description. Dual modality imaging is a technique available in the newest imaging equipment that combines different types of imaging techniques to simultaneously evaluate functional structure and physiology. Traditional single-mode structural imaging includes ultrafast computed tomography (CT) and magnetic resonance imaging (MRI). Traditional functional imaging that evaluates the physiology occurring in tissues includes positive emission tomography (PET) and single-photon emission computed tomography (SPECT). Dual mode imaging combines one of the structural imaging techniques with one of the functional imaging techniques and data are acquired by one machine containing both the x-ray component and the radionuclide detector during only one procedure. After both sets of images are acquired, computer software then merges the data and fuses the images to give results that are more sensitive and specific than a single procedure alone, and that overcomes many limitations of each single procedure. In addition, simultaneous imaging can provide improved attenuation correction, anatomic mapping, and overcomes issues with the body being positioned differently for tests taken at two separate times.

Professional Considerations

1. Consent form IS required.

Risks

See risks described in each separate mode of imaging to be combined in the specific equipment to be used listed under 2-A below.

Contraindications

See contraindications described in each separate mode of imaging to be combined in the equipment to be used listed under 2-A below.

Precautions

See contraindications described in each separate mode of imaging to be combined in the equipment to be used listed under 2-A below.

---

2. Preparation:
   A. See separate preparation information, depending on the modalities combined in the dual-mode imaging equipment:
      i. *Magnetic resonance imaging, Diagnostic*

      ii. *Positron emission tomography, Diagnostic*
      iii. *Single photon emission computed tomography, Brain, Diagnostic*
      iv. *Ultrafast computed tomography, Diagnostic*
   B. Document clinical indications on the test requisition. This helps guide the interpreter to provide the most relevant test interpretation, and it also is essential for many types of procedure reimbursement.
3. Procedure:
   A. The client is positioned supine on the scanning table. See procedure for individual led listing
4. Postprocedure care:
   A. Assess the venous access site for infiltration.
5. Client and family teaching:
   A. You will have to hold breath for several seconds.
   B. It is important to lie still for the test.
   C. A sensation of burning may be felt from the injection of the contrast.
6. Factors that affect results:
   A. See individual tests as described in 2-A. Factors that affect the results for all tests are considerably reduced by the dual mode imaging technique.
7. Other data:
   A. GE Medical Systems manufactures the Discovery VH Hawkeye, Discovery VI Positrace, and Discovery LS imaging systems. Siemens Medical manufactures the Biography imaging system. Phillips Medical Systems manufactures the Gemini imaging system.

D-XYLOSE

(see Xylose, Blood; Xylose, Urine; D-Xylose absorption test, Diagnostic; Xylose tolerance test, Diagnostic)

EAR, ROUTINE, CULTURE

(see Culture, Routine, Specimen)

EASTERN EQUINE ENCEPHALITIS VIRUS TITER, SPECIMEN

Norm. Titer <1:10.

Positive. A fourfold increase in titer between acute and convalescent specimens supports the diagnosis of eastern equine encephalitis.

Negative. Normal finding or bacterial infection.

Description. Eastern equine encephalitis is an inflammation of the brain caused by an arbovirus that attacks the central nervous system. The mode of transmission to humans is through the bite of a mosquito of the genus *Culex*. High risk when in contact with deciduous wetlands.

Professional Considerations
1. Consent form NOT required.
2. Preparation:
   A. Tube: Red topped, red/gray topped, or gold topped.
   B. Assess for fever and symptoms of meningitis and meningoencephalitis, including convulsions, abnormal reflexes, extremity rigidity, and bulging of the fontanelle in infants. In children, assess for headache, drowsiness of 2-3 days, nausea, and vomiting. In adults, assess for frontal headache, photophobia, nausea, and vomiting.
3. Procedure:
   A. Draw a 7-mL blood sample.
4. Postprocedure care:
   A. Send the specimen to the laboratory immediately.
   B. Draw a convalescent sample 14 days later.
5. Client and family teaching:
   A. The convalescent sample will be drawn in 2 weeks to see if the treatment is working.
   B. The mortality in the United States is 65-75%. Survivors often have significant neurologic disabilities.
6. Factors that affect results:
   A. Failure to collect a convalescent sample will result in the inability to show a rising of antibody titer between the acute and convalescent phases of the disease.
7. Other data:
   A. Common hosts include mosquitoes, birds, ducks, fowl, and horses.
   B. MRI is a sensitive test to identify early radiographic signs including involvement of the basal ganglia and thalamus.

EBCT
(see Computed tomography of the body, Diagnostic)

ECG
(see Electrocardiography, Diagnostic)

ECHINOCOCCOSIS SEROLOGIC TEST, BLOOD

Norm. IHA 1:2-1:64.

Usage. Echinococcosis.

Description. Echinococcosis is a tapeworm infection common among clients in contact with sheep or cattle. Any member of the dog family may serve as a definitive host for the adult tapeworm. Dogs are infected by feeding on the offal of domestic animals or on animal parts at butchering time. Children are at a high risk of ingesting eggs excreted by dogs because of their close contact with their pet dogs. Humans are the intermediate host. The eggs become blood borne and form cysts in the liver and other parts of the body such as the heart, lungs, and bone. It may take 5-20 years for a cyst to grow large enough to cause symptoms. Common in persons associated with goats or sheep or who live in Turkey or in Muslim communities of southern Israel.

Professional Considerations
1. Consent form NOT required.
2. Preparation:
   A. Tube: Red topped, red/gray topped, or gold topped.
   B. Obtain recent history for possible animal contact.
3. Procedure:
   A. Draw a 7-mL blood sample.
4. Postprocedure care:
   A. Surgical resection of the cyst is the treatment of choice.
   B. Aspiration of the cyst contents should not be attempted for a diagnosis because of the danger of rupture and leakage of the contents. This could cause an acute allergic reaction, anaphylactic shock, or dissemination of the infection.

5. **Client and family teaching:**
   A. Results are normally available within 72 hours.
   B. Treatment with benzimidazole compounds (mebendazole, albendazole) may take years or decades.
6. **Factors that affect results:**
   A. False-positive results may occur in clients with a history of cirrhosis, collagen disease, systemic lupus erythematosus, or schistosomiasis.
7. **Other data:**
   A. Positive titers occur in 35%-50% of cases with hydatid lung cysts and in 85% with hydatid liver cysts.
   B. Removal of the cyst does not dramatically lower the antibody titer. It may persist for years.

ECHOCARDIOGRAPHY (ECHO, HEART SONOGRAM, HEART ULTRASONOGRAM), DIAGNOSTIC

Norm. No abnormalities.

Usage. Atrial septal defect, aortic stenosis or regurgitation, atrial tumors, bradycardia, cardiac tamponade, cardiomyopathy, congenital heart disease, effusion (pericardial), embolization of artery, endocarditis, idiopathic hypertrophic subaortic stenosis, lymphoma metastasis, Marfan syndrome, mitral regurgitation or stenosis, mitral valve prolapse, myocardial infarction post evaluation for wall-motion abnormalities, myocarditis, panic disorder, patent ductus arteriosus, pericarditis, subacute bacterial endocarditis (SBE), transposition of the great arteries, tricuspid atresia, ventricular septal defect, and other cardiac defects.

Description. Echocardiography is a noninvasive, acoustic imaging procedure that determines the size, shape, position, thickness, and movements of the heart valves, walls, and chambers during each cardiac cycle. It records the echoes created by the deflection of short pulses of an ultrasonic beam off the cardiac structures onto an oscilloscope. The time required for the ultrasonic beam to be reflected back to the transducer from differing densities of tissue is converted by a computer to an electrical impulse displayed on an oscilloscopic screen to create a two-dimensional picture of the heart in different projections. The resolution of the oscilloscope recording obtained is determined by the frequency of the beam. Lower frequencies penetrate further but provide less resolution than higher frequencies do. Echocardiography can also be performed transesophageally (TEE) with the transmitter inserted into the esophagus similar to an endoscope. This gives a clearer view of the valves and endocardium, especially in the presence of obesity or severe chronic obstructive pulmonary disease (COPD).

Professional Considerations
1. Consent form NOT required.
2. **Preparation:**
   A. The client should disrobe above the waist or wear a gown.
3. **Procedure:**
   A. With the client in a supine or recumbent position, conductive gel is placed over the third and fourth intercostal spaces to the left of the sternum.
   B. A transducer is angled directly over the intercostal spaces or beneath the xiphoid process to direct ultrasonic waves that are displayed on the oscilloscopic machine and printed in the M (motion) mode on a recorder.
   C. The client may also be placed on the left side to obtain a different view of the heart and may occasionally be asked to perform certain maneuvers or to inhale amyl nitrite (a gas with a slightly sweet odor) to record changes in heart function.
   D. For a transesophageal echocardiogram, the throat is anesthetized with spray, and the transducer is passed orally into the esophagus. (See *Transesophageal ultrasonography, Diagnostic,* for more information).
4. **Postprocedure care:**
   A. Remove the conductive gel from the skin.
   B. For a transesophageal echocardiogram, oral fluids must be held until the local anesthetic is no

longer in effect and the gag reflex has returned.

5. **Client and family teaching:**
   A. The procedure takes 30-60 minutes, can be performed at the bedside, and is painless.
   B. Remain as still as possible.
   C. Results are normally available within 24 hours.

6. **Factors that affect results:**
   A. Thick chests, COPD, obesity, or chest wall abnormalities or scar tissue, or dressings may alter the display of ultrasonic waves on the recorder.
   B. Better resolution can be obtained for children than for adults because their thinner, less dense chest wall enables use of a higher-frequency, shorter-wavelength sound.
   C. Improper placement of the transducer.

7. **Other data:**
   A. Very sensitive test in detecting pericardial effusion.
   B. Side effects of amyl nitrite, which has a short duration of action, are dizziness, flushing, and tachycardia.
   C. See also *Stress test, Pharmacologic, Diagnostic; Transesophageal ultrasonography, Diagnostic.*

ECHOENCEPHALOGRAPHY
(see Brain ultrasonography, Diagnostic)

ECHOGRAPHY / ECHOGRAM
(see Abdominal aorta ultrasonography, Diagnostic; Brain ultrasonography, Diagnostic; Breast ultrasonography, Diagnostic; Echocardiography, Diagnostic; Eye and orbit ultrasonography, Diagnostic; Gallbladder and biliary system ultrasonography, Diagnostic; Gynecologic ultrasonography, Diagnostic; Kidney ultrasonography, Diagnostic; Liver ultrasonography, Diagnostic; Gallbladder and biliary system ultrasonography, Diagnostic; Obstetric ultrasonography, Diagnostic; Pancreas ultrasonography, Diagnostic; Prostate ultrasonography, Diagnostic; Spleen ultrasonography, Diagnostic; Thyroid ultrasonography,

Diagnostic; Transesophageal ultrasonography, Diagnostic; or Urinary bladder ultrasonography, Diagnostic)

ECSTASY
(see Amphetamines, Blood)

EEG
(see Electroencephalography, Diagnostic)

EGD
(see Esophagogastroduodenoscopy, Diagnostic)

EKG
(see Electrocardiography, Diagnostic)

EKG, SIGNAL-AVERAGED, DIAGNOSTIC
(see Signal-averaged electrocardiography, Diagnostic)

ELECTROCARDIOGRAPHY (ECG, EKG), DIAGNOSTIC

Norm. Normal sinus rhythm, no dysrhythmias.

Usage. Anesthesia, angina pectoris, anxiety, atrial septal defect, beriberi, bradycardia, carbon monoxide poisoning, chest pain, coarctation of the aorta, congestive heart failure, dysrhythmias, effusion (pericardial), emergency monitoring, endocarditis, heart murmur, ischemia, myocardial infarction (MI), pacemaker function, palpitations, panic disorder, patent ductus arteriosus, pericarditis, preoperative evaluation, pulmonic stenosis, respiratory distress, surgery, syncope, tetralogy of Fallot, transposition of the great arteries, tricuspid atresia, ventricular hypertrophy, ventricular septal defect, and yellow fever.

Description. Recording of the heart's electrical current using electrodes from 12 different leads: bipolar limb leads I, II, III; augmented limb leads aV_R, aV_L, aV_F; and precordial chest leads V_1-V_6. The heart's electrical activity takes three

forms on the ECG: the P-wave, which signifies atrial depolarization; the QRS complex, which signifies ventricular depolarization; and the T-wave, which signifies ventricular repolarization. This test identifies conduction abnormalities and dysrhythmias, monitors recovery from MI, and helps evaluate the effectiveness of cardiac medications. Single-lead tracings monitor the presence and type of electrical conduction during cardiac emergencies and during insertion of a temporary transvenous pacemaker.

Professional Considerations

1. Consent form NOT required.
2. **Preparation:**
   A. The client should disrobe above the waist.
   B. Cleanse the skin where the electrodes will be placed by rubbing it lightly with an alcohol wipe and then scraping gently with the edge of an electrode.
   C. Check the paper supply.
3. **Procedure:**
   A. *Single-channel recording:*
      i. The client is positioned supine.
      ii. Five electrodes are placed over clean fleshy skin with the conductor ends pointing upward. Electrodes are positioned on the right arm, the left arm, the right leg, and the left leg; the lead is sequentially repositioned for 6-second recording at locations V_1-V_6 on the chest.
      iii. The machine is turned on, and the recording is begun.
      iv. In nonautomatic machines, turn the lead selector to lead I and run it for 6 seconds for each lead from I through aV_F. Then turn the lead selector to neutral and determine the proper placement for leads V_1-V_6 before recording. The position of V_1 is at the fourth intercostal space, right sternal border. V_2 is at the fourth intercostal space, left sternal border. V_3 is midway between V_2 and V_4. V_4 is at the left midclavicular line at the fifth intercostal space. V_5 follows V_4 in a straight line over the fifth intercostal space to the anterior axillary line, and V_6 follows V_5 in a straight line over the fifth intercostal space to the left midaxillary line.
      v. The procedure takes 15 minutes.
      vi. During emergencies, three electrodes can be placed for monitoring: the white lead on the right upper chest, the black read on the left upper chest, and the red lead on the lower left lateral chest.
   B. *Simultaneous 12-channel recording:*
      i. The client is positioned supine.
      ii. The limb leads are connected to electrodes, and each is attached to a limb.
      iii. Leads V_1-V_6 are connected to electrodes and attached to the chest wall in the locations described under procedure A.
      iv. The machine is activated, and a simultaneous recording of all 12 channels is printed automatically by the electrocardiograph machine.
      v. The procedure takes 5-10 minutes.
4. **Postprocedure care:**
   A. Label the ECG with name, room number, date, time, and episodes of chest pain during the procedure.
   B. Remove the electrodes and cleanse the skin of any residual conductive gel.
5. **Client and family teaching:**
   A. You should not move or talk during the procedure.
6. **Factors that affect results:**
   A. Body movement, poor skin cleansing, or improper electrode placement produces an artifact, which may necessitate repeating the test.
   B. The results should be interpreted in comparison with prior electrocardiograms, if available.
7. **Other data:**
   A. MI produces three changes on the ECG: elevated ST indicates formation of ischemia and then the T-wave flattens and becomes inverted with an enlarged Q-wave appearing, which indicates necrosis.
   B. See also *Holter monitor, Diagnostic; Signal-averaged electrocardiography, Diagnostic.*

E

C. The abbreviation "EKG" is often spoken and written instead of the more proper "ECG" to decrease confusion with "EEG" (electroencephalogram).

ELECTROENCEPHALOGRAPHY (EEG), DIAGNOSTIC

Norm. Normal electrical brain activity as recorded by the EEG instrument.

Usage. Used as a diagnostic tool in the diagnosis of Alzheimer's disease (declining D alpha values), attention-deficit/hyperactivity disorder (ADHD), different central nervous system disorders including tumors, infections, and various encephalopathic states. Special use involves the characterization of various types of seizure disorders and also the determination of the anatomic locus of seizure activity within the brain (the "seizure focus"). The EEG is also of value in the determination of central nervous system death ("brain death"). It is occasionally helpful in establishing the diagnosis of various neurosensory disorders when used in its applied forms (the recording of "visual evoked" and "auditory evoked potentials").

Description. Using a special cap, electroconductive gel, and electrodes, an EEG recording of the electrical potentials of the cerebral cortex of the brain is taken and subsequently analyzed to determine the presence or absence of various waveform activities.

Professional Considerations

1. Consent form NOT required.
2. **Preparation:**
   A. See *Client and family teaching.*
   B. Although portable EEG equipment is available, the test is generally conducted in an EEG lab by a neurologist or an EEG technician.
   C. Sedative drugs and prolonged fasting (hypoglycemia) can influence the test and should be avoided if possible.
3. **Procedure:**
   A. The client is placed in a recumbent position in a darkened room.
   B. A cap with numerous plastic electrode locators is placed on the client's head, and the openings in

the electrode locators are filled with electroconductive gel.
   C. Electrodes are inserted through the locators into proximity with the client's scalp. (It is not necessary to shave or puncture the scalp to accomplish this step.)
   D. EEG recordings are made in the supine position. The client may be asked to perform various physical maneuvers during the test; occasionally recordings are made during sleep.
4. **Postprocedure care:**
   A. Electrodes and EEG cap are removed and the gel is wiped from the scalp.
5. **Client and family teaching:**
   A. Pretest orientation with a description of the method used to attach the electrodes is important.
   B. Shaving of the scalp hair is not necessary for this test.
   C. Hair should be free of products such as gel or hair spray, which could interfere with conductivity to the electrodes.
   D. It is important to lie still throughout the test.
   E. If the EEG is used as an adjunct in the determination of brain death, a detailed description of the test and the rationale behind its use in this setting should be given to the family.
   F. The procedure may take up to 2 hours.
6. **Factors that affect results:**
   A. Hypoglycemia (prolonged fasting) may decrease response time, leading to an abnormal pattern.
   B. Certain sedative drugs.
   C. Caffeine causes significant reduction of total EEG power at frontoparieto-occipital central electrode positions of both hemispheres when subjects have their eyes open.
   D. Oily hair or hair spray interferes with the recording because it reduces conductivity to the electrodes.
   E. Sleep, motor activity on the part of the client, muscle tension, and various external sensory stimuli may interfere with the waveform patterns and prolong the test.
7. **Other data:**
   A. Prolonged (semiambulatory) EEG recordings may be valuable

in the management of certain clients with epilepsy.
B. The EEG may be used as an evaluation tool in the management of anesthesia and sedation.
C. A single negative EEG finding should not rule out a seizure disorder. Serial or repeated EEG tracings are necessary.
D. See also *Visual evoked potentials, Diagnostic.*

ELECTROLYTES PANEL (EP), BLOOD

Norm. See individual test listings: *Bicarbonate, Chloride, CO$_2$, Potassium, and Sodium.*

Usage. See individual test listings.

Description. The Electrolytes Panel is a term defined by The Centers for Medicare and Medicaid Services (CMS) in the United States to indicate a group of tests for which a bundled reimbursement is available. The panel is one of several that replace the multichannel

tests, such as SMA-6. The panel is disease oriented, meaning that payment through Medicare is available only when the test is used to diagnose and monitor a disease and payment is not available when the test is used for screening purposes in clients who have no signs and symptoms. All the tests in the panel must be carried out when a BMP is ordered.

Professional Considerations
1. Consent form NOT required.
2. Preparation:
   A. Tube: Red topped, red/gray topped, or gold topped.
   B. Do NOT draw specimens during hemodialysis.
3. Procedure:
   A. Draw a 5-mL blood sample.
4. Postprocedure care:
   A. None.
5. Client and family teaching:
   A. See individual test listings.
6. Factors that affect results:
   A. See individual test listings.
7. Other data:
   A. See individual test listings.

ELECTROLYTES, PLASMA OR SERUM
(see also Anion gap, Blood; Carbon dioxide, Blood; Chloride, Serum; Potassium, Serum; Sodium, Plasma or Serum)

Norm:

		SI UNITS
Anion Gap	7-17 mEq/L	7-17 mmol/L
Carbon Dioxide, Total Content		
Adults	22-30 mEq/L or 38-50 mm Hg	22-30 mmol/L
Panic levels	<15 mEq/L or >50 mEq/L	<15 mmol/L >50 mmol/L
Neonates-2 years	32-44 mm Hg	
Children >2 years	22-26 mEq/L	22-26 mmol/L
Chloride		
Children and adults	97-107 mEq/L	97-107 mmol/L
Premature infants	95-110 mEq/L	95-110 mmol/L
Full-term infants	96-106 mEq/L	96-106 mmol/L
Panic levels	<80 mEq/L or >115 mEq/L	<80 mmol/L >115 mmol/L

		SI UNITS
Potassium		
Adults	3.5-5.3 mEq/L	3.5-5.3 mmol/L
Premature Infants		
Cord blood	5.0-10.2 mEq/L	5.0-10.2 mmol/L
2 Days	3.0-6.0 mEq/L	3.0-6.0 mmol/L
Full-term Newborn		
Cord blood	5.6-12.0 mEq/L	5.6-12.0 mmol/L
Newborn	3.7-5.0 mEq/L	3.7-5.0 mmol/L
Infants	4.1-5.3 mEq/L	4.1-5.3 mmol/L
Children	3.4-4.7 mEq/L	3.4-4.7 mmol/L
Panic Levels		
Adults	<2.5 mEq/L	<2.5 mmol/L
	or >6.6 mEq/L	or >6.6 mmol/L
Newborn	<2.5 mEq/L	<2.5 mmol/L
	or >8.1 mEq/L	or >8.1 mmol/L
Sodium		
Adults	136-145 mEq/L	136-145 mmol/L
Umbilical cord	116-166 mEq/L	116-166 mmol/L
Infants	139-146 mEq/L	139-146 mmol/L
Children	138-145 mEq/L	138-145 mmol/L

Usage. Evaluate the four electrolytes at once and compare their relative values. Evaluate acid-base balance and determine the anion gap $[Na^+ - (Cl^- + HCO_3^-)]$. Serum sodium levels <133 mEq/L seen in cerebral salt wasting syndrome.

Description. The electrolyte panel is a series of tests performed on one tube of blood. The tests commonly included are *Anion gap, Blood; Carbon dioxide, Blood; Chloride, Serum; Potassium, Serum;* and *Sodium, Plasma or Serum.* See individual test listings for further description.

Professional Considerations
1. Consent form NOT required.
2. **Preparation:**
   A. Tube: Red topped, red/gray topped, or gold topped.
   B. Do not allow the client to clench-unclench the hand before blood drawing.
   C. Do NOT draw specimens during hemodialysis.
3. **Procedure:**
   A. Collect the specimen without a tourniquet or quickly after tourniquet application, to prevent stasis.
   B. Using a 20-gauge or larger needle, draw a 5-mL blood sample.

C. Do not aspirate strongly or push plunger into the vacuum tube too forcefully.
4. **Postprocedure care:**
   A. Write the collection time on the laboratory requisition.
   B. Transport the specimen to the laboratory within 15 minutes.
5. **Client and family teaching:**
   A. Do NOT clench-unclench the fist before blood drawing.
   B. Results are normally available within 24 hours.
6. **Factors that affect results:**
   A. Hemolysis of the specimen abnormally elevates the potassium level and invalidates results.
   B. Hypoalbuminemia lowers anion gap.

   Adjustment of anion gap (with albumin concentrations in grams per liter) = Observed anion gap + 0.25 × [(Normal albumin) (Observed albumin)]

   If the albumin is given in g/dL, the factor is 2.50.
7. **Other data:**
   A. Cognitive status assessed by the Mini-Mental State Examination correlates to serum sodium and serum chloride levels in the elderly.
   B. See individual test listings.

ELECTROLYTES, URINE
(see also Chloride, Urine; Potassium, Urine; Sodium, Urine)

Norm:

		SI UNITS
Chloride		
Adults	110-250 mEq/24 hours or 9 g/L	110-250 mmol/day
Children	15-115 mEq/L	15-115 mmol/L
Potassium		
Adults (intake dependent)	25-123 mEq/24 hours	25-123 mmol/day
Children	17-57 mEq/24 hours	17-57 mmol/day
Sodium		
Adults	75-200 mEq/24 hours	75-200 mmol/day
Children		
Newborn	14-40 mEq/24 hours	14-40 mmol/day
6-10 years		
Females	20-69 mEq/24 hours	20-69 mmol/day
Males	41-115 mEq/24 hours	41-115 mmol/day
10-14 years		
Females	48-168 mEq/24 hours	48-168 mmol/day
Males	63-177 mEq/24 hours	63-177 mmol/day

Usage. Evaluate renal function and fluid volume status by noting the amount of each electrolyte excreted and determine the anion gap $[(Na^+ + K^+) - Cl^-]$. A ratio of urine sodium to urine chloride of >1.16 identifies 51.6% of persons with bulimia nervosa.

Description. Urine electrolyte testing involves a series of tests performed on a sample of urine. The urine specimen may be random or a timed 12-hour or 24-hour urine. Tests commonly included are *Chloride, Urine; Potassium, Urine;* and *Sodium, Urine.* See individual test listings for further description.

Professional Considerations
1. Consent form NOT required.
2. Preparation:
   A. Obtain a specimen container or 3-L container without preservatives or a pediatric urine collection device or bag and tape, depending on whether the sample is to be a random sample or a 24-hour urine collection.
   B. Write the beginning time of the collection on the laboratory requisition and the specimen container.
   C. Note the diuretic or glucocorticoid therapy on the laboratory requisition.
3. Procedure:
   A. Obtain a random fresh urine specimen from a void or a urinary catheter drainage bag.
   B. For a 24-hour specimen, discard the first morning urine specimen.
   C. Save all the urine voided for 24 hours in a refrigerated, clean, 3-L container without preservatives. Document the quantity of the urine output during the specimen-collection period. Include urine voided at the end of the 24-hour period. For catheterized clients, keep the drainage bag on ice and empty the urine into the collection container hourly.
   D. Pediatric or infant specimen collection:
      i. Place the child in a supine position with the knees flexed and the hips externally rotated and abducted.
      ii. Cleanse, rinse, and thoroughly dry the perineal area.
      iii. To prevent the child from removing the collection device or bag, a diaper may be placed over the genital area.

E

iv. *Females:* Tape the pediatric collection device or bag to the perineum. Starting at the area between the anus and vagina, apply the device or bag in an anterior direction.

v. *Males:* Place the pediatric collection device or bag over the penis and scrotum and tape it to the perineal area.

vi. Empty the collection device or bag into the refrigerated collection container hourly.

4. **Postprocedure care:**
   A. For a 24-hour specimen, compare the urine quantity in the specimen container with the urinary output record for the test. If the specimen contains less urine than what was recorded as output, some of the sample may have been discarded, invalidating the test.
   B. Document the quantity of urine and the collection ending time on the laboratory requisition.
   C. Send the specimen to the laboratory and refrigerate it.
   D. See also individual test listings.

5. **Client and family teaching:**
   A. Save all the urine voided in the 24-hour period and urinate before defecating to avoid loss of urine. Avoid contaminating the urine with toilet tissue or stool. If any urine is accidentally discarded, discard the entire specimen and restart the collection the next day.

6. **Factors that affect results:**
   A. All the urine voided for the 24-hour period must be included in the 24-hour specimen to avoid a falsely low result.
   B. For spot urine testing, potassium levels are higher at night than in the morning, and sodium levels are higher in the morning than at night.
   C. See also individual test listings.

7. **Other data:**
   A. Urine osmolality is often requested at the same time as urine electrolytes.
   B. See also individual test listings.

ELECTROMYELOGRAPHY
(see Electromyography and nerve conduction studies, Diagnostic)

ELECTROMYOGRAPHY (EMG) AND NERVE CONDUCTION STUDIES (ELECTROMYELOGRAM), DIAGNOSTIC

Norm. Electromyelogram: no electrical activity at rest. A variety of abnormal electrical patterns produced by diseased muscles at rest and during activity exist and may allow diagnosis of specific myopathy. Nerve conduction studies: normal nerve conduction varies depending on the nerve studied but is in the range 40-70 m/sec.

Usage. Nerve conduction studies combined with electromyography can provide useful clues to the existence of neuromuscular disease, primary myopathy and neuropathic states. Specific disease states that are diagnosed with these techniques include carpal tunnel syndrome, myasthenia gravis, various forms of myositis, Guillain-Barré syndrome, and the myopathies.

Description. *Electromyogram:* One or more needles are inserted into the muscle to be studied. Electrodes are also attached to the skin. Recordings are made at rest after an interval has elapsed subsequent to the needle insertion. Recordings are repeated during a period of voluntary muscle contraction by the client. *Nerve conduction study:* Electroconductive gel is applied over the nerve to be studied. Electrodes are attached to the nerve to be studied, and an electric current is applied so that velocity measurements can be made. This process can be performed for both motor and sensory nerves.

Professional Considerations
1. Consent form IS required.

Risks
Bleeding, interference with pacemaker function, infection at the site of needle insertion.

Contraindications
History of bleeding disorder or chronic anticoagulation therapy, pacemaker.

2. **Preparation:**
   A. Client will bathe or shower the day of the test.

B. Avoid skin cosmetic products.

C. The physician ordering the tests may ask the client to avoid tobacco and caffeine for several hours before the procedures.

D. Fasting before the tests is not necessary.

3. Procedure:

A. *Electromyography:* The procedure may be performed with the client either in the sitting or in the supine position. Electrodes are inserted into the muscle of interest and recordings are made at rest and during voluntary contraction of the muscle. The test takes from 30 minutes to an hour to complete.

B. *Nerve conduction study:* A conductive gel is applied to the skin over the nerve of interest, and electrodes are attached at either end of the segment to be studied. An electric current is applied to the nerve segment, and the conduction velocity is measured.

4. Postprocedure care:

A. The conductive gel is cleaned from the skin.

B. Hospitalized clients may require transport from the testing location back to their rooms.

C. Local application of ice or a cold pack may alleviate postprocedure pain associated with EMG needle placement.

5. Client and family teaching:

A. The needles used in the EMG procedure are disposable, and the risk of infection is consequently minimal.

B. Pain may occur during and after insertion of the EMG needles. This is generally minor, and a local anesthetic is not usually given. Minor discomfort may be associated with the nerve conduction procedure.

6. Factors that affect results:

A. Cooperation of the client.

B. Drugs that affect neuromuscular conduction.

7. Other data:

A. These techniques may be helpful in the early detection of subclinical diabetic neuropathy.

B. Portable equipment is available and can be used in the performance of these procedures.

C. This application has primarily been used in the workplace to screen large numbers of workers for carpal tunnel syndrome.

ELECTROMYOGRAPHY (EMG), DIAGNOSTIC

(see Electromyography and nerve conduction studies, Diagnostic)

ELECTRON BEAM CT

(see Computed tomography of the body, Diagnostic)

ELECTRON MICROSCOPY (CARDIOMYOPATHY, NERVE TISSUE, SMALL BOWEL MUCOSA), DIAGNOSTIC

Norm. No abnormality or disease noted.

Usage. Doxorubicin HCl (Adriamycin) cardiotoxicity, cardiomyopathy, Hand-Schüller-Christian disease, liver disease, neuropathy, renal disease, tumors, and Whipple's disease.

Description. An examination of a thin section of tissue for microscopic evaluation. Used to define tumor classification when light microscopy is insufficient.

Professional Considerations

1. Consent form NOT required for this test.

2. Preparation:

A. Prepare for the surgical excision.

B. Obtain a sterile container filled with 0.9% saline.

3. Procedure:

A. Obtain a fresh unfixed tissue specimen and place it into a container of 0.9% saline.

4. Postprocedure care:

A. Deliver the specimen to the laboratory immediately so that the proper fixative can be applied.

5. Client and family teaching:

A. Results are normally available within 72 hours.

6. Factors that affect results:

A. Specimens should NOT be placed into formalin.

7. Other data:

A. Useful in diagnosing or differentiating leukemia or lymphoma,

sarcoma, endocrine, and brain tumors.
B. This is an expensive and time-consuming procedure.

ELECTRONYSTAGMOGRAPHY (EYE MOVEMENT, ENG) TEST, DIAGNOSTIC

Norm. Normal eye movement free of nystagmus.

Usage. Brain lesion, dizziness (not valuable in community-derived sample of dizzy elderly subjects >65 years old), falls in elderly over 65 years of age (best fall indicator is ocular motor battery), unilateral hearing loss, neurotoxicity related to antiepileptic drugs, nystagmus, tinnitus, and vertigo.

Description. Technique for recording eye movements allowing exact quantification of physiologic and pathologic nystagmus. The test picks up subtle spontaneous nystagmus and also helps differentiate peripheral from central nystagmus. The battery of tests includes visual ocular control, the search for pathologic nystagmus with fixation and with eyes open in darkness, and measurement of induced physiologic nystagmus (caloric and rotational). The test can be helpful in identifying a vestibular lesion and localizing it within the peripheral and central pathways. It also provides serial tracings to compare a client's pattern over time.

Professional Considerations
1. Consent form NOT required.

Risks
Water caloric test: perforation of the eardrum.

Contraindications
In clients with pacemakers or with a perforated eardrum.

2. **Preparation:**
   A. None.
3. **Procedure:**
   A. Small electrodes are taped to the skin on either side of each eye.
   B. Tests include calibration, gaze nystagmus, pendulum tracking, optokinetics, positional tests, and water caloric test.

i. *Calibration test:* The client holds head straight and fixed and follows with the eyes a stylus, from the right side to the middle and then to the left side.
ii. *Gaze nystagmus test:* The client must close his or her eyes and perform an arithmetic task for 30 seconds while eye motion is recorded. Then eye motion is recorded with the eyes open and fixed looking straight ahead.
iii. *Pendulum tracking:* A 20-second eye motion recording is made as the client looks straight ahead and follows a pendulum with the eyes. This is followed by a 30-second recording of eye motion as the client stares straight ahead with the eyes closed.
iv. *Optokinetics test:* Two 30-second recordings of eye motion are made as the client stares straight ahead and then follows a target across the visual field from right to left and then from left to right.
v. *Positional tests:* A 5-second baseline recording of eye motion is obtained, followed by a recording of eye motion as the client follows the following nine commands:
   a. "With head erect and eyes forward, turn your head quickly to the right."
   b. "With head erect and eyes forward, turn your head quickly to the left."
   c. "Sit erect with eyes closed and quickly lie flat on your back with your eyes still closed."
   d. "Sit up quickly from the lying position with your eyes closed."
   e. "Lie on your back with your eyes closed and quickly turn your body and head to the right."
   f. "Lie on your back with your eyes closed and turn your body and head to the left."
   g. "Sit erect with your eyes forward and closed and lay your head back quickly so

that it hangs over the back of the chair."

h. "Quickly pick up your head from over the back of the chair to the erect position."

i. "Quickly put your head back to the right so that it hangs over the back right side of the headrest on the chair and then repeat this by putting your head to the left so that it hangs over the back left side of the headrest on the chair."

vi. *Water caloric test:* The client is positioned at a 30-degree head-of-bed elevation with the eyes closed. Water is instilled directly into the ear canal so that it hits the tympanic membrane, while eye motion is simultaneously recorded. This is followed by a 60-second recording with the eyes open and a final recording with the eyes closed until nystagmus disappears or for 3 minutes.

4. Postprocedure care:
   A. Remove electrodes.
   B. Assess for dizziness, nausea, or weakness.

5. Client and family teaching:
   A. The test takes less than 1 hour.
   B. The client must be cooperative and able to follow commands to ensure the accuracy of the test results.

6. Factors that affect results:
   A. CNS stimulants will increase eye movement, and depressants will decrease eye movement.
   B. Poor eyesight.
   C. Loose electrodes.
   D. Requires considerable cooperation on the part of the client and skill on the part of the operator in conducting and interpreting the test.

7. Other data:
   A. Results are reported as normal, borderline, or abnormal.

ELECTROPHYSIOLOGIC STUDY (EPS), DIAGNOSTIC

Norm. Negative for ability to induce dysrhythmias. Normal cardiac conduction system mapping. No reentrant pathways identified.

Usage. To document the anatomy and physiologic substrates of episodic dysrhythmias by reproducing them so that the mechanism can be identified. Helps diagnose cardiac conduction defects, circus reentry, ectopic foci, syncope of unexplained cause, tachydysrhythmias, and ventricular preexcitation syndromes; evaluates the effectiveness of antidysrhythmic medications or ablation; helps determine proper choice of a pacemaker; maps the cardiac conduction system before ablation; determines the need for an implanted defibrillator to prevent sudden cardiac death; and records intracardiac electrocardiograms.

Description. Electrophysiologic study involves the introduction of an electrode catheter under fluoroscopy through a peripheral vein or artery and into the cardiac chambers or sinuses and the performance of programmed electrical stimulation of the heart. Clients who may require EPS include survivors of sudden cardiac death, those with syncope with other than cardiac causes ruled out, and clients with dysrhythmias. Clients who usually require repeat EPS are those who have undergone antidysrhythmic therapy or catheter ablation since the last study. EPS is usually performed in a special laboratory or operating room by a cardiologist, with a specially trained registered nurse and a technician in attendance, certified in ACLS (Advanced Cardiac Life Support).

Professional Considerations
1. Consent form IS required.

Risks
Arterial injury (rare), cardiac perforation or rupture, cerebrovascular accident, fatal dysrhythmias, death, hemorrhage (rare), infection, insertion-site hematoma, major venous thrombosis, myocardial infarction, pericardial effusion, pulmonary embolus.

Contraindications
Bleeding disorders, thrombocytopenia. Sedatives are contraindicated in clients with central nervous system depression.

2. **Preparation:**
   A. Antidysrhythmic drugs are usually discontinued for several days before the test, when tolerated, for initial EPS. For evaluation of effectiveness of antidysrhythmic therapy, drug levels should reach a steady state before EPS. This may take several days or even a few weeks for drugs such as amiodarone.
   B. The client should fast from food overnight and from fluids for 4 hours before the test.
   C. Establish intravenous access.
   D. If left ventricular stimulation that requires an arterial EPS route is planned, preheparinization may be prescribed.
   E. Have emergency cart and defibrillator or cardioverter readily available.
   F. A sedative may be prescribed.
   G. Obtain baseline vital signs. Monitor vital signs and level of consciousness continuously throughout the procedure. Observe respiratory status closely throughout the procedure, especially if a sedative is administered.

3. **Procedure:**
   A. The client is positioned on the procedure table, and the peripheral pulses distal to the insertion site are marked. The location and baseline quality of the pulses are documented.
   B. A baseline electrocardiogram is obtained. The leads are left in place for continuous cardiac monitoring.
   C. The insertion site is cleansed with povidone-iodine solution, allowed to dry, and draped.
   D. An introducer (sheath, Cordis) catheter is introduced, using the Seldinger technique, through a femoral, brachial, subclavian, or jugular vein. An arterial approach is used for stimulation of the left ventricle. A size 5F, 6F, or 7F electrode catheter is advanced under fluoroscopy to the heart.
   E. Intracardiac electrocardiograms are recorded.
   F. After proper catheter position is verified, the following or any combination may be performed, depending on the purpose of the study (an amnestic such as midazolam may be administered before induction of dysrhythmias):
      i. Mapping of the electrical system and pathways, with characterization of the electrical properties of the cardiac conduction system.
      ii. Measurement of conduction times, refractory periods, and recovery times of different portions of the heart.
      iii. Pacing of the atria may be performed, and extra stimuli may be added at specific intervals, to evaluate whether they can stimulate dysrhythmias.
      iv. Attempts to induce dysrhythmias by delivery of a small electrical charge to specific locations of the chamber walls.
      v. Overdrive pacing.
      vi. Antidysrhythmic drug effectiveness may be evaluated by administration of the drug to terminate stimulated dysrhythmias.
   G. Induced dysrhythmias that are poorly tolerated (that is, cause hypotension, loss of consciousness) may be terminated by overdrive pacing, cardioversion, or defibrillation.
   H. The catheter is removed, and pressure is applied to the site for 10 minutes, or at least until 10 minutes after bleeding stops. A pressure dressing is placed over the site.

4. **Postprocedure care:**
   A. Assess and document the following every 15 minutes × 4, then every 30 minutes × 4, then hourly × 4, and then every 4 hours until 24 hours after the procedure.
      i. Vital signs.
      ii. Insertion site for bleeding or hematoma.
      iii. Color, motion, temperature, sensation, and the presence and quality of pulses in the extremity distal to the insertion site as compared to baseline value, and the opposite extremity. Notify the physician for any changes from baseline assessment.
   B. If deep sedation was used, follow institutional protocol for postsedation monitoring. Typical monitoring includes continuous ECG monitoring and pulse oximetry, with continual assessments (every 5-15 minutes) of airway,

vital signs, and neurologic status until the client is lying quietly awake, is breathing independently, and responds appropriately to commands spoken in a normal tone.

C. For bleeding at insertion site, apply firm pressure for 10 minutes. If bleeding continues after 10 minutes, continue holding pressure, and notify physician.

D. A sandbag may be placed over the insertion site for several hours.

E. Maintain continuous electrocardiographic monitoring and observe for dysrhythmias for at least 24 hours.

F. Resume diet.

G. If antidysrhythmic drugs were administered during EPS or begun after EPS, observe cardiac monitor pattern for their effect.

5. **Client and family teaching:**
    A. Fast from food from midnight the night before the procedure. Fluids may be taken up to 4 hours before the test, but no caffeine is permitted.
    B. The procedure takes up to 8 hours.
    C. Because this procedure can be frightening, good explanations are necessary. Inform the client of the following information: you will have to lie as motionless as possible on your back, and feelings of flushing, anxiousness, dizziness, and palpitations are common during EPS. EPS will cause abnormal heart rhythms, and the doctors, nurses, and technicians are skilled at quickly treating these rhythms. The procedure may take 1-8 hours. After EPS, you must lie with the extremity distal to the insertion site motionless for several (usually 8) hours, and a sandbag may be in place over the site. Vital signs, the insertion site, and affected extremity circulation will be checked frequently after EPS.

6. **Factors that affect results:**
    A. Antidysrhythmic drugs that are not completely cleared from the body before initial EPS may result in a falsely normal study.

7. **Other data:**
    A. Subsequent treatment based on EPS findings may include antidysrhythmic drugs, ablation,

implantation of an implantable cardioverter defibrillator (ICD), implantation of a rapid atrial pacemaker (overdrive pacing), combinations of the above, or other techniques.

B. Blacks have significantly lower rates of utilization of EPS and ICD procedures and higher subsequent mortality rates (Alexander et al, 2002).

C. EPS can elicit latent atrial flutter or tachycardia in clients with refractory atrial fibrillation.

D. See also *HIS bundle electrophysiology, Diagnostic.*

EMG
(see Electromyography and nerve conduction studies, Diagnostic)

ENDOMETRIUM, ANAEROBIC, CULTURE

Norm. No growth of anaerobic bacteria.

Positive. Actinomycosis, endometriosis, and pelvic inflammatory disease.

Description. The endometrium is the interior uterine mucosal layer formed of epithelium. This is the uterine layer that proliferates and sheds in response to hormonal effects throughout the menstrual cycle. Because the uterus is an anaerobic environment, anaerobic endometrial infections may cause symptoms of severe abdominal pain and bloating, menstrual irregularities, and infertility problems. Endometrial culture is performed when any of the above are suspected.

Professional Considerations
1. Consent form NOT required.
2. **Preparation:**
    A. Obtain disinfectant, a sterile syringe, a vaginal speculum, and an anaerobic transport tube.
3. **Procedure:**
    A. Place the client in the dorsal lithotomy position with feet in the stirrups and drape her for comfort and privacy.
    B. Insert the vaginal speculum, disinfect the cervix; then, using a sterile syringe, aspirate material through the cervical os.

C. Expel air bubbles from the syringe and place the collected material into the anaerobic tube.
4. Postprocedure care:
   A. Provide a sanitary pad for the client for minor bleeding.
   B. Transport the specimen to the laboratory within 30 minutes.
   C. Include the site of the specimen and list any recent antibiotic therapy on the laboratory requisition.
5. Client and family teaching:
   A. A feeling of pelvic cramping similar to a strong menstrual cramp is normally felt during insertion of the aspiration tube through the cervix. Prostaglandin inhibitors, such as ibuprofen or naproxen sodium, will lessen the discomfort and may be taken before or after the procedure, or at both times.
   B. Minor spotting on a sanitary pad is normal during the 24 hours after the procedure.
   C. Notify the physician for excessive bleeding or purulent drainage, increasing pelvic pain, or fever >101° F (38.3° C).
   D. Take showers, rather than tub baths, for 3-4 days.
   E. Do not have sexual relations for 7 days after the procedure.
   F. Results are normally available within 72 hours.
6. Factors that affect results:
   A. Do not refrigerate the sample(s).
7. Other data:
   A. This test is not optimal for fungus culture.
   B. Actinomycosis may be associated with endometritis and pelvic inflammatory disease from use of IUD contraception.

ENDOMYSIAL ANTIBODY(EMYA), SERUM

Norm. No endomysial antibody detected.

Usage. Noninvasive measure for screening and diagnosis of celiac sprue and duodenal villous atrophy (78% sensitivity). May be used with jejunal biopsy, a definitive diagnostic standard.

Description. Indirect immunofluorescent test that measures endomysial antibodies that react against the endomysial component of smooth muscle in the duodenum and jejunum. With a positive endomysial antibody titer there is a suggested association between celiac disease and sclerosing cholangitis, primary biliary cirrhosis, autoimmune connective tissue disease, insulin-dependent diabetes mellitus, or inflammatory bowel disease. It has approximately 80% sensitivity and 95% specificity in untreated clients.

Professional Considerations
1. Consent form NOT required.
2. Preparation:
   A. Tube: Red topped or red/gray.
3. Procedure:
   A. *Adults:* Draw a 4-mL blood sample.
   B. *Children:* Draw a 2-mL blood sample.
4. Postprocedure care:
   A. None.
5. Client and family teaching:
   A. Test results will be available in a few days.
   B. Dietary therapy with removal of all foods containing wheat, rye, and barley gluten.
6. Factors that affect results:
   A. Current or recent cigarette smoking associated with EMA-negative status.
7. Other data:
   A. The serum is stable for 7 days if refrigerated and 1 year if frozen.
   B. Celiac Sprue Association telephone: 1-402-558-0600 (USA).

ENDOSCOPIC RETROGRADE CHOLANGIOPANCREATOGRAPHY (ERCP), DIAGNOSTIC

Norm. Patent bile ducts, duodenal papilla, pancreatic ducts, and gallbladder.

Usage. Determine the cause of cirrhosis, evaluate jaundice, obtain tissue samples from the pancreatobiliary tree, diagnose cholangitis, pancreatic cancer, pancreatitis, pancreatic cysts, pancreatic ductal lesions, pancreas divisum, and papillary stenosis. After the ERCP, by endoscopy, cysts can be drained, stones can be removed from the common bile duct, and stents can be placed across biliary or pancreatic strictures.

Description. Endoscopic retrograde cholangiopancreatography (ERCP) is the radiographic viewing of the hepatobiliary tree and pancreatic ducts through an endoscope using contrast medium injected through the ampulla of Vater. ERCP is used for detection of common bile duct stones when the probability for this condition is high. A newer test, endoscopic ultrasound (EUS) is also used for detection of stones in the common bile duct. EUS is less risky because it does not involve exposure to radiation. See *Endoscopic ultrasound, Diagnostic.*

Professional Considerations
1. Consent form IS required.

Risks
Cholangitis, dysrhythmias, hemorrhage, pancreatitis, perforation of intestine, peritonitis, sphincter of Oddi dysfunction.

Contraindications
Anticoagulant therapy, bleeding disorders, thrombocytopenia, renal insufficiency. Sedatives are contraindicated in clients with central nervous system depression.

Precautions
During pregnancy, risks of cumulative radiation exposure to the fetus from this and other previous or future imaging studies must be weighed against the benefits of the procedure. Although formal limits for client exposure are relative to this risk:benefit comparison, the United States Nuclear Regulatory Commission requires that the cumulative dose equivalent to an embryo/fetus from occupational exposure not exceed 0.5 rem (5 mSv). Radiation dosage to the fetus is proportional to the distance of the anatomy studied from the abdomen and decreases as pregnancy progresses. For pregnant clients, consult the Radiologist/Radiology Department to obtain estimated fetal radiation exposure from this procedure.

2. **Preparation:**
   A. A kidney-ureter-bladder (KUB) flat-plate radiograph of the abdomen is taken to determine the absence of barium.
   B. See *Client and family teaching.*
   C. Obtain a topical anesthetic, sedative, and endoscope.
   D. Establish intravenous access.
   E. Antibiotic prophylaxis beforeERCP results in fewer cases of cholangi-

tis in clients with obstructive jaundice (Thompson et al, 2002).
3. **Procedure:**
   A. A topical anesthetic is applied to the oropharyngeal area.
   B. Sedatives are given intravenously.
   C. The client is placed in the left lateral position.
   D. The endoscope is inserted through the esophagus to the stomach and then into the duodenum.
   E. The client is then placed in the prone position, the papilla is cannulated with a catheter, and contrast dye is injected into the pancreatic or bile ductal system.
   F. Several radiographs are taken, and then biopsy specimens may be taken if desired.
4. **Postprocedure care:**
   A. The client should have nothing by mouth until the gag reflex returns.
   B. If deep sedation was used, follow institutional protocol for postsedation monitoring. Typical monitoring includes continuous ECG monitoring and pulse oximetry, with continual assessments (every 5-15 minutes) of airway, vital signs, and neurologic status until the client is lying quietly awake, is breathing independently, and responds appropriately to commands spoken in a normal tone.
   C. Assess for the complications of urinary retention and intraabdominal hematoma.
   D. Transient rise in serum liver enzymes is common up to 24 hours after ERCP.
5. **Client and family teaching:**
   A. Fast from food and fluids for 12 hours before and after the procedure until the gag reflex returns.
   B. The procedure takes approximately 1 hour.
6. **Factors that affect results:**
   A. Retained barium can obstruct viewing.
7. **Other data:**
   A. Up to 95% of the pancreatic duct and 85% of the biliary duct can be visualized by an experienced physician.
   B. Useful in differentiating surgical from medical jaundice.
   C. Therapeutic ERCP has a significantly higher complication rate (4.6%) and higher mortality rate

E

(0.5%) when compared to diagnostic ERCP.

D. Magnetic resonance cholangiopancreatography (MRCP) may make diagnostic ERCP obsolete and is more effective in the evaluation of intrahepatic stones. ERCP is more sensitive in detecting common bile duct stones than is computed tomography cholangiography.

E. For detection of pancreatobiliary malignant obstruction, MRCP, ERCP, and EUS provided similar diagnostic results.

F. Factors that may indicate the presence of gall stones include clinical jaundice or elevated bilirubin, liver function tests, and common bile duct dilation (identified via ultrasound).

ENDOSCOPIC ULTRASONOGRAPHY (EUS), DIAGNOSTIC

Norm. Requires interpretation. Lipomas image as bright and echogenic. Tumors are usually dark and hypoepogenic, often with irregular borders.

Usage. Gastrointestinal (GI) cancer staging; imaging of lymph node metastasis from the GI tract to help determine TNM staging; screening for cancer in clients with Barrett's esophagus; screening for recurrence of GI cancer of all types. Provides guidance for fine-needle aspiration biopsies of the abdominal organs and lymph nodes. More sensitive than upper GI endoscopy for diagnosing varices. Evaluation for the presence of stones in the common bile duct. More accurate than any other tests for detection of pancreatic cancer. Some therapeutic uses are also being investigated.

Description. One of the newest uses for ultrasonography involves taking ultrasound images from within the GI tract. EUS improves diagnostic accuracy by reducing artifacts caused that occur from anatomic structures and gas when imaging from the exterior of the body. Because the ultrasound probe is much closer to the area being examined, higher frequency ultrasound can be used, which normally is not an option when imaging from greater distances. Higher frequencies can provide clearer images of smaller areas and better detail

of the layers of the GI tract, which are often the site where cancer begins.

Professional Considerations
1. Consent form IS required.

Risks
Vasovagal bradycardia and drug-induced tachycardia are likely dysrhythmias; esophageal perforation; bleeding; transient hypoxemia; oversedation.

Contraindications
Esophageal obstructions, stenosis, fistula, or dysphagia; history of radiation therapy to the esophagus or surrounding area (mediastinum); acute penetrating chest injuries. Neonates and young children are not candidates because of the unavailability of specially sized scopes. Sedatives are contraindicated in clients with central nervous system depression and in clients who cannot tolerate lying flat.

2. Preparation:
   A. See *Client and family teaching.*
   B. Document clinical indications on the test requisition. This helps guide the interpreter to provide the most relevant test interpretation.
   C. Start an IV infusion at KVO (keep vein open) rate for administration of sedation or emergency medications.
   D. Remove dentures and glasses. Have the client void before the procedure.
   E. Obtain local anesthetic spray.
   F. A drying agent is typically given to reduce secretions (that is, glycopyrrolate 0.1 to 0.2 mg IV). Some clients require a small IV dose of an antianxiety agent (such as midazolam or diazepam). Prophylactic antibiotics are usually given if the client has a prosthetic valve.

3. Procedure:
   A. The client is monitored continuously: heart rate and rhythm by cardiac monitor, blood pressure by noninvasive monitor, and O_2 by pulse oximetry.
   B. Position the client in the left lateral decubitus position.
   C. Topical anesthesia per physician preference is used to numb the throat and suppress the gag reflex. This may be repeated several times during the procedure.

D. The client should be awake enough to follow commands but drowsy. This procedure may also be performed on a fully anesthetized or intubated client.

E. The client is asked to open the mouth and flex the neck forward in a chin-to-chest position.

F. The lidocaine-lubricated probe is inserted, and the client is asked to swallow.

G. A small flexible tube equipped with an ultrasonic probe and camera at the tip is inserted through the mouth or rectum and advanced into the GI tract. Ultrasonic images are taken at points appropriate to the clinical indications for the procedure.

H. The nurse remains with the client to monitor respiratory status, vital signs, and cardiac rhythm and to assess the need for further sedation or suctioning.

4. **Postprocedure care:**
   A. Continue assessment of respiratory status. If deep sedation was used, follow institutional protocol for postsedation monitoring. Typical monitoring includes continuous ECG monitoring and pulse oximetry with continual assessments (every 5-15 minutes) of airway, vital signs, and neurologic status until client reaches level 3, 2, or 1 on the Ramsay Sedation scale.
   B. Once the gag reflex has returned, the client can resume fluids. Full diet is not recommended until 3 hours after procedure.

5. **Client and family teaching:**
   A. This procedure involves having a narrow, flexible tube inserted through your mouth and esophagus into your stomach and small intestine and having an ultrasound picture taken from inside the body.
   B. Fast for 6-8 hours before the test. Medications may be taken with a small amount of water as directed by the physician. You will have to remove your dentures and eyeglasses, but you should keep your hearing aid on so that you can hear the physician's instructions.
   C. You will be given a sedative for the procedure. You should arrange for someone to drive you home because you may be drowsy

after the procedure and will not be permitted to drive.
   D. Do not eat or drink for 4-6 hours before the procedure. Take any prescription medications with a small sip of water.
   E. Bowel preps may be ordered for lower EUS.
   F. The test takes about 45 minutes.
   G. The tongue and throat may feel swollen after the topical anesthetic; the mouth and lips will feel sticky and dry if a drying agent is used. Do not eat or drink after the procedure until the numbness is gone.
   H. Home-going instructions: Promptly report persistent sore throat, dysphagia, stiff neck, and epigastric, substernal or abdominal pain that worsens with breathing or movement.

6. **Factors that affect results:**
   A. None found.

7. **Other data:**
   A. None found.

ENTAMOEBA HISTOLYTICA, SEROLOGIC TEST, BLOOD

Norm. Negative, IHA titer <1:128, CF titer <1:8.

Positive. Diarrhea (inflammatory or HIV related), dysentery, liver abscess, lung abscess, perianal ulcers, perineal ulcers, salpingitis. A fourfold rise in titer supports the diagnosis of *Entamoeba* infection.

Negative. Bacterial infection of the intestines.

Description. *Entamoeba histolytica* is a protozoon that causes intestinal disease transmitted in infected food and water by flies and by direct contact causing acute diarrhea. Abscesses may form on the liver (75% found in right lobe), lungs, and brain, causing death. Prevalence in the United States is lowest in winter (22%-27%) and highest between July and October (36%-43%). This test cannot distinguish between amoebic liver abscess and intestinal amebiasis.

Professional Considerations
1. Consent form NOT required.
2. **Preparation:**
   A. See *Client and family teaching.*

B. Tube: Red topped, red/gray topped, or gold topped.
3. **Procedure:**
   A. Draw a 7-mL blood sample.
4. **Postprocedure care:**
   A. Resume previous diet.
   B. Draw convalescent sample 14-21 days after acute sample.
5. **Client and family teaching:**
   A. Fast from food and fluids from midnight until after the test has been completed.
   B. *Entamoeba histolytica* amebiasis is treated with metronidazole 750 mg TID for 10 days (for extra intestinal form) or paromomycin 30 mg/kg in 3 divided doses for 7 days or diloxanide 500 mg TID for 10 days (for intraluminal and extra intestinal trophozoites), except during pregnancy.
   C. Return in 2-3 weeks to have a follow-up sample drawn. This will help determine whether the infection is responding to treatment.
6. **Factors that affect results:**
   A. Ulcerative colitis may cause false-positive results.
7. **Other data:**
   A. 99% of serologic test results are positive 1 week after infection and may remain positive for as long as 2 years after curative therapy.
   B. *Entamoeba histolytica* amebiasis is a reportable disease in most areas.

EOS, BLOOD
(see Differential leukocyte count, Peripheral blood)

EOSINOPHIL COUNT, BLOOD
(see Differential leukocyte count, Peripheral blood)

EOSINOPHIL SMEAR, SPECIMEN

Norm. No eosinophils.

Usage. Evaluate allergic airway inflammation in clients with asthma.

Description. Eosinophils are found in increased numbers in the sputum of clients with allergic airway inflammation. An induced sputum is a useful noninvasive method for studying the inflammation.

Professional Considerations
1. Consent form NOT required.
2. **Preparation:**
   A. Obtain two glass slides, a sterile applicator, and a sterile container.
3. **Procedure:**
   A. Obtain a sputum specimen in a sterile container or induce a sputum specimen by giving the client an aerosol inhalation treatment with 0.9% saline and then encouraging him or her to cough.
4. **Postprocedure care:**
   A. The requisition must state the site of the specimen.
5. **Client and family teaching:**
   A. Deep coughs are necessary to produce sputum, rather than saliva. To produce the proper specimen, take several breaths in, without fully exhaling each, and then expel sputum with a "cascade cough" and catch the sputum in the container.
   B. Results are normally available in 24 hours.
6. **Factors that affect results:**
   A. Reject slides received in cytologic fixative.
   B. Theophylline inhibits eosinophilic activity.
7. **Other data:**
   A. Over 80% eosinophils in relation to total neutrophils are suggestive of asthma.
   B. GM-CSF is responsible for increased survival of eosinophils in the airways of asthmatics, thereby decreasing lung function.

EP
(see Protoporphyrin, Free erythrocyte, Blood; Electrolytes panel, Blood)

EPHEDRINE
(see Amphetamines, Blood)

EPINEPHRINE, BLOOD
(see Catecholamines, Plasma)

EPS, DIAGNOSTIC
(see Electrophysiologic study, Diagnostic)

EPSTEIN-BARR VIRUS (EBV), SEROLOGY, BLOOD

Norm. Negative, no virus found.

Increased. Autoimmune thyroiditis, breast carcinoma, Burkitt's lymphoma, dysplasia, Epstein-Barr virus, gastric adenocarcinoma, head and neck tumors, HIV, Hodgkin's disease, hyperplasia, infectious hepatitis, infectious mononucleosis, lung carcinoma, lymphocytic leukemia, lymphoepithelioma, nasopharyngeal carcinoma, non-Hodgkin's lymphoma, post transplant lymphoproliferative disorders in lung transplant, prostatic intraepithelial cancer, sarcoidosis, and systemic lupus erythematosus.

Description. Epstein-Barr virus is a B-lymphocyte human herpesvirus that is the causative agent of infectious mononucleosis. The mode of transmission is through direct contact with the saliva of an infected client. Signs and symptoms, after a 4- to 8-week incubation period, include malaise, anorexia, chills, fever, cervical lymphadenopathy, pharyngitis, splenomegaly, hepatitis, and peripheral atypical lymphocytosis. An Epstein-Barr virus panel includes four antibody levels: IgM VCA (viral capsid antigen), IgG VCA, EA (early antigen), and EBNA (Epstein-Barr nuclear antigen). The pattern of reactivity is helpful in distinguishing recent primary infection, reactivated infection, or remote inactive infection. Individual laboratories will give their reference range with the test results.

Professional Considerations
1. Consent form NOT required.
2. Preparation:
   A. Tube: Red topped, red/gray topped, or gold topped.
   B. Write the date of the onset of illness on the laboratory requisition.
3. Procedure:
   A. Draw a 3-mL blood sample.
4. Postprocedure care:
   A. Refrigerate the serum after separation.
5. Client and family teaching:
   A. Results are normally available within 72 hours.
6. Factors that affect results:
   A. Cytomegalovirus in clients who have had organ transplants will cause a positive result for EBV serology.

B. Posttransfusion reactions of blood and blood products will cause a temporary increase in EBV serologic features.
C. False-positive results occur in clients with collagen vascular disease such as rheumatoid arthritis, leukemia, lymphoma, or HIV.
7. **Other data:**
   A. Up to 20% of people are negative for heterophil antibodies (*Monospot screen, Blood*) with infectious mononucleosis.
   B. In the presence of clinical findings of infectious mononucleosis with negative heterophil and specific viral antibody tests, primary cytomegalovirus infection should be considered.
   C. Antibody titers for EBV are needed only if there is a question of a false-positive result on the Monostat rapid slide test for EBV.
   D. Many people with chronic fatigue syndrome present with high antibody titers for EBV, but these are probably unrelated to the disease process.
   E. IgG avidity assay is a supplementary test that distinguishes between acute and past infections better than lysate immunoblot banding does.
   F. See also *Monospot screen, Blood.*

ERCP
(see Endoscopic retrograde cholangiopancreatography, Diagnostic)

ERGONOVINE MALEATE TEST, DIAGNOSTIC

Usage. Aids in the diagnosis of coronary spasm during coronary arteriography, echocardiography, and electrophysiologic studies in clients with variant angina and no major occlusions of the coronary arteries.

Description. Ergonovine maleate (Ergotrate) stimulates contractions of vascular smooth muscle. It is administered during the cardiac procedure to produce and evaluate the effects of the resulting coronary artery spasm. The IV initial phase half-life is 1-5 minutes. The terminal phase half-life is 0.5-2.0 hours. This drug is no longer commercially available in the United States.

Professional Considerations
1. Consent form IS required.

Risks
Adverse drug effects may occur with ergonovine: nausea and vomiting, dizziness, headache, tinnitus, diaphoresis, palpitations, transient chest pain, dyspnea, thrombophlebitis, hematuria, water intoxication, nasal congestion, diarrhea, and allergic phenomena, including shock. Ergonovine-induced hypertension has been accompanied by headaches, severe dysrhythmias, seizures, and cerebrovascular accidents. Hypotension has also been reported. See also individual procedures for procedure-specific risks.

Contraindications or Precautions
Previous allergy to ergot, hypertension, pregnancy, toxemia, untreated hypocalcemia. Use Ergonovine with extreme caution in the presence of renal or hepatic dysfunction, coronary artery disease, peripheral vascular disease, or sepsis. See also individual procedures for procedure-specific contraindications.

2. Preparation:
   A. See the listing for the procedure that is being performed.
3. Procedure:
   A. 0.1-0.4 mg of ergonovine maleate is given slowly intravenously with dilution.
4. Postprocedure care:
   A. See the specific procedure for postprocedure care.
   B. Observe for adverse drug effects (listed under *Risks*).
5. Client and family teaching:
   A. Inform the client about the approximate time length of the procedure that will be used with ergonovine administration.
6. Factors that affect results:
   A. None found.
7. Other data:
   A. Hypertension may occur if the client is given the IV dose too rapidly or without dilution or if ergonovine is used along with a regional anesthetic or vasoconstrictor.
   B. This drug is also used to stimulate contractions of the uterus to prevent and treat postpartum and postabortion hemorrhage caused by uterine atony.
   C. Ergonovine test is not necessary for diagnosis of coronary artery spasm if client's exercise test or thallium perfusion scan is negative. Use of ^{123}I-MIBG SPECT scan is feasible under these circumstances.

ERYTHROCYTE, BLOOD
(see Red blood cells, Blood)

ERYTHROCYTE PROTOPORPHYRIN (EP), BLOOD
(see Protoporphyrin, Free erythrocyte, Blood)

ERYTHROCYTE SEDIMENTATION RATE, BLOOD
(see Sedimentation rate, Erythrocyte, Blood)

ERYTHROPOIETIN (EPO), SERUM

Norm. 7-36 milli-immunochemical units/mL.

Increased. Absolute erythrocytosis, aplastic anemia, acute lymphocytic leukemia, cerebellar hemangioblastomas, chronic obstructive pulmonary disease, hepatoma, high altitudes, hypoxia, kidney transplant rejection, myelodysplastic syndromes, nephrectomy, nephroblastoma, pheochromocytoma, pregnancy, renal cancer, renal cysts, and sickle-cell anemia (thrombotic events). Drugs include hydroxyurea treatment in sickle cell disease.

Decreased. Acute neuropsychiatric porphyrias, autoimmune diseases, cancer, Hodgkin's disease, polycythemia rubra vera, and renal failure (chronic). Hemoperfusion with polymyxin B–immobilized fiber (PMX-F). EPO declines with repeated chemotherapy and in lead toxicity if blood values of lead are >32 mg/dL.

Description. Erythropoietin is a glycoprotein produced in the peritubular cells in the renal cortex of the kidney. It is released in response to renal hypoxia and stimulates the formation and development of erythrocytes in the bone marrow.

In healthy persons there is an inverse correlation between serum Epo and hematocrit: an exponential increase in Epo levels occurs as hematocrit decreases.

Professional Considerations
1. Consent form NOT required.
2. **Preparation:**
   A. Tube: Red topped, red/gray topped, or gold topped.
3. **Procedure:**
   A. Draw a 5-mL blood sample.
4. **Postprocedure care:**
   A. Note on the laboratory requisition the amount of oxygen delivery because oxygen influences erythrocyte function.
5. **Client and family teaching:**
   A. The results are normally available within 24 hours.
6. **Factors that affect results:**
   A. Morning values are higher than afternoon values because of the diurnal rhythm of secretion.
   B. Blood donation increases serum values.
7. **Other data:**
   A. Useful in differentiating primary from secondary polycythemia.
   B. May not reliably detect ectopic erythropoietin-like substances, and so neoplasia cannot be excluded.
   C. Can be used as a measure of oxygenation in critically ill clients.

ESOPHAGEAL ACIDITY TEST (TUTTLE TEST), DIAGNOSTIC
Norm:

Esophageal pH:	>5.0
Esophageal reflux pH:	≤5.0

Usage. Helps diagnose gastroesophageal reflux.

Description. A test that evaluates the integrity of the esophageal sphincter by measuring the pH of gastric and esophageal contents using a pH electrode attached to an esophageal catheter introduced through the mouth and esophagus. This test may be performed with esophageal manometry.

Professional Considerations
1. Consent form IS required.

Risks
Aspiration and chemical bronchitis, vasovagal response.

Contraindications
Clients at high risk for poor tolerance of a vasovagal reaction (that is, clients with known cardiac instability).

2. **Preparation:**
   A. See *Client and family teaching.*
   B. Verify that the client has fasted.
   C. Obtain a gastric catheter with a pH electrode, and 300 mL of 0.1%N hydrochloric acid (HCl).
   D. Establish intravenous access. Have a 0.9% saline and atropine on hand for use in the event a vasovagal response occurs.
   E. The client should void just before the test.
3. **Procedure:**
   A. Place the client in a high Fowler's position.
   B. Assess for vasovagal reaction, dysrhythmia, cyanosis, or coughing during the procedure.
   C. Introduce the catheter with a pH electrode through the mouth to the back of the throat. Instruct the client to swallow, perform the Valsalva maneuver, or lift the legs to stimulate reflux to catheter level, and then determine the pH.
   D. If the pH is normal, pass the catheter into the stomach, instill 300 mL of 0.1%N HCl over 3 minutes, and repeat item 3B.
4. **Postprocedure care:**
   A. Assess vital signs every 30 minutes × 2. Extend assessments as needed if the client was treated for a vasovagal reaction during the procedure.
5. **Client and family teaching:**
   A. Fast from midnight before the test and avoid smoking for 24 hours before the test.
   B. Do not drink alcohol for 24 hours before the test.
   C. The physician may want you to stop taking adrenergic blockers, antacids, anticholinergics, cimetidine, cholinergics, corticosteroids, and reserpine for 24 hours before the test. Check with your doctor before stopping any of your medicine.

D. You must swallow a catheter with a small electrode attached, which will measure the amount of acid in your esophagus and stomach. After the measurements are taken, the electrode will be slowly pulled out of your stomach.
E. The test takes 30 minutes or less.
F. The results are immediately available.

6. Factors that affect results:
A. Antacids, anticholinergics, and cimetidine may decrease pH. Adrenergic blockers, cholinergics, corticosteroids, ethyl alcohol (ethanol), and reserpine may increase pH.

7. Other data:
A. None.

ESOPHAGEAL MANOMETRY, DIAGNOSTIC

Norm.
"Congruent esophageal pressures bilaterally; smooth progression of motility and peristalsis in a proximal-to-distal pattern, absence of spasm.
Diurnal variations in distal and proximal pressure amplitudes, distal duration, and propulsive contractions.
Median proportion of propulsive waves: 56%.
Median proportion of simultaneous waves: 10%.
No significant difference in the elderly population." (Adamek et al, 1994)

Usage. Assessment and diagnosis of achalasia, dysphagia, esophageal reflux, spasm, and motility abnormalities, hiatal hernia.

Description. In esophageal manometry, a multilumen esophageal catheter is introduced through the mouth and oropharynx into the esophagus, and pressures along the esophagus are measured as the client performs a series of swallowing maneuvers. The test helps identify locations of abnormal contractions and peristalsis in the esophagus as well as areas of increased pressure that would indicate esophageal spasm. The test may be performed with the esophageal acidity (Tuttle) test and the acid perfusion (Bernstein) test. It has been used extensively in the research setting in the study of esophageal motility

disorders and is less commonly used in the clinical setting.

Professional Considerations
1. Consent form IS required.

Risks
Vasovagal reaction, dysrhythmia, cyanosis, or coughing.

Contraindications
Clients at high risk for poor tolerance of a vasovagal reaction (that is, clients with known cardiac instability).

2. Preparation:
A. Verify that the client has fasted.
B. The client should void just before the test.
C. Obtain a gastric catheter, a swallowing sensor, water, and a syringe.

3. Procedure:
A. Place the client in a high Fowler's position.
B. Introduce the catheter through the mouth to the back of the throat. Instruct the client to swallow the catheter several times until it has passed into the esophagus to the proper level.
C. Reposition the client in a supine position.
D. Attach the swallowing sensor to the client's neck.
E. The client is then asked to swallow small amounts of water injected into the mouth with a syringe, and the esophageal pressures are measured. This is followed by several dry swallows with corresponding pressure measurements.

4. Postprocedure care:
A. Assess vital signs every 30 minutes × 2. Extend assessments as needed if the client was treated for a vasovagal reaction during the procedure.
B. Observe for cholinergic side effects: bradycardia, dizziness, diaphoresis, flushing, muscle cramping, nausea, urinary urgency, and vomiting.

5. Client and family teaching:
A. Fast from midnight before the test and avoid smoking for 24 hours before the test.
B. Do not drink alcohol or take adrenergic blockers, antacids, anticholinergics, cimetidine, cholinergics, corticosteroids, and reserpine for 24 hours before the test.

C. Arrange for transportation home because you will not be allowed to drive for 12-24 hours after receiving edrophonium chloride.

D. You must swallow a catheter with a small electrode attached. You will then be asked to swallow several times, first with small amounts of water injected into the mouth and then without water. The catheter and neck sensor will measure the pressures in the esophagus as you swallow. After the measurements are taken, the catheter will be slowly pulled out of the stomach.

E. The test takes 30 minutes or less.

F. Irritation of nose and throat are common problems for up to 8 hours post procedure.

6. **Factors that affect results:**
   A. None.

7. **Other data:**
   A. See also *Acid perfusion test, Diagnostic; Esophageal acidity test, Diagnostic.*

ESOPHAGEAL RADIOGRAPHY, DIAGNOSTIC

Norm. Normal size and normal peristalsis.

Usage. Achalasia, esophageal varices, esophagitis, locating a foreign body, gastrointestinal (GI) bleeding, guidance for balloon dilatation of stricture, head and neck cancer, impaction, hiatus hernia, polyps.

Description. A radiographic and fluoroscopic examination of the esophagus for patency, structure, and motility. When examined with the stomach, duodenum, and upper jejunum, this test is known as an upper GI series.

Professional Considerations
1. Consent form IS required.

Risks
This procedure carries minimal risks.

Contraindications
Dysphagia, ileus.

Precautions
During pregnancy, risks of cumulative radiation exposure to the fetus from this and other previous or future imaging studies must be weighed against the benefits of the procedure. Although formal limits for client exposure are relative to this risk:benefit comparison, the United States Nuclear Regulatory Commission requires that the cumulative dose equivalent to an embryo/fetus from occupational exposure not exceed 0.5 rem (5 mSv). Radiation dosage to the fetus is proportional to the distance of the anatomy studied from the abdomen and decreases as pregnancy progresses. For pregnant clients, consult the Radiologist/Radiology Department to obtain estimated fetal radiation exposure from this procedure.

2. **Preparation:**
   A. Verify that the client has fasted.

3. **Procedure:**
   A. A plain radiograph of the esophagus is taken in the supine position.
   B. Barium sulfate, approximately 400 mL, is then swallowed with the client in a standing position in front of the fluoroscope, and radiographs are again taken.
   C. Follow-up radiographs at 24 hours may be performed.
   D. The procedure takes 45 minutes.

4. **Postprocedure care:**
   A. Resume diet.
   B. Observe for passage of barium in the stool for 2-3 days.
   C. A laxative may be needed to evacuate barium.
   D. Encourage the oral intake of fluids to help prevent barium impaction.

5. **Client and family teaching:**
   A. Fast from food and fluids from midnight on, before the test.
   B. Drink 4-6 glasses of water per day (unless contraindicated) for 2-3 days after the test to promote barium excretion. Barium stools will look grayish white. Notify health care provider if unable to pass barium in stool within 3 days.
   C. Results are normally available within 24 hours.

6. **Factors that affect results:**
   A. Retained barium from a previous examination interferes with the quality of the radiographic images.

7. **Other data:**
   A. Esophageal varices are difficult to identify and are usually a sign of liver cirrhosis.
   B. Barium comes in flavors but is still described as unpleasant to swallow.

E

ESOPHAGOGASTRO-DUODENOSCOPY (EGD), DIAGNOSTIC

Norm. Normal upper gastrointestinal tract (that is, esophageal mucosa is smooth and pink, with visible submucosal blood vessels; stomach mucosa is composed of continuous, deeper red rugal folds; duodenal lining is covered with villi). All surfaces are free of ulcers, varices, bleeding, and lesions.

Usage. Biopsy, cancer, dysphagia, esophagitis, gastric ulcers, hiatal hernia, Mallory-Weiss tear, odynophagia (painful swallowing), postoperative examination of the gastrointestinal (GI) tract, and upper GI bleeding.

Description. Visualization of the esophagus, stomach, and upper duodenum with a fiberoptic scope that has a lighted mirror lens on the end. EGD is less sensitive than endoscopic ultrasound for detection of varices of the esophagus and stomach. See *Endoscopic ultrasound, Diagnostic.*

Professional Considerations
1. Consent form IS required.

Risks
Gastrointestinal perforation and hemorrhage, aspiration, infection, respiratory arrest, death.

Contraindications
Zenker's diverticulum or large aortic aneurysm. Sedatives are contraindicated in clients with central nervous system depression.

Precautions
During pregnancy, risks of cumulative radiation exposure to the fetus from this and other previous or future imaging studies must be weighed against the benefits of the procedure. Although formal limits for client exposure are relative to this risk:benefit comparison, the United States Nuclear Regulatory Commission requires that the cumulative dose equivalent to an embryo/fetus from occupational exposure not exceed 0.5 rem (5 mSv). Radiation dosage to the fetus is proportional to the distance of the anatomy studied from the abdomen and decreases as pregnancy progresses. For pregnant clients, consult the radiologist/radiology department to obtain estimated fetal radiation exposure from this procedure.

2. Preparation:
   A. Verify that the client has fasted.
   B. The client should urinate and attempt to defecate before the procedure to increase comfort.
   C. The client should remove dentures, partial plates, and jewelry.
   D. Assess for allergies to anesthetics.
   E. Establish intravenous access.
   F. Obtain specimen containers, one with 95% ethyl alcohol, the other with 10% formaldehyde; an endoscope; and an intravenous sedative.
   G. Measure and record heart rate, blood pressure, and respiratory rate.
   H. Attach electrodes for continuous ECG monitoring and initiate continuous-pulse oximetry measurement.
   I. Atropine may be prescribed to dry secretions before the test.
   J. Infusion of erythromycin before EGD reduces the need for second-look endoscopy in clients with upper GI bleeding.

3. Procedure:
   A. A topical, bitter-tasting anesthetic is applied to the throat and a mouth guard inserted if the client has teeth.
   B. Intravenous sedation is given.
   C. The endoscope is inserted into the esophagus and slowly advanced to the duodenum.
   D. Air is instilled to distend any area to aid in visualization.
   E. Biopsy specimens or photos may be taken.

4. Postprocedure care:
   A. If deep sedation was used for the procedure, follow institutional protocol for postsedation monitoring. Typical monitoring includes continuous ECG monitoring and pulse oximetry, with continual assessments (every 5-15 minutes) of airway, vital signs, and neurologic status until the client is lying quietly awake, is breathing independently, and responds appropriately to commands spoken in a normal tone.
   B. Resume previous diet after the gag reflex returns and sedation has worn off, usually 2 hours after the procedure.

C. Observe for signs of perforation: pain, fever, dyspnea, tachycardia, cyanosis, and pleural effusion.
5. **Client and family teaching:**
   A. Ambulatory clients should arrange for transportation home because they will not be allowed to drive for 12 hours after the procedure.
   B. Fast from food and fluids for 8 hours before the test.
   C. You may receive medication to dry secretions during the test, and this will cause a dry mouth. Sedation may also be used to cause a relaxed state, which may or may not result in sleeping through the test. After a local anesthetic is sprayed into the back of the throat, you will be positioned lying on the side, and the flexible scope will be inserted through the mouth. Suction will remove any draining saliva. Pressure may be felt as the scope advances through the esophagus into the stomach. Feelings of bloating but not pain are common.
   D. The procedure lasts about 40 minutes.
   E. Results are normally available within 24 hours.
   F. Complications in elderly include arrhythmia, elevated blood pressure over 50 mm Hg, increased pulse rate, and decreased oxygen saturation.
6. **Factors that affect results:**
   A. If the client moves excessively during the procedure, the risk of perforation is increased.
7. **Other data:**
   A. Emergency EGD diagnostic accuracy is 80-85%.

ESR
(see Sedimentation rate, Erythrocyte, Blood)

ESTERASE STAIN, DIAGNOSTIC

Norm. Descriptive interpretation by hematologist.

Usage. Granulocytic sarcoma, leukemia.

Description. Stain of bone marrow to distinguish normal and leukemic cells of neutrophils, monocytes, and their precursors.

Professional Considerations
1. Consent form NOT required.
2. **Preparation:**
   A. Obtain glass slides, a lancet, a capillary tube, and a bone marrow tray.
3. **Procedure:**
   A. Obtain a bone marrow specimen and a fingerstick collection for peripheral blood smear.
4. **Postprocedure care:**
   A. Assess the bone marrow aspiration site for bleeding or hematoma.
   B. The client must lie flat for 1-2 hours after the procedure.
   C. Send the specimen slides to the laboratory immediately.
5. **Client and family teaching:**
   A. Bone marrow aspiration is very painful but only for a brief moment.
   B. Results are normally available within 24 hours.
6. **Factors that affect results:**
   A. Poor bone marrow sample will decrease the amount or quality of the cells, leading to inaccurate interpretation.
7. **Other data:**
   A. Staining of fresh specimens enhances assessment.
   B. See also Bone marrow aspiration analysis, Specimen, for professional considerations related to the bone marrow aspiration procedure.
   C. Mitomycin-C may be a suitable agent for inhibiting RPE proliferation in vivo.

ESTRADIOL, SERUM

Norm:

	SI UNITS	
Menstruating Females		
Early cycle	20-170 pg/mL	73-626 pmol/L
Midcycle	70-500 pg/mL	258-1840 pmol/L
Late cycle	45-340 pg/mL	166-1251 pmol/L
Postmenopausal	6.44-18 pg/mL	18.4-66 pmol/L

Continued

		SI UNITS
Females Taking Oral Contraceptives	12-50 pg/mL	44-184 pmol/L
Adult Males	10-50 pg/mL	37-184 pmol/L
Prepubertal Males	2-8 pg/mL	11-29 pmol/L

Increased. Adrenal tumors, breast cancer risk, cirrhosis, gynecomastia in males, hyperthyroidism, in vitro fertilization success of ovulation induction and pregnancy (fourth day of gonadotropin therapy), Klinefelter syndrome, liver tumors, ovarian neoplasm, polycystic ovary syndrome.

Decreased. Amenorrhea, anorexia nervosa, hypopituitarism, infertility, menopause, osteoporosis, ovarian hypofunction, pituitary disease, and polycystic ovary syndrome.

Description. Estradiol is an estrogenic hormone secreted by the ovary and by the placenta that acts on the mucosa of the uterus to stimulate endometrial growth in preparation for the progestational stage. Other actions include follicle-stimulating hormone (FSH) suppression and luteinizing hormone (LH) stimulation. Estradiol levels help evaluate ovarian function, menstrual abnormalities, feminization disorders, and estrogen-producing tumors. Estradiol production diminishes or stops during menopause. Ozcakir et al (2002) found that the estradiol level at the time of intrauterine insemination did not seem to affect the pregnancy rate in nonandrologic and nonperitubal factor infertility.).

Professional Considerations
1. Consent form NOT required.
2. Preparation:
   A. Tube: Red topped, red/gray topped, or gold topped.

3. Procedure:
   A. Draw a 3-mL blood sample.
4. Postprocedure care:
   A. Write the collection time and the client's sex and present menstrual cycle phase on the laboratory requisition.
   B. Transport the specimen to the laboratory immediately for spinning and freezing within 1 hour.
5. Client and family teaching:
   A. Results are normally available within 24 hours.
6. Factors that affect results:
   A. Reject the specimen if the client has had a radioactive scan within 7 days.
   B. Highest levels occur 1 day before the LH surge and again after corpus luteum formation.
   C. Drugs that may falsely elevate results include ampicillin, cortisone (large doses), diethylstilbestrol, hydrochlorothiazide, meprobamates, phenazopyridine, prochlorperazine, and tetracyclines.
   D. An herb that may falsely elevate results includes Cascara sagrada (*Rhamnus purshiana*).
7. Other data:
   A. The specimen is stable at room temperature for 1 week, in a frost-free refrigerator for 1 year, and in a nondefrosting freezer for 3 years.
   B. This test should not be used to evaluate fetal well-being because it does not measure estriol.

ESTRADIOL RECEPTOR AND PROGESTERONE RECEPTOR IN BREAST CANCER, DIAGNOSTIC

Norm:

		SI UNITS
Negative	<6 fmol/mg cytosol protein	<6 nmol/kg cytosol protein
Borderline	6-10 fmol/mg cytosol protein	6-10 nmol/kg cytosol protein
Positive	>10 fmol/mg cytosol protein	>10 nmol/kg cytosol protein

Usage. Used to predict response to hormonal therapy in clients with breast cancer.

Description. Estrogen receptors and progesterone receptors are intracellular proteins that specifically bind estrogens and progesterones. The establishment of receptor status in clients with breast cancer is crucial because they are the most predictive factor for the response to hormonal therapies for primary and metastatic breast cancer. They are the only tumor markers recommended for routine clinical use in breast cancer by the Tumor Marker Panel of the American Society of Clinical Oncology. Clients whose tumors express the estrogen and progesterone receptors respond more often and have longer disease-free and overall survival when treated with hormonal therapy. Although receptor status is important in determining which clients are likely to benefit from endocrine therapy, estrogen and progesterone receptor status is only a weak predictor of long-term relapse and mortalities and are not to be used alone to assign a client to a particular prognostic grouping. It should be noted that breast cancers that are initially hormone dependent might progress to a hormone-independent form, despite the continued expression of the receptor. This may limit the long-term usefulness of the hormonal therapies. Historically these receptors were measured by means of biochemical assays, but there are now highly specific monoclonal antibodies and immunohistochemical techniques available to assess estrogen and progesterone receptor status. When receptor status is determined using biochemical assays, sampling error may occur if the sample does not contain enough tumor, if there is significant desmoplastic response or if there is a delay in the processing of the specimen. A value of less than 3 fmol/mg is considered negative when measured by the biochemical assay. Using the immunocytochemical assay, which measures the concentration of receptors by staining them with monoclonal antibodies, avoids sampling error. An additional advantage to the monoclonal assay is the ability to assay formalin-fixed, paraffin-embedded tissue. Most labs have chosen 10-20% positive cells as the cutoff for receptor positivity, though recent studies have suggested that clients whose tumors contain as few as 1% weakly positive cells

have significantly improved disease-free and overall survival when treated with hormonal therapy. Clients with a negative receptor status have at most an 8% chance of response to hormonal therapy.

Professional Considerations

1. Consent form IS required for biopsy. See *Biopsy, Site-specific, Specimen,* for procedure-specific risks and contraindications.
2. Preparation:
   A. *Biochemical assay or frozen-tissue immunoassay:* Obtain a 60-mg solid tumor biopsy bottle (fluorescent pink), a waxed cardboard container or plastic tube without fixative, and a needle biopsy tray.
   B. *Immunohistochemistry on paraffin block:* Obtain biopsy bottle containing 10% formalin and biopsy tray. Use of fixatives other than 10% formalin may not yield satisfactory results.
3. Procedure:
   A. Local anesthetic is not used because it may destroy receptors and lead to a false-negative result.
   B. A 0.5-1.0 mg solid tumor tissue is removed, with care being taken to remove excess fat and blood, both of which may lead to false-positive results.
   C. *Biochemical assay or frozen-tissue immunoassay:* The tissue is immediately cut into small pieces and assayed. If the assay is unable to be performed immediately, the tissue should be frozen on dry ice, in a cryostat, or in liquid nitrogen within 20 minutes of collection. The specimen will be rejected if thawed or formalin fixed. Specimen should not be placed in foil, gauze, or fixative.
   D. *Immunohistochemistry on paraffin block:* Tissue is placed in 10% formalin for not longer than 48 hours, preferably 12-24 hours. A paraffin block is then made on which an immunoassay to measure concentration of receptors may be performed.
4. Postprocedure care:
   A. Apply a dry, sterile dressing to the biopsy site.
   B. Mild analgesics may be used for postprocedure pain.
   C. Depending on where assay is performed, results may not be available for several days.

E

5. **Client and family teaching:**
   A. A small sample of breast tissue will be removed with a hollow needle. The breast will not be numbed with an anesthetic because this can cause false-negative results, and so there will be discomfort for a short time. The procedure takes a few minutes and leaves no scar.
   B. Use mild analgesia for postprocedure pain if needed.

C. Results may not be available for several days.
6. **Factors that affect results:**
   A. Specimens not frozen within 20 minutes will falsely decrease results.
   B. Antiestrogen preparations taken within the last 2 months may cause a negative estradiol receptor response.
7. **Other data:**
   A. 50-70% of breast cancers are positive.

ESTRIOL, SERUM, 24-HOUR URINE

Norm:

	TOTAL ESTRIOL	SI UNITS

Serum

A diurnal pattern is present, with the highest levels occurring in the mid- to late afternoon.

Weeks of Pregnancy

30-32	31-330 ng/mL	108-1145 nmol/L
34-36	45-350 ng/mL	156-902 nmol/L
36-38	48-570 ng/mL	167-1978 nmol/L
40	95-460 ng/mL	330-1596 nmol/L

Urine

Week 30 of pregnancy	6-18 mg/24 hours	21-62 µmol/24 hours
Week 35 of pregnancy	9-28 mg/24 hours	31-97 µmol/24 hours
Week 40 of pregnancy	13-42 mg/24 hours	45-146 µmol/24 hours
Females, nonpregnant	0-54 mg/24 hours	0-188 µmol/24 hours
Males	0.3-2.4 mg/24 hours	1.0-8.2 µmol/24 hours
Children	0.3-2.4 mg/24 hours	1.0-8.2 µmol/24 hours
Panic level	4 ng/mL or 40% below the average of two prior values	

Increased. Feminizing tumors, true precocious puberty, liver cirrhosis, and multiple pregnancy. Drugs include oxytocin.

Decreased. Anencephaly, abortion, anemia, choriocarcinoma, diabetes mellitus, erythroblastosis fetalis, fetal adrenal aplasia, fetal Down syndrome, fetal growth retardation, fetal encephalopathy, gynecomastia, hepatic disease, hemoglobinopathy, hydatidiform mole, intrauterine death, menopause, neural tube defects, postmaturity, preeclampsia, Rh immunization, and Smith-Lemli-Opitz syndrome. Drugs include betamethasone, corticosteroids (large doses), dexamethasone, diuretics, glutethimide, estrogens, mandelamine,

meprobamate, penicillins, phenazopyridine, phenolphthalein, probenecid, and senna (*Cassia* species). Herbs or natural remedies include cascara sagrada (*Rhamnus purshiana*).

Description. Estriol is an estrogen synthesized in the placenta by a fetal hormone. Serum estriol levels are used to evaluate fetal and placental function for abnormalities such as growth retardation and fetal death. Low serum estriol has been associated with increased risk for X-linked ichthyosis. Estriol levels must be evaluated in consideration of the number of weeks gestation because levels vary during pregnancy. Because serum levels fluctuate throughout the day, serial levels over time are used to evaluate the status of the fetus and the placenta.

Professional Considerations
1. Consent form NOT required.
2. Preparation:
   A. Tube: Red topped, red/gray topped, or gold topped.
   B. Obtain a clean, 3-L container without preservative.
3. Procedure:
   A. *Serum test:* Draw a 5-mL blood sample.
   B. *Urine test:*
      i. Discard the first morning urine specimen.
      ii. Begin to time a 24-hour urine collection.
      iii. Save all the urine voided for 24 hours in a clean, 3-L container. Document the quantity of urine output during the specimen collection period. Include the urine voided at the end of the 24-hour period.
4. Postprocedure care:
   A. Mix the 24-hour urine specimen gently and obtain a 100-mL aliquot to send to the laboratory.
5. Client and family teaching:
   A. Discard the first specimen of the morning, and then save all the urine voided in a 24-hour period and urinate before defecation to avoid loss of urine. If any urine is accidentally discarded, discard the entire specimen and restart the collection the next day.

B. Results are normally available within 24 hours after completion of the urine collection.
C. Refer pregnant clients with low serum estriol levels for genetic counseling.
6. Factors that affect results:
   A. Draw serum levels at the same time of the day for each sample.
   B. Reject the specimen if the client has had a radioactive scan within 48 hours.
   C. Levels are higher in Asian and black women compared to Hispanic and white women.
7. Other data:
   A. Single values are not so meaningful as a trend in a series of measurements.
   B. Reductions of estradiol by decreasing dietary fat intake by 12% decreases the risk for breast cancer in women.

ESTROGEN RECEPTOR ASSAY, TISSUE SPECIMEN
(see Estradiol receptor and progesterone receptor in breast cancer, Diagnostic)

ESTROGENS, NONPREGNANT, 24-HOUR URINE
(see Estrogens, Serum and 24-Hour urine)

ESTROGENS, SERUM, AND 24-HOUR URINE

Norm:

	TOTAL ESTROGENS	SI UNITS
Serum	**pg/mL**	**ng/L**
Premenopausal females	60-400	60-400
Postmenopausal females	<130	<130
Males	10-130	10-130
Children	<25	<25
24-Hour Urine *Adult Females*	**g/g Creatinine**	**mg/mol Creatinine**
Follicular phase	7-65	0.79-7.35
Midcycle peak	32-104	3.62-11.75
Luteal phase	8-135	0.90-15.26
Adult Males	4-23	0.45-2.60

Increased in Serum. Amenorrhea, fibrocystic disease, feminizing tumors, corpus luteum cyst, hypogonadism in males, and Stein-Leventhal syndrome. Drugs include, chlortetracycline, estrogens, levodopa, oral contraceptives, phenothiazines, tetracyclines, and vitamins. Herbs or natural remedies include cascara sagrada (*Rhamnus purshiana*).

Increased in Urine. Adrenocortical tumor, HIV-positive males, ovarian or testicular tumors, and virilization. Drugs include acetazolamide (in pregnant women), cascara, clomiphene, chlortetracycline, corticotropin, hydrochlorothiazide (in pregnant women), levodopa, phenothiazines, testosterone, tetracyclines, and vitamins.

Decreased in Serum. Amenorrhea, anorexia nervosa, dysmenorrhea, infertility, menopause, menorrhagia, menstruation, metrorrhagia, osteoporosis, psychogenic stress, and Turner syndrome. Drugs include acetazolamide, glucose, hydrochlorothiazide, phenothiazines, tetracyclines, and vitamins. Herbs or natural remedies include cascara sagrada (*Rhamnus purshiana*).

Decreased in Urine. Amenorrhea, breast cancer risk factor, menopause, ovarian dysfunction, and Simmonds' disease. Drugs include acetazolamide, glucose, hydrochlorothiazide, phenothiazines, senna, tetracyclines, and vitamins. Herbs or natural remedies include cascara sagrada (*Rhamnus purshiana*).

Description. Estrogen is a hormone produced in the ovaries, testes, placenta, and adrenals that influences the development and maintenance of the female sex organs. Estrogen levels in females fluctuate in predictable amounts throughout the menstrual cycle, with the highest amounts produced during ovulation and the levels greatly decreasing during the latter phase of the cycle. Decreasing estrogen and rising progesterone levels signal the body that pregnancy has not occurred and leads to sloughing of the uterine lining. Serum and urine tests may be performed independently.

Professional Considerations
1. Consent form NOT required.

2. Preparation:
   A. Tube: Red topped, red/gray topped, or gold topped. Also obtain ice.
   B. Obtain urine collection bottle containing 10-mL glacial acetic acid or boric acid.
   C. Screen client for the use of herbal preparations or natural remedies such as ginseng.
3. Procedure:
   A. *Serum:* Draw a 1.5-mL blood sample. Place the specimen on ice.
   B. Discard the first morning void, and then collect all the urine voided in a refrigerated, 24-hour urine bottle containing glacial acetic acid. For catheterized clients, keep the drainage bag on ice and empty the bag into a refrigerated collection container hourly.
4. Postprocedure care:
   A. Write the client's age, sex, and current menstrual cycle phase on the laboratory requisition. For urine samples, document the quantity of urine output and the ending time for the 24-hour collection on the laboratory requisition.
   B. Place the blood or urine specimen on ice. Deliver to the laboratory within 30 minutes after the collection has been completed.
5. Client and family teaching:
   A. Discard the first specimen of the morning, and then save all the urine voided in a 24-hour period and urinate before defecation to avoid loss of urine. If any urine is accidentally discarded, discard the entire specimen and restart the collection the next day.
   B. Results are normally available within 48 hours.
6. Factors that affect results:
   A. Reject the specimen if the client has received a radioactive scan within the last 48 hours.
   B. An incomplete urine specimen may cause falsely decreased results.
   C. Herbs and natural remedies with additive effects to estrogens include ginseng.
7. Other data:
   A. Do NOT use this test in pregnant females or to assess fetal well-

being because it does not measure estriol.

B. Risk for coronary artery disease is decreased by exposure to estrogen.

C. Ingestion of alcohol by postmenopausal women who are on estrogen replacement therapy may increase their risk for breast cancer.

ETHANOL
(see Alcohol, Blood; Toxicology, Volatiles group by GLC, Blood or Urine)

ETHCHLORVYNOL, BLOOD

Norm. Negative.

		SI UNITS
Therapeutic level	5-10 µg/mL	35-70 µmol/L
Toxic level	>20 µg/mL	>138 µmol/L
	or >40 mg/L	or >280 mmol/L
Panic level	>25 µg/mL	>175 µmol/L

Panic Level Symptoms and Treatment

Symptoms. Nausea, vomiting, hypotension, bradycardia, respiratory depression, hypothermia, coma.

Treatment:
Note: Treatment choice(s) depend on client history and condition and episode history.
Monitor for noncardiogenic pulmonary edema.
Protect airway and support breathing.
Perform gastric lavage with warm tap water or normal saline if the client is treated soon after ingestion.
Give activated charcoal.
Seizure precautions: use phenobarbital or diazepam or restart ethchlorvynol, and then taper off drug if convulsions occur.
Administer resin or charcoal hemoperfusion if comatose.
(Note: Hemodialysis and peritoneal dialysis will NOT remove ethchlorvynol from the bloodstream.)
Provide cardiovascular and respiratory support of symptoms.

Usage. Drug abuse and overdose.

Description. A nonbarbiturate sedative-hypnotic drug that is absorbed through the gastrointestinal tract and metabolized in the liver, with a half-life

of up to 20 hours. Duration of action is 5 hours.

Professional Considerations
1. Consent form NOT required.
2. **Preparation:**
   A. Tube: Red topped or red/gray top.
   B. Do NOT use alcohol wipe at venipuncture site.
   C. The specimen MAY be drawn during hemodialysis.
3. **Procedure:**
   A. Cleanse the site with povidone-iodine solution, and then draw a 5-mL blood sample.
4. **Postprocedure care:**
   A. Monitor cardiovascular, respiratory, and neurologic status for symptoms of overdose and provide support as needed.
5. **Client and family teaching:**
   A. For accidental overdose, teach client and family about proper dosing and side effects as well as interactions of the drug with alcohol and the signs for which medical attention must be sought.
   B. For intentional overdose, refer the client and family for psychiatric counseling and crisis intervention.
   C. Referrals to appropriate rehabilitation centers and therapeutic community programs should be offered to all addicted clients who may be interested.
   D. If activated charcoal was given for elevated levels, the client should drink 4-6 glasses of water

each day for 2 days to prevent constipation. The activated charcoal will cause stools to be black for a few days.

6. **Factors that affect results:**
   A. Peak blood levels occur 1.0-1.5 hours after ingestion.
   B. The refrigerated specimen remains stable at 0-6° C for several days.

7. **Other data:**
   A. Sedative effects are potentiated by alcohol.

B. Ethchlorvynol interacts with monoamine oxidase (MAO) inhibitors, tricyclic antidepressants, alcohol, barbiturates, central nervous system depressants, and oral anticoagulants. Transient delirium reported when used concurrently with amitriptyline.

C. Intravenous use may precipitate pleural effusion.

ETHOSUXIMIDE, BLOOD

Norm. Negative.

	TROUGH	**SI UNITS**
Therapeutic level	40-110 µg/mL	280-780 µmol/L
Panic level	>200 µg/mL	>1420 µmol/L

Overdose Symptoms and Treatment

Symptoms. Nausea, vomiting, lethargy.

Treatment:
Note: Treatment choice(s) depend on client history and condition and episode history.
Give activated charcoal slurry.
Administer saline cathartic unless client has an ileus.
Give sorbitol cathartic.
Perform gastric lavage if soon after ingestion.
Protect airway and support breathing.
Administer neurologic checks every hour.
Forced diuresis is not helpful.
Hemodialysis WILL remove ethosuximide.

Increased. Drug abuse and overdose.

Decreased. Absence of ethosuximide use and convulsions during ethosuximide use.

Description. Anticonvulsant used in the treatment of petit mal seizures. Depresses motor cortex and elevates central nervous system threshold to stimuli. Absorbed from the gastrointestinal (GI) tract. Half-life of 40-60 hours in adults and 30-50 hours in children. Metabolized by the liver and excreted slowly in the urine. Steady-state levels are reached after 8-12 days in adults and 6-10 days in children.

Professional Considerations
1. Consent form NOT required.
2. **Preparation:**
   A. Tube: Green topped, red/gray topped, or gold topped.
   B. Do NOT draw during hemodialysis.
3. **Procedure:**
   A. Draw a 1-mL TROUGH blood sample.
   B. Obtain serial measurements at the same time each day.
4. **Postprocedure care:**
   A. Monitor for overdose symptoms and provide support as needed.
5. **Client and family teaching:**
   A. Results are normally available within 24 hours.
   B. Seek medical attention if early warning signs of drug overdose are noted: fatigue, drowsiness, confusion, difficulty waking up, slurred speech, unsteady gait.
   C. If activated charcoal was given for elevated levels, the client should drink 4-6 glasses of water each day for 2 days to prevent constipation. The activated charcoal will cause stools to be black for a few days.
   D. Refer clients with overdose for crisis intervention.
   E. Referrals to appropriate rehabilitation centers and therapeutic community programs should be offered to all addicted clients who may be interested.

6. **Factors that affect results:**
   A. Peak levels occur 2-4 hours after dose.
7. **Other data:**
   A. Adverse effects include gastric disturbances, lymphadenopathy, psychiatric disorders, and a lupus-like syndrome.
   B. Neurotoxic interaction with valproate is possible.
   C. Hypersensitivity to succinimides may cause adverse reactions, including pancytopenia, dizziness, myopia, vaginal bleeding, urticaria, swelling of tongue, and hirsutism.
   D. Research, using rats, shows that estrogen increases EEG episodes of seizures.

ETHYL ALCOHOL
(see Alcohol, Blood or toxicology, Volatiles group by GLC, Blood or Urine)

ETHYLENE GLYCOL, SERUM AND URINE

Norm. Serum and urine: Negative.

		SI UNITS
Serum panic level	>2 mEq/L	>2 mmol/L
Serum lethal level	>30 mEq/L	>30 mmol/L

Poisoning Symptoms and Treatment

Symptoms:
1. Within the first hour, the client appears drunk, followed by coma with convulsions.
2. First 12 hours, hypertension and an elevation in leukocytes occur.
3. Within 12-24 hours, cardiopulmonary failure, acute renal failure, and metabolic acidosis (with increased anion gap and osmolal gap) occur. Other symptoms include abdominal pain and tetany.

Treatment:
Note: Treatment choice(s) depend on client history and condition and episode history.
Hemodialysis is the treatment of choice. Both hemodialysis and peritoneal dialysis WILL remove ethylene glycol.
Fomepizole has been found to be effective as an antidote to ethylene glycol and can eliminate the need for dialysis, except in clients with renal problems or levels above 50 mg/dL. Administer IV loading dose of 15 mg/kg followed by maintenance dose of 10 mg/kg every 12 hours × 4, followed by 15 mg/kg every 12 hours to reach therapeutic fomepizole level >8.6 mg/mL. Continue until ethylene glycol concentrations are undetectable. Dosing frequency must be increased if dialysis is also used.
Monitor for hyperventilation secondary to acidemia.

Usage. Evaluation for ethylene glycol poisoning; monitoring response to treatment for ethylene glycol poisoning.

Description. Ethylene glycol is a compound contained in antifreeze and other automotive products that, when ingested and metabolized, causes toxicity to the body. After ingestion, oxalic acid is excreted by the kidneys, causing oxalate crystals in the urine, acidosis, tetany, and renal failure. The minimum lethal dose is approximately 100 mL, but any amount ingested may produce toxic symptoms. Half-life is 3 hours without treatment, 2.5 hours with dialysis, and 17 hours with concomitant orally administered ethyl alcohol.

Professional Considerations
1. Consent form NOT required.
2. **Preparation:**
   A. *Serum:* Tube: Gray topped, red/gray topped, or gold topped.
   B. Do NOT draw during hemodialysis.

C. *Urine:* Obtain a clean specimen container.
3. **Procedure:**
   A. *Serum:* Draw a 1-mL blood sample.
   B. *Urine:* Obtain a random urine sample in a clean container.
4. **Postprocedure care:**
   A. Store the blood or urine sample at 4° C.
   B. Observe for seizures or coma, and assess for renal failure.
5. **Client and family teaching:**
   A. Explain the possible side effects of ethylene glycol ingestion (described above) and that the client will require intensive care monitoring for up to 48 hours or longer.
6. **Factors that affect results:**
   A. An uncooperative client may require catheterization to obtain a urine specimen.
   B. Ethylene glycol is rapidly metabolized; therefore, levels may not be obtainable. In this case, examination of urine under a Wood's lamp may reveal oxalate crystals characteristic of the metabolism of ethylene glycol.
7. **Other data:**
   A. Ethyl glycol can also be detected in gastric secretions.
   B. Highest known concentration that a person survived is 1889 mg/dL.

ETOH, BLOOD
(see Alcohol, Blood or toxicology, Volatiles group by GLC, Blood or Urine)

EUGLOBULIN CLOT LYSIS, BLOOD

Norm. Lysis in 1.5-4 hours.
Panic level: 100% lysis in 1 hour.

Panic Level Symptoms and Treatment

Symptoms. Bleeding from wounds, phlebotomy sites, or intracerebrally, or all three.

Treatment:
Note: Treatment choice(s) depend on client history and condition and episode history.

Discontinue any drugs (listed below) contributing to shortened lysis time.
Place the client on bleeding precautions.
Monitor neurologic status for signs of intracerebral bleeding.

Usage. Urokinase and streptokinase monitoring.

Increased or Longer Lysis Time. Diabetes mellitus type 2 in women, dialysis (hemodialysis, continuous ambulatory peritoneal), polycystic ovary syndrome.

Decreased or Shortened Lysis Time. Disseminated intravascular coagulation (DIC), fibrinolysis, hemorrhage, pancreatic or pulmonary surgery, and pyrogen reactions. Drugs include asparaginase, clofibrate, dextran, epinephrine, misoprostol, streptokinase, and urokinase.

Description. Euglobulin clot lysis gives a measure of fibrinogen activity by measuring plasminogen and plasminogen activator, which are proteins important in preventing fibrin clot formations.

Professional Considerations
1. Consent form NOT required.
2. **Preparation:**
   A. Tube: 2.7-mL blue topped or a 4.5-mL blue topped and a control tube and a waste tube or syringe. Also obtain a container of ice.
   B. Schedule the test with the laboratory before drawing blood because the sample must be centrifuged within 30 minutes of obtaining it.
3. **Procedure:**
   A. Avoid taking the sample from an extremity into which intravenous fluids are infusing.
   B. Withdraw 2 mL of blood into a syringe or vacuum tube. Remove the syringe or tube, leaving the needle in place. Attach a second syringe, and draw two blood samples, one in a citrated blue-topped tube and the other in a control tube. The sample quantity should be 2.4 mL for a 2.7-mL tube and 4.0 mL for a 4.5-mL tube. Place the specimens immediately into a container of ice.
4. **Postprocedure care:**
   A. Deliver specimens to the laboratory for processing within 30 minutes.

5. **Client and family teaching:**
   A. Avoid strenuous physical activity for 1 hour before sampling.
6. **Factors that affect results:**
   A. Aminocaproic acid (Amicar) neutralizes urokinase and streptokinase.
   B. Lysis time may be shortened in clients who have exercised within the last hour.
   C. Venipuncture that is rough, including pumping the fist or massaging the vein, may shorten lysis time.
7. **Other data:**
   A. Heparin does not affect results.
   B. See also *Diluted whole blood clot lysis, Blood.*

EUS, DIAGNOSTIC
(*see Endoscopic ultrasonography, Diagnostic*)

EXACTECH, DIAGNOSTIC
(*see Glucose monitoring machines, Diagnostic*)

EXCRETION FRACTION OF FILTERED SODIUM, BLOOD AND URINE

Norm. 1-2 excretion fraction (F).

Increased. Acute tubular necrosis, renal failure, uremia, and urinary obstruction. Drugs include diuretics.

Decreased. Azotemia, glomerulonephritis, and hepatorenal syndrome.

Description. A sensitive and specific test for acute tubular necrosis that requires assays of both urine and serum sodium and creatinine. The excretion fraction is calculated by the equation:

Excretion fraction (F) =
[(Urine sodium/Plasma sodium) × (Plasma creatinine/Urine creatinine)] × 100

Professional Considerations
1. Consent form NOT required.
2. **Preparation:**
   A. Tube: Red topped, red/gray topped, or gold topped. Also obtain a urine cup.
   B. List diuretics on the laboratory requisition.

3. **Procedure:**
   A. Obtain a 10-mL random urine specimen.
   B. Draw a 7-mL blood sample.
4. **Postprocedure care:**
   A. Send specimens to the laboratory within 2 hours.
5. **Client and family teaching:**
   A. Results are normally available within 12 hours.
6. **Factors that affect results:**
   A. See individual tests (*Sodium, Plasma, Urine; Creatinine, Plasma, Urine*).
7. **Other data:**
   A. Timed specimens are not required.

EXCRETORY UROGRAPHY
(*see Intravenous pyelography, Diagnostic*)

EXERCISE STRESS TEST
(*see Stress/exercise test*)

EXOPHTHALMOMETRY TEST, DIAGNOSTIC

Norm. 12-20 mm. Eyes differ by <3 mm.

Usage. Cellulitis, enophthalmos, exophthalmos, periostitis, retinoblastoma, thyroid disease, tumors of the eye, and xanthomatosis.

Description. Measures the amount of forward protrusion of the eye by means of an exophthalmometer. The exophthalmometer is a horizontal, calibrated bar with movable 45-degree mirrors on both sides.

Professional Considerations
1. Consent form NOT required.
2. **Preparation:**
   A. If previous examination results are available, calibrate the bar to the baseline reading.
3. **Procedure:**
   A. Position client upright, facing the examiner, with eyes on the same level.
   B. Hold the horizontal bar of the exophthalmometer in front of the client's eyes and parallel to the floor.
   C. Move the two concave carriers against the lateral orbital margins and record the reading.

D. Measure each eye separately.
E. Have the client fixate his or her right eye on your left eye. Using the locked inclined mirrors, superimpose the apex of the right cornea on the scale, and record the reading.
F. Repeat the procedure with the client's left eye fixated on the examiner's right eye and record the reading.
4. **Postprocedure care:**
A. For abnormal results, refer to a specialist.
5. **Client and family teaching:**
A. The test is painless.
6. **Factors that affect results:**
A. Failure to set calibrated bar at baseline value.
7. **Other data:**
A. Use of steroids may contribute to exophthalmos.

EXTRACTABLE NUCLEAR ANTIGEN (ENA COMPLEX), SERUM

(see Anti-SM test, Diagnostic; Anti-RNP test, Diagnostic)

EYE AND ORBIT ULTRASONOGRAPHY (EYE AND ORBIT ECHOGRAMS, EYE AND ORBIT SONOGRAMS), DIAGNOSTIC

Norm. Negative for foreign body, cyst, inflammation, tumor, retinal detachment, or optic nerve atrophy. Orbit is of proper size, shape, and concavity.

Usage. Alternative to direct ophthalmoscopic visualization of the interior of the eye when cataract, fundal opacity, or vitreous hemorrhage is present; detection of intraocular foreign body or tumor; detection of retrobulbar optic nerve, optic nerve atrophy, or optic nerve tumor; differentiation of intraocular melanoma; eye measurement before lens implant; and evaluation of fundal abnormalities, intactness of retina, and the vitreous humor.

Description. Evaluation of the eye and orbit by the creation of an oscilloscopic picture from the echoes of high-frequency sound waves passing over the eye and eyelid (acoustic imaging). The time required for the ultrasonic beam to be reflected back to the transducer from differing densities of tissue is converted by a computer to an electrical impulse displayed on an oscilloscopic screen to create both a linear waveform and a two-dimensional dot-pattern picture of the structures. The B-scan mode is used to evaluate the optic disc, and the A-scan mode is used to evaluate optic nerve disease. Water immersion of the eye may also be used with the eye ultrasonogram to enhance images of the anterior part of the globe. The immersion of the transducer in water lifts it away from the eye, while still preventing air from obscuring the image. The transducer provides the best picture when it is at least 5-8 mm away from the structures being imaged. A newer method, ultrasound biomicroscopy, is able to provide even better images of the relationship of the structures of the anterior globe of the eye than conventional immersion ultrasonography.

Professional Considerations
1. Consent form NOT required.
2. **Preparation:**
A. A sedative or general anesthetic may be used for children being evaluated for retinoblastoma or other purposes. The child should fast from food and fluids for 4 hours if general anesthesia will be used.
B. Remove metal objects such as eyeglasses or jewelry from the client's head and neck.
C. Obtain anesthetic eye drops and conductive gel. If water immersion is to be performed, obtain an ocular drape and 0.9% sterile saline.
3. **Procedure:**
A. The client is positioned supine in bed or on a procedure table.
B. After anesthetic eye drops are administered, a transducer coated with conductive gel is slowly passed over a clear, methylcellulose eye form applied to the eye to form an airtight seal. The resulting waveform provides eye measurements and helps delineate the presence of abnormal tissue or structure.
C. The eye cup is removed and the eyelid closed. The gel-coated transducer is then slowly passed over the eyelid. A two-dimensional image of the eye and orbit are displayed on the oscilloscope.
D. *Water immersion* (sometimes performed):

i. A waterproof drape is fastened around the orbit.

ii. After anesthetic drops are instilled, the eyelid is retracted, and the eye is flooded with warm, sterile 0.9% saline.

iii. The transducer is immersed into the water and moved slowly across the eye.

iv. The client may be asked to move the eye in specific directions.

v. The water is then drained and the drape removed.

E. The procedure takes less than 30 minutes. Permanent photographs of the oscilloscopic recordings are made.

4. **Postprocedure care:**

A. Remove conductive gel from the eyelid(s) after the anesthetic effects have worn off (to prevent corneal damage).

B. If general anesthesia was administered, monitor vital signs every 15 minutes × 4, then every 30 minutes × 2, and then hourly × 4. Additional monitoring typically includes continuous ECG monitoring and pulse oximetry, with continual assessments (every 5-15 minutes) of airway, vital signs, and neurologic status until the client is lying quietly awake, is breathing independently, and responds appropriately to commands spoken in a normal tone.

5. **Client and family teaching:**

A. The procedure is noninvasive, painless, and poses no risk; it is important for you to relax the eyelid during the procedure.

B. You may hear an echo that sounds like repetitious humming or a musical note as the eye structures reflect the ultrasonic beam.

C. Avoid rubbing your eyes until the anesthetic effects have worn off (about ½ hour). Infants or small children may need to be restrained during this time.

6. **Factors that affect results:**
   A. None found.

7. **Other data:**
   A. None found.

EYE CULTURE AND SENSITIVITY, DIAGNOSTIC
(see Conjunctivae, Routine, Culture)

EYE RADIOGRAPHY (X-RAY FILM OF THE EYE), DIAGNOSTIC

Norm. Normal, no foreign bodies or masses.

Usage. Foreign bodies, fractures, and tumors.

Description. An invasive radiographic examination of the eye performed to determine the location of foreign body, tumor mass, or fracture of the orbit.

Professional Considerations
1. Consent form IS required.

Risks
Allergic reaction to contrast media (itching, hives, rash, tight feeling in the throat, shortness of breath, bronchospasm, anaphylaxis, death); renal toxicity from contrast medium.

Contraindications
Previous allergy to iodine, shellfish, or contrast media; pregnancy, if iodinated contrast medium is used (because of radioactive iodine crossing the blood-placental barrier); renal insufficiency.

Precautions
During pregnancy, risks of cumulative radiation exposure to the fetus from this and other previous or future imaging studies must be weighed against the benefits of the procedure. Although formal limits for client exposure are relative to this risk:benefit comparison, the United States Nuclear Regulatory Commission requires that the cumulative dose equivalent to an embryo/fetus from occupational exposure not exceed 0.5 rem (5 mSv). Radiation dosage to the fetus is proportional to the distance of the anatomy studied from the abdomen and decreases as pregnancy progresses. For pregnant clients, consult the Radiologist/Radiology Department to obtain estimated fetal radiation exposure from this procedure.

2. **Preparation:**
   A. Have emergency equipment readily available.

3. **Procedure:**
   A. After the client's head is immobilized, he or she is asked to stare at a fixed point.

D

E

B. Oxygen is injected between the capsule and sclera to detect a foreign body or into the muscle cone to detect masses.

C. Iodine contrast may also be injected and radiography taken within 15 minutes because of the quick absorption rate.

D. The total examination takes 40 minutes.

E. For more precise localization, magnetic resonance imaging (MRI) is used.

4. Postprocedure care:
   A. Medicate for pain if required.

5. Client and family teaching:
   A. A head immobilizer will be used because any movement will blur the radiographic images. If needed, numbing medicine will be used to minimize discomfort during the procedure.

6. Factors that affect results:
   A. Motion of the client during radiography obscures the results.
   B. Artifacts in the film holder may cast shadows.

7. Other data:
   A. Meningiomas and papillomas are tumors that usually displace the eye.
   B. Rounding of inferior rectus muscle indicates orbital fracture.

FACTOR, FITZGERALD (HIGH MOLECULAR WEIGHT KININOGEN), PLASMA

Norm. Activated partial thromboplastin time (APTT) normal or 25-35 seconds (ellagic acid [$C_{14}H_6O_8$] activation products) or 30-45 seconds (diatomaceous earth activation products) after mixing the sample with plasma known to be deficient for the Fitzgerald factor.

Increased. Congenital deficiency of the Fitzgerald factor, factor XI (sometimes), factor XII deficiency (sometimes), and high-molecular-weight kininogen deficiency. Drugs include bishydroxycoumarin, heparin calcium, heparin sodium, and warfarin sodium.

Decreased. Not applicable.

Description. Fitzgerald factor deficiency is a rare, autosomal recessive trait affecting the intrinsic pathway of coagulation that results in an abnormal APTT and coagulation time without other factor deficiencies. Fitzgerald factor interferes with plasminogen activation, immune pathway activation, and generation of the vasoactive polypeptide bradykinin. The client is asymptomatic for bleeding.

Professional Considerations

1. Consent form NOT required.
2. **Preparation:**
   A. Preschedule this test with the laboratory.
   B. Tube: 2.7- or 4.5-mL blue topped. Also obtain ice.
3. **Procedure:**
   A. Withdraw 2 mL of blood into a syringe or vacuum tube. Remove the syringe or tube, leaving the needle in place. Attach a second syringe, and draw a 2.4-mL sample in a 2.7-mL tube or a 4.0-mL sample in a 4.5-mL tube. Place the specimens immediately in a container of ice.
   B. Gently tilt the tube five or six times to mix.
4. **Postprocedure care:**
   A. Place the specimen on ice immediately.
   B. Write the collection time on the laboratory requisition.
   C. Transport the specimen to the laboratory immediately, discard the ice, and refrigerate the specimen. The sample should be centrifuged and refrigerated within 1 hour of collection. Freeze the plasma if the test will not be performed within 24 hours of specimen collection.
5. **Client and family teaching:**
   A. The client should not have warfarin therapy for 2 weeks or heparin therapy for 2 days before the test.
   B. Results are normally available within 24 hours.
6. **Factors that affect results:**
   A. Failure to discard the first 1-2 mL of blood may result in specimen contamination with tissue thromboplastin.
   B. Reject hemolyzed or clotted specimens, specimens not completely mixed, tubes partially filled with blood, specimens diluted or contaminated with heparin, specimens not placed on ice, or specimens received more than 1 hour after collection.

7. **Other data:**
   A. Compare results to prior PTT and APTT.
   B. See *Activated partial thromboplastin time and partial thromboplastin time, Plasma; Activated partial thromboplastin substitution test.*

FACTOR, FLETCHER (PREKALLIKREIN), PLASMA

Norm. Activated partial thromboplastin time (APTT) normal or 30-45 seconds (diatomaceous earths activator) after mixing the sample with plasma known to be deficient for the Fletcher factor.

Increased. Fletcher factor deficiency, hepatic disease, prekallikrein deficiency, and uremia. Drugs include bishydroxycoumarin, heparin sodium, heparin calcium, and warfarin sodium.

Decreased. Not applicable.

Description. Rare condition of prolonged APTT and prekallikrein deficiency. The APTT shortens only after prolonged contact activation. The deficiency is believed to be inherited as an autosomal recessive trait in which the client is asymptomatic for bleeding. Fletcher factor is believed to function as a necessary component in the activation of factor XI and XII. To detect a deficient Fletcher factor, an APTT test is conducted on the sample and then repeated with a diatomaceous earth activator and lengthened incubation time from 3 to 10 minutes. The deficiency is suggested if the second APTT test is corrected.

Professional Considerations
1. Consent form NOT required.
2. **Preparation:**
   A. Preschedule this test with the laboratory.
   B. Tube: 2.7-mL or 4.5-mL blue topped. Also obtain ice.
3. **Procedure:**
   A. Withdraw 2 mL of blood into a syringe or vacuum tube. Remove the syringe or tube, leaving the needle in place. Attach a second syringe, and draw a 2.4-mL sample in a 2.7-mL tube or a 4.0-mL sample in a 4.5-mL tube. Place the specimens immediately in a container of ice.
   B. Gently tilt the tube five or six times to mix.
4. **Postprocedure care:**
   A. Place the specimen on ice immediately.
   B. Write the collection time on the laboratory requisition.
   C. Transport the specimen to the laboratory immediately, discard the ice, and refrigerate the specimen. The sample should be centrifuged and refrigerated within 1 hour of collection. Freeze the plasma if the test will not be performed within 24 hours of collection.
5. **Client and family teaching:**
   A. The client should not have warfarin therapy for 2 weeks or heparin therapy for 2 days before the test.
   B. Results are normally available within 24 hours.
6. **Factors that affect results:**
   A. Failure to discard the first 1-2 mL of blood may result in specimen contamination with tissue thromboplastin.
   B. Reject hemolyzed or clotted specimens, specimens not completely mixed, tubes partially filled with blood, specimens not received on ice, specimens diluted or contaminated with heparin, or specimens received more than 1 hour after collection.
   C. Ellagic acid activation products should not be used for this test.
7. **Other data:**
   A. Compare results to prior PT and APTT.
   B. See *Activated partial thromboplastin time and partial thromboplastin time, Plasma; Activated partial thromboplastin substitution test.*

FACTOR I, PLASMA
(see Fibrinogen, Plasma)

FACTOR II (PROTHROMBIN), BLOOD
(see Prothrombin time, Blood)

FACTOR V (LABILE FACTOR, PROACCELERIN, AC-GLOBULIN), BLOOD

Norm. 50%-150% of normal (control sample) activity. Half-life is 12-36 hours.

Increased. Not applicable.

Decreased. Alpha-globulin deficiency, disseminated intravascular coagulation, factor V deficiency, factor V inhibitors (circulating), fibrinogenolysis, HELLP syndrome, hepatic disease, labile factor deficiency, leukemia (acute), parahemophilia, postoperatively, proaccelerin deficiency, and radioactive phosphorus therapy. Drugs include anisindione, bishydroxycoumarin, carbimazole, dicumarol, phenprocoumon, and warfarin sodium.

Description. Factor V is a vitamin K–dependent glycoprotein synthesized in the liver. It is part of the prothrombin-converting complex that functions in the extrinsic pathway of blood clotting. Specifically it is a cofactor that accelerates the conversion of prothrombin to thrombin. Factor V deficiency is an inherited, autosomal recessive condition that occurs with equal frequency in men and women. The symptoms can be mild to severe and include bruising easily, frequent nosebleeds, menorrhagia, and prolonged bleeding after traumatic episodes, including operative and dental procedures. One performs the test by first performing a prothrombin time (PT) on the client's plasma. A factor V–deficient plasma substrate is then mixed with the client's plasma and the degree of correction in the PT is determined and compared to the degree of correction obtained by normal plasma. The *Factor V Leiden mutation*, newly identified in the 1990s, is a molecular defect in factor V, which makes it resistant to anticoagulant activation by protein C. The Leiden mutation is identified by performing an activated protein C resistance test and confirming an abnormal result with DNA evaluation for the Leiden mutation. See *Protein C, Blood.*

Professional Considerations
1. Consent form NOT required.
2. **Preparation:**
   A. Preschedule this test with the laboratory.
   B. Tube: 2.7- or 4.5-mL blue topped. Also obtain ice.
3. **Procedure:**
   A. Withdraw 2 mL of blood into a syringe or vacuum tube. Remove the syringe or tube, leaving the needle in place. Attach a second syringe, and draw a 2.4-mL sample in a 2.7-mL tube or a 4.0-mL sample in a 4.5-mL tube. Place the specimens immediately in a container of ice.
   B. Gently tilt the tube five or six times to mix.
4. **Postprocedure care:**
   A. Place the specimen on ice immediately.
   B. For clients with coagulopathy, hold pressure over the sampling site for at least 5 minutes and observe the site closely for development of a hematoma.
   C. Write the collection time on the laboratory requisition.
   D. Take the iced specimen to the laboratory immediately because factor V is labile in drawn blood samples.
5. **Client and family teaching:**
   A. The client should not have warfarin therapy for 2 weeks or heparin therapy for 2 days before the test.
   B. Results are normally available within 24 hours.
   C. Seek medical attention for signs of bleeding (that is, hematoma, bleeding of gums, wounds, petechiae, confusion, changing level of consciousness).
6. **Factors that affect results:**
   A. Failure to discard the first 1-2 mL of blood may result in specimen contamination with tissue thromboplastin.
   B. Reject hemolyzed or clotted specimens, specimens not completely mixed, tubes partially filled with blood, specimens not on ice, specimens diluted or contaminated with heparin, or specimens received more than 2 hours after collection.
   C. Some drugs that may cause shortened prothrombin time include meprobamate, barbiturates, ethchlorvynol, glutethimide, oral contraceptives, and vitamin K.
   D. Some drugs that may cause prolonged prothrombin time include antibiotics, chloral hydrate, hydroxyzine hydrochloride, hydroxyzine pamoate, iothiouracil, methylthiouracil, phenylbutazone, phenyramidol, phosphorus (toxicity), propylthiouracil, salicylates, sulfonamides, tolbutamide, and vitamin A.

7. **Other data:**
   A. The coagulation-factor roman numerals identify order of discovery rather than their order in the stages of clot formation.
   B. Platelet transfusion is a common treatment.
   C. See *Activated partial thromboplastin time and partial thromboplastin time, Plasma; Activated partial thromboplastin substitution test.*

FACTOR VII (STABLE FACTOR, PROCONVERTIN, AUTOPROTHROMBIN I), BLOOD

Norm. 50%-150% of normal (control sample) activity. Half-life is 6 hours.

Increased. Pregnancy (late) and thromboembolism, uremia. Drugs include oral contraceptives.

Decreased. Factor VII deficiency, hemorrhagic disease of the newborn, hepatic carcinoma, hepatitis, jaundice (obstructive), kwashiorkor, menstrual cycle, proconvertin autoprothrombin I deficiency, stable factor deficiency, and vitamin K deficiency. Drugs include anisindione, bishydroxycoumarin, dicumarol (dicoumarin), metformin, phenprocoumon, and warfarin sodium. Diet including olive oil.

Description. Factor VII is a vitamin K–dependent beta globulin synthesized in the liver. It is activated in the extrinsic pathway during blood clotting and in turn activates tissue thromboplastins, with excess amounts of factor VII present in serum and plasma when clotting is completed. Both forms of the rare factor VII deficiency are autosomal recessive and affect both males and females. Bleeding symptoms may be severe, including cerebral hemorrhage. One performs the test by first performing a prothrombin time (PT) on the client's plasma. A factor VII–deficient plasma substrate is then mixed with the client's plasma, and the degree of correction in the PT is determined and compared to the degree of correction obtained by normal plasma.

Professional Considerations
1. Consent form NOT required.
2. **Preparation:**
   A. Preschedule this test with the laboratory.
   B. Tube: 2.7-mL or 4.5-mL blue topped.
3. **Procedure:**
   A. Withdraw 2 mL of blood into a syringe or vacuum tube. Remove the syringe or tube, leaving the needle in place. Attach a second syringe, and draw a 2.4-mL sample in a 2.7-mL tube or a 4.0-mL sample in a 4.5-mL tube. Place the specimen immediately in a container of ice.
   B. Gently tilt the tube five or six times to mix.
4. **Postprocedure care:**
   A. For clients with coagulopathy, hold pressure over the sampling site for at least 5 minutes and observe the site closely for development of a hematoma.
   B. Write the collection time on the laboratory requisition.
   C. Transport the specimen to the laboratory immediately. Centrifuge and leave the specimens at room temperature.
5. **Client and family teaching:**
   A. The client should not have coumarin therapy for 2 weeks before the test.
   B. Results are normally available within 24 hours.
   C. Seek medical attention for signs of bleeding (that is, hematoma, bleeding of gums, wounds, petechiae, confusion, changing level of consciousness).
6. **Factors that affect results:**
   A. Failure to discard the first 1-2-mL of blood may result in specimen contamination with tissue thromboplastin.
   B. Reject hemolyzed or clotted specimens, specimens not completely mixed, tubes partially filled with blood, specimens not refrigerated, or specimens received more than 2 hours after collection.
   C. Cold temperatures activate factor VII. Do not refrigerate or freeze the plasma.
   D. Drugs that may cause shortened PT include barbiturates, ethchlorvynol, glutethimide (Dorimide), meprobamate, oral contraceptives, and vitamin K.
   E. Some drugs that may cause prolonged prothrombin time include antibiotics, chloral hydrate, hydroxyzine hydrochloride, hydroxy-

zine pamoate, iothiouracil, methyl-thiouracil, phenylbutazone, phosphorus (toxicity), propylthiouracil, salicylates, tolbutamide, and vitamin A.
7. Other data:
   A. After separation of plasma, factor VII is stable for 4 days at 25°-37° C.
   B. The coagulation-factor roman numerals identify order of discovery rather than their order in the stages of clot formation.
   C. See *Prothrombin time.*

FACTOR VIII (ANTIHEMOPHILIA FACTOR, AHF), BLOOD

Norm. 50%-150% of normal (control sample) activity.

Mild deficiency	5%-25%
Moderately severe deficiency	1%-5%
Severe deficiency	<1%
Von Willebrand's disease	1%-50%
Plasma level	≈100 µg/L

Increased. Coronary artery disease, exercise, hyperthyroidism, hypoglycemia, macroglobulinemia, myocardial infarction (factor VIII antigen), pregnancy, and surgery. Drugs include oral contraceptives and sudden discontinuance of bishydroxycoumarin and warfarin sodium.

Decreased. Disseminated intravascular coagulation, factor VIII inhibitor (from childbirth, multiple myeloma, neoplasms, penicillin allergy, rheumatoid arthritis, or systemic lupus erythematosus), fibrinolysis, hemophilia A, and von Willebrand's disease.

Description. Factor VIII is a glycoprotein believed to be made up of two components that are easily dissociated. One component contains von Willebrand factor (vWf), newly recognized as the initiator of platelet adhesion in combination with collagen and glycoprotein Ib. The second component contains factor VIII Ag, a protein antigen, and factor VIII (measured by this test), which refers to the coagulant activity. Factor VIII is the antihemophilia (A) factor essential for thromboplastin generation in stage I of the intrinsic coagulation pathway. Factor VIII deficiency is usually transmitted as a sex-linked, reces-

sive condition. One performs this test by first performing a partial thromboplastin time (PTT) on the client's plasma. A factor VIII–deficient plasma substrate is then mixed with the client's plasma, and the degree of correction in the PTT is determined and compared to the degree of correction obtained by normal plasma.

Professional Considerations
1. Consent form NOT required.
2. Preparation:
   A. Preschedule this test with the laboratory.
   B. Tube: 2.7- or 4.5-mL blue topped. Also obtain ice.
3. Procedure:
   A. Withdraw 2 mL of blood into a syringe or vacuum tube. Remove the syringe or tube, leaving the needle in place. Attach a second syringe, and draw a 2.4-mL sample in a 2.7-mL tube or a 4.0-mL sample in a 4.5-mL tube. Place the specimen immediately in a container of ice.
   B. Gently tilt the tube five or six times to mix.
4. Postprocedure care:
   A. For clients with coagulopathy, hold pressure over sampling site for at least 5 minutes and observe site closely for development of a hematoma.
   B. Transport the specimen to the laboratory immediately, discard the ice, and refrigerate the specimen. The sample should be centrifuged and refrigerated within 1 hour. Freeze the plasma if the test will not be performed within 24 hours of collection.
5. Client and family teaching:
   A. The client should not have warfarin therapy for 2 weeks or heparin therapy for 2 days before the test.
   B. Results are normally available within 24 hours.
6. Factors that affect results:
   A. Failure to discard the first 1-2 mL of blood may result in specimen contamination with tissue thromboplastin.
   B. Reject hemolyzed or clotted specimens, specimens not completely mixed, tubes partially filled with blood, specimens not on ice, or

specimens received more than 1 hour after collection.

7. **Other data:**
    A. The coagulation-factor roman numerals identify order of discovery rather than their order in the stages of clot formation.
    B. There is currently less-than-optimal standardization of this test.
    C. Previous terminology used for factor VIII includes factor VIIIC, AHG, and AHF.
    D. Factor VIII is stable in polyvinyl-chloride bags for continuous infusion by ambulatory minipump.
    E. See also *Activated partial thromboplastin time and partial thromboplastin time, Plasma; Activated partial thromboplastin substitution test, Diagnostic.*

FACTOR VIII R:AG, BLOOD
(see von Willebrand factor antigen, Blood)

FACTOR IX (CHRISTMAS FACTOR, HEMOPHILIC FACTOR B, PLASMA THROMBOPLASTIN COMPONENT, PTC), BLOOD

Norm. 50%-150% of normal (control sample) activity. Plasma level about 4 mg/L. Half-life is 20 hours.

Increased. Drugs include hormone replacement therapy.

Decreased. Hemophilia B (Christmas disease), hepatic disease, nephrotic syndrome, and vitamin K deficiency. Drugs include anisindione, bishydroxy-coumarin, dicumarol (dicoumarin), heparin calcium, heparin sodium, phenprocoumon, and warfarin sodium.

Description. Factor IX is a vitamin K–dependent beta globulin essential in stage I of the intrinsic coagulation system as an influence on the amount of thromboplastin available. It is deficient in the inherited, sex-linked disease of hemophilia B, with bleeding symptoms similar to hemophilia A but usually milder. Factor IX deficiency may also be acquired in severe hepatic dysfunction. One performs the test by first performing a partial thromboplastin time (PTT) on the client's plasma. A factor IX–defi-

cient plasma substrate is then mixed with the client's plasma, and the degree of correction in the PTT is determined and compared to the degree of correction obtained by normal plasma.

Professional Considerations
1. Consent form NOT required.
2. **Preparation:**
    A. Preschedule this test with the laboratory.
    B. Tube: 2.7- or 4.5-mL blue topped. Also obtain ice.
3. **Procedure:**
    A. Withdraw 2 mL of blood into a syringe or vacuum tube. Remove the syringe or tube, leaving the needle in place. Attach a second syringe, and draw a 2.4-mL sample in a 2.7-mL tube or a 4.0-mL sample in a 4.5-mL tube.
    B. Gently tilt the tube five or six times to mix.
4. **Postprocedure care:**
    A. Place the specimen on ice immediately.
    B. For clients with coagulopathy, hold pressure over the sampling site for at least 5 minutes and observe the site closely for development of a hematoma.
    C. Write the collection time on the laboratory requisition.
    D. Transport the specimen to the laboratory immediately. The specimen should be centrifuged and refrigerated within 2 hours, where it will remain stable for several weeks.
5. **Client and family teaching:**
    A. The client should not have coumarin therapy for 2 weeks or heparin therapy for 2 days before the test.
    B. Results are normally available within 24 hours.
    C. Seek medical attention for signs of bleeding (that is, hematoma, bleeding of gums, wounds, petechiae, confusion, changing level of consciousness).
6. **Factors that affect results:**
    A. Reject hemolyzed or clotted specimens, specimens not completely mixed, tubes partially filled with blood, specimens not refrigerated, specimens diluted or contaminated with heparin, or specimens received more than 2 hours after collection.

F

B. Failure to discard the first 1-2 mL of blood may result in specimen contamination with tissue thromboplastin.

7. **Other data:**
   A. The coagulation-factor roman numerals identify order of discovery rather than their order in the stages of clot formation.
   B. Treatment with factor IX can result in anaphylaxis and nephrotic syndrome.
   C. See also *Activated partial thromboplastin time and partial thromboplastin time, Plasma; Activated partial thromboplastin substitution test, Diagnostic.*

FACTOR X (STUART-PROWER FACTOR), BLOOD

Norm. 50%-150% of normal (control sample) activity. Plasma level about 12 mg/L. Half-life is 30-50 hours.

Increased. Normal pregnancy. Drugs include oral contraceptives.

Decreased. Factor X deficiency, hepatic disease, and vitamin K deficiency. Drugs include anisindione, bishydroxycoumarin, dicumarol (dicoumarin), phenprocoumon, and warfarin sodium.

Description. A vitamin K–dependent proenzyme alpha globulin active in both the intrinsic and extrinsic coagulation pathways. Factor X deficiency can be inherited and also acquired in severe hepatic dysfunction and causes usually mild bleeding and prolonged prothrombin time (PT) and activated partial thromboplastin time (APTT). One performs the test by first performing a PT on the client's plasma. A factor X–deficient plasma substrate is then mixed with the client's plasma, and the degree of correction in the PT is determined and compared to the degree of correction obtained by normal plasma.

Professional Considerations
1. Consent form NOT required.
2. **Preparation:**
   A. Preschedule this test with the laboratory.
   B. Tube: 2.7- or 4.5-mL blue topped.
3. **Procedure:**
   A. Withdraw 2 mL of blood into a syringe or vacuum tube. Remove the syringe or tube, leaving the needle in place. Attach a second syringe, and draw a 2.4-mL sample in a 2.7-mL tube or a 4.0-mL sample in a 4.5-mL tube.
   B. Gently tilt the tube five or six times to mix. Place the specimen immediately in a container of ice.
4. **Postprocedure care:**
   A. For clients with coagulopathy, hold pressure over the sampling site for at least 5 minutes and observe the site closely for development of a hematoma.
   B. Transport the specimen to the laboratory immediately. The specimens should be left at room temperature, with the stopper in place until tested within 24 hours.
5. **Client and family teaching:**
   A. The client should not have coumarin therapy for 2 weeks or heparin therapy for 2 days before the test.
   B. Results are normally available within 24 hours.
   C. Seek medical attention for signs of bleeding (that is, hematoma, bleeding of gums, wounds, petechiae, confusion, changing level of consciousness).
6. **Factors that affect results:**
   A. Failure to discard the first 1-2 mL of blood may result in specimen contamination with tissue thromboplastin.
   B. Reject hemolyzed or clotted specimens, specimens not completely mixed, tubes partially filled with blood, specimens diluted or contaminated with heparin, or specimens received more than 2 hours after collection.
   C. Some drugs that may cause shortened prothrombin time include barbiturates, ethchlorvynol, glutethimide, meprobamate, oral contraceptives, and vitamin K.
   D. Some drugs that may cause prolonged prothrombin time include antibiotics, chloral hydrate, hydroxyzine hydrochloride, hydroxyzine pamoate, iothiouracil, methylthiouracil, phenylbutazone, phosphorus (toxicity), propylthiouracil, salicylates, tolbutamide, and vitamin A.
7. **Other data:**
   A. The coagulation-factor roman numerals identify order of discov-

ery rather than their order in the stages of clot formation.

B. See *Activated partial thromboplastin time and partial thromboplastin time, Plasma.*

FACTOR XI (PLASMA THROMBOPLASTIN ANTECEDENT, PTA), BLOOD

Norm. 65%-135% of normal (control sample) activity. Plasma level about 7 mg/dL. Half-life is 40-80 hours.

Increased. Not applicable.

Decreased. Congenital heart disease, factor XI deficiency (common in Ashkenazi Jews), hepatic disease, newborns (transient), pregnancy, and vitamin K deficiency. Drugs include anisindione, bishydroxycoumarin, dicumarol (dicoumarin), heparin calcium, heparin sodium, phenprocoumon, and warfarin sodium.

Description. Factor XI is a beta globulin active in stage I of the intrinsic coagulation pathway and missing, defective, or deficient in hemophilia C, an inherited, autosomal recessive deficiency that occurs in both sexes and causes prolonged coagulation evidenced by mild bleeding after surgical procedures. One performs the test by first performing a partial thromboplastin time (PTT) on the client's plasma. A factor XI–deficient plasma substrate is then mixed with the client's plasma, and the degree of correction in the PTT is determined and compared to the degree of correction obtained by normal plasma.

Professional Considerations
1. Consent form NOT required.
2. **Preparation:**
   A. Preschedule this test with the laboratory.
   B. Tube: 2.7- or 4.5-mL blue topped. Also obtain ice.
3. **Procedure:**
   A. Withdraw 2 mL of blood into a syringe or vacuum tube. Remove the syringe or tube, leaving the needle in place. Attach a second syringe, and draw a 2.4-mL sample in a 2.7-mL tube or a 4.0-mL sample in a 4.5-mL tube.
   B. Gently tilt the tube five or six times to mix.

4. **Postprocedure care:**
   A. Place the specimen on ice immediately.
   B. For clients with coagulopathy, hold pressure over the sampling site for at least 5 minutes and observe the site closely for development of a hematoma.
   C. Write the collection time on the laboratory requisition.
   D. Transport the specimen to the laboratory immediately, discard the ice, and refrigerate the specimens. The sample should be centrifuged and refrigerated within 2 hours.
5. **Client and family teaching:**
   A. The client should not have warfarin therapy for 2 weeks or heparin therapy for 2 days before the test.
   B. Results are normally available within 24 hours.
   C. Seek medical attention for signs of bleeding (that is, hematoma, bleeding of gums, wounds, petechiae, confusion, changing level of consciousness).
6. **Factors that affect results:**
   A. Failure to discard the first 1-2 mL of blood may result in specimen contamination with tissue thromboplastin.
   B. Reject hemolyzed or clotted specimens, specimens not completely mixed, tubes partially filled with blood, specimens not refrigerated, specimens diluted or contaminated with heparin, or specimens received more than 2 hours after collection.
   C. The test for factor XI deficiency must be performed on a freshly collected specimen.
   D. Freezing the specimen may falsely elevate results.
7. **Other data:**
   A. The coagulation-factor roman numerals identify order of discovery rather than their order in the stages of clot formation.
   B. Factor XI concentrate use is associated with the development of venous thromboembolic disease.
   C. See also *Activated partial thromboplastin time and partial thromboplastin time, Plasma; Activated partial thromboplastin substitution test, Diagnostic.*

F

FACTOR XII (HAGEMAN FACTOR), BLOOD

Norm. 50%-150% of normal (control sample) activity. Plasma level: 23-47 mg/mL. Half-life is 52-60 hours.

Increased. After alcohol intake or exercise, high risk for coronary heart disease.

Decreased. Factor XII deficiency, nephrotic syndrome, and pregnancy. Diet including olive oil or sunflower oil.

Description. Factor XII is a beta globulin or gamma globulin enzyme, the active form of which initiates the intrinsic coagulation pathway. Its deficiency is inherited as an autosomal recessive defect with bleeding symptoms usually absent and causes a prolonged partial thromboplastin time (PTT). One performs the test by first performing a PTT on the client's plasma. A factor XI–deficient plasma substrate is then mixed with the client's plasma, and the degree of correction in the PTT is determined and compared to the degree of correction obtained by normal plasma.

Professional Considerations
1. Consent form NOT required.
2. Preparation:
   A. Preschedule this test with the laboratory.
   B. Tube: 2.7- or 4.5-mL blue topped. Also obtain ice.
3. Procedure:
   A. Withdraw 2 mL of blood into a syringe or vacuum tube. Remove the syringe or tube, leaving the needle in place. Attach a second syringe, and draw a 2.4-mL sample in a 2.7-mL tube or a 4.0-mL sample in a 4.5-mL tube.
   B. Gently tilt the tube five or six times to mix.
4. Postprocedure care:
   A. Place the specimen on ice immediately.
   B. For clients with coagulopathy, hold pressure over the sampling site for at least 5 minutes and observe the site closely for development of a hematoma.
   C. Write the collection time on the laboratory requisition.
   D. Transport the specimen to the laboratory immediately, discard the ice, and refrigerate the specimen. The sample should be centrifuged and refrigerated within 2 hours. Freeze the plasma if the test will not be performed within 24 hours of collection.
5. Client and family teaching:
   A. The client should not have warfarin therapy for 2 weeks or heparin therapy for 2 days before the test.
   B. Results are normally available within 24 hours.
   C. Seek medical attention for signs of bleeding (that is, hematoma, bleeding of gums, wounds, petechiae, confusion, changing level of consciousness).
6. Factors that affect results:
   A. Failure to discard the first 1-2 mL of blood may result in specimen contamination with tissue thromboplastin.
   B. Reject hemolyzed or clotted specimens, specimens not completely mixed, tubes partially filled with blood, specimens not refrigerated, specimens diluted or contaminated with heparin, or specimens received more than 2 hours after collection.
7. Other data:
   A. The coagulation-factor roman numerals identify order of discovery rather than their order in the stages of clot formation.
   B. See also *Activated partial thromboplastin time and partial thromboplastin time, Plasma; Activated partial thromboplastin substitution test, Diagnostic.*

FACTOR XIII (FIBRIN-STABILIZING FACTOR, CLOT UREA SOLUBILITY), BLOOD

Norm. Clot is insoluble in 5 M urea for at least 24 hours. Half-life of factor XIII is 100 hours.

Increased. Factor XIII is more often increased than decreased in most clients.

Decreased. Agammaglobulinemia, Crohn's disease, factor XIII deficiency, hepatic disease, hyperfibrinogenemia, lead poisoning, malaria (*Plasmodium falciparum*), multiple myeloma, postoperatively, and ulcerative colitis.

Description. Factor XIII is an alpha globulin that, in its active form, stabilizes fibrin clots. Its deficiency is a rare, inherited, autosomal recessive condition that may result in symptoms ranging from abnormal bleeding from cuts and bleeding in joints to cerebral hemorrhage and infant death from umbilical cord hemorrhage. One performs the test by adding calcium chloride to the sample and clotting the mixture at 37° C for $\frac{1}{2}$ hour and then placing the clot in 5 M urea and observing hourly for clot dissolution. Clots from clients with factor XIII deficiency will dissolve within 1-3 hours.

Professional Considerations
1. Consent form NOT required.
2. **Preparation:**
   A. Tube: 2.7- or 4.5-mL blue topped. Also obtain ice.
3. **Procedure:**
   A. Withdraw 2 mL of blood into a syringe or vacuum tube. Remove the syringe or tube, leaving the needle in place. Attach a second syringe, and draw a 2.4-mL sample in a 2.7-mL tube or a 4.0-mL sample in a 4.5-mL tube. Place the specimens immediately in a container of ice.
   B. Gently tilt the tube five or six times to mix.
4. **Postprocedure care:**
   A. Place the specimens on ice immediately.
   B. For clients with coagulopathy, hold pressure over the sampling site for at least 5 minutes and observe the site closely for development of a hematoma.
   C. Write the collection time on the laboratory requisition.
   D. Transport the specimens to the laboratory immediately, discard the ice, and refrigerate the specimens.
5. **Client and family teaching:**
   A. The client should not have warfarin therapy for 2 weeks or heparin therapy for 2 days before the test.
   B. Results are normally available within 24 hours.
   C. Seek medical attention for signs of bleeding (that is, hematoma, bleeding of gums, wounds, petechiae, confusion, changing level of consciousness).

6. **Factors that affect results:**
   A. Reject hemolyzed or clotted specimens, specimens not completely mixed, tubes partially filled with blood, specimens not refrigerated, specimens diluted or contaminated with heparin, or specimens received more than 2 hours after collection.
   B. The presence of only 1% of normal levels of factor XIII is enough to provoke a normal test result.
7. **Other data:**
   A. The coagulation-factor Roman numerals identify order of discovery rather than their order in the stages of clot formation.
   B. Factor XIII is used as a treatment for scleroderma and status post coronary surgery to decrease bleeding and reduce the need for blood transfusions. It is a useful supplementation (5000 units initially, followed by 20 IU/kg body weight three times a day for up to 3 weeks) in the treatment of acute graft-versus-host disease of the bowel poststem cell transplantation. Used to prevent development of leakage syndrome and myocardial edema in children undergoing surgery for congenital heart conditions.

FAST MRI
(*see Magnetic resonance imaging, Diagnostic*)

FASTING BLOOD SUGAR
(*see Glucose, Blood*)

FAT, SEMIQUANTITATIVE, STOOL
Norm:

Neutral fat	<50 globules/HPF
Fatty acids	<100 globules/HPF

Increased. Amyloidosis, beta-lipoprotein deficiency, bile salt deficiency, blind loop syndrome, celiac disease, cystic fibrosis, diarrhea, diverticulosis, enteritis, hepatobiliary disease, hypogammaglobulinemia, increased peristalsis, ingestion of castor oil or mineral oil, intestinal fistula, lymphangiectasis, lymphoma, pancreatic disease (cancer, chronic pancreatitis, enzyme deficiency, mucoviscoidosis), postoperatively (bowel resection), sprue, Whipple's disease, and Zollinger-Ellison syndrome.

Decreased. Persons fed medium-chain-triglyceride-enriched formula.

Description. Fecal fat is measured to aid diagnosis of conditions causing poor absorption of dietary fat, resulting in steatorrhea.

Professional Considerations
1. Consent form NOT required.
2. Preparation:
   A. Obtain a clean plastic specimen container and a clean toilet-seat urine collection container.
   B. The client is to ingest 60 g of fat a day for 3-6 days.
   C. Avoid use of suppositories, oily lubricants, or mineral oil in the perianal or genital areas for 3 days before and during specimen collection.
3. Procedure:
   A. Collect 20 mL of stool in a clean glass or plastic container.
4. Postprocedure care:
   A. Cleanse the anal area.
5. Client and family teaching:
   A. Explain the need to avoid use of rectal, vaginal, or genital-area oils, lubricants, or suppositories for 3 days before the test. The client should urinate before defecating and then defecate sample into the urine collection container and transfer the stool sample to the specimen container with a wooden spatula.
   B. Results may take several days.
6. Factors that affect results:
   A. Send fresh random stool samples to the laboratory within 2 hours.
7. Other data:
   A. Bedtime laxatives may be needed for constipated clients.
   B. Some malabsorption syndromes such as tropical sprue may not show increased fecal fat.

FDP, BLOOD
(*see Fibrinogen breakdown products, Blood*)

FEBRILE AGGLUTININS, SERUM

Norm. Negative, or less than a four-fold rise in titer between acute and convalescent samples.

Normal Dilutions:

Salmonella antibody	<1:80
Brucella antibody	<1:80
Francisella antibody	<1:40
Rickettsia antibody	<1:40

Usage. Suspected infection with *Brucella*, *Francisella* (tularemia), *Proteus*, *Rickettsia* (Rocky Mountain spotted fever, typhus), *Salmonella* (paratyphoid, salmonellosis, and typhoid). Chronic granulomatous disease.

Description. Febrile agglutination tests are performed to identify the cause of febrile illnesses. Bacterial antibodies to the above organisms will agglutinate in vitro if present in the serum.

Professional Considerations
1. Consent form NOT required.
2. Preparation:
   A. Tube: Red topped, red/gray topped, or gold topped.
3. Procedure:
   A. Draw a 10-mL blood sample and label it as the acute sample. Repeat the test every 3-5 days. Draw the final sample in 10-14 days and label it as the convalescent sample.
4. Postprocedure care:
   A. Send the specimens to the laboratory immediately.
5. Client and family teaching:
   A. Two samples must be taken about 2 weeks apart to identify a trend in levels that can pinpoint the cause of the fever. The client may be treated empirically before the second sample is taken.
6. Factors that affect results:
   A. Reject hemolyzed specimens.
   B. Chronic exposure to or vaccination against the above-mentioned organisms may cause high titers.
   C. Immunosuppressed clients may be infected but have low or negative titers.
   D. Antibiotic therapy causes low initial titers.
   E. *Brucella* antigen skin tests may elevate titers.

F. Many cross-reactions are possible.

7. **Other data:**
A. Results are given in the highest dilution in which a positive reaction with the antigen occurs.
B. A blood culture for the above organisms should be performed concurrently.
C. Failure rate is 22% when tularemia is being treated with streptomycin antibiotic. Retreatment with ciprofloxacin is recommended followed by ofloxacin if needed.
D. Oculoglandular tularemia is an uncommon conjunctivitis caused by a tick or insect bite and is most common in the state of Arkansas, USA.

FECAL FAT, QUANTITATIVE, 72-HOUR, STOOL

Norm:

Adult, 60 g of fat/day diet	2-6 g/24 hours, or <20% of total solids, or 7-21 mmol/day
Adult, fat-free diet	<4 g/day
Breast-fed infant	<1 g/day
Child up to 6 years old	<2 g/day

Increased. Amyloidosis, beta-lipoprotein deficiency, bile salt deficiency, blind loop syndrome, celiac disease, Crohn's disease, cystic fibrosis, diarrhea, diverticulosis, enteritis, Graves' disease, hepatobiliary disease, hypogammaglobulinemia, increased peristalsis, ingestion of castor oil or mineral oil, intestinal fistula, lymphangiectasis, lymphoma, pancreatic disease (cancer, chronic pancreatitis, enzyme deficiency, mucoviscoidosis), postoperatively (bowel resection), sprue (celiac), Whipple's disease, and Zollinger-Ellison syndrome. Drugs include lanreotide and orlistat (Xenical). Dietary intake of >40 g of olestra per day increased levels to that of steatorrhea clients.

Description. Fecal fat is measured to aid diagnosis of conditions causing poor absorption of dietary fat resulting in steatorrhea. The value of this test is that the amount of dietary fat intake is known and used in evaluation of the results.

Professional Considerations
1. Consent form NOT required.
2. **Preparation:**
A. Obtain 500-mL clean plastic containers, dry ice, and a clean toilet-seat urine collection container.
3. **Procedure:**
A. Collect all stools, using a urine collection container in the toilet, on the fourth, fifth, and sixth days of the specified diet and place the stools in the clean plastic containers.
B. Keep the specimen containers refrigerated during the collection period.
4. **Postprocedure care:**
A. Freeze the specimens on dry ice if the testing will not be performed within 24 hours.
B. Record the date and time of each specimen collected.
5. **Client and family teaching:**
A. The client is to ingest 50- to 150-g of fat per day for 3-6 days.
B. Avoid suppositories, oily lubricants, or mineral oil in the perianal or genital areas for 3 days before and during collection.
C. Avoid contaminating the stool with urine or toilet paper.
D. Results may take several days.
6. **Factors that affect results:**
A. Reject specimens submitted in improper containers such as cartons, coffee cans, or plastic bags.
B. False-negative results are most commonly caused by failure to collect all stools.
C. False-positive results are caused by dietary ingestion of olestra found in some potato chips.
7. **Other data:**
A. Bedtime laxatives may be needed for constipated clients.
B. Some clients with malabsorption syndromes such as tropical sprue may not show increased fecal fat excretion.

FECAL LEUKOCYTES, STOOL, DIAGNOSTIC

Norm. No leukocytes present.

Usage. Determine the type of diarrhea, invasive or noninvasive, to the mucosa of the colon. If no fecal leukocytes are present in the stool specimen, an antidiarrheal medication can be given. If fecal leukocytes are present, an antidiarrheal medication should not be given. The results of this test will be readily available, whereas a culture will take several days.

Description. The presence of fecal leukocytes in the stool indicates that the cause of the diarrhea is an organism such as Shiga toxin-producing *E. coli* or process that is breaking the mucosal barrier of the colon, such as *Salmonella, Shigella, Amoeba, Campylobacter, Helicobacter,* or *Yersinia* infections, Crohn's disease, and chronic inflammatory bowel disease. Fecal leukocytes are usually not present in infectious processes that do not invade the mucosa, such as "viral enteritis," toxin-mediated diarrhea, or infections with noninvasive *E. coli.* The absence of blood and fecal leukocytes usually means that the diarrhea process is transient and can be treated symptomatically. *Clostridium difficile* may or may not be associated with leukocytes in the stool (fecal leukocyte stain is 14% sensitive and 90% specific); so, if it is suspected, a stool culture should be sent and no antidiarrheal agent given until the results are back and negative.

Professional Considerations
1. Consent form is NOT required.
2. Preparation:
   A. Obtain a stool specimen container.
3. Procedure:
   A. Instruct the client to collect a stool sample, or use a bedpan so that the sample can be obtained.
   B. Send the specimen to the laboratory.
4. Postprocedure care:
   A. Keep the rectal area as clean and as dry as possible to prevent skin breakdown.

B. If diarrhea is frequent, encourage fluids and check serum electrolytes for abnormalities.
5. Client and family teaching:
   A. Avoid contaminating the stool with toilet tissue or urine.
   B. Results are normally available within 48 hours.
6. Factors that affect results:
   A. None.
7. Other data:
   A. Stool cultures should be obtained from all clients with fecal leukocytes to differentiate acute infection from inflammatory bowel syndrome. In the absence of fecal leukocytes, stool cultures are usually negative.

FENFLURAMINE
(*see Amphetamines, Blood*)

FERRIC CHLORIDE TEST, DIAGNOSTIC

Norm. No color change when the diagnostic reagent (ferric chloride) is added to the urine.

Usage. Of value in the diagnosis of epidemic dropsy, certain drug intoxications (salicylates and phenothiazines) and in the diagnosis of several inborn errors of amino acid metabolism (phenylketonuria, maple syrup urine disease, and alcaptonuria). Also occasionally used to detect melanin in the urine.

Description. A spot urine sample is obtained. Ferric chloride solution is added to the urine sample, and characteristic color changes occur depending on the pathologic condition present (that is, purple with salicylates, purple-pink with phenothiazines, gray with melanin, etc.).

CONDITION	COLOR CHANGE IN URINE
Alcoholism	Red or red-brown
Alkaptonuria	Blue or green, fades quickly
Diabetes	Red or red-brown
Drug ingestion	
Acetophenetidines	Red
Aminosalicylic acid	Red-brown
Antipyrines	Red

CONDITION	COLOR CHANGE IN URINE
Drug ingestion—cont'd	
Cyanates	Red
Phenol derivative	Violet
Phenothiazines	Purple-pink
Salicylates	Stable purple
Histidinemia	Green or blue-green
Maple syrup urine disease	Blue
Phenylketonuria	Blue or blue-green, fades to yellow
Starvation	Red or red-brown
Tyrosinosis	Green, fades in seconds
Other products	
Alpha-ketobuturic acid	Purple, fades to red-brown
Bilirubin	Blue-green
ortho-Hydroxyphenylacetic acid	Mauve
ortho-Hydroxyphenylpyruvic acid	Red
Pyruvic acid	Deep gold-yellow or green
Xanthurenic acid	Deep green, later brown

Professional Considerations

1. Consent form NOT required.
2. Preparation:
   A. Several drugs can influence the test and cause a color change when the ferric chloride reagent is added to the urine. These include salicylates (aspirin and related drugs) and phenothiazine-related compounds. These should be avoided if possible before the test.
   B. Fasting is not required before the test, and no other pretest preparation is necessary.
3. Procedure:
   A. Urine is collected from the client into a clean container and submitted to the diagnostic laboratory for analysis.
   B. In the laboratory ferric chloride is added to the urine sample, and the technician waits for a color change to occur.
4. Postprocedure care:
   A. No special postprocedure care of the client is required.
5. Client and family teaching:
   A. The client and appropriate family members should be oriented as to the rationale behind the test before it is performed.
   B. Several of the conditions diagnosed with this test represent inborn errors of metabolism.
   C. Genetic counseling may be indicated once the diagnosis of these disorders is established.
6. Factors that affect results:
   A. Preparation and storage of the ferric chloride reagent.
   B. Ingestion of certain drugs (salicylates and phenothiazines) may cause a color change when the ferric chloride is added to the urine sample.
7. Other data:
   A. The ferric chloride test is rather insensitive because it relies on a gross (qualitative) color change observed by a technician. Other more sensitive tests (including chromatography) may be helpful in the diagnosis of several of the disorders listed above.

FERRITIN, SERUM

Norm:

		SI UNITS
Adult Females		
≤40 years	11-122 ng/mL	11-122 µg/L
>40 years	12-263 ng/mL	12-263 µg/L

Continued

		SI UNITS
Adult Males	15-200 ng/mL	15-200 μg/L
Children		
Newborn	25-200 ng/mL	25-200 μg/L
1 month	200-600 ng/mL	200-600 μg/L
2-5 months	50-200 ng/mL	50-200 μg/L
6 months	7-140 ng/mL	7-140 μg/L
1-15 years	7-140 ng/mL	7-140 μg/L

Increased. Anemia (chronic, hemolytic, megaloblastic, pernicious, sideroblastic), carcinoma (generalized, hepatic), cirrhosis, hemochromatosis (idiopathic), hepatic disease (acute, chronic), hepatic necrosis, hepatitis, hepatoma, Hodgkin's disease, hyperthyroidism, inflammation (chronic), iron intake (excessive dietary or by blood transfusion), leukemia, jaundice (obstructive), multiple myeloma, polycythemia, renal disease (chronic), rheumatoid arthritis, respiratory infection (upper) with fever, siderosis, thalassemia (major, minor), and tissue trauma. Drugs include alcohol (wine ethanol), ascorbic acid (women only), iron, and hormonal contraceptives.

Decreased. Acid peptic disease, adenoma of GI tract, anemia (iron deficiency), colon cancer, hemodialysis, IgG-positive people, inflammatory bowel disease, pregnancy, rigorous athletic training, and surgery (gastrointestinal).

Description. An iron-storing protein manufactured in the liver, spleen, bone marrow, tumor cells, and sites of inflammation. Evaluation of ferritin levels is most often performed in the differential diagnosis of several types of anemia. Serum ferritin has been found to be more specific and sensitive and specific than serum transferrin receptor for differentiating iron-deficiency anemia from anemia of chronic disease in elderly clients with anemia. However, in infants, serum ferritin is less accurate in identifying iron deficiency than is serum transferrin receptor and the serum transferrin receptor:serum ferritin ratio.

Professional Considerations
1. Consent form NOT required.

2. **Preparation:**
   A. Tube: Red topped, red/gray topped, or gold topped.
3. **Procedure:**
   A. Draw a 1-mL blood sample.
4. **Postprocedure care:**
   A. Centrifuge and freeze samples.
5. **Client and family teaching:**
   A. Results may not be available for several days.
6. **Factors that affect results:**
   A. Reject specimens if the client had a radioactive scan within 48 hours before specimen collection.
7. **Other data:**
   A. Hemolyzed samples are acceptable.
   B. Ferritin <50 ng/mL is predictive of a serious GI tract pathologic condition.
   C. Elevated ferritin levels a few hours after cerebral vascular accident (CVA) and weeks after the CVA are predictive of a poor prognosis.

FETAL FIBRONECTIN (fFN, ONCOFETAL FIBRONECTIN), SPECIMEN

Norm. >0.050 μg/mL

Usage. Assay indicated for use with other clinical information as an aid to rapidly assess the risk of preterm delivery in symptomatic and asymptomatic pregnant women between 24 and 34 weeks of completed gestation.

Description. Qualitative test for the detection of fetal fibronectin (fFN) in cervicovaginal secretions. fFN can be detected in cervicovaginal secretions of women throughout pregnancy by use of a monoclonal antibody–based immunoassay. fFN is elevated in cervicovaginal secretions during the first 24 weeks of pregnancy but diminishes between

24 and 34 weeks in normal pregnancies. The significance of its presence in the vagina during the first 24 weeks of pregnancy is not understood. However, it may simply reflect the normal growth of the extravillous trophoblast population and the placenta. Detection of fFN in cervicovaginal secretions between 24 and 34 completed weeks of gestation is reported to be associated with preterm delivery in symptomatic and asymptomatic pregnant women. Ninety-nine percent of pregnant women with signs and symptoms of preterm delivery who test negatively for fFN do not deliver within the next 14 days. A positive fFN result is the single best predictor of impending delivery.

Professional Considerations
1. Consent form NOT required.

Contraindications
Symptomatic women with one or more of the following conditions: advanced cervical dilatation (>3 centimeters), rupture of amniotic membranes, cervical cerclage, moderate or gross vaginal bleeding, OR *asymptomatic* women with one or more of the following conditions: multiple gestations, cervical cerclage, placenta previa (partial or complete), sexual intercourse in the preceding 24 hours.

---

2. **Preparation:**
   A. See *Client and family teaching.*
   B. Obtain a polyester-fiber (Dacron) swab, sterile gloves, speculum.
   C. The client should disrobe below the waist.
   D. Position the client recumbent on a gynecologic examination table in the lithotomy position and drape for comfort and privacy.
3. **Procedure:**
   A. *Note:* Specimen must be obtained before digital examination.
   B. Cervicovaginal swab: Collection from *symptomatic* women:
      i. Insert a sterile speculum into the vagina. You should collect the specimen from the posterior fornix of the vagina during a sterile speculum examination by slightly rotating the Dacron swab for approximately 10 seconds to absorb the cervicovaginal secretions. Remove swab

and immerse Dacron tip into buffered collection tube. Break the swab shaft even with the top of the tube. Align the shaft of the swab with the hole inside the tube cap and push the cap down tightly to seal the tube.
   C. Cervicovaginal swab: Collection from *asymptomatic* women:
      i. Insert a sterile speculum into the vagina. You should collect the specimen from either the posterior fornix of the vagina or the ectocervical region of the external cervical os during a sterile speculum examination by slightly rotating the Dacron swab for approximately 10 seconds to absorb the cervicovaginal secretions. Remove swab and immerse Dacron tip into buffered collection tube. Break the swab shaft even with the top of the tube. Align the shaft of the swab with the hole inside the tube cap, and push the cap down tightly to seal the tube.
4. **Postprocedure care:**
   A. Write the client's age, the reason for the study, calculated gestational weeks on the lab requisition.
   B. Document any signs or symptoms of preterm delivery in the client's record.
   C. Send specimen to the laboratory immediately.
5. **Client and family teaching:**
   A. It is customary practice for the physician to discuss with the client the purpose of the procedure and risks associated with the procedure. Arrangements for discussing the results of the test should be made by the client's physician.
6. **Factors that affect results:**
   A. A positive fetal fibronectin result may be observed for clients who have experienced cervical disruption caused by but not limited to events such as sexual intercourse, digital cervical examination, or vaginal probe ultrasonography.
   B. Care must be taken not to contaminate the swab or cervicovaginal secretions with lubricants, soaps, or disinfectants (such as

K-Y Jelly, povidoneiodine solution [Betadine], hexachlorophene). Lubricants or creams may physically interfere with absorption of the specimen onto the the the swab. Soaps or disinfectants may interfere with the antibody-antigen reaction.

C. Cotton swabs absorb the fetal fibronectin and are not acceptable for this assay.

D. Results obtained from pregnant women who have had intercourse within the previous 24 hours before collection are difficult to interpret.

E. Test interference from the following components has not been ruled out: douches, white blood cells, bacteria, and bilirubin.

F. Results should be interpreted with caution when a specimen is obtained from a client with unconfirmed gestational age.

G. Rupture of membranes should be ruled out before the assay is performed, since fFn is found in both amniotic fluid and the fetal membranes.

7. **Other data:**

A. Other research studies in fFN testing have been done in the field of embryo and trophoblast implantation.

B. "Oncofetal" fibronectin was the name given to the molecule by researchers Matsuura and Hakomori (1985) who discovered the FDC-6 antibody; they originally demonstrated the antibody's capability of binding to tumor cells and tissues. The company marketing the "fetal" fibronectin test (which uses the FDC-6 antibody), dropped the "onco" portion of the test name to avoid raising concern that the test or reasons for use has any association with cancer.

FETAL HEMOGLOBIN (HbF), BLOOD

Norm:

Adults 0-2% of total hemoglobin

Children

Newborn	60-90% of total hemoglobin
1-5 months	<75% of total hemoglobin
6-12 months	<5% of total hemoglobin
1-20 years	<2% of total hemoglobin

Increased. Anemia (aplastic, megaloblastic, nonhereditary refractory normoblastic, pernicious, refractory, sickle cell, spherocytic), anorexia nervosa, bone marrow metastasis, bulimia nervosa, diabetes, Down syndrome, erythroleukemia, hereditary persistence of fetal hemoglobin, hyperthyroidism, hypothyroidism, infants (small for gestational age, chronic intrauterine anoxia, developmental abnormalities), leukemia, lymphoma, macroglobulinemia, multiple myeloma, myelofibrosis, paroxysmal nocturnal hemoglobinuria, post cord blood stem cell transplant, pregnancy (fetal blood leakage into mother's blood), spherocytosis, sudden infant death syndrome (SIDS), thalassemia (beta major, minor), thyrotoxicosis, trisomy 13-15, D trisomy, and trisomy 21. Drugs include anticonvulsants.

Decreased. Multiple chromosome abnormality (C/D translocation).

Description. HbF, the hemoglobin present during fetal development, contains a polypeptide globin chain that is different from that in adult hemoglobin. It composes most of the hemoglobin of a newborn's red blood cells. Over the first 6 months of life, most of the fetal hemoglobin is replaced by adult hemoglobin, though a small portion of HbF may persist throughout the life span. This test is most often used to differentiate thalassemia and other hemoglobinopathies in which abnormalities may be found in the polypeptide globin chains.

Professional Considerations

1. Consent form NOT required.
2. **Preparation:**
   A. Tube: Lavender topped or green topped.

```

3. **Procedure:**
A. Draw a 2-mL blood sample.
4. **Postprocedure care:**
A. None.
5. **Client and family teaching:**
A. Results may take several days.
6. **Factors that affect results:**
A. Reject specimens older than 4 days at room temperature.

7. **Other data:**
A. Sample is stable at room temperature for 4 days.

**FETAL HEMOGLOBIN STAIN**
*(see Betke-Kleihauer stain, Diagnostic)*

## FETAL MONITORING, EXTERNAL, DIAGNOSTIC

**Norm.** Fetal heart rate (FHR) and variability normal.
FHR 120-160 bpm
FHR variability 5-25 bpm

**Usage.** Monitoring FHR and uterine contractions, evaluation of fetal effects of stressed and nonstressed situations, assessment of the need for internal fetal monitoring, and monitoring of fetal well being during the oxytocin challenge test.

**Description.** A noninvasive test in which an electronic transducer is placed on the pregnant abdomen to amplify the FHR while a cardiotachometer records FHR and pressure sensors record uterine contractions. External fetal monitors record fluctuations in the baseline FHR and detect variability between beats. This test is able to detect FHR accelerations and decelerations in response to uterine contractions.

**Professional Considerations**
1. Consent form NOT required.
2. **Preparation:**
A. Obtain a fetal heart monitor and an electroconductive gel.
B. Cleanse the transducer and transducer connections.
3. **Procedure:**
A. The client is placed in a semi-Fowler's or left lateral position with the abdomen exposed.
B. The transducer is coated with electroconductive gel and strapped over the abdominal area with the most distinct fetal heart tones. For active labor, this is the fundus.
C. The alarm limits for FHR are set, and test recordings are started to ensure that the system is functioning properly.

D. For active labor, baseline FHR is recorded and calculated over a 10-minute period and then monitored continuously as labor progresses. The recording is evaluated for abnormalities in FHR and FHR response to contractions, drugs, or maternal position.
E. Transducer location may need adjustment in response to fetal movement in utero.
4. **Postprocedure care:**
A. Weekly external fetal monitoring is indicated for diabetes, hypertension, fetal growth retardation, and pregnancy over 42 weeks of gestation.
5. **Client and family teaching:**
A. For antepartal testing, the client should eat a full meal just before the test.
B. The test poses no risk of harm to the client or the fetus.
6. **Factors that affect results:**
A. Maternal position may cause fetal distress. The left-side lying position best promotes oxygen delivery to the fetus.
B. Maternal obesity may interfere with the adequacy of recordings.
C. Artifact may result from poor transducer connections, or dried electroconductive gel on the transducer.
7. **Other data:**
A. Events that cause changes in the FHR recordings during active labor are handwritten on the graphic recording. These include maternal movement, administration of drugs, and procedures.

F
```

FETAL MONITORING, EXTERNAL, CONTRACTION STRESS TEST (CST) AND OXYTOCIN CHALLENGE TEST (OCT), DIAGNOSTIC

Norm. Fetal heart rate (FHR) and variability normal.

FHR   110-160 bpm
FHR variability   5 bpm: minimal variability
                        6-25 bpm: moderate variability
                        <25 bpm: pronounced variability

Usage. To stimulate labor, to evaluate fetal responses to contractions. CST/OCT administered as a result of nonreactive non-stress test (NST). CST is one measure used to evaluate the quality of placental perfusion and fetal well-being. This test is usually conducted after 32 weeks of gestation.

Description. A noninvasive procedure in which the fetus is electronically monitored and uterine contractions are stimulated. A regular contraction pattern is achieved for the purpose of evaluating fetal responses and making predictions regarding fetal outcome to labor.

Interpretation of CST/OCT:

Negative = No decelerations during entire procedure; long-term viability (LVT) is present. Uterine contractions have no adverse effect on fetus (deceleration). Is predictive of continued fetal well-being for 7 days.

Positive = At least half of contractions obtained are accompanied by late decelerations. Prognosis is poor in the presence of decreased LTV. Vigorous management is indicated.

Equivocal = Test needs to be repeated within 24 hours.

Hyperstimulation = >4 contractions in 10 minutes, or contractions lasting longer than 90 seconds, or <60 seconds between contractions.

Suspicious = Late decelerations present in less than half of contractions. LTV usually present.

Unsatisfactory = Quality of tracing too poor to provide accurate interpretation.

Professional Considerations

1. Consent form is NOT required, but maternal permission should be obtained. Client needs to be informed that the effect of the oxytocin may induce labor.

Contraindications
Preterm labor, placenta previa.

2. **Preparation:**
   A. Complete a 20-minute monitor strip for a baseline FHR and uterine activity. Observe fetal movement and changes in FHR.
   B. Test must be conducted in an intrapartal unit in the event of nonreassuring outcomes that require immediate interventions.

3. **Procedure:**
   A. For exogenous oxytocin release by oxytocin (Pitocin) infusion, begin an intravenous infusion of either lactated Ringer's, dextrose with saline, or normal saline. Add oxytocin piggyback IV infusion at 0.5 milliunits (mU)/minute. Test period conducted until client achieves three uterine contractions, each lasting 40 seconds, within 10-minutes. Increase oxytocin rate per protocol until contraction pattern is achieved.
   B. For endogenous oxytocin release, see *Client and family teaching.*

4. **Postprocedure care:**
   A. Continue to observe and document fetal patterns and changes in uterine activity. Watch for uterine hyperstimulation.
   B. Discontinue oxytocin, monitor client's blood pressure and pulse until contractions have subsided.

5. **Client and family teaching:**
   A. For endogenous oxytocin release by nipple stimulation, instruct client to brush or massage a nipple until contractions begin, or for 10 minutes. If no contractions after 10 minutes, ask client to brush or message other nipple.

6. **Factors that affect results:**
   A. CST/OCT has a <2% false-negative rate and a >50% false-positive rate.

7. **Other data:**
   A. CST/OCT is more sensitive to fetal oxygen reserves than the NST is.

B. In the presence of variable decelerations, regardless of outcomes

of test, amniotic fluid infusion may be indicated.

FETAL MONITORING, EXTERNAL, NON–STRESS TESTING (NST), DIAGNOSTIC

Norm. Fetal heart rate (FHR) and variability normal.
FHR   110-160 bpm
FHR variability   5 bpm: minimal variability
                           6-25 bpm: moderate variability
                           <25 bpm: pronounced variability

Usage. Monitoring FHR and uterine patterns under normal, nonstressful circumstances during late pregnancy (third trimester). This test is able to detect FHR accelerations as associated with fetal movement. In the presence of uterine contractions, decelerations may be observed.

Description. A noninvasive test in which an electronic transducer is placed on the pregnant abdomen to amplify the FHR while a cardiotachometer records FHR and a pressure sensor (tocomanometer) records any uterine contractions. A baseline FHR is determined, fetal movements are recorded, and any change in FHR associated with movement is evaluated.

Interpretation of NST:

Reactive = At least 2 accelerations during 20 minutes.
Nonreactive = None of the reactive criteria met; long-term variability minimal.
Unsatisfactory = Unable to obtain adequate tracing; fetal patterns are borderline for criteria. Reschedule testing as indicated by condition.

Professional Considerations
1. Consent form NOT required. Client agreement is recommended.
2. **Preparation:**
   A. Obtain a fetal heart monitor and an electroconductive gel.
   B. Cleanse the transducer, tocomanometer, and monitor connections with alcohol pads.
3. **Procedure:**
   A. The client is instructed to empty her bladder and then is placed in a left lateral or semi-Fowler's position (with left hip roll) with the abdomen exposed. Use Leopold's maneuvers to deter-

mine fetal outline. Palpate fetal spine and locate occiput. The most distinct fetal heart tones are obtained over area of the fetal shoulders (usually lower left or lower right quadrant).
B. The transducer is coated with electroconductive gel and strapped over the location of fetal heart tone.
C. The alarm limits for FHR are set, and a baseline heart rate over a 2-minute period is determined.
D. Assess uterine fundus to locate area where contractions are best palpated and not affected by fetal position. Strap tocomanometer over this area.
E. Client is monitored for a minimum of 30 minutes. During this time, monitor will electronically record any fetal movements, including kicking. If monitor does not have this capacity, client will be asked to press a button each time a movement is felt in order to record activity.
F. Fetus should exhibit accelerations during a 20-minute period. Acceleration is defined as an increase of 15 bpm over fetal baseline rate, lasting 15 seconds.
4. **Postprocedure care:**
   A. Weekly external fetal monitoring is indicated for diabetes, hypertension, fetal growth retardation, and pregnancy over 42 weeks of gestation.
   B. In the event of a nonreactive result, client will be scheduled for a contraction stress test (CST)/oxytocin challenge test (OCT).
5. **Client and family teaching:**
   A. For antepartal testing, the client should eat a full meal just before the test.

B. The test poses no risk or harm to the client or the fetus.

6. **Factors that affect results:**
   A. False-positive result associated with inadequate testing time, maternal hypotension, and maternal medications.

B. False-negative result associated with improper placement of monitoring devices.

7. **Other data:**
   A. None.

FETAL MONITORING, INTERNAL, DIAGNOSTIC

Norm. Fetal heart rate (FHR) and variability normal.

FHR	110-160 bpm
FHR variability	5 bpm: minimal variability
	6-25 bpm: moderate variability
	<25 bpm: pronounced variability

Maternal Contractions and Intrauterine Pressure during Labor:

Prelabor	<3 contractions over 10 minutes
	25-40 mm Hg contraction pressure
First stage	<6 contractions over 10 minutes
	8-12 mm Hg baseline pressure
	30-40 mm Hg contraction pressure
Second stage	1 contraction about every 2 minutes
	10-20 mm Hg baseline pressure
	50-80 mm Hg contraction pressure

Usage. Monitoring of beat-to-beat variability of FHR and rate and pressure monitoring of uterine contractions during labor. Often used as an adjunct to external fetal monitoring. More accurate than external fetal monitoring, especially in cases of maternal obesity. Internal monitoring is less affected by fetal or maternal movement than external monitoring is.

Description. During this invasive monitoring procedure, a sterile fetal scalp electrode and a uterine catheter are inserted through the vaginal canal for the purpose of FHR and uterine-contraction measurements during labor after 3-cm cervical dilatation and rupture of membranes. Internal monitoring is recommended over external monitoring for a better assessment of the effects of labor on the fetus and to provide interpretation of quality of contraction pattern.

Professional Considerations
1. Consent form IS required.

Risks
Maternal uterine perforation; intrauterine infection; and fetal scalp infection, abscess, or hematoma.

Contraindications
Active genital herpes.

Precaution
Test should be performed only when the fetal presenting part is the head.

2. **Preparation:**
   A. Obtain an antiseptic solution, sterile gloves, a fetal scalp electrode and guide, a pressure catheter for intrauterine contraction monitoring, a catheter guide, a transducer, a fetal heart monitor, and a topical antibiotic.
   B. Ascertain that membranes are ruptured and that the presenting part is the fetal head.
3. **Procedure:**
   A. The client is placed in a dorsal lithotomy position.
   B. The perineal area is cleansed with antiseptic solution.
   C. A sterile vaginal examination is performed to measure cervical dilatation and identify a fetal scalp location over bone for electrode placement.

D. The electrode is guided through the vaginal canal and cervical os and gently screwed into place on the fetal scalp.

E. The electrode wires are connected to the fetal monitor. Correct placement and functioning of the system are verified when a FHR signal is demonstrated by the fetal monitor.

F. The pressure-sensitive catheter for monitoring uterine contractions is then guided into place, through the cervix, a shallow distance to the uterus. The distal end is connected to a pressure transducer for continuous monitoring of intrauterine pressure. The monitor is calibrated to zero for a uterine pressure baseline value.

G. Continue monitoring FHR and contraction pattern as with external monitoring.

4. Postprocedure care:
A. Cleanse the fetal scalp electrode site with antiseptic at the time of delivery.
B. Document observed laceration(s) of the baby's scalp.

5. Client and family teaching:
A. Explain procedure to client. Internal fetal monitoring poses risks (listed above) but provides much better assessment of how well the fetus is tolerating the labor process than external fetal monitoring does.

6. Factors that affect results:
A. Drugs that affect the sympathetic and parasympathetic nervous systems may influence FHR.
B. The maternal position may cause fetal distress. The left side-lying position best promotes oxygen delivery to the fetus.

7. Other data:
A. Internal scalp electrode may be inserted and removed by a registered nurse who has received specialized preparation in this skill or a physician. The intrauterine pressure catheter may be inserted only by a physician.

FETOSCOPY, DIAGNOSTIC

Norm.
Normal fetal development. Absence of neural tube defects.

Usage. Diagnosis of malformation of the fetus. Detection of neural tube defect. Blood samples may be obtained to test for sickle cell anemia and hemophilia.

Description. Fetoscopy is an endoscopic procedure that allows direct examination of the fetus by means of the fetoscope.

Professional Considerations
1. Consent form IS required.

Risks
Abortion or premature labor; amnionitis (antibiotics may be given prophylactically to prevent this complication).

Contraindications
Anteriorly placed placenta, bleeding disorder, hypertensive crisis, incompetent cervix, history of spontaneous abortion or premature labor.

2. Preparation:
A. To prevent excessive fetal activity during the procedure, the mother may be given meperidine (Demerol), which crosses the placenta and quiets the fetus.
B. Obtain a local anesthetic and a fetoscopy tray.

3. Procedure:
A. The abdominal wall of the mother is anesthetized with a local anesthetic.
B. An ultrasound examination is then used to locate the fetus and placenta.
C. A small incision is made in the abdominal wall, and the fetoscope is inserted through the abdominal wall into the amniotic cavity. The fetus is visualized for obvious malformations, such as neural tube defects.

4. Postprocedure care:
A. Apply a dry, sterile dressing to the fetoscopy site.

5. Client and family teaching:
A. This procedure poses risks (listed above).
B. A local anesthetic will be used to prevent pain. The client will feel pressure as the fetoscope is inserted.
C. The test takes about 40 minutes.

6. Factors that affect results:
A. Excessive movement of the mother may obscure results.

F

7. **Other data:**
   A. None.

FETUS EXAMINATION AFTER DEATH
(see Autopsy, Diagnostic)

FIBRIN BREAKDOWN PRODUCTS, BLOOD
(see Fibrinogen breakdown products, Blood)

FIBRIN DEGRADATION FRAGMENT
(see d-Dimer, Blood)

FIBRIN DEGRADATION PRODUCTS, BLOOD
(see Fibrinogen breakdown products, Blood)

FIBRIN SPLIT PRODUCTS, PROTAMINE SULFATE TEST, BLOOD

Norm. Negative test.

Positive Test. Deep vein thrombosis, disseminated intravascular coagulation (DIC), infarcts, Kasabach-Merrit syndrome, postoperative blood vessel clots, and pulmonary embolism.

Description. Protamine sulfate added to the blood sample helps differentiate between conditions producing secondary fibrinolysin (positive test) and conditions producing primary fibrinolysin (negative test). It is primarily used as a screening test for DIC, which produces secondary fibrinolysin.

Professional Considerations
1. Consent form NOT required.
2. **Preparation:**
   A. Tube: Blue topped.
   B. Perform this test before implementing heparin therapy.
3. **Procedure:**
   A. Draw a 3-mL blood sample.
4. **Postprocedure care:**
   A. For clients with coagulopathy, hold pressure over the sampling site for at least 5 minutes and observe the site closely for development of a hematoma.
   B. Write the collection time on the laboratory requisition.
   C. Do NOT shake the tube or place it on ice.
   D. Transport the specimen to the laboratory immediately for incubation.
5. **Client and family teaching:**
   A. Results are normally available within 2 hours.
   B. Seek medical attention for signs of bleeding (that is, hematoma, bleeding of gums, wounds, petechiae, confusion, changing level of consciousness).
6. **Factors that affect results:**
   A. Reject hemolyzed specimens or specimens received more than 2 hours after collection.
   B. Drugs that may produce a false-positive result include heparin calcium and heparin sodium.
7. **Other data:**
   A. Assess for signs of shock from bleeding: tachycardia, hypotension, and clammy cold skin.

FIBRIN STABILIZING FACTOR, BLOOD
(see Factor XIII, Blood)

FIBRINOGEN (FACTOR I), PLASMA

Norm. Quantitative is 150-400 mg/dL (1.5-4.0 g/L, SI units).
Lower values can occur in newborns.

Increased. Arthritis (rheumatoid), familial paroxysmal peritonitis (familial Mediterranean fever, periodic disease), hepatitis, infection (acute), and menstruation.

Decreased. Abortion (septic, missed), anemia (acquired hemolytic), burns (severe), carcinoma (prostate, lung, metastasis), circulating fibrinogen inhibitors, cirrhosis, coagulation factor deficiency, congenital fibrinogen disorders (afibrinogenemia, hypofibrinogenemia, dysfibrinogenemia), cryoglobulinemia, disseminated intravascular coagulation (DIC), eclampsia, embolism (amniotic fluid, fat, meconium), leukemia, lymphoma, macroglobulinemia, multiple myeloma, septicemia, shock, snakebite, thrombotic thrombocytopenic purpura, transfusion reaction, and trauma. Drugs include asparaginase, bezafibrate, perindopril, phenobarbital drug poisoning, streptokinase, ticlopidine, and urokinase. Elevation slows or stops with the administration of glycoprotein IIB/IIIA inhibitors.

Description. Fibrinogen (factor I) is a heat-stable, complex polypeptide that converts to the insoluble polymer of fibrin after thrombin enzymatic action and combines with platelets to clot the blood. Synthesized in the liver, fibrinogen increases in diseases associated with tissue damage or inflammation. There is some evidence that it may be useful as a predictor of arteriosclerotic disease. One performs this test by adding thrombin to the client's plasma and measuring the amount of time taken for clotting to occur at standard dilutions. The amount of fibrin is then calculated based on the thrombin clotting time.

Professional Considerations
1. Consent form NOT required.
2. Preparation:
   A. Tube: 2.7- or 4.5-mL blue topped.
3. Procedure:
   A. Withdraw 2 mL of blood into a syringe or vacuum tube. Remove the syringe or tube, leaving the needle in place. Attach a second syringe and draw two blood samples, one in a citrated blue-topped tube and the other in a control tube. The sample quantity should be 2.4-mL for a 2.7-mL tube and 4.0 mL for a 4.5-mL tube. Draw a 5-mL blood sample in a sodium citrate–anticoagulated blue-topped tube.
4. Postprocedure care:
   A. For clients with coagulopathy, hold pressure over sampling site for at least 5 minutes and observe site closely for development of a hematoma.
   B. Transport the specimens to the laboratory immediately for spinning. The specimens are then stable for 3 days when refrigerated.
5. Client and family teaching:
   A. Seek medical attention for signs of bleeding (that is, hematoma, bleeding of gums, wounds, petechiae, confusion, changing level of consciousness).

6. Factors that affect results:
   A. Reject hemolyzed specimens or tubes partially filled with blood.
7. Other data:
   A. Active bleeding or administration of a blood transfusion within 1 month before the test invalidates results.
   B. Normally a prothrombin time and an activated partial thromboplastin time can also be performed on this specimen.
   C. See also *Activated partial thromboplastin time, and thromboplastin time, Plasma.*

FIBRINOGEN BREAKDOWN PRODUCTS (FIBRIN DEGRADATION PRODUCTS, FDP), BLOOD

Norm. 2-10 µg/mL. Panic range: >40 µg/mL.

Increased. Abruptio placentae, aneurysm, blood transfusion reaction, brain damage, burns, carcinomatosis, cirrhosis (alcoholic), congenital heart disease, deep vein thrombosis, disseminated intravascular coagulation, internal bleeding (newborns), intrauterine death, myocardial infarction, organ rejection (renal transplant), parturition, postcesarean birth, preeclampsia, pregnancy (third trimester), pulmonary embolism, pulmonary infarction, renal disease, respiratory distress (newborns), rheumatoid arthritis, sepsis, shock, squamous cell carcinoma of the oral cavity, subdural hematoma, sunstroke, surgical complications, and tissue damage (extensive). Drugs include barbiturates (large doses causing coma), megestrol acetate (high-dose), oral contraceptives containing desogestrel (DSG), streptokinase, and urokinase.

Decreased. Not clinically significant.

Description. Seven split products result from splitting fibrin or fibrinogen as a result of attack by plasmin during dissolution of fibrin clots. These split products, labeled A, B, C, D, E, X, and Y, indicate recent clotting activity. Greatly increased amounts interfere with hemostatic plug formation and indicate abnormal amounts of fibrinolysis. Levels over 40 mg/mL are highly suggestive of disseminated intravascular coagulation.

Professional Considerations
1. Consent form NOT required.
2. Preparation:
   A. Tube: 2.7- or 4.5-mL blue topped. Also obtain ice.
3. Procedure:
   A. Withdraw 2 mL of blood into a syringe or vacuum tube. Remove the syringe or tube, leaving the needle in place. Attach a second syringe, and draw a 2.4-mL sample in a 2.7-mL tube or a 4.0-mL sample in a 4.5-mL tube. Place the specimens immediately in a container of ice.
   B. Gently tilt the tube until a clot forms.
4. Postprocedure care:
   A. For clients with coagulopathy, hold pressure over the sampling site for at least 5 minutes and observe the site closely for development of a hematoma.
   B. Place the specimens on ice.
5. Client and family teaching:
   A. Results are normally available within 4 hours.
   B. Seek medical attention for signs of bleeding (that is, hematoma, bleeding of gums, wounds, petechiae, confusion, changing level of consciousness).
6. Factors that affect results:
   A. Reject specimens of non-clotted blood.
   B. Reject specimens if the tube is mixed vigorously.
   C. If heparin is to be administered, do so after this specimen is drawn.
7. Other data:
   A. This test does not distinguish between conditions producing primary fibrinolysin activity and those producing secondary fibrinolysin activity.

FIBRINOLIGASE, BLOOD
(see Factor XIII, Blood)

FIBRINOPEPTIDE A (FPA), BLOOD

Norm. 0.6-1.9 mg/mL

Increased. Cellulitis, disseminated intravascular coagulation, infection, leukemia, systemic lupus erythematosus.

Decreased. Elevation slows or stops with the administration of glycoprotein IIB/IIIA inhibitors.

Description. A peptide involved in thrombus formation after vascular endothelial damage occurs and a platelet plug develops. Thromb cleaves to fibrinopeptide A and B from fibrinogen that is circulating in the blood and forms soluble fibrin monomer complexes, which become the base on which a fibrin clot builds. The presence of increased fibrinopeptide A indicates that coagulation is occurring.

Professional Considerations
1. Consent form NOT required.
2. Preparation:
   A. Tube: 2.7- or 4.5-mL blue topped.
3. Procedure:
   A. Withdraw 2 mL of blood into a syringe or vacuum tube. Remove the syringe or tube, leaving the needle in place. Attach a second syringe, and draw two blood samples, one in a citrated blue-topped tube and the other in a control tube. The sample quantity should be 2.4-mL for a 2.7-mL tube and 4.0 mL for a 4.5-mL tube. Draw a 5-mL blood sample in a sodium citrate–anticoagulated blue-topped tube.
4. Postprocedure care:
   A. For clients with coagulopathy, hold pressure over sampling site for at least 5 minutes and observe site closely for development of a hematoma.
   B. Transport the specimens to the laboratory immediately for spinning. The specimens are then stable for 3 days when refrigerated.
5. Client and family teaching:
   A. Seek medical attention for signs of bleeding (that is, hematoma, bleeding of gums, wounds, petechiae, confusion, changing level of consciousness).
6. Factors that affect results:
   A. Reject hemolyzed specimens or tubes partially filled with blood.
7. Other data:
   A. See also *Soluble fibrin monomer complex, Serum.*

FIBROBLAST SKIN CULTURE

Norm. Requires interpretation.

Usage. Gardner syndrome, hereditary tyrosinemia (type 1), Hurler syndrome, Marfan syndrome, and mucopolysaccharidosis.

Description. Fibroblasts, large stellate spindle-shaped connective tissue cells, are common in developing or repairing tissues, where they are associated with protein and collagen synthesis. The test is used to help identify gene coding for genetic diseases through cytogenetic study.

Professional Considerations
1. Consent form IS required.

Risks
Bleeding, infection.

Contraindications
None.

2. Preparation:
   A. Obtain povidone-iodine solution, a sterile needle, a knife, and a sterile container.
3. Procedure:
   A. Cleanse the site to be biopsied with povidone-iodine solution and allow it to dry.
   B. Raise the skin with a sterile needle.
   C. Excise a 2-gram skin snip just below the needle with the knife.
   D. Place the skin snip in a sterile container.
4. Postprocedure care:
   A. Send the skin biopsy without fixative to the laboratory.
5. Client and family teaching:
   A. The test involves taking a tiny sample of skin for testing, Pain is minimal enough that a local anesthetic is often not needed.
6. Factors that affect results:
   A. None.
7. Other data:
   A. A scleral punch may also be used for the biopsy.

FLAT-PLATE RADIOGRAPHY OF ABDOMEN (KIDNEY-URETER-BLADDER, KUB, SCOUT FILM), DIAGNOSTIC

Norm. Normal-sized kidneys as judged by radiopaque renal outlines, no abdominal calcifications, no abdominal free air, no evidence of intramural bowel gas, no evidence of bowel distention to indicate possible obstruction or ileus, no rib or pelvic fractures, no evidence of nephrolithiasis or cholelithiasis.

Usage. A screening abdominal radiograph used to rule out acute abdominal disease processes to include colonic perforation, obstruction, or ileus. Occasionally helpful in the diagnosis of cholelithiasis and nephrolithiasis. At times helpful in establishing the diagnosis of chronic pancreatitis (in this disorder abdominal calcifications can be seen occasionally on KUB film).

Description. A plain abdominal film exposed from anterior to posterior (AP) with the client in the supine position. The lower portion of the radiograph displays the superior portion of the symphysis pubis, and the superior portion of the film shows the upper margins of the renal shadows.

Precautions
During pregnancy, risks of cumulative radiation exposure to the fetus from this and other previous or future imaging studies must be weighed against the benefits of the procedure. Although formal limits for client exposure are relative to this risk:benefit comparison, the United States Nuclear Regulatory Commission requires that the cumulative dose equivalent to an embryo/fetus from occupational exposure not exceed 0.5 rem (5 mSv). Radiation dosage to the fetus is proportional to the distance of the anatomy studied from the abdomen and decreases as pregnancy progresses. For pregnant clients, consult the radiologist/radiology department to obtain estimated fetal radiation exposure from this procedure.

Professional Considerations
1. Consent form NOT required.
2. Preparation:
   A. The radiograph may be taken either in the x-ray department or in the client's room with portable equipment.
   B. No special preparation of the client is necessary before the radiography.
3. Procedure:
   A. The client is placed in the supine position.
   B. Radiographic shields are placed over the gonadal areas.

F

C. The client is asked to expire and hold his or her breath. The film is exposed at the end of expiration.

4. **Postprocedure care:**
   A. No special postprocedure care is required. The client may require transport back to his or her nursing care unit if the film is done in the radiology department.

5. **Client and family teaching:**
   A. The risk of malignancy from plain abdominal radiographic procedures is minimal.
   B. Radiographic damage to the gonads is prohibited by abdominal shielding of these areas during the radiographic procedure.

6. **Factors that affect results:**
   A. Respiration artifact (the client breathing during exposure of the radiograph).
   B. Inappropriate positioning of the radiograph cassette leading to abdominal areas missed when the film is exposed.
   C. Underexposure or overexposure of the film.

7. **Other data:**
   A. The KUB is considered to be a screening procedure. More powerful diagnostic radiologic procedures (computed tomography, magnetic resonance imaging scans, barium studies) may be required to establish the diagnosis.

FLECAINIDE, PLASMA OR SERUM

Norm. Negative.

		SI UNITS
Therapeutic trough	0.2-1.0 μg/mL	0.5-2.4 μmol/L
Panic level	>1.0 μg/mL	>2.4 μmol/L

Overdose Symptoms and Treatment

Symptoms. Overdose will produce effects that are extensions of pharmacologic effects. AV nodal escape rhythms and prolongation of QRS and QT intervals. ECG abnormalities associated with overdose have included bradycardia, atrioventricular block, regular ventricular tachycardia with a right bundle branch that progressed to polymorphous tachycardia, substantial prolongation of the PR and QT intervals, widened P waves. Sudden death may occur.

Treatment:
Note: Treatment choice(s) depend on client history and condition and episode history.
Symptomatic and supportive care with ECG, blood pressure, and respiratory monitoring. There is no specific antidote.
Hemodialysis will NOT remove flecainide.

Increased. Hepatic or renal dysfunction. Drugs include amiodarone, cimetidine, and propranolol.

Decreased. Drugs include phenobarbital and rifampin.

Description. Flecainide is a class 1C antidysrhythmic used for ventricular dysrhythmias and reducing atrial defibrillation threshold in clients treated with low-energy internal atrial cardioversion. It is metabolized and excreted by the liver and kidneys, with a half-life of 20 hours and steady-state levels reached by 3-5 days after therapy is started. Safe to take during pregnancy.

Professional Considerations
1. Consent form NOT required.
2. **Preparation:**
   A. If the client is also taking propranolol or quinidine, indicate this on the laboratory requisition.
   B. Tube: Red topped, red/gray topped, gold topped, or green topped.
   C. MAY be drawn during hemodialysis.
3. **Procedure:**
   A. Draw the blood sample just before the next scheduled dose.
   B. Draw a 2-mL blood sample.
4. **Postprocedure care:**
   A. Send the specimen to the laboratory promptly. Serum or plasma must be separated within 2 hours.

5. **Client and family teaching:**
   A. Results are normally available within 24 hours.
   B. Refer clients with intentional overdose for crisis intervention.
6. **Factors that affect results:**
   A. Propranolol and quinidine cause unreliable results when the spectrofluorometric method is used.
   B. Refer clients with intentional overdose for crisis intervention.
7. **Other data:**
   A. Plasma levels >1.2 μg/mL in clients with renal dysfunction are associated with serious side effects and sudden death.

B. Administration in persons with implanted AAIR pacemaker due to sick sinus syndrome can cause failure of pacing.
C. Can cause diffuse infiltrative lung disease. Treatment includes discontinuation of flecainide and prednisone treatment.
D. Interaction of flecainide with topical timolol maleate and verapamil includes bradycardia.

FLEXIBLE SIGMOIDOSCOPY
(see Sigmoidoscopy, Diagnostic)

FLUCYTOSINE, SERUM

Norm:

		SI UNITS
Therapeutic level	25-100 μg/mL	195-775 μmol/L
Panic level	>125 μg/mL	>970 μmol/L

Panic Level Symptoms and Treatment

Symptoms. Panic levels correlate poorly with clinical symptoms. May have adverse effects on renal, hepatic, and hematopoietic systems and include acute cerebellopathy.

Treatment:
Note: Treatment choice(s) depend on client history and condition and episode history.
Flucytosine can be eliminated by hemodialysis (50%), peritoneal dialysis, and, in part, hemofiltration.

Usage. Monitoring for therapeutic and toxic levels of the drug.

Description. An orally effective, systemic antifungal drug that is a secondary agent often used with amphotericin B for treating serious, deep-seated mycotic infections caused by *Candida* and *Cryptococcus* species. Is less effective but less toxic than amphotericin B. Ancobon is well absorbed, well distributed throughout the body, and the majority is excreted unchanged by the kidneys. Half-life is 3-6 hours.

Professional Considerations
1. Consent form NOT required.
2. **Preparation:**
   A. Tube: Red topped, red/gray topped, or gold or green topped.
   B. Do NOT draw during hemodialysis.
3. **Procedure:**
   A. Draw a 5-mL blood sample 2 hours after oral administration for peak levels and immediately before oral administration for trough levels.
4. **Postprocedure care:**
   A. None.
5. **Client and family teaching:**
   A. Inform the client or the family of the rationale for the test.
   B. Results are normally available in 24 hours.
   C. Refer clients with intentional overdose for crisis intervention.
6. **Factors that affect results:**
   A. Ancobon half-life may increase up to 200 hours in clients with renal failure.
7. **Other data:**
   A. There is a 57% failure rate when flucytosine is used alone for treatment.
   B. 68% clinical response for treatment of cryptococcal meningitis in persons with AIDS using amphotericin B and flucytosine.

F

C. Flucytosine can be combined with both amphotericin B and fluconazole.

FLUORESCEIN ANGIOGRAPHY (EYE FUNDUS), DIAGNOSTIC

Norm. No leakage of dye from blood vessels of the retina during any of the following phases.

Filling stage. Begins 12-15 seconds after dye injection; noted when retinal vessels begin filling with dye.

Choroidal flush. The retina fluoresces and appears evenly mottled throughout the capillaries.

Arterial stage. Noted when arteries begin to fill with dye.

Arteriovenous stage. Noted when arteries have filled with dye and veins begin to fill with dye.

Venous stage. The arteries have emptied, and the veins have become filled and then emptied.

Late stage. $\frac{1}{2}$-1 hour after injection, the dye has circulated throughout the body, and recirculation of the retinal vessels can be seen.

Usage. Evaluation of retinopathy, tumors, retinal circulation abnormalities (occlusion, stenosis, dilatation, aneurysm, arteriovenous shunt), or papilledema. Identification of leakage and retinal thickening for subsequent laser treatment.

Description. A radiographic examination of the retinal vasculature after rapid injection of fluorescein dye. Fluorescein angiography provides rapid and direct acquisition of sequential images of the vasculature and the ability to manipulate the fluorescein images with the computer. For example, the processor can adjust for fluorescein leakage into the vitreous, cataracts, or cloudy corneas. It also provides the ability to display fluorescein images and color fundus images for comparison during laser treatment. The rapidly available images are also used to help explain the disease process to the client being examined.

Professional Considerations
1. Consent form IS required.

Risks
Allergic reaction (itching, hives, rash, tight feeling in the throat, shortness of breath, bronchospasm, anaphylaxis, death), or seizure reaction to sodium fluorescein.

Contraindications
Previous allergy to sodium fluorescein; clients who are unable to keep their eyes open for the test.

Precautions
During pregnancy, risks of cumulative radiation exposure to the fetus from this and other previous or future imaging studies must be weighed against the benefits of the procedure. Although formal limits for client exposure are relative to this risk:benefit comparison, the United States Nuclear Regulatory Commission requires that the cumulative dose equivalent to an embryo/fetus from occupational exposure not exceed 0.5 rem (5 mSv). Radiation dosage to the fetus is proportional to the distance of the anatomy studied from the abdomen and decreases as pregnancy progresses. For pregnant clients, consult the radiologist/radiology department to obtain estimated fetal radiation exposure from this procedure.

2. **Preparation:**
   A. Obtain mydriatic eye drops and 5% or 10% sodium fluorescein.
   B. Administer mydriatic eye drops as prescribed 15-30 minutes before the test.
   C. Insert a heparin lock intravenously.
   D. Have emergency equipment, including diazepam or phenytoin, available in case of allergic or seizure reaction.

3. **Procedure:**
   A. Dilating eye drops are administered.
   B. The client's chin and forehead rest against the fundus camera, and one arm is extended to the side.
   C. The client is instructed to open the eyes very wide, close the mouth, and look forward. The client can blink normally.
   D. Baseline fundus photographs are taken.
   E. Fluorescein dye is injected quickly and may cause facial flushing or nausea.

F. Photographs of the fundus of the eye are taken every second for 25-45 seconds. Late-phase photographs are taken 30 minutes later, if needed.
4. **Postprocedure care:**
 A. Discontinue the heparin lock.
5. **Client and family teaching:**
 A. Clients with glaucoma should omit mydriatic eye drops the day of the test.
 B. Do not drive for at least 2 hours after the test.
 C. Protective eyewear may be necessary for at least 2 hours after the test if the environment is bright or sunny.
 D. Yellow discoloration of the skin and urine is normally present for up to 2 days.
6. **Factors that affect results:**
 A. Cataracts may interfere with fundal view.
7. **Other data:**
 A. None.

FLUORESCEIN MENISCUS TEST
(see Schirmer tearing eye test, Diagnostic)

FLUORESCENT RABIES ANTIBODY (FRA), SPECIMEN

Norm. Negative. Requires interpretation.

Positive. Rabies.

Description. The rabies rhabdovirus causes an acute viral infection of the central nervous system of a variety of animals characterized by neurotropic ribonucleic acid (RNA) viral presence in the saliva, urine, feces, brain, and spinal cord. This virus is occasionally transmitted to humans by an infected skunk, squirrel, cat, bat, dog, or other animal, and is 99% fatal if symptoms appear before treatment is instituted. The serum of a human bitten by a rabid animal is examined by immunofluorescence to detect a significant serum antibody rise. This test can be used for antemortem diagnosis in clients who have never received rabies vaccine or passive antibody.

Professional Considerations
1. Consent form NOT required.
2. **Preparation:**
 A. Tube: Red topped, red/gray topped, or gold topped

3. **Procedure:**
 A. Draw a 7-mL human blood sample and send it to the laboratory along with animal brain. (See *Animals and rabies, Negri bodies.*)
4. **Postprocedure care:**
 A. None.
5. **Client and family teaching:**
 A. Results are normally available in 24 hours.
 B. Both preexposure and postexposure prophylaxis is available against rabies.
6. **Factors that affect results:**
 A. None.
7. **Other data:**
 A. Animal survival for 10 days makes rabies unlikely.
 B. Rabies is a reportable disease in most areas, as are animal bites.
 C. Rabies can also be detected by reverse transcriptase-PCR method using saliva, CSF, and skin biopsy samples from the client.

FLUORESCENT TREPONEMAL ANTIBODY–ABSORBED DOUBLE-STAIN (FTA-Abs DS) TEST, SERUM

Norm. Nonreactive.

Usage. Serologic confirmation of syphilis when nontreponemal tests are positive.

Description. Syphilis is a complex, sexually transmitted disease characterized by a wide range of symptoms that imitate other diseases and is caused by the organism *Treponema pallidum*. This test provides the most sensitive detection of treponemal antibodies for syphilis in all stages. It differentiates biologic false-positive results from true syphilis-positive results and can help diagnose syphilis when definite clinical signs are present but other tests are negative. This test is positive in the treponemal diseases of bejel, pinta, syphilis, and yaws. Before testing, the serum is treated to remove antibodies that could cause false-positive results. The technique involves using fluorescence microscopy with special filters that decrease the amount of natural fluorescence from the background of the specimen. Fluorescein-conjugated antibodies to IgG are added as a counterstain to the stained specimen, and the treponemes are identified as they fluoresce in combination with the antibodies.

Professional Considerations

1. Consent form NOT required.
2. Preparation:
   A. Tube: Red topped, red/gray topped, or gold topped.
3. Procedure:
   A. Draw a 3-mL blood sample.
4. Postprocedure care:
   A. None.
5. Client and family teaching:
   A. Results are normally available in 24 hours.
   B. If testing positive:
      i. Notify all sexual contacts from the last 90 days (if early stage) to be tested for syphilis.
      ii. Syphilis can be cured with antibiotics. These may worsen the symptoms for the first 24 hours.
      iii. Do not have sex for 2 months and until after repeat testing has confirmed that the syphilis is cured. Use condoms after that for 2 years. Return for repeat testing every 3-4 months for the next 2 years to make sure the disease is cured.
      iv. Do not become pregnant for 2 years because syphilis can be transmitted to the fetus.
      v. If left untreated, syphilis can damage many body organs, including the brain, over several years.
6. Factors that affect results:
   A. Reject hemolyzed specimens or chylous serum samples.
   B. False-positive results may be caused by antinuclear antibodies, drug abuse, elevated or abnormal globulins, pregnancy, or systemic lupus erythematosus (beaded pattern).
7. Other data:
   A. This test may remain positive indefinitely for clients previously infected with syphilis. Thus it is not useful for monitoring clinical response to treatment for syphilis.
   B. Borderline results necessitate repeating the test.

FLUOROSCOPY, DIAGNOSTIC

Norm. Requires interpretation. Usually there is symmetric, synchronous pulmonary and diaphragmatic motion. Diaphragmatic excursion = 2-4 cm. Absence of calcification in the coronary arteries.

Usage. Assessment of diaphragmatic function; localization of lung mass for percutaneous biopsy, mediastinal mass, pleural effusion, pleural lesion, and pulmonary disease; screening tool for detection of coronary artery disease; infrequent applications of fluoroscopy other than that of the chest include gastrointestinal imaging, venography, myelography, and genitourinary fluoroscopy.

Description. A radiographic examination of pulmonary motion using a fluoroscopic screen containing calcium tungstate crystals, which fluoresce when struck by x rays. When the x ray passes through the body, dense areas allow less radiation to pass through onto the fluoroscopic screen than less dense areas do. The resulting pattern of light and dark areas aids in the diagnosis of pathophysiologic conditions. Fluoroscopy can reveal subtle nodular or parenchymal calcifications and coronary artery calcifications better than regular radiographs. The test takes about 5 minutes and includes less than 1 minute of x-ray exposure.

Professional Considerations

1. Consent form IS required.

Risks

Radiation exposure, radiodermatitis, infection.

Contraindications

Pregnancy and during breast-feeding.

Precautions

During pregnancy, risks of cumulative radiation exposure to the fetus from this and other previous or future imaging studies must be weighed against the benefits of the procedure. Although formal limits for client exposure are relative to this risk:benefit comparison, the United States Nuclear Regulatory Commission requires that the cumulative dose equivalent to an embryo/fetus from occupational exposure not exceed 0.5 rem (5 mSv). Radiation dosage to the fetus is proportional to the distance of the anatomy studied from the abdomen and decreases as pregnancy progress. For pregnant clients, consult the radiologist/radiology department to obtain estimated fetal radiation exposure from this procedure.

2. **Preparation:**
   A. The client should remove all upper body clothing, jewelry, and metal items.
3. **Procedure:**
   A. The client stands with the chest between the x-ray tube and the fluoroscopic screen.
   B. Remove electrocardiographic monitoring leads and patches containing metal snaps and safety pins. Move invasive lines out of the fluoroscopic field if possible.
   C. Wear a lead apron if remaining in the room.
   D. Proceed with fluoroscopy. The client turns in different projections for the procedure.
4. **Postprocedure care:**
   A. None.
5. **Client and family teaching:**
   A. Inform the client or family of the rationale for the test.
   B. The client must remove all jewelry or metal objects from the trunk of the body.

C. The client must not be pregnant.
D. Results will be available after the examination of the procedure results by a radiologist.
E. In women who are breast-feeding, formula should be substituted for breast milk for 1 or more days after the procedure.
6. **Factors that affect results:**
   A. Metallic objects may interfere with the quality of films obtained by fluoroscopy.
7. **Other data:**
   A. A videotape of the film may be made for later examination.
   B. Fluoroscopy delivers more radiation than a chest radiograph does.

FLUOXETINE
(see Selective serotonin reuptake inhibitors, Blood)

FLUPHENAZINE
(see Phenothiazines, Blood)

FLURAZEPAM, SERUM

Norm. Negative.

	THERAPEUTIC RANGES	SI UNITS
Hydroxyethylflurazepam metabolite	0-4 ng/mL	0-9 nmol/L
n-Desalkylflurazepam metabolite	10-140 ng/mL	21-300 nmol/L
Flurazepam panic level	>2000 ng/mL	>4300 nmol/L

Panic Level Symptoms and Treatment

Symptoms. Dizziness, somnolence, impaired coordination, slurred speech, confusion, coma, and diminished reflexes. Hypotension, respiratory depression, and apnea may occur if the dose has been large.

Treatment:
Note: Treatment choice(s) depend on client history and condition and episode history.
Gastric lavage is not recommended, but should be considered if within 1 hour of ingestion and if ingestion of additional lethal substance is suspected. Use warm tap water or 0.9% saline.

Administer activated charcoal if within 4 hours of ingestion or if symptoms are present. Repeat as necessary, because benzodiazepines undergo hepatic recirculation.
Monitor for central nervous system depression.
Protect airway. Support breathing with oxygen and mechanical ventilation, if necessary.
Flumazenil is not recommended for routine use in benzodiazepine overdose. Flumazenil has been used as a competitive antagonist to reverse the profound effects of benzodiazepine overdose. Use of flumazenil is contraindicated if concomitant tricyclic antidepressants were taken or in

dependence states because of the risk of causing seizures from lowering of the seizure threshold and because it may precipitate symptoms of benzodiazepine withdrawal. Flumazenil may not completely reverse benzodiazepine effects. Close monitoring for re-sedation is required and repeated doses may be needed.
Do NOT use barbiturates.
Do NOT induce emesis.
Forced diuresis or hemodialysis will NOT remove benzodiazepines. to any significant extent. No information was found on whether peritoneal dialysis will remove these drugs.

Positive. Drug abuse, overdose, and seizures.

Negative. Absence of drug in serum.

Description. Flurazepam is a schedule-IV, long-acting benzodiazepine anxiolytic and hypnotic used for the treatment of insomnia and irregular sleeping habits. Flurazepam depresses the central nervous system and relaxes the skeletal muscles. It is absorbed from the gastrointestinal tract within 1 hour, metabolized by the liver, and excreted via the kidneys, with a half-life of up to 100 hours.

Professional Considerations
1. Consent form NOT required.
2. **Preparation:**
   A. Tube: Red topped, red/gray topped, or gold topped.
   B. MAY be drawn during hemodialysis.
3. **Procedure:**
   A. Draw a 5-mL blood sample.
4. **Postprocedure care:**
   A. None.
5. **Client and family teaching:**
   A. Inform the client or family of the rationale for the test.
   B. Results are normally available within 24 hours.
   C. If activated charcoal was given for elevated levels, the client should drink 4-6 glasses of water each day for 2 days to prevent constipation. The activated charcoal will also cause stools to be black for a few days.

D. Refer clients with intentional overdose for crisis intervention.
E. Referrals to appropriate rehabilitation centers and therapeutic community programs should be offered to all addicted clients who may be interested.
6. **Factors that affect results:**
   A. Stable at room temperature with considerable breakdown at 240 days.
7. **Other data:**
   A. See also *Benzodiazepines, Plasma and Urine.*

FLURAZEPAM HYDROCHLORIDE
(see Benzodiazepines, Plasma and Urine)

FMT
(see Schirmer tearing eye test, Diagnostic)

FOAM STABILITY INDEX, AMNIOTIC FLUID

Norm. Fetal lung maturity indicated by ≥ 0.47.
Fetal lung immaturity indicated by ≤ 0.46.

Usage. Foam Stability Index (FSI) of amniotic fluid uncontaminated by blood or meconium provides a direct measure of fetal lung maturity by determining the amount of surfactant in amniotic fluid and thus helps determine the risk for respiratory distress syndrome (RDS) or hyaline membrane disease. The test helps the clinician decide whether to delay delivery of the fetus. The test is commonly done before repeat cesarean delivery when gestational age is uncertain and for other indications including medical or obstetrical conditions such as severe maternal hypertension, renal disease, or preterm labor. Results indicating immaturity of the fetal lungs may lead to delay of delivery through use of tocolytics to suppress preterm labor or postponement of elective delivery.

Description. Pulmonary surfactant is measured in the amniotic fluid by noting the ability of the fluid to form a stable surface film that can support a ring of foam around a test tube. Proteins, bile acids, and salts of free fatty acids also will form a stable foam; these are removed from the foam by adding ethanol, which competes with these substances for a position in the surface foam. A fixed volume of amniotic fluid is mixed with a solution of 95% ethanol in increasing volumes, and the largest fraction of ethanol in which the amniotic fluid is capable of supporting a ring of bubbles 360 degrees around the tube is recorded; this fraction is the FSI.

Professional Considerations
1. Consent form IS required for the amniocentesis. See *Amniocentesis and amniotic fluid analysis, Diagnostic.*
2. **Preparation:**
   A. See *Amniocentesis and amniotic fluid analysis, Diagnostic.*
3. **Procedure:**
   A. See *Amniocentesis and amniotic fluid analysis, Diagnostic.*
4. **Postprocedure care:**
   A. See *Amniocentesis and amniotic fluid analysis, Diagnostic.*
5. **Client and family teaching:**
   A. This test evaluates fetal lung maturity but is only sensitive in 86% of cases.
   B. Test results are quickly available.
6. **Factors that affect results:**
   A. Amniotic fluid must be obtained via amniocentesis; fluid from vaginal pool not acceptable.

B. Fluid must be collected in clean, untreated tubes.
C. Amniotic fluid contaminated with blood or meconium gives a false lung maturity result.
D. Amniotic fluid must be tested immediately or refrigerated at 4° C.
E. Test must be performed with fluid between 20° and 25° C.
7. **Other data:**
   A. This test has up to a 50% false-maturity and false-immaturity result.
   B. Test results are interpreted as "mature" versus "immature" when there is actually a continuum of maturity
   C. Artificial surfactant and antenatal corticosteroids have decreased RDS mortality and thus have lessened the need for fetal maturity testing. However, the American College of Obstetrics and Gynecology recommends pulmonary maturity testing for all planned elective deliveries at less than 39 weeks of amenorrhea.
   D. An older, unstandardized form of this test was called the Shake Test.

FOLEY CATHETER TIP, CULTURE
(see Foreign body, Routine, Culture)

FOLIC ACID, RED BLOOD CELLS, BLOOD

Norm. Folate present in packed cells (ng/mL).

		SI UNITS
Adults		
≤60 years	95-503 ng/mL	215-1132 nmol/L
>60 years	150-450 ng/mL	340-1020 nmol/L

Increased. Folic acid supplements, myelodysplastic syndrome.

Decreased. Alcoholism, anemia (pure vitamin B_{12} deficiency, hemolytic megaloblastic, pernicious, sickle cell), blind loop syndrome, celiac disease, coronary artery disease, Crohn's disease, dermatitis herpetiformis, diet (inadequate intake), folate coenzyme dysfunction, hepatic disease, lactation (without increased dietary folate), leukopenia, hemodialysis, hyperthyroidism, infants, iron and folate deficiency, leukemia (acute myelomonocytic), malabsorption syndromes, malignancy, malnutrition, mania, myeloproliferative disease, myelosclerosis, neoplastic diseases, pregnancy (without increased dietary folate), renal failure, sprue (tropical, nontropical), thrombocytopenia, and vitamin B_{12} deficiency. Drugs include aminopterin, anticoagulants (chronic), anticonvulsants, chloroquine hydrochloride, chloroquine phosphate, ethyl alcohol (ethanol), glutethimide, hydroxychloroquine sulfate, isoniazid, methotrexate, oral contraceptives (long-term), phenytoin, phenytoin sodium, primaquine phosphate, pyrimethamine, quinacrine hydrochloride, quinine sulfate, smoking cigarettes, and sulfonamides.

Description. Folic acid (folate) is a vitamin and amino acid needed for normal functioning of red and white blood cells. It is formed by bacteria in the intestines, stored in the liver, and found in foods such as eggs, milk, leafy vegetables, yeast, liver, and fruits. Folate is absorbed in the jejunum and functions in the metabolism of amino acids and nucleotides, affecting all tissues that undergo a large amount of cell multiplication. Folate deficiency causes megaloblastic anemia and eventually leukopenia and thrombocytopenia. Folic acid is believed to play a role in birth defects such as spina bifida, anencephaly, and orofacial clefts. Symptoms of deficiency take about 3 months to appear and can be caused by inadequate intake, increased body demand, or folate antagonism by drugs. Red blood cells contain more folate than the serum does, and this measurement of folic acid is less sensitive to recent dietary intake of folic acid than the serum folic acid test is.

Professional Considerations
1. Consent form NOT required.
2. Preparation:
   A. Tube: Red topped, red/gray topped, or gold topped, and lavender topped; and ascorbic acid.

3. Procedure:
   A. Draw a 5-mL blood sample in a red-topped tube.
   B. Draw a 5-mL blood sample in a lavender-topped tube.
   C. Prepare a hemolysate by adding 0.5 mL of EDTA blood to 4.5 mL of ascorbic acid and freeze immediately.
4. Postprocedure care:
   A. Protect the specimen from light by inserting it into a paper bag.
5. Client and family teaching:
   A. Results are normally available within 24 hours.
6. Factors that affect results:
   A. Reject specimens if the client had a radioactive scan within 48 hours before specimen collection.
   B. Bacterial contamination of the specimen may invalidate the results.
   C. A standard multivitamin increases RBC-folate levels in clients on hemodialysis.
7. Other data:
   A. The same specimen from step 3-A may be used for serum folic acid level.
   B. The recommended dietary intake of folate is 400 mg/day.
   C. RBC folate is higher is white men and women compared to African-American men and women or Mexican-American men and women, respectively.

FOLIC ACID (VITAMIN B$_9$), SERUM

Norm:

		SI UNITS
Adults		
≤60 years	1.8-9 ng/mL	4.1-20.4 nmol/L
>60 years	1.2-12 ng/mL	4.1-27.2 nmol/L

Increased. Folic acid supplements.

Decreased. Alcoholism, Alzheimer disease, anemia (pure vitamin B$_{12}$ deficiency, hemolytic, megaloblastic, pernicious, sickle cell), bacterial overgrowth, blind loop syndrome, celiac disease, Crohn's disease, dermatitis herpetiformis, diet (inadequate intake), folate coenzyme dysfunction, hemolytic processes or conditions, hepatic disease, lactation (without increased dietary folate), leukopenia, hemodialysis, hyper-thyroidism, insufficient dietary intake, infants, iron and folate deficiency, jejunal diseases, leukemia (acute myelomonocytic), malabsorption syndromes, malignancy, malnutrition, myeloproliferative disease, myelosclerosis, neoplastic diseases, pregnancy (without increased dietary folate), renal failure, short bowel syndrome, sprue (tropical, nontropical), stroke, thrombocytopenia, and vitamin B$_{12}$ deficiency. Drugs include alcohol, aminopterin, anticoagulants (chronic), anticonvulsants, chloroquine hydrochloride, chloroquine phosphate, ethyl alcohol, glutethimide, hydroxychloroquine sulfate, isoniazid, methotrexate, oral contraceptives (long-term), phenytoin, phenytoin sodium, primaquine primidone, phosphate, pyrimethamine, quinacrine hydrochloride, quinine sulfate, sulfonamides, and triamterene.

Description. Folic acid (folate) is a vitamin and amino acid needed for normal functioning of red and white blood cells. It is formed by bacteria in the intestines, stored in the liver, and found in foods such as eggs, milk, leafy vegetables, yeast, liver, and fruits. Folate is absorbed in the jejunum and functions in the metabolism of amino acids and nucleotides, affecting all the tissues that undergo a large amount of cell multiplication. Folate deficiency causes megaloblastic anemia and eventually leukopenia and thrombocytopenia. Folic acid is believed to play a role in birth defects such as spina bifida, anencephaly, and orofacial clefts as well as reducing cardiovascular morbidity and mortality. Symptoms of deficiency take about 3 months to appear and can be caused by inadequate intake, increased body demand, or folate antagonism by drugs. Serum contains less folate than the red blood cells do. This measurement of folic acid is more sensitive to recent dietary intake of folic acid than the red blood cell folic acid test is.

Professional Considerations
1. Consent form NOT required.
2. **Preparation:**
   A. Tube: Red topped, red/gray topped, or gold topped.
   B. See *Client and family teaching.*
3. **Procedure:**
   A. Draw a 1-mL blood sample before any injections of vitamin B_{12}.

4. **Postprocedure care:**
   A. Protect the specimen from light by inserting it into a paper bag.
   B. Transport the specimen to the laboratory and refrigerate the serum until tested.
   C. If the specimen will not be tested within 24 hours, the serum should be frozen at $-10°$ C and protected from light.
5. **Client and family teaching:**
   A. Do not eat food 8 hours before sampling. Water is permitted.
   B. Results are normally available within 24 hours.
6. **Factors that affect results:**
   A. Reject hemolyzed specimens and samples not frozen or not protected from light.
   B. Hemolysis falsely elevates results.
   C. Drugs that are folate antagonists, such as methotrexate and pentamidine, and cigarette smoking, antacids, anticonvulsants, and NSAIDS may induce a deficiency state.
   D. Levels may decrease in clients taking oral contraceptives.
7. **Other data:**
   A. The same specimen may be used for one portion of the red blood cell folic acid level test.
   B. Levels fall below normal 21-28 days after deficiency begins.
   C. Most women still receive less folate than the 0.4 mg/day recommended. Women of childbearing age need 400 µg/day intake of folic acid.
   D. Folic acid supplements reduce methotrexate gastrointestinal side effects in clients with rheumatoid arthritis.
   E. In the United States, since 1998, flour is enriched with folic acid to help prevent birth defects and decrease coronary artery disease.

FOLLICLE-STIMULATING HORMONE (FSH, FOLLITROPIN), SERUM

Norm. Normal ranges will vary among laboratories and are dependent on which international system of measurement is used.

		SI UNITS
Adult Females		
Premenopausal	4-30 mIU/mL	4-30 IU/L
Follicular phase	2-25 mIU/mL	2-25 IU/L
Midcycle peak	10-90 mIU/mL	10-90 IU/L
Luteal phase	2-25 mIU/mL	2-25 IU/L

Continued

		SI UNITS
Adult Females—cont'd		
Pregnant	Low to undetectable	
Menopausal	40-250 mIU/mL	40-250 IU/L
Postmenopausal	40-250 mIU/mL	40-250 IU/L
Adult Males	4-25 mIU/mL	4-25 IU/L
Children, Prepubertal	5-13 mIU/mL	5-13 IU/L

Increased. Acromegaly (early), amenorrhea (primary), anorchism, castration, endometrial ablation, gonadal failure, hyperpituitarism, hypogonadism, hypothalamic tumor, hysterectomy, Klinefelter syndrome, male climacteric, menopause, menstruation, orchidectomy, ovarian failure, pituitary tumors, precocious puberty, premature menopause, seminiferous tubule failure, seminoma, Stein-Leventhal syndrome (polycystic ovary syndrome), testicular agenesis, testicular destruction (caused by radiation or mumps orchitis), testicular failure, testicular feminization syndrome (complete), and Turner syndrome (primary hypogonadism). Drugs include excessive cigarette smoking.

Decreased. Adrenal hyperplasia, amenorrhea (secondary), anorexia nervosa, anovulatory menstrual cycle, delayed puberty, hypogonadotropinism, hypophysectomy, hypothalamic dysfunction, neoplasm (adrenal, ovarian, testicular), panhypopituitarism, and prepubertal child. Drugs include chlorpromazine, estrogens, oral contraceptives, progesterone, and testosterone.

Description. When released from the anterior pituitary gland, folliclestimulating hormone (FSH) in women promotes maturation of the ovarian follicle, which produces estrogen. As levels of estrogen rise, luteinizing hormones are produced. Together, FSH and luteinizing hormone induce ovulation. In men, FSH produces spermatogenesis, and the luteinizing hormone stimulates the secretion of androgens. This test aids in the differential diagnosis of hypogonadism, infertility, menstrual disorders, and precocious puberty.

Professional Considerations
1. Consent form NOT required.
2. **Preparation:**
   A. Tube: Red topped, red/gray topped, or gold topped or lavender topped.
3. **Procedure:**
   A. Draw a 1-mL blood sample between 6 and 7 AM.
4. **Postprocedure care:**
   A. Write the beginning date of the female's last menstruation on the laboratory requisition.
   B. Send the specimen to the laboratory immediately for separation and freezing of serum.
5. **Client and family teaching:**
   A. Results are normally available within 24 hours.
   B. Repeating of the test is often required to ensure an accurate diagnosis.
6. **Factors that affect results:**
   A. Reject hemolyzed specimens or if the client had a radioactive scan within 48 hours.
   B. Radionuclides cause a falsely decreased FSH level.
   C. Values should be compared with the norms for the laboratory performing the test.
7. **Other data:**
   A. Several daily specimens are recommended because of episodic release of FSH from the pituitary gland.

FOLLICLE-STIMULATING HORMONE (FSH, FOLLITROPIN), URINE

Norm:

		SI UNITS
Adult Females	3-12 IU/24 hours	3-12 IU/day
Follicular phase	2-15 IU/24 hours	2-15 IU/day
Midcycle peak	8-60 IU/24 hours	8-60 IU/day

		SI UNITS
Adult Females—cont'd		
Luteal phase	2-10 IU/24 hours	2-10 IU/day
Menopausal	35-100 IU/24 hours	35-100 IU/day
Adult Males	2-18 IU/24 hours	>2-18 IU/day
>61 years	>2-18 IU/24 hours	
Female Children		
Neonate-12 months	<1.4 IU/24 hours	<1.4 IU/day
12 months-8 years	<4.0 IU/24 hours	<4.0 IU/day
9-10 years	1-4 IU/24 hours	1-4 IU/day
11-12 years	1-8 IU/24 hours	1-8 IU/day
13-14 years	1-10 IU/24 hours	1-10 IU/day
Male Children		
Neonate-12 months	<1.4 IU/24 hours	<1.4 IU/day
12 months-8 years	<4.5 IU/24 hours	<4.5 IU/day
9-10 years	1-5 IU/24 hours	1-5 IU/day
11-12 years	1.5-5 IU/24 hours	1.5-5 IU/day
13-14 years	2-12 IU/24 hours	2-12 IU/day

Increased. Acromegaly (early), amenorrhea (primary), anorchism, castration, gonadal failure, hyperpituitarism, hypogonadism, hypothalamic tumor, hysterectomy, Klinefelter syndrome, male climacteric, menopause, menstruation, orchiectomy, ovarian failure, pituitary tumors, precocious puberty, premature menopause, seminiferous tubule failure, seminoma, Stein-Leventhal syndrome (polycystic ovary syndrome), testicular agenesis, testicular destruction (caused by radiation or mumps orchitis), testicular failure, testicular feminization syndrome (complete), and Turner syndrome (primary hypogonadism).

Decreased. Adrenal hyperplasia, amenorrhea (secondary), anorexia nervosa, anovulatory menstrual cycle, delayed puberty, hypogonadotropinism, hypophysectomy, hypothalamic dysfunction, nonconceptive cycles, neoplasm (adrenal, ovarian, testicular), panhypopituitarism, and prepubertal child. Drugs include chlorpromazine, estrogens, oral contraceptives, progesterone, and testosterone.

Description. When released from the anterior pituitary gland, follicle-stimulating hormone (FSH) in women promotes maturation of the ovarian follicle, which produces estrogen. As levels of estrogen rise, luteinizing hormones are produced. Together, FSH and luteinizing hormone induce ovulation. In men, FSH produces spermatogenesis, and luteinizing hormone stimulates the secretion of androgens. Urine FSH levels are more useful than serum levels because a 24-hour collection will reflect both the peaks and lows of the episodic FSH secretion. This urine test aids in the differential diagnosis of hypogonadism, infertility, menstrual disorders, and precocious puberty.

Professional Considerations
1. Consent form NOT required.
2. **Preparation:**
   A. Obtain a 3-L container with boric acid additive.
   B. Write the beginning time of the collection on the laboratory requisition.
3. **Procedure:**
   A. Discard the first morning urine specimen.
   B. Collect all the urine voided in a 24-hour period in a refrigerated, 3-L container to which 10 g of boric acid has been added. Document the quantity of urine output during the collection period. Include the urine voided at the end of the 24-hour period. For catheterized clients, keep the drainage bag on ice and empty urine into the collection container hourly.
4. **Postprocedure care:**
   A. Write the total amount of urine in the 24-hour sample on the laboratory requisition.
   B. Gently mix the container and send a 50-mL aliquot to the lab.
   C. Best storage is at 4° C without any additive.

5. **Client and family teaching:**
   A. Save all the urine voided in the 24-hour period and urinate before defecating to avoid loss of urine. If any urine is accidentally discarded, discard the entire specimen and restart the collection the next day.
   B. Results are normally available within 24 hours.
   C. A repeat of the test is required to ensure an appropriate diagnosis.
6. **Factors that affect results:**
   A. Radionuclides cause a falsely decreased FSH level.
7. **Other data:**
   A. Several 24-hour urine specimens are recommended because of episodic release of FSH from the pituitary gland.

FOLLITROPIN, SERUM
(see Follicle-stimulating hormone, Serum)

FOLLITROPIN, URINE
(see Follicle-stimulating hormone, Urine)

FOREIGN BODY, ROUTINE, CULTURE

Norm. No growth.

Usage. Aids diagnosis of infection caused by invasive lines, catheters, and other foreign bodies. Part of the work-up for suspected septic processes in clients on hyperalimentation or with other invasive lines. Determination of sensitivity of line-sepsis microorganisms to antibacterial therapy.

Description. Includes the culturing of heart valves, dialysis catheters, Swan-Ganz or other central line tip, and intrauterine devices. Test also includes culture of indwelling urinary catheters. Nosocomial urinary tract infections associated with the presence of indwelling urinary catheters account for up to 40% of urinary tract infections.

Professional Considerations
1. Consent form NOT required.
2. **Preparation:**
   A. Obtain povidone-iodine solution, a sterile container or a red-topped tube, and sterile gloves.
   B. For urinary catheter tip culture, obtain sterile scissors, a 20-mL

syringe, and a sterile specimen cup or red-topped tube.
3. **Procedure:**
   A. *Invasive lines:*
      i. Remove the line site dressing.
      ii. Cleanse the line insertion site and surrounding skin with povidone-iodine and allow to dry.
      iii. Remove the invasive line, taking care not to contaminate the distal portion with skin or other objects.
      iv. Insert the tip (distal end) into a sterile, red-topped tube or sterile container. Cut the distal 1.5-inch tip with sterile scissors, allowing the tip to drop into the container.
   B. *Indwelling urinary catheter:*
      i. Remove the water filling the balloon of the catheter using a syringe.
      ii. Remove the catheter, using sterile gloves and being careful not to contaminate the tip.
      iii. While holding the tip over or inside a sterile container, cut off at least 1 inch with sterile scissors and allow the tip to fall into the container.
      iv. Close the container.
4. **Postprocedure care:**
   A. Write the type of catheter and the removal site on the requisition.
   B. Write the collection time on the laboratory requisition.
   C. Transport the specimen to the laboratory within 1 hour.
   D. Do not refrigerate or incubate the specimen.
5. **Client and family teaching:**
   A. Specimen collection is usually painless.
   B. Incubation of the culture may take 24-48 hours.
6. **Factors that affect results:**
   A. Reject specimens if received more than 2 hours after collection.
   B. Contamination of the urinary catheter specimen with the external genital area may obscure the validity of the results. This is a frequent occurrence in the collection of the tip.
7. **Other data:**
   A. Irritation of the urethra is minimized by total deflation of the balloon, which holds from 5 to 30 mL of sterile water.

B. Most ingested foreign bodies are found within 24 hours and are common in Southeast Asia and Singapore as otolaryngologic emergencies. Few require culture.

FPA
(*see Fibrinopeptide A, Blood*)

FRA, SPECIMEN
(*see Fluorescent rabies antibody, Specimen*)

FRACTIONAL EXCRETION OF SODIUM IN URINE, DIAGNOSTIC
(*see Renal indices, Diagnostic*)

FRACTIONAL URINE, SPECIMEN
(*see Urinalysis, Fractional, Urine*)

FREE CALCIUM, SERUM
(*see Calcium, Ionized, Blood*)

FREE METANEPHRINES
(*see Metanephrines, Total, 24-Hour urine, and Free, Plasma*)

FREE PSA, SERUM
(*see Prostate-specific antigen, Serum*)

FREI SKIN TEST FOR LYMPHOGRANULOMA VENEREUM, DIAGNOSTIC

Norm. Negative.

Usage. Aids in the diagnosis of lymphogranuloma venereum (LGV).

Description. Lymphogranuloma venereum is a sexually transmitted disease caused by *Chlamydia trachomatis* of immunotypes L1-L3, resulting in suppurative inguinal adenitis several days to several weeks after exposure. The most common mode of transmission is through sexual contact. The Frei test is not diagnostically specific. Clients with the disease become positive at about 3 weeks after the initial infection.

Professional Considerations
1. Consent form NOT required.

Risks
Allergic reaction to LGV injection; infection.

Contraindications
Previous allergy to chicken eggs.

2. **Preparation:**
   A. Obtain a 1-mL syringe with a needle and LGV antigen for intradermal injection.
3. **Procedure:**
   A. Inject intradermally 0.1 mL of heat-inactivated, egg-grown LGV.
   B. Inject a control substance made from a normal yolk sac at another intradermal site.
   C. Read the skin test in 48-72 hours. The test is positive if the test site has a raised papular area $\geq 6 \times 6$ mm and the control site reaction is $\leq 5 \times 5$ mm.
4. **Postprocedure care:**
   A. List the injection site location on the client's record.
5. **Client and family teaching:**
   A. Results will be available in 48-72 hours.
6. **Factors that affect results:**
   A. *Chlamydia* infections that share the same group antigen will produce a positive Frei test.
7. **Other data:**
   A. Licensed Frei test antigens are not available commercially in the United States.
   B. Clients testing positive will always test positive on any future Frei tests.
   C. Delayed positive reactions are possible for several days.

FROZEN TISSUE SECTION, DIAGNOSTIC

Norm. Interpreted by pathologist.

Usage. Rapid diagnosis on biopsied tissue while surgery is in progress.

Description. The rapid freezing and slicing of tissue for pathologic examination and interpretation. Using frozen tissue section samples as a basis for diagnosis, though NOT 100% accurate, has consistently proved to be a highly accurate method for *rapid* diagnosis. This method may also be used for fluorescent microscopy and for identification of fats and enzymes undetectable by other methods.

Professional Considerations

1. Consent form IS required for the procedure used to obtain the specimen. See *Biopsy, site-specific, Specimen*, for procedure-specific risks and contraindications.
2. **Preparation:**
   A. Preoperative teaching involving the type of procedure required for the sampling to proceed.
   B. See *Client and family teaching*.
3. **Procedure:**
   A. Place the moistened, fixed or unfixed tissue on a freezing microtome table.
   B. Allow carbon dioxide to enter the table through the side perforations.
   C. Freeze the tissue and slice it into thin sections by means of the cryostat.
   D. Attach the frozen section to a glass slide.
   E. Stain the nucleus of the cells with a hematoxylin dye.
   F. Stain the cytoplasm of the cells with eosin dye.
   G. Examine the slide microscopically and interpret.
4. **Postprocedure care:**
   A. See individual procedure listings.
5. **Client and family teaching:**
   A. Preparation for the procedure is necessary.
   B. Fast from food and fluids for 12 hours before the procedure.
   C. Call the physician for signs of infection at the procedure site: increasing pain, redness, swelling, purulent drainage, or for fever >101° F (38.2° C).
   D. Supply information on possible support groups available for the diagnosis.
6. **Factors that affect results:**
   A. Poor tissue sample.
7. **Other data:**
   A. Microscopic examination is often able to confirm a diagnosis of a specific lesion.
   B. Frozen sections have been reported as false-positive and false-negative results. A fresh section is best for accuracy.

FRUCTOSAMINE, SERUM

Norm. Normal ranges vary according to method.

Adult

Nondiabetic	1.5-2.7 mmol/L
Diabetic	>2.0-5.0 mmol/L

Child 5% below adult levels

Usage. Evaluate diabetic control, reflecting glucose concentrations over a shorter time period (2-3 weeks) than that represented by glycated hemoglobin (hemoglobin A_{1C}) (4-8 weeks). Can be used as an index of longer-term control than glucose levels especially in diabetic clients with abnormal hemoglobin, in clients with gestational diabetes, and in children with type 1 diabetes.

Professional Considerations

1. Consent form is NOT required.
2. **Preparation:**
   A. Tube: Red topped, red/gray topped, or gold topped.
   B. See *Client and family teaching*.
3. **Procedure:**
   A. Draw a 5-mL blood sample.
4. **Postprocedure care:**
   A. None.
5. **Client and family teaching:**
   A. Abstain from food and drink 12 hours before the test.
   B. Results are normally available within 24 hours.
6. **Factors that affect results:**
   A. Albumin levels <3.0 g/dL may falsely lower fructosamine concentrations.
7. **Other data:**
   A. Hemoglobin, ascorbic acid, and ceruloplasmin inhibit fructosamine generation.
   B. Fructosamine >285 mmol/L associated with 4.3-fold increase in cardiovascular mortality.

FRUCTOSE CHALLENGE TEST, DIAGNOSTIC

Norm. Lack of significant change in serum glucose, phosphorus, and magnesium after intravenous fructose administration. Lack of a fall in serum glucose after an oral fructose load. Normal plasma fructose is <10 mg/dL or <6 mmol/L (SI units).

Usage. The intravenous fructose challenge test and an oral fructose challenge test are used in the evaluation of several inherited disorders of fructose metabolism including essential fructosuria, hereditary fructose intolerance, and fructose-1,6-diphosphatase deficiency, and to aid in the diagnosis of steatohepatitis.

Description. Fructose disorders all are inherited as autosomal recessive traits. Essential fructosuria is a clinically benign disorder. Fructose-1,6-diphosphatase deficiency is a clinically severe and often terminal illness in the newborn that is frequently diagnosed by clinical clues that do not involve fructose-loading tests. Hereditary fructose intolerance is a disorder, seen in children as well as adults, that is caused by a deficiency of fructose-1-phosphate aldolase. This condition, characterized by an aversion to sweet foods, may be diagnosed by use of the intravenous fructose challenge test. In this test, a weight-based dose of intravenous fructose is administered intravenously, and serial blood and urine samples are obtained.

Professional Considerations
1. Consent form IS required.

Risks
Profound hypoglycemia is likely to occur in clients with hereditary fructose intolerance.

Contraindications
Known fructose intolerance. Ancillary medical conditions in which hypoglycemia would impose unacceptable risk to the client (certain forms of cardiac and neurologic disease).

2. **Preparation:**
    A. See *Client and family teaching.*
    B. Insert an indwelling intravenous catheter for the administration of fructose, for obtaining blood samples, and if the emergent administration of intravenous glucose is needed.
    C. Insert an indwelling urinary catheter if urine samples will be measured.
    D. Obtain 10 red-topped, red/gray-topped, or gold-topped tubes.
    E. Obtain blood glucose monitoring machine and associated supplies.
    F. Obtain parenteral glucose solution ($D_{50}W$).
    G. Have emergency equipment readily available.
3. **Procedure:**
    A. The client is positioned recumbent.

B. Draw a 7-mL baseline blood sample for serum glucose, fructose, potassium, phosphorus, magnesium, and urate determination.
C. If urine testing will be included, collect a 2-hour baseline urine sample for urate, phosphorus, lactate, alanine, magnesium, and fructose.
D. Administer 200 mg/kg (body weight) of 20% fructose solution intravenously over a 1-minute period for children or over a 2-minute period for adults.
E. Repeat step B above drawn immediately after the injection and then at 5, 10, 15, 20, 30, 45, 60, 90, and 120 minutes after the fructose infusion.
F. Urine measurements of fructose, lactate, alanine, magnesium, and phosphorus are occasionally performed during the fructose challenge test.
G. Serum glucose is monitored frequently during the test with cutaneous blood glucose monitoring.
4. **Postprocedure care:**
    A. Write beginning and ending times of each urine collection on the laboratory requisition.
    B. Perform cutaneous blood glucose measurement frequently and observe closely for signs of hypoglycemia for several hours after the test.
    C. Discontinue urinary catheter.
    D. Discontinue intravenous catheter once it is determined that hypoglycemia is no longer a risk.
5. **Client and family teaching:**
    A. Consume a diet free of fructose and sucrose during the 3 weeks before the test.
    B. This test is needed to help diagnose hereditary fructose intolerance. This is a condition in which modifying your diet to reduce fructose in your food can improve your prognosis.
    C. This test may cause you to feel hypoglycemic. If this occurs, it will be quickly treated.
6. **Factors that affect the test:**
    A. Accurately timed and labeled serum and urine samples are essential.
    B. Abnormally low fructose levels may result if the urine specimen is not tested when it is still fresh.

C. Timed studies of this type are often best performed on special diagnostic areas where the personnel are familiar with the diagnostic procedure.

7. **Other data:**
   A. Hereditary fructose intolerance is associated with hypoglycemia after intravenous fructose administration. Other phenomena observed in these clients during the test include a rise in serum magnesium and uric acid, a fall in serum phosphorus, and a decrease in urine phosphorus excretion after the fructose administration.
   B. Infants fed with a sucrose-containing formula that is hydrolyzed to fructose will exhibit more severe symptoms than breast-fed infants, who are usually asymptomatic, because lactose is not catabolized by the fructose enzyme.
   C. Liver biopsy specimens examined for metabolites of fructose may also be used for diagnosis of hereditary fructose intolerance.
   D. Treatment for hereditary fructose intolerance is a fructose-free and sucrose-free diet.

FSH, SERUM

(see Follicle-stimulating hormone, Serum)

FSH, URINE

(see Follicle-stimulating hormone, Urine)

FT4

(see Thyroid test: Thyroxine Free, Serum)

FTA-ABS, SERUM

(see Fluorescent treponemal antibody absorption, Serum)

FUNCTIONAL MRI

(see Magnetic resonance imaging, Diagnostic)

FUNGAL ANTIBODY SCREEN, BLOOD

Norm. Negative.

Usage. Rapid detection of antifungal antibodies. Monitoring effectiveness of therapy for fungal infections.

Description. Fungi are slow-growing, eukaryotic organisms that can grow on living and nonliving organic materials and are subdivided into yeasts and molds. Only a few fungi species infect humans. Normal host defense mechanisms limit the damage they cause superficially. Viral serologic testing for fungal antibodies aids in the diagnosis of aspergillosis, blastomycosis, coccidioidomycosis, *Cryptococcus* antigen, fungal infections, histoplasmosis, and *Sporothrix* antibodies. Antibodies to fungi may be found soon after infection and rise as the infection progresses. Diagnosis of a fungal infection is confirmed when the convalescent sample demonstrates a rise in titer from the acute sample.

Professional Considerations
1. Consent form NOT required.
2. **Preparation:**
   A. Tube: Red topped, red/gray topped, or gold topped.
   B. See *Client and family teaching.*
3. **Procedure:**
   A. Draw a 10-mL blood sample.
   B. Acute and convalescent samples are required. Obtain the acute sample as soon as possible after onset. Draw the convalescent sample in 1-2 weeks.
4. **Postprocedure care:**
   A. Send the specimen to the laboratory for immediate separation and freezing of the serum.
5. **Client and family teaching:**
   A. Fast for 12 hours before the test.
   B. A repeat specimen is required in 1-2 weeks.
   C. The treatment will usually be started prophylactically.
6. **Factors that affect results:**
   A. Reject hemolyzed specimens, tubes partially filled with blood, or specimens received more than 2 hours after collection.
   B. Recent fungal antigen skin tests may cause falsely high results.
   C. Blastomycosis and histoplasmosis antigens may cross-react to cause falsely high results. Cystic fibrosis may cause false-positive results for coccidioidomycosis.
   D. False-negative results may be caused by immunosuppression from mycoses.
7. **Other data:**
   A. Factors that predispose clients to fungal infectious by lowering the

normal host defense mechanisms include administration of broad-spectrum antibiotics, invasive lines, poor nutritional status, parenteral nutrition, surgery, trauma, long-term use of steroids, and chemotherapy for cancer treatment. Other significant risk factors are age over 60 years and staying in an intensive care unit.

FUNGIZONE, BLOOD
(see Amphotericin B, Blood)

FUNGUS, CEREBROSPINAL FLUID, CULTURE
(see Cerebrospinal fluid, Routine, Culture and cytology, Specimen)

FV LEIDEN
(see Factor V, Blood and Prothrombin C, Blood)

G6PD, BLOOD
(see Glucose-6-phosphate dehydrogenase, Quantitative and Screen, Blood)

GALACTOKINASE, BLOOD

Norm:

Adults   12.1-39.7 mU/g Hb

Children
2-18 years   11.0-53.6 mU/g Hb
<2 years   11.0-150.0 mU/g Hb
Infants   3-4 times adult values

Increased. Not clinically significant.

Decreased. Galactokinase deficiency, galactosemia, and juvenile cataracts.

Description. Galactokinase is an enzyme that functions in the metabolism of galactose to glucose in the liver, a deficiency of which may result in galactosemia. Galactokinase deficiency is one of three forms of galactosemia, an autosomal recessively transmitted inborn error of metabolism characterized by the inability to convert galactose into glucose with mutations found in the GALK1 gene. This form of galac-

tosemia results in the appearance of infantile or childhood cataracts.

Professional Considerations
1. Consent form NOT required.
2. **Preparation:**
   A. Preschedule this test with the laboratory.
   B. Tube: Green topped, and a container of ice.
3. **Procedure:**
   A. Draw a 7-mL blood sample.
4. **Postprocedure care:**
   A. Place the specimen on ice immediately.
   B. Write the collection time on the laboratory requisition.
   C. Send the specimen to the laboratory within 2 hours. Keep the specimen on ice until tested.
5. **Client and family teaching:**
   A. Results are normally available within 24 hours.
   B. Diet counseling is strongly recommended if the test is positive.
   C. Stress the importance of follow-up examination.
   D. Refer clients with positive results for genetic counseling.
6. **Factors that affect results:**
   A. Reject specimens that were not placed on ice or were not received in the laboratory within 2 hours after collection.
7. **Other data:**
   A. Homozygotes have a form of galactosemia with cataracts but without mental retardation or liver disease.

GALACTOSE-1-PHOSPHATE, BLOOD

Norm. <1 mg% of galactose-1-phosphate per 100 mL of lysed packed red blood cells. 18.5-28.5 U/g hemoglobin.

Increased. Transferase deficiency (classical) galactosemia.

Description. Galactose-1-phosphate is a metabolite that results after the action of galactokinase on galactose. It is found in red blood cells, subsequently converted to glucose-l-phosphate by galactose-l-phosphate uridyltransferase, and used for energy by the body. In clients with galactosemia who are ingesting milk and milk products, the level of galactose-l-phosphate rises and may become toxic. This test is used to monitor the dietary compliance of clients with galactosemia.

Professional Considerations
1. Consent form NOT required.
2. Preparation:
   A. Preschedule this test with the laboratory.
   B. Tube: Green topped.
3. Procedure:
   A. Draw a 2-mL blood sample and gently invert the tube three times.
4. Postprocedure care:
   A. Write the collection time on the laboratory requisition.
   B. Refrigerate specimens until tested.

5. **Client and family teaching:**
   A. Results are normally available within 24 hours.
   B. If results are positive, the client and family will require diet counseling regarding a galactose-free diet.
   C. Galactose toxicity may cause failure to thrive, liver dysfunction, mental retardation, and vomiting or diarrhea.
6. **Factors that affect results:**
   A. Reject specimens received in the laboratory more than 3 hours after collection.
7. **Other data:**
   A. None.

GALACTOSE-1-PHOSPHATE URIDYLTRANSFERASE, ERYTHROCYTE, BLOOD

Norm:

		SI UNITS
Adult	5.9-9.5 µmol/hr/mL	98-158 U/L
Heterozygote	2.0-4.8 µmol/hr/mL	33-80 U/L
Homozygote	0.0 µmol/hr/mL	0.0 U/L
Other norms		
Normal	18-28 U/g Hb	
Possible carrier state	5-18.5 U/g Hb	

Increased. Not applicable.

Decreased. Galactose-1-phosphate uridyltransferase deficiency and transferase-deficiency (classical) galactosemia.

Description. Galactose-1-phosphate uridyltransferase is an enzyme active in the metabolism of galactose to glucose in the liver. It catalyzes the conversion of galactose-1-phosphate into glucose-1-phosphate. Deficiency of galactose-1-phosphate uridyltransferase is the most common cause of galactosemia. In this test, measurements of this enzyme are performed on the hemolysate of washed erythrocytes.

Professional Considerations
1. Consent form NOT required.
2. Preparation:
   A. Tube: Green topped, and a container of ice.
3. Procedure:
   A. Draw a 2-mL blood sample and then gently invert the tube three times.
4. Postprocedure care:
   A. Place the specimen immediately on ice.

5. **Client and family teaching:**
   A. If the results are positive, the client and family will require diet counseling regarding a galactose-free diet.
6. **Factors that affect results:**
   A. Reject the specimen if it contains recently transfused blood to avoid a possible false-negative result.
   B. Reject hemolyzed specimens or specimens not received on ice.
7. **Other data:**
   A. Treat galactosemia with a lactose-free diet.
   B. See also *Galactose-1-phosphate uridyltransferase, Qualitative, Blood.*

GALACTOSE-1-PHOSPHATE URIDYLTRANSFERASE, QUALITATIVE, BLOOD

Norm. Negative.

Positive. Transferase-deficiency (classical) galactosemia.

Description. A qualitative screen for galactosemia and differential diagnosis of milk intolerance in the newborn. This enzyme catalyzes the conversion of galactose-1-phosphate into glucose-1-phosphate in the liver. Galactosemia is an autosomal recessively transmitted inborn error of metabolism characterized by the inability to convert galactose into glucose. This causes deposits of galactose-1-phosphate in body tissues, resulting in vomiting, diarrhea, failure to thrive, liver dysfunction, splenomegaly, and cataracts in the infant. Symptoms appear a few days after a milk diet is started. Deficiency of galactose-1-phosphate uridyltransferase is the most common form of galactosemia. Early detection of galactosemia enables institution of a lactose-free diet and avoidance of complications of galactose toxicity. The test involves examining specially treated filter paper with a drop of dried blood under fluorescent lights after timed exposure to ultraviolet radiation. In a negative test (enzyme present), the blood fluoresces. In a positive test (enzyme absent), the blood will not fluoresce.

Professional Considerations
1. Consent form NOT required.
2. Preparation:
   A. Preschedule this test with the laboratory.
   B. Write the client's birth date on the laboratory requisition.
   C. Obtain a galactosemia-screening filter paper.
3. Procedure:
   A. Obtain three drops of blood from an infant heelstick on the lateral curvature of the heel.
   B. Place each drop in a circle on galactosemia-screening filter paper and allow to dry.
   C. Heparinized blood may also be used (green-topped tube).
4. Postprocedure care:
   A. Apply a dressing to the heel-stick site.
   B. Label the filter paper with the client's name and identification.
   C. Store the specimen at room temperature. Protect it from heat if it is transferred to an outside laboratory.
5. Client and family teaching:
   A. Results are normally available within 24 hours.

B. If results are positive, the family will require diet counseling regarding a galactose-free diet.
6. Factors that affect results:
   A. This test should be performed during the first 3 days after the infant is born.
   B. False-negative results may occur up to 3 months after blood transfusion if the Beutler-Baluda screening method is used.
7. Other data:
   A. Treat galactosemia with a lactose-free diet.
   B. Blood testing is considered more reliable than urine testing in screening for galactosemia.
   C. Positive results should be confirmed with a quantitative galactose-1-phosphate uridyltransferase measurement.

GALACTOSE, SCREENING TEST FOR GALACTOSEMIA, URINE

Norm. <10 mg/dL. Galactostix has a lower limit of sensitivity of 100 mg/dL.

Increased. Galactokinase deficiency, galactose-1-phosphate uridyltransferase deficiency, and galactosemia.

Description. A urine screen for galactosemia and differential diagnosis of milk intolerance in the newborn after a positive Benedict's or Clinitest result and a negative glucose oxidase test for glucose. Urine galactose measurements are performed by chromatography.

Professional Considerations
1. Consent form NOT required.
2. Preparation:
   A. Obtain a clean container with a lid, pediatric urine collection device, and tape.
3. Procedure:
   A. Obtain at least a 10-mL random urine specimen in a clean container.
   B. Place the infant supine, with the knees flexed and the hips externally rotated and abducted.
   C. Cleanse, rinse, and thoroughly dry the perineal area.
   D. To prevent the child from removing the collection device, a diaper may be placed over the genital area.

E. *Females:* Tape the pediatric collection device to the perineum. Starting at the area between the anus and vagina, apply the device in an anterior direction.

F. *Males:* Place the pediatric collection device over the penis and scrotum and tape it to the perineal area.

4. **Postprocedure care:**
   A. Send the specimens to the laboratory and refrigerate them if not tested immediately.

5. **Client and family teaching:**
   A. If the results are positive, the family will require diet counseling regarding a galactose-free diet.
   B. Results are normally available within 24 hours.

6. **Factors that affect results:**
   A. None found.

7. **Other data:**
   A. Blood testing is more reliable than urine testing in screening for galactosemia.
   B. Positive results should be confirmed with a quantitative galactose-1-phosphate uridyltransferase measurement.
   C. See also *Galactose-1-phosphate uridyltransferase, Qualitative, Blood.*

GALACTOSE TOLERANCE TEST, DIAGNOSTIC
(see Galactose loading test, Diagnostic)

GALLBLADDER SERIES
(see Cholecystography radiography, Diagnostic)

GALLBLADDER AND BILIARY SYSTEM ULTRASONOGRAPHY, DIAGNOSTIC

Norm:

Gallbladder

Appearance	Sonolucent; free of sludge or stones
Location	Anterior to the right kidney, lateral to the pancreas and duodenum
Shape	Circular on transverse scans
	Pear shaped on longitudinal scans
	7-10 cm long and 2-3 cm wide with a capacity of 30-50 mL
Walls	Sharply defined and smooth, 1-2 mm thick

Cystic Duct

Appearance	Not sonolucent because of lumen; Heister's valves visible
Shape	Serpentine

Common Bile Duct

Shape	Linear; internal diameter <6 mm

Hepatic Duct

Lumen	Internal diameter <4 mm

Usage. Diagnosis of cholelithiasis and cholecystitis and differential diagnosis of the cause of jaundice (obstructive versus nonobstructive).

Description. Evaluation of the gallbladder, cystic duct, and common bile duct by the creation of an oscilloscopic picture from the echoes of high-frequency sound waves passing over these areas. The time required for the ultrasonic beam to be reflected back to the transducer from differing densities of tissue is converted by a computer to an electrical impulse displayed on an oscilloscopic screen to create a three-dimensional picture of the gallbladder and biliary duct system. This test is used when cholecystography cannot confirm a suspected diagnosis. The presence of sludge causes low-level echoes in the interior of the gallbladder. Acute cholecystitis causes the walls to appear thickened and sonolucent because of edema. Cholelithiasis is demonstrated by a dilated interior, with shadows present. Biliary tree gas causes shadows. Polyps appear as sharply defined masses, whereas carcinoma appears as a poorly defined mass. In obstructive jaundice, dilatation of the gallbladder and biliary duct system is detected.

Professional Considerations
1. Consent form NOT required.

Risks
If sincalide is given: infection.

Contraindications
Administration of sincalide is contraindicated in pregnancy and in children.

2. **Preparation:**
   A. See *Client and family teaching*.
   B. Some scans may require intravenous access.
3. **Procedure:**
   A. The client is positioned supine and instructed to hold his or her breath during the scans.
   B. A lubricated transducer is passed slowly over the right upper quadrant of the abdomen with transverse scans (moving from the midline to the right side) taken every 1 cm from the xiphoid process to the right subcostal area.
   C. As the gallbladder borders are identified, they are marked on the client's skin.
   D. Longitudinal and oblique scans are then taken every 5 mm between the marked borders of the gallbladder.
   E. The client is then turned to a steep, left lateral decubitus position, and the scan is repeated from the right costal margin.
   F. The client may then be positioned upright to observe for a movement of suspected stones away from the walls of the gallbladder or cystic duct.
   G. If contractility of the gallbladder is to be evaluated, intravenous sincalide may be injected or a fatty meal may be ingested, and the scan is repeated in 30 minutes.
   H. Photographs are taken of the oscilloscopic display.
4. **Postprocedure care:**
   A. Remove the lubricant from the skin.
   B. Resume previous diet.
5. **Client and family teaching:**
   A. Consume a diet free of fat the day before the test.
   B. Fast for 8-12 hours before the ultrasonography, but drink plenty of fluids.
   C. It is important to lie as motionless as possible during the ultrasonography.
6. **Factors that affect results:**
   A. Gallstones appear as shadows when well mixed with bile, but if the gallbladder is full of stones, shadows are difficult to detect.
   B. Sincalide may cause nausea. Movement during nausea may interfere with results.
   C. Dehydration interferes with adequate contrast between organs and body fluids.
   D. Very small stones (<1-2 mm) in the gallbladder must be differentiated from polyps by repositioning of the client. The stones will move downward with gravity, whereas polyps will remain stable.
   E. The more abdominal fat present, the greater is the attenuation (reduction in sound-wave amplitude and intensity), which interferes with the clarity of the picture.
7. **Other data:**
   A. Gallbladder cancer cannot usually be diagnosed by sonography.

GALLBLADDER SCAN
(see Hepatobiliary scan, Diagnostic)

GALLIUM SCAN
(see Gallium scan of bone, brain, breast, or liver, Diagnostic)

GALLIUM SCAN OF BONE, DIAGNOSTIC

Norm. Normal patterns of bone gallium uptake as interpreted by a nuclear medicine physician.

Usage. Detection of osteomyelitis, joint infections, and metastatic bone neoplasms (Wilms' tumor).

Description. Nuclear medicine scan using gallium-67 citrate to localize inflammatory lesions of the bone, bone marrow, and cartilage. Although the bones normally take up the gallium-67 citrate, abnormal areas of inflammation or tumors appear as areas of increased uptake of the radiopharmaceutical.

Professional Considerations
1. Consent form IS required.

Risks
Allergic reaction to the radiopharmaceutical (itching, hives, rash, tight feeling in the throat, shortness of breath, bronchospasm, anaphylaxis, death), infection.

Contraindications
Previous allergic reaction to the same radiopharmaceutical. This test is usually contraindicated during pregnancy and breast-feeding.

2. Preparation:
   A. Inject the client with a gallium-67 citrate radiopharmaceutical intravenously 48-72 hours before the test. *Exception:* For the detection of acute inflammatory lesions, scan at 6-24 hours and then again at 48-72 hours.
   B. If the pelvis is to be scanned, the bladder should be emptied completely just before the procedure.
   C. See *Client and family teaching.*
3. Procedure:
   A. The client is positioned under the gamma (Anger) camera or a scintillation camera.
   B. Serial images are obtained anteriorly and posteriorly while an uptake probe and detector head measure the radiation emissions.
   C. The client must lie motionless throughout the scan.
4. Postprocedure care:
   A. See *Client and family teaching.*
5. Client and family teaching:
   A. Increase oral intake of fluids, where not contraindicated, beginning 24 hours before the scan.
   B. The scan takes 30-60 minutes and is painless.
   C. The camera will make clicking noises during the scan.
   D. It is important to lie motionless during the scan.
   E. Drink 6-8 glasses of water and other fluids each day for 2 days after the test (unless contraindicated).
   F. Results are normally available 24 hours after the completion of the scan.

6. Factors that affect results:
   A. Lesions that are <1-2 cm in size will not be detectable with a gallium scan.
   B. False-positive results may be obtained in the presence of leukopenia.
7. Other data:
   A. Gallium is excreted by the kidney and colon in 24-48 hours.
   B. This test does not distinguish between benign and malignant lesions.
   C. Health care professionals working in a nuclear medicine area must follow federal standards set by the Nuclear Regulatory Commission. These standards include precautions for handling the radioactive material and monitoring of potential radiation exposure.

GALLIUM SCAN OF BRAIN, DIAGNOSTIC

Norm. Normal pattern of brain-tissue gallium uptake as interpreted by a nuclear medicine physician.

Usage. Screening and localizing intracranial neoplasms, identification of cerebrovascular accident or tumor recurrence after surgical excision, and differentiation of localized inflammations of central nervous system (abscesses).

Description. A nuclear medicine scan in which radiopharmaceutical gallium-67 or gallium-68 is injected intravenously and a scintillation camera is used to obtain photographs of the meninges and brain soft tissue 24-48 hours later. The gallium is transported to the brain tissue via cerebrospinal fluid and plasma, where it binds to the transferrin receptor sites of soft-tissue cells of neutrophilic lactoferrin. Tumors and inflammatory lesions frequently contain large concentrations of these two proteins. A positive scan will have distinct patterns of gallium uptake that differ from normal tissue uptake. For example, neoplasms will appear as dense areas with increased gallium uptake, whereas inflammatory lesions (most frequently abscesses) appear on the scan as well-localized areas of increased gallium uptake that are encapsulated. Finally, cerebral hemorrhages will differ from normal gallium uptake, appearing as irregular, diffuse areas of uptake. This is attributable to the vascular occlusion and tissue damage associated with cerebrovascular accidents.

Professional Considerations
1. Consent form IS required.

Risks
Allergic reaction to the radiopharmaceutical (itching, hives, rash, tight feeling in the throat, shortness of breath, bronchospasm, anaphylaxis, death), infection.

Contraindications
Previous allergic reaction to the same radiopharmaceutical. This procedure is usually contraindicated during pregnancy and breast-feeding.

2. **Preparation:**
   A. The client is injected intravenously with radiopharmaceutical gallium-67 or gallium-68 from 6 to 48 hours before the scan.
   B. See *Client and family teaching.*
3. **Procedure:**
   A. The client is positioned under the scintillation camera, and serial images are obtained from anterior, posterior, lateral, and, occasionally, vertex views.
   B. The client must lie motionless throughout the scan.
4. **Postprocedure care:**
   A. See *Client and family teaching.*
5. **Client and family teaching:**
   A. Increase oral intake of fluids, where not contraindicated, beginning 24 hours before the scan.
   B. The scan takes 30-60 minutes and is painless.
   C. The camera may touch the body and will make a clicking noise during the scan.
   D. It is important to lie motionless during the scan.
   E. Drink 6-8 glasses of water and other fluids each day for 2 days after the test (unless contraindicated).
   F. Results are normally available 24 hours after the completion of the scan.
6. **Factors that affect results:**
   A. Lesions <1-2 cm in size may not be detectable with a gallium scan.
   B. Lesions located at the base of the brain, such as pituitary adeno-

mas, may be difficult to detect because of the increased vascularity of the area and the difficulty in positioning the camera for clear images.
   C. False-positive results may be obtained in the presence of leukopenia.
   D. Pediatric neoplasms will most frequently appear intrafrontally, whereas adult neoplasms will most often be located supratentorially.
7. **Other data:**
   A. Gallium is excreted by the kidney and colon in 24-48 hours.
   B. Gallium scanning does not differentiate malignant from benign tumors.
   C. Health care professionals working in a nuclear medicine area must follow federal standards set by the Nuclear Regulatory Commission. These standards include precautions for handling the radioactive material and monitoring of potential radiation exposure.

GALLIUM SCAN OF BREAST, DIAGNOSTIC

Norm. Normal pattern of breast gallium uptake as interpreted by a nuclear medicine physician.

Usage. Detection and location of tumor or inflammatory lesions of the breast, evaluation of lymphomas, and identification of recurrent tumors after chemotherapy or radiation therapy.

Description. Nuclear medicine scan using gallium-67 citrate to localize neoplasms and inflammatory lesions of the breast tissues and lymph nodes. It is believed that the gallium binds to the transferrin and lactoferrin circulating in plasma and soft tissue. Tumors and lesions containing neutrophils also have a large concentrations of these two beta globulins, causing the gallium clearance to be slower than that in normal tissue. Therefore these abnormalities appear on the scan as abnormally large concentrations of gallium uptake.

Professional Considerations
1. Consent form IS required.

G

Risks

Allergic reaction to the radiopharmaceutical (itching, hives, rash, tight feeling in the throat, shortness of breath, bronchospasm, anaphylaxis, death), infection.

Contraindications

Previous allergic reaction to a radiopharmaceutical. This procedure is usually contraindicated during pregnancy and breast-feeding.

2. Preparation:
   A. The client is injected with a gallium-67 citrate radiopharmaceutical intravenously 48-72 hours before the scan.
   B. See *Client and family teaching.*
3. Procedure:
   A. The client is positioned either erect or recumbent under a gamma (Anger) camera or rectilinear scanner in the nuclear medicine department.
   B. Serial images are obtained anteriorly and posteriorly, and occasional lateral views may be required.
   C. The client must lie motionless during the scan.
4. Postprocedure care:
   A. See *Client and family teaching.*
5. Client and family teaching:
   A. Increase intake of fluids, where not contraindicated, beginning 24 hours before the scan.
   B. The camera will make clicking noises during the scan.
   C. It is important to lie motionless during the scan.
   D. Drink 6-8 glasses of water and other fluids per day for 2 days after the scan.
6. Factors that affect results:
   A. Breast tissue has an increased affinity for gallium uptake during pregnancy, lactation, and menarche. These conditions may produce a false-positive result.
   B. Drugs that may cause false-positive results include oral contraceptives.
   C. Lesions <1-2 cm in size may not be detectable with a gallium scan.
7. Other data:
   A. Gallium is excreted by the kidney and colon in 24-48 hours.
   B. Gallium scanning does not differentiate malignant from benign tumors.

C. The scan takes 30-60 minutes to perform.
D. Health care professionals working in a nuclear medicine area must follow federal standards set by the Nuclear Regulatory Commission. These standards include precautions for handling the radioactive material and monitoring of potential radiation exposure.

GALLIUM SCAN OF LIVER, DIAGNOSTIC

Norm. Symmetric patterns of liver gallium uptake. Requires interpretation.

Usage. Detection of hepatomas, abscesses, biopsy sites, and alcoholic cirrhoses and evaluation of recurrent lymphomas or tumors after chemotherapy and radiation therapy.

Description. Nuclear medicine scan of the liver using gallium-67 citrate radiopharmaceutical. Normal liver tissue will absorb gallium in a symmetric fashion. Abscesses appear as a "rim sign," heavily concentrated areas of gallium uptake surrounding a cold center. The cold center is an area where no inflammation exists. Abscesses are rich with lactoferrin in the neutrophils, and gallium appears to bind to the lactoferrin, making the abscess visible. Tumors appear as heavily concentrated areas of gallium with normal symmetric gallium uptake in the surrounding liver tissue.

Professional Considerations
1. Consent form IS required.

Risks
Allergic reaction to radiopharmaceutical (itching, hives, rash, tight feeling in the throat, shortness of breath, bronchospasm, anaphylaxis, death), infection.

Contraindications
Previous allergic reaction to a radiopharmaceutical. This procedure is usually contraindicated during pregnancy and breast-feeding.

2. Preparation:
   A. The client is injected with a gallium-67 citrate radiopharmaceutical intravenously 48-72 hours before the scan.

B. See *Client and family teaching.*
3. **Procedure:**
   A. The client is positioned either erect or recumbent under a gamma (Anger) camera or rectilinear scanner in the nuclear medicine department.
   B. Serial images are obtained anteriorly and posteriorly, and occasionally lateral views may be required.
   C. The client must lie motionless during the scan.
4. **Postprocedure care:**
   A. See *Client and family teaching.*
5. **Client and family teaching:**
   A. Increase oral intake of fluids, where not contraindicated, 24 hours before the scan.
   B. A clear-liquid diet may be prescribed for the day before the test.
   C. Cleansing enemas may be prescribed the morning before the test.
   D. The camera will make clicking noises during the scan.
   E. The scan takes 30-60 minutes to perform.
   F. Drink 6-8 glasses of water and other fluids per day for 2 days

(where not contraindicated) after the scan.
6. **Factors that affect results:**
   A. Normal hepatic gallium uptake may obscure the detection of abnormal para-aortic nodes in Hodgkin's disease, resulting in a false-negative scan.
   B. Localization of neutrophils labeled with gallium into fresh operative sites and inflamed peritoneum limit their usefulness in clients who have recently undergone surgery.
7. **Other data:**
   A. Gallium is excreted by the kidney and colon in 24-48 hours.
   B. Gallium scanning does not differentiate malignant from benign tumors.
   C. Health care professionals working in a nuclear medicine area must follow federal standards set by the Nuclear Regulatory Commission. These standards include precautions for handling the radioactive material and monitoring of potential radiation exposure.

GAMMA GLOBULIN (IgG, QUANTITATIVE IgG), PLASMA

Norm:

		SI UNITS
Adults	550-1750 mg/dL	5.5-17.5 g/L
Children		
Pediatric cord blood	660-1800 mg/dL	6.6-18 g/L
Newborn	831-1231 mg/dL	8.3-12.3 g/L
1-3 months	311-549 mg/dL	3.1-5.5 g/L
4-6 months	241-613 mg/dL	2.4-6.1 g/L
7-12 months	442-880 mg/dL	4.4-8.8 g/L
13-24 months	553-971 mg/dL	5.5-9.7 g/L
2-3 years	709-1075 mg/dL	7.1-10.8 g/L
3-5 years	701-1257 mg/dL	7.0-12.6 g/L
6-8 years	667-1179 mg/dL	6.7-11.8 g/L
9-11 years	889-1359 mg/dL	8.9-13.6 g/L
12-16 years	822-1170 mg/dL	8.2-11.7 g/L

Increased. AIDS, chronic granulomatous infections, cystic fibrosis of the pancreas, hepatitis (chronic), hyperimmunization, infection, juvenile rheumatoid arthritis, Laënnec's cirrhosis, multiple myeloma (IgG myeloma), myxoma of left atrium of heart, nonimmune chronic idiopathic neutropenia in adults, pulmonary tuberculosis, serum protein monoclonal gammopathy, Sjögren syndrome, and systemic lupus erythematosus. Drugs include aminophenazone, anticonvulsants, asparaginase, ethotoin, hydralazine hydrochloride, mephenytoin, methadone, oral contraceptives, phenylbutazone, phenytoin, and phenytoin sodium prompt.

Decreased. Agammaglobulinemia, heavy chain disease, IgA myeloma, leukemia (chronic lymphocytic), lymphoid aplasia, macroglobulinemia, nephrotic syndrome, and type I dysgammaglobulinemia. Drugs include cancer chemotherapeutic agents, dextrans, methylprednisolone, methylprednisolone acetate, methylprednisolone sodium succinate, and phenytoin.

Description. Protein IgG is the major immunoglobulin of blood that possesses antibody activity against viruses, some bacteria, and toxins. It is the only immunoglobulin that crosses the placenta. Used to evaluate humoral immunity, monitor therapy in IgA G myeloma, and evaluate clients, especially those with a propensity to infections.

Professional Considerations
1. Consent form NOT required.
2. Preparation:
   A. See *Client and family teaching.*
   B. Tube: Red topped, red/gray topped, or gold topped.
3. Procedure:
   A. Draw a 5-mL blood sample.
4. Postprocedure care:
   A. Note vaccinations, immunizations, or toxoid administration within the previous 6 months on the laboratory requisition.
   B. Note administration of blood products within the previous 6 weeks on the laboratory requisition.
   C. Send the specimen to the laboratory immediately.
5. Client and family teaching:
   A. Do not eat or drink, except for water, for 12 hours before sampling.
   B. Results are normally available within 24 hours.
6. Factors that affect results:
   A. Vaccination, immunization, and toxoid administration within 6 months before the test may affect results.
   B. Receipt of blood products within 6 weeks before the test may affect results.
   C. Drug or radiation treatment for cancer may cause decreased results.
7. Other data:
   A. Electrophoresis is a more precise measurement for gamma globulins.

GAMMA-GLUTAMYLTRANSFERASE, BLOOD

(see Gamma-glutamyltranspeptidase, Blood)

GAMMA-GLUTAMYLTRANSPEPTIDASE (GGTP, GAMMA-GLUTAMYLTRANSFERASE), BLOOD

Norm:

Adult females	4-25 U
	9-31 mU/mL
	3.5-13 IU/L
	3-33 U/L at 37° C
Adult males	7-40 U
	12-38 mU/mL
	4-23 IU/L
	9-69 U/L at 37° C
Children	
Cord blood	190-270 U/L at 37° C
Premature infants	<140 U/L at 37° C
1-3 days	56-233 U/L at 37° C
4-21 days	0-130 U/L at 37° C
3-12 weeks	4-120 U/L at 37° C
3-6 months, female	5-35 U/L at 37° C
3-6 months, male	5-65 U/L at 37° C
>6 months, female	15-85 IU/L at 37° C
>6 months, male	5-55 IU/L at 37° C
1-15 years	0-23 U/L at 37° C

Usage. Evaluation of progression of liver disease and hepatic metastasis, screening for alcoholism, and as legal evidence in rape.

Increased. Acetaminophen toxicity, alcoholism, alpha$_1$-antitrypsin deficiency, biliary atresia, cholecystitis (caused by biliary obstruction), cholestasis (intrahepatic), cirrhosis (biliary, Laënnec's), congestive heart failure, fatty liver, hepatic carcinoma (metastatic), hepatitis (acute, chronic), home parenteral nutrition associated cholestasis, jaundice (obstructive), Kawasaki disease, lipoid nephrosis, liver disease, mononucleosis-like syndrome (MLS), myocardial infarction, obesity (extreme), pancreatic carcinoma, pancreatitis (acute), primary biliary cirrhosis, renal carcinoma, and systemic lupus erythematosus. Drugs include glutethimide, high dose 5-FU arterial infusion chemotherapy, methaqualone, phenobarbital, phenytoin, phenytoin sodium, and rosiglitazone.

Decreased. Not clinically significant.

Description. GGTP is a biliary excretory enzyme that assists in the transfer of amino acids and peptides across cellular membranes. It is found in the liver, kidneys, pancreas, brain, heart, salivary glands, and prostate gland. Progression of carcinoma is associated with increasing levels, and regression of carcinoma is associated with decreasing GGTP levels.

Professional Considerations
1. Consent form NOT required.
2. **Preparation:**
   A. See *Client and family teaching.*

B. Tube: Red topped, red/gray topped, or green topped.
3. **Procedure:**
   A. Draw a 1-mL blood sample.
4. **Postprocedure care:**
   A. The specimen may be frozen.
5. **Client and family teaching:**
   A. Fast, except for drinking water, for 8 hours and. refrain from drinking alcohol for 24 hours before the test.
6. **Factors that affect results:**
   A. Reject hemolyzed specimens.
   B. Elevation may occur with phenytoin or phenobarbital therapy; one of the alternative tests, leucine aminopeptidase (LAP), or 5′-nucleotides, is preferable.
   C. *Echinacea* taken for 8 weeks or longer may cause hepatotoxicity.
7. **Other data:**
   A. The stability of specimens is as follows: room temperature, 5 days; refrigerated, 7 days; frozen −4° F (−20° C), 90 days.
   B. GGTP is more accurate than alkaline phosphatase for hepatic disease because it is unaffected by abnormalities of skeletal muscles.

GAMMA-HYDROXYBUTYRIC ACID (GHB, GAMMA-HYDROXYBUTYRATE, LIQUID ECSTASY), BLOOD OR URINE

Norm. Negative.

POSSIBLE OUTCOME IN AVERAGE-SIZED ADULTS	INGESTION AMOUNT	SERUM OR PLASMA LEVEL	URINE LEVEL
Euphoria	100 mg		1100 mg/L
Coma	4 g (just under 1 teaspoon)	>2.5 mmol/L	
Death possible	10 g		

Overdose Symptoms and Treatment

Clients who receive supportive treatment commonly regain consciousness spontaneously up to 5 hours after ingestion of GHB. Left untreated, GHB overdose of over 10 g can lead to death.

Symptoms

Agitation or aggression (more common in daily users).

Amnesia occurs in 13%.
Ataxia.
Central nervous system depression (somnolence progressing to coma) occurs in 66%. Coma can occur when a 2- to 4-g dose (about ½ to 1 teaspoon) is ingested in an adult of average size.
Cardiovascular depression (such as bradycardia).
Emesis is possible.

Hypothermia often occurs when another substance is coingested.
Nystagmus.
Respiratory depression, respiratory acidosis.
Hypotension.
Hypothermia.
Emergence phenomenon as the client regains consciousness may include agitation, myoclonus, confusion, and combativeness.

Treatment:
Note: Treatment choice(s) depend on client history and condition and episode history.
Frequent neurologic checks.
Aspiration precautions.
Airway support, including oxygen and rapid-sequence intubation and mechanical ventilation as needed.
Continuous cardiac monitoring.
Use atropine, neostigmine, or physostigmine if symptomatic bradycardia is present or worsening.
Establish intravenous access.
Stimulate client frequently.
Consider what treatment is needed for possible coingested substances.
Most clients who recover have no further symptoms and can be discharged after being observed for 6 hours.
Naloxone, flumazenil, and anticonvulsants all have been shown NOT to reduce GHB levels or symptoms in humans.
Withdrawal symptoms of visual hallucinations, tachycardia, tremor, nystagmus and diaphoresis have been successfully treated with administration of benzodiazepines and phenobarbital (Schneir et al, 2001).

Usage. Determining drugs of abuse used in clients with overdose symptoms or central nervous system depression where the cause is unknown.

Description. GHB is a drug used legally outside of the United States as a sedative adjunct to anesthesia, in treating alcohol-withdrawal syndrome, and in treating narcolepsy. It is also sold and used worldwide as an illegal "street drug" and has been used for weight loss or muscle production and date rape. In the human body, GHB is a naturally occurring derivative of GABA and is believed to have an inhibitory role in neurotransmission and to help regulate sleep cycles, temperature regulation, and glucose metabolism. When large doses are ingested, GHB causes a feeling of euphoria accompanied by central nervous system depression progressing to coma. GHB levels may indicate ingestion of either GHB or its precursor drug gamma-butyrolactone (GBL). GHB is water soluble and rapidly metabolized, having an onset of 15-30 minutes orally and 2-15 minutes IV, duration of 3 hours, and a half-life of 27 minutes. The drug is excreted rapidly in urine in <10 hours. It is metabolized to succinic acid and carbon dioxide, with the majority of GHB leaving the body in expired carbon dioxide. GBL has a longer half-life because of its solubility in lipids and thus may have a longer duration of action. Although GHB is regulated by law, GBL is not and is sold in over-the-counter body-building supplements. In this test, a sample of blood or urine is tested using gas chromatography–mass spectrometry methods.

Professional Considerations
1. Consent form IS usually required because specimens may be used as legal evidence.
2. **Preparation:**
   A. Tube: red topped, green topped, or blue topped.
   B. Obtain clean specimen container for urine collection.
   C. Obtain a container of ice.
3. **Procedure:**
   A. Obtain a 3-mL blood sample or a ≥7-mL random or straight-catheterized urine specimen. Place sample immediately on ice.
4. **Postprocedure care:**
   A. Write the client's name, the date, exact time of collection, and specimen source on the laboratory requisition. Sign, and have the witness sign, the laboratory requisition.
   B. Transport the specimen to the laboratory immediately in a sealed plastic bag marked as legal evidence. All clients handling the specimen should sign and mark the time of receipt on the laboratory requisition.
   C. Freeze specimen if sent off site for testing.

5. **Client and family teaching:**
   A. Refer client and family or significant others for follow-up counseling and/or crisis intervention services. Offer drug abuse recovery resources as appropriate.
   B. Survivors of sexual assault should be referred to appropriate crisis-counseling agencies as well as for gynecologic follow-up examination.
   C. Because clients with overdose often are unaware of the dangers of GHB, educate client about this.
6. **Factors that affect results:**
   A. At 12 hours after ingestion, GHB can no longer be detected in urine.
7. **Other data:**
   A. People who ingest GHB recreationally are often found to have taken more than one toxic substance.
   B. Many states have enacted laws reclassifying GHB as a controlled substance.
   C. In the United States, report GHB cases to the Drug Enforcement Administration in Washington, DC, (202) 307-7207 for blood values >5µg/mL and urine values >10 µg/mL.
   D. Production of GHB increases with time after death in postmortem liver.

GAS VENTILATION LUNG SCAN, DIAGNOSTIC

Norm. Radioactive gas is distributed equally in both lungs with normal "wash-in" and "wash-out" phases.

Usage. Used with a lung perfusion scan to diagnose, identify, and evaluate regions of lung tissue that are not ventilated during respirations. Some conditions in which this may occur include pulmonary embolism, chronic obstructive pulmonary disease, and parenchymal disease (bronchogenic carcinoma).

Description. A nuclear medicine scan in which the client inhales air mixed with radiolabeled gas (xenon 133) through a mask. A gamma (Anger) camera images the gas distribution of the posterior lung fields through three phases: phase 1 is the "wash-in" phase in which the buildup of radioactive gas occurs. In phase 2, equilibrium occurs. Phase 3 is the "wash-out" phase, in which the gas is removed from the lungs. Decreased areas of ventilation will appear lighter with longer than normal wash-out phases.

Professional Considerations
1. Consent form NOT required.

Risks
Dizziness, fetal damage.

Contraindications
In clients who are unable to follow directions.

Precautions
During pregnancy, risks of cumulative radiation exposure to the fetus from this and other previous or future imaging studies must be weighed against the benefits of the procedure. Although formal limits for client exposure are relative to this risk:benefit comparison, the United States Nuclear Regulatory Commission requires that the cumulative dose equivalent to an embryo/fetus from occupational exposure not exceed 0.5 rem (5 mSv). Radiation dosage to the fetus is proportional to the distance of the anatomy studied from the abdomen and decreases as pregnancy progresses. For pregnant clients, consult the radiologist/radiology department to obtain estimated fetal radiation exposure from this procedure.

2. **Preparation:**
   A. Obtain baseline vital signs and continue to monitor vital signs every 10-15 minutes.
   B. Remove jewelry and metal objects.
3. **Procedure:**
   A. The client is positioned erect or supine throughout the scan.
   B. The client inhales a mixture of air and radioactive xenon-133 gas through a mask and holds his or her breath for 20 seconds. For mechanically ventilated clients, krypton-85 gas should be substituted for xenon 133.
   C. The client's chest is scanned with a gamma camera as he or she exhales.
4. **Postprocedure care:**
   A. None.
5. **Client and family teaching:**
   A. The test is painless and takes about 15-30 minutes.
   B. Results are normally available after interpretation by a radiologist.
6. **Factors that affect results:**
   A. An improperly fitting or loose seal on the ventilation mask

G

interferes with the proper mixing of air and gas and allows radioactive gas to contaminate the surrounding air.

7. **Other data:**
   A. None.

GASTRIC ACID ANALYSIS TEST (PEPTAVLON STIMULATION TEST), DIAGNOSTIC

Norm. Within normal limits.

BASAL (PRESTIMULATION) ACID OUTPUT (BAO) IS THE GASTRIC ACID SECRETED WITHOUT STIMULATION:		SI UNITS
Adult Female		
Normal	1-4 mEq/hour	1-4 mmol/hour
Duodenal ulcer	3-8 mEq/hour	3-8 mmol/hour
Gastric carcinoma	0-3 mEq/hour	0-3 mmol/hour
Gastric ulcer	1-3 mEq/hour	1-3 mmol/hour
Atrophic gastritis	0 mEq/hour	0 mmol/hour
Pernicious anemia	0 mEq/hour	0 mmol/hour
Zollinger-Ellison syndrome	>20 mEq/hour	>20 mmol/hour
Adult Male		
Normal	2-5 mEq/hour	2-5 mmol/hour
Duodenal ulcer	5-10 mEq/hour	5-10 mmol/hour
Gastric carcinoma	0-3 mEq/hour	0-3 mmol/hour
Gastric ulcer	1-5 mEq/hour	1-5 mmol/hour
Atrophic gastritis	0 mEq/hour	0 mmol/hour
Pernicious anemia	0 mEq/hour	0 mmol/hour
Zollinger-Ellison syndrome	>20 mEq/hour	>20 mmol/hour

MAXIMUM (STIMULATED) ACID OUTPUT (MAO) IS THE GASTRIC ACID OUTPUT AFTER STIMULATION (SUM OF FOUR 15-MINUTE SPECIMENS):		
Adult Female		
Normal	7-15 mEq/hour	7-15 mmol/hour
Duodenal ulcer	10-20 mEq/hour	10-20 mmol/hour
Gastric carcinoma	0-5 mEq/hour	0-5 mmol/hour
Gastric ulcer	5-15 mEq/hour	5-15 mmol/hour
Atrophic gastritis	0 mEq/hour	0 mmol/hour
Pernicious anemia	0 mEq/hour	0 mmol/hour
Zollinger-Ellison syndrome	35-60 mEq/hour	35-60 mmol/hour
Adult Male		
Normal	5-26 mEq/hour	5-26 mmol/hour
Duodenal ulcer	15-35 mEq/hour	15-35 mmol/hour
Gastric carcinoma	0-20 mEq/hour	0-20 mmol/hour
Gastric ulcer	10-20 mEq/hour	10-20 mmol/hour
Atrophic gastritis	0 mEq/hour	0 mmol/hour
Pernicious anemia	0 mEq/hour	0 mmol/hour
Zollinger-Ellison syndrome	35-60 mEq/hour	35-60 mmol/hour

BAO:MAO RATIO		
Normal	1:2.5-1:5.0	0.3-0.6
Gastric ulcer/gastric carcinoma		20%
Gastric ulcer/duodenal ulcer		20-40%
Duodenal ulcer/Zollinger-Ellison		40-60% syndrome
Zollinger-Ellison syndrome		>60%

PEAK ACID OUTPUT (PAO) IS 2 × TOTAL VALUES OF THE TWO HIGHEST 15-MINUTE MAO SAMPLES; BAO:PAO RATIO	SI UNITS
Adult Female	0.23
Adult Male	0.29

Usage. Diagnosing and evaluating atrophic gastritis, duodenal ulcer, gastric carcinoma, gastric ulcer, Ménétrier's disease, pernicious anemia, postoperative stomal ulcer, and Zollinger-Ellison syndrome.

Increased. Duodenal ulcer, gastric ulcers in some cases, *Helicobacter pylori* infection, peptic ulcer disease, pyloric ulcer, and Zollinger-Ellison syndrome. Drugs include adrenergic blockers, alseroxylon, caffeine, calcium salts, cholinergics, corticosteroids, deserpidine, ethyl alcohol (ethanol), rescinnamine, and reserpine.

Decreased. Achlorhydria, anemia (pernicious), gastric atrophy, gastric neoplasm, gastric ulcer, and gastritis. Drugs include antacids, anticholinergics, beta-blocking agents, cimetidine, famotidine, nizatidine, ranitidine hydrochloride, and tricyclic antidepressants.

Description. Gastric acid consists of hydrochloric acid (HCl), electrolytes, and mucus and is colorless and very acidic, with a pH of <2.5. It is normally secreted by the parietal cells of the stomach in response to the presence of gastrin during the gastric phase of digestion. In the presence of tumors, ulcerative disease, or pernicious anemia, the rate of gastric acid secretion can be accelerated or diminished. The Peptavlon (pentagastrin) stimulation test involves a 1-hour aspiration of stomach secretions. A basal and four 15-minute collections are made after subcutaneous injection of Peptavlon. Peptavlon normally stimulates gastric acid secretion within 10 minutes, with peaks occurring at approximately 30 minutes. By measuring the rate and volume of gastric acid secretion in response to Peptavlon, one can evaluate gastric function. Pernicious anemia and atrophic gastritis result in hyposecretion of gastric acid. Hypersecretion and the rate of secretion can indicate location and type of ulcerative disease, Zollinger-Ellison syndrome, and the need for surgical intervention.

Professional Considerations
1. Consent form NOT required.
2. **Preparation:**
   A. See *Client and family teaching.*
   B. Obtain a Levin tube, lubricant, 8 clean plastic containers without preservative, a Toomey syringe, suction equipment, a marker or grease pencil, and Peptavlon (pentagastrin).
   C. Prepare the suction apparatus and tubing.
3. **Procedure:**
   A. Position the client sitting or lying on the left side.
   B. Insert a Levin tube with a radiopaque tip through the client's nose or mouth into the stomach. Position the Levin tube tip in the lumen below the stomach fundus and confirm the placement by radiography or fluoroscopy.
   C. Reposition the client to a sitting position and wait at least 10 minutes before proceeding further.
   D. Apply low continuous suction to the Levin tube. At 15 and 30 minutes, withdraw two specimens with a Toomey syringe and discard the aspirate.
   E. Begin continuous aspiration of gastric contents, using the syringe, for a total of 60 minutes. Collect the aspirate into the collection containers (labeled 1, 2, 3, 4), using a new collection container every 15 minutes until the basal acid output collection is complete.
   F. Administer Peptavlon 6 mg/kg of body weight subcutaneously and begin post stimulation collections, as in step 3E, immediately. The post stimulation collection should continue for 1 hour. Observe for hypersensitivity reaction.

G

4. **Postprocedure care:**
   A. Send all 8 containers identified as basal or post stimulation to the laboratory for analysis.
   B. Remove the Levin tube.
   C. Refrigerate the specimens if testing will be delayed more than 4 hours.
   D. Resume previous diet.
   E. Observe for nausea and vomiting.
5. **Client and family teaching:**
   A. Fast from food after the evening meal the day before testing and from water for 1 hour before the test.
   B. Do not smoke or chew gum, and avoid stressful situations for 4 hours before the test.
   C. The test involves the insertion of a tube through the nose into the stomach and periodic removal of the stomach contents with a syringe through the tube. The test may cause symptoms of indigestion because a drug that stimulates gastric acid secretion is given. Mild, temporary discomfort may be experienced during the tube insertion.
   D. The test takes more than 3 hours. Bring reading material or other diversional activity.
6. **Factors that affect results:**
   A. Histamine antagonists or anticholinergics and antacids should be discontinued 72 and 12 hours before the test. If, however, the objective is to test the effectiveness of a histamine antagonist on acid secretions, the drugs should be continued, and the basal output of gastric acid should be performed 1 hour after administration of a morning dose.
   B. Stimuli that may increase gastric acid production include smoking, the sight or odor of food, or stimuli that cause the client to become angry, fearful, or depressed.
7. **Other data:**
   A. Peptavlon use in children is not indicated.
   B. The test must be used with caution in conditions of esophageal varices, esophageal diverticula, esophageal stenosis, malignant neoplasm of the esophagus, aortic aneurysm, gastric hemorrhage, and congestive heart failure.

GASTRIC ACID SECRETION TEST (GASTRIC ACID STIMULATION TEST), DIAGNOSTIC

Norm. Within normal limits.

BASAL (PRESTIMULATION) ACID OUTPUT (BAO) IS THE GASTRIC ACID SECRETED WITHOUT STIMULATION:		SI UNITS
Adult Female		
Normal	1-4 mEq/hour	1-4 mmol/hour
Duodenal ulcer	3-8 mEq/hour	3-8 mmol/hour
Gastric carcinoma	0-3 mEq/hour	0-3 mmol/hour
Gastric ulcer	1-3 mEq/hour	1-3 mmol/hour
Atrophic gastritis	0 mEq/hour	0 mmol/hour
Pernicious anemia	0 mEq/hour	0 mmol/hour
Zollinger-Ellison syndrome	>20 mEq/hour	>20 mmol/hour
Adult Male		
Normal	2-5 mEq/hour	2-5 mmol/hour
Duodenal ulcer	5-10 mEq/hour	5-10 mmol/hour
Gastric carcinoma	0-3 mEq/hour	0-3 mmol/hour
Gastric ulcer	1-5 mEq/hour	1-5 mmol/hour
Atrophic gastritis	0 mEq/hour	0 mmol/hour
Pernicious anemia	0 mEq/hour	0 mmol/hour
Zollinger-Ellison syndrome	>20 mEq/hour	>20 mmol/hour

MAXIMUM (STIMULATED) ACID OUTPUT (MAO) IS THE GASTRIC ACID OUTPUT AFTER STIMULATION (SUM OF FOUR 15-MINUTE SPECIMENS):

Adult Female

Normal	7-15 mEq/hour	7-15 mmol/hour
Duodenal ulcer	10-20 mEq/hour	10-20 mmol/hour
Gastric carcinoma	0-5 mEq/hour	0-5 mmol/hour
Gastric ulcer	5-15 mEq/hour	5-15 mmol/hour
Atrophic gastritis	0 mEq/hour	0 mmol/hour
Pernicious anemia	0 mEq/hour	0 mmol/hour
Zollinger-Ellison syndrome	35-60 mEq/hour	35-60 mmol/hour

Adult Male

Normal	5-26 mEq/hour	5-26 mmol/hour
Duodenal ulcer	15-35 mEq/hour	15-35 mmol/hour
Gastric carcinoma	0-20 mEq/hour	0-20 mmol/hour
Gastric ulcer	10-20 mEq/hour	10-20 mmol/hour
Atrophic gastritis	0 mEq/hour	0 mmol/hour
Pernicious anemia	0 mEq/hour	0 mmol/hour
Zollinger-Ellison syndrome	35-60 mEq/hour	35-60 mmol/hour

BAO:MAO RATIO

Normal	1:2.5-1:5	0.3-0.6
Gastric ulcer/gastric carcinoma		20%
Gastric ulcer/duodenal ulcer		20-40%
Duodenal ulcer/Zollinger-Ellison syndrome		40-60%
Zollinger-Ellison syndrome		>60%

PEAK ACID OUTPUT (PAO) IS 2 × TOTAL VALUES OF THE TWO HIGHEST 15-MINUTE MAO SAMPLES; BAO:PAO RATIO

	SI UNITS
Adult Female	0.23
Adult Male	0.29

Usage. Diagnosis and evaluation of duodenal ulcer, gastric carcinoma, gastric ulcer, pernicious anemia, postoperative stomal ulcer, and Zollinger-Ellison syndrome.

Increased. Duodenal ulcer, gastric ulcers in some cases, peptic ulcer disease, pyloric ulcer, and Zollinger-Ellison syndrome. Drugs include adrenergic blockers, alseroxylon, caffeine, calcium salts, cholinergics, corticosteroids, deserpidine, ethyl alcohol (ethanol), rescinnamine, and reserpine.

Decreased. Achlorhydria, anemia (pernicious), gastric atrophy, gastric neoplasm, gastric ulcer, and gastritis. Nasojejunal feeding tubes in mechanically ventilated clients. Drugs include antacids, anticholinergics, beta-blocking agents, cimetidine, famotidine, nizati-dine, ranitidine hydrochloride, and tricyclic antidepressants.

Description. Gastric acid is secreted by the parietal cells of the stomach in response to neurologic and hormonal stimulation. Gastric acid is secreted during the gastric phase of digestion and aids in the breakdown of proteins and in the absorption of vitamin B_{12}, folic acid, and iron. It consists of hydrochloric acid (HCl), electrolytes, enzymes, and mucus. It is colorless and very acidic, with a pH of <2.5. In the presence of tumors, ulcerative disease, or pernicious anemia, the rate of gastric acid secretion by the parietal cells can be altered. A diagnostic gastric acid stimulation test involves aspirating and collecting basal and maximal acid outputs. Histalog (betazole, a histamine analog) or histamine diphosphate is injected intramuscularly to stimulate gastric acid secretion. By measurement of the rate and volume of gastric acid, gastric function can be evaluated.

Professional Considerations
1. Consent form NOT required.

Risks
Allergic reaction to injection (itching, hives, rash, tight feeling in the throat, shortness of breath, bronchospasm, anaphylaxis, death).

Contraindications
Positive skin test. Use of histamine diphosphate is contraindicated for clients who have a history of asthma, paroxysmal hypertension, urticaria, or other allergic conditions. Histalog (betazole hydrochloride) has a lower incidence of side effects than histamine diphosphate has.

2. **Preparation:**
   A. Perform a skin test to determine hypersensitivity by injecting 0.1 mL of Histalog or histamine diphosphate subcutaneously. Wait 30 minutes for a reaction to occur. If the wheal exceeds 10 mm in diameter, do not perform the stimulation portion of this test.
   B. Obtain a Levin tube, lubricant, 8-12 clean plastic containers without preservative, a Toomey syringe, suction equipment, a marker or grease pencil, and histamine diphosphate or Histalog.
   C. Prepare suction apparatus and tubing.
   D. See *Client and family teaching.*
3. **Procedure:**
   A. Position the client sitting or lying on the left side.
   B. Insert a Levin tube with a radiopaque tip through the client's nose or mouth into the stomach. Position the tube tip in the lumen below the stomach fundus and confirm the placement by radiography or fluoroscopy.
   C. Reposition the client to a sitting position and wait at least 10 minutes before proceeding further.
   D. Apply low continuous suction to the Levin tube. At 15 and 30 min-

utes, withdraw two specimens with a Toomey syringe and discard the aspirate.
   E. Begin continuous aspiration of the gastric contents, using the syringe, for a total of 60 minutes. Collect the aspirate into the collection containers (labeled 1, 2, 3, 4), using a new collection container every 15 minutes until basal acid output collection is complete.
   F. Administer Histalog (betazole hydrochloride) 0.5 mg/kg of body weight, or histamine diphosphate 0.1 mg/kg of body weight, intramuscularly, and begin post stimulation collections, as in step 3E, immediately. Observe for hypersensitivity reaction.
   G. Post stimulation collection should continue for 1 hour (4 specimens) if histamine diphosphate was used, or for 2 hours (8 specimens) if Histalog was used.
4. **Postprocedure care:**
   A. Send all 8-12 containers, identified as basal or poststimulation, to the laboratory.
   B. Remove the Levin tube.
   C. Resume previous diet.
   D. Observe for nausea and vomiting.
5. **Client and family teaching:**
   A. Fast from food for 12 hours and from water for 1 hour before the procedure.
   B. Do not smoke or chew gum, and avoid stressful situations for 4 hours before the test.
   C. The test involves the insertion of a tube through the nose into the stomach and periodic removal of the stomach contents with a syringe through the tube. The test may cause symptoms of indigestion because a drug that stimulates gastric acid secretion is given. Mild, temporary discomfort may be experienced during tube insertion. Lidocaine jelly may be used as lubricant to decrease discomfort of tube insertion.
   D. The test takes more than 2 hours.
   E. Results are normally available within 24 hours.
6. **Factors that affect results:**
   A. Histamine antagonists or anticholinergics and antacids should be discontinued 72 and 12 hours,

respectively, before the test. If, however, the objective is to test the effectiveness of a histamine antagonist on acid secretions, the drugs should be continued, and the basal output of gastric acid should be performed 1 hour after administration of a morning dose.

B. Stimuli that may increase gastric acid production include smoking, the sight or odor of food, or stimuli that cause the client to become angry, fearful, or depressed.

C. Peak acid output after Histalog may not occur until the second hour after administration.

7. **Other data:**
A. None.

GASTRIC ANALYSIS, SPECIMEN

Norm:

Bile	Absent or minimal
Mucus	Appears evenly mixed
Blood	Absent or scant
Fasting acidity	2.5 mEq/L
Quantity produced	62 mL/hour
pH	1.0-2.5

Usage. Anemia (pernicious), stomach pain and burning, ulcers, and Zollinger-Ellison syndrome. Can also determine the presence of *Helicobacter pylori*.

Description. This test analyzes the contents of the stomach for acidity, appearance, and volume.

Professional Considerations
1. Consent form NOT required.

Risks
Complications of nasogastric tube insertion include bleeding, dysrhythmias, esophageal perforation, laryngospasm, and decreased mean pO_2.

Contraindications
Esophageal varices.

2. **Preparation:**
A. The client should fast for 12 hours.
B. The client should not smoke tobacco or chew gum for 6 hours.
C. Obtain a nasogastric tube, a lubricant, a Toomey syringe, and a clean container.

3. **Procedure:**
A. Pass a nasogastric tube into the stomach.
B. Aspirate all gastric contents into a clean container.
C. Remove the nasogastric tube.

4. **Postprocedure care:**
A. Refrigerate the sample if not tested within 4 hours.

5. **Client and family teaching:**
A. Fast for 12 hours, and do not chew gum or smoke cigarettes for 6 hours before the test.
B. The test involves the insertion of a tube through the nose into the stomach and removal, with a syringe, of the gastric contents through the tube. The insertion may be uncomfortable and may cause a pressure like feeling or may cause you to gag and cough. You will be asked to take sips of water and swallow to make the tube insertion easier. Removal of the stomach contents causes no pain.
C. Further tests may be indicated, based on the results of this analysis.

6. **Factors that affect results:**
A. Stimuli that may increase gastric acid production include chewing gum, smoking, the sight or odor of food, or stimuli that cause the client to become angry, fearful, or depressed.
B. Drugs that may increase gastric acid production include adrenergic blockers, caffeine, calcium salts, cholinergics, corticosteroids, ethyl alcohol (ethanol), and reserpine.
C. Drugs that may decrease gastric acid production include antacids, anticholinergics, beta-blocking agents, cimetidine, famotidine, nizatidine, ranitidine hydrochloride, and tricyclic antidepressants.
D. Use of Hemoccult slides, as opposed to Gastroccult slides, may lead to a false-negative result if the pH of the gastric secretion is <4.

7. **Other data:**
A. Small amounts of bile may be present because of gagging during insertion of the nasogastric tube.
B. Scant amounts of blood may be present because of trauma during insertion of the nasogastric tube.

G

GASTRIC ANALYSIS, BASAL NOCTURNAL ACID OUTPUT, DIAGNOSTIC

Norm:

BASAL ACID OUTPUT (BAO)		SI UNITS
Adult Female		
Normal	1-4 mEq/hour	1-4 mmol/hour
Duodenal ulcer	3-8 mEq/hour	3-8 mmol/hour
Gastric carcinoma	0-3 mEq/hour	0-3 mmol/hour
Gastric ulcer	1-3 mEq/hour	1-3 mmol/hour
Atrophic gastritis	0 mEq/hour	0 mmol/hour
Pernicious anemia	0 mEq/hour	0 mmol/hour
Zollinger-Ellison syndrome	>20 mEq/hour	>20 mmol/hour
Adult Male		
Normal	2-5 mEq/hour	2-5 mmol/hour
Duodenal ulcer	5-10 mEq/hour	5-10 mmol/hour
Gastric carcinoma	0-3 mEq/hour	0-3 mmol/hour
Gastric ulcer	1-5 mEq/hour	1-5 mmol/hour
Atrophic gastritis	0 mEq/hour	0 mmol/hour
Pernicious anemia	0 mEq/hour	0 mmol/hour
Zollinger-Ellison syndrome	>20 mEq/hour	>20 mmol/hour

Usage. Aids diagnosis of pernicious anemia, duodenal or stomal ulcer, Ménétrier's disease, and Zollinger-Ellison syndrome.

Increased. Duodenal ulcer, gastric ulcers in some cases, peptic ulcer disease, pyloric ulcer, and Zollinger-Ellison syndrome. Drugs include adrenergic blockers, alseroxylon, caffeine, calcium salts, cholinergics, corticosteroids, deserpidine, ethyl alcohol (ethanol), rauwolfia, rescinnamine, and reserpine.

Decreased. Achlorhydria, anemia (pernicious), gastric atrophy, gastric neoplasm, gastric ulcer, and gastritis. Drugs include antacids, anticholinergics, beta-blocking agents, cimetidine, famotidine, nizatidine, ranitidine hydrochloride, and tricyclic antidepressants.

Description. Basal nocturnal acid output is the rate of secretion of acid by the stomach when the client is calm and resting, after a 12-hour fast, and at least 24 hours after the last dose of medications that increase or decrease gastric acid. It is measured in millimoles of titratable acidity per hour.

Professional Considerations
1. Consent form NOT required.

Risks
Complications of nasogastric tube insertion include bleeding, dysrhythmias, esophageal perforation, laryngospasm, and decreased mean pO_2.

Contraindications
In clients with esophageal varices, evaluate risk versus benefit in severely thrombocytopenic clients at risk for hemorrhage.

2. **Preparation:**
   A. See *Client and family teaching.*
   B. Obtain a Levin tube, a lubricant, four clean plastic containers without preservative, a Toomey syringe, suction equipment, and a marker or grease pencil.
   C. Prepare the suction apparatus and tubing.
3. **Procedure:**
   A. Position the client sitting or lying on the left side.
   B. Insert a Levin tube with a radiopaque tip through the client's nose or mouth into the stomach. Position the tube tip in the lumen below the stomach fundus and confirm the placement by radiography or fluoroscopy.

C. Reposition to a sitting position. Wait at least 10 minutes before proceeding further.

D. Apply low, continuous suction to the Levin tube. At 15 and 30 minutes, withdraw two specimens with a Toomey syringe and discard the aspirate.

E. Begin continuous aspiration of gastric contents using the syringe, for a total of 60 minutes. Collect the aspirate into the collection containers (labeled 1, 2, 3, 4), using a new collection container every 15 minutes until basal acid output collection is complete.

4. Postprocedure care:
   A. Send all four sequentially labeled containers to the laboratory.
   B. The specimens should be refrigerated if not tested within 4 hours.
   C. Remove the nasogastric tube.
   D. Resume previous diet.

5. Client and family teaching:
   A. Fast for 12 hours, and do not chew gum or smoke cigarettes during the 6 hours before the test.
   B. The test takes about 2 hours. Bring reading material or other diversions.
   C. The test involves the insertion of a tube through the nose into the stomach and removal, with a syringe, of the gastric contents through the tube. The insertion may be uncomfortable and may cause a pressure like feeling or cause you to gag and cough. You will be asked to take sips of water and swallow to make the tube insertion easier. Removal of the stomach contents causes no pain.

6. Factors that affect results:
   A. Reject specimens if contaminated with bile.
   B. Stimuli that may increase gastric acid production include smoking, the sight or odor of food, or stimuli that cause anger, fear, or depression.
   C. The amount of gastric acid increases as body weight increases.

7. Other data:
   A. This test is sometimes followed by stimulation of gastric acid production with pentagastrin or histamine. See also *Gastric acid*

analysis test, Diagnostic; Gastric acid stimulation test, Diagnostic.

GASTRIC ASPIRATE, ROUTINE, CULTURE

Norm. Negative. No growth.

Usage. Aids in the diagnosis pulmonary as well as gastrointestinal infections.

Positive. Growth of microorganisms may be secondary to carcinoma or to puncture of the stomach with concomitant peritonitis or intra-abdominal abscess.

Description. One performs this test by withdrawing a small sample of gastric aspirate through a nasogastric tube and culturing the sample for the growth of microorganisms.

Professional Considerations
1. Consent form NOT required.

Risks
Complications of nasogastric tube insertion include bleeding, dysrhythmias, esophageal perforation, laryngospasm, and decreased mean pO_2.

Contraindications
Esophageal varices.

2. Preparation:
   A. Obtain a nasogastric tube, a lubricant, a sterile syringe, and a sterile specimen tube.
3. Procedure:
   A. Pass a nasogastric tube into the stomach.
   B. Using a sterile syringe, aspirate a minimum of 2 mL of gastric contents into the sterile tube.
   C. Remove the nasogastric tube.
4. Postprocedure care:
   A. Write the collection time on the laboratory requisition.
   B. Send the sample to the laboratory within 30 minutes.
5. Client and family teaching:
   A. The test involves the insertion of a tube through the nose into the stomach and removal, with a syringe, of the gastric contents through the tube. The insertion

G

may be uncomfortable and may cause a pressure like feeling or cause you to gag and cough. You will be asked to take sips of water and swallow to make the tube insertion easier. Removal of the stomach contents causes no pain.

B. Do not swallow sputum just before or during the procedure. Suction will be provided to help remove sputum from the back of the mouth.

C. Results are normally available within 48 hours.

6. **Factors that affect results:**
   A. Reject specimens received more than 30 minutes after collection.

7. **Other data:**
   A. The esophagus and stomach are the two usually sterile areas of the gastrointestinal tract.
   B. Clients who are unable to expectorate sputum may swallow it, thus contaminating their gastric aspirate.

GASTRIC CYTOLOGY, SPECIMEN

(see Cytologic study of gastrointestinal tract, Diagnostic)

GASTRIC PH, SPECIMEN

Norm. 1.0-2.5.

Increased. Duodenal ulcer, evaluation after vagotomy, marginal ulcer, peptic ulcer disease, and Zollinger-Ellison syndrome.

Decreased. Achlorhydria, hypochlorhydria, and pernicious anemia.

Description. Gastric pH expresses hydrogen-ion concentration of the gastric contents. It is a reflection of the amount of hydrochloric acid (HCl) produced by the parietal cells of the stomach in response to gastrin stimulation.

Professional Considerations
1. Consent form NOT required.

Risks
Complications of nasogastric tube insertion include bleeding, dysrhyth-

mias, esophageal perforation, laryngospasm, and decreased mean pO_2.

Contraindications
Esophageal varices.

2. **Preparation:**
   A. Obtain a nasogastric tube, a lubricant, a syringe, a clean container, and a pH Test-Tape.
   B. See *Client and family teaching*.

3. **Procedure:**
   A. Pass a nasogastric tube into the stomach.
   B. Aspirate a minimum of 2 mL of gastric contents into the clean container.
   C. Dip the pH Test-Tape into the specimen and compare the color change with that on the Test-Tape container.
   D. Remove the nasogastric tube.

4. **Postprocedure care:**
   A. None.

5. **Client and family teaching:**
   A. Do not eat for 8 hours before the test. Do not smoke cigarettes or chew gum for 4 hours before the test. Avoid stressful situations during the 4 hours immediately before the test.
   B. The test involves the insertion of a tube through the nose into the stomach and removal, with a syringe, of the gastric contents through the tube. The insertion may be uncomfortable and may cause a pressure like feeling or cause you to gag and cough. You will be asked to take sips of water and swallow to make the tube insertion easier.

6. **Factors that affect results:**
   A. Stimuli that may increase gastric acid production include smoking, the sight or odor of food, or stimuli that cause anger, fear, or depression.
   B. Postprandial time with acidic pH in stomach is significantly increased in clients with chronic pancreatitis.

7. **Other data:**
   A. Gastric carcinoma is associated with decreased acidity.

GASTRIN, SERUM

Norm:

		SI UNITS
Fasting		
≤60 years	<100 pg/mL	<47.7 pmol/L
	or <200 pg/mL	<95.4 pmol/L
>60 years		
Upper 15% of population	100-800 pg/mL	47.7-381.6 pmol/L
Postprandial	95-250 pg/mL	45.3-119.2 pmol/L
Zollinger-Ellison	≤60,000 pg/mL	≤28,620 pmol/L
syndrome	Often 100-500 pg/mL	Often 47.7-238.3 pmol/L

Increased. Achlorhydria, anemia (pernicious), atrophic gastritis, carcinoma (of the body of the stomach), duodenal ulcer, elderly clients, gastric ulcer, G-cell hyperplasia (antrum of the stomach), hypercalcemia (chronic), hyperparathyroidism, hypochlorhydria, pancreatic neuroendocrine tumor, peptic ulcer disease (with Zollinger-Ellison syndrome), pyloric obstruction with gastric distension, renal disease (chronic, end-stage), sarcoidosis, short-bowel syndrome, status post vagotomy, uremia, and Zollinger-Ellison syndrome. Drugs include acetylcholine chloride, calcium carbonate, calcium chloride, cholinergics, insulin, and lansoprazole.

Decreased. Drugs include anticholinergics and tricyclic antidepressants.

Description. Gastrin is a hormone secreted by the G-cells of the antrum of the stomach and by the pancreatic islets of Langerhans. Its secretion is stimulated by alkalinity, by distension of the stomach antrum, by vagal stimulation (such as chewing, tasting, or smelling), and by the presence of peptides, amino acids, alcohol, or calcium in the stomach. Its secretion is inhibited by gastric acidity by a negative-feedback system. Gastrin is absorbed into the blood and returned to the stomach, where it stimulates the secretion of gastric acid under the mediation of histamine. Other effects of gastrin include increased gastrointestinal motility and stimulation of insulin, pepsin, and intrinsic factor secretion. Catabolism of gastrin occurs in the kidneys. Serum gastrin measurement is accomplished by radioimmunoassay.

Professional Considerations
1. Consent form NOT required.
2. **Preparation:**
   A. See *Client and family teaching.*
   B. Tube: Red topped, red/gray topped, or gold topped.
3. **Procedure:**
   A. Draw a 2-mL blood sample.
4. **Postprocedure care:**
   A. Write the collection time on the laboratory requisition.
5. **Client and family teaching:**
   A. Fast from food for 12 hours and from alcohol for 24 hours before the test.
   B. Do not chew gum or smoke cigarettes for 4 hours before the test.
   C. Results are normally available within 24 hours.
6. **Factors that affect results:**
   A. Reject hemolyzed specimens, specimens drawn in anticoagulated tubes, or specimens not received in the laboratory within 30 minutes after collection.
   B. Reject grossly lipemic samples, which may yield falsely elevated serum gastrin values as determined by radioimmunoassay.
   C. Food, especially high-protein food, causes an increase in gastrin secretion.
   D. Hypoglycemia caused by insulin increases gastrin secretion.
   E. Drugs that may indirectly cause increased gastrin secretion in response to drug suppression of gastric acidity include antacids, beta-blocking agents, cimetidine, famotidine, nizatidine, and ranitidine hydrochloride.
   F. Drugs that may indirectly cause depressed gastrin secretion in response to drug-stimulated

increased gastric acidity include adrenergic blockers, alseroxylon, caffeine, calcium salts, corticosteroids, deserpidine, ethyl alcohol (ethanol), rauwolfia, rescinnamine, and reserpine.

7. Other data:
A. 15-26% of clients with Zollinger-Ellison syndrome have Wermer syndrome: hyperparathyroidism, islet cell tumors, pituitary tumors, Cushing syndrome, and hyperthyroidism.

GASTROINTESTINAL CANCER ANTIGEN
(see CA 19-9, Blood)

GASTROSCOPY OR GASTRODUODENOJEJUN-OSCOPY (GJD), DIAGNOSTIC

Norm. Cardiac and pyloric sphincters are intact. Rugal folds of the stomach are continuous. No blood or lesions are detected. Blood vessels are not visible.

Usage. Detection of gastric cancer, gastric ulcer, gastritis, hiatal hernia, and Mallory-Weiss tears; investigation of unexplained weight loss or dysphagia; and to obtain brushings of gastric mucosa to help determine infectious states such as *Helicobacter pylori* infection.

Description. Gastroscopy involves the insertion through the esophagus of a lighted flexible fiberoptic endoscope into the stomach and upper portion of the small intestine, with concurrent visual examination of the mucosal lining for active bleeding sites, varices, ulcers or perforations, lesions, or tears. The procedure takes approximately 30 minutes. Gastroduodenojejunoscopy involves advancing the instrument further into the small intestine to evaluate the integrity of the jejunum as well as any structural or obstructive abnormalities.

Professional Considerations
1. Consent form IS required.

Risks
Gastrointestinal perforation and hemorrhage, peritonitis, aspiration, respiratory arrest, death.

Contraindications
Thrombocytopenia. Sedatives are contraindicated in clients with central nervous system depression.

2. Preparation:
A. See *Client and family teaching.*
B. Dentures should be removed.
C. A sedative may be prescribed.
D. Obtain baseline vital signs.
E. Follow facility policy and procedure for clients receiving conscious sedation.
F. Obtain a blood pressure cuff, lidocaine spray, a suction machine and tubing, an endoscope, pulse oximetry, and a gastroscopy cart. A cardiac monitor may be required with some clients.

3. Procedure:
A. A blood pressure cuff is left in place on the client's arm, and vital signs along with pulse oximetry are monitored on an individual basis throughout the procedure.
B. The mouth and oropharynx are anesthetized locally.
C. Oral secretions are suctioned or allowed to drain out as they accumulate.
D. The client is placed in a left lateral position with the head tilted forward.
E. As the endoscope is advanced into the esophagus, the head is slowly tilted back.
F. The esophagus and cardiac sphincter are examined as the endoscope is advanced. The endoscope is rotated clockwise as it is advanced into the stomach and the stomach lining, and the cardiac and pyloric sphincters are examined. The scope is advanced through the pylorus into the duodenal bulb and beyond the bulb apex into the second portion of the pH duodenum. Advancement can continue into the jejunum as well. Photographs of suspicious areas and biopsy specimens or brushings may also be taken. Sclerotherapy is commonly performed during this procedure if active bleeding is noted. Polypectomies are also common. The endoscope is slowly withdrawn.

4. Postprocedure care:
A. Fasting is required until the gag reflex returns.

B. Continue assessment of respiratory status. If deep sedation was used, follow institutional protocol for postsedation monitoring. Typical monitoring includes continuous ECG monitoring and pulse oximetry, with continual assessments (every 5-15 minutes) of airway, vital signs, and neurologic status until the client is lying quietly awake, is breathing independently, and responds to commands spoken in a normal tone.
C. Observe for symptoms of complications, which may include hypotension, pallor, tachycardia (from bleeding), shoulder, neck, back, or abdominal pain (from perforation), or tachypnea and rales caused by pulmonary edema after thoracic perforation.
D. Use of topical and injected local anesthetics has been associated with methemoglobinemia in rare instances. Consider this condition in clients exhibiting signs and symptoms of hypoxia refractory to oxygen therapy.

5. **Client and family teaching:**
   A. Fast from food and fluids for 8-12 hours before the procedure.
   B. Arrange for someone else to drive you home because clients receiving sedation should not drive until 24 hours later.
   C. It is important to swallow when asked as the endoscope is being inserted through the mouth and advanced into the stomach.

6. **Factors that affect results:**
   A. The client must be able to swallow.

7. **Other data:**
   A. This test is to be performed with caution in clients with perforated ulcer, aortic aneurysm, recent bleeding esophageal varices, or Zenker's diverticulum.
   B. Complications of this procedure include esophageal, thoracic, gastric, or diaphragmatic perforation.

GCT
(*see Gastric challenge test, Diagnostic*)

GEMINI IMAGING, DIAGNOSTIC
(*see Dual modality imaging, Diagnostic*)

GENITAL, BACILLUS *HAEMOPHILUS DUCREYI,* CULTURE

Norm. No growth

Usage. Distinguishes genital chancroid from other genital ulcerations such as syphilis, herpes genitalis, lymphogranuloma venereum, granuloma inguinale, and traumatic ulcer.

Description. The causative agent of the chancroid genital ulcer, *Haemophilus ducreyi*, is a nonmotile, gram-negative bacillus transmitted by direct sexual contact. It is more common in warm climates than in cold climates and is contagious until completely healed.

Professional Considerations
1. Consent form NOT required.
2. **Preparation:**
   A. Obtain one or more of the following culture media: agar supplemented with IsoVitale X, agar with CVA enrichment, agar with vancomycin (3 mg/L).
3. **Procedure:**
   A. Cleanse the ulcer and the area surrounding it with three culture kit towelettes. Cleanse the ulcer from front to back, and discard each towelette after one pass from front to back.
   B. Swab the base of the ulcer with a sterile cotton swab, and transfer the culture directly onto one or more culture media.
4. **Postprocedure care:**
   A. Transport the culture to the laboratory immediately.
5. **Client and family teaching:**
   A. Describe the procedure above if the client is to collect the specimen independently.
   B. Results are normally available in 48 hours.
6. **Factors that affect results:**
   A. For successful growth, inoculation of the culture medium must be performed immediately.
   B. The isolation rate is improved when more than one type of medium is used.
7. **Other data:**
   A. If the results are negative, the test should be repeated because of common difficulty in growing *H. ducreyi*.

G

GENITAL, *CANDIDA ALBICANS*, CULTURE

Norm. No growth of *Candida*. Normal flora present.

Usage. Candidiasis (moniliasis), urethritis, and vulvovaginitis.

Description. *Candida albicans* is a fungus that is often part of the normal human skin flora but may also be transmitted sexually. It may cause infections of the skin, nails, and mucous membranes and may also cause a disseminated infection in debilitated individuals. Predisposing factors for *C. albicans* infections include diabetes mellitus, infection with human immunodeficiency virus, general debilitation, and broad-spectrum antibiotic therapy. *C. albicans* is a common cause of vaginitis in females.

Professional Considerations
1. Consent form NOT required.
2. Preparation:
   A. Obtain three or four towelettes, a Culturette or sterile cotton swab, and a red-topped tube.
3. Procedure:
   A. Collect the specimen by cleansing the vulva and peritoneal area with three or four culture kit or microbiologic towelettes. Cleanse the area from front to back and discard each towelette after one pass from front to back. Alternatively, swab the urethral orifice, vulva, or vagina with a sterile cotton swab and place it into a sterile tube.
4. Postprocedure care:
   A. Document the specimen source and site, the symptoms, recent antibiotic therapy, and the collection time on the laboratory requisition.
   B. Send the specimen to the laboratory within 2 hours.
5. Client and family teaching:
   A. Results are normally available within 24-48 hours.
   B. *C. albicans* infection is curable with oral and topical medication. The medication must be continued for the full course of treatment to cure the infection.
   C. Future prevention for *C. albicans* infection should include avoidance of nylon pantyhose and underwear and, if the client is diabetic, maintenance of normal blood glucose levels.
   D. Do not have sexual relations until your physician confirms that the infection is gone.
   E. Do not use feminine hygiene sprays or douche during the treatment.
6. Factors that affect results:
   A. Results may be negative if antibiotic therapy was started before specimen collection.
   B. Results are invalidated if the specimen is refrigerated.
7. Other data:
   A. At least 48 hours are required for results.
   B. Consider testing for sexually transmitted diseases because *Candida* colonization has been associated with *Trichomonas vaginalis*.

GENITAL, *NEISSERIA GONORRHOEAE*, CULTURE

Norm. All sites negative for *Neisseria gonorrhoeae*.

Vaginal culture	Normal flora
Vulval culture	Normal flora
Urethral culture	Normal flora
Prostatic fluid culture	No growth
Endocervical culture	No growth

Usage. Cervicitis, dysuria, endometritis, epididymitis, gonorrhea, menstrual irregularities, pelvic inflammatory disease, pelvic peritonitis, perihepatitis, proctitis, prostatitis, salpingitis, urethral stricture, urethritis, vaginitis, and vulvovaginitis.

Description. *N. gonorrhoeae* is a pyogenic, gram-negative, oxidase-positive coccus that is an obligate parasite of humans. It is the causative organism of the sexually transmitted infection gonorrhea. *N. gonorrhoeae* inhabits the mucous membranes of the genital tract and may also be found in the oral mucosa of clients who engage in oral sex and the rectum of clients who engage in anal sex. Symptoms include dysuria, purulent urethral discharge, proctitis, and pharyngitis. Females are often asymptomatic. Left untreated, gonorrhea leads to skin lesions, arthritis, meningitis, and reproductive problems. *N. gonorrhoeae* is most often found in the urethra of males and the cervix and perineum of females.

Professional Considerations
1. Consent form NOT required.
2. **Preparation:**
   A. Wait 1 hour after urination to collect urethral specimens.
   B. Obtain three or four towelettes, a Culturette or cotton swab, and culture media (Transgrow, Jembec, or Thayer-Martin).
3. **Procedure:**
   A. Collect the specimen with a Culturette swab and either place it in a Culturette tube, then squeeze the tube tip to release the ampule of medium or the specimen may also be inoculated directly onto culture media.
   B. A rectal culture may also be collected for suspected gonorrheal proctitis by insertion of a sterile Culturette swab into the rectum. The swab should be held in place for 15 seconds and then removed and placed into the Culturette tube.
4. **Postprocedure care:**
   A. Write the specimen source and site, time of collection, sex, age, symptoms, and recent antibiotic therapy on the laboratory requisition.
   B. Transport the specimen to the laboratory within 1 hour. If it was inoculated directly onto Thayer-Martin medium, transport the specimen to the laboratory imme-

diately and insert it into a carbon dioxide incubator.
5. **Client and family teaching:**
   A. Review the specimen collection procedure with the client.
   B. Results are normally available within 48 hours.
   C. Gonorrhea infection is treatable with antibiotics.
   D. If the results are positive, provide the client with the appropriate information on sexually transmitted diseases.
      i. Notify all sexual partners from the last 90 days to be tested for gonorrhea infection.
      ii. Do not have sexual relations until your physician confirms that the infection is gone.
   E. Do not use feminine hygiene sprays or douche during the treatment.
   F. Wear underpants and pantyhose that have a cotton lining in the crotch.
   G. Take showers instead of tub baths until the infection is gone.
6. **Factors that affect results:**
   A. Reject specimens received more than 30 minutes after collection.
   B. Do not refrigerate samples. *N. gonorrhoeae* is easily destroyed by cold.
7. **Other data:**
   A. The sensitivity pattern of *N. gonorrhoeae* is ceftriaxone 100%, azithromycin 100%, tetracycline 65.7%, penicillin 40%, and ciprofloxacin 5.7%.

GENTAMICIN, BLOOD

Norm:

		SI UNITS
Peak therapeutic level	6-10 µg/mL	12-20 µmol/L
Peak panic level	>12 µg/mL	>24 µmol/L
Trough therapeutic level	<2 µg/mL	<4 µmol/L
Trough panic level	>2 µg/mL	>4 µmol/L

Overdose Symptoms and Treatment

Both sustained peak levels and trough levels that are high can be toxic.

Symptoms. Loss of hearing, acute tubular necrosis.

Treatment:
Note: Treatment choice(s) depend on client history and condition and episode history.
Both hemodialysis and peritoneal dialysis WILL remove gentamicin.

Usage. Evaluation of appropriateness of dosing during gentamicin therapy.

Description. Gentamicin is an aminoglycoside antibiotic effective against gram-positive and gram-negative bacteria, including *Pseudomonas aeruginosa*, *Klebsiella*, *Proteus*, *Escherichia*, and *Serratia*. It is excreted by the kidney, with accumulation in renal tubular cells. The half-life is 2-3 hours, with steady-state levels reached in 10-15 hours in clients with normal renal function. Gentamicin has a narrow range of therapeutic value. Thus, it is important to monitor gentamicin levels throughout therapy, beginning from the time it reaches a steady state. In clients with baseline renal impairment, monitoring should be initiated sooner than recommended in this procedure.

Professional Considerations
1. Consent form NOT required.
2. **Preparation:**
   A. Tube: Red topped, red/gray topped.
   B. Write any recent antibiotic therapy on the laboratory requisition.
   C. Do NOT draw during hemodialysis.
3. **Procedure:**
   A. For every 8-hour gentamicin administration, levels should be measured after dose number 5. For every 12-hour dosing, levels should be measured after dose number 3.
   B. Draw a 1-mL blood sample. Draw a trough specimen just before the gentamicin dose. Draw a peak specimen 30 minutes to 3 hours after completion of the intravenous dose or 15-60 minutes after completion of the intramuscular dose.
4. **Postprocedure care:**
   A. Label the tube and laboratory requisition with the specimen collection time and indicate whether it is a peak or trough specimen.
   B. Send the specimen promptly to the laboratory. The sample should be spun within 1 hour, with the serum then frozen or refrigerated until testing.
5. **Client and family teaching:**
   A. The test helps determine whether the antibiotic is being given at the safe and effective dose.

B. The trough level is drawn before the antibiotic dose, and the peak level is drawn after the dose.
   C. Results are normally available within 24 hours.
6. **Factors that affect results:**
   A. Increased results may be attributable to gentamicin nephrotoxicity.
   B. Serum separator gel tubes can absorb serum gentamicin and falsely decrease obtained levels.
7. **Other data:**
   A. Daily creatinine and beta$_2$-microglobulin levels should be monitored during gentamicin therapy.
   B. Gentamicin nephrotoxicity is more likely to occur when other nephrotoxic drugs are administered during gentamicin therapy.
   C. Neonates receiving gentamicin should have their hearing assessed before starting therapy and then every day until therapy is completed. Hearing testing should be performed on adults if possible before starting therapy. If the client can cooperate, Weber, Rinne, and whisper testing can be done at the bedside or clinic to assess and monitor hearing status. Notify client to report tinnitus, vertigo, or hearing loss immediately to the prescribing clinician or nurse. Intake and output should be monitored closely throughout gentamicin therapy.
   D. Controlled mechanical ventilation has been shown to decrease levels of gentamicin.

GGTP, BLOOD
(see Gamma-glutamyltranspeptidase, Blood)

GHB
(see Gamma-hydroxybutyric acid, Blood or Urine)

GHRELIN, PLASMA

Norm. 77.52-98.06 pg/mL
22.94-29.03 fmol/mL (SI Units)

Increased.[*] Bulimia nervosa, weight-loss. (Exception: Ghrelin levels do not increase when weight is reduced in people who have had gastric bypass surgery.)

Decreased.[*] Obesity, Short bowel syndrome, status post gastric bypass. Drugs include growth hormone.
[*]Note: Increased and Decreased sections above summarize findings from research. Since Ghrelin has been discovered only recently, many studies have not yet been replicated.

Description. Ghrelin is a growth-hormone releasing peptide found in the stomach and in many other organs and tissues throughout the body. This peptide's function in the stomach is best understood, but its function throughout the rest of the body is still being studied. Ghrelin levels have been shown to increase before meals, causing an increase in glucose level, which increases the appetite. Ghrelin also stimulates the release of insulin from the islet cells of the pancreas. Ghrelin levels decrease after meals, possibly in response to increased plasma glucose. In those on weight-reduction diets, Ghrelin baseline levels have been found to increase (Cummings et al, 2002). This effect indicates a potential role of Ghrelin in weight regain experienced by many dieters. Other effects of Ghrelin include stimulating the release of adrenocorticotropic hormone, epinephrine, and glucose.

Professional Considerations
1. Consent form IS required.

2. **Preparation:**
   A. Tube: 2.7- or 4.5-mL blue topped.
3. **Procedure:**
   A. Withdraw 2 mL of blood into a syringe or vacuum tube. Remove the syringe or tube, leaving the needle in place. Attach a second syringe, and draw two blood samples, one in a citrated blue-topped tube and the other in a control tube. The sample quantity should be 2.4 mL for a 2.7-mL tube and 4.0 mL for a 4.5-mL tube. Draw a 5-mL blood sample in a sodium citrate anticoagulated blue-topped tube.
4. **Postprocedure care:**
   A. Transport the specimens to the laboratory immediately for spinning and refrigeration.
5. **Client and family teaching:**
   A. Results may not be available for at least 3 days.
6. **Factors that affect results:**
   A. Reject hemolyzed specimens or tubes partially filled with blood.
   B. Use of heparin anticoagulant can cause falsely high values.
7. **Other data:**
   A. Ghrelin is being studied for possible vasodilatory effects.

GICA
(see CA 19-9, Blood)

GILCHRIST'S SKIN TEST
(see Blastomycosis skin test, Diagnostic)

GLOBULIN, PLASMA

Norm:

		SI UNITS
Total		2.5 g of protein
Alpha$_1$	0.1-0.4 g/dL	1-5% of total
Alpha$_2$	0.4-1.0 g/dL	4.6-14% of total
Beta	0.5-1.5 g/dL	7.3-15% of total
Gamma	0.5-1.7 g/dL	8-21% of total

Increased Alpha$_1$ Globulin. Burns, carcinomatosis, focal episodes as a result of tumors, chemical injury, dehydration, diabetes mellitus, glomerulonephritis, Hodgkin's disease, inflammation (acute), lymphoma, necrosis, pregnancy, trauma, and ulcerative colitis. Drugs include estrogens.

Increased Alpha$_2$ Globulin. Acute infection, adrenal insufficiency, allergies, asthma, burns (haptoglobin, ceruloplasmin), carcinomatosis, chemical injury (haptoglobin, ceruloplasmin), Cushing syndrome, dehydration, diabetes mellitus (advanced), focal episodes as a result of tumors (haptoglobin, ceruloplasmin), Hodgkin's disease, hypernephroma, hyperparathyroidism, hyperthyroidism, hypoalbuminemia, infarction (haptoglobin, ceruloplasmin), inflammation (haptoglobin, ceruloplasmin), leukemia (myelogenous), lymphoma, myxedema, necrosis (haptoglobin, ceruloplasmin), nephrotic syndrome, nephrosis, peritonitis (familial paroxysmal), pregnancy, rheumatic fever, rheumatoid arthritis, sarcoidosis, systemic lupus erythematosus, trauma (haptoglobin, ceruloplasmin), and ulcerative colitis. Drugs include adrenocorticosteroids (haptoglobin) and estrogens (ceruloplasmin).

Increased Beta Globulin. Biliary cirrhosis, chickenpox, chronic iron deficiency anemia (transferrin), carcinoma (complement), cirrhosis, Cushing's disease (complement), dehydration, diabetes mellitus, dysproteinemia (familial, idiopathic), hepatitis (viral), hypercholesterolemia, hyperparathyroidism, hypothyroidism, macroglobulinemia, malignant hypertension (complement), nephrosis, nephrotic syndrome, nonfasting specimen, pregnancy (transferrin), obstructive jaundice, polyarteritis nodosa (complement), and sarcoidosis.

Increased Gamma Globulin. Amyloidosis, aortic arch syndrome, bacterial endocarditis, carcinoma, chickenpox, Crohn's disease, chronic inflammations, chronic lymphocytic leukemia, cirrhosis, congestive heart failure, cryoglobulinemia, cystic fibrosis, dehydration, Hashimoto's disease, hepatitis (viral), Hodgkin's disease, hypergammaglobulinemia, infection, leukemia (myelocytic, monocytic, myelogenous), liver disease, lymphogranuloma venereum, macroglobulinemia, malignant lymphoma, myasthenia gravis, multiple myeloma, myxedema, myxoma of left heart atrium, obstructive jaundice, polymyositis, retroperitoneal fibrosis, rheumatic fever, rheumatoid arthritis, sarcoidosis, systemic lupus erythematosus, temporal arteritis, tertiary syphilis, toxoplasmosis, trichinosis, tuberculo-

sis, visceral larva migrans, and Waldenström's macroglobulinemia.

Decreased Alpha₁ Globulin. Alpha₁-antitrypsin deficiency, hepatitis (viral), malabsorption, nephrotic syndrome, scleroderma, and starvation.

Decreased Alpha₂ Globulin. Hepatitis (viral), liver disease (haptoglobin), malabsorption, malnutrition (ceruloplasmin), megaloblastic anemia (haptoglobin), nephrotic syndrome (ceruloplasmin), protein-losing enteropathy (ceruloplasmin), red blood cell hemolysis (haptoglobin), scleroderma, starvation, and Wilson's disease (ceruloplasmin). Drugs include estrogens (haptoglobin).

Decreased Beta Globulin. Atransferrinemia (transferrin), autoimmune disease, malabsorption, protein malnutrition (transferrin), scleroderma, starvation, steatorrhea, systemic lupus erythematosus, and ulcerative colitis.

Decreased Gamma Globulin. Asthma, allergies, amyloidosis, Bruton's disease, Cushing syndrome, heavy chain disease, hyperglycinemia, hypogammaglobulinemia, leukemia (lymphocytic), lymphoma, malabsorption, nephrosis, nephrotic syndrome, malabsorption, protein-losing enteropathy, scleroderma, starvation, steatorrhea, thymic tumor, and ulcerative colitis.

Description. Globulins are plasma proteins formed mainly in the liver, but also in the lymphatic and reticuloendothelial systems. There are three types of proteins in the family of globulins: alpha, beta, and gamma. Alpha₁ globulin comprises alpha₁-antitrypsin, alpha₁-acid glycoprotein, alpha-fetoprotein, cortisol-binding protein, and thyroxine-binding globulin. Alpha₂ globulin comprises haptoglobin, alpha₂-macroglobulin, and ceruloplasmin. Beta globulin comprises transferrin, beta-lipoprotein, and complement components. Gamma globulin comprises IgG, IgA, IgM, IgD, and IgE antibodies. Functions served by the globulins include buffers in acid-base balance; transporters of constituents of blood such as lipids, vitamins, hormones, iron, copper, and enzymes; and antibody activity.

Professional Considerations
1. Consent form NOT required.
2. Preparation:
   A. See *Client and family teaching*.
   B. Tube: Red topped, red/gray topped, or gold topped.
   C. Do NOT draw specimen during hemodialysis.
3. Procedure:
   A. Draw a 7-mL blood sample.
4. Postprocedure care:
   A. Vaccinations and immunizations within the previous 6 months should be noted on the laboratory requisition.
   B. Blood product administration or antitoxin administration within the previous 6 weeks should be noted on the laboratory requisition.
5. Client and family teaching:
   A. Fast for 8 hours before the test.
6. Factors that affect results:
   A. Reject hemolyzed specimens.
7. Other data:
   A. The globulin level may be estimated by subtraction of albumin from total protein.

GLOMERULAR BASEMENT MEMBRANE ANTIBODY, SERUM

Norm. Negative.

Positive. Antiglomerular basement membrane disease including glomerulonephritis (crescentic) and Goodpasture syndrome. Positive in systemic vasculitis presenting as pulmonary-renal syndrome.

Description. Antibodies specific for the glomerular basement membrane (GBM) bind to specific antigens, causing an immune response leading to various anti-GBM diseases. This test identifies the presence of circulating GBM antibodies and is positive in 87% of clients with anti-GBM–associated Goodpasture syndrome and 60% of clients with anti-GBM–associated glomerulonephritis. Goodpasture syndrome is a rare disease characterized by necrotizing glomerulonephritis and hemorrhagic pneumonitis, which may result in renal failure and death.

Professional Considerations
1. Consent form NOT required.
2. Preparation:
   A. See *Client and family teaching*.
   B. Tube: Red topped, red/gray topped, or gold topped.
3. Procedure:
   A. Draw a 4-mL blood sample.
4. Postprocedure care:
   A. Transport the specimen to the laboratory immediately.
   B. Freeze the serum if the test is not run immediately.
5. Client and family teaching:
   A. Fast (except for water) for 8 hours before the test.
6. Factors that affect results:
   A. Antibiotic administration may produce a false-negative result.
   B. Up to 20% of results may be false negative.
7. Other data:
   A. In addition to a specimen of blood, a kidney or lung biopsy may also be evaluated for the presence of the antibody.

GLUCAGON, PLASMA

Norm. Norms vary by laboratory.

		SI UNITS
Big glucagon	34-192 pg/mL	34-192 ng/L
Proglucagon	<28 pg/mL	<28 ng/L
Glucagon	2-60 pg/mL	2-60 ng/L
Small glucagon	8-54 pg/mL	8-54 ng/L
Adult	20-100 pg/mL	20-100 ng/L
Cord blood	0-215 pg/mL	0-215 ng/L
Newborn-3 days	0-1750 pg/mL	0-1750 ng/L
4 days-14 years	0-148 pg/mL	0-148 ng/L

Increased. Acromegaly, burns, cirrhosis, Cushing syndrome, diabetes mellitus (average 1525 ± 578 pg/mL [1525 ± 578 ng/L]), diabetic ketoacidosis, familial hyperglucagonemia, glucagonoma (levels >900 pg/mL [900 ng/L, SI units]), hyperosmolality, hypoglycemia, Japanese encephalitis, pancreatic islet cell lesion, pancreatitis (acute, severe), pheochromocytoma, postoperatively, renal failure (average 500-580 pg/mL, 500-580 ng/L), stress, trauma, and uremia. Drugs include amino acids, cholecystokinin-pancreozymin, danazol, fructose infusion, gastrin, glucocorticoids, insulin, nifedipine, and sympathomimetic amines. Diet high in fat.

Decreased. Cystic fibrosis, hypoglycemia (related to chronic pancreatitis), idiopathic glucagon deficiency, insulinoma, neoplastic replacement of pancreas, pancreatitis (chronic), and status post pancreatectomy. Drugs include atenolol, pindolol, propranolol, and secretin. Treatments include acupuncture.

Description. Glucagon is a peptide hormone manufactured in and secreted by the alpha-cells of the pancreatic islets of Langerhans. Hypoglycemia, beta-adrenergics, and amino acids stimulate the secretion of glucagon, whereas increasing insulin levels inhibit its secretion. Glucagon increases blood glucose by increasing the breakdown of glycogen to glucose and stimulates activity of phosphorylase, the enzyme that initiates the first step in gluconeogenesis. This test is most often used as an aid in the diagnosis of glucagonoma, an alpha-islet–cell neoplasm occurring most often in females after menopause, and hypoglycemia caused by chronic pancreatitis or idiopathic glucagon deficiency.

Professional Considerations
1. Consent form NOT required.
2. Preparation:
   A. See *Client and family teaching.*
   B. Tube: Lavender topped, and ice.
3. Procedure:
   A. Draw a 10-mL blood specimen into a chilled tube.

B. Place the specimen immediately on ice.
4. Postprocedure care:
   A. Send the specimen to the laboratory immediately.
   B. Current administration of insulin or catecholamines, or both, should be noted on the laboratory requisition.
5. Client and family teaching:
   A. Fast for 10-12 hours before test.
   B. Because exercise and stress elevate plasma glucagon levels, the client should be relaxed and recumbent for 30 minutes before the test.
6. Factors that affect results:
   A. Results are invalidated if the client had a radioactive scan within 48 hours.
   B. Reject hemolyzed specimens.
   C. Prolonged fasting, stress, or current use of insulin or catecholamines may elevate glucagon levels.
7. Other data:
   A. Because of the influence on glucagon secretion, serum insulin and glucose should also be measured.
   B. This test should not be performed for poorly controlled diabetics.
   C. Stimulation or suppression tests may be needed to confirm a diagnosis of idiopathic glucagon deficiency or hypoglycemia caused by chronic pancreatitis.

GLUCOCHEK, DIAGNOSTIC
(*see Glucose monitoring machines, Diagnostic*)

GLUCOMETER, DIAGNOSTIC
(*see Glucose monitoring machines, Diagnostic*)

GLUCOSCAN, DIAGNOSTIC
(*see Glucose monitoring machines, Diagnostic*)

GLUCOSE, BLOOD

Norm. Dependent on time and content of last meal. In normal clients, glucose levels return to the fasting level (given in these norms) within 2 hours after the last meal.

WHOLE BLOOD		SI UNITS
Adults	60-89 mg/dL	3.3-4.9 mmol/L
>60 years	68-98 mg/dL	3.8-5.4 mmol/L
Children		
Cord blood	38-82 mg/dL	2.1-4.6 mmol/L
Premature infant	17-51 mg/dL	0.9-2.8 mmol/L
Neonate	25-51 mg/dL	1.4-2.8 mmol/L
Newborn to 24 hours	34-51 mg/dL	1.9-2.8 mmol/L
Newborn >24 hours	42-68 mg/dL	2.3-3.8 mmol/L
Child	51-85 mg/dL	2.8-4.7 mmol/L

SERUM		
Adults	70-105 mg/dL	3.9-5.8 mmol/L
>60 years	80-115 mg/dL	4.4-6.4 mmol/L
Children		
Cord blood	45-96 mg/dL	2.5-5.3 mmol/L
Premature infants	20-60 mg/dL	1.1-3.3 mmol/L
Neonates	30-60 mg/dL	1.7-3.3 mmol/L
Newborn to 24 hours	40-60 mg/dL	2.2-3.3 mmol/L
Newborn >24 hours	50-80 mg/dL	2.8-4.4 mmol/L
Child	60-100 mg/dL	3.3-5.5 mmol/L

Note: Whole-blood glucose values are about 15% less than serum glucose values because of greater dilution.

PANIC LEVELS		
Adults	<40 mg/dL or >700 mg/dL	<2.2 mmol/L or >38.6 mmol/L
Neonates	<30 mg/dL or >300 mg/dL	<1.6 mmol/L >16.0 mmol/L

G

Panic Level Symptoms and Treatment—Increased

Symptoms. Abdominal pain, fatigue, muscle cramps, nausea, polyuria, thirst, and vomiting.

Treatment:
Note: Treatment choice(s) depend on client history and condition and episode history.
Subcutaneous or intravenous injection of insulin per sliding scale. Intravenous insulin is typically administered by continuous infusion for panic levels accompanied by reduced level of consciousness. Hourly adjustments are based on subsequent blood glucose measurements.

Hourly neurologic checks.
Hourly intake and output.
Monitor for hypokalemia as side effect of treatment.

Panic Level Symptoms and Treatment—Decreased

Symptoms. Confusion, headache, hunger, irritability, nervousness, restlessness, sweating, and weakness.

Treatment
Note: Treatment choice(s) depend on client history and condition and episode history.
Administer oral form of glucose followed by oral ingestion of carbohydrates. For neonates or unconscious clients, give IV glucose or IV/IM glucagon.

Increased. Acromegaly, anesthesia, burns, carbon monoxide poisoning, cerebrovascular accident, convulsions, Cushing's disease, Cushing syndrome, cystic fibrosis, diabetes mellitus, eclampsia, encephalitis, erectile dysfunction, gigantism, hemochromatosis, hemorrhage, hyperosmolar hyperglycemic nonketotic coma (HHNK), hyperthyroidism, hyperpituitarism, hyperadrenalism, hypertension, hypervitaminosis A (chronic), infections, injury, malnutrition (chronic), meningitis, myocardial infarction, obesity, pancreatic carcinoma, pancreatic insufficiency, pancreatitis (chronic) pheochromocytoma, pituitary adenoma, pregnancy, shock, subarachnoid hemorrhage, stress, trauma, and Wernicke's encephalopathy. Drugs include anabolic steroids, androgens, arginine, ascorbic acid, asparaginase, aspirin, baclofen, benzodiazepines, bisacodyl (prolonged use), chlorpromazine, chlorthalidone, cimetidine, clonidine, corticosteroids, corticotropin, dextran, dextrothyroxine, diazoxide, disopyramide phosphate, epinephrine, epinephrine bitartrate, epinephrine borate, epinephrine hydrochloride, estrogens, ethacrynic acid, furosemide, glucose infusions, haloperidol, imipramine, isoproterenol hydrochloride, heparin calcium, heparin sodium, hydralazine hydrochloride, indomethacin, isoniazid, levodopa, levothyroxine sodium/T4, lithium carbonate, magnesium hydroxide (prolonged high doses), mercaptopurine, methimazole, methyldopa, methyldopa (hydrochloride), nalidixic acid, nicotine, nicotinic acid, oral contraceptives, oxazepam, para-aminosalicyclic acid, phenolphthalein, phenytoin, phenytoin sodium, progestins, promethazine hydrochloride, propranolol (in diabetics), propylthiouracil, protease inhibitors, reserpine, ritodrine hydrochloride, terbutaline sulfate, tetracyclines, thiazides, thyroglobulin, thyroid, tolbutamide (SMA methodology), and triamterene.

Decreased. Addison's disease, adrenal medulla unresponsiveness, alcoholism, carcinoma (adrenal gland, stomach, fibrosarcoma), cirrhosis, cretinism, diabetes mellitus (early), dumping syndrome, exercise, fever, Forbes' disease (type-III glycogen deposition disease), fructose intolerance, galactosemia, glucagon deficiency, hepatic phosphorylase deficiency (type-VI glycogen storage disease), hepatitis, hyperinsulinemia, hypopituitarism, hypothermia, hypothyroidism, infant of diabetic mother, insulin overdose (factitious hypoglycemia), insulinoma, kwashiorkor, leucine sensitivity, malnutrition, maple syrup urine disease, muscle phosphofructokinase deficiency (type-VII glycogen storage disease), myxedema, pancreatic islet cell tumor, pancreatitis, postoperatively (after gastrectomy or gastroenterostomy), postprandial hypoglycemia, Reye syndrome, Simmonds' disease, vomiting, von Gierke's disease (type-I glycogen storage disease), Waterhouse-Friderichsen syndrome, and Zetterstrom syndrome. Drugs include allopurinol, amphetamines, aspirin, beta-adrenergic blockers, caffeine, cerivastatin, chlorpropamide, clofibrate, edetate disodium, ethyl alcohol (ethanol), gatifloxacin, guanethidine sulfate, isoniazid, insulin, isocarboxazid, marijuana, nitrazepam, oral hypoglycemic agents, para-aminosalicylic acid, pargyline hydrochloride, phenacetin, phenazopyridine, phenelzine sulfate, phenformin, propranolol (in diabetics), and tranylcypromine sulfate. Herbs or natural remedies include zhi[1]mu[3] ('know-mother', *Anemarrhena asphodeloides*, an herb) and shi[2]gao[1] ('stone-plaster', calcium sulfate, gypsum) taken in combination; xuan[2]shen[1] ('black ginseng', *Scrophularia ningpoensis*, figwort) and cang[1]zhu[2] ('green-shu/zhu herb', *Atractylodes lancea*, var. ovata) taken in combination; shan[1]yao[4] ('mountain-medicine', *Dioscorea batatas*, potato yam) and huang[2]qi[2] ('yellow-old 60', *Astragalus reflexistipulus*, or *A. hoantchy*, yellow vetch) taken in combination; and karela (*Momordica charantia*, balsam apple) taken in combination with chlorpropamide. Herbs or natural remedies include teas (decoctions, infusions) containing chromium, karela, ginseng, guar gum, meshasringi (*Gymnema sylvestre*, mesha shringi, Indian milkweed vine), methi (fenugreek leaves), tundika (*Coccinia indica*).

Description. Glucose is a monosaccharide found naturally occurring in fruits. It is also formed from the digestion of carbohydrates and the conversion of glycogen by the liver and is the body's main source of cellular energy. Glucose is essential for brain and erythrocyte function. Excess glucose is stored as glycogen in the liver and muscle cells. Hormones influencing glucose metabolism include insulin, glucagon, thyroxine, somatostatin, cortisol, and epinephrine. Fasting glucose levels are used to help diagnose diabetes mellitus and hypoglycemia. A randomly timed test for glucose is usually performed for routine screening and nonspecific evaluation of carbohydrate metabolism. The American Diabetes Association criteria for diagnosis of diabetes mellitus include a fasting plasma glucose level of >126 mg/dL (7 mmol/L).

Professional Considerations
1. Consent form NOT required.
2. Preparation:
   A. See *Client and family teaching.*
   B. Tube: Red topped, red/gray topped, or gold topped or gray topped.
   C. Observe for signs of hypoglycemia (weakness, slurred speech, confusion, somnolence, pallor, palpitations, convulsions) in fasting clients.
   D. Screen client for the use of herbal preparations or natural remedies such as chromium, karela, ginseng, guar gum, *meshasringi, methi,* and *tundika.*
3. Procedure:
   A. Draw a 1-mL blood sample.
4. Postprocedure care:
   A. Send the sample to the laboratory for immediate spinning. If transport is delayed, refrigerate the sample.
   B. The time of the client's last pretest meal, the sample collection time, and the time of the last pretest insulin or oral hypoglycemic agent (if applicable) should be noted on the laboratory requisition.

5. Client and family teaching:
   A. Fast (except for water) for 8-12 hours before collection for fasting specimen.
   B. Withhold morning insulin or oral hypoglycemic agent until after fasting blood sample has been drawn.
   C. Refer newly diagnosed diabetics for diabetic teaching and long-term medical follow-up care.
   D. Resume diet after the fasting specimen has been drawn.
   E. Watch for signs of hypoglycemia (listed on p. 599) and hyperglycemia (listed on p. 599). Teach appropriate intervention.
6. Factors that affect results:
   A. Reject specimens received more than 1 hour after collection to prevent falsely low results.
   B. Falsely decreased glucose values may occur when the glucose oxidase/peroxidase procedure is used or if the client has recently taken acetaminophen or oxycodone.
7. Other data:
   A. Spun samples are stable for 8 hours.
   B. In a client with diabetes, the blood specimen should be drawn before insulin treatment or administration of oral hypoglycemic drugs.
   C. Factitious hypoglycemia by unprescribed or excessive use of sulfonylureas is biochemically indistinguishable from insulinoma. Factitious hypoglycemia has also been reported by unprescribed and intentionally excessive use of insulin.
   D. Revised American Diabetes Association 1999 guidelines for the diagnosis of diabetes call for a diagnosis of diabetes when fasting plasma blood glucose is 126 mg/dL or higher.

GLUCOSE, 2-HOUR POSTPRANDIAL, SERUM

Norm:

		SI UNITS
Newborn to 50 years	65-140 mg/dL	3.6-7.7 mmol/L
50-60 years	65-150 mg/dL	3.6-8.3 mmol/L
>60 years	65-160 mg/dL	3.6-8.8 mmol/L
American Diabetes Association diagnosis of diabetes (after 75 g glucose load)	>200 mg/dL	>11 mmol/L

Usage. Screening for diabetes mellitus and assessing control of hyperglycemia.

Increased. Acromegaly, anoxia, anxiety, brain tumor, cirrhosis, convulsive disorders, Cushing's disease, Cushing syndrome, diabetes mellitus, dumping syndrome (after gastrectomy), hepatic disease (chronic), hyperlipoproteinemia, hyperthyroidism, infarction (myocardial, cerebral), lipoproteinemias, malnutrition, malignancy, nephrotic syndrome, pancreatitis, pheochromocytoma, preeclampsia, pregnancy, sepsis, and stress (physical, emotional). Drugs include those discussed under *Glucose, Blood.*

Decreased. Addison's disease, adrenal insufficiency, anterior pituitary insufficiency, congenital adrenal hyperplasia, hepatic insufficiency, hyperinsulinism, hypoglycemia, hypopituitarism, hypothyroidism, insulinoma, islet cell adenoma, malabsorption syndrome, myxedema, steatorrhea, and von Gierke's disease. Drugs include those discussed under *Glucose, Blood.*

Description. The 2-hour postprandial glucose test is the measurement of serum glucose 2 hours from the beginning of a meal containing a specific amount of carbohydrate. In normal clients, glucose should return to fasting levels within 2 hours after the ingestion of the test meal.

Professional Considerations
1. Consent form NOT required.
2. **Preparation:**
   A. See *Client and family teaching.*
   B. Tube: Gray topped, and test meal.
3. **Procedure:**
   A. Draw a 5-mL blood sample 2 hours after beginning ingestion of the designated test meal.

4. **Postprocedure care:**
   A. Refrigerate specimens not sent to the laboratory within 1 hour.
5. **Client and family teaching:**
   A. Eat a high-carbohydrate (200-300 g) diet for 3 days before the test.
   B. Fast (except for water) for 8-12 hours and abstain from alcohol for 36 hours before the test.
   C. When possible, drugs affecting the results should be stopped 3-21 days before the test.
   D. Insulin and oral hypoglycemic agents should be withheld the morning of the test.
   E. Eat a meal containing 75-100 g of carbohydrate within 20 minutes during the testing period.
   F. Avoid strenuous activity, caffeine, and nicotine after the meal until the sample is drawn.
6. **Factors that affect results:**
   A. Falsely increased values may occur with strenuous activity, inhalation of nicotine, ingestion of caffeine during the test and in 10% of healthy elderly without a pathologic process.
   B. Falsely decreased glucose values may occur with acetaminophen and oxycodone when the glucose oxidase/peroxidase procedure is used.
   C. Stresses caused by acute illness, infection, pregnancy, or surgery invalidate the results.
7. **Other data:**
   A. An abnormally elevated test indicates the need for a glucose tolerance test.

GLUCOSE, CEREBROSPINAL FLUID, SPECIMEN
(*see Cerebrospinal fluid, Glucose, Specimen*)

GLUCOSE, QUALITATIVE, SEMIQUANTITATIVE, URINE

Norm. Negative.

FIVE-DROP METHOD		TWO-DROP METHOD	
Negative	Blue-green	Negative	Blue-green
0.25%	Green	Trace	Dark green
0.5%	Olive-green	0.5%	Green
0.75%	Brown-green	1%	Olive-green
1%	Gold	2%	Brown-green
2%	Orange	3%	Gold
		>5%	Orange

Positive. Adrenal disorders, central nervous system disease, diabetes mellitus, eclampsia, Fanconi syndrome, glomerulonephritis, glucose administration, heavy metal poisoning, hepatic disease, hyperalimentation, infections, nephrosis, pregnancy, presence of reducing substances and sugars other than glucose in the urine (copper-reduction method only), thyroid disorders, total parenteral nutrition, and toxic renal tubular disease. Drugs include ammonium chloride, asparaginase, carbamazepine, corticosteroids, dextrothyroxine sodium, indomethacin, isoniazid, lithium carbonate, nicotinic acid, phenothiazines, and thiazide diuretics.

Negative. Negative results occur with Clinistix when sugars other than glucose are present in the urine.

Description. A random urine specimen is tested by either copper reduction (Clinitest) or by the enzymatic glucose oxidase method (Clinistix) for the presence of glucose. Semiquantitative determination includes reagent strips called R-strip and T-strip.

Clinitest is a copper-reduction tablet test used to detect melituria and to detect and monitor urine glucose and nonglucose sugar levels. Urine sugar up to 2% may be measured with the five-drop method, and up to 5% may be measured with the two-drop method. Copper-reduction methods are helpful when the test purpose is to detect both glucose and nonglucose sugars present in the urine, as in metabolic disease or parenteral nutrition administration.

Clinistix test is a qualitative dipstick method of urine glucose testing that involves an oxidation reaction between urine, impregnated enzymes, and a chromogen, resulting in a color change proportional to the amount of glucose present in the urine. Clinistix is classified as a glucose oxidase method of urine glucose testing. The advantage of glucose oxidase methods over copper-reduction tests is that this method is specific for glucose and unaffected by other sugars and reducing substances.

Professional Considerations
1. Consent form NOT required.
2. Preparation:
   A. Clinitest:
      i. Obtain a 50-mL clean plastic container, a test tube, a dropper, and urine test tablets.
      ii. Dark blue tablets should be discarded. Use only fresh tablets, which are light blue and flecked with dark blue.
      iii. Avoid touching the tablets. To avoid burns, wash the affected area quickly if skin contact occurs.
      iv. A fresh-voided, postprandial specimen is recommended.
   B. Clinistix:
      i. For a Clinistix test, obtain a 50-mL clean plastic container and urine test strips.
      ii. Keep the Clinistix bottle tightly capped. Open the bottle to quickly remove a reagent strip and then recap it before performing test.
      iii. Light exposure and moisture speed the degradation of Clinistix. Inspect the strip before use, even if the contents of bottle have not expired. If the strip is darkened, discard it and the bottle from which it was taken.
3. Procedure:
   A. Have the client completely empty the bladder and then drink at least 8 ounces of fluid; 30 minutes later, have him or her void at least 20 mL of urine into a clean plastic container. A fresh specimen may be taken from a urinary drainage bag. Refrigerate the specimen if it is not tested promptly.
   B. Clinitest:
      i. Five-drop method: Add 5 drops of urine to a clean test tube and rinse the dropper with water. Then add 10 drops of water to a test tube.
      ii. Add one Clinitest tablet to this mixture.
      iii. Recap the Clinitest jar tightly.
      iv. Observe the color changes during the boiling phase. Be careful because the tube is hot!
      v. Glucose >2 g/dL causes a rapid color change to orange during the boiling phase. If this occurs, the test should be repeated as above, using 2 drops instead of 5 drops of urine and comparing results

G

to the Clinitest color chart for the two-drop test.

vi. 15 seconds after the boiling stops, agitate the test tube and immediately compare the mixture color to the Clinitest color chart. Record the results as shown in the table on page 602.

C. Clinistix test:

i. Dip the Clinistix reagent strip into the urine, making sure to completely immerse the test pad for 2 seconds.

ii. While removing the strip, slide the pad side against the edge of the container.

iii. Exactly 30 seconds after removal of the strip from the urine, compare the color of the test pad to the colors on the bottle.

iv. Record the results as either negative, light, medium, or dark.

4. **Postprocedure care:**

A. Discard the specimen and the reagent strip, if used. Rinse the test tube, if used, with water.

5. **Client and family teaching:**

A. New diabetics must learn home glucose testing, which may be with or without a machine.

B. Do not contaminate the urine specimen with stool or toilet tissue.

C. For home monitoring, provide the written instructions and a flow sheet so that the client can record the test results.

D. Watch for signs of hyperglycemia and hypoglycemia (see *Glucose, Blood,* for symptoms and treatment).

6. **Factors that affect results:**

A. Failure to perform the test on a fresh or refrigerated specimen invalidates the results.

B. Copper-reduction method (Clinitest):

i. The color charts for the two-drop and five-drop methods are different and must be used with the appropriate test.

ii. Failure to protect tablets from moisture can result in false findings and possibly an explosion.

iii. Use of discolored or dark blue tablets invalidates the results.

iv. The presence of radiographic contrast medium in the urine may cause false-negative results.

v. Reducing substances that cause a false-positive test include aminosalicylic acid, ampicillin, ampicillin sodium, ascorbic acid, camphor, cephalosporins, chloral hydrate, chloramphenicol, chloroform, creatinine, formaldehyde, fructose, galactose, glucosamine, glucuronic acid, homogentisic acid, isoniazid, ketones, levodopa, maltose, menthol, metolazone, nitrofurantoin, nitrofurantoin sodium, penicillin G benzathine, penicillin G potassium, pentose, phenol, salicylates, streptomycin sulfate, tetracyclines, turpentine, and uric acid.

C. Glucose oxidase method (Clinistix):

i. Clinistix strips must be compared with the color chart on the bottle from which they were taken.

ii. Use of darkened strips or those exposed to prolonged moisture or air invalidates the results.

iii. Drugs that may cause false-negative results with Clinistix include ascorbic acid, levodopa, methyldopa, methyldopate hydrochloride, phenazopyridine, and salicylates.

7. **Other data:**

A. If the client is receiving ascorbic acid, hydrochlorites, levodopa, peroxides, phenazopyridine, or salicylates, use Clinitest tablets.

B. Other available glucose oxidase urine testing strips include Diastix, n-Multistix, and Tes-Tape.

C. These tests are now used less frequently to monitor urine glucose in clients with diabetes because of the availability of more precise techniques for blood glucose self-monitoring and blood testing for hemoglobin A_{1C}.

D. See also *Benedict's Test, Diagnostic.*

GLUCOSE, QUANTITATIVE, 24-HOUR, URINE

Norm. ≤100 mg/24 hours (≤5.6 mmol/day, SI units).

Increased. Adrenal disorders, central nervous system disease, diabetes mellitus, eclampsia, Fanconi syndrome, glomerulonephritis, glucose administration, heavy-metal poisoning, hepatic disease, hyperalimentation, infections, nephrosis, pregnancy, thyroid disorders, and toxic renal tubular disease. Drugs include ammonium chloride, asparaginase, carbamazepine, corticosteroids, dextrothyroxine sodium, indomethacin, isoniazid, lithium carbonate, nicotinic acid, phenothiazines, and thiazide diuretics.

Description. A quantitative measurement of urine glucose may detect glucose spillage into the urine that occurs intermittently and thus may not be detected by random urine glucose measurement. The enzymatic glucose oxidase method is used to detect the presence and amount of glucose. However, the test is performed in the laboratory on an aliquot of a 24-hour urine collection, and the results are reported as numeric values.

Professional Considerations

1. Consent form NOT required.
2. Preparation:
   A. Obtain a 3-L, 24-hour urine collection bottle containing toluene preservative.
   B. For pediatric collections, also obtain a pediatric urine-collection device and tape.
   C. Write the beginning time of collection on the laboratory requisition.
3. Procedure:
   A. *Adult collection:*
      i. Discard the first morning-urine specimen.
      ii. Save all the urine voided for 24 hours in a refrigerated, clean, 3-L container to which toluene preservative has been added. For catheterized clients, keep the drainage bag on ice and empty the urine into the refrigerated collection container hourly.
      iii. Document the quantity of urine output during the col-

lection period. Include the urine voided at the end of the 24-hour period.
   B. *Pediatric collection:*
      i. Place the child in a supine position with the knees flexed and the hips externally rotated and abducted.
      ii. Cleanse, rinse, and thoroughly dry the perineal area.
      iii. To prevent the child from removing the collection device, a diaper may be placed over the genital area.
      iv. *Females:* Tape the pediatric collection device to the perineum. Starting at the area between the anus and vagina, apply the device in the anterior direction.
      v. *Males:* Place the pediatric collection device over the penis and scrotum and tape it to the perineal area.
      vi. After each void, empty the collection device into a refrigerated, 3-L container to which toluene preservative has been added.
4. Postprocedure care:
   A. Refrigerate the specimen until it is tested.
   B. Compare the urine quantity in the specimen container with the urinary output record for the test. If the specimen contains less urine than what was recorded as output, some of the sample may have been discarded, invalidating the test.
   C. Document the quantity of urine output and the ending time on the laboratory requisition.
   D. Send the specimen to the laboratory for measurement.
5. Client and family teaching:
   A. Save all the urine voided in the 24-hour period and urinate before defecating to avoid loss of urine. If any urine is accidentally discarded, discard the entire specimen and restart the collection the next day.
6. Factors that affect results:
   A. All the urine voided for the 24-hour period must be included to avoid a falsely low result.
   B. Drugs that may cause false-negative results with Clinistix include ascorbic acid, levodopa,

G

methyldopa, methyldopate hydrochloride, phenazopyridine, and salicylates.

C. Failure to refrigerate the specimen throughout the collection period decreases accuracy of the results because of bacterial growth.

7. Other data:

A. This test aids in the regulation of diet and medication in clients with diabetes mellitus.

B. Because of the problem with incomplete urine collections, laboratories sometimes check the

creatinine present in the urine to validate that the sample represents a full 24 hours.

GLUCOSE, SEMIQUANTITATIVE, URINE

(see Glucose, Qualitative, Semiquantitative, Urine)

GLUCOSE ALERT, DIAGNOSTIC

(see Glucose monitoring machines, Diagnostic)

GLUCOSE CHALLENGE TEST (GCT, O'SULLIVAN TEST, 50-G 1-HR GLUCOSE TOLERANCE TEST, ORAL GLUCOSE SCREENING), DIAGNOSTIC

Norm. (Serum)

SI UNITS		
Normal	< 130 mg/dL (<7.2 mmol/L)	
Elevated	≥130 mg/dL (≥7.2 mmol/L)	Has 90% sensitivity for gestational DM
Elevated	>140 mg/dL (>7.8 mmol/L)	Has 80% sensitivity for gestational DM

Usage. Screening during pregnancy for gestational diabetes mellitus (GDM).

High-risk pregnant women should be screened at initial visit, if negative, repeat at 24-28 weeks or if symptoms occur. High-risk characteristics include member of high-risk ethnic group, age over 30 years, obesity (>20% above ideal body weight), previous history of GDM, glucosuria, strong family history of diabetes (first-degree relative), previous impaired oral glucose tolerance test, previous baby with >9-lb birth weight.

Average risk pregnant women should be screened at 24-28 weeks of gestation.

Increased. Acromegaly, anoxia, anxiety, brain tumor, cirrhosis, convulsive disorders, Cushing's disease, Cushing syndrome, diabetes mellitus, dumping syndrome (after gastrectomy), hepatic disease (chronic), hyperlipoproteinemia, hyperthyroidism, infarction (myocardial, cerebral), lipoproteinemia, malnutrition, malignancy, nephritic syndrome, pancreatitis, pheochromocytoma, preeclampsia, pregnancy, sepsis, and stress (physical, emotional). Drugs include those administered in the *Glucose tolerance test, Blood.*

Decreased. Addison's disease, adrenal insufficiency, anterior pituitary insufficiency congenital adrenal hyperplasia, celiac disease, hepatic insufficiency, hyperinsulinism, hypoglycemia, hypopituitarism, hypothyroidism, insulinoma, islet cell adenoma, malabsorption syndrome, myxedema, steatorrhea, pancreatic islet cell hyperplasia, sprue, and von Gierke's disease. Drugs include those administered in the *Glucose tolerance test, Blood.*

Description. Glucose is a monosaccharide formed from the digestion of carbohydrates and the conversion of glycogen by the liver and is the body's main source of cellular energy. The glucose challenge test is most commonly used to screen for gestational diabetes. It should NOT be confused with the oral glucose tolerance test. If absorption from the gut has been normal, pregnant women with a level below the cutoff have a low risk of developing GDM. Those with glucose levels at or above the cutoff are at higher risk and should have an oral glucose tolerance test for definitive diagnosis.

Professional Considerations

1. Consent form NOT required.

2. **Preparation:**
   A. Tube: Gray-top.
   B. See *Client and family teaching.*
3. **Procedure:**
   A. Client should completely ingest 50 g of glucose solution within 5 minutes. (In some cases, jelly bean candy has been used instead of the glucose solution; however, this method can result in lower test sensitivity.)
   B. Note the time the client completed drinking the solution.
   C. Draw a 5-mL venous blood sample.
4. **Postprocedure care:**
   A. Label the tube "50-g glucose" and the time it was ingested.
   B. Current administration of medications known to affect the test results should be noted on the laboratory requisition.
   C. Send blood sample to the laboratory immediately or refrigerate.
5. **Client and family teaching:**
   A. It is not necessary to fast for this test.
   B. No eating, smoking, drinking, or exercise is permitted during the test period. You will be asked to remain seated during the test period.
   C. This tests usually takes 60-90 minutes.
6. **Factors that affect results:**
   A. Eating, smoking, drinking, or exercise during the test period invalidate the results.
   B. Caffeine interferes with the accuracy of the results. Sips of water may be allowed.
   C. Stresses caused by acute illness, pregnancy, or surgery invalidate the results.

D. There is debate regarding the time of day that the GCT should be done. Some evidence indicates that pregnant women having the test in the afternoon were twice as likely to have a positive result than women tested in the morning.
7. **Other data:**
   A. There is debate regarding whether all women should be screened at 24-28 weeks. Arguments for screening all women are that 1%-2% of women with no risk factors develop GDM. The American Diabetic Association indicates that women with low risk of gestational diabetes mellitus do not require glucose testing. Low-risk pregnant women meet all of the following requirements: age: <25 years, body mass index of 25 or less, member of ethnic group with a low prevalence of GDM, no known diabetes in first-degree relatives, no history of abnormal glucose tolerance, no history of poor obstetric outcome.
   B. There is debate regarding the most appropriate cut-off level for continued diagnostic criteria. The 130 mg/dL level provides more false-positive results and increased cost of continued testing; however, the some feel that the maternal and fetal risk associated with GDM merits this level. Since the cost-benefit ratio of diagnosing GDM remains unresolved, either the 130 mg/dL or 140 mg/dL threshold is considered acceptable.

GLUCOSE MONITORING MACHINES, DIAGNOSTIC

Norm. Whole-blood glucose values are about 15% less than serum glucose values as a result of greater dilution.

WHOLE BLOOD		SI UNITS
Adults	60-89 mg/dL	3.3-4.9 mmol/L
>60 years	68-98 mg/dL	3.8-5.4 mmol/L
Children		
Cord blood	38-82 mg/dL	2.1-4.6 mmol/L
Premature infant	17-51 mg/dL	0.9-2.8 mmol/L
Neonate	25-51 mg/dL	1.4-2.8 mmol/L
Newborn to 24 hours	34-51 mg/dL	1.9-2.8 mmol/L
Newborn >24 hours	42-68 mg/dL	2.3-3.8 mmol/L
Child	51-85 mg/dL	2.8-4.7 mmol/L

Usage. Chronic glucose monitoring for diabetes mellitus, monitoring for hypoglycemia in newborn, and bedside whole-blood glucose analysis.

Description. Blood glucose monitoring is generally considered to be more reliable for diabetic glucose monitoring than urine glucose levels. This is particularly true for clients with an abnormally low renal threshold for glucose reabsorption after glomerular filtration. The term "glucose monitoring machines" encompasses a variety of reflectance meters that can be used to quickly quantitate whole blood glucose levels. In general, the technique involves applying a drop of capillary or venous blood to a reagent strip, blotting the drop after a specific time period, inserting the strip into the reflectance meter, and then following the manufacturer's recommended steps for processing. The result is generally obtained within 2 to 3 minutes and has been estimated to cost as little as $1/20$ of a "stat." laboratory glucose measurement. Home meters need to be verified at regular intervals, as $1/3$ of readings deviated significantly in one study (Henry et al, 2001).

Professional Considerations
1. Consent form NOT required.
2. **Preparation:**
   A. Verify that the client's hematocrit level is within the range for which the specific brand of machine is designed to be accurate. If the hematocrit is outside the required range, perform the Glucose Blood test instead of this test.
   B. Verify that the machine has been calibrated within the time requirements specified by the manufacturer.
   C. Obtain an alcohol wipe, a 2.5-mm lancet (or a needle and a syringe), a reagent strip, a cotton ball, a reflectance meter, sterile gauze, and a capillary tube if heelstick blood will be used.
   D. Read the instructions for the specific reflectance meter to be used.
3. **Procedure:**
   A. *Fingerstick capillary method:*
      i. Cleanse the lateral aspect of the pad of the finger with an alcohol wipe and allow the area to dry.
      ii. Using a 2.5-mm lancet, puncture the lateral aspect of the pad of the finger. Wipe the first drop of blood away with sterile gauze.
      iii. Holding the puncture site dependent, allow a second, large drop of blood to accumulate and drop onto the reagent strip, making sure there is enough blood to completely cover the pad of the reagent strip. The pad of the finger may be very gently and repeatedly pressed to encourage blood flow, but avoid milking the finger.
      iv. Follow directions for the specific reflectance meter being used.
   B. *Heelstick capillary method:*
      i. Prewarming the heel is not necessary.
      ii. Avoid puncturing over previous puncture sites or puncturing the posterior curvature of the heel.
      iii. Cleanse an area on the medial or lateral plantar surface of the heel with 70% alcohol and allow the area to dry.
      iv. Using a 2.5-mm lancet, puncture the heel until a free flow of blood is obtained. Wipe the first drop of blood away with sterile gauze.
      v. Holding the puncture site dependent, allow a second, large drop of blood to accumulate and drop onto the reagent strip, making sure that there is enough blood to completely cover the pad of the reagent strip. Avoid milking the heel.
      vi. Follow the directions for the specific reflectance meter being used.
   C. *Venous method:*
      i. Obtain a 1-mL venous blood sample in a syringe or green-topped tube.
      ii. Completely cover the pad of the reagent strip with a drop of the blood specimen.
      iii. Follow the directions for the specific reflectance meter being used.

4. **Postprocedure care:**
   A. Hold pressure to the site until the bleeding stops. Leave puncture sites open to the air to heal.
5. **Client and family teaching:**
   A. Teach the newly diagnosed client with diabetes how to perform a fingerstick and use a reflectance meter.
   B. Watch for signs of hyperglycemia and hypoglycemia (see *Glucose, Blood*, for symptoms and treatment).
   C. Bring a home reflectance meter to office appointments with the physician so that technique and machine calibration may be assessed.
6. **Factors that affect results:**
   A. After the skin is cleansed with alcohol, the skin must be allowed to dry completely before the puncture is performed.
   B. Failure to completely cover the reagent area with blood may cause inaccurate results.
   C. Using too little or too much blood may cause inaccurate results. Cotton, rather than gauze, should be used for blotting the strip.
   D. Failure to follow timing instructions exactly as recommended by the manufacturer may cause inaccurate results.

E. The most accurate and reliable results are obtained when the reflectance meter is calibrated according to the schedule recommended by the manufacturer.
F. Instruments used for monitoring of hypoglycemia in newborns must have the calibration adjusted for this purpose.
G. For glucose levels >400 mL/dL, accuracy of Chemstrip bG and the Accu-Chek reflectance meter has been shown to improve when a 1-mL specimen of heparinized blood is diluted with 2 mL of 0.9% saline and the corresponding result is multiplied by 3 to correct for dilution.
H. Vigorous milking of the heel or finger may cause falsely low results because of dilution of the specimen with interstitial fluid.
I. Many conditions and drugs affect glucose levels. (See *Glucose, Blood.*)
7. **Other data:**
   A. In normal clients, blood glucose levels return to fasting levels within 2 hours postprandially.
   B. Glucose monitoring machine: competency of the operator may be evaluated by assessment of results of control solutions.
   C. Incidence of significant error ranges from 6% to 76%.

GLUCOSE TOLERANCE TEST (GTT), BLOOD

Norm (serum levels):

INTRAVENOUS GTT		SI UNITS
Fasting	70-105 mg/dL	3.9-5.8 mmol/L
5 minutes	300-400 mg/dL	16.5-22.0 mmol/L
30 minutes	180-200 mg/dL	9.9-11.0 mmol/L
1 hour	160-180 mg/dL	8.8-9.9 mmol/L
2 hours	≤140 mg/dL	≤7.7 mmol/L
≥3 hours	70-105 mg/dL	3.9-5.8 mmol/L

ORAL GTT		
Fasting	70-105 mg/dL	3.9-5.8 mmol/L
30 minutes	150-160 mg/dL	8.3-8.8 mmol/L
1 hour	160-170 mg/dL	8.8-9.4 mmol/L
1.5 hours	145-155 mg/dL	8.0-8.5 mmol/L
2 hours	≤120 mg/dL	≤6.6 mmol/L
3 hours	70-105 mg/dL	3.9-5.8 mmol/L

Usage. Evaluation of clients with symptoms of diabetic complications but with fasting glucose levels <140 mg/dL and screening during pregnancy for gestational diabetes (a single 1-hour cut-off of 8.9 mmol/L or 160 mg/dL).

Increased Results (Decreased Glucose Tolerance). Acromegaly, aldosteronism (primary), central nervous system lesions, Cushing syndrome, cystic fibrosis, diabetes mellitus, Forbes' disease (type-III glycogen deposition disease, debrancher deficiency, limit dextrinosis), gigantism, hemochromatosis, hepatic damage (severe), hyperlipidemia (types III, IV, V), hyperthyroidism, Louis-Bar syndrome, myocardial infarction, neoplasm, pancreatic tumor (islet cell), pancreatitis (chronic), pheochromocytoma, pregnancy, uremia, and von Gierke's disease (type-I glycogen storage disease, glucose-6-phosphatase deficiency). Drugs include anabolic steroids, androgens, arginine, ascorbic acid, asparaginase, aspirin, baclofen, benzodiazepines, bisacodyl (prolonged use), chlorpromazine, chlorthalidone, cimetidine, clonidine, corticosteroids, corticotropin, dextran, dextrothyroxine, diazoxide, disopyramide phosphate, epinephrine, epinephrine bitartrate, epinephrine borate, epinephrine hydrochloride, estrogens, ethacrynic acid, furosemide, glucose infusions, haloperidol, imipramine, isoproterenol hydrochloride, heparin calcium, heparin sodium, hydralazine hydrochloride, indomethacin, isoniazid, levodopa, levothyroxine sodium, lithium carbonate, magnesium hydroxide (prolonged high doses), mercaptopurine, methimazole, methyldopa, methyldopate hydrochloride), nalidixic acid, nicotine, nicotinic acid, oral contraceptives, oxazepam, *para*-aminosalicylic acid, phenolphthalein, phenytoin, phenytoin sodium, progestins, promethazine hydrochloride, propranolol (in diabetics), propylthiouracil, reserpine, ritodrine hydrochloride, terbutaline sulfate, tetracyclines, thiazides, thyroglobulin, thyroid, tolbutamide (SMA methodology), and triamterene.

Decreased Results (Increased Glucose Tolerance). Addison's disease (oral GTT only), celiac disease (oral GTT only), hepatic disease, hypoglycemia, hypoparathyroidism (oral GTT only), hypothyroidism (oral GTT only), islet cell adenoma, malabsorption (oral GTT only), narcotic addiction, pancreatic islet cell hyperplasia, and sprue (oral GTT only). Drugs include allopurinol, amphetamines, beta-adrenergic blockers, caffeine, chlorpropamide, clofibrate, edetate disodium, ethyl alcohol (ethanol), guanethidine sulfate, isoniazid, insulin, isocarboxazid, marijuana, nitrazepam, oral hypoglycemic agents, *para*-aminosalicyclic acid, pargyline hydrochloride, phenacetin, phenazopyridine, phenelzine sulfate, phenformin, propranolol (in diabetics), and tranylcypromine sulfate.

Description. Glucose is a monosaccharide formed from the digestion of carbohydrates and the conversion of glycogen by the liver and is the body's main source of cellular energy. The glucose tolerance test is most commonly used to aid in the diagnosis of diabetes mellitus. If blood glucose levels peak at higher than normal levels at 1 and 2 hours (after injection or ingestion of glucose) and are slower than normal to return to fasting levels, diabetes mellitus is confirmed.

Professional Considerations
1. Consent form NOT required.
2. **Preparation:**
   A. See *Client and family teaching.*
   B. Tubes: Gray topped × 6-7.
   C. Label each tube as shown in the table on p. 611.
3. **Procedure:**
   A. Begin the test between 7 and 9 AM.
   B. Draw a 1-mL venous blood sample.
   C. *Intravenous GTT:* Inject a standardized intravenous solution of 0.5 g/kg of body weight of 50% glucose, or 50 mL of 50% glucose intravenously over 4 minutes.
   D. *Oral GTT:* Adults should completely ingest a solution containing 75-100 g of glucose within 5 minutes.

TUBE NO	INTRAVENOUS GTT	ORAL GTT
1	Fasting	Fasting
2	5 minutes	30 minutes
3	30 minutes	1 hour
4	1 hour	1.5 hours
5	2 hours	2 hours
6	3 hours	3 hours
7	4 hours	4 hours

For children, the dosages are as follows:

<18 months:	2.5 g/kg
18 months-3 years:	2.0 g/kg
3 years-12 years:	1.75 g/kg
>12 years:	1.25 g/kg (100-g limit)

   E. Repeat step 3B at the following precise time intervals after infusion or ingestion of glucose is started.

   F. If evaluating for postprandial hypoglycemia, draw an additional sample at 4 hours.

4. **Postprocedure care:**

   A. Current administration of medications known to affect the test results should be noted on the laboratory requisition.

   B. Send blood samples to the laboratory immediately or refrigerate them.

5. **Client and family teaching:**

   A. Eat a high-carbohydrate (200-300 g) diet for 3 days before testing.

   B. Avoid alcohol, coffee, and smoking for 36 hours before testing.

   C. Fast (except for water) for 10-16 hours.

   D. When possible, drugs affecting results should be stopped 3-21 days before the test.

   E. Insulin and oral hypoglycemic agents should be withheld the morning of the test.

   F. Avoid strenuous exercise for 8 hours before and after the test.

   G. Because the test requires multiple blood samples, suggest bringing a book or other quiet diversion to the test because it usually requires a minimum of 3 hours.

   H. Alert the client to the symptoms of hypoglycemia and tell him or her to report these symptoms immediately.

6. **Factors that affect results:**

   A. No eating, smoking, or exercise is permitted during the testing period. Caffeine interferes with the accuracy of the results.

   B. Water may be given to help ease the collection of urine specimens.

   C. Failure to adhere to a high-carbohydrate diet for 3 days before the test may produce abnormally increased results.

   D. Stresses caused by acute illness, pregnancy, or surgery invalidate the results.

   E. Slight increases are normal in clients over 50 years of age (up to 1 mg/dL per year of age over 50).

   F. When the glucose oxidase/peroxidase procedure is used, falsely decreased glucose values may occur when the client has recently taken acetaminophen or oxycodone.

7. **Other data:**

   A. This test usually takes 3-5 hours.

   B. 10 mL of urine for glucose measurement may also be collected at the same time as the blood samples.

   C. The intravenous glucose tolerance testing method is recommended for clients who may have impaired or erratic intestinal absorption of glucose.

   D. The oral glucose tolerance test has been shown to be unreliable for use in the evaluation of reactive hypoglycemia.

   E. In a client with non–insulin-dependent diabetes (type 1), fasting serum glucose levels may be within normal range, but insufficient secretion of insulin after ingestion of carbohydrates causes serum glucose to increase

G

sharply and return to normal slowly.

F. If a client develops severe hypoglycemia during the test, draw a blood sample, record the time on the laboratory requisition, and discontinue the test. Have the client ingest an oral form of glu-cose or administer intravenous glucose according to the physician's orders.

G. 2-hour glucose level is better than fasting level alone in identifying older adults at increased risk of major incident cardiovascular events (Smith et al, 2002).

GLUCOSE-6-PHOSPHATE DEHYDROGENASE (G6PD, G-6-PD), QUANTITATIVE, BLOOD

Norm. Norms vary according to the test method used:
140-280 U/billion cells
125-280 U/dL packed red blood cells
8.6-18.6 U/g hemoglobin
4.5-10.8 U/g hemoglobin

ZINKHAM METHOD (30° C)		SI UNITS
Newborn	7.8-14.4 U/g Hb	0.50-0.93 U/mol Hb
	226-418 U/10^{12} Ercs	0.23-0.42 U/L Ercs
	2.65-4.90 U/mL Ercs	2.65-4.90 kU/L Ercs
Adult	5.5-9.3 U/g Hb	0.35-0.60 U/mol Hb
	160-270 U/10^{12} Ercs	0.16-0.27 U/L Ercs
	1.87-3.16 U/mL Ercs	1.87-3.16 kU/L Ercs

"Ercs" means 'electronic counters'.

Increased. Anemia (pernicious, megaloblastic), hepatic coma, hyperthyroidism, leptospirosis, myocardial infarction, and Werlhof's disease (idiopathic thrombocytopenic purpura).

Decreased. Anemia (congenital nonspherocytic hemolytic), favism, congenital G6PD deficiency, and nonimmunologic hemolytic disease of the newborn. Drugs include cefoperazone/sulbactam, gentamicin sulfate, netilmicin sulfate and tocopherol acetate. Herbicide 4-chlorophenoxy-acetic acid (4-CPA).

Description. Glucose-6-phosphate dehydrogenase (G6PD) is an enzyme normally present in the erythrocytes. This enzyme is part of the pentose phosphate pathway that metabolizes glucose and functions to protect cells from damage by oxidizing agents. This test measures G6PD levels in red blood cells, thereby detecting deficiencies of this enzyme. G6PD deficiency is a sex-linked genetic disorder found mostly in males that results in hemolysis of erythrocytes, producing anemia after the receipt of certain drugs. Drugs that may precipitate hemolytic episodes in affected individuals include acetanilid, acetylphenylhydrazine, antipyrine, ascorbic acid, aspirin, chloramphenicol, nalidixic acid, naphthalene, nitrofurantoin, nitrofuran, pentaquine, phenacetin, phenylhydrazine, primaquine, probenecid, quinacrine, quinidine, quinine, sulfonamides, and vitamin K. Other precipitants include diabetic acidosis, fava bean ingestion, infections (viral, bacterial), and septicemia.

Professional Considerations
1. Consent form NOT required.

2. **Preparation:**
   A. Tube: Lavender topped, blue topped, or green topped.
3. **Procedure:**
   A. Draw a 3-mL blood sample.
   B. Invert the tube gently several times to mix the sample.
   C. Handle the sample gently to prevent hemolysis.
4. **Postprocedure care:**
   A. Recent blood transfusion or current or recent ingestion of antimalarials, aspirin, fava beans, nitrofurantoin, phenacetin, sulfonamides, or vitamin K should be noted on the laboratory requisition.
5. **Client and family teaching:**
   A. Refer the client with elevated levels for long-term medical follow-up care.
   B. Clients testing positive should receive thorough disease teaching, including which drugs place the client at risk for a hemolytic episode.
   C. Refer clients testing positive for genetic counseling.
6. **Factors that affect results:**
   A. Reject hemolyzed specimens to avoid false-negative results.
   B. False-negative results may occur after a blood transfusion or a hemolytic episode.
7. **Other data:**
   A. Several methods are available to test for G6PD deficiency. The method used by the particular laboratory determines the type of blood tube used.
   B. G6PD deficiency is demonstrated most frequently in African Americans, Greeks, Sardinians, and Sephardic Jews.

GLUCOSE-6-PHOSPHATE DEHYDROGENASE (G6PD, G-6-PD) SCREEN, BLOOD

Norm. Enzyme activity detected.

Increased. Not applicable.

Decreased. Anemia (congenital nonspherocytic hemolytic), favism, congenital G6PD deficiency, and nonimmunologic hemolytic disease of the newborn.

Description. G6PD is an enzyme normally present in erythrocytes. This enzyme is part of the pentose phosphate pathway that metabolizes glucose and functions to protect cells from damage by oxidizing agents. This test measures G6PD levels in red blood cells, thereby detecting deficiencies of this enzyme. G6PD deficiency is a sex-linked genetic disorder found mostly in males that results in hemolysis of erythrocytes, producing anemia after the receipt of certain drugs. Drugs that may precipitate hemolytic episodes in affected individuals include acetanilid, acetylphenylhydrazine, antipyrine, ascorbic acid, aspirin, chloramphenicol, nalidixic acid, naphthalene, nitrofurantoin, nitrofuran, pentaquine, phenacetin, phenylhydrazine, primaquine, probenecid, quinacrine, quinidine, quinine, sulfonamides, and vitamin K. Other precipitants include diabetic acidosis, fava bean ingestion, infections (viral, bacterial), and septicemia.

Professional Considerations
1. Consent form NOT required.
2. **Preparation:**
   A. Tube: Lavender topped.
3. **Procedure:**
   A. Draw a 2-mL blood sample.
   B. Invert the tube gently several times to mix the sample.
   C. Handle the sample gently to prevent hemolysis.
4. **Postprocedure care:**
   A. Recent blood transfusion or current or recent ingestion of antimalarials, aspirin, fava beans, nitrofurantoin, phenacetin, sulfonamides, or vitamin K should be noted on the laboratory requisition.
5. **Client and family teaching:**
   A. Results are normally available within 24 hours.
   B. Clients testing positive should receive thorough disease teaching, including which drugs place the client at risk for a hemolytic episode.

G

C. Refer clients testing positive for genetic counseling.

6. Factors that affect results:
   A. Reject hemolyzed specimens to avoid false-negative results.
   B. False-negative results may occur after a blood transfusion or a hemolytic episode.

7. Other data:
   A. G6PD deficiency is demonstrated most frequently in African Americans, Greeks, Sardinians, and Sephardic Jews.

GLUTETHIMIDE, BLOOD

Norm:

		SI UNITS
Therapeutic	2-6 µg/mL	9-28 µmol/L
Toxic level	>20 µg/mL	>92 µmol/L
Panic level	>30 µg/mL	>135 µmol/L

Overdose Symptoms and Treatments

Symptoms. Central nervous system depression, cerebral edema, hypotension, paralysis, respiratory depression, spasticity, and tachycardia. Death may occur at doses over 30 µg/mL.

Treatment:
Note: Treatment choice(s) depends on client history and condition and episode history.
Gastric lavage of water and caster oil in a 1:1 mix because glutethimide is soluble in lipids.
Hemodialysis will NOT but hemoperfusion WILL remove glutethimide.

Usage. Glutethimide abuse and glutethimide overdose.

Description. Glutethimide is a schedule-III, piperidine-derivative, nonbarbiturate sedative-hypnotic with actions similar to barbiturates used for temporary insomnia, preoperative sedation, and during stage 1 of labor. It is primarily stored in fat tissue, hydroxylized in the liver, and excreted primarily by the kidneys, with a biphasic half-life of 5-22 hours.

Professional Considerations
1. Consent form NOT required.

2. Preparation:
   A. Tube: Red topped, red/gray topped, or gold topped, black topped, or lavender topped.
   B. MAY be drawn during hemodialysis.

3. Procedure:
   A. Draw a 7-mL blood sample.

4. Postprocedure care:
   A. Observe closely for symptoms of overdose. This includes continuous ECG and airway monitoring, frequent neurologic checks, and vital sign measurement every 15-60 minutes.

5. Client and family teaching:
   A. Be alert for symptoms of overdose (see 4-A, above) and seek medical attention if they occur.
   B. Refer clients with intentional overdose for crisis intervention.
   C. Referrals to appropriate rehabilitation centers and therapeutic community programs should be offered to all addicted clients who may be interested.

6. Factors that affect results:
   A. Serial measurements for glutethimide are recommended because of the variable release of the drug from adipose tissue.

7. Other data:
   A. Mortality rate is highest in glutethimide intoxication in suicidal poisonings.

GLYCOSYLATED HEMOGLOBIN (GHB, GLYCOHEMOGLOBIN, Hb A$_{1A}$, Hb A$_{1B}$, Hb A$_{1C}$), BLOOD

Norm:

	PERCENTAGE OF TOTAL Hb
Total of Hb A$_{1a}$, Hb A$_{1b}$, and Hb A$_{1c}$	5.5-8.8
Diabetes under control	7.5-11.4
Diabetes less well controlled	11.5-15
Diabetes out of control	>15
Ketoacidosis	14.3-20
High-performance liquid chromatography	
Hb A$_{1a}$	1.8
Hb A$_{1b}$	0.8
Hb A$_{1c}$	3.5–6.0

Increase. Diabetes mellitus, glycosouria, hyperglycemia, and polycystic ovary syndrome.

Decrease. See 6-C, below, *Factors that affect results*.

Description. Glycoslated hemoglobin is blood glucose bound to hemoglobin (Hb) and includes forms Hb A$_{1a}$, Hb A$_{1b}$, and Hb A$_{1c}$. Hb A$_{1c}$ is formed as hemoglobin, is gradually glycosylated throughout the 120-day red blood cell life span, and forms the largest portion of the three glycosylated Hb fractions. The amount of glycosylated hemoglobin found and stored in erythrocytes depends on the amount of glucose available. Hb A$_{1c}$ is a reflection of how well blood glucose levels have been controlled for up to the previous 4 months. Hyperglycemia in diabetics is usually a cause of an increase in Hb A$_{1c}$.

Professional Considerations:
1. Consent form NOT required.
2. **Preparation:**
   A. Tube: Lavender topped, green topped, or gray topped.
3. **Procedure:**
   A. Draw a 5-mL blood sample.
   B. Invert the tube gently several times to mix the sample.
4. **Postprocedure care:**
   A. Send the specimen to the laboratory for prompt spinning.

5. **Client and family teaching:**
   A. The test evaluates the effectiveness of diabetes therapy over a period of several months, and so more samples will be needed in the future.
   B. The client should maintain his or her prescribed medication or diet regimen between physician visits.
6. **Factors that affect results:**
   A. Reject hemolyzed specimens.
   B. Falsely increased values may be attributable to fetal-maternal transfusion, hemodialysis, hereditary persistence of fetal hemoglobin, neonates, and pregnancy.
   C. Falsely decreased values may be attributed to anemia (hemolytic, pernicious, sickle cell); chronic loss of blood; effects of splenectomy; renal failure (chronic); and thalassemias or drug use of monoclonal antibodies.
7. **Other data:**
   A. Glycoslated hemoglobin cannot be used to monitor control of diabetic clients with chronic renal failure because levels are significantly lower due to shortened erythrocyte survival.

GONORRHOEAE CULTURE

(see Genitals, Neisseria gonorrhoeae, Culture)

GRAM STAIN, DIAGNOSTIC
Norm:

Body fluid, drainage, or wound   Interpretation required
Urine   No organisms detected

Usage

Diagnostic. Anthrax meningitis (CSF), cough (sputum sample), effusion (abdominal or pleural), empyema, gonorrhea, impetigo, *Legionella*, tuberculosis, and wounds.

Sputum. Cough (productive), fever, infections, and pneumonia.

Urine. Cystitis and urethritis.

Description. Gram-staining divides bacteria into two groups according to their staining properties: gram negative and gram positive. The staining involves placing drops of crystal violet dye onto the specimen sample, washing off the violet stain, and flooding the smear with an iodine solution followed by a 95% ethyl alcohol (ethanol) solution. Gram-positive cells remain blue, and gram-negative cells are decolorized by the alcohol. The specimen is then stained with a red dye called "safranin O," which colors the gram-positive cells red and leaves the gram-negative cells appearing purple. The cell wall structure is the basis of the Gram reaction. Gram staining of specimens aids in decision making for early, broad-spectrum antibiotic therapy. Gram stain is 67.9% sensitive for detection of bacteria in blood cultures.

Professional Considerations
1. Consent form NOT required.
2. Preparation:
   A. *Diagnostic:* Obtain a sterile container or swab.
   B. *Sputum:* Obtain a sterile sputum container or suction tubing, suction source, and sputum trap.
   C. *Urine:* Obtain a sterile container and clean-catch urine specimen collection kit, or a straight catheter or a syringe and needle if the specimen will be collected from an indwelling catheter.
   D. See *Client and family teaching.*

3. Procedure:
   A. *Diagnostic:*
      i. Obtain the specimen using a sterile technique and a sterile container or swab.
      ii. Avoid contamination of the sample with surrounding tissue.
   B. *Sputum:*
      i. Collect an early-morning sputum sample into a sterile sputum container.
      ii. Specimens are of best quality when obtained by being suctioned directly into a sputum trap.
      iii. For expelled specimens, have the client sit up, take two or three deep breaths without fully exhaling each, and then cough expulsively to mobilize the sputum from the respiratory tract directly into the sterile specimen container.
   C. The clean-catch urine technique must be used to decrease the risk of specimen contamination. See clean-catch collection instructions in the test *Body fluid, Routine, Culture.*
4. Postprocedure care:
   A. Write the specimen source, the diagnosis, and recent antibiotic therapy on the laboratory requisition.
   B. Place the specimen in the refrigerator if not delivered to microbiology area immediately after collection.
5. Client and family teaching:
   A. *Sputum:* Cough the specimen directly into the container and avoid holding the sputum in the mouth. Deep coughs are necessary to produce sputum, rather than saliva. To produce the proper specimen, take several breaths in, without fully exhaling each, and then expel sputum with a "cascade cough."

B. *Urine:* See clean-catch collection instructions in the test *Body fluid, Routine, Culture.*
6. **Factors that affect results:**
   A. Epithelial cells will appear in the specimen if it is contaminated with mucosal surfaces.
   B. Saliva contamination of sputum specimens invalidates the results.
7. **Other data:**
   A. Gram-staining is not useful for identifying species of bacteria but can be suggestive of certain broad species.
   B. A culture and sensitivity study of the specimen should also be performed to confirm the diagnosis and proper choice of antibiotic.
   C. Compared to Gram stain of vaginal secretions, the cervical Papanicolaou smear has fair sensitivity (55%) and excellent positive predictive value (96%) in the diagnosis of bacterial vaginosis.

GRANULOCYTE, BLOOD
(*see Differential leukocyte count, Peripheral blood*)

GROWTH HORMONE (SOMATOTROPIN, GH), BLOOD

Norm:

		SI UNITS
Adults, Female	<10 ng/mL	<440 pmol/L
>60 years	1-14 ng/mL	44-616 pmol/L
Adults, Male	≤5 ng/mL	≤220 pmol/L
>60 years	0.4-10 ng/mL	18-440 pmol/L
Children		
Cord blood	10-50 ng/mL	440-2200 pmol/L
Newborn	15-40 ng/mL	660-1760 pmol/L
Child	<20 ng/mL	<880 pmol/L

Increased. Acromegaly, anorexia nervosa, deep sleep states, infants, gigantism, hypoglycemia, hyperpituitarism, starvation, and surgery. Drugs include arginine, beta-adrenergic blockers, estrogens, gamma-hydroxybutyrate (GHB) (which can increase levels up to 40 ng/mL), gamma-butyryl lactone (GBL), glucagon, levodopa, and oral contraceptives. Herbs or natural remedies include St. John's wort (*Hypericum perforatum, calycinum,* and *persortum*), which contains hypericin.

Decreased. Congenital growth hormone deficiency, congenital pituitary hypoplasia, dwarfism, failure to thrive, growth hormone deficiency, hyperglycemia, hypothalamic degeneration, hypopituitarism, lesion (pituitary or hypothalamus), and pituitary fibrosis or calcification. Drugs include corticosteroids, phenothiazines, and selective serotonin reuptake inhibitors (SSRI).

Description. Growth hormone (GH) is a polypeptide anterior pituitary hormone essential for bodily growth. GH synthesis and release is controlled by the hypothalamus through growth hormone–releasing factor (GHRF) and growth hormone release–inhibiting hormone (GHRIH). GH stimulates the production of RNA and protein synthesis and mobilizes fatty acids and insulin. It is influenced by several drugs as well as exercise and stress.

Professional Considerations
1. Consent form NOT required.
2. **Preparation:**
   A. See *Client and family teaching.*
   B. Tube: Red topped, red/gray topped, or gold topped.
   C. Have the client recline for 30 minutes before sampling.
   D. Screen client for the use of herbal preparations or natural remedies such as St. John's wort.

3. **Procedure:**
   A. Draw a 1-mL blood sample.
4. **Postprocedure care:**
   A. Write the collection time and client's recent activity (sleeping, eating, resting, walking) on the laboratory requisition.
   B. Current administration of corticosteroids or phenothiazines should be noted on the laboratory requisition.
   C. Transport the specimen to the laboratory immediately. The serum should be separated into a plastic container and frozen until testing.
5. **Client and family teaching:**
   A. Fast and limit physical activity for 10-12 hours before the test.
   B. A second blood sample may have to be drawn the next day for comparison to the first sample.
6. **Factors that affect results:**
   A. Reject specimens if the client had a radioactive scan within the previous 48 hours.
   B. Growth hormone in serum samples is unstable at room temperature.
7. **Other data:**
   A. Serial measurements are recommended because of the episodic release of growth hormone.
   B. This test may be performed as part of a GH-stimulation test, using arginine, glucose, glucagon, levodopa, insulin-induced hypoglycemia, or other methods.

GUTHRIE TEST FOR PHENYLKETONURIA, DIAGNOSTIC

Norm. Negative or <3 mg/dL.

Usage. Neonatal screening for phenylketonuria (PKU).

Description. The Guthrie test is a bacterial inhibition assay in which elevated levels of phenylalanine cause growth of the bacterium *Bacillus subtilis* around the blood sample. If growth occurs around the bacterium, the diagnosis of PKU is suggested; further blood testing is needed to confirm the diagnosis.

Phenylketonuria is an autosomal recessive inherited disorder with a frequency of one in 10,000 live births. This condition is caused by a deficiency of the enzyme phenylalanine hydroxylase, which leads to an accumulation of phenylalanine in the blood and deficiency of tyrosine in the blood. Resultant symptoms include neurologic conditions such as mental retardation, microcephaly, seizures, and hyperactivity, as well as eczema, growth retardation, and a musty odor. If treatment with a restricted phenylalanine diet is begun early, these symptoms can be minimized and even prevented.

PKU testing is performed in the newborn period on a metabolic screening filter paper. Although states vary in the panel of conditions they test, all states test for PKU.

Professional Considerations

1. Consent form NOT required.
2. **Preparation:**
   A. Obtain supplies: 2.0-2.5 lancet, alcohol wipe, gauze pads, gloves, and blood collection form (filter paper) with completed information.
3. **Procedure:**
   A. Warm heel for 3-5 minutes with warm, wet cloth or heel warmer with foot lowered below the heart to increase blood flow.
   B. Clean heel with alcohol wipe and dry with sterile gauze.
   C. Puncture the lateral third of the plantar surface of the heel. Wipe first drop of blood away with gauze pad and, when another large drop of blood collects, lightly touch the filter paper, making sure to fill the designated circle completely. Fill in all circles on the filter paper in the same manner.
4. **Postprocedure care:**
   A. Place pressure on the heel for 5-10 minutes, and then cover with sterile gauze or a bandage.
   B. Allow the form to dry on a flat surface for a minimum of 4 hours and mail to the laboratory within 24 hours.
5. **Client and family teaching:**
   A. Inform parents that the sample is sent to the state laboratory and that they will be informed of an abnormal result within 2 weeks.
   B. When positive results are found, call the family immediately,

repeat the test, and institute a low-phenylalanine diet with consultations to a nutritionist and geneticist.
6. **Factors that affect results:**
   A. Method of sample collection: Samples must be carefully collected. The heel should not be squeezed excessively, blood spots on the filter paper should not be touched, the sample should be air-dried, and the sample should not be applied with a capillary tube.
   B. Factors that produce false-negative results:
      i. *Protein intake:* Child must have had 24 hours of protein feedings (either breast milk or formula) in order for the test to be valid.
      ii. *Antibiotic use:* Test should be repeated if child had been taking antibiotics when the sample was collected.
   C. Factors that produce false-positive results: goat milk intake, total parenteral nutrition, severe illness, layering of blood on test paper.
7. **Other data:**
   A. Test should be performed, if possible, before a transfusion.
   B. Each circle on the filter paper needs to be completely filled.
   C. If the baby is <48 hours old at the time of collection, a repeat sample should be obtained within the first week of life.

GYNECOLOGIC ULTRASONOGRAPHY (GYNECOLOGIC ECHOGRAM, GYNECOLOGIC SONOGRAM, PELVIC SONOGRAM, PELVIC ULTRASOUND), DIAGNOSTIC

Norm. Normal size, shape, and position of pelvic structures (uterus, ovaries, fallopian tubes); negative for cyst, foreign body, stones, or tumor.

Usage. Evaluation of the size, shape, and position of bladder, ovaries, vagina, and uterus; detection of pelvic cyst, ectopic pregnancy, endometrial abnormalities, foreign body (such as intrauterine device), hydatidiform mole, stones, or masses; differentiation of solid from liquid masses; infertility work-up (monitoring the ovarian follicle or screening for uterine cavity abnormalities); monitoring of pelvic tumor response to therapy; and transvaginal sonography have an added advantage of providing information regarding the cervical and uterine vascular supplies.

Description. Gynecologic ultrasonography (ultrasound) is the evaluation of the pelvic structures by the creation of an oscilloscopic picture from the echoes of high-frequency sound waves passing over the pelvic area (acoustic imaging). The time required for the ultrasonic beam to be reflected back to the transducer from differing densities of tissue is converted by a computer to an electrical impulse displayed on an oscilloscopic screen to create a three-dimensional picture of the pelvic contents. Both transabdominal and transvaginal methods may be used. Traditional transabdominal methods are more helpful for the evaluation of large cysts and fibroids, whereas the newer, transvaginal method is more specific for ruling out ectopic pregnancy or evaluating endometrial abnormalities. Transvaginal methods have also been shown to provide better depictions of the fine structures and individual organs of the pelvic cavity and are better tolerated by the subject because a full bladder is not required. Gynecologic ultrasonography may be used as an adjunct to the pelvic bimanual examination in women who are at risk for ovarian cancer.

Professional Considerations
1. Consent form NOT required.
2. Preparation:
   A. This test should be performed before intestinal barium tests or after the barium is cleared from the system.
   B. The client should disrobe below the waist or wear a gown.
   C. Obtain ultrasonic gel.
   D. See *Client and family teaching.*
3. Procedure:
   A. *Transabdominal method:*
      i. The client is positioned supine in bed or on a procedure table.
      ii. The pelvic area is covered with ultrasonic gel, and a

lubricated transducer is passed slowly and firmly over the lower abdomen at a variety of angles and at 1- to 2-cm intervals.

iii. The client may be repositioned to a right or slight left decubitus position so that better pictures of the ovaries or the adnexal area may be obtained.

iv. A water enema may be administered if more specific evaluation of the adnexal area is required.

v. Photographs are taken of the oscilloscopic pictures.

vi. The procedure takes less than 30 minutes.

B. *Transvaginal method:*

i. The client is positioned in the dorsal lithotomy position or on a conventional examination table, with a pillow supporting the hips.

ii. A sterile, nonreservoir condom containing ultrasonic gel is placed over the transducer, and air bubbles are worked out of it. The condom is then coated with a sterile lubricant.

iii. The client or the examiner may insert the transducer into the vagina until it touches the posterior or anterior walls.

iv. The transducer is rotated 90 degrees against the vaginal vault to obtain sagittal and coronal scans of the uterus. The probe is pulled back 2-3 cm to examine the cervix. Using identified landmarks, the ovaries and fallopian tubes are pictured. All possible angles are scanned. The client may be repositioned slightly to facilitate imaging.

4. **Postprocedure care:**

A. Remove the lubricant from the skin.

B. Allow the client to void.

C. Disinfect the transducer probe by soaking in glutaraldehyde solution for 10 minutes.

5. **Client and family teaching:**

A. The procedure is painless and carries no risks.

B. If transabdominal ultrasonography is to be performed, drink 1 quart of water during the hour before the test, and refrain from voiding during this time. The full bladder provides an acoustic window for imaging.

C. If transvaginal ultrasonography is to be performed, fast from fluids for 4 hours before the procedure, and void just before the procedure.

6. **Factors that affect results:**

A. Dehydration interferes with adequate contrast between organs and body fluids.

B. Intestinal barium or gas obscures results by preventing proper transmission and deflection of the high-frequency sound waves. This problem is particularly pronounced with pelvic ultrasonography as the result of the proximity of the large bowel.

C. The more abdominal fat present, the greater is the attenuation (reduction in sound-wave amplitude and intensity), which interferes with the clarity of the transabdominal picture.

D. Transvaginal techniques are not adequate for very large masses.

7. **Other data:**

A. Further studies may include tomography or other radiographic imaging.

HAGEMAN FACTOR, BLOOD
(see Factor XII, Blood)

HALOPERIDOL, SERUM

Norm. Negative.

Therapeutic level	3-20 µg/L
Panic level	>25 µg/L

Panic Level Symptoms and Treatment

Symptoms. Hypotension, sedation with respiratory depression severe enough to cause a shocklike state, severe extrapyramidal neuromuscular reactions (dystonia, hyperreflexia, and oculogyric crises), and rhabdomyolysis with hypertonia as part of neuroleptic malignant syndrome (NMS).

Treatment:

Note: Treatment choice(s) depend on client history and condition and episode history.

Ipecac may be used to induce vomiting, with due regard for haloperidol's antiemetic properties and aspiration hazards. Induction of vomiting is contraindicated in clients with no gag reflex or with central nervous system depression or excitation. Gastric lavage may also be used, followed by activated charcoal and saline cathartics. Intravenous diphenhydramine (Benadryl) can be used to treat extrapyramidal symptoms.

Hemodialysis and peritoneal dialysis will NOT remove haloperidol.

Usage. Periodic monitoring for therapeutic levels in clients receiving haloperidol. Screening for haloperidol toxicity or overdose.

Description. Haloperidol is a butyrophenone that acts as an antipsychotic, sedative, and antiemetic. It depresses the central nervous system, directly acts on the chemoreceptor trigger zone (CTZ), and inhibits catecholamines. This drug is used in agitation, schizophrenia, and the manic phase of manic-depressive psychosis and to manage vocal utterances in Gilles de la Tourette syndrome. It is absorbed in the gastrointestinal tract, concentrates in the liver, and is excreted in the urine and in bile. Has been known to induce torsades de pointes.

Professional Considerations:
1. Consent form NOT required.
2. **Preparation:**
   A. Tube: Red topped, red/gray topped, or gold topped.
   B. May require assistance if the client is uncooperative.
   C. MAY be drawn during hemodialysis.
3. **Procedure:**
   A. Obtain a 3-mL blood sample.
4. **Postprocedure care:**
   A. Refrigerate the specimen.
5. **Client and family teaching:**
   A. For periodic monitoring, it is not necessary to restrict food or fluids.

B. If activated charcoal was given for elevated levels, the client should drink 4-6 glasses of water each day for 2 days to prevent constipation. The activated charcoal will also cause stools to be black for a few days.
C. Refer clients with intentional overdose for crisis intervention.
D. Referrals to appropriate rehabilitation centers and therapeutic community programs should be offered to all clients who may be interested.
6. **Factors that affect results:**
   A. Therapeutic norms are not well established; laboratory values vary among clients on equal doses.
   B. Significant lowering of serum haloperidol occurs with the coadministration of carbamazepine and/or barbiturates.
   C. Drugs which may cause increased levels include Fluoxetine.
7. **Other data:**
   A. For consistency, collect the specimen at least 12 hours after the last dose (trough level).
   B. Extrapyramidal effects occur frequently during the first few days and are dose related though they can occur even with small doses.
   C. Diphenhydramine may interfere with some methods used to measure haloperidol.

HAM TEST (ACIDIFIED SERUM TEST), BLOOD

Norm. Negative, <5% lysis.

Usage. Paroxysmal nocturnal hemoglobinuria (PNH) or the PNH abnormality.

Description. For the Ham test, a blood sample is taken from the client, mixed with his or her own serum and with a sample of serum from an ABO-compatible donor, acidified, and examined for lysis. The presence of lysis in the client's own serum is definitive in the diagnosis of PNH. This rare condition, in which hemoglobin is found in the urine during and after sleep, is believed to be related to red blood cell hypersensitivity to higher levels of carbon dioxide and a resulting decrease in the plasma pH, though the cause of this disease is unknown.

Professional Considerations:
1. Consent form NOT required.
2. **Preparation:**
   A. Tube: Lavender topped.
3. **Procedure:**
   A. Draw a 7-mL blood sample.
4. **Postprocedure care:**
   A. Defibrinate the sample immediately.
5. **Client and family teaching:**
   A. Results are normally available within 24 hours.
6. **Factors that affect results:**
   A. Hemolysis of the specimen invalidates results.

B. Transfusion of red blood cells within the last 3 weeks may cause false-negative results.
C. False-positive results may occur in dyserythropoietic anemia, spherocytosis, aplastic anemia, and leukemia.
7. **Other data:**
   A. PNH has been a candidate for myeloproliferative disease occurring in 55-65% of cases of myeloid metaplasia and primary myelofibrosis.

HAPTOGLOBIN (Hp), SERUM

Norm:

		SI UNITS
Adult	40-240 mg/dL	0.4-2.40 g/L
Newborn	5-48 mg/dL	0.05-4.8 g/L

Usage. Serves as an index of hemolysis, investigates hemolytic transfusion reactions, identifies suspected ahaptoglobinemia, and helps establish proof of paternity.

Increase. Abscess, burns, acute rheumatic disease, arterial disease, biliary obstruction, infection, inflammation, malignancies, myocardial infarction, peptic ulcer, pneumonia, pregnancy tissue necrosis, tuberculosis, and ulcerative colitis. Drugs include corticosteroids and oral contraceptives.

Decrease. Ahaptoglobinemia, artificial heart valve implantation, G6PD deficiency, hemolysis (intravascular or extravascular), hemolytic anemia, liver disease, malarial infestation, megaloblastic anemia, mononucleosis (infectious), sickle cell anemia, systemic lupus erythematosus (SLE), thalassemia, tissue hemorrhage, and transfusion reaction (hemolytic). Drugs include estrogens.

Description. Haptoglobin is an alpha$_2$ globulin that combines with hemoglobin that has been released as the result of red blood cell destruction. Its primary function is to preserve the body's iron stores from being excreted in the urine. Haptoglobin can be depleted rapidly by any condition that destroys red blood cells.

Professional Considerations:
1. Consent form NOT required.
2. **Preparation:**
   A. Tube: Red topped, red/gray topped, or gold topped.
3. **Procedure:**
   A. Draw a 1-mL blood sample.
4. **Postprocedure care:**
   A. Report abnormal vital signs on the laboratory requisition.
   B. Deliver the specimen to the laboratory immediately, taking care not to shake it.
5. **Client and family teaching:**
   A. Results may not be available for several days.
   B. Call the physician if noting symptoms of hemolysis, which include back pain, chills, distended neck veins, fever, flushing, hypotension, tachycardia, and tachypnea.
6. **Factors that affect results:**
   A. Hemolysis of the specimen invalidates results.
   B. Specimen contact with peroxidase or other oxidants may falsely elevate the result.
7. **Other data:**
   A. Do not consider this test alone for diagnosing.
   B. Haptoglobin levels rise to normal by 4 months of age.

C. In about 1% of the population (4% of blacks), haptoglobin is permanently absent (congenital ahaptoglobinemia).

HAWKEYE IMAGING, DIAGNOSTIC
(see Dual modality imaging, Diagnostic)

HB, BLOOD
(see Hemoglobin, Blood)

HBDH
(see Hydroxybutyrate dehydrogenase, Blood)

hCFH-rp
(see BTA test for bladder cancer, Diagnostic)

HCO₃, SERUM
(see Bicarbonate, Serum)

HCG
(see Human chorionic gonadotropin, Beta-subunit, Serum or Pregnancy Test, Serum and Urine)

HCT, BLOOD
(see Hematocrit, Blood)

HCY
(see Homocysteine, Plasma or Urine)

HCYSU
(see Homocysteine, Plasma or Urine)

HDL, HDL-C
(see High-density lipoprotein cholesterol, Blood)

HEAD-UP TILT TABLE TEST
(see Tilt table test, Diagnostic)

HEARING TEST FOR LOUDNESS—RECRUITMENT, DIAGNOSTIC
(see Audiometry test, Diagnostic)

HEART SCAN, DIAGNOSTIC

Norm

Technetium-99m stannous pyrophosphate (radiolabeled PYP). No evidence of myocardial ischemia.

Thallium 201. No evidence of myocardial ischemia or infarction.

Multigated blood pool study (MUGA). Normal (55-65%) ejection fraction, symmetric contraction of the left ventricle.

Nitroglycerin MUGA. Normal (55-65%) ejection fraction, symmetric contraction of the left ventricle.

Sestamibi or sestamibi-dipyridamole exercise testing and scan. No evidence of diminished perfusion, ischemia, or infarction.

Usage. Aneurysm, angina, cardiomegaly, coronary artery disease, myocardial infarction, and presurgical evaluation.

Dipyridamole injection. Replaces the treadmill portion of the test for clients with chronic lung disease, peripheral vascular disease, impaired mobility, medication therapy that prevents demonstration of maximal exercise effort (calcium-channel blockers, beta-adrenergic blockers), or post–myocardial infarction risk stratification.

Description. Heart scan encompasses any of several noninvasive scans that involve radiopharmaceutical injection.

The *PYP scan* is used to determine the occurrence, extent, and prognosis of myocardial infarction. Technetium-99m stannous pyrophosphate is believed to combine with the calcium in damaged myocardial cells, forming a spot on the scan. Such spots appear within 12 hours of infarction, are most prominent 48-72 hours after an infarction, and disappear within 1 week. A spot that does not disappear indicates continued myocardial damage.

The *thallium-201 scan* is used to show myocardial perfusion, location, and extent of acute or chronic myocardial infarction, coronary artery disease, or effectiveness of angioplasty, angina therapy, or grafted coronary arteries. An analog of potassium, this radionuclide is absorbed into healthy tissue while avoiding damaged tissue, forming spots on the scan. Ischemic areas (which eventually absorb isotope) can be differentiated from infracted areas (which never absorb isotope) by repeating of the scan within 5 minutes. May be performed under stress. Thallium scans are often combined with dipyridamole administration (described below) because this causes greater thallium uptake and improved quality of images and accuracy of diagnoses. The combination is used for clients who are unable to perform exercise treadmill or bicycle testing in conjunction with their scan.

The *MUGA scan* is used to assess the function of the left ventricle and show myocardial wall abnormalities. Once the isotope is injected, the heart appears as a map with all four chambers, and the great vessels are visualized simultaneously. A series of images are taken during systole (low isotope in left ventricle) and diastole (high isotope in left ventricle). These can be shown like a movie or superimposed to show the left ventricular function, and the ejection fraction can be calculated. May be performed under stress.

The *nitroglycerin scan* is an additional feature of the MUGA scan. Another series of images is taken to evaluate the effectiveness of sublingual nitroglycerin administration. May be performed under stress.

The *sestamibi exercise testing and scan* is used to evaluate cardiac perfusion before and after a treadmill exercise test. The injected radiopharmaceutical ^{99m}Tc-pertechnetate (sestamibi) is taken up by ischemic or infarcted cardiac cells that did not improve in perfusion with exercise and is seen as a "hot spot" in nuclear imaging.

The *sestamibi-dipyridamole stress test and scan* is used in clients who cannot walk on a treadmill or pedal a bicycle because of physical mobility limitations. Dipyridamole is an antiplatelet drug used in nuclear medicine for its coronary artery vasodilatory action. It causes increased endogenous adenosine levels, which causes an effect on the perfusion of the heart muscle similar to that of an exercise test. For this test, the cardiac perfusion is compared in scans taken before and after the tracer and dipyridamole injections. Because the areas that vasodilate can draw blood flow from less-perfused areas, the test can cause ischemia and infarction. Thus this test carries specific risks related

to the radiopharmaceutical administered and requires a cardiologist to be present in many institutions.

The *single-photon emission computed tomography (SPECT)* scan is a newer nuclear medicine procedure in which the radiopharmaceutical technetium-99m hexamethyl propylene amine oxime is injected intravenously. This substance decomposes and remains for several hours in the heart and other tissues, where it can be detected with the SPECT camera. The camera sends images to a computer that can reproduce visual images, or "slices," of the heart along several planes. An advantage of SPECT imaging over older nuclear medicine scans is that it can produce clear, more accurate images.

Professional Considerations
1. Consent form IS required.

Risks
Persantine (dipyridamole): chest pain (angina), ECG changes, ischemia, including infarction, bronchospasm, nausea, vomiting, hypotension, headache, dyspnea, facial flushing.
Radiopharmaceutical or radiolabeled albumin: allergic reaction (itching, hives, rash, tight feeling in the throat, shortness of breath, bronchospasm, anaphylaxis, death).
Treadmill testing: cardiac ischemia, including myocardial infarction, dysrhythmias, hypotension, hypertension, dizziness.

Contraindications
Clients who are unable to lie motionless for the scan; women who are breastfeeding; previous allergic reaction to radiopharmaceutical or radiolabeled albumin if use is planned.

Dipyridamole. Previous allergy to dipyridamole; unstable cardiac status; allergy to aminophylline (which is used as an antidote to adverse effects of dipyridamole); aminophylline or pentoxifylline taken within the last 48 hours; severe asthma or bronchospasm.

Relative contraindications, dipyridamole. Congestive heart failure, status post heart transplantation, bilateral carotid artery disease, days 1-3 after acute myocardial infarction.

Treadmill testing. Active unstable angina, recent significant changes in

ECG, alcohol intoxication, uncontrolled dysrhythmias, chest pain, acute infection, cardiac inflammation (myocarditis, pericarditis), acute congestive heart failure, coronary insufficiency syndrome, digitalis toxicity, heart blocks (2°, 3°), thrombophlebitis, recent pulmonary embolism, inability to walk on a treadmill or pedal a bicycle.

Precautions

During pregnancy, risks of cumulative radiation exposure to the fetus from imaging studies must be weighed against the benefits of the procedure. Although formal limits for client exposure are relative to this risk:benefit comparison, the United States Nuclear Regulatory Commission requires that the cumulative dose equivalent to an embryo/fetus from occupational exposure not exceed 0.5 rem (5 mSv). Radiation dosage to the fetus is proportional to the distance of the anatomy studied from the abdomen and decreases as pregnancy progresses. For pregnant clients, consult the radiologist/radiology department to obtain estimated fetal radiation exposure from any of these procedure.

2. **Preparation:**
   A. Assess for history of hypersensitivity to radioactive dyes.
   B. Have emergency equipment readily available. This includes aminophylline to counteract the side effects of dipyridamole if the dipyridamole test is to be performed.
   C. For scans conducted with stress testing, obtain a baseline 12-lead ECG.
   D. See *Client and family teaching.*
3. **Procedure:**
   A. *PYP:* Technetium-99m stannous pyrophosphate (20 mCi) is injected 2-3 hours before the test. Images are taken from different angles, with a total of 30-60 minutes being taken.
   B. *Thallium 201:* Resting imaging takes place within the first few hours of cardiac symptoms. The radionuclide is injected, and scanning begins within 5 minutes. For stress scanning, an intravenous line is started, and a blood pressure cuff and ECG leads are attached. After 15 minutes on a treadmill or bicycle, the

client is injected with radioactive thallium; 15 minutes later, imaging occurs for 1 hour, with a repeat scan performed within the next 24 hours. A thallium-201 dose is 1.5-3 mCi.
   C. *Thallium-dipyridamole:* ECG and blood pressure are monitored continuously throughout this scan. After the resting image is taken and the radionuclide is injected, dipyridamole is injected intravenously over 4 minutes. Some clients may be asked to perform mild exercise, which improves blood flow through the coronary arteries, increases uptake of the thallium, and reduces the side effects of the dipyridamole. Thallium is then injected about 4 minutes later, when peak coronary blood flow is expected, and the final scan is taken. Aminophylline may be infused prophylactically or in response to adverse side effects of the dipyridamole. The client may then return for redistribution imaging in about 4 hours.
   D. *MUGA:* 15-20 mCi of ^{99m}Tc-pertechnetate is tagged to serum albumin or red blood cells; 1 minute after injection, imaging begins. The client should be in a supine position though he or she may be asked to exercise. The procedure takes 1 hour.
   E. *Nitroglycerin:* A cardiologist assesses a baseline MUGA scan, injects nitroglycerin, takes another scan, and repeats this procedure until blood pressure reaches desired level.
   F. *Sestamibi exercise testing and scan:* After a 12-lead ECG machine is attached to chest electrodes, the nuclear medicine technician injects the tracer and completes a resting scan, which lasts approximately 30 minutes. The ECG and blood pressure are then measured continuously as the client completes the exercise portion of the test on a treadmill. Heart rate, blood pressure, and ECG are recorded every 1-2 minutes during each 3-minute stage. If vital signs and ECG have remained stable, the nuclear medicine technician then injects additional

H

tracer 1 minute before the client comes off the treadmill. The final scan of another 30 minutes is then completed.

G. *Sestamibi-dipyridamole stress test and scan:* After a 12-lead ECG machine is attached to chest electrodes, the nuclear medicine technician injects the tracer and completes a resting scan, which lasts approximately 30 minutes. The client is instructed to perform isometric hand grips until dipyridamole injection to help prevent the drug's side effects. The ECG and blood pressure are then measured continuously as a dose of dipyridamole is injected over 4 minutes. 2-7 minutes later, the nuclear medicine technician injects the sestamibi tracer. The side effects of persantine may include chest pain, dysrhythmias, nausea, vomiting, bronchospasm, headache, flushing, or dizziness and hypotension. The side effects may be treated with intravenous aminophylline, which acts as an adenosine receptor agonist. 30 minutes after the tracer injection, the final scan is completed.

H. *Single-photon emission computed tomography (SPECT) scan:* The client is transported to the nuclear medicine department, positioned supine on the scanning table, and left to rest quietly for approximately 10 minutes. A radiopharmaceutical is injected intravenously and allowed to circulate. The SPECT scan is then taken while the client lies motionless.

4. **Postprocedure care:**
   A. Monitor the pulse, blood pressure, and respirations every 15 minutes × 2.
   B. For scans that involved stress testing or administration of dipyridamole, the client is monitored until vital signs or ECG patterns, or both, return to baseline values.

5. **Client and family teaching:**
   A. Do not take drugs or drink caffeine-containing beverages for 6 hours before testing (24 hours for the SPECT scan).
   B. Some tests take several hours. Bring reading material or other diversional activity.

C. *PYP, thallium 201, dipyridamole:* Fast for 4 hours before the test.
   D. *Dipyridamole:* Do not take drugs containing aminophylline for 48 hours before the test.
   E. *Thallium-201, MUGA, nitroglycerin:* Report fatigue, pain, or shortness of breath immediately, particularly if stress (exercise) is used.
   F. You may be asked to move into different positions during the scan.
   G. Drink plenty of fluids for 24 hours after the procedure.

6. **Factors that affect results:**
   A. Digitalis and quinidine alter contractility. Notation should be made on the chart.
   B. Bundle branch block, left ventricular hypertrophy, or hypokalemia.
   C. Thallium-201 scans may produce false-negative results in clients with single-vessel disease.
   D. MUGA does not give positive results for 24 hours after myocardial infarction (MI), and so it cannot be used to diagnose acute MI.
   E. Radionuclides or radioactive tracers with long half-lives from recent scans will interfere with the quality of the images.

7. **Other data:**
   A. The larger the perfusion defect, the poorer the prognosis.
   B. Abnormalities of the heart scan may indicate the need for further studies or cardiac catheterization.
   C. Health care professionals working in a nuclear medicine area should wear a film badge at waist level (the level closest to the client).
   D. Technetium half-life is 6 hours. Thallium half-life is 73 hours.
   E. Health care professionals working in a nuclear medicine area must follow federal standards set by the Nuclear Regulatory Commission. These standards include precautions for handling the radioactive material and monitoring of potential radiation exposure.
   F. MUGA scan is used to monitor cardiac function in clients receiving cardiotoxic antineoplastic chemotherapy.
   G. See also *Stress/exercise test, Diagnostic; Stress test, Pharmacologic, Diagnostic.*

HEART SHUNT SCAN, DIAGNOSTIC

Norm. Normal pulmonary transit time and chamber-filling sequence.

Usage. Determines improper shunting of blood in heart disorders, especially in children.

Description. The heart shunt scan is an angiography study to examine the transit of a bolus of technetium-99m into the jugular vein. Images are taken to follow the bolus on its journey through the heart chambers to visualize any abnormal shunting of blood between chambers.

Professional Considerations
1. Consent form IS required.

Risks
Infection.

Contraindications
During pregnancy or breast-feeding.

2. Preparation:
   A. Have emergency equipment readily available.
3. Procedure:
   A. With the client positioned in a 20-degree Fowler's position, radionuclide is injected into the external jugular vein.
   B. Scanning is performed for approximately 45 minutes.
4. Postprocedure care:
   A. Assess the venipuncture site for bleeding, hematoma.
   B. Observe the client carefully for up to 60 minutes after the study

for a possible (anaphylactic) reaction to the radionuclide.
   C. Wear rubber gloves when discarding urine that is voided up to 24 hours after the procedure. Wash the gloved hands with soap and water before removing the gloves. Wash the ungloved hands after the gloves have been removed.
5. Client and family teaching:
   A. Meticulously wash the hands with soap and water after each void for 24 hours.
6. Factors that affect results:
   A. None.
7. Other data:
   A. This test is specific for left-to-right shunt and right-to-left shunt.
   B. Health care professionals working in a nuclear medicine area should wear a film badge at waist level (the level closest to the client).
   C. Health care professionals working in a nuclear medicine area must follow federal standards set by the Nuclear Regulatory Commission. These standards include precautions for handling the radioactive material and monitoring of potential radiation exposure.
   D. Technetium half-life is 6 hours.

HEART SONOGRAM, DIAGNOSTIC
(see Echocardiography, Diagnostic)

HEART ULTRASOUND
(see Echocardiography, Diagnostic)

HEAVY METALS, BLOOD AND 24-HOUR URINE

Norm:

BLOOD		SI UNITS
Antimony	0.052 ± 0.019 µg/dL	4.35 ± 1.6 nmol/L
Arsenic	2-23 µg/L	0.03-0.31 µmol/L
Chronic poisoning	100-500 µg/L	1.33-6.65 µmol/L
Acute poisoning	600-9300 µg/L	7.98-124 µmol/L
Bismuth	0.1-3.5 µg/L	0.5-16.7 nmol/L
Cadmium		
Smokers	0.6-3.9 µg/L	5.3-34.7 nmol/L
Nonsmokers	0.3-1.2 µg/L	2.7-10.7 nmol/L
Toxic	100-3000 µg/L	0.9-26.7 µmol/L

Continued

BLOOD		SI UNITS
Cobalt	0.11-0.45 µg/L	1.9-7.6 nmol/L
Copper		
Infants	20-70 µg/dL	3.1-11 µmol/L
Child, 6 years	90-190 µg/dL	14.1-29.8 µmol/L
Child, 12 years	80-160 µg/dL	12.6-25.1 µmol/L
Adult male	70-140 µg/dL	11.0-22.0 µmol/L
Adult female	80-155 µg/dL	12.6-24.3 µmol/L
Pregnant	118-302 µg/dL	18.5-47.4 µmol/L
Lead		
Child	<25 µg/dL	<1.21 µmol/L
Adult	<40 µg/dL	<1.93 µmol/L
Industry exposure	<60 µg/dL	<2.90 µmol/L
Toxic concentration	≥100 µg/dL	≥4.83 µmol/L
Toxic concentration in children	≥25 µg/dL	≥1.21 µmol/L
Mercury	≤0.06 µg/mL	≤0.3 nmol/L
Selenium	58-234 µg/L	0.74-2.97 µmol/L
Thallium	<0.5 µg/dL	<24.5 nmol/L
Toxic concentration	10-800 µg/dL	0.5-39.1 µmol/L
Zinc	70-150 µg/dL	10.7-23 µmol/L

24-HOUR URINE		SI UNITS
Antimony	<10 µg/L	<82.1 µmol/L
Toxic concentration	≥10 µg/L	≥82.1 µmol/L
Arsenic	5-50 µg/L	0.067-0.665 µmol/L
Chronic poisoning	50-5000 µg/L	0.67-66.5 µmol/L
Acute poisoning	1000-20,000 µg/L	13.3-266 mmol/L
Bismuth	0.3-4.6 µg/L	1.4-22 nmol/L
Cadmium	0.5-4.7 µg/L	4.4-41.8 nmol/L
Industrial exposure	10-580 µg/L	0.09-5.16 µmol/L
Cobalt	1-2 µg/L	17-34 nmol/L
Copper	2-80 µg/L	0.03-1.26 µmol/L
Lead	<80 µg/L	<0.39 µmol/L
Industrial exposure	<120 µg/L	<0.58 µmol/L
Mercury		
Adult	≤10 µg/24 hours	<0.05 µmol/L
Toxic concentration	>50 µg/24 hours	>0.25 µmol/L
Selenium	7-160 µg/L	0.09-2.03 µmol/L
Toxic concentration	>400 µg/L	>5.08 µmol/L
Thallium	<2 µg/L	<9.8 nmol/L
Toxic concentration	1-20 mg/L	4.9-97.8 µmol/L
Zinc	150-1200 µg/L	2.3-18.4 µmol/L
Toxic concentration	>1200 µg/L	>18.4 µmol/L

Toxic or Poisoning Symptoms and Treatment

Symptoms:

Antimony: Vomiting.

Arsenic: Gastric pain, vomiting, diarrhea, convulsions, coma, and death in acute poisoning; and diarrhea, scaling and pigmentation of skin, hair loss, and peripheral neuropathy in chronic poisoning.

Bismuth: Weakness, decreased appetite, fever, halitosis, black gum line, rheumatic type pain, and renal damage.

Cadmium: Pneumonia, pulmonary edema, and cardiovascular collapse from inhalation; violent gastrointestinal symptoms from acute ingestion; and osteomalacia and renal dysfunction from chronic ingestion.

Cobalt: Thyroid gland hyperplasia, giant cell pneumonitis, hypersensitivity pneumonitis, pulmonary fibrosis, bronchiolitis obliterans, cardiomyopathy, nerve damage, and myxedema.

Copper: Nausea, vomiting, headache, diarrhea, and abdominal pain, Wilson's disease, Indian childhood cirrhosis, noncaseating granuloma, pulmonary fibrosis.

Lead: Anorexia, abdominal pain, vomiting, irritability, and apathy.

Mercury: Fatigue, headache, loss of memory, apathy, emotional instability, paresthesia, ataxia, deafness, dysarthria, visual deterioration, dysphagia, coma, and death.

Nickel: Contact dermatitis, irritability of gastrointestinal and respiratory systems, diffuse interstitial pneumonitis and cerebral edema with severe poisoning. Little data to support carcinogenic potential. Treatment: sodium diethyldithiocarbamate (investigational chelating agent).

Selenium: Garlic smell in breath and urine, metallic taste, headaches, nausea, vomiting, pneumonia, and pulmonary edema.

Thallium: Ataxia, pulmonary edema, vomiting, constipation, restlessness, delirium, and coma.

Vanadium: Rhinitis, wheezing, nasal hemorrhage, conjunctivitis, cough, sore throat, and chest pain.

Zinc: Cough, chest discomfort, tachycardia, hypertension, gastrointestinal irritation, nausea, vomiting, diarrhea, and metallic taste in mouth.

Treatment:

Note: Treatment choice(s) depend on client history and condition and episode history.

Antidotes for heavy-metal poisoning include BAL (British antilewisite, dimercaprol), deferoxamine, dimercaprol, and EDTA. Heavy metals respond to hemodialysis or hemoperfusion in varying degrees (poor to well).

Usage. Screening for heavy-metal toxicity from overexposure, ingestion, or occupational exposure. Disorders for individual metals found under test listings for individual metals. Drugs that may further increase some values include carbamazepine, estrogens, oral contraceptives, penicillamine, phenobarbital, phenytoin, and sodium salts.

Description. Heavy metals include antimony, arsenic, bismuth, cadmium, cobalt, copper, lead, mercury, nickel, selenium, thallium, vanadium, and zinc.

Antimony exposure occurs in miners, smelters, and ore-refinery workers.

Arsenic is found naturally in food and the environment as well as in pesticides.

Bismuth exposure occurs in workers in cosmetic, disinfectant, and pigment industries. It may also occur as a result of treatment for syphilis.

Cadmium accumulates in the lungs, liver, and kidneys by exposure to food, water, air, and cigarette smoke.

Cobalt, a component of vitamin B_{12}, is found in most foods. It is also used to treat some resistant anemias and some radiosensitive malignancies. Occupational exposure occurs with glass and ceramic pigmentation, electroplating, chemical and petroleum industries, grinding and sharpening of hard metal tools, and animal-feed manufacturing.

Copper is a trace element found in normal diets. It is one of the few heavy metals that are potentially harmful at low levels as well as at toxic levels. Toxic levels may be caused by the use of copper IUDs, ingestion of contaminated substances, electroplating, metal reclamation, roasting, crushing, smelting, and fungicide exposure. The biliary tract is the primary route of elimination. Gastrointestinal symptoms occur around whole blood levels near 3 mg of Cu per liter. Treatment is by chelating agents ($CaNa_2$-EDTA, BAL) or fungicide exposure.

Lead is absorbed into the body by the ingestion of lead-containing paint or after industrial exposure (bone lead levels are higher in men in blue-collar occupations). Exposure adversely affects a child's academic achievement and reduces cognitive abilities in exposed adults.

Mercury is found in fungicides, industrial processes, and fish (living in polluted water). It can also be ingested in the form of mercury salts. High mercury levels have been noted among dental workers.

H

Nickel is ubiquitous in soil, water, and many foods. Nickel does not accumulate in humans, and acute toxicity is usually related to exposure to nickel carbonyl. Current data are insufficient to indicate risk of carcinogenesis from nickel exposure.

Selenium is a metal used for the activity of human glutathione peroxidase. Exposure occurs as a result of the manufacture of glass, paints, dyes, electronic equipment, fungicides, rubber, and semiconductors.

Thallium is present in cosmetics, pesticides, and some medications. It is absorbed through intact skin and mucous membranes.

Vanadium is a corrosion-resistant metal that does not occur in nature. The primary source of exposure is from the diet. Occupational exposure occurs during boiler-cleaning operations as a result of the generation of vanadium oxide dust. The kidneys are the primary routes of excretion. Toxicity overall is low.

Zinc is a trace metal important for cellular growth and metabolism. Toxicity can occur from industrial exposure and consumption of acidic food or beverages from galvanized containers.

Professional Considerations

1. Consent form NOT required.
2. **Preparation:**
   A. *Blood:*
      i. Tube: Metal-free tube containing EDTA anticoagulant.
      ii. Do NOT draw specimens during hemodialysis.
   B. *24-hour urine:*
      i. Obtain a 3-L, plastic, acid-washed collection container. Use a plastic bedpan or urinal for voided specimens.
      ii. Write the beginning date and the time of collection on the container and the laboratory requisition.
3. **Procedure:**
   A. *Blood:* Draw a 10-mL blood sample.
   B. *24-hour urine:* Save all the urine in a 3-L plastic, acid-washed container for 24 hours.
4. **Postprocedure care:**
   A. Do NOT spin blood.
   B. *24-hour urine:* Record the total volume and the ending time of collection on the specimen container and label the container with the client information.
   C. Refrigerate the specimen(s).

5. **Client and family teaching:**
   A. *24-hour urine:* Save all the urine voided for the next 24 hours and urinate before defecating to avoid contaminating the urine specimen with stool. If any urine is accidentally discarded, discard the entire specimen and restart the collection the next day.
6. **Factors that affect results:**
   A. A diet high in heavy metals may elevate results.
   B. Occupational exposure may elevate results.
   C. A recent seafood diet may cause increased arsenic values.
   D. A diurnal variation exists such that the highest copper levels are found in the morning.
   E. Copper levels are 8%-12% higher in blacks.
   F. Drugs that may further increase some values include dimercaprol, loop diuretics (intravenous), naproxen, penicillamine, sodium chloride, and thiazide diuretics.
7. **Other data:**
   A. Make sure the specimen for the 24-hour urine is not voided into a metal bedpan or urinal.
   B. Urine is the preferred specimen for arsenic if symptoms are present or in acute exposure.
   C. Supplemental vanadyl sulfate, used by some athletes to enhance weight training, can increase vanadium levels.
   D. Many asymptomatic occupationally exposed workers have elevated vanadium levels.
   E. Except for lead and cadmium, evidence is lacking on toxicity levels.
   F. In the absence of acute toxicity, serial testing is usually more informative when applied in context with physical examination and knowledge of exposure history.
   G. Blood lead levels have been correlated with higher levels of serum total cholesterol and high-density lipoprotein.
   H. Increased intake of ascorbic acid has been shown to decrease blood lead level
   I. See also *Arsenic, Blood; Arsenic, Urine; Cadmium, Serum and 24-Hour urine; Copper, Serum; Copper, Urine; Lead, Blood and Urine; Mercury, Blood; Mercury, 24-Hour urine; Thallium, Serum; Thallium, 24-Hour urine; Zinc, Blood.*

HEINZ BODY STAIN, DIAGNOSTIC

Norm. Negative.

Positive. G6PD deficiency, Heinz-body anemia, hemolytic anemia, homozygous beta-thalassemia, and after splenectomy. Drugs include acetanilid, aminosalicylic acid, analgesics, aniline, antipyretics, chlorates, hydroxylamine, naphthalene, nitrobenzene, phenol derivatives, phenolhydrazine, phenothiazines, phenylsemicarbazide, pyridine, resorcin, salicylazosulfidine, sodium sulfoxone, sulfapyridine, sulfones, tolbutamide, and large doses of vitamin K.

Negative. No Heinz body identified.

Description. Heinz bodies are small, irregular particles of denatured hemoglobin within mature red blood cells. These appear when stained with methyl violet or cresyl blue but not under Wright-stained preparations. The presence of Heinz bodies in a stained specimen indicates an abnormal hemoglobin structure.

Professional Considerations
1. Consent form NOT required.
2. **Preparation:**
   A. Tube: Lavender topped.
   B. Contact the laboratory to arrange for testing.
3. **Procedure:**
   A. Draw a 3.5-mL blood sample.
   B. Invert the tube gently several times to adequately mix the sample and the anticoagulant.
4. **Postprocedure care:**
   A. Refrigerate the specimen.
   B. Current administration of antimalarials, furazolidone, nitrofurantoin, phenacetin, procarbazine, or sulfonamides should be noted on the laboratory requisition.
5. **Client and family teaching:**
   A. Results are normally available within 24-48 hours.
6. **Factors that affect results:**
   A. Hemolysis or clotting of the specimen invalidates the results.
   B. Antimalarials, furazolidone (in infants), nitrofurantoin, phenacetin, procarbazine, and sulfonamides can cause false-positive results.

7. **Other data:**
   A. Heinz bodies per cell vary from 1 to 20.
   B. G6PD deficiency often affects Dutch, German, or French individuals.

HELICAL CT, DIAGNOSTIC
(*see Computed tomography of the body, Diagnostic*)

HELICOBACTER PYLORI ANTIGEN TEST, STOOL

Norm. Negative for the presence of *H. pylori* antigens.

Usage. Provides earlier evaluation than the urea breath test of the success of treatment for *H. pylori* infection.

Description. See *Urea Breath Test, Diagnostic*. The *H. pylori* stool antigen test is one of the newest tests developed to evaluate for the persistence of the bacteria and detects the *H. pylori* antigen that is shed in the stool of clients with active *H. pylori* infection. A positive test as early as 7 days after the completion of treatment indicates that the treatment was *not* successful. This test's early usefulness is as sensitive and specific as the urea breath test, which should not be performed for at least 4-6 weeks after treatment, for evaluation of treatment success.

Professional Considerations
1. Consent form IS required.
2. **Preparation:**
   A. Obtain a clean container.
3. **Procedure:**
   A. Obtain a small sample of stool in a clean, dry container.
   B. The stool is smeared on a microplate coated with *H. pylori* antibodies, incubated, and the resulting color change is compared to a chart. The greater the degree of color change, the greater the amount of *H. pylori* antigen in the stool sample.
4. **Postprocedure care:**
   A. None.
5. **Client and family teaching:**
   A. Do not take Omeprazole, Lansoprazole, or Pantoprazole within 14 days before the test.

H

B. Do not take bismuth mixtures (e.g., Pepto Bismol) within 1 month before the test.
C. Test results are normally available in about 3 hours.
6. **Factors that affect results:**
   A. Recent intake of bismuth-containing compounds (Pepto Bismol) or lansoprazole may cause false-negative results.
7. **Other data:**
   A. See also *Campylobacter-like–organism test, Specimen; Helicobacter pylori, Quick office serology, Serum and Titer, Blood;* and *Urea breath test, Diagnostic.*

HELICOBACTER PYLORI QUICK OFFICE SEROLOGY, SERUM AND TITER, BLOOD

Norm. Negative.

Usage. Duodenal ulcers, gastric cancer, gastric ulcers, gastritis (chronic), lymphoma (stomach), and peptic ulcers.

Description. *H. pylori* are S- or C-shaped, gram-negative bacilli with a smooth outer coat and two to four unipolar flagella. These organisms were first detected in the stomachs of clients with gastritis *circa* 1990 and have now been shown to be the major cause of active chronic gastritis. In addition, the evidence that *H. pylori* play a major role in the pathophysiology of duodenal and peptic ulcers and possibly gastric ulcers is compelling. An association between *H. pylori* and gastric cancer and lymphoma of the stomach may also exist. There is no known natural reservoir for *H. pylori* in the environment, but it is believed that these organisms are spread by the fecal-oral or oral-oral route. The Quick Office Serology test may be performed in the physician's office in 20 minutes on serum, providing a yes-or-no answer to the presence of IgA and IgG antibodies to *H. pylori*. Laboratory-based serology tests are more specific than office-based tests in that they quantitate antibody levels, providing titers so that antibody levels can be monitored after therapy. An elevated antibody level indicates active or recent infection. Because antibodies remain in

the blood long after the infection is eradicated, this test cannot evaluate response to treatment. Instead, the *urea breath test* should be used to confirm eradication after treatment. (See *Urea breath test, Diagnostic.*)

Professional Considerations
1. Consent form NOT required.
2. **Preparation:**
   A. Tube: Red topped, red/gray topped, or gold topped.
3. **Procedure:**
   A. Draw a 3-mL blood sample.
4. **Postprocedure care:**
   A. If shipping the sample to an off-site laboratory, keep the specimen cool with frozen coolant from April through October and with refrigerated coolant from November through March.
5. **Client and family teaching:**
   A. Because serologic tests may remain positive for many months after successful treatment for *H. pylori*, other tests are also recommended for evaluating progress (endoscopy or breath test).
6. **Factors that affect results:**
   A. Serologic testing alone is associated with high false-positive rates because of past infection without active disease.
7. **Other data:**
   A. These tests require 1 mL of serum.
   B. *H. pylori* affects about 20% of clients younger than 40 years and 50% of those older than 60 years.
   C. *H. pylori* is uncommon in young children.
   D. More than 90% of duodenal ulcers are caused by *H. pylori*.
   E. See also *Campylobacter-like organism test, Specimen.*

HELLP (HEMOLYSIS, ELEVATED LIVER ENZYMES, LOW PLATELETS) SYNDROME PANEL, SERUM

Norm. Blood pressure within normal limits or below 160/110 mm Hg. Complete blood count (CBC) and liver enzymes within normal limits.

Usage. Laboratory studies of blood values and liver enzymes will confirm diagnosis of syndrome. Serves as a foundation for client care.

Description. Pregnancy-related syndrome associated with severe cases of pregnancy-induced hypertension (PIH)/preeclampsia, occurring in 4%-12% of these clients. Pathophysiologic cause of syndrome is unknown. Persistent hypertension results in a decrease in intrinsic vasodilators (prostacyclin and nitric oxide) and increased production of vasopressors such as thromboxane. A chain of events leads to widespread vasospasms, acute renal failure, pulmonary edema, ascites, pleural effusion, ARDS, and/or multiple-organ damage.

Hepatic dysfunction caused by vasospasms affects:

- metabolism of free fatty acids → increased plasma levels of fatty acids → aberrations in membranes of red blood cells (RBCs).
- liver function, namely, AST (formerly SGOT), ALT (formerly SGPT), LDH.
- endothelial integrity, platelet adherence, fibrin deposits. Increased sensitivity to angiotensin II, associated with PIH, heightens effect of angiotensin II on cells, causing them to contract. Increased prostacyclin (vasodilator and aggregation inhibitor) contributes to platelet "stickiness."

Lab values associated with HELLP syndrome:

ALT (SGPT) >50 U/L
AST (SGOT) >72 U/L
Bilirubin >1.2 mg/dL
BUN >10mg/dL
Cr >2 mg/dL
Hct <32%
Hgb <10 mg/dL
LDH >350 IU/L
Plasma fibrinogen <300 mg/dL
PLT <100,000/mm
PT/PTT prolonged
Uric acid >10 mg/dL

Signs or symptoms associated with HELLP syndrome:

Blood pressure: 160/110 mm Hg or systolic >30 mm Hg or diastolic >15 mm Hg over baseline value
Dependent edema that progresses to nondependent edema of upper arms, upper legs, abdomen, face, and neck
Epigastric pain, right upper abdominal quadrant tenderness
Hemolytic anemia: fatigue, pallor, dyspnea
Jaundice
Proteinuria: +4
Pulmonary edema

Professional Considerations:
1. Consent form NOT required.
2. **Preparation:**
   A. Tube: Red topped, red/gray topped, or gold topped for liver function tests.
   B. Do NOT draw during hemodialysis.
   C. Lavender-topped tube for platelets.
   D. Obtain intravenous access for possible blood product infusion(s).
   E. Obtain baseline vital signs.
3. **Procedure:**
   A. Draw a 4-mL blood sample.
   B. Management with fresh-frozen plasma and packed RBCs. Avoid platelet transfusion because platelet consumption will occur.
   C. Monitor vital signs frequently.
4. **Postprocedure care:**
   A. Specimen may be refrigerated but not frozen.
   B. For clients with HELLP syndrome, the critical period is 24 hours postpartum. During this time, the client's condition often worsens before improvement is seen.
5. **Client and family teaching:**
   A. Results available within an hour.
   B. Clients with HELLP syndrome usually deliver by cesarean section and need to receive therapeutic blood components.
   C. Mother is very ill and her condition will be of concern for at least 48 hours after delivery.
   D. Condition of the baby will depend on gestational age at time of delivery, effects of uteroplacental insufficiency (associated with PIH), and maternal hemorrhage before delivery.
6. **Factors that affect results:**
   A. Delivery of fetus will correct preeclampsia. HELLP syndrome is complicated by disseminated

H

intravascular coagulation (DIC) and potential liver rupture.
    B. Hemolysis affects serum laboratory results for liver function.
7. **Other data:**
    A. Usually develops between 20 and 37 weeks of gestation. Maternal mortality can be as high as 60%.

HEMAGGLUTINATION TREPONEMAL TEST FOR SYPHILIS (HATTS), SERUM

Norm. Titer <1:160.

Usage. Serologic confirmation of syphilis when nontreponemal antibody tests are positive.

Description. Syphilis is a complex, sexually transmitted disease characterized by a wide range of symptoms that imitate other diseases and is caused by the organism *Treponema pallidum*. In this test, the client's serum is heat treated and mixed with *T. pallidum*–sensitized turkey red blood cells, incubated, and compared with a control. A positive result occurs when agglutination occurs in the test sample but not in the control. Positive results will occur in treponemal diseases of bejel, pinta, syphilis, and yaws.

Professional Considerations
1. Consent form NOT required.
2. **Preparation:**
    A. See *Client and family teaching.*
    B. Tube: Red topped, red/gray topped, or gold topped.
3. **Procedure:**
    A. Draw a 7-mL blood sample.
4. **Postprocedure care:**
    A. Send the specimen to the laboratory and refrigerate it until it is tested.
    B. All cases of syphilis should be reported to the Centers for Disease Control and Prevention in Atlanta, Georgia, at their telephone: 404-639-2206.
    C. Sexual contacts should be notified in the event of positive results.
5. **Client and family teaching:**
    A. Fast overnight before the test.
    B. Refer clients with elevated titers for medical management, which

is necessary to slow or prevent the sequelae of syphilis.
    C. If testing positive:
        i. Notify all sexual contacts from the last 90 days (if in the early stage) to be tested for syphilis.
        ii. Syphilis can be cured with antibiotics. These may worsen the symptoms for the first 24 hours.
        iii. Do not have sex for 2 months and until after repeat testing has confirmed that the syphilis is cured. Use condoms after that for 2 years. Return for repeat testing every 3-4 months for the next 2 years to make sure the disease is cured.
        iv. Do not become pregnant for 2 years because syphilis can be transmitted to the fetus.
        v. If left untreated, syphilis can damage many body organs, including the brain, over several years. Neurosyphilis (late stage) is very difficult to treat with currently available regimens.
6. **Factors that affect results:**
    A. False-positive results may be attributable to infectious mononucleosis, leprosy, or systemic lupus erythematosus.
    B. False-negative results may occur in clients with AIDS. Treponemal antigen tests demonstrate greater accuracy in detecting late-stage infection in clients with HIV.
7. **Other data:**
    A. This test may remain positive indefinitely for clients previously infected with syphilis. Thus it is not useful for monitoring clinical response to treatment for syphilis.
    B. Benzathine penicillin G is the drug of choice to treat syphilis. Severe disease or immunosuppressed clients may require intravenous therapy. Consider doxycycline, ceftriaxone, or tetracycline with PCN allergy.
    C. Serial quantitative cardiolipin antigen testing is used for monitoring treatment response.
    D. False-positive results have been reported in IV drug users infected with HIV and hepatitis B virus.

HEMATOCRIT (HCT), BLOOD

Norm:

		SI UNITS
Females		
Adult	35-47%	0.35-0.47
Pregnant	30-46%	0.30-0.46
Adult Males	42-52%	0.42-0.52
Children		
Neonates	42-68%	0.42-0.68
3 months	29-54%	0.29-0.54
1-2 years	35-44%	0.35-0.44
6-10 years	31-43%	0.31-0.43
Panic Levels	<15% or <60%	<0.15 or >0.60

Panic Level Symptoms and Treatment—Increased

Note: Treatment choice(s) depend on client history and condition and episode history.

Cause	Symptoms	Possible Treatments
Hemoconcentration	Decreased pulse pressure and volume, decreased skin turgor, decreased venous filling, dry mucous membranes, low central venous pressure, orthostatic hypotension, tachycardia, thirst and weakness	Administer IV fluids. Monitor hematocrit. Stop or reduce dose of diuretics if they are contributors condition.
True polycythemia overtransfusion	Extremity pain and redness, facial flushing, irritability, anasarca decreasing QRS voltage with severe Fluid overload	Administer IV fluids. Monitor hematocrit. Observe for signs of thrombosis. Perform bloodletting by venipuncture (phlebotomy).

Panic Level Symptoms and Treatment—Decreased

Cause	Symptoms	Possible Treatments
Hemodilution	Rales, anxiety, edema, hypertension, jugular venous distension, restlessness, and shortness of breath	Administer diuretics. Restrict sodium. Restrict fluids. Monitor hematocrit and intake and output. Administer oxygen.
Blood loss	Hypotension, bleeding, hypoxia	Identify and treat cause of bleeding. Give isotonic fluids. Give isotonic fluids. Perform blood transfusion. Administer omeprazole (if blood loss is caused by bleeding esophageal varices). Protect airways; administer oxygen as needed

H

Increased. Addison's disease, blood doping (autologous transfusion to improve athletic performance), burns (severe), dehydration (severe), diabetes mellitus, diarrhea, eclampsia, erythrocytosis, hemorrhage, hemoconcentration, pancreatitis (acute), polycythemia, shock, and tetralogy of Fallot. Any condition that increases red blood cells (RBCs).

Decreased. Anemia, bone marrow hyperplasia, burns (severe), cardiac decompensation, cirrhosis, congestive heart failure, cystic fibrosis, fatty liver, fluid overload, hemolytic reactions to chemicals or drugs or prosthetics, hemorrhage, hydremia of pregnancy, hyperthyroidism, hypothyroidism, idiopathic steatorrhea, intestinal obstruction (late), leukemia, overhydration, pancreatitis (hemorrhagic), pneumonia, and pregnancy. Also, conditions that decrease RBCs. Drugs include acetaminophen, acetohexamide, aminosalicylic acid, amphotericin, antimony potassium tartrate, antineoplastic agents, antibiotics, atabrine hydrochloride, chloramphenicol, chloroquine hydrochloride or phosphate, doxapram hydrochloride, ethosuximide, ethotoin, furazolidone, haloperidol, hydralazine hydrochloride, indomethacin, isocarboxazid, isoniazid, mefenamic acid, mephenytoin, mercurial diuretics, metaxalone, methaqualone, methsuximide, methyldopa, methyldopate hydrochloride, nitrates, nitrofurantoin, novobiocin sodium, oleandomycin, oxyphenbutazone, paramethadione, pargyline hydrochloride, penicillins, phenacemide, phenelzine sulfate, phenobarbital, phensuximide, phenylbutazone, phenytoin sodium, phytonadione, primidone, radioactive agents, rifampin, spectinomycin hydrochloride, sulfonamides, tetracyclines, thiazide diuretics, thiocyanates, thiosemicarbazones, tolazamide, tolbutamide, tranylcypromine sulfate, trimethadione, tripelennamine hydrochloride, troleandomycin, valproic acid, vegetarian diet, vitamin A, and zidovudine (AZT).

Description. Hematocrit is the percentage of red blood cells in a volume of whole blood.

Professional Considerations
1. Consent form NOT required.

2. **Preparation:**
   A. Tube: Lavender-topped or heparinized capillary tube with a red band on the anticoagulant end.
   B. Do NOT draw during hemodialysis.
3. **Procedure:**
   A. Draw a 3.5-mL blood sample from an extremity that does not have intravenous fluids infusing into it to avoid hemodiluted samples. Do not leave the tourniquet in place for longer than 1 minute during collection.
   B. For a capillary puncture (fingers, toes, heels), establish a free flow of blood to minimize dilution with tissue fluid. Fill the capillary tube from the red-banded end to about two-thirds capacity and seal this end with clay.
   C. For a central venous access device temporarily stop all fluids infusing through ports, prepare injection port with povidone-iodine solution or alcohol, using only 10-mL syringes flush with 10 mL of 0.9% NaCl, and immediately withdraw 10 mL of discard blood. Withdraw required blood volume with new syringes and transfer specimen to appropriate tubes. Flush port with 10 mL of 0.9% NaCl. (Refer to your facility's policy and procedure manual or obtain related current standards from Intravenous Nursing Society, Oncology Nursing Society, or North American Vascular Access Network.) Flush solutions and discard volumes may vary by client population and published guidelines.
4. **Postprocedure care:**
   A. Invert the tube gently 10 times to mix.
   B. Refrigerate the sample after 10 hours. Do not freeze it.
5. **Client and family teaching:**
   A. Results are normally available within less than 24 hours.
6. **Factors that affect results:**
   A. Hemolysis of the specimen invalidates results.
   B. Results are elevated with dehydration or leukocytosis over 100 $\times 10^9$/L.
   C. False elevations occur with glucose >400 mg/dL.
   D. Obtain the specimen before bath, shower, or massage because these

can cause a temporary rise in the value.

E. High altitude may increase the value.

F. Level may measure as normal, even in the condition of blood loss, because of compensatory mechanisms and/or overlying conditions such as dehydration.

7. **Other data:**
A. The hematocrit value is approximately three times the value of the hemoglobin.
B. Hematocrit does not detect iron deficiency in infants, but ferritin

level will for those 9-18 months of age.

C. Consider hemoglobin levels with pulse oximetry—if hemoglobin is low and oxygen saturation is 100%, oxygenation could be clinically significantly inadequate.

D. Clients older than 64 years with a hematocrit less than 39% should be treated routinely using preoperative storage of autologous blood.

HEMOCCULT, STOOL
(see Occult Blood, Stool)

HEMOGLOBIN (Hb, Hgb), BLOOD

Norm:

		SI UNITS
Females	12-15 g/dL	7.45-9.31 mmol/L
Pregnant	10-15 g/dL	6.3-9.9 mmol/L
Males	13.6-17.2 g/dL	8.44-10.67 mmol/L
Children		
Neonates	14-27 g/dL	8.69-16.76 mmol/L
3 months	10-17 g/dL	6.21-10.55 mmol/L
1-2 years	9-15 g/dL	5.58-9.31 mmol/L
6-10 years	11-16 g/dL	6.82-9.92 mmol/L
Panic Levels	<5 g/dL	<3.10 mmol/L
	>20 g/dL	>12.41 mmol/L

Panic Level Symptoms and Treatment—Increased. See *Hematocrit, Blood*

Panic Level Symptoms and Treatment—Decreased. See *Hematocrit, Blood*

Increased. Burns (severe), congestive heart failure, chronic obstructive pulmonary disease (COPD), dehydration, diarrhea, erythrocytosis, hemorrhage, hemoconcentration, high altitudes, intestinal obstruction (late), polycythemia vera, snorers, and thrombotic thrombocytopenic purpura. Also conditions that increase red blood cells (RBCs). Drugs include gentamicin and methyldopa.

Decreased. Andersen's disease, anemia (iron deficiency), carcinomatosis, cirrhosis, cystic fibrosis, fat emboli,

fatty liver, fluid retention, hemorrhage, hemolysis, hemolytic reaction to chemicals or drugs or prosthetics, Hodgkin's disease, hydremia of pregnancy, hyperthyroidism, hypervitaminosis A, hypothyroidism, idiopathic steatorrhea, intravenous overload, leukemia, lymphoma, platelet apheresis, pregnancy, renal cortical necrosis, sarcoidosis, severe hemorrhage, systemic lupus erythematosus, tetralogy of Fallot, and transfusion of incompatible blood. Also, conditions that decrease RBCs. Drugs include antibiotics, antineoplastic agents, Apresoline (hydralazine HCl with hydrochlorothiazide), aspirin, hydantoin derivatives, indocin, monoamine oxidase inhibitors, primaquine, rifampin, sulfonamides, and tridione, vegetarian diet, and zidovudine (AZT).

Description. Hemoglobin is the oxygen-carrying pigment of the RBCs. It is composed of amino acids that form a single protein called "globin" and a compound called "heme." Heme contains iron atoms and the red pigment porphyrin. Each erythrocyte contains approximately 300 million molecules of hemoglobin.

Professional Considerations

1. Consent form NOT required.
2. Preparation:
   A. Tube: Lavender-topped or heparinized capillary tube with a red band on the anticoagulant end.
   B. Do NOT draw specimen during hemodialysis.
3. Procedure:
   A. Draw a 3.5-mL blood sample from an extremity that does not have intravenous fluids infusing into it. Do not leave the tourniquet in place for longer than 1 minute during collection.
   B. For capillary puncture (fingers, toes, heels), establish a free flow of blood to minimize dilution with tissue fluid. Fill the capillary tube from the red-banded end to about two-thirds capacity and seal this end with clay.
   C. Central venous catheter—see *Hematocrit.*
4. Postprocedure care:
   A. Invert the tube gently 10 times to mix it.
   B. The specimen is stable at room temperature for 10 hours; then refrigerate it for up to 18 hours total.
5. Client and family teaching:
   A. Results are normally available within less than 24 hours.
6. Factors that affect results:
   A. Hemolysis of the specimen invalidates the results.
   B. Results are falsely elevated by lipemic samples and leukocytosis >30×10^9/L.
   C. Obtain the specimen before bath, shower, or massage because these can cause a temporary rise in value.
   D. High altitude may increase the value.
   E. The mean hemoglobin in blacks is 0.4-1.0 g/dL lower than that in whites after the first decade of life.
7. Other data:
   A. The hemoglobin value is approximately one third the value of the hematocrit.
   B. Recent animal studies of hemoglobin have indicated that it may play a role in blood pressure regulation by carrying and releasing "super–nitric oxide," a form of gas that causes relaxation of muscle cells in peripheral blood vessels.

HEMOGLOBIN A$_1$A

(see Glycosylated hemoglobin, Blood)

HEMOGLOBIN A$_1$B

(see Glycosylated hemoglobin, Blood)

HEMOGLOBIN A$_1$C

(see Glycosylated hemoglobin, Blood)

HEMOGLOBIN A$_2$, BLOOD

Norm:

		SI UNITS (MASS FRACTION)
Cord blood	0-1.8%	0-0.018
Birth to 6 months	0-3.5%	0-0.035
>6 months	1.5-3.5%	0.015-0.035
Beta-thalassemia		
Trait	3.7-6.5%	0.037-0.065
Sickle cell trait	1.7-4.5%	0.017-0.045

Increased. Anemia (megaloblastic) and beta-thalassemia (homozygous).

Decreased. Anemia (iron deficiency, microcytic, sideroblastic), alpha-thalassemia, beta-thalassemia, erythroleukemia, hemoglobin A_2-Monreale mutation, and hemoglobin H disease.

Description. Hemoglobin A_2 is a normally present hemoglobin component constituting 2%-3% of the normally present hemoglobin. This test is used to help differentiate hemoglobin abnormalities.

Professional Considerations
1. Consent form NOT required.
2. Preparation:
   A. Tube: Lavender topped.
3. Procedure:
   A. Draw a 2-mL blood sample, without hemolysis.
4. Postprocedure care:
   A. Invert the tube gently 10 times to mix.
5. Client and family teaching:
   A. Results are normally available within 24-48 hours.
6. Factors that affect results:
   A. Hemolysis or clotting of the specimen invalidates the results.
   B. Clients with both beta-thalassemia and iron deficiency may demonstrate normal HbA$_2$ and may need to be retested after taking iron supplements.
   C. In clients who have received recent blood transfusions, the results may be unreliable.
7. Other data:
   A. HbA$_2$ cannot be measured in the presence of HbC, HbE, or HbO.

HEMOGLOBIN ELECTROPHORESIS, BLOOD

Norm:

		SI UNITS (HB FRACTION)
Hemoglobin A	>95%	>0.95
Infants	10%-30%	0.10-0.30
Hemoglobin A_2	3-4%	0.03-0.04
Hemoglobin F	<1%	<0.01
Neonates	70%-80%	0.70-0.80
1 month	70%	0.70
2 months	50%	0.50
3 months	25%	0.25
6 months-1 year	3%	0.03
Hemoglobin C	Absent	
Hemoglobin D	Absent	
Hemoglobin E	Absent	
Hemoglobin H	Absent	
Hemoglobin S	Absent	

Usage. Heinz-body anemia, hemoglobin C disease (trait = 45%, disease >90%), hemolytic anemia (HbD and HbE), microcytic anemia, sickle cell anemia (HbS: trait = 20%-40%, disease = 80%-100%), and thalassemia minor (HbH).

Description. A screening procedure in which the hemoglobin molecules migrate in solution in response to electrical currents such that the different components and their percentages can be determined.

Hemoglobins A, A_2, and F are types of hemoglobin that are found normally in the body.

Hemoglobin C causes red blood cells to sickle at times because of osmotic fragility. It occurs in 2%-3% of the black population.

Hemoglobins D and E rarely occur by themselves though the anemias are without symptoms. When either occurs in combination with sickle cell anemia or thalassemia, the disease takes a more serious form.

Hemoglobin H is known to develop many inclusion bodies within the red blood cell, resulting in a damaged cell membrane and premature cell death (40 days). It also disrupts transport of oxygen to tissues by binding with rather than releasing the oxygen.

Hemoglobin S is the most common of the abnormal hemoglobin traits, occurring in 10% of the black population. Its presence results in a sickling distortion of the red blood cells in response to reduced oxygen levels.

Professional Considerations
1. Consent form NOT required.
2. **Preparation:**
   A. Tube: Lavender topped.
3. **Procedure:**
   A. Draw a 2.5-mL blood sample.
4. **Postprocedure care:**
   A. Deliver the specimen to the laboratory immediately because abnormal hemoglobins are unstable.
   B. Recent (within the past 4 months) blood transfusion(s)

should be noted on the laboratory requisition.
5. **Client and family teaching:**
   A. The client should wear a medical identification tag if chronic anemia is present.
   B. If the sickle cell trait or the disease is present, offer genetic counseling.
6. **Factors that affect results:**
   A. Red blood cell transfusion within the previous 4 months may mask or reduce the presence of abnormal hemoglobins.
   B. Hemoglobins A_2, C, and S may be decreased in iron deficiency.
   C. False-negative tests occur in hemoglobin S with clients with polycythemia or in those less than 3 months of age.
7. **Other data:**
   A. More than 350 variants of Hb have been recognized.
   B. Changes in the proportion of normal types of hemoglobin may imply a hemolytic disease.

HEMOGLOBIN (FREE), PLASMA AND QUALITATIVE, URINE

Norm:

Urine. Negative.

BLOOD		SI UNITS
Normal	<3 mg/dL	<0.47 μmol/L
Hemoglobinemia	>10 mg/dL	>1.55 μmol/L
Intravascular hemolysis	>30 mg/dL	>4.65 μmol/L
Hemoglobinuria occurs at	>150 mg/dL	>23.25 μmol/L
Cherry-red plasma occurs at	>200 mg/dL	>31 μmol/L

Increased in Plasma. Autoimmune hemolytic anemia, burns, cold hemagglutins, disseminated intravascular coagulation, falciparum malaria, intravascular hemolysis, leptospirosis, lupus erythematosus, paroxysmal nocturnal hemoglobinuria, septicemia, sickle cell anemia, thrombosis, transfusion reaction, and traumatic hemolysis. Drugs include analgesics, antimalarials, cinchona alkaloids, nitrofurantoins, sulfonamides, and sulfones.

Positive in Urine. Autoimmune hemolytic anemia, blackwater fever, bladder irrigation, burns, *Clostridium perfringens* infection, disseminated intravascular coagulation, hemolytic anemia, kidney infarctions, malaria, paroxysmal nocturnal hemoglobinuria, poisonings, pregnancy, transfusion reaction, and transurethral prostatectomy. Drugs include arsenic, bacitracin, ciprofloxacin, coumadin, cyclophosphamide, fenoprofen, gold salts, indomethacin, mebendazole, nitrofurantoin, phenacetin, phenothiazines, phenylbutazone, polymyxin B, quinine, and suprofen.

Description. Free hemoglobin is hemoglobin that escapes from erythrocytes during intravascular hemolysis. A small amount of hemoglobin is normally present, but it is raised in the bloodstream and urine after massive hemolysis.

Professional Considerations
1. Consent form NOT required.
2. **Preparation:**
   A. Tube: Red topped, red/gray topped, or gold topped, and green topped for plasma sample.
   B. Obtain a sterile plastic specimen container for the urine sample.
   C. If the female client is menstruating, reschedule the urine test.
3. **Procedure:**
   A. *Plasma:* Do NOT draw from an extremity with intravenous solution infusing. Draw the blood sample using an 18-gauge needle with an attached infusion tubing as follows:
      i. Gently place the tourniquet around the upper arm. Follow this with venipuncture of the antecubital vein with as little trauma as possible.
      ii. Release the tourniquet and clamp the tubing as soon as flashback occurs.
      iii. Collect 3 mL of blood in the red-topped tube. Remove the top from the green-topped tube, and collect 5 mL of blood. Replace the top of the heparinized green-topped tube.
      iv. Clamp the tubing, withdraw the needle, and apply pressure to the venipuncture site.
   B. *Urine:* Obtain a 20-mL random urine specimen in a sterile plastic container.
4. **Postprocedure care:**
   A. *Plasma:* Send the specimen to the laboratory immediately. The plasma must be separated from the cells within 1-2 hours.
   B. *Urine:*
      i. Do not shake the specimen.
      ii. Dip a commercial dipstick in the urine and match the stick with a color block or chart, or send the stick to the laboratory immediately.
      iii. Refrigerate the specimen if the test is not performed within 1 hour.
5. **Client and family teaching:**
   A. Urinate before defecating and avoid contaminating the urine with toilet tissue.
6. **Factors that affect results:**
   A. Hemolysis of blood specimens invalidates the results. The specimen-collection procedure is critical because any damage to red blood cells can produce falsely elevated results.
   B. False-positive urine results may occur if the specimen is contaminated with menstrual blood.
   C. Ascorbic acid (or medications containing ascorbic acid as a preservative, such as antibiotics) may cause false-negative urine tests by inhibiting reagent activity.
   D. Bromides, copper, iodides, and oxidizing agents cause false-positive urine tests.
7. **Other data:**
   A. If plasma hemoglobin levels are increased, encourage periods of rest to preserve usable hemoglobin.
   B. Free hemoglobin can often be detected in the urine when red blood cells cannot because they lyse in strongly alkaline or dilute urine.
   C. The urine test is often part of a routine analysis.

HEMOGLOBIN PROFILE, ARTERIAL OR VENOUS, BLOOD
(see CO-oximeter profile, Arterial or venous, Blood)

HEMOGLOBIN, UNSTABLE, HEAT-LABILE TEST, BLOOD

Norm. <5% (<0.05 factor, SI units).

Increased. Heinz-body anemia and iron deficiency anemia.

Description. Unstable hemoglobin is a type of hemoglobin, normally absent, that precipitates faster than normal hemoglobin. After precipitation, unstable hemoglobin forms Heinz bodies, inclusions attached to erythrocyte membranes that increase the fragility of the red blood cell and lead to hemolysis. In Heinz-body and iron deficiency anemia, a small percentage of hemoglobin becomes denatured when subjected to acid and heated to 50° C.

Professional Considerations
1. Consent form NOT required.
2. **Preparation:**
   A. Tubes: Two lavender topped.

3. Procedure:
   A. Draw a 3.5-mL blood sample in each of both tubes.
4. Postprocedure care:
   A. Invert the tube 10 times gently to mix the specimen.
5. Client and family teaching:
   A. Results are normally available within 24 hours.
6. Factors that affect results:
   A. Reject specimens received more than 3 hours after collection.
7. Other data:
   A. The test should be run with a normal control.

HEMOGLOBIN, UNSTABLE, ISOPROPANOL PRECIPITATION TEST, BLOOD

Norm. Negative. No precipitation at 40 minutes.

Positive. Heinz-body anemia and slight opacity at 10 minutes in the presence of hemoglobin H.

Description. Unstable hemoglobin is a type of hemoglobin, normally absent, that precipitates faster than normal hemoglobin. After precipitation, unstable hemoglobin forms Heinz bodies, inclusions attached to erythrocyte membranes that increase the fragility of the red blood cell and lead to hemolysis. Unstable hemoglobin is detectable when subjected to isopropanol.

Professional Considerations
1. Consent form NOT required.
2. Preparation:
   A. Inform the laboratory of the time the specimen will be arriving.
   B. Tube: Lavender topped.
3. Procedure:
   A. Draw a 2-mL blood sample.
4. Postprocedure care:
   A. Invert the sample gently 10 times to mix.
   B. Send the specimen to the laboratory immediately because the test must be run on fresh blood.
5. Client and family teaching:
   A. Results are normally available within 24 hours.
6. Factors that affect results:
   A. The presence of hemoglobin F may cause a false-positive result.

7. Other data:
   A. More sensitive than heat denaturization.

HEMOPHILIC FACTOR B, BLOOD
(see Factor IX, Blood)

HEMOSIDERIN STAIN (SIDEROCYTE STAIN), URINE

Norm. Negative.

Positive. Burns, cold hemagglutins, hemochromatosis, hemolytic anemia, hemosiderosis, megaloblastic anemia, paroxysmal nocturnal hemoglobinuria, pernicious anemia, renal tubular cell disintegration, sickle cell anemia, thalassemia major, and transfusions (multiple).

Description. Hemosiderin are iron-storage granules normally found in the liver cytoplasm, spleen, and bone marrow. Hemosiderin granules are not normally found in the urine because they are absorbed by the renal tubules. They appear in hemolytic processes, iron overload, and renal tubular damage. This test involves the microscopic examination of urine sediment for coarse granules of hemosiderin, which stain blue when potassium ferrocyanide is added to the sample.

Professional Considerations
1. Consent form NOT required.
2. Preparation:
   A. Obtain a sterile plastic specimen container.
3. Procedure:
   A. Collect the first 50 mL of the first morning void in a sterile plastic container.
4. Postprocedure care:
   A. Refrigerate the specimens.
5. Client and family teaching:
   A. There are no restrictions before the test.
6. Factors that affect results:
   A. Hemosiderin is not detected in alkaline urine.
7. Other data:
   A. Hemosiderin can also be present in pancreatitis with the breakdown of cells in the intraperitoneal cavity.

B. A liver or bone marrow biopsy is necessary for confirmation of primary hemochromatosis.

HEPATIC FUNCTION PANEL (HFP), BLOOD

Norm. See individual test listings: *Alanine aminotransferase, Albumin, Alkaline phosphatase, Aspartate aminotransferase, and Bilirubin (Total and Direct)*.

Usage. See individual test listings.

Description. The HFP is a term defined by The Centers for Medicare and Medicaid Services (CMS) in the United States to indicate a group of tests for which a bundled reimbursement is available. The panel is disease oriented, meaning that payment through Medicare is available only when the test is used to diagnose and monitor a disease and payment is not available when the test is used for screening purposes in clients who have no signs and symptoms. All the tests in the panel must be carried out when a BMP is prescribed.

Professional Considerations
1. Consent form NOT required.
2. Preparation:
   A. Tube: Red topped, red/gray topped, or gold topped and one blue topped
   B. Do NOT draw specimens during hemodialysis.
3. Procedure:
   A. Draw a 3- to 5-ml blood sample in each tube.
4. Postprocedure care:
   A. None.
5. Client and family teaching:
   A. See individual test listings.
6. Factors that affect results:
   A. See individual test listings.
7. Other data:
   A. See individual test listings.

HEPATITIS A ANTIBODY, IgM AND IgG (HAV-ab), BLOOD

Norm. Negative.

Positive. Hepatitis A and jaundice.

Description. IgM is a marker for the hepatitis A virus that appears 2-4 weeks after exposure and is detectable for only 4-8 weeks. It does differentiate between an acute infection and a past or preexisting infection. IgG replaces IgM, and these antibodies persist for life, providing immunity from reinfection of hepatitis A. Hepatitis A is usually transmitted through the fecal-oral route.

Professional Considerations
1. Consent form NOT required.
2. Preparation:
   A. See *Client and family teaching*.
   B. Tube: Red topped, red/gray topped, or gold topped.
   C. Screen the client for the use of herbal preparations or natural remedies such as Chinese *jin^1 bu^{2}huan^4* ('gold-inconvertible', Jin Bu Huan Anodyne Tablets, patent medicine with misidentified constituents: essence of *t'ienchi [tianqi]* flowers, "Noto-ginseng"; also *kombucha;* also *Lycopodium serratum,* or club moss; but with plant alkaloid levo-tetrahydropalmatine, a potent neuroactive substance) and Bougainvillea Wild (Nyctaginaceae: *Bougainvillaea*).
3. Procedure:
   A. Draw a 2-mL blood sample.
4. Postprocedure care:
   A. Remove the serum and freeze it if the blood will not be tested within 7 days.
5. Client and family teaching:
   A. Results may not be available for several days.
   B. A person cannot be infected more than once with hepatitis A.
   C. Hepatitis A can be prevented by good handwashing. Wash your hands well with soap and water and with rapid scrubbing action after urinating or defecating.
   D. Do not drink alcohol, beer, or wine or take medicine that contains acetaminophen or paracetamol for 3 weeks, or as specified by your physician.
6. Factors that affect results:
   A. If using the radioimmunoassay technique, injection of radionuclides within the last week may falsely elevate results.
   B. Herbs or natural remedies that may cause hepatitis include Chinese *in bu huan* (see above).
   C. Herbs or natural remedies that decrease hepatitis are Bougainvillea Wild (Nyctaginaceae).

H

7. **Other data:**
   A. This test requires 2 mL of serum.
   B. The serum is stable at room temperature for 7 days and indefinitely if frozen.
   C. In the United States, although over 50% of the population is positive for anti-HAV IgG, it is clinically insignificant.
   D. The presence of anti-HAV IgG does not rule out acute hepatitis B or non-A, non-B hepatitis.
   E. Screening for HAV and HBV is recommended with elevated serum transaminase levels.

HEPATITIS B CORE ANTIBODY (ANTI-HBc), BLOOD

Norm. Negative.

Positive. Hepatitis B.

Description. Hepatitis B core antibody is the antibody marker that arises 1-2 weeks after contraction of the hepatitis B virus, rises during the chronic phase of the illness, and remains present for life. It is the most reliable test to determine the presence of hepatitis B infection in the absence of hepatitis B surface antibody and hepatitis B surface antigen.

Professional Considerations
1. Consent form NOT required.
2. **Preparation:**
   A. Tube: Red topped, red/gray topped, or gold topped.
   B. Screen the client for the use of herbal preparations or natural remedies such as Chinese $jin^1bu^2huan^4$ ('gold-inconvertible', Jin Bu Huan Anodyne Tablets, patent medicine with misidentified constituents: essence of *t'ienchi [tianqi]* flowers, "Noto-ginseng"; also *kombucha;* also *Lycopodium serratum,* or club moss; but with plant alkaloid levo-tetrahydropalmatine, a potent neuroactive substance), and Bougainvillea Wild (Nyctaginaceae: *Bougainvillaea*).
3. **Procedure:**
   A. Draw a 3-mL blood sample.
4. **Postprocedure care:**
   A. Remove the serum and freeze it if the blood will not be tested within 7 days.

5. **Client and family teaching:**
   A. Results may not be available for several days.
   B. Hepatitis B can be spread by blood and other body fluids, including the sharing of needles and sexual contact. An infected mother can pass the infection on to her baby.
   C. To help prevent spreading hepatitis B, wash your hands well with soap and water and use rapid scrubbing action after urinating or defecating.
   D. Do not drink alcohol, beer, or wine or take medicine that contains acetaminophen or paracetamol for 3 weeks, or as specified by your physician.
6. **Factors that affect results:**
   A. If the radioimmunoassay technique is used, the injection of radionuclides within the last week may falsely elevate results.
   B. Herbs or natural remedies that may cause hepatitis include Chinese *jin bu huan* (see above).
   C. Herbs or natural remedies that decrease hepatitis are Bougainvillea Wild (Nyctaginaceae).
7. **Other data:**
   A. The serum is stable at room temperature for 7 days and indefinitely if frozen.

HEPATITIS B e ANTIBODY (ANTI-HBe, HBeAb), SERUM

Norm. Negative.

Positive. Hepatitis B.

Description. Hepatitis B e antibody is a serum marker for hepatitis B that appears 8-16 weeks after infection and indicates resolution of acute infection. The presence of this antibody in clients with chronic positive hepatitis B surface antigen indicates an asymptomatic, healthy carrier.

Professional Considerations
1. Consent form NOT required.
2. **Preparation:**
   A. See *Client and family teaching.*
   B. Tube: Red topped, red/gray topped, or gold topped.
   C. Screen the client for the use of herbal preparations or natural

remedies such as jin¹bu²huan⁴ ('gold-inconvertible', Jin Bu Huan Anodyne Tablets, patent medicine with misidentified constituents: essence of *t'ienchi [tianqi]* flowers, "Noto-ginseng"; also *kombucha*; also *Lycopodium serratum,* or club moss; but with plant alkaloid levo-tetrahydropalmatine, a potent neuroactive substance) and Bougainvillea Wild (Nyctaginaceae: *Bougainvillaea*).
3. Procedure:
   A. Draw a 2-mL blood sample.
4. Postprocedure care:
   A. Remove the serum and freeze it if the blood will not be tested within 7 days.
5. Client and family teaching:
   A. Results may not be available for several days.
6. Factors that affect results:
   A. If the radioimmunoassay technique is used, injection of radionuclides within the previous week may falsely elevate results.
   B. An herb or natural remedy that may cause hepatitis includes Chinese *jin bu huan* (see above).
   C. An herb or natural remedy that decreases hepatitis is Bougainvillea Wild (Nyctaginaceae: *Bougainvillaea*).
7. Other data:
   A. The serum is stable at room temperature for 7 days and indefinitely if frozen.
   B. The test is more meaningful when measured in conjunction with hepatitis B e antigen.
   C. The test should be prescribed only in clients with documented recent infection of hepatitis B.

HEPATITIS B e ANTIGEN (HBeAg), BLOOD

Norm. Negative.

Positive. Hepatitis B.

Description. Usually appearing within 4-12 weeks of infection, hepatitis B e antigen is one of the first indicators of hepatitis B infection, usually preceding symptoms and representing the greatest threat of transmission. It is usually pres-

ent for only 3-6 weeks. Persistence of the antigen for greater than 3 months is suggestive of chronic liver disease.

Professional Considerations
1. Consent form NOT required.
2. Preparation:
   A. Tube: Red topped, red/gray topped, or gold topped.
   B. Screen the client for the use of herbal preparations or natural remedies such as Chinese *jin bu huan* and Bougainvillea Wild.
3. Procedure:
   A. Draw a 2-mL blood sample.
4. Postprocedure care:
   A. Remove the serum and freeze it if the blood will not be tested within 7 days.
5. Client and family teaching:
   A. Results may not be available for several days.
6. Factors that affect results:
   A. If the radioimmunoassay technique is used, injection of radionuclides within the previous week may falsely elevate results.
   B. An herb or natural remedy that may cause hepatitis includes Chinese *jin bu huan* (see above).
   C. An herb or natural remedy that decreases hepatitis is Bougainvillea Wild (Nyctaginaceae: *Bougainvillaea*).
7. Other data:
   A. The serum is stable at room temperature for 7 days and indefinitely if frozen.
   B. Clients with chronic positive tests should also be tested for the hepatitis B e core antibody, which indicates that the client is an asymptomatic, healthy carrier.
   C. A hepatitis B vaccine is available and recommended for health care workers who may come into contact with blood and body fluids.

HEPATITIS B SURFACE ANTIBODY (HBsAB), BLOOD

Norm. Negative.

Positive. Hepatitis B.

Description. This marker appears 2-16 weeks after hepatitis B surface antigen has disappeared. It usually represents clinical recovery and immunity to the virus. It will also be present during passive transfer in blood by transfusion or by administration of hepatitis B immune globulin (HBIG). Presence of the hepatitis B surface antibody along with the hepatitis B surface antigen indicates a poor prognosis.

Professional Considerations

1. Consent form NOT required.
2. Preparation:
   A. Tube: Red topped, red/gray topped, or gold topped.
   B. Screen the client for the use of herbal preparations or natural remedies such as Chinese *jin bu huan* and Bougainvillea Wild (Nyctaginaceae: *Bougainvillaea*).
3. Procedure:
   A. Draw a 3-mL blood sample.
4. Postprocedure care:
   A. Remove the serum and freeze it if the blood will not be tested within 7 days.
5. Client and family teaching:
   A. Results may not be available for several days.
6. Factors that affect results:
   A. If the radioimmunoassay technique is used, injection of radionuclides within the previous week may falsely elevate results.
   B. An herb or natural remedy that may cause hepatitis includes *jin bu huan* (see above).
   C. An herb or natural remedy that decreases hepatitis is Bougainvillea Wild (Nyctaginaceae: *Bougainvillaea*).
7. Other data:
   A. The serum is stable at room temperature for 7 days and indefinitely if frozen.
   B. There is a high prevalence of positive tests among intravenous drug abusers.

HEPATITIS B SURFACE ANTIGEN (HBsAG:HAA), BLOOD

Norm. Negative.

Positive. Hepatitis B.

Description. The hepatitis B surface antigen usually appears between 4 and 12 weeks of infection. It is indicative of active hepatitis B, either acute or chronic. It is the earliest indicator of hepatitis B, often preceding clinical symptoms. Presence of the hepatitis B surface antibody along with the hepatitis B surface antigen indicates a poor prognosis.

This test, required by the Food and Drug Administration when clients wish to donate blood, has helped reduce the incidence of hepatitis.

Professional Considerations

1. Consent form NOT required.
2. Preparation:
   A. Tube: Red topped, red/gray topped, or gold topped.
   B. Screen the client for the use of herbal preparations or natural remedies such as Chinese *jin bu huan* and Bougainvillea Wild (Nyctaginaceae: *Bougainvillaea*).
3. Procedure:
   A. Draw a 2-mL blood sample.
4. Postprocedure care:
   A. Remove the serum and freeze it if the blood will not be tested within 7 days.
5. Client and family teaching:
   A. If the client is giving blood, explain the donation procedure.
   B. Results may not be available for several days.
6. Factors that affect results:
   A. If the radioimmunoassay technique is used, injection of radionuclides within the previous week may falsely elevate results.
   B. An herb or natural remedy that may cause hepatitis includes Chinese *jin bu huan* (see above).
   C. An herb or natural remedy that decreases hepatitis is Bougainvillea Wild (Nyctaginaceae: *Bougainvillaea*).
7. Other data:
   A. The serum is stable at room temperature for 7 days and indefinitely if frozen.
   B. This test does not screen for hepatitis A, hepatitis C, or non-A, non-B viruses.
   C. HBsAG may also be present in more than 5% of clients with Down syndrome, hemophilia, Hodgkin's disease, and leukemia.
   D. When HBsAG is found in donor blood, it must be discarded because it carries a 40-70% chance of transmitting hepatitis.

E. Report confirmed viral hepatitis to public health authorities.

HEPATITIS C ANTIBODY, SERUM

Norm. Negative.

Positive. Hepatitis C and non-A, non-B hepatitis.

Description. An assay to identify antibodies of the IgG class to the hepatitis C virus, a newly identified gene to a ribonucleic acid (RNA) virus that does not have the qualities of either hepatitis A or hepatitis B; 20% of posttransfusion hepatitis falls into this category. Causes include intravenous drug use and abuse, transfusions, dialysis, and needle sticks.

Professional Considerations
1. Consent form NOT required.
2. Preparation:
   A. Tube: Red topped, red/gray topped, or gold topped.
   B. Screen the client for the use of herbal preparations or natural remedies such as Chinese *jin bu huan* and Bougainvillea Wild (Nyctaginaceae: *Bougainvillaea*).
3. Procedure:
   A. Draw a 2-mL blood sample.
4. Postprocedure care:
   A. Remove the serum and freeze it if the blood will not be tested within 7 days.
5. Client and family teaching:
   A. If the client is giving blood, explain the donation procedure.
   B. Results may not be available for several days.
6. Factors that affect results:
   A. If the radioimmunoassay technique is used, injection of radionuclides within the previous week may falsely elevate results.
   B. An herb or natural remedy that may cause hepatitis includes Chinese *jin bu huan* (see above).
   C. An herb or natural remedy that decreases hepatitis is Bougainvillea Wild (Nyctaginaceae: *Bougainvillaea*).
7. Other data:
   A. This test requires 0.5 mL of serum.
   B. The serum is stable at room temperature for 7 days and indefinitely if frozen.

C. Notify public health authorities if the test results are positive.
D. Up to now, there has been no commercially available serologic test to detect hepatitis C antigen (HCAg).

HEPATITIS C GENOTYPE (HCV GENOTYPE), SERUM

Norm. Negative

Usage. Genotyping of the hepatitis C virus (HCV)–affected RNA is utilized, in conjunction with a client's clinical presentation and other laboratory findings, to determine a treatment plan and a client's prognosis and to assist in identifying a cause for clients with a diagnosis of hepatitis C.

Increased. Identification of hepatitis C genotype subtype 1a, 1b,

Decreased. 1c, 2a, 2b, 2c, 3a, 3b, 4a-h, 5a, and 6a.

Positive. Individual tests may yield additional genotypes.

Description. HCV is a genus from the family of Flaviviridae. Its RNA is single stranded and has heterogeneous subtypes. Nucleic acid sequencing determines the type and subtype of the viral genome. Treatment decisions are based on the specific genotype identified in the affected HCV RNA. Clients with chronic HCV are at a greater risk for development of cirrhosis and hepatocellular carcinoma. Genotype I runs a more severe course and has a faster progression.

Professional Considerations
1. Consent form NOT required.
2. Preparation:
   A. Tube: Lavender or gold top.
   B. Specimens may not be drawn during hemodialysis.
   C. Screen the client for the use of herbal preparations or natural remedies such as Chinese *jin*[1]*bu*[2]*huan*[4] ('gold-inconvertible', Jin Bu Huan Anodyne Tablets, patent medicine with misidentified constituents: essence of *t'ienchi [tianqi]* flowers, "Notoginseng"; also *kombucha*; also

H

Lycopodium serratum, or club moss; but with plant alkaloid levo-tetrahydropalmatine, a potent neuroactive substance) and Bougainvillea Wild (Nyctaginaceae: *Bougainvillaea*).

3. Procedure:
   A. Collect 2 mL of blood (minimum 0.5 mL).
   B. Transport specimen in ice immediately to laboratory.
4. Postprocedure care:
   A. None.
5. Client and family teaching:
   A. A complete history should be obtained before testing to identify possible causes of HCV.
   B. Treatment options should be explained to client on receipt of the results. Special attention to the possible side effects of the antiviral agents should be provided.
6. Factors that affect results:
   A. Qualitative (detect circulating HCV RNA) and quantitative (measure the circulating HCV RNA) should be completed before genotyping. (Samples containing less than 1000 RNA copies/mL may not be suitable for genotype testing.)
   B. HCV genotyping is not effective in clients with mixed hepatitis types (hepatitis A and B); the test will be read as indeterminate.
   C. Heparinized collection tubes or clients receiving heparin will render the test invalid and will be read as indeterminate.
   D. An herb or natural remedy that may cause hepatitis includes Chinese *jin bu huan* (see above).
   E. An herb or natural remedy that decreases hepatitis is Bougainvillea Wild (Nyctaginaceae: *Bougainvillaea*).
7. Other data:
   A. Genotypes 1 and 4 are associated with more complicated disease and are less responsive to interferon treatment as compared to genotypes 2 and 3, especially in African Americans with chronic hepatitis C.
   B. Antiviral agent ribavirin may be an adjunctive therapy option in chronic HCV and may be considered in more complicated cases in addition to treatment with interferon.

C. Non-A, non-B HCV is most frequently the origin of parenterally induced hepatitis.

HEPATITIS DELTA ANTIBODY (TOTAL ANTI-HDV), SERUM

Norm. Negative.

Positive. Hepatitis D.

Description. An assay to identify total (that is, predominantly IgG) antibodies to the hepatitis D virus. Hepatitis D is an incomplete virus requiring the presence of HBsAg of the hepatitis B virus for replication and expression. It infects only clients concurrently infected with hepatitis B virus or those who have a preexisting hepatitis B virus infection. Hepatitis D virus is most common among intravenous drug abusers, hemophiliacs, and clients who have received multiple blood transfusions. It is a more severe form of hepatitis than hepatitis B alone, accounting for a higher incidence of chronic hepatitis and cirrhosis.

Clinically, hepatitis D virus cannot be distinguished from other types of hepatitis. Serologic tests must be positive for hepatitis B virus and total anti-HDV to make a diagnosis of hepatitis D. Hepatitis D virus is not a reportable disease in most of the United States at the present time.

Professional Considerations

1. Consent form NOT required.
2. Preparation:
   A. Tube: Red topped, red/gray topped, or gold topped.
   B. Screen the client for the use of herbal preparations or natural remedies such as Chinese *jin[1]bu[2]huan[4]* ('gold-inconvertible', Jin Bu Huan Anodyne Tablets, patent medicine with misidentified constituents: essence of *t'ienchi [tianqi]* flowers, "Noto-ginseng"; also *kombucha;* also *Lycopodium serratum,* or club moss; but with plant alkaloid levo-tetrahydropalmatine, a potent neuroactive substance) and Bougainvillea Wild (Nyctaginaceae: *Bougainvillaea*).
3. Procedure:
   A. Draw a 3-mL blood sample.

4. **Postprocedure care:**
   A. Remove the serum and freeze it if the blood will not be tested within 7 days.
5. **Client and family teaching:**
   A. Results may not be available for several days.
6. **Factors that affect results:**
   A. If the radioimmunoassay technique is used, injection of radionuclides within the previous week may falsely elevate results.
   B. Clients with lipemia or high-titer rheumatoid factor may have false-positive results.
   C. An herb or natural remedy that may cause hepatitis includes Chinese *jin bu huan* (see above).
   D. An herb or natural remedy that decreases hepatitis is Bougainvillea Wild (Nyctaginaceae: *Bougainvillaea*).
7. **Other data:**
   A. This test requires 2 mL of serum.
   B. Serum is stable at room temperature for 7 days and indefinitely if frozen.
   C. Blood is potentially infectious during all phases of active infection.
   D. Clients who test positive for HBsAg are at risk for hepatitis D; however, immunity to hepatitis B virus provides immunity to hepatitis D virus.
   E. Mortality is 30% in chronic cases.
   F. In rare cases, HBsAg may be transiently undetectable in serum, resulting in an erroneous diagnosis of non-A, non-B hepatitis, unless specific testing for hepatitis D is performed.
   G. Up to now, there has been no commercially available serologic test to detect hepatitis D antigen (HDAg).

HEPATOBILIARY SCAN (HIDA SCAN), DIAGNOSTIC

Norm. Negative. Requires interpretation by a radiologist.

Normal anatomy and physiology of liver, spleen, and biliary tract as determined by a radiologist. Normal distribution of injectate: 86% in reticuloendothelial system (RES) of liver, 6% in spleen, 8% in RES of bone marrow.

Hepatobiliary (scan after IV injection of ^{99m}Tc-dimethylacetic acid): First-hour images show liver, cardiac, and vascular activity; gallbladder (GB) and common bile duct/bowel activity seen by 60 minutes. GB uptake should precede bowel visualization. An inflamed gallbladder will not take up radionuclide. In the presence of biliary tree obstruction, no radionuclide will be visualized beyond the point of obstruction.

Liver-spleen (scan after IV injection of technetium-99m radionuclide): Uniform uptake throughout liver and spleen. Decreased uptake, or "cold spots," seen in areas with space-occupying lesions such as in Caroli's disease. Increased blood flow to the liver will be evidenced by increased radionuclide uptake, or "hot spots."

Usage. Used to visualize biliary tract and to detect acute acalculous, acute cholecystitis and calculous cholecystitis (caused by obstruction of cystic ducts), hepatocellular disease, gallbladder disease, jaundice, liver cancer, liver metastasis, obstruction, and perihepatic abscess; used to study biliary kinetics (biliary dyskinesia, gallbladder ejection fraction); evaluates patency of biliary system and cystic duct, including post surgically, and nonspecifically demonstrates focal disease as "cold spots" of non uptake of the radionuclide. Evaluation of pediatric jaundice (choledochocyst; biliary atresia versus neonatal hepatitis); congenital bronchobiliary fistula; conditions causing increased flow to the liver will appear as "hot spots."

Description. The hepatobiliary scan is a radionuclide study that demonstrates hepatic parenchyma, extrahepatic bile ducts, gallbladder, and normal passage into the intestines as well as the position, size, and shape of the liver. Intravenously injected HIDA, a radionuclide, travels through the liver into the biliary system, enabling gamma camera imaging of the entire hepatobiliary system. The cells of the liver absorb the radionuclide within 30 minutes and can be observed on the scan before it is redeposited in the bloodstream and excreted. Dye is excreted in the bile, stored briefly in the gallbladder, and eliminated through the intestine, all within 4 hours. Failure of the dye to appear in the intestines is indicative of obstruction.

Professional Considerations
1. Consent form IS required.

Risks
Infection.

Contraindications
During pregnancy or breast-feeding; in children.

2. Preparation:
   A. Establish intravenous access.
   B. Have emergency equipment readily available.
   C. See *Client and family teaching*.
3. Procedure:
   A. The client is injected with radionuclide (usually ^{99m}Tc-IDA, the dose calculated by body weight) intravenously 30 minutes before the scan.
   B. Delay imaging for 6-48 hours after injection for clients known to have hepatocellular disease.
   C. The client is positioned supine on the scanning table during the scan.
   D. A gamma camera is placed over the right upper quadrant of the abdomen.
   E. Scintiphotos are obtained at 15, 30, 60, and 90 minutes after injection of the radiopharmaceutical.
   F. The procedure is repeated at 2-6 hours and 24 hours if obstruction is suspected or when the biliary system was not visualized.
4. Postprocedure care:
   A. For 24 hours after the procedure wear rubber gloves when discarding urine. Wash the gloved hands with soap and water before removing the gloves. Wash the hands again after the gloves have been removed.
5. Client and family teaching:
   A. Fast from food and fluids for 4-6 hours before the scan.

B. The scan takes 1.0-1.5 hours.
C. Report any sensations that might indicate an allergic reaction such as itching or difficulty in breathing.
D. Meticulously wash the hands with soap and water after each void for 24 hours after the procedure.
E. Results are normally available from the physician within 24 hours.
6. Factors that affect results:
   A. The scan must be performed promptly after the injection because radionuclides have a short transit time through the liver.
   B. Do not schedule any other radionuclear scans within 24 hours of this scan.
   C. If client has just eaten, the gallbladder will be contracted and may not fill with HIDA, giving a false-positive study for acute cholecystitis. If the client has not eaten for many hours, the gallbladder may be full of bile or sludge and may not fill with HIDA, also giving a false-positive study.
   D. Total parenteral nutrition may also result in impaired visualization of the gallbladder.
   E. The presence of barium in the intestinal tract may inhibit gallbladder visualization.
7. Other data:
   A. Health care professionals working in a nuclear medicine area must follow federal standards set by the Nuclear Regulatory Commission. These standards include precautions for handling the radioactive material and monitoring potential radiation exposure.

HER-2/*neu* ONCOGENE (C-*erb*-S, HUMAN EPIDERMAL GROWTH FACTOR), SPECIMEN

Norm. Normally present in cell membranes as a single DNA copy. Must be interpreted by a pathologist.

Positive. Presence of either or both molecular genetic alterations:

Gene amplification	Multiple DNA copies, characterized by in situ fluorescence hybridization
Gene overexpression	Characterized by membrane immunostaining by immunohistochemistry

Negative. Absence of gene amplification or overexpression.

Usage. Determination of genetic abnormalities in effort to predict client response to hormonal therapy, adjuvant chemotherapy, and monoclonal antibody therapy.

Increased (Overexpressed). Brain cancer, breast cancer (predictive of poor short-term prognosis but can benefit from Herceptin therapy), colorectal cancer (predicts poor survival), malignant mesothelioma, non–small-cell lung cancer, ovarian cancer, and endometrial carcinoma, uterine serous papillary carcinoma.

Description. HER-2/*neu* is a gene that codes for a transmembrane tyrosine kinase. Amplification of the gene product is noted in up to 30% of breast, ovarian, and endometrial carcinomas. High levels of the gene product are associated with low estrogen and progesterone receptor concentration, and clients have little or no response to hormonal therapy. HER-2/*neu* overexpression is a phenotypic marker for comedocarcinoma, a subtype of intraductal carcinoma with necrosis. It is associated with increased risk of relapse and decreased survival time. Breast cancer clients with overexpression of HER-2/*neu* have a better response to doxorubicin HCl (Adriamycin)-based chemotherapy regimens. The predictive value of HER-2/*neu* is true only with node-positive disease. In clients with endometrial carcinoma, HER-2/*neu* is also associated with shorter overall survival. Testing for HER-2/*neu* overexpression is useful when one is predicting which clients will have a response to monoclonal antibodies directed against HER-2/*neu*. HER-2/*neu* is measured by several techniques including gene amplification, mRNA level, and immunohistochemical staining. Immunohistochemistry may be performed on serum, plasma, and fresh or paraffin-embedded tissue, but fresh tissue is the specimen of choice.

Professional Considerations. (See *Biopsy, Site-specific,* for technique steps for obtaining the tissue specimen.) The considerations that follow are specific to the correct processing of tissue to maximize accurate results.

1. Consent IS required if biopsy is performed; see *Biopsy, Site-specific, Specimen,* for risks and contraindications.
2. Preparation:
   A. Obtain solid-tumor biopsy bottle for tissue specimen (fluorescent pink).
   B. If paraffin block is to be made, obtain container with 10% formalin.
3. Procedure:
   A. Obtain tissue specimen by desired procedure or draw blood and place in appropriate container.
   B. Cut tissue into small pieces and quick freeze on dry ice, in cryostat, or in liquid nitrogen within 20 minutes of collection. Place in biopsy bottle or formalin if paraffin block to be made.
   C. If paraffin block is to be assayed, it must be fixed for 12-24 hours, not to exceed 48 hours.
4. Postprocedure care:
   A. Apply clean, sterile dressing to biopsy site.
   B. Assess the site and vital signs for signs of bleeding. The frequency may vary with the physician. Generally, assess every 15 minutes the first hour, every 30 minutes the second hour, and then every hour × 4.
   C. Observe for signs of infection (fever, chills, hypotension, tachycardia, inflammation at site) for 24-48 hours.
5. Client and family teaching:
   A. Provide emotional support to the client awaiting results.
   B. If biopsy confirms cancer, additional tests will be prescribed to determine appropriate treatment.
   C. Results may not be available for several days.
6. Factors that may affect results:
   A. Dried specimens must be discarded.
   B. Frozen tissue thawed.
   C. Use of fixative other than 10% formalin.
   D. Reagents with a high degree of sensitivity and specificity to HER-2/*neu* in paraffin-embedded tissues should be selected for this test, or the sensitivity of the reagent used should be characterized to correctly interpret the significance of the test results. Studies have shown wide variability in the efficacy of the various antibody reagents currently in use. The use of more than one antibody (that is,

H

antibody "cocktails") may also improve immunostaining.

7. Other data:
   A. The use and application of this test are still investigational, and the test is not yet routinely prescribed. Therefore testing is likely to be performed on archival tissue samples, making the preprocedural and intraprocedural steps above not applicable.
   B. Clients showing amplification may qualify for clinical trials using murine monoclonal antibodies, produced against the HER-2/*neu* receptor to inhibit tumor cell replication.
   C. Further studies of HER-2/*neu* amplification and overexpression promise to give insights into possible prevention, detection, and treatment strategies of cancers in which these genetic alterations occur.

HEROIN, URINE

Norm. Negative.

Positive. With heroin use the urine is >2 ng/mL.

> **Overdose Symptoms and Treatment**
>
> Symptoms. Bradycardia, euphoria, flushing, itching, hypotension, hypothermia, respiratory depression.
>
> Treatment:
> Note: Treatment choice(s) depend on client history and condition and episode history.
> Naloxone (Narcan).
> Hemodialysis will NOT remove heroin.

Description. Heroin (diacetylmorphine), a drug of abuse, is made from morphine. The half-life is 1.7-4.5 hours. Heroin is rapidly metabolized back into morphine, and up to 67% of the dose is excreted in the urine as morphine or morphine glucuronides; 50% is excreted in the urine in the first 8 hours and 90% in the first 24 hours.

Professional Considerations

1. Consent form NOT required unless results may be used as legal evidence.
2. Preparation:
   A. Obtain clean urine cup.
   B. If the specimen may be used as legal evidence, have the specimen collection witnessed.
3. Procedure:
   A. Obtain 50 mL of random urine in a clean container.
4. Postprocedure care:
   A. Store samples at −20° C.
   B. If the specimen may be used as legal evidence, write the client's name, date, exact time of collection, and specimen source on the laboratory requisition. Sign, and have the witness sign, the laboratory requisition. Transport the specimen to the laboratory immediately in a sealed plastic bag marked as legal evidence. All clients handling the specimen should sign and write the time of receipt on the laboratory requisition.
5. Client and family teaching:
   A. Refer clients with intentional overdose for crisis intervention.
   B. Referrals to appropriate rehabilitation centers and therapeutic community programs should be offered to all addicted clients who may be interested.
6. Factors that affect results:
   A. False-positive results occur if the client ingested 20 mg of codeine cough syrup or 5-15 g of poppy seeds 24 hours before the sample was obtained.
   B. Heroin is eliminated from the system in 2 days, but quinine, which is a nonnarcotic used as a diluent, may stay in the system for up to 1 week.
7. Other data:
   A. Street heroin is generally 5-10% actual heroin, with the usual euphoric dose taken by abusers equivalent to 10-20 mg of morphine.
   B. Common complications of overdose are pulmonary edema, endocarditis, *Clostridium botulinum* infection, and septicemia.

HERPES CULTURE, SPECIMEN
(*see Viral culture, Specimen*)

HERPES CYTOLOGY, SPECIMEN

Norm. Negative.

Positive. Genital herpes, herpes virus infection, meningitis, and vaginitis.

Description. Herpes simplex virus types 1 and 2 are two similar viruses but differ slightly in structure. Herpes simplex virus type 1 is generally found in the respiratory tract, eyes, or mouth (cold sores), and herpes simplex virus type 2 is found in the genitourinary tract (transmitted by sexual contact, or during childbirth for infants). Both viruses have been isolated in both locations. Cytology is the examination of cells under a microscope to establish the presence of the virus, which is seen as multinucleated epithelial cells with enlarged atypical nuclei. This can be performed using a Papanicolaou test and has an average sensitivity of 45-50%.

Professional Considerations
1. Consent form NOT required.
2. **Preparation:**
   A. Obtain a sterile tongue depressor or swab, slides, and a 95% ethyl alcohol (ethanol) fixative.
3. **Procedure:**
   A. Scrape the lesion with the sterile tongue depressor.
   B. Spread the scrapings evenly on the slide with the tongue depressor, or roll the specimen onto the slide using the swab.
4. **Postprocedure care:**
   A. Fix the slide with the 95% ethyl alcohol fixative.
   B. Deliver the specimen to the laboratory within 1 hour.
   C. The final report for a negative culture takes 5 days.
5. **Client and family teaching:**
   A. If the client is pregnant, a cesarean section may be required if the virus is still present at the time of delivery. The risk of miscarriage is higher than normal in women infected with genital herpes.
   B. Pain from sores may be treated with mild analgesics, warm baths, or wet tea bags held over the site.
   C. Safe sex practices to prevent transmission to partner(s):
      i. Notify all sexual partners to be tested for the virus.
      ii. Do not have sex when blisters or sores are present. These usually take about 4 weeks to clear up completely.
      iii. Use a condom during all sexual activity, even if sores are not present. Spermicides con-

taining nonoxynol-9 help kill the herpesvirus.
   D. Antivirals may reduce viral shedding and relieve skin discomfort.
   E. Lesions of confused clients should be covered with a dressing to prevent autoinoculation (spread from one site to another).
6. **Factors that affect results:**
   A. Air drying or improper fixative will cause the laboratory to reject the specimen.
   B. Smears with heavy inflammatory exudate are difficult to interpret because of the nonspecific staining technique.
7. **Other data:**
   A. Viral serologic testing is more definitive, but serologic testing in herpes simplex virus is of little practical importance in clients with HIV because most are seropositive.
   B. 50% of active lesions may not demonstrate herpes inclusions.
   C. Lesions that are dry may be moistened with saline before being scraped.

HERPES SIMPLEX ANTIBODY, BLOOD

Norm. Negative, <0.25 by ELISA, or <1:10.

Positive. 1:10–1:100 indicates infection within 7 days; 1:100–1:500 current-to-late infection; >1:500 established latent infection.

Usage. Genital herpes, herpes simplex, and herpes zoster virus infection.

Description. See *Herpes cytology, Specimen,* for description of the virus characteristics. Peak antibody levels are reached 4-6 weeks after inoculation with the virus and decline and stabilize thereafter. The serum sample is incubated onto a solid phase, and enzyme activity is quantitated and compared to a set of controls.

Professional Considerations
1. Consent form NOT required.
2. **Preparation:**
   A. Tube: Red topped, red/gray topped, or gold topped.
3. **Procedure:**
   A. Draw a 10-mL blood sample.

4. Postprocedure care:
   A. Deliver the sample to the laboratory within 1 hour.
5. Client and family teaching:
   A. See *Herpes cytology, Specimen.*
6. Factors that affect results:
   A. Hemolysis of the specimen invalidates the results.
   B. Herpes simplex virus type 1, herpes simplex virus type 2, and varicella zoster may cross-react, but the antibody rise in the infecting virus usually exceeds that of the other antibodies.
7. Other data:
   A. Diagnosis of a current infection should not be made based on the results of a single serum analysis. Collection of two samples, 10-14 days apart, is recommended.

HERPES VIRUS ANTIGEN, DIRECT FLUORESCENT ANTIBODY, SPECIMEN

Norm. Negative.

Usage. Cervicitis, encephalitis, and herpes simplex.

Description. See *Herpes cytology, Specimen,* for description of the characteristics of the virus. If emergent diagnosis is necessary (such as encephalitis), this is the most rapid and sensitive test if cytology findings are negative. The specimen is examined by immunofluorescence or immunoperoxidase technique.

Professional Considerations
1. Consent form NOT required.
2. Preparation:
   A. Obtain a sterile swab and a sterile specimen container or Culturette.
3. Procedure:
   A. Collect the specimen from the infected site as described above.
   B. Do NOT place the specimen in a fixative.
4. Postprocedure care:
   A. Send the sample to the laboratory immediately or freeze it. This includes operative specimens and spinal fluid specimens.
   B. This test should be performed immediately, day or night, and the laboratory should be notified of arriving specimens.
5. Client and family teaching:
   A. See *Herpes cytology, Specimen.*
   B. Results are normally available within 24 hours.
6. Factors that affect results:
   A. Specimens will be rejected if placed in fixative.
   B. Inflammatory exudate on specimens will cause nonspecific color development of the immunoperoxidase reagent.
7. Other data:
   A. None.

HETEROPHIL AGGLUTININS, BLOOD

Norm. Negative.

Positive. Cytomegalic inclusion disease (by cytomegalovirus), infectious mononucleosis (by Epstein-Barr virus), serum sickness, and toxoplasmosis.

Description. A heterophil antibody is capable of reacting with an antigen that is completely unrelated to the antigen originally stimulating its formation. This infectious mononucleosis screening procedure tests for the presence of agglutinins (indicated by clumping) reacting to the red blood cells of horses or sheep. Infectious mononucleosis is a viral infection characterized by fatigue, anorexia, swollen glands, fever, and sore throat. Symptoms may continue for up to 6 weeks. Mode of transmission is through person-to-person transmission of saliva through kissing, sneezing, or coughing. Generally, this test is positive 3-10 days after infection, peaks within 3 weeks, and can remain elevated for up to 1 year.

Professional Considerations
1. Consent form NOT required.
2. Preparation:
   A. Tube: Red topped, red/gray topped, or gold topped or lavender topped.
3. Procedure:
   A. Draw a 2.5-mL blood sample.
4. Postprocedure care:
   A. None.
5. Client and family teaching:
   A. For clients testing positive:

i. Drink plenty of fluids and eat a balanced diet, even if not hungry or thirsty.
ii. Use saltwater gargle for sore throat.
iii. Use the antipyretic recommended by the physician for fever.
iv. Get plenty of rest during the febrile period. Then limit physical activity for 5 weeks.
v. Isolation is not necessary, but avoid coughing or sneezing on or near other persons as well as kissing other persons until cleared by the physician.

6. **Factors that affect results:**
   A. Hemolysis of the specimen invalidates the results.
   B. This test may be falsely negative because of the occasional delay in the appearance of the agglutinins in the first 4 weeks after infection, despite the presence of clinical symptoms.
   C. False-positive results (<2%) have been reported with Hodgkin's disease, lymphoma, acute lymphocytic leukemia, infectious hepatitis, pancreatic cancer, cytomegalovirus, Burkitt's lymphoma, rheumatoid arthritis, malaria, and rubella.

7. **Other data:**
   A. With infectious mononucleosis, heterophil antibodies appear in 60% of clients within 2 weeks and in 90% within 4 weeks. Most titers decline in 3-6 months.
   B. 10% of true adult Epstein-Barr virus mononucleosis cases have negative heterophil agglutinins; the virus occurs more frequently in children. Epstein-Barr virus antibodies may occur in these cases.
   C. See also *Epstein-Barr virus, Serology, Blood.*

HETEROPHIL SCREEN
(*see Monospot screen, Blood*)

HFP
(*see Hepatic function panel, Blood*)

HIDA SCAN, DIAGNOSTIC
(*see Hepatobiliary scan, Diagnostic*)

HIGH-DENSITY LIPOPROTEIN (HDL) CHOLESTEROL (HDL-C), BLOOD

Norm:

HIGH-DENSITY LIPOPROTEIN CHOLESTEROL				
	MALE		**FEMALE**	
AGE (YEARS)	mg/dL	**SI UNITS** mmol/L	mg/dL	**SI UNITS** mmol/L
Adults				
20-24	30-63	0.78-1.63	33-79	0.85-2.04
25-29	31-63	0.80-1.63	37-83	0.96-2.15
30-34	28-63	0.72-1.63	36-77	0.93-1.99
35-39	29-62	0.75-1.60	34-82	0.88-2.12
40-44	27-67	0.70-1.73	34-88	0.88-2.28
45-49	30-64	0.78-1.66	34-87	0.88-2.25
50-54	28-63	0.72-1.63	37-92	0.96-2.38
55-59	28-71	0.72-1.84	37-91	0.96-2.35
60-64	30-74	0.78-1.91	38-92	0.98-2.38
65-69	30-75	0.78-1.94	35-96	0.91-2.48
>70	31-75	0.80-1.94	33-92	0.85-2.38

Continued

HIGH-DENSITY LIPOPROTEIN CHOLESTEROL

AGE (YEARS)	MALE		FEMALE	
	mg/dL	SI UNITS mmol/L	mg/dL	SI UNITS mmol/L
Children				
Cord blood	6-53	0.16-1.37	13-56	0.34-1.45
5-9 years	38-75	0.98-1.94	36-73	0.93-1.89
10-14 years	37-74	0.96-1.91	37-70	0.96-1.81
15-19 years	30-63	0.78-1.63	35-74	0.91-1.91

Note: Levels for African Americans are approximately 10 mg/dL (0.26 mmol/L, SI units) higher than those listed.

Increased. Alcoholism, chronic hepatitis, biliary cirrhosis (primary), familial hyperalphalipoproteinemia. Drugs include chlorinated hydrocarbons, cimetidine, cyclofenil, estrogens (alone or with progesterone), ethyl alcohol (ethanol), lovastatin, niacin, nicotinic acid, phenytoin, and terbutaline. Herbs or natural remedies: flaxseed, soybean, soy sauce.

Decreased. Arteriosclerosis, bacterial infections, cholestasis, coronary heart disease, hypercholesterolemia, hypertriglyceridemia, hypolipoproteinemia, liver disease, obesity (often), polycystic ovary syndrome (PCOS), renal disease, Tangier's disease, type-IV hyperlipoproteinemia, metabolic syndrome, and viral infections. Drugs include androgens, beta-adrenergic blockers, and intravenous immunoglobulin (IVIG). Diet high in carbohydrates.

Description. High-density lipoprotein (HDL) is a type of cholesterol carried by alpha-lipoprotein. HDL is believed to help protect against the risk of coronary artery disease and has been shown to be inversely related to the risk of coronary heart disease. HDL <35 mg/dL for men and <40 mg/dL for women are risk factors for coronary heart disease.

Professional Considerations
1. Consent form NOT required.
2. **Preparation:**
   A. See *Client and family teaching.*
   B. Tube: Lavender topped (2 tubes for lipid profile).
3. **Procedure:**
   A. Draw a 7-mL blood sample.
4. **Postprocedure care:**
   A. Resume previous diet.
5. **Client and family teaching:**
   A. Fast for 12-14 hours before sampling. Water is permitted.
   B. For clients with low levels, provide information regarding the reduction of modifiable risk factors, that is, smoking, obesity, and physical inactivity.
   C. A low-cholesterol diet includes avoidance of butter, lard, palm oil, coconut oil, pastries, waffles, avocados, olives, liver, bacon, sausage, luncheon meats, hot dogs, red meat, whole milk, cream, ice cream, and chocolate.
6. **Factors that affect results:**
   A. A diet high in carbohydrates or polyunsaturated fats or with smoking decreases the results.
7. **Other data:**
   A. For every 5 mg/dL decrease in HDL below the mean, the risk of coronary heart disease increases by 25%.
   B. See also *Cholesterol, Blood; Low-density lipoprotein cholesterol, Blood.*

HIGH-MOLECULAR-WEIGHT KININOGEN, PLASMA
(see Factor, Fitzgerald, Plasma)

HIGH-RESOLUTION CT, DIAGNOSTIC
(see Computed tomography of the body, Diagnostic)

HIGH-SENSITIVITY CRP
(see C-Reactive protein, Serum)

HIS BUNDLE ELECTROGRAPHY, DIAGNOSTIC

Norm. Atrial-to-His (A–H) interval = 50-120 msec; His-to-ventricular (H–V) activation = 35-55 msec.

Usage. Antidysrhythmic drug evaluation, precise location of bundle branch block, bypass tract physiology evaluation, decision making about pacemaker implant, syncope evaluation, and differentiation of true AV (atrioventricular) block from concealed AV extrasystoles.

Description. His bundle electrography is the use of a bipolar catheter electrode system during right-sided heart catheterization for recording activity of rhythm and conduction in the bundle of His located in the heart. This test provides information on intra-atrial and intraventricular conduction that is not available with regular electrocardiography.

Professional Considerations
1. Consent form IS required.

Risks
Dysrhythmias, phlebitis, pulmonary emboli, thromboemboli, and hemorrhage.

Contraindications
Clients with coagulopathy and acute pulmonary embolism.

2. **Preparation:**
   A. Have emergency medication available for use in case a dysrhythmia develops.
   B. See *Client and family teaching.*
3. **Procedure:**
   A. A catheter is introduced through the femoral vein and guided by fluoroscopy to the right ventricle.
   B. Leads I, II, and III placed on the limbs are recorded simultaneously with two intracardiac bipolar electrograms. One is in the high right atrium (HRA), and the other is over the septal leaflet of the tricuspid valve to record the bundle of His (HBE). The first deflection of the HBE represents right atrial activity. The second deflection represents His bundle activity. The third deflection represents ventricular activation.
4. **Postprocedure care:**
   A. Monitor vital signs and lower extremity pulses and observe and palpate for hematoma at the catheter site every 15 minutes × 4 and then hourly × 4.
   B. Maintain the extremity in extension until the frequent monitoring period has passed.

   C. Assess the catheter site for bleeding every 30 minutes for 4 hours.
5. **Client and family teaching:**
   A. Fast from food and fluids for at least 6 hours.
   B. The test takes 1-3 hours.
   C. Results are available immediately.
6. **Factors that affect results:**
   A. Poor catheter positioning.
7. **Other data:**
   A. See also *Cardiac catheterization, Diagnostic,* for other care required.

HISTAMINE STIMULATION TEST, DIAGNOSTIC
(see Gastric acid secretion, Gastric acid stimulation, Diagnostic)

HISTOPATHOLOGY, SPECIMEN

Norm. Requires interpretation by pathologist.

Usage. *Histologic diagnosis:* Abortion, abscess, achlorhydria, ache vulgaris, actinomycosis, alcoholism, amenorrhea, amyloidosis, appendicitis, arthritis (osteo-), brain tumors, cancers, cardiomyopathy, cervicitis, cholecystitis, cirrhosis, Crohn's disease, Cushing syndrome, cystitis, cytomegalovirus, dermatitis, diverticulitis, diverticulosis, duodenal ulcer, echinococcosis, ectopic pregnancy, eczema, emphysema, endometritis, epididymitis, esophagitis, esophagoscopy, fever of undetermined origin, fibrocystic breast disease, C-cell hyperplasia, ganglioneuroblastoma, gangrene, gastric ulcer, gastritis, genital herpes, giardiasis, glycogen storage disease, gynecomastia, hairy-cell leukemia, Hashimoto's thyroiditis, hemochromatosis, hepatitis, Hirschsprung's disease, histoplasmosis, Hodgkin's disease, hyperaldosteronism, hydatidiform mole, hyperparathyroidism, idiopathic thrombocytopenic purpura, infertility, insulinoma, intraductal breast papilloma, jaundice, kidney stone, Legionnaires' disease, leprosy (Hansen's disease), lymphogranuloma venereum, melanoma, metastasis, myocarditis, necrotizing granulomas (histoplasmosis), nephrolithiasis, neuropathy, pancreatitis, pelvic inflammatory disease, pemphigus, peptic ulcer, pericarditis, peripheral neuropathy, peritonitis, pleurisy, psoriasis, Reye syndrome, renal infarction, rubeola, sarcoidosis, scleroderma, sinusitis, Sjögren syndrome, stress ulcers, tumors, ulcerative colitis, vasculitis, Whipple's disease, and xerostomia.

Description. Specimen or tissue disorder involving gross and microscopic examination of biopsy sample and diagnosis by a qualified pathologist.

Professional Considerations
1. Consent form NOT required.
2. **Preparation:**
   A. Obtain a sterile container and fixative or formalin.
   B. The requisition must include the operative diagnosis and the site of the specimen.
3. **Procedure:**
   A. The tissue or fluid sample is obtained by means of local or general anesthesia.
   B. Label the specimen with the client's name, age, sex, room number, and operative diagnosis; the source of the specimen; and the surgeon and other physicians desiring a copy of the pathology report.
4. **Postprocedure care:**
   A. Fresh tissue is fixed in phosphate-buffered formalin (5-20 times the bulk of the specimen) or submitted directly to a responsible party on saline-soaked sterile gauze.
   B. Deliver the specimen to the laboratory within 1 hour.
5. **Client and family teaching:**
   A. The diagnosis will take 1 day or more.
   B. See *Biopsy, Site-specific, Specimen*.
6. **Factors that affect results:**
   A. Poor sampling technique or contamination.
   B. A sample that has become dried out will impair interpretation.
7. **Other data:**
   A. Tissue fixed in formalin CANNOT be used for bacteriology, electron microscopy, estrogen or progesterone receptors, or histochemistry study.
   B. See also *Biopsy, Site-specific, Specimen*.

HISTOPLASMOSIS SEROLOGY, BLOOD

Norms. Immunodiffusion test.

Negative. Complement fixation titer: <1:4 (normal finding).

Positive. Histoplasmosis.
Complement fixation titer: Fourfold rise in titer indicates current infection.
Suspicious for infection: 1:8-1:16; diagnostic for active infection: >1:32.
Immunodiffusion test: Presence of H (active) and M (active, recent, or past) bands indicate infection.

Description. *Histoplasma capsulatum* is a soil saprobic fungus that resides in the intestines of birds and bats and causes a common respiratory, noncommunicable, infection called "histoplasmosis." *H. capsulatum* spores are inhaled, enter the bloodstream, and spread through the reticuloendothelial system, causing breathing difficulty and enlargement of the spleen and lymph nodes. The antibody titers are usually elevated 6 weeks after infection, last weeks or months, and decline quickly, though they may remain elevated for up to 1 year.

Professional Considerations
1. Consent form NOT required.
2. **Preparation:**
   A. Tube: Red topped, red/gray topped, or gold topped.
   B. Obtain travel history to identify exposure in high-risk endemic areas.
   C. Ascertain if the client has been exposed to droppings of bats, chickens, pigeons, starlings, or blackbirds.
   D. The sample should be drawn before the histoplasmosis skin test.
3. **Procedure:**
   A. *Immunodiffusion:* Draw a 1-mL blood sample.
   B. *Complement fixation:* Draw a 2-mL blood sample.
4. **Postprocedure care:**
   A. No special care required.
5. **Client and family teaching:**
   A. Signs and symptoms of histoplasmosis include flulike symptoms,

pleuritic pain, pericarditis, pancy-topenia, and hepatosplenomegaly.

B. HIV-positive clients should avoid travel to endemic areas (in the United States, these include the middle, central, and south central states).

C. Follow-up specimens should be drawn at 2- to 3-week intervals to identify fluctuating antibody levels.

D. A 3% solution of formalin sprayed on contaminated soil will destroy the fungi.

6. **Factors that affect results:**

A. False-positive results can occur with aspergillosis, blastomycosis, and coccidioidomycosis.

B. A recent histoplasmosis skin test may falsely elevate titer.

7. **Other data:**

A. One third of all cases are in infants.

B. Histoplasmosis can cause pleural effusion.

C. Serum LDH levels of 600 IU/L or greater are suggestive of histoplasmosis.

HISTOPLASMOSIS SKIN TEST, DIAGNOSTIC

Norm. Negative as evidenced by no induration and erythema <5 mm in diameter.

Positive. Histoplasmosis.

Description. (See *Histoplasmosis, Serology.*) Skin tests become positive 2-3 weeks after infection and remain positive in 90% of the infected population for life.

Professional Considerations

1. Consent form NOT required.

2. **Preparation:**

A. Travel history should be included as part of the client's health history to determine exposure to high-incidence endemic areas.

B. Obtain an alcohol wipe; a needle; a syringe; and histoplasmin, an antigen prepared from culture (usually commercially prepared).

3. **Procedure:**

A. Histoplasmin is injected intradermally.

B. Record the location of the injection for reading.

C. The injection should follow a blood draw for serum titer.

4. **Postprocedure care:**

A. Read the test in 24-48 hours. An area of erythema and induration of >5 mm diameter is indicative of a positive reaction.

5. **Client and family teaching:**

A. See *Histoplasmosis, Serology, Blood.*

6. **Factors that affect results:**

A. Test may be falsely negative in 50% of people with disseminated histoplasmosis and 10% of people with cavitary histoplasmosis.

B. False-negative results may occur because of depressed immunologic status or steroid therapy.

C. False-positive results may occur in people with blastomycosis (30%) or coccidioidomycosis (40%).

7. **Other data:**

A. Acutely ill clients may not have a positive skin reaction.

B. This test is not recommended because of the difficult interpretation and because it may cause the serology test to be falsely positive.

HIV BATTERY
(*see Acquired immunodeficiency syndrome evaluation battery, Diagnostic*)

HIV ORAL TEST
(*see Oral mucosal transudate, Specimen*)

HIV-1 P24 ANTIGEN
(*see Acquired immunodeficiency syndrome evaluation battery, Diagnostic*)

HLA
(*see Human leukocyte antigen, Blood*)

HLA B-27
(*see Human leukocyte antigen B-27, Blood*)

HOLLANDER (BASAL GASTRIC SECRETION) TEST, DIAGNOSTIC

Norm.
Complete vagotomy: No acid secretion observed within 45 minutes of insulin-induced hypoglycemia.

Incomplete vagotomy: Acid secretion is >20 mmol/L if total acid output is >2 mmol/hour.

Usage. Evaluate the effectiveness of a vagotomy.

Description. The Hollander test, usually performed 3-6 months after a surgical vagotomy, involves injection of insulin intravenously into a client with an otherwise normal blood glucose. The vagus nerve responds to hypoglycemia by stimulating gastric acid secretion. Thus, in the presence of hypoglycemia, increased acid production indicates an incomplete vagotomy, and absence of acid production indicates a complete vagotomy.

Professional Considerations
1. Consent form IS required.

Risks
Hypoglycemic seizures, strokes, myocardial infarction, and deaths have been reported during this test. Complications of nasogastric tube insertion include bleeding, dysrhythmias, esophageal perforation, laryngospasm, and decreased mean pO_2.

Contraindications
Hypoglycemia, coronary artery disease, or cerebrovascular disease.

2. Preparation:
   A. The client should have patent intravenous access.
   B. Obtain regular insulin, a nasogastric tube and an irrigation syringe, a needle, a syringe, a fluoridated gray-topped tube, and an ampule of dextrose 50.
   C. See *Client and family teaching.*
3. Procedure:
   A. Insert the nasogastric tube, aspirate gastric contents, and place these in a container to measure.
   B. Inject an intravenous bolus of 0.1-0.2 U/kg of body weight of regular insulin. After the blood glucose falls to <50 mg/dL (usually within 30 minutes), the gastric contents should be aspirated.
   C. If postinsulin gastric acid production exceeds the reinjec-

tion amount of gastric acid, the vagotomy is likely incomplete.
4. Postprocedure care:
   A. Monitor vital signs every 15 minutes × 4 and then every hour × 4. Monitor closely and treat for complications (listed in section 5C below).
   B. Monitor blood glucose every hour × 2. Provide food sources of glucose as needed if hypoglycemic symptoms appear.
5. Client and family teaching:
   A. Fast from food for 12 hours and from liquids for 8 hours before the test.
   B. Do not smoke for 8 hours before the test.
   C. A nasogastric tube will be inserted through your nose into your stomach. Insertion may be uncomfortable and cause a pressure like feeling or cause you to gag and cough. You will be asked to take sips of water and swallow to make tube insertion easier.
6. Factors that affect results:
   A. None.
7. Other data:
   A. None.

HOLTER MONITOR, DIAGNOSTIC

Norm. No dysrhythmias.

Usage. Brugada syndrome, cardiomyopathy, cerebral ischemia, dysrhythmias (detection), mitral valve prolapse, pacemaker function, palpitations, and syncope.

Description. A Holter monitor is a portable, miniaturized electrocardiographic amplifier coupled to a magnetic recorder. It is used to obtain a permanent recording of continuous electrocardiographic activity of a client for an extended period of time, such as 24-48 hours. The client wears the monitor continuously and must record all activity and symptoms experienced at the specific times of occurrence throughout the monitoring period. The resulting electrocardiographic recording is analyzed for abnormalities and correlated with the documented activities and symptoms to help diagnose or rule out abnormalities such as those listed under *Usage.*

Professional Considerations

1. Consent form NOT required.
2. **Preparation:**
   A. Explain purpose to client or family.
   B. Obtain a diary and a pen or pencil, electrodes, and a Holter monitor.
   C. The electrodes must be applied to skin free of hair (shaved) that has been cleansed with acetone.
   D. See *Client and family teaching.*
3. **Procedure:**
   A. Assess for paper-roll availability with each monitor.
   B. Maintain a diary of movements to assist the diagnostician in evaluating the heart rhythm.
4. **Postprocedure care:**
   A. Remove all electrodes.
5. **Client and family teaching:**
   A. This monitor is used to identify abnormal heart rhythms that may occur for brief periods of time. Keeping a complete diary of times, activities, and sensations throughout monitoring helps pinpoint the cause of symptoms and the effect of activities on the heart.
   B. Avoid bathing (other than sponge bath), magnets, metal detectors, high-voltage areas, and electric blankets because these may interfere with recording.
6. **Factors that affect results:**
   A. An incomplete diary interferes with accurate interpretation of findings.
   B. Failure to apply electrodes correctly may cause an artifactual or incomplete signal.
7. **Other data:**
   A. None.

H

HOMOCYSTEINE, PLASMA (HCY) OR URINE (HCYSU)

Norm. *Note:* Studies are underway to establish reference levels. Norms below were taken from the findings of a variety of these initial studies. Higher homocysteine levels are almost always associated with low folate and vitamin B_{12} levels.

	SI UNITS
Plasma	
From the Hordaland Homocysteine Study:	
Norms in nonsmoking adults, 40-42 years of age with high folate intake and who drink less than 1 cup of coffee per day	3.0-4.8 μmol/L
Findings from Other Studies:	
Preterm infants up to 48 hours of age	3.5-4.1 μmol/L
Term infants	4.8-7.4 μmol/L
12-19 years of age	
Male	4.3-9.9 μmol/L
Female	3.3 to 7.2 μmol/L
20-59 years	
Male	6.5-11.3 μmol/L
Female	5.35-9.95 μmol/L
>59 years	
Male	5.9 to 15.3 μmol/L
Female	4.9 to 11.6 μmol/L
Urine	0-9 μmol/g of creatinine

Increased. Alcohol ingestion, Alzheimer's disease, atherosclerosis, cancer, cardiovascular disease, homocysteinuria, hypothyroidism, hypovolemia, inherited metabolic defects, psoriasis, renal failure (chronic), schizophrenia, vitamin deficiency (ascorbic acid-C, cobalamin-B_{12}, folate-B_9, pyridoxine-B_6, folate).

Decreased. Hyperthyroidism. Drugs include folic acid 5 mg daily.

Description. Homocysteine is an amino acid that results from the metabolism of methionine by the B vitamins cobalamin, folate, pyridoxine, and riboflavin. The breakdown of methionine to homocysteine is counterbalanced by choline and betaine, coenzymes that convert homocysteine back into methionine. Although the exact function of homocysteine is not known, it is postulated that it may cause damage to vascular endothelium or have a part in the causation of thrombi. It is known that a high homocysteine level signals risks in several areas. Homocysteinuria is an inherited disease in which persons who lack the enzymes that help control homocysteine levels demonstrate severe cardiovascular disease at a young age. Hyperhomocystinemia has been established in recent years as an independent risk factor for cardiovascular disease, including atherosclerosis, carotid artery stenosis, coronary artery disease, stroke, peripheral vascular disease, and venous thrombosis. Elevated levels are also associated with fetal neural tube defects, recurrent spontaneous abortion, placental infarction, and reduced cognitive functioning in the elderly and are considered to be a uremic toxin. Because firmly established reference ranges do not yet exist, homocysteine may often not be measured. Instead, physicians measure vitamin levels and, when vitamin deficiencies are found, infer elevated homocysteine levels. In other situations, homocysteine levels may be used as a functional test to determine folate deficiency because there exists an inverse relationship between the two values. The plasma test is best for this purpose and for assessment of cardiovascular risk. The urine homocysteine test should NOT be used in clients with renal failure, although it has been.

Professional Considerations
1. Consent form NOT required.
2. Preparation:
   A. *For plasma test:* Tube: Lavender topped.
   B. Obtain a clean, random urine specimen container and ice for urine test.
3. Procedure:
   A. *For plasma test:* Collect a 2-mL blood sample.
   B. *For urine test:* Collect a random urine sample from the second morning void. Place specimen immediately on ice.
4. Postprocedure care:
   A. Send specimen to the lab immediately.
   B. Process immediately (that is, within 30 minutes) to separate plasma. Specimen may be stored refrigerated or frozen up to 48 hours.
5. Client and family teaching:
   A. Fast from food and fluids for 8 hours before the test.
6. Factors that affect results:
   A. Levels are higher in smokers, coffee drinkers, diabetics, and persons who are obese or hypertensive than in the general population.
   B. Levels correctly directly with age and are higher in males than in females and in black women than in white women.
   C. Falsely increased values will result if specimen is allowed to sit without separation of the plasma because the red blood cells will continue to manufacture homocysteine in vitro.
7. Other data:
   A. Folic acid and vitamins B_{12} and B_6 supplementation are used to treat hyperhomocystinemia.

HOMOVANILLIC ACID (HVA), 24-HOUR URINE

Norm. Measures of HVA and measures of creatinine as follows:

	μg HVA/MG OF CREATININE	SI UNITS μmol HVA/mol CREATININE
Adults	0.25-2.5 or <8 mg/24 hours	1-14 10-35 mol/24 hours
Children		
<1 year	1.2-35	7-192
1 year	4-23	22-126
2-4 years	0.5-14	3-77
5-9 years	0.5-9	3-49
10-14 years	0.25-12	1-66
15-18 years	0.5-2	3-11

Increased. Brain tumor, ganglioneuroblastoma, occupational manganese exposure, neuroblastoma, and pheochromocytoma. Drugs include aminosalicylic acid, disulfiram, levodopa, methocarbamol, reserpine, and robaxin.

Decreased. Not clinically significant. Drugs include aminosalicylic acid, levodopa, methocarbamol, and monoamine oxidase inhibitors.

Description. Homovanillic acid is the major terminal metabolite of dopamine, one of the three catecholamines produced in the brain. Dopamine is broken down by the liver and excreted in the urine as homovanillic acid. Elevated levels can occur as a result of catecholamine-secreting tumors. Because urinary HVA levels fluctuate with creatinine excretion, results are normalized to the amount of creatinine present in the urine sample.

Professional Considerations

1. Consent form NOT required.
2. **Preparation:**
   A. Obtain a clean, 3-L container without preservative.
   B. Write the beginning time of collection on the laboratory requisition.
   C. See *Client and family teaching.*
3. **Procedure:**
   A. Discard the first morning urine specimen.
   B. Save all urine voided for 24 hours in a refrigerated, clean, 3-L container to which 20 mL of hydrochloric acid (HCl) preservative has been added. Document the quantity of urine output during the collection period. Include the urine voided at the end of the 24-hour period. For catheterized clients, keep the drainage bag on ice and empty urine into the collection container hourly.
4. **Postprocedure care:**
   A. Compare the urine quantity in the specimen container with the urinary output record for the test. If the specimen contains less urine than what was recorded as output, some of the sample may have been discarded, thus invalidating the test.
   B. Document the quantity of urine output and the ending time for the collection period on the laboratory requisition.
   C. Send the entire 24-hour urine specimen immediately to the laboratory for testing.
5. **Client and family teaching:**
   A. Avoid large doses of aspirin, coffee, tea, chocolate, caffeine, phenothiazine, antihypertension agents, fruit, and any vanilla-containing substances for 48 hours before urine collection.
   B. If taking levodopa meditation, the physician may discontinue this medication for 2 weeks before the test.
   C. Save all the urine voided in the 24-hour period and urinate before defecating to avoid loss of urine. If any urine is accidentally discarded, discard the entire specimen and restart the collection the next day.
6. **Factors that affect results:**
   A. Falsely-elevated results may occur with excessive physical exercise or emotional stress.

7. Other data:
   A. Homovanillic acid is usually measured simultaneously with metanephrine, normetanephrine, and vanillylmandelic acid to assist in differential diagnosis.

HORMONAL EVALUATION, CYTOLOGIC, SPECIMEN

Norm. Requires interpretation based on clinical status. Maturation index is reported as percentages of parabasal, intermediate, and superficial cells.

Usage. Amenorrhea, feminizing tumor, ovarian dysfunction, pituitary dysfunction, and virilizing tumor.

Description. Microscopic evaluation of cellular composition of the surface layers of the vaginal squamous epithelium, which reflects the balance of estrogen and progesterone.

Professional Considerations
1. Consent form NOT required.
2. Preparation:
   A. Obtain drapes, a sterile wooden spatula, a glass slide, and a fixative spray or 95% ethyl alcohol (ethanol).
   B. The client should disrobe below the waist.
   C. See *Client and family teaching.*
3. Procedure:
   A. Position the client in the dorsal lithotomy position, and drape her for privacy and comfort.
   B. Use lubricating gel sparingly because excess will interfere with the cytologic examination.
   C. Excess glove powder should be removed before the spatula is handled because starch granules make slide interpretation difficult.
   D. Scrape the lateral vaginal wall with a sterile wooden spatula.

4. Postprocedure care:
   A. Transfer the secretions to a glass slide and fix them with 95% ethyl alcohol or spray fixative.
   B. Include on the laboratory requisition the date of the last menstrual period and history of radiation therapy or gynecologic surgery.
5. Client and family teaching:
   A. Do not douche for 24 hours before obtaining the smear.
   B. The test is painless and takes only a moment.
6. Factors that affect results:
   A. A dried specimen caused by failure to apply fixative is cause for specimen rejection.
   B. Agents that cause misleading desquamation include cortisone, digitalis, estrogen, and tetracycline suppositories.
7. Other data:
   A. This test has limited value when applied to an individual because there is a great variation in normal values and between counters.

HPRL
(*see Prolactin, Serum*)

HPV
(*see Human papillomavirus, Specimen*)

HRCT
(*see Computed tomography of the body, Diagnostic*)

hsCRP
(*see C-Reactive protein, Serum*)

hTAU ANTIGEN, CSF
(*see Tau Test, CSF*)

HUMAN CHORIONIC GONADOTROPIN (HCG), BETA-SUBUNIT, SERUM

Norm:

		SI UNITS
Beta subunit	<2 ng/mL or <5 mIU/mL	<2 μg/L <5 IU/L

Increased. Cancer (bladder, chorio-carcinoma, colon, esophageal squamous cell, germ cell, hepatoma, leiomyosarcoma, lung, ovarian, pancreas, stomach, testicular), eclampsia, ectopic pregnancy, erythroblastosis fetalis, gynecomastia, hydatidiform mole, hyperreaction luteinalis, insulinoma, osteolytic meningioma, pregnancy and seminoma.

Decreased. Abortion and ectopic pregnancy.

Description. Human chorionic gonadotropin is a glycoprotein hormone with alpha and beta subunits, which are normally produced by a developing placenta and may be produced by some germ cell tumors. The alpha sequence is identical to the follicle-stimulating hormone, luteinizing hormone, and thyroid-stimulating hormone, and it can cause a false-positive pregnancy test if not tested along with the beta-subunit. This test can detect pregnancy in as little as 1 week after conception. Serial monitoring is used to help determine gestational age. The beta-subunit is often used to follow the status of neoplasms after surgery or chemotherapy. Elevated levels have been associated with a poor outcome in clients with colorectal cancer.

Professional Considerations
1. Consent form NOT required.
2. Preparation:
   A. Tube: Red topped, red/gray topped, or gold topped.
   B. For females, write the date of the last menstrual cycle on the laboratory requisition.
3. Procedure:
   A. Obtain a 1-mL blood sample.
4. Postprocedure care:
   A. Send the sample to the laboratory immediately. The sample can be kept at 2°-8° C for up to 24 hours. Additional delay in processing would require that the serum be frozen.
5. Client and family teaching:
   A. If the test is being used to determine pregnancy, results are normally available within 2 hours.
   B. Additional samples will be drawn periodically to help determine fetal gestational age.
6. Factors that affect results:
   A. False-positive tests result from hemolyzed, lipemic, or icteric serum.
   B. If the test is to be performed using radioimmunoassay, a radionuclide scan within 1 week of the test may falsely elevate results.
   C. EDTA (ethylenediaminetetraacetate solution) and heparin anticoagulants decrease plasma levels and may cause false-negative results.
   D. Values increase more slowly in ectopic than in normal pregnancies.
7. Other data:
   A. Does not eliminate the possibility of pregnancy if results are low or borderline.
   B. False-positive results have resulted in unnecessary treatment with chemotherapy for suspected malignancy. One can confirm or exclude positive hCG tests by obtaining a quantitative urine hCG test. Assistance can be obtained from the hCG Reference Service when accuracy of results is questionable. (The hCG Reference Service is located at Yale University, New Haven, CT 06520, USA.)
   C. See also *Pregnancy test, Routine, Serum.*

HUMAN CHORIONIC GONADOTROPIN (HCG, PREGNANCY TEST), SERUM
(see Pregnancy test, Routine, Serum)

HUMAN EPIDERMAL GROWTH FACTOR
(see HER-2/neu oncogene, Specimen)

HUMAN IMMUNODEFICIENCY VIRUS
(see Acquired immunodeficiency syndrome evaluation battery, Diagnostic)

HUMAN LEUKOCYTE ANTIGEN (HLA) B-27, BLOOD

Norm. Requires clinical correlation.

Positive. Ankylosing spondylitis (Marie-Strumpell disease), arthritis (rheumatoid), congenital adrenal hyperplasia, Goodpasture syndrome, narcolepsy, pemphigus, Reiter syndrome, and thyroiditis (subacute).

Negative. Normal finding.

Description. See *Human leukocyte antigen typing, Blood,* for description of the HLA antigen. The presence of B-27 antigen is highly correlated with ankylosing spondylitis and rheumatoid arthritis.

Professional Considerations
1. Consent form NOT required.
2. Preparation:
   A. Tube: Green topped.
   B. Preschedule this test with the laboratory.
3. Procedure:
   A. Draw a 10-mL blood sample.
4. Postprocedure care:
   A. Send the specimen to the laboratory immediately; do not freeze it.
5. Client and family teaching:
   A. Results are normally available within 24 hours.
6. Factors that affect results:
   A. The test must be performed on live lymphocytes. If the cells have died, a new sample must be drawn.
7. Other data:
   A. Clients who are HLA B-27 positive have a 120 times greater chance of developing ankylosing spondylitis than clients who are negative.

HUMAN LEUKOCYTE ANTIGEN (HLA) TYPING (TISSUE TYPING), BLOOD

Norm. Interpretation required for tissue typing and determination of histocompatibility match or nonmatch.

Usage. Paternity testing and transplants (to determine histocompatibility); selection of platelet donors for immunized clients.

Description. Human leukocyte antigens (HLAs) are glycoproteins found on all nucleated cells. They result from four closely linked genes on chromosome 6 and are important to histocompatibility complement, and immune response. The antigens are divided into A, B, C (Class I, derived from T cells), D, and DR (D-related, Class II, derived from B cells). There are multiple antigens of each type, meaning that the combinations of antigens that identify any individual are infinite. The HLA are inherited as two sets (one from each parent) of six antigens. This test is most commonly used in bone marrow and renal transplantation. The antigens must match for transplantation to occur without organ rejection.

Professional Considerations
1. Consent form NOT required.
2. Preparation:
   A. Preschedule this test with the laboratory. The sample should be drawn before or 72 hours after a blood product transfusion.
   B. *For donor specimen:* Tube: Two green-topped tubes.
   C. *For recipient specimen:* Tube: Red topped, red/gray topped, or gold topped.
3. Procedure:
   A. *Donor specimen:* Completely fill two green-topped tubes with blood (7 mL each).
   B. *Recipient specimen:* Completely fill a red-topped tube with 7 mL of blood.
4. Postprocedure care:
   A. Send the specimen to the laboratory for immediate testing.
   B. Do not refrigerate or freeze the specimen or place the specimen on ice.
5. Client and family teaching:
   A. Encourage the client to express concerns regarding illness (such as awaiting a suitable donor, symptom management).
6. Factors that affect results:
   A. Refrigeration of or delay in processing specimens may result in inadequate lymphocytes for accurate testing.
7. Other data:
   A. Samples that have been used for cross-matching should be frozen and stored for 1 year.
   B. Bone marrow transplant clients or clients receiving chemotherapy with HLA-B51 or HLA-B52 who develop an infection at time of WBC nadir may develop ARDS.
   C. See also *Human leukocyte antigen B-27, Blood.*

HUMAN PAPILLOMAVIRUS (HPV) IN SITU HYBRIDIZATION, SPECIMEN

Norm. Determination (by histopathologist) of absence of genetic changes consistent with the human papillomavirus.

Usage. Used to confirm HPV infection and to determine HPV type.

Description. Human papillomaviruses are DNA viruses that are known to cause Bowen's extragenital disease; warts; condyloma accuminatum; intraepithelial neoplasia; and anogenital, cervical, or oropharyngeal cancers. There are more than 70 different types of HPV, with about 20 of these types being associated with genital warts. Most genital warts are associated with the "low-risk" HPV types 6 and 11. Invasive carcinoma of the cervix, vulva, anus, and penis are associated with HPV types 16, 18, 33, 35, and 39. Endocervical carcinoma is associated with HPV 18. Although these specific associations exist, only a small proportion of HPV 16 and 18 lesions actually progress to a malignancy. In situ hybridization is a technique used to both confirm the presence of the HPV virus in a specimen and to type the HPV. DNA from the specimen is placed on a nitrocellulose membrane and fixed. The membrane can then be hybridized to a DNA sample of known sequence that is radioactively labeled. If the pathogenic DNA is present in the sample (such as HPV type 18), the sample DNA will hybridize to the known DNA, producing a double-stranded DNA segment. The radioactive label is incorporated into the double-stranded DNA segment, allowing this segment to be detected by autoradiography.

Professional Considerations

1. Consent form IS required for the procedure used to obtain the specimen.

Risks

Bleeding, infection.

Contraindications

Bleeding disorder or anticoagulated state.

2. **Preparation:**
   A. Schedule collection from a female client when she is not menstruating, preferably 1 week after menses (especially important if a Pap smear is also being obtained).
   B. A special collection kit is obtained from the laboratory that will be doing the hybridization. For *Detection and typing, HPV probe,* it is necessary to use the HPV collection kit (supplied by Roche).
   C. Cervical swabs or biopsy specimens may be obtained from female client; urethral swabs are obtained from male clients.
   D. Specimen collection cannot be performed after colposcopy if acetic acid is used.
   E. If biopsy specimen is obtained, specimen should be approximately 3 mm in diameter. Specimen should immediately be placed in transport tube and frozen at $-20°$ C. If cervical (female) or urethral (male) swab is obtained, it is placed in a collection tube and may be stored at room temperature for up to 7 days.

3. **Procedure:**
   A. *In situ hybridization:*
      i. Assist the client to the lithotomy position.
      ii. A colposcope may be used to visualize the cervix and is inserted through the unlubricated speculum.
      iii. Tissue sample(s) removed from any visible lesion(s) or doctor-selected site(s); enough for a minimum of eight 5-μm sections.
   B. *DNA probe:*
      i. *Male:* Collect cells from the urethra using a swab. Place the collection device in the HPV transport tube for shipment to the lab.
      ii. *Female:* Collect cervical cells from the endocervical canal and the exocervix using the HPV collection kit. Place a swab in the transport tube for shipment to the lab.

4. **Postprocedure care:**
   A. Tissue: Submit the biopsy (frozen), 3 mm in diameter, in an HPV collection tube. Biopsy

H

specimens must be shipped frozen at −20° C.

B. Swab the cervix with silver nitrate to control bleeding after biopsy, and the examiner may insert a tampon if bleeding persists.

C. The tissue must be fixed with formalin solution immediately and then embedded in paraffin within 72 hours. Embed in paraffin in a way that the tissue section will fit into a 10-mm circle. The specimen must not remain in formalin beyond 72 hours.

D. Complete the filling out of the requisition, noting the number and appearance of tissue samples.

5. **Client and family teaching:**
   A. Rest for 8-24 hours after procedure, avoiding heavy lifting or strenuous exercise.
   B. Avoid douching and intercourse for 2 weeks or as directed by the physician.
   C. An odorous, gray-green vaginal discharge is normal and may occur for up to 3 weeks after procedure.
   D. Some bleeding will occur normally, but inform the doctor if heavy bleeding (heavier than menstrual clots) occurs.
   E. Mild discomfort during and after the procedure is normal. Take a nonaspirin analgesic as needed.
   F. Results may not be available for several days.

6. **Factors that affect results:**
   A. Improperly fixed tissue cannot be used for this test.
   B. An inadequate amount of tissue would cause specimen rejection.
   C. Specimen has become thawed out.
   D. Specimen was obtained after acetic acid application to biopsy or swab site.

7. **Other data:**
   A. A DNA probe is used to aid in the diagnosis of sexually transmitted HPV infections, distinguishing between infections with types associated with low-grade squamous intraepithelial lesions (LSIL), types 6, 11, 42, 43, or 44, and types associated with SIL of all grades, including high-grade (HSIL), types, 16, 18, 31, 33, 35, 45, 51, 52, and 56.

B. The polymerase chain reaction test for HPV detection can identify 9 specific types of the virus but is currently for *investigational use only*. Specimen collection and before and after care are essentially the same as for the in situ hybridization method.

HUMAN PROLACTIN
(see Prolactin, Serum)

HUMAN TUMOR STEM-CELL ASSAY, DIAGNOSTIC

Norm. Growth or inhibition of growth of tumor cells.

Usage. Determine the sensitivity or resistance of an individual's tumor cells to an anticancer drug.

Description. An in vitro test to determine responsiveness of tumor cells to specific drugs. A specimen of tumor is obtained from the individual. The cells are enzymatically dissociated, centrifuged, and placed into suspensions. Different anticancer drugs are added to each sample before being placed onto agar plates. The plates are examined microscopically twice each week for at least 2-3 weeks when cell growth is likely to have occurred. Growth of the cells implies resistance to the drug or irradiation, and lack of growth indicates some anticancer effect.

Professional Considerations
1. Consent form NOT required but IS required for the procedure used to obtain the specimen. See individual procedure for risks and contraindications.
2. **Preparation:**
   A. Prepare surgical instruments for tissue removal.
3. **Procedure:**
   A. Cells from the tumor are obtained and enzymatically dissociated in the laboratory.
   B. The cells are examined microscopically twice a week for 2-3 weeks.
4. **Postprocedure care:**
   A. Apply a sterile dressing to the incision site.

B. Observe the site for bleeding and symptoms of infection for 24-48 hours.

C. See *Biopsy, Site-specific, Specimen.*

5. **Client and family teaching:**
   A. Results take approximately 3 weeks but can help the physician select the treatment regimen most likely to be effective in destroying cancer cells.

6. **Factors that affect results:**
   A. Approximately 50% of tumors are unsuitable for in vitro growth, making the test difficult to interpret.

7. **Other data:**
   A. Prediction of drug sensitivity is 40-90% correct, and prediction of drug resistance is 90-95% correct.

HYDROCEPHALUS RADIOLOGIC EVALUATION, DIAGNOSTIC

Norm. Absence of hydrocephalus.

Usage. Diagnosis of hydrocephalus and whether it is communicating or noncommunicating.

Description. Under computed tomography, radionuclide (usually technetium 99m) is tagged to albumin and injected into a lumbar puncture site. The radionuclide then travels upward into the brain, where it can be observed in terms of the amount of fluid and whether the fluid is able to travel into the ventricles (communicating). Noncommunicating hydrocephalus prevents the radionuclide from traveling into the ventricles.

Professional Considerations
1. Consent form IS required.

Risks
Increased intracranial pressure; allergic reaction to radiolabeled albumin (itching, hives, rash, tight feeling in the throat, shortness of breath, bronchospasm, anaphylaxis, death).

Contraindications
Previous allergy to radiolabeled albumin; increased intracranial pressure.

2. **Preparation:**
   A. Remove all metal objects from the client's head.
   B. Obtain a lumbar puncture tray.
   C. ACT scan is typically performed to rule out increased intracranial pressure before lumbar puncture in critically ill clients or those with changed mental status.

3. **Procedure:**
   A. Radiolabeled human serum albumin is given to demonstrate the flow of CSF from the point of the lumbar puncture up into the cranium.

4. **Postprocedure care:**
   A. Assess vital signs every 15 minutes × 4.
   B. Observe the client carefully for up to 60 minutes after the study for a possible (anaphylactic) reaction to the radionuclide.
   C. For 24 hours wear rubber gloves when discarding urine after the procedure. Wash the gloved hands with soap and water before removing the gloves. Wash the ungloved hands after gloves are removed.

5. **Client and family teaching:**
   A. The test takes 1-2 hours.
   B. Meticulously wash hands with soap and water after each void for 24 hours.

6. **Factors that affect results:**
   A. None.

7. **Other data:**
   A. Health care professionals working in a nuclear medicine area must follow federal standards set by the Nuclear Regulatory Commission. These standards include precautions for handling the radioactive material and monitoring of potential radiation exposure.
   B. Technetium half-life is 6 hours.

HYDROXYBUTYRATE DEHYDROGENASE (HBDH), BLOOD

Norm. 140-350 IU/L.

Increased. Anemia (hemolytic or megaloblastic), hepatic cellular damage, leukemia, lymphoma, malignant melanoma, muscular dystrophy, myocardial infarction, nephrotic syndrome, and orthopedic hip surgery.

Decreased. Not clinically significant.

Description. Enzyme similar to lactate dehydrogenase 1 (LD1), which is found in the brain, heart muscle, kidney, and red blood cells. It is most generally used to diagnose myocardial infarction though levels may also be elevated when there is damage to other organs. HBDH levels are more specific and last longer than CK, AST, and total LD for diagnosing myocardial infarction. HBDH levels rise within 8-10 hours of infarction, peak in 48-96 hours, and remain abnormal for 16-18 days. This test is primarily used in small laboratories where the complete LD isoenzyme battery is unavailable or because it is less costly and simpler to perform than LD electrophoresis.

Professional Considerations
1. Consent form NOT required.
2. **Preparation:**
   A. Tube: Red topped, red/gray topped, or gold topped.
3. **Procedure:**
   A. Draw a 7-mL blood sample, without hemolysis.
4. **Postprocedure care:**
   A. Do not freeze the specimen.
5. **Client and family teaching:**
   A. Results are normally available within 24 hours.
6. **Factors that affect results:**
   A. Specimens may be falsely negative if frozen because enzyme activity is lost.
   B. Traumatic venipuncture or hemolysis causes false-positive results.
7. **Other data:**
   A. HBDH is stable at room temperature for 5 days and for 10 days refrigerated.

17-HYDROXYCORTICOSTEROIDS (17-OHCS), 24-HOUR URINE

Norm:

		SI UNITS
Adult Female	2.5-10 mg/24 hours	6.9-27.6 µmol/24 hours
Adult Male	4.5-12 mg/24 hours	12.4-33.1 µmol/24 hours
Child		
0-1 year	0.5-1 mg/24 hours	1.4-2.8 µmol/24 hours
<12 years	1-4.5 mg/24 hours	2.8-12.4 µmol/24 hours

Increased. Acetonuria, acromegaly, Cushing syndrome, fructosuria, glucosuria, hirsutism, hypertension (severe), insomnia, obesity, pregnancy, stress, and virilization. Drugs include acetazolamide, ACTH, ascorbic acid, Atarax (hydroxyzine HCl), cephalothin, cefoxitin, chloral hydrate, chlordiazepoxide, chlorpromazine, colchicine, cortisone acetate, digitalis glycosides, Doriden (glutethimide), erythromycin, etryptamine (alpha-ethyltryptamine), glutethimide, gonadotropins, hydrocortisone, hydroxyzine, iodides, mandelamine, meprobamate, methenamine, methicillin, methyprylon, oleandomycin, paraldehyde, quinine, quinidine, spironolactone, and troleandomycin.

Decreased. Addison's disease, anorexia nervosa, congenital adrenal hyperplasia, hypopituitarism, and hypothyroidism. Drugs include Apresoline (hydralazine HCl), carbamazepine, corticosteroids, dextropropoxyphene, estrogens, medroxyprogesterone, meperidine, morphine, oral contraceptives, pentazocine, phenergan, phenothiazines, phenytoin, reserpine (high doses), salicylates, and thiazide diuretics.

Description. 17-hydroxycorticosteroids are carbon compounds that have a dihydroxyacetone group on the 17th carbon. In urine, the primary 17-OHCSs are breakdown products of cortisone and hydrocortisone, which can be used as a measure of their production (adrenocortical function).

Professional Considerations
1. Consent form NOT required.

2. **Preparation:**
   A. Obtain a 3-L plastic container with acetic, boric, or hydrochloric acid (HCl) additive.
   B. Write the beginning time of collection on the laboratory requisition.
   C. See *Client and family teaching.*
3. **Procedure:**
   A. Discard the first morning-urine specimen.
   B. Save all the urine voided for 24 hours in a clean, 3-L container (on ice) to which acetic acid, boric acid, or HCl preservative has been added. Document the quantity of urine output during the collection period. Include the urine voided at the end of the 24-hour period. For catheterized clients, keep the drainage bag on ice and empty urine into the collection container hourly.
4. **Postprocedure care:**
   A. Compare the urine quantity in the specimen container with the urinary output record for the test. If the specimen contains less urine than what was recorded as output, some of the sample may have been discarded, thus invalidating the test.
   B. Document the quantity of urine output and the ending time for the collection period on the laboratory requisition.
   C. Send the entire 24-hour urine specimen to the laboratory for testing. Refrigerate or freeze the specimen after collection.
5. **Client and family teaching:**
   A. Stop all medications 24 hours before the collection of urine (with physician's approval).
   B. Inform the physician ordering the test of any prescription or over-the-counter medications being taken.
   C. Save all urine voided in the 24-hour period and urinate before defecating to avoid loss of urine. If any urine is accidentally discarded, discard the entire specimen and restart the collection the next day.
   D. Resume medications after the 24-hour urine collection has been completed.
6. **Factors that affect results:**
   A. Increases in 17-OHCS can be caused by acute illness.

   B. Methyprylon may interfere with the absorbance of both urinary 17-ketosteroids using the Holtorff Koch modification of the Zimmerman reaction, and 17-hydroxycorticosteroids, using the modified Glenn-Nelson technique
7. **Other data:**
   A. Urinary free cortisol and serum cortisol are more sensitive and specific tests.
   B. The specimen is stable up to 45 days if properly acidified and refrigerated.

5-HYDROXYINDOLEACETIC ACID (5-HIAA), QUANTITATIVE, 24-HOUR URINE

Norm. *Qualitative:* Negative.
  Quantitative: 1-10 mg/24 hours (5.2-52 µmol/24 hours, SI units).

Increased. Carcinoid tumors (foregut and midgut) (when dietary sources of 5-HIAA are eliminated before testing), celiac sprue, diarrhea, endocarditis, ganglioneuroblastoma, toxemia of pregnancy, and tropical sprue. Drugs include acetaminophen, atenolol, cisplatin (peaks 6 hours after induction), diazepam, fluorouracil, glyceryl guaiacolate, melphalan, mephenesin, methenasin carbamate, methocarbamol, naproxen, oxprenolol, phenacetin, pindolol, and reserpine.

Decreased. Carcinoid tumors (rectal), depression, Hartnup's disease, mastocytosis, nonmetastatic carcinoid tumors, phenylketonuria, and small intestine resection diarrhea. Drugs include acetic acid, corticotropin, dihydroxyphenol-acetic acid, ethyl alcohol (ethanol), formaldehyde, gentisic acid, homo-gentisic acid, imipramine, isoniazid, lanreotide, levodopa, methenamine, methyldopa, monoamine oxidase (MAO) inhibitors, phenothiazines, salicylates, and sulfasalazine.

Description. 5-HIAA is a primary urinary metabolite of serotonin. Under normal conditions, serotonin is produced in the gastrointestinal tract and acts as a vasoconstrictor. Approximately 5% of serotonin is converted to 5-HIAA and excreted in the urine. Increased

H

urinary 5-HIAA is reflective of overproduction of serotonin, which occurs with carcinoid tumors.

Professional Considerations
1. Consent form NOT required.
2. Preparation:
   A. Obtain a 3-L plastic container to which 12 g of boric acid or 25 mL of hydrochloric acid (HCl) has been added.
   B. Write the beginning time of collection on the laboratory requisition.
   C. See *Client and family teaching.*
3. Procedure:
   A. Discard the first morning-urine specimen.
   B. Save all the urine voided for 24 hours in a refrigerated, clean, 3-L container to which 12 g of boric acid or 24 mL of HCl has been added. Document the quantity of urine output during the collection period. Include the urine voided at the end of the 24-hour period. For catheterized clients, keep the drainage bag on ice and empty urine into the collection container hourly.
4. Postprocedure care:
   A. Compare the urine quantity in the specimen container with the urinary output record for the test. If the specimen contains less urine than what was recorded as output, some of the sample may

have been discarded, thus invalidating the test.
   B. Document the quantity of urine output and the ending time for the collection period on the laboratory requisition.
   C. Send the entire 24-hour urine specimen to the laboratory for testing.
5. Client and family teaching:
   A. Avoid the following foods 5 days before the test: bananas, avocados, plums, eggplant, tomatoes, plantain (a hard banana), pineapples, and walnuts. These are sources of 5-HIAA.
   B. Save all the urine voided in the 24-hour period and urinate before defecating to avoid loss of urine. If any urine is accidentally discarded, discard the entire specimen and restart the collection the next day.
6. Factors that affect results:
   A. Falsely elevated results may be caused by the ingestion of foods containing serotonin within 48 hours before specimen collection. Examples are avocados, bananas, eggplant, red plums, and tomatoes.
7. Other data:
   A. Carcinoid tumors may cause increased excretion of tryptophan, 5-hydroxytryptophan, and histamine.

17-HYDROXYPROGESTERONE, BLOOD

Norm:

		SI UNITS
Adult Male	50-250 ng/dL	1.5-7.5 nmol/L
Adult Female		
Follicular phase	20-100 ng/dL	0.6-3.0 nmol/L
Midcycle peak	100-250 ng/dL	3.0-7.5 nmol/L
Luteal peak	100-500 ng/dL	3.0-15.5 nmol/L
Children		
Cord blood	900-5000 ng/dL	27.3-151.5 nmol/L
Newborn	7-77 ng/dL	0.2-2.3 nmol/L
Child	3-90 ng/dL	0.1-2.7 nmol/L
Puberty, male	3-175 ng/dL	0.1-5.3 nmol/L
Puberty, female	3-265 ng/dL	0.1-8.0 nmol/L

Increased. Congenital adrenal hyperplasia, germinoma, hirsutism, ovarian tumors, polycystic ovary syndrome (PCOS), and virilization.

Decreased. Not clinically significant.

Description. 17-Hydroxyprogesterone (17-OHP), which is derived from progesterone, is the metabolic precursor of 11-deoxycortisol in cortisol biosynthesis. Elevated levels generally occur as a result of 21-hydroxylase or 11-hydroxylase deficiency. 17-OHP is converted and excreted as pregnanetriol.

Professional Considerations
1. Consent form NOT required.
2. Preparation:
   A. Tube: Red topped, red/gray topped, or gold topped; and ice.

3. Procedure:
   A. Draw a 1.5-mL blood sample. Place the sample immediately on ice.
4. Postprocedure care:
   A. Deliver the sample to the laboratory within 30 minutes for immediate testing.
5. Client and family teaching:
   A. Results are normally available within 24 hours.
6. Factors that affect results:
   A. Recent radionuclide administration (within 48 hours) may cause false-positive results if the test is performed using radioimmunoassay technique.
7. Other data:
   A. Measurement of 11-deoxycortisol may help differentiate between 11- and 21-hydroxylase deficiencies.

HYDROXYPROLINE, TOTAL, 24-HOUR URINE

Norm:

		SI UNITS
Adults		
18-21 years	20-55 mg/day	0.15-0.42 μmol/day
22-40 years	15-42 mg/day	0.11-0.32 μmol/day
41-55 years	15-43 mg/day	0.11-0.33 μmol/day
Children		
1-5 years	20-65 mg/day	0.15-0.49 μmol/day
6-10 years	35-99 mg/day	0.27-0.75 μmol/day
11-14 years	63-180 mg/day	0.48-1.37 μmol/day

Increased. Acromegaly, Albright syndrome, bone cancer, bone metastasis, bone osteopenia, burns, congenital hypophosphatasia, diabetes mellitus, growth spurts, healing fracture, hyperparathyroidism, hyperpituitarism, hyperthyroidism, Marfan syndrome, multiple myeloma, osteomalacia, osteomyelitis, Paget's disease of the bone, psoriasis, and rickets. Drugs include growth hormone, parathyroid hormone, phenobarbital, and sulfonylureas.

Decreased. Hypoparathyroidism, hypopituitarism, hypothyroidism, malnutrition, and muscular dystrophy. Drugs include acetylsalicylic acid, antineoplastic agents, ascorbic acid, calcitonin, calcium gluconate, corticosteroids, diphosphonate, ergocalciferol, estradiol, estriol, glucocorticoids, mithramycin, and propranolol.

Description. Hydroxyproline is an amino acid found in collagen. Excretion of hydroxyproline in the urine is a useful measure of collagen turnover. It reflects bone resorption and is therefore a good test for monitoring the status of Paget's disease.

Professional Considerations
1. Consent form NOT required.
2. Preparation:
   A. Obtain a clean, 3-L container without preservative.
   B. Write the beginning time of collection on the laboratory requisition.
   C. See *Client and family teaching*.
3. Procedure:
   A. Discard the first morning urine specimen.
   B. Save all the urine voided for 24 hours in a refrigerated, clean, 3-L container. Document the quantity of urine output during the

collection period. Include the urine voided at the end of the 24-hour period. For catheterized clients, keep the drainage bag on ice and empty urine into the collection container hourly.

4. Postprocedure care:
   A. Compare the urine quantity in the specimen container with the urinary output record for the test. If the specimen contains less urine than what was recorded as output, some of the sample may have been discarded, thus invalidating the test.
   B. Document the quantity of urine output and the ending time for the collection period on the laboratory requisition.
   C. Send the entire 24-hour urine specimen to the laboratory for testing and refrigerate it.

5. Client and family teaching:
   A. Avoid gelatin-containing foods and red meat, poultry, and fish 48 hours before urine collection.
   B. Save all the urine voided in the 24-hour period and urinate before defecating to avoid loss of urine. If any urine is accidentally discarded, discard the entire specimen and restart the collection the next day.

6. Factors that affect results:
   A. Meat and gelatin may produce false-positive results.

7. Other data:
   A. Normal range is higher in infancy, childhood, and adolescence, especially during growth spurts.
   B. There is a diurnal variation in excretion, with higher levels excreted at night.

5-HYDROXYTRYPTAMINE, PLASMA

(see Serotonin, Plasma)

HYPERSENSITIVITY PNEUMONITIS SEROLOGY, BLOOD

Norm. Negative.

Positive. Asthma and farmer's lung. Workplace related to cockatiel exposure, methotrexate exposure, mold exposure, mushroom farming, naphthylene-

1,5-diisocyanate (NDI), working in the machining industry. Drugs include anthrax vaccination, loxoprofen.

Description. Hypersensitivity pneumonitis (extrinsic allergic alveolitis) is an inflammatory, interstitial pneumonia that results from an immunologic reaction in response to a variety of inhaled antigens. These antigens usually include organisms such as *Aspergillus fumigatus, Micropolyspora faeni,* or *Thermoactinomyces vulgaris.*

Professional Considerations
1. Consent form NOT required.
2. Preparation:
   A. Tube: Red topped, red/gray topped, or gold topped.
3. Procedure:
   A. Obtain a 7-mL blood sample.
4. Postprocedure care:
   A. None.
5. Client and family teaching:
   A. Results are normally available within 48 hours.
6. Factors that affect results:
   A. Reject hemolyzed, chylous, or contaminated samples.
7. Other data:
   A. A client with no symptoms may produce a positive test, whereas a client with symptoms may produce a negative test. Careful correlation of clinical symptoms and laboratory results is a must.

HYPERVENTILATION TEST

Norm. No elevation in ST segment of ECG.

Usage. Provocative noninvasive diagnostic study used to identify coronary vasospasm as a causal agent in clients with variant angina and as an adjuvant test for epilepsy.

Positive. The hyperventilation test is positive when one of these conditions is present on the ECG. ST-segment elevation ≥ 0.2 mV in two leads of the ECG during or after the test. ST-segment depression ≥ 0.1 mV in two leads after the completion of the test. Inverted U-wave not present on the baseline ECG.

Description. Hyperventilation causes cellular alkalosis, which in turn promotes movement of calcium ions intracellularly, which leads to an increase in the tone of vascular smooth muscle in the coronary vasculature. The intent of this study is to induce vasoconstriction in the coronary arteries to determine alterations in myocardial tissue perfusion and oxygenation demonstrated on the ECG. Hyperventilation can facilitate induction of supraventricular tachycardia (SVT).

Professional Considerations
1. Consent form IS required.
2. **Preparation:**
   A. Test is best performed during the early morning hours between 0600 and 0800.
   B. Vasodilators should not be administered 24-48 hours before the test.
3. **Procedure:**
   A. Baseline ECG.
   B. Respirations of 35-40 per minute × 6 minutes.
   C. Arterial blood gas measurement should be completed at the end of the test to confirm an adequate alkalotic state (pH ≥7.55).
4. **Postprocedure care:**
   A. Encourage client to rest after procedure.
5. **Client and family teaching:**
   A. Obtain a medical history before the test. Clients who have a history of pulmonary disease may be adversely affected or unable to tolerate the test and should be excluded.
   B. Inform client to hold vasoactive medications before test.
   C. Encourage client to verbalize any discomfort throughout and after the test.
   D. Chest pain or ECG changes may not occur until completion of the 6 minutes of hyperventilation.
   E. Dysrhythmias may occur, most commonly in test-positive clients.
6. **Factors that affect results:**
   A. None
7. **Other data:**
   A. Calcium-channel blockers may be prescribed for clients having a positive hyperventilation test. Beta-adrenergic blockers should not be prescribed for clients having a positive hyperventilation test.

HYSTEROSALPINGOGRAPHY (UTEROSALPINGOGRAPHY), DIAGNOSTIC

Norm. Normal uterine cavity and fallopian tubes.

Usage. Identification of adhesions of peritoneum, hydrosalpinx, infertility, pelvic abscess or infection, tubal abnormality, tubal pregnancy, tubal ligation, and uteroileal fistula confirmation.

Description. Using serial fluoroscopic radiographs, contrast media (usually water-soluble diatrizoate or iothalamate) is inserted through the cervix so that the uterus, fallopian tubes, and lumens can be visualized. If laparoscopy is also used, the pelvic peritoneal space can be visualized. The test is used to identify malformations, foreign bodies, trauma, and fallopian-tube patency as well as fistulas or adhesions.

Professional Considerations
1. Consent form IS required.

Risks
Allergic reaction to dye (itching, hives, rash, tight feeling in the throat, shortness of breath, bronchospasm, anaphylaxis, death); renal toxicity from contrast medium; uterine perforation; vascular injection of dye; and infection.

Contraindications
Previous allergy to iodine, shellfish, or radiographic dye; renal insufficiency; cervicitis; vaginal bleeding or infection; suspected pregnancy; and cardiopulmonary compromise.

2. **Preparation:**
   A. The test should be performed in the first part of the menstrual cycle.
   B. Administer cleansing enemas.
   C. Have emergency equipment readily available.
   D. The client should disrobe and wear a gown and void just before the procedure.
   E. Obtain a speculum, a uterine cannula, and dye (diatrizoate or iothalamate).
   F. Measure and document baseline vital signs.
   G. See *Client and family teaching.*

3. Procedure:
   A. The client is positioned in the lithotomy position on a tilt table or regular procedure table.
   B. A speculum is inserted into the vagina.
   C. Under fluoroscopy, 6-10 mL (in 3-mL increments) of dye is injected into the cervical opening with a uterine cannula to fill the uterine cavity and fallopian tubes. The table is tilted (or the client is moved) to various positions to enable gravitational flow of the dye through the uterus and the fallopian tubes.
   D. Radiographs are taken 8-24 hours later to help delineate delayed emptying when oily contrast medium is used.
4. Postprocedure care:
   A. Assess for signs of gross bleeding or vaginal discharge.
   B. Monitor vital signs every 15 minutes × 2 and then every 30 minutes × 2.
   C. Small amounts of bloody vaginal discharge may be present up to 2 days postoperatively.
5. Client and family teaching:
   A. Take the prescribed laxative the night before the procedure. Cleansing enemas will be given before the procedure.
   B. It is normal to experience cramping, similar to menstrual cramps, and dizziness during the procedure. Taking prostaglandin inhibitors such as ibuprofen before or after the procedure will lessen the cramping discomfort.
   C. The procedure lasts about 45 minutes.
   D. Avoid vaginal douching and sexual intercourse for 2 weeks after the procedure.
6. Factors that affect results:
   A. A normal fallopian tube may appear strictured if there is too much traction or if there is tubal spasm.
   B. Fallopian tubes may appear normal in the presence of adhesions if too much traction is applied.
7. Other data:
   A. See also Rubin's test, Diagnostic.

HYSTEROSCOPY, DIAGNOSTIC

Norm. Uterine cavity normal.

Usage. Asherman syndrome, endocervical biopsy, fibroid removal, hysterectomy, infertility, intrauterine adhesions, IUD or foreign body removal, septate uteri, and uterine arterial bleeding location.

Description. A 4-mm hysteroscope (telescope type of instrument) is inserted vaginally into the uterus to view the disorder within the uterine cavity that is sometimes missed by hysterosalpingography or curettage.

Professional Considerations
1. Consent form IS required.

Risks
Allergic reaction to Hyskon (32% solution of dextran 70 suspended in glucose) (itching, hives, rash, tight feeling in the throat, shortness of breath, bronchospasm, anaphylaxis, death); renal toxicity from contrast medium. Risks include infection, perforation, and a 1-3% chance of developing PID. Possible life-threatening complications include disseminated intravascular coagulation (DIC) and acute respiratory distress syndrome (ARDS).

Contraindications
Previous allergy to Hyskon (if use is planned). Hysteroscopy is contraindicated in pelvic inflammatory disease (PID), inflamed cervix, and purulent vaginal discharge.

2. Preparation:
   A. Schedule after menstrual bleeding has ceased and before ovulation.
   B. Have emergency equipment readily available.
   C. Have the client void before the procedure.
3. Procedure:
   A. A hysteroscope is inserted vaginally through the cervix into the uterus after the use of a speculum.
   B. Carbon dioxide or Hyskon is instilled to distend the uterine cavity.
   C. The interior walls of the uterus are closely examined for abnormalities, lesions, or bleeding, and photographs or biopsy specimens may be taken.
4. Postprocedure care:
   A. Assess for side effects from the use of carbon dioxide to distend

the uterine cavity: shoulder pain, diaphoresis, nausea, and postoperative bleeding.
   B. Assess for side effects of Hyskon: pulmonary edema, coagulation defects, and anaphylaxis.
5. **Client and family teaching:**
   A. The procedure takes less than 30 minutes.
   B. It is normal to experience cramping, similar to menstrual cramps, and dizziness during the procedure. Taking prostaglandin inhibitors such as ibuprofen before or after the procedure will lessen the cramping discomfort.
   C. Carbon dioxide side effects (listed in section 4A above) may last for a few days. Use a mild analgesia to relieve discomfort.
   D. Immediately report any nausea, pain, shortness of breath, or any other symptoms of discomfort after the procedure.
   E. Avoid vaginal douching and sexual intercourse for 2 weeks after the procedure.
6. **Factors that affect results:**
   A. None found.
7. **Other data:**
   A. Hysteroscopy did not improve on the sensitivity of D & C in the detection of endometrial hyperplasia or carcinoma.
   B. Paracervical anesthesia fails to reduce pain during outpatient hysteroscopy and endometrial biopsy.

IBUPROFEN, BLOOD

Norm:

		SI UNITS
Therapeutic level	10-50 μg/mL	49-243 μmol/L
Toxic level	100-700 μg/mL	485-3395 μmol/L

Overdose Symptoms and Treatment

Note: Treatment choice(s) depend on client history and condition and episode history.

Symptoms. The amount of ibuprofen ingested does not correlate well with symptoms. Ibuprofen overdose usually produces minimal symptoms of toxicity and is rarely fatal. Onset of symptoms generally occurs within 4 hours after ingestion, and clients with normal renal function usually recover completely within 24 hours with supportive care. Typical signs and symptoms include mild gastrointestinal symptoms such as nausea, anorexia, vomiting, abdominal pain. Other signs and symptoms that may occur include gastrointestinal hemorrhage (especially in the elderly), headache, CNS depression (light-headedness, drowsiness, lethargy, coma), seizures, nystagmus, diplopia, tinnitus, hyperventilation, rash, hypotension, bradycardia, hypoprothrombinemia, hypothermia, hepatic failure, apnea, respiratory depression, and cardiac arrest. Renal insufficiency and secondary acute renal failure are generally reversible with supportive therapy.

Treatment of Overdose in Adults

Ingestion of <100 mg/kg	Encourage intake of milk or water to decrease gastrointestinal toxicity.
Ingestion of >100 mg/kg	Empty the stomach by emesis using ipecac syrup or gastric lavage. (*Do NOT induce vomiting* in clients with a decreased level of consciousness, an absent or depressed gag reflex, or a client with a history of a seizure disorder.) After gastric emptying, a saline cathartic should be given.

| **Laboratory Monitoring** | Renal function studies (BUN, creatinine, urinalysis): baseline and repeated in 1-2 weeks, ABG, CBC, liver function studies. |

Management of Specific Symptoms

Hypotension	Typically managed with IV fluids and dopamine if needed.
Seizures (recurrent)	Controlled with IV diazepam, followed by barbiturates.
Symptomatic	Atropine. bradycardia
Severe metabolic	May be treated with sodium bicarbonate. acidosis (pH <7.10)
Renal failure	Dopamine, dobutamine.

The effectiveness of urine alkalinization to enhance urinary excretion is controversial.

Hemodialysis is not effective in the treatment of toxicity because of the high degree of protein binding of the drug.

Monitor for hematuria and proteinuria.

Observe and assess vital signs and neurologic status of symptomatic adults for 24 hours.

Asymptomatic adults should be observed for 4 hours.

Safety considerations and psychiatric consultation are indicated in intentional overdose.

Treatment of Overdose in Children

Amount Ingested	**Treatment**
<100 mg/kg	Generally unlikely to result in toxicity Home observation Caregiver education regarding signs and symptoms to monitor for any dangers of childhood poisoning
100-200 mg/kg	Empty the stomach by emesis and observe for 4 hours. (*Do NOT induce vomiting* in clients with a decreased LOC, an absent or depressed gag reflex, a child who ingested >400 mg/kg, or a client with a history of a seizure disorder.)
200-400 mg/kg	Gastric decontamination, followed by cathartic. Observe at least 4 hours.
>400 mg/kg	Immediate gastric lavage. Observe child carefully for seizure activity.

Usage. Ibuprofen blood levels are not generally indicated; however, they may be useful to identify drug concentrations when overdose, misuse, toxicity is suspected. Monitoring therapeutic levels in long-term ibuprofen use or when high doses are used in children with cystic fibrosis.

Description. Ibuprofen is a nonsteroidal anti-inflammatory drug (NSAID) that is also used for its antipyretic and analgesic activity. Its anti-inflammatory action is believed to be attributable to the inhibition of the synthesis or release of prostaglandins and to its antipyretic effect because of its action on the hypothalamus, with heat dissipation increased as a result of vasodilatation and increased peripheral blood flow. Ibuprofen is rapidly absorbed from the gastrointestinal tract and is 99% protein bound. It is metabolized in the liver and almost completely excreted in the urine 24 hours after ingestion. Half-life is 2-4 hours, with peak blood levels reached in 1-2 hours, though it may take up to 2 weeks to achieve therapeutic response for chronic inflammatory problems.

Ibuprofen is used for rheumatoid arthritis and osteoarthritis, musculoskeletal disorders, fever, primary dysmenorrhea, gout, and dental pain. It can increase bleeding time by inhibiting platelet aggregation, though this action is reversible within 24 hours after the medication is discontinued. High-performance liquid chromatography is used to establish ibuprofen blood levels.

Professional Considerations

1. Consent form NOT required.
2. **Preparation:**
   A. Tube: Red topped. Plasma may be acceptable from tubes with heparin (green topped), EDTA (lavender topped), or sodium fluoride/potassium oxalate (gray topped). Use of gel tubes (red/gray topped) is NOT advised.
3. **Procedure:**
   A. Draw blood from opposite arm if client is receiving ibuprofen intravenously. Draw a 3-mL blood sample.
   B. Refrigerated samples can be used for up to 2 weeks.
4. **Postprocedure care:**
   A. If toxic levels are found, withhold the drug and notify the physician.
5. **Client and family teaching:**
   A. If overdose is suspected, prepare the client and family for supportive treatment outlined above.
   B. If overdose or toxicity occurred in child, instruct the child's parents or caregiver in safe, accurate administration of ibuprofen and review safety issues regarding prevention of accidental poisoning.
   C. Refer clients with intentional overdose for crisis intervention.
6. **Factors that affect results:**
   A. None found.
7. **Other data:**
   A. "Stat" ibuprofen blood levels are not widely available and are not frequently used in overdose or suspected toxicity cases. Since blood levels are not readily available during the relevant initial 4-hour period and there is little correlation between ibuprofen blood levels and symptoms, the management of ibuprofen overdose focuses on symptom management.
   B. Ibuprofen blood levels are not generally monitored during routine ibuprofen therapy. Thera-

peutic response is monitored by evaluation of the degree of symptom relief.
   C. Ibuprofen may decrease renal function because of the inhibition of renal prostaglandin synthesis. This is especially important in clients with decreased renal function or congestive heart failure, since renal prostaglandins may have a role in supporting renal perfusion in these clients. Serum BUN and creatinine levels should also be monitored in clients with impaired renal function, heart failure or hepatic dysfunction, those receiving nephrotoxic drug concomitantly, dehydrated clients, and geriatric clients.
   D. Liver-function studies should be monitored in long-term ibuprofen therapy.

IgA
(see Immunoglobulin A, Serum)

IgD
(see Immunoglobulin D, Serum)

IgE
(see Immunoglobulin E, Serum)

IgG
(see Immunoglobulin G, Serum)

IgM
(see Immunoglobulin M, Serum)

^{125}I-LABELED FIBRINOGEN (FIBRINOGEN UPTAKE) LEG SCAN, DIAGNOSTIC

Norm. No evidence of thrombi. No areas of abnormal concentration in the deep veins of the lower legs.

Usage. Used to monitor the development and progression of deep vein thromboses. Longitudinal screening for clients at risk for thrombotic processes.

Positive. Deep vein thrombosis, thrombophlebitis, and thrombosis.

Negative. Normal finding. Also negative after the active clotting process has stopped.

Description. Fibrinogen (factor I) is a complex polypeptide that converts to the insoluble polymer of fibrin after thrombin enzymatic action and combines with platelets to clot the blood. The ^{125}I-labeled fibrinogen leg scan is an invasive, nuclear medicine test involving the intravenous injection of radionuclide-labeled fibrinogen (fibrinogen labeled with radioactive iodine) and scanning with a well counter for subsequent incorporation of the radioactive material into a thrombus. The scan measures increased surface radioactivity (>20%), which indicates uptake by thrombi in the leg(s). The test is most useful in detecting actively forming thromboses of the calf; 85% of positive results are seen within the first 24 hours after the calf is injected with iodine 125.

Professional Considerations
1. Consent form IS required.

Risks
Infection, allergic reaction to radio labeled fibrinogen (itching, hives, rash, tight feeling in the throat, shortness of breath, bronchospasm, anaphylaxis, death).

Contraindications
Anticoagulant therapy, bleeding disorders, thrombocytopenia, during pregnancy or breast-feeding, previous allergy, radio labeled albumin.

2. **Preparation:**
   A. Ten drops of Lugol's solution in juice are given to block thyroid gland uptake of the radioactive tracer.
   B. Establish 18-gauge intravenous access.
   C. Have emergency equipment readily available.
   D. Assess for swelling in the calf, tenderness, and cyanosis of the skin.
   E. Assess for Homan's sign. Once it is determined to be positive, do NOT repeat Homan's sign assessment.
   F. Elevate the legs during the imaging procedure, which takes about 10 minutes.

3. **Procedure:**
   A. The client's legs are elevated during scanning to prevent pooling of blood in the veins of the legs.
   B. ^{125}Iodine-labeled fibrinogen is injected intravenously, and serial scans are performed on each leg 1, 4, 24, and 48 hours afterward. Surface radioactivity may be measured daily for as long as 2 days.
   C. The extremity is marked in segments along the course of the vein tract.
   D. Areas of fibrinogen incorporation into a thrombus are detected with the counter as areas exhibiting increased radioactivity, indicating increased concentration of radioactive tracer.

4. **Postprocedure care:**
   A. Maintain bed rest if thrombi are detected.
   B. Do not wash off markings on the extremity.
   C. Assess the venipuncture site for infiltration.
   D. Assess for swelling in the calf, tenderness, and cyanosis of the skin.
   E. Observe the client carefully for up to 60 minutes after the study for a possible (anaphylactic) reaction to the radionuclide.
   F. For 24 hours after the procedure, wear rubber gloves when discarding urine. Wash the gloved hands with soap and water before removing the gloves. Wash the ungloved hands after the gloves have been removed.

5. **Client and family teaching:**
   A. This test involves several leg scans after the client receives an intravenous tracer that shows up on the scan. Scanning may continue for up to 2 days after the injection.
   B. The test poses no risk of radioactive damage to the client.
   C. Maintain bed rest until deep venous thrombosis (DVT) has been ruled out.
   D. Meticulously wash hands with soap and water after each void for 24 hours.

6. **Factors that affect results:**
   A. False-negative results may occur where active clot formation is completed, but the thrombus still remains.
   B. Usually 1-2 days are required for enough radiolabeled fibrinogen

to be incorporated into the clot before the clot can be detected.

C. Thrombi of the pelvis are difficult to detect with this test.

D. False-positive results may occur in clients with bacterial inflammatory conditions of the lower extremities.

E. A radioactive test within the previous 24 hours invalidates the results.

F. Up to 72 hours may elapse before the results become positive.

7. **Other data:**
A. Other tests to detect DVT are Doppler ultrasonography, venography, thermography, perfusion lung scan, gas ventilation lung scan, and pulmonary angiography.

B. This test is insensitive to upper thigh and pelvic vein thrombosis.

C. Rate of thrombosis is significantly less with laparoscopic intervention only.

D. Health care professionals working in a nuclear medicine area must follow federal standards set by the Nuclear Regulatory Commission. These standards include precautions for handling the radioactive material and monitoring of potential radiation exposure.

E. Iodine-125 half-life is 60 days.

IMIPRAMINE

(see Tricyclic antidepressants, Plasma or Serum)

IMMUNE COMPLEX ASSAY, BLOOD

Norm:
Complexes not detected.
C1q binding: <13%.
Raji cell assay: <50 g of aggregated human gamma globulin equivalents (AHG).

Positive. Arthritis (rheumatoid), biliary cirrhosis, dengue fever, disseminated gonorrhea, endocarditis, glomerulonephritis, Hansen's disease (leprosy), Hodgkin's disease, leukemia, malaria, malignant melanoma, pulmonary fibrosis, schistosomiasis, serum hepatitis, serum sickness, Sjögren syndrome, and systemic lupus erythematosus (SLE).

Description. Complements are proteins, which, when activated, assist the cell lysis function of antibodies. Activation of complement by an antigen-antibody response is called the "classical pathway." Complement activation independent of antibody, initiated by complement binding to the surfaces of infectious organisms, is known as the "alternative pathway." Both pathways ultimately result in the complement cascade's formation of the membrane attack complex (MAC). This radioimmunoassay (RIA) test is helpful in diagnosing autoimmune and infectious inflammatory disease processes.

Professional Considerations
1. Consent form NOT required.
2. **Preparation:**
A. Tube: Red topped, red/gray topped, or gold topped.
3. **Procedure:**
A. Draw a 2-mL blood sample.
4. **Postprocedure care:**
A. Write the collection time and date on the laboratory requisition.
5. **Client and family teaching:**
A. Results are normally available within 2 days.
6. **Factors that affect results:**
A. Reject specimens received more than 1 hour after collection.
B. Certain cryoglobulins, cold agglutinins, rheumatoid factors, and paraproteins may cause false-positive results.
7. **Other data:**
A. There are specific assays to measure different populations of immune complexes.
B. Also see Raji cell and C1q binding assays.
C. Clinical information and physical findings may be the first sign of an immune complex disorder.
D. See also *TA90 Immune Complex Assay, Serum.*

IMMUNOELECTROPHORESIS, SERUM AND URINE

Norm:

Serum:	No abnormal proteins present.
Urine:	No abnormal proteins present; requires pathologist's interpretation.

Usage. Dysproteinemia, Hodgkin's disease, humoral immune deficiency, multiple myeloma, renal failure, and Waldenström's macroglobulinemia.

Description. A sample of serum or urine is placed on a slide containing agar gel, and an electrical current is passed through the gel, causing separation according to different electrical charges in each immunoglobulin: IgG, IgA, IgM, IgD, and IgE. Each immunoglobulin develops a band that has a certain curvature, position, and intensity of color. Abnormalities in any immunoglobulin cause the band for that precipitation to be displaced, bowed, lighter in color, thicker, or absent. After protein electrophoresis, antisera to immunoglobulins G, A, and M and to kappa and lambda light chains are applied to a urine sample to confirm and identify a suspected monoclonal protein or the presence of Bence Jones proteins (free kappa or lambda light chains).

Professional Considerations
1. Consent form NOT required.
2. Preparation:
   A. *For serum:* Tube: Red topped, red/gray topped, or gold topped. *For urine:* Sterile urine collection container.
   B. Record any vaccinations or immunizations within the previous 6 months on the laboratory requisition.
   C. Record any blood or blood component therapy within the previous 6 weeks on the laboratory requisition.
3. Procedure:
   A. *For serum test:* Draw a 1-mL blood sample.
   B. *For urine test:* Obtain a 12-mL urine sample in a sterile container.
4. Postprocedure care:
   A. Refrigerate the urine; send it to the laboratory within 2 hours.
5. Client and family teaching:
   A. Results are normally available within 24 hours.
6. Factors that affect results:
   A. Anticoagulants, anticonvulsants, hydralazine, oral contraceptives, and phenylbutazone affect the thickness of the bands, causing difficult interpretation in serum tests.

B. Chemotherapy and radiation treatments affect color and thickness of the bands, adding difficulty to the interpretation of the serum test.
7. Other data:
   A. This is a valuable initial screening tool for identifying diseases with altered protein fractions.
   B. The urine test cannot be performed if urine protein is <60 mg/L or if urine protein electrophoresis is normal.

IMMUNOFLUORESCENCE, SKIN BIOPSY, SPECIMEN

Norm. Requires interpretation.

Positive. Collagen disease, dermatitis herpetiformis, immune complex glomerulonephritis, immune disorders of the lung, lupus, malignant lymphoma, multiple myeloma, pemphigus, Waldenström's macroglobulinemia, Wegener's granulomatosis.

Negative. Keratinized tissue.

Description. This procedure uses fluorescent light to visualize tissue and subepidermal blood vessels for the presence of complement, immunoglobulins, and immune complexes containing antibodies and their antigens. Immune complexes are present in many autoimmune diseases and identification of their presence in skin specimens can help to differentiate a diagnosis.

Professional Considerations
1. Consent form IS required for the procedure used to obtain the specimen. See *Biopsy, site-specific, Specimen*, for procedure-specific risks and contraindications.
2. Preparation:
   A. Obtain covered saline-soaked gauze or filter paper, a punch biopsy instrument, ice or a Petri dish, and a local anesthetic.
   B. The container must be labeled with the client's identification information and the date.
3. Procedure:
   A. Local anesthetic may be injected into the biopsy site.
   B. A 3-mm punch biopsy of tissue is collected and placed on ice or in a Petri dish containing 0.9% saline.

4. **Postprocedure care:**
   A. Send the moistened tissue sample to the laboratory immediately to be quickly frozen in liquid nitrogen.
   B. The site may be left open to air or covered with a dry, sterile dressing.
5. **Client and family teaching:**
   A. Keep the site clean and dry and report any signs of infection, such as redness, pain (severe) for more than 24 hours, swelling, or purulent drainage.
   B. Keep the site covered with a Band-Aid or gauze for 2 days, and then leave the site open to air.
   C. Call the physician if there is bleeding amounting to more than a small area on the dressing, or bleeding that won't stop after pressure is applied for 5-10 minutes.
   D. Use a mild analgesic as prescribed, if necessary, for site tenderness.
6. **Factors that affect results:**
   A. Reject specimens in a fixative or any that have dried out.
7. **Other data:**
   A. Failure to detect IgG may be attributed to an infectious or inflammatory process in the sampled tissue.
   B. Repeated biopsies may be necessary for diagnosis of dermatitis herpetiformis.
   C. Skin biopsy in combination with histopathologic examination yields the best diagnostic results.
   D. Submit an additional specimen in formalin for light microscopy.

IMMUNOGLOBULIN A (IgA), SERUM

Norm:

		SI UNITS
Adults	90-400 mg/dL	0.9-4.00 g/L
Children		
Newborn	0-5 mg/dL	0-0.05 g/L
Infants, 25% of adult	0-11 mg/dL	0-0.11 g/L
1-3 months	7-34 mg/dL	0.07-0.34 g/L
4-6 months	10-46 mg/dL	0.10-0.46 g/L
7-12 months	19-55 mg/dL	0.19-0.55 g/L
13-24 months	26-74 mg/dL	0.26-0.74 g/L
25-36 months	34-108 mg/dL	0.34-1.08 g/L
3 years, 50% of adult		
3-5 years	66-120 mg/dL	0.66-1.20 g/L
6-8 years	79-169 mg/dL	0.79-1.69 g/L
9-11 years	71-191 mg/dL	0.71-1.91 g/L
12-16 years	85-211 mg/dL	0.85-2.11 g/L
>16 years	90-400 mg/dL	0.9-4.00 g/L

Increased. Arthritis (rheumatoid), autoimmune disorders, Berger's disease, carcinoma, cirrhosis, chronic infections, dysproteinemia, Henoch-Schönlein purpura, multiple myeloma, polio, sinusitis, and Wiskott-Aldrich syndrome.

Decreased. Bruton's disease, burns, congenital IgA deficiency, hereditary ataxia telangiectasia, humoral immunodeficiency, hypogammaglobulinemia, nephrotic syndrome, and protein-losing enteropathies. Drugs include carbamazepine, dextran, estrogens, gold, methylprednisolone, oral contraceptives, penicillamine, phenytoin, and valproic acid.

Description. Immunoglobulin A (IgA) exists in both serum and secretory forms. IgA is the antibody effective against viruses and certain bacteria such as *Clostridium tetani*, *Corynebacterium diphtheriae,* and *Escherichia coli.* With an area of response localized primarily to mucosal membranes, it is the main immunoglobulin in colostrum, saliva, tears, and secretions of the bronchial, genitourinary, gastrointestinal, and respiratory tracts. Ig A has been found in receptors on alveolar macrophages and on leukocytes and is most recently thought to perform a broad protective function in the respiratory tract. It protects by neutralizing invading viruses at the apical surface of endothelium after infection. In the blood, IgA normally constitutes 10%-15% of client's total serum immunoglobulins.

Professional Considerations
1. Consent form NOT required.
2. Preparation:
   A. Tube: Red topped, red/gray topped, or gold topped.
   B. Write the client's age on the laboratory requisition.
3. Procedure:
   A. Draw a 1-mL blood sample.
4. Postprocedure care:
   A. Refrigerate the specimen if it is not processed immediately.
5. Client and family teaching:
   A. Results are normally available within 24 hours.
6. Factors that affect results:
   A. Reject hemolyzed or turbid samples.
7. Other data:
   A. IgA does not cross the placenta.
   B. Clients with congenital IgA deficiency may develop anaphylaxis if transfused with blood products containing IgA.
   C. Secretory IgA is under investigation for production rate in response to varying conditions. More than one recent study has found an increase in production of salivary IgA after subjects performed progressive relaxation techniques.

IMMUNOGLOBULIN A (IgA) ANTIBODIES, SERUM

Norm. Antibody not present (negative).

Positive. Anaphylactic transfusion reaction in IgA-deficient individual; Disease-specific IgA antibodies indicate past infection.

Description. Antibody formed against IgA when IgA is introduced into the bloodstream of a client with a congenital IgA deficiency. The Ig A is recognized as a foreign antigen, with resultant action of IgG antibodies attacking it, causing anaphylaxis. Testing for IgA antibodies should be performed in all anaphylactic transfusion reactions. A particle gel immunoassay method being tested shows promise for rapid, sensitive, and reproducible detection of IgA antibodies, which can help to quickly confirm IgA transfusion reaction. Other uses for IgA antibody testing are to determine whether a client has had a past infection from a specific organism, such as *Chlamydia pneumoniae*, measles, polio, or *Toxoplasma gondii*.

Professional Considerations
1. Consent form NOT required.
2. Preparation:
   A. Tube: Red topped, red/gray topped, or gold topped.
3. Procedure:
   A. Draw a 7-mL blood sample.
4. Postprocedure care:
   A. Give the client a wallet card, specifying the IgA deficiency.
5. Client and family teaching:
   A. If the test is positive, any future blood transfusions must be IgA deficient or else a severe allergic reaction will occur.
6. Factors that affect results:
   A. Temperature of specimen not held at 37° C.
7. Other data:
   A. None.

IMMUNOGLOBULIN D (IgD), SERUM

Norm. Composes <1% of client's serum immunoglobulins.

		SI UNITS
Adult	0-8.0 mg/dL	5-30 µg/L
Newborn	<1.0 mg/dL	<10 µg/L

Increased. Chronic infections, connective tissue disease, dysproteinemia, and IgD myeloma.

Decreased. Acquired immunodeficiency syndromes. Drugs include phenytoin.

Description. Immunoglobulin D is a protein that may act as an autoimmune antibody in clients with collagen disease. The true biologic function of IgD is unknown but is suspected to play a role in the induction of humoral response and tolerance. The utility of this test is limited, since abnormal findings are rare.

Professional Considerations
1. Consent form NOT required.
2. **Preparation:**
   A. Tube: Red topped, red/gray topped, or gold topped.
   B. Write the client's age on the laboratory requisition.

3. **Procedure:**
   A. Draw a 1-mL blood sample.
4. **Postprocedure care:**
   A. None.
5. **Client and family teaching:**
   A. Results are normally available within 24 hours.
6. **Factors that affect results:**
   A. A chylous serum sample invalidates the results.
7. **Other data:**
   A. 75% of IgD is in the intravascular compartment.
   B. 90% of multiple myelomas are of the IgD type.

IMMUNOGLOBULIN E (IgE), SERUM

Norm:

	IU/mL	U/mL	SI UNITS µg/L
Adults	3-423	4.2-592	10-1421
15-20 years	6.8-39.6	1.5-384	3.60-921.6
21-40 years	20.3-36.5	0.9-239	2.20-573.6
41-60 years	26-53	1.2-324	2.90-777.6
61-87 years	16.2-43.8	0.7-197	1.70-472.8
Children			
Cord blood	0.1-1.5	0.1-2	0.24-4.8
6 weeks	0.1-2.8	0.1-4	0.24-9.6
6 months	0.9-28	0.1-56	0.24-134.4
1 year	1.1-10.2	0.1-83	0.24-199.2
4 years	2.4-34.8	0.4-144	0.96-345.6
10 years	0.3-215	1.9-421	4.56-1010.4
14 years	1.9-159	1.6-456	3.84-1094.4

Increased. Alcohol intake (moderate or more), asthma, allergic rhinitis, atopic dermatitis, bronchopulmonary aspergillosis, eczema, food and (some) drug allergies, hay fever, IgE myeloma, insect sting allergy, occupations with high exposure to hairdressing chemicals, latex allergy, paracoccidioidomycosis, parasitic infections, pemphigoid, periarteritis nodosa, postoperatively (early phase, correlating with severity of surgical injury), sinusitis, visceral leishmaniasis, and Wiskott-Aldrich syndrome. Drugs include gold compounds. Herbal or natural remedies include documented reactions to garlic or *Echinacea*.

Decreased. Advanced carcinoma, alcoholics (after ethanol abstinence), agammaglobulinemia, ataxia-telangiectasia, and IgE deficiency. Drugs include phenytoin sodium. Herbal or natural remedies include *shoseiryu-to* ('minor blue dragon combination', *syo-seiryu-to, xiao³-qing¹long²-tang¹*, composed of *Pinellia, ma²huang²* [yellow vetch], peony, licorice, cinnamon bark, wild ginger [*Asarum*], schizandra [*Schisandra*], and ginger [*Panax*]).

Description. Immunoglobulin E is the antibody protein primarily responsible for allergic reactions such as hay fever, asthma, and allergies to foods and drugs, as well as atopic reactions such as latex allergies. When inhaled or ingested, IgE comes into contact with and activates the mast cells in the respiratory and gastrointestinal tracts and causes a histamine response in the body.

Professional Considerations
1. Consent form NOT required.
2. Preparation:
   A. Tube: Red topped, red/gray topped, or gold topped.
   B. Write the client's age on the laboratory requisition.
3. Procedure:
   A. Draw a 1-mL blood sample.
4. Postprocedure care:
   A. Handle the tube carefully because hemolysis invalidates the test.
5. Client and family teaching:
   A. IgE is elevated in approximately half the people with allergies.
6. Factors that affect results:
   A. The test should not be performed if the client has undergone a radionuclide scan within the previous 72 hours.
B. Levels increase during allergic reactions and disease processes above, and decrease as symptoms subside and clinical conditions improve.
7. Other data:
   A. 50% of IgE is intravascular.
   B. Normal IgE levels do not exclude allergic phenomena.
   C. IgE normally constitutes <0.1% of the client's immunoglobulins.
   D. Among investigational treatments being studied for allergic conditions are an anti-IgE therapy using immunoglobulin directed against IgE and the use of disodium cromoglycate is for reduction of IgE production.

IMMUNOGLOBULIN G (IgG), SERUM

Norm. Normally constitutes 75% of client's total immunoglobulins.

		SI UNITS
Adults	565-1765 mg/dL	5.65-17.65 g/L
Children		
Cord	650-1600 mg/dL	6.5-16.0 g/L
1 month	250-900 mg/dL	2.5-9.0 g/L
2-5 months	200-700 mg/dL	2.0-7.0 g/L
6-9 months	220-900 mg/dL	2.2-9.0 g/L
10-12 months	290-1070 mg/dL	2.9-10.7 g/L
1 year	340-1200 mg/dL	3.4-12.0 g/L
2-3 years	420-1200 mg/dL	4.2-12.0 g/L
4-6 years	460-1240 mg/dL	4.6-12.4 g/L
>6 years	650-1600 mg/dL	6.5-16.0 g/L

Increased. Infections (chronic or recurrent), liver disease (chronic), malignancies (lymphomas), multiple myeloma, pulmonary tuberculosis, rheumatoid arthritis, sarcoidosis, Waldenström syndrome, and systemic lupus erythematosus. The IgG titer is usually elevated in clients with *Helicobacter pylori,* indicating active infection.

Decreased. Acquired immunodeficiency syndrome, aplastic anemia, humoral immunodeficiency, and Wiscott-Aldrich syndrome.

Description. Immunoglobulin G, constituting 75% of all immunoglobulins in the bloodstream, possesses antibody activity against viruses, some bacteria, and toxins. IgG is able to cross the placenta and provide immunity to a developing fetus. It also serves as an activator of the complement system. IgG levels increase in response to infection and remain elevated, even if the infection becomes chronic. IgG is also important in autoimmune diseases because many of the autoantibodies belong in this class. This test evaluates humoral immunity and monitors therapy in IgG myeloma. Various forms of IgG assays are designed to pinpoint disease-specific IgG antibodies for a variety of infections.

Professional Considerations
1. Consent form NOT required.

2. **Preparation:**
   A. Tube: Red topped, red/gray topped, or gold topped.
   B. Write the client's age on the laboratory requisition.
3. **Procedure:**
   A. Draw a 1-mL blood sample.
4. **Postprocedure care:**
   A. None required.
5. **Client and family teaching:**
   A. Results are normally available within 24 hours.
6. **Factors that affect results:**
   A. Specimens should be stored at 37° C.
7. **Other data:**
   A. IgG is the only immunoglobulin that crosses the placenta.

B. Laboratory-based serology titers should be obtained to quantitate the antibody level and establish a baseline when treatment for *H. pylori* is planned. This allows for follow-up after therapy, which if successful, will usually show a consistent fall in IgG titer levels.

IMMUNOGLOBULIN G (IgG) SYNTHESIS RATE, CEREBROSPINAL FLUID, SPECIMEN

(see Cerebrospinal fluid, Immunoglobulin G, Immunoglobulin G ratio and Immunoglobulin G index, Immunoglobulin G synthesis rate, Specimen)

IMMUNOGLOBULIN M (IgM), SERUM

Norm. Normally constitutes 5-10% of the client's total immunoglobulins.

		SI UNITS
Adults	35-375 mg/dL	0.35-3.75 g/L
Children		
Cord	0-19 mg/dL	0-0.19 g/L
1-3 months	7-78 mg/dL	0.07-0.78 g/L
3-6 months	19-72 mg/dL	0.19-0.72 g/L
6-12 months	21-104 mg/dL	0.21-1.04 g/L
1-2 years	19-148 mg/dL	0.19-1.48 g/L
2-3 years	40-151 mg/dL	0.40-1.51 g/L
3-5 years	28-142 mg/dL	0.28-1.42 g/L
5-8 years	30-162 mg/dL	0.30-1.62 g/L
8-12 years	24-161 mg/dL	0.24-1.61 g/L
12-16 years	26-221 mg/dL	0.26-2.21 g/L
Pregnancy	IgM development during pregnancy occurs at an increase of 0.5 mg/dL per week of gestation.	

Increased. Biliary cirrhosis, cutaneous leishmaniasis, Cytomegalovirus, collagen vascular disease, dysproteinemia, infection (bacterial, parasitic), Leptospirosis, Lyme disease, reticulosis, rheumatoid arthritis, sarcoidosis, toxoplasmosis, trypanosomiasis parasite, and Waldenström's macroglobulinemia. Drugs include chlorpromazine.

Decreased. Humoral immunodeficiency, hypogammaglobulinemia, multiple myeloma IgA or IgG, and protein-losing enteropathy. Drugs include carbamazepine and dextran.

Description. Immunoglobulin M is the first antibody to appear after an antigen enters the body and is active against gram-negative organisms and rheumatoid factors. IgM forms the natural antibodies such as those to the ABO blood groups. The IgM molecule is too large to cross the placenta; thus it does not help provide fetal immunity to antigens. If levels are elevated in cord blood samples, it may indicate that the infant was infected before birth with organisms that can cause birth defects, such as *Toxoplasma gondii*, cytomegalovirus, or togavirus (causing rubella). This test is used to screen for congenital infections and to help diagnose and monitor infections.

Professional Considerations
1. Consent form NOT required.
2. Preparation:
   A. Tube: Red topped, red/gray topped, or gold topped.
3. Procedure:
   A. Draw a 1-mL blood sample.
4. Postprocedure care:
   A. None.
5. Client and family teaching:
   A. Results are normally available within 24 hours.
6. Factors that affect results:
   A. Specimen storage at a temperature other than 37° C may cause falsely decreased results.
   B. IgM responses may remain positive in for up to 20 years after a client has had Lyme disease.
7. Other data:
   A. None.

INDENTATION TONOMETRY
(see Tonometry test for glaucoma, Diagnostic)

INDICAN, URINE

Norm. <220 μmol in 24 hours, or negative.

Positive. Hartnup's disease and ileal dysfunction.

Negative. Normal protein catabolism or intestinal absorption.

Description. Indican is a tryptophan metabolite that is excreted mostly in the feces but also in small amounts in the urine as a result of absorption and detoxification of indole produced by bacterial action on tryptophan in the intestines. The presence of indican in the urine indicates amino acid malabsorption.

Professional Considerations
1. Consent form NOT required.
2. Preparation:
   A. Obtain a sterile plastic container.
   B. A sample from a first-morning void or an aliquot of a 24-hour collection is preferred.
3. Procedure:
   A. Collect at least a 6-mL or a random urine specimen in a sterile plastic container.
4. Postprocedure care:
   A. Transport the specimen to the laboratory within 1 hour after collection and refrigerate until testing.
5. Client and family teaching:
   A. Results are normally available with 24 hours.
6. Factors that affect results:
   A. Results are invalid if the urine is not delivered to the laboratory within 1 hour after collection.
7. Other data:
   A. Increased indican may cause the urine specimen to blacken in color over time.

INDIRECT ANTIGLOBULIN TEST
(see Coombs' test, Indirect, Serum)

INFECTIOUS MONONUCLEOSIS SCREENING TEST, BLOOD
(see Heterophil agglutinins, Blood)

INFERTILITY SCREEN, SPECIMEN

Norm:

Multiplex polymerase chain reaction test:	Negative
Antisperm antibody test:	Negative for sperm agglutinating antibody.
Semen analysis:	
pH	7.12-8.0 (average 7.7)
Volume	2-6 mL (0.002-0.006 L, SI units)
Count	50-200 million/mL
Liquification time	Within 30 minutes of collection
Motility	60%-80% are motile
Morphology	>70% are of normal shape

Usage. Evaluation for possible causes of infertility.

Description. The infertility screen includes test of sperm function, antisperm antibody detection, and a genetic test to detect deletion of the Y chromosome long arm DAZ (deleted in azoospermia) gene. This screen may be done alone or as part of a full infertility evaluation that narrows down causes of infertility into the following common categories: abnormal sperm function, abnormal ovulation, tubal dysfunction, antisperm antibodies, and genetic causes. *For evaluation of sperm function,* semen is analyzed for the presence, number, volume, motility, morphology, and liquification time of sperm. *To test for the presence of antisperm antibodies,* spermatozoa, cervical mucus, and both male and female serum are analyzed using an enzyme-linked immunoabsorbent assay, mixed antiglobulin reaction (MAR) with or without immunobead-binding tests, which can identify IgG, IgA, and IgM anti–sperm antibodies. These antibodies have been linked to infertility and are believed to interfere with the interaction of the sperm and the egg and to block the sperm from passing through cervical mucus. *Genetic testing* includes identifying microdeletions from specific regions of the Y chromosome and identification of a congenital bilateral absence of the vas deferens, which is associated with the cystic fibrosis gene. Microdeletions are present to a greater extent in azoospermic men than in men with less severe spermatogenic infertility. Microdeletions reduce fertility. *Other testing* commonly included in infertility evaluation includes ovulation evaluation, laparoscopy, hysterosalpingography, the Sims-Huhner test, and postcoital testing. Less common testing methods sometimes used include hormonal testing, pelvic ultrasonography, hysteroscopy, cervical cultures, and endometrial biopsy.

Professional Considerations
1. Consent form NOT required.
2. Preparation:
   A. Obtain for each partner, a tube: Red topped, red/gray topped, or gold topped.
   B. Obtain a clean, plastic container.
   C. See *Client and family teaching.*
   D. If the semen is to be collected on site, provide privacy for the male client.
   E. See *Client and family teaching.*
3. Procedure:
   A. Obtain a 7-mL blood sample from each partner.
   B. Obtain a fresh semen specimen from male. The specimen should be collected by masturbation, without using a condom or lubricants.
4. Postprocedure care:
   A. Explain that repeat testing may be necessary.
   B. Write the semen collection time on the laboratory requisition, and send the specimen to the laboratory within 2 hours of collection.
5. Client and family teaching:
   A. Do not have intercourse or masturbate for 48 hours before specimen collection.
   B. Collect a fresh semen specimen in a plastic cup. The specimen may be collected by masturbation at the institution or at home, but it must be collected by masturbation. Do not use a condom or a lubricant, other than saliva.
   C. Keep track of the time the semen was collected.
   D. After collecting the specimen, keep the container of semen warm by putting it in a pocket next to the body.
   E. If the specimen is collected at home, it must be delivered to the laboratory within 1 hour.
   F. Consult with your physician before using natural or herbal remedies or medicines because some have been shown to impair the activity of or damage sperm as well as oocytes.
   G. Clients with positive genetic tests should be referred for follow-up genetic counseling.
6. Factors that affect results:
   A. Reject semen specimens more than 2 hours old.
   B. Heavy tobacco smoking and heavy coffee consumption may decrease the number of motile spermatozoa. However, one recent study found that sperm motility increased significantly

with coffee drinking and with smoking when evaluated in infertile couples.

C. Use of coital lubricants reduces sperm motility.

D. The presence of antisperm antibodies has been shown to affect sperm linearity, but not sperm motility.

7. **Other data:**

A. Repeat testing may be necessary because results vary with samples.

B. One study (Haugen et al, 1998) of 207 men found semen pH levels consistently above the WHO upper limit of 8.0.

C. There is some preliminary research, now being carried out more fully through the U.S. National Institutes of Health, that implicates calcium-channel blockers taken by the male as causes of failure to conceive, when all other findings are normal.

D. The infertility rate is about 15%, with the most frequent cause being of genetic origin in the male.

E. See also *Semen analysis, Specimen.*

INFLUENZA A AND B TITER, BLOOD

Norm. Less than a fourfold increase in titer in paired sera. Less than 1:8 titer indicates previous exposure.

Positive. Influenza.

Negative. Bacterial infections.

Description. Influenza viruses are typed for epidemiologic surveys. Both viruses, A and B, cause major epidemics every 2-4 years, as antigenic shifts occur, leaving the population susceptible to reinfection by a different strain. Virus B usually is sporadic and local, whereas virus A spreads rapidly and to all population areas.

Professional Considerations
1. Consent form NOT required.

2. **Preparation:**
   A. Tube: Red topped, red/gray topped, or gold topped.
3. **Procedure:**
   A. Draw a 7-mL blood sample at the onset of symptoms.
   B. Draw a convalescent sample 14 days later.
4. **Postprocedure care:**
   A. None.
5. **Client and family teaching:**
   A. Return in 2 weeks for a second sample to be drawn. This helps monitor recovery.
   B. Annual influenza vaccinations are recommended in the latter portions of each year for the elderly, health care workers, and others at high risk for exposure to the influenza virus.
6. **Factors that affect results:**
   A. Failure to collect a convalescent sample limits the value of the acute sample results.
   B. Immune response to the vaccine is less in those that have received previous influenza vaccination than in those receiving it for the first time.
   C. The immune response to the influenza vaccine is significantly impaired in clients who have received liver transplants.
7. **Other data:**
   A. Serologic diagnosis is not necessary during an epidemic but is valuable for epidemiologic purposes.
   B. Influenza vaccination is typically not very effective in those age 80 years and over. One study found immune response in this population to be enhanced in those given nutritional supplementation.
   C. Intranasal vaccines have been found equivalent to the intramuscular route in stimulating the immune response.

INHIBITION LEVEL, ANTIBIOTIC
(see Schlichter test, Specimen)

INR
(see Prothrombin time and International Normalized Ratio, Serum)

INSULIN AND INSULIN ANTIBODIES, BLOOD

Norm. Free insulin: fasting: ≤25 µU/mL (<179 pmol/L, SI units).
  Insulin level via radioimmunoassay:

ADULT		SI UNITS
Adult, fasting level	<17 µU/mL or 1.00 mg/L	42-243 pmol/L
Newborn	3-20 µU/mL	21-139 pmol/L
Infant	<13 µU/mL	≤89 pmol/L
Prepubertal child	<13 µU/mL	≤89 pmol/L
Panic levels	>30 µU/mL	>290 pmol/L
Last trimester, amniotic fluid	11.3 µU/mL	78 pmol/L

Insulin Antibodies. Undetectable to less than 4% when using either bovine or porcine insulin as a reagent. Insulin antibodies have been shown to occur more frequently with aging and in females than in males.

Panic Level Symptoms and Treatment

Symptoms. Diaphoresis, dizziness, faintness, pallor, weakness, progressing to stupor and seizures.

Treatment:
Note: Treatment choice(s) depend on client history and condition and episode history.
Administer 50% dextrose in water ($D_{50}W$) by 50-mL IV injection, followed by carbohydrate and protein foods.
Follow with $D_{10}W$ infusion if NPH or other long-acting insulin was taken.
Administer glucagon IV if the client has normal liver function.
Take bedside or laboratory glucose measurement hourly.
If serum potassium level is low or cardiac dysrhythmias are present, give KCl infusion.
Hemodialysis and peritoneal dialysis will NOT remove insulin.

Increased Insulin. Acromegaly, Beckwith-Wiedemann syndrome, beta-cell adenoma, Cushing syndrome, dystrophia myotonica, familial fructose and galactose intolerance, hyperinsulinism, hypoglycemia, insulin-resistance syndromes, insulinoma, liver disease, non–insulin-dependent diabetes mellitus, metabolic syndrome, nesidioblastosis, obesity, overdose of insulin, pancreatic islet cell lesion, and pheochromocytoma. Drugs include albuterol, calcium gluconate in the newborn, estrogen, fructose, glucagon, glucose, insulin, levodopa, medroxyprogesterone, oral contraceptives, prednisolone, quinine, quinidine, spironolactone, sucrose, terbutaline, tolazamide, and tolbutamide.

Decreased Insulin. Diabetes mellitus, hyperglycemia, hypopituitarism, and pancreatectomy-induced diabetes. Drugs include beta-adrenergic blockers, asparaginase, calcitonin, cimetidine, diazoxide, ethacrynic acid, ethyl alcohol (ethanol), ether, furosemide, metformin, nifedipine, phenformin, phenobarbital, phenytoin, and thiazide diuretics.

Positive Insulin Antibodies. Factitious hypoglycemia, autoimmune insulin syndrome (AIS).

Negative Insulin Antibodies. Normal finding. Also negative in insulinoma.

Description. Insulin is a hormone that regulates carbohydrate metabolism. It is produced in the pancreas by the beta cells of the islets of Langerhans of the pancreas, and its rate of secretion is determined primarily by the level of blood glucose. The radioimmunoassay test measures endogenous insulin by using a series of tubes containing a fixed amount of antibody label and an aliquot of standard, control, or unknown. The client's unlabeled antigen in the blood competes with labeled antigen for antibody-binding sites. The percentage of antigen bound to antibody is related to the total antigen present and is reflected by the distribution of a radioactive label. Low immunoreactive insulin levels have been associated with a higher risk of developing degenerative diseases such as atherosclerosis, hypertension, and dyslipidemia. *Insulin antibodies*, also referred to as anti–insulin-Ab, may be present in either diabetics treated for several weeks or more with conventional insulin. These antibodies may also be present in persons who have never received insulin but have autoimmune insulin syndrome (AIS), a rare condition characterized by hyperinsulinemia and hypoglycemia. For diabetics, this test may be used with C-peptide to determine whether hypoglycemia is caused by insulin abuse. Insulin antibodies are transferred through the placenta and are present in 30-50% of children at the time of diagnosis before beginning insulin therapy.

Professional Considerations
1. Consent form NOT required.
2. **Preparation:**
   A. Tube: Red topped, red/gray topped, or gold topped. Also obtain ice.
   B. Specimens MAY be drawn during hemodialysis.
   C. See *Client and family teaching.*
3. **Procedure:**
   A. Draw a 7-mL blood sample. Place the sample immediately on ice.
4. **Postprocedure care:**
   A. Resume diet and any medications held prior to the test.
   B. Assess the client for signs of hypoglycemia, which could occur as a response to fasting.
5. **Client and family teaching:**
   A. This test is used to evaluate for insulin-producing neoplasm (islet cell tumor, insulinoma) or to evaluate insulin production in diabetes mellitus.
   B. Fast from food and fluids (except water) for 8 hours before the test
   C. Do not take insulin before the test.
   D. Review the procedure used to obtain the blood sample, including the fact that some discomfort may be experienced when the needle enters the skin.

6. **Factors that affect results:**
   A. Reject specimens if the client had a radioactive scan within 7 days before the test.
   B. Hemodialysis destroys insulin.
   C. Specimen hemolysis invalidates the results.
   D. Falsely elevated results have been found when insulin antibodies are present in the blood when the radioimmunoassay testing method is used. More accurate results are obtained when the immunoradiometric assay testing method is used if insulin antibodies are suspected.
   E. Values are higher in plasma samples than in serum.
   F. Elevated results have been found in men with elevated c-reactive protein levels.
7. **Other data:**
   A. Serum insulin level is commonly prescribed with serum glucose to confirm functional hypoglycemia, uncontrolled insulin-dependent diabetes mellitus, or fasting hypoglycemia of unknown cause.
   B. The norms and standardization of the test method vary widely by laboratory.
   C. Undetectable in amniotic fluid during the first trimester.
   D. Complete absence of insulin during the last trimester of pregnancy is associated with intrauterine death.
   E. Some studies evaluating the relationship of C-reactive protein, glucose, and Hb_{1ac} indicate a possible role of inflammation in insulin resistance.
   F. When insulin antibodies are present, the test of choice is C-peptide to determine whether exogenous insulin administration is being abused. If C-peptide levels are not elevated, endogenous insulin secretion has not increased.

INSULIN-LIKE GROWTH FACTOR-I (IgF-I), BLOOD

Norm:

		SI UNITS
Adult Females	24-253 ng/mL or 0.4-2 U/mL	24-253 m/L or 400-2000 U/L
Adult Males	43-178 ng/mL or 0.7-1.7 U/mL	43-178 m/L 700-1700 U/L

		SI UNITS
Children		
0-2 Years		
Female	14-60 ng/mL	14-60 m/L
Male	14-56 ng/mL	14-56 m/L
3-5 Years		
Female	18-97 ng/mL	18-97 m/L
Male	13-81 ng/mL	13-81 m/L
6-9 Years		
Female	34-137 ng/mL	34-137 m/L
Male	29-108 ng/mL	29-108 m/L
10-12 Years		
Female	66-215 ng/mL	66-215 m/L
Male	44-207 ng/mL	44-207 m/L
13-15 Years		
Female	192-347 ng/mL	192-347 m/L
Male	98-319 ng/mL	98-319 m/L
16-18 Years		
Female	132-305 ng/mL	132-305 m/L
Male	136-293 ng/mL	136-293 m/L

Increased. Acromegaly, diabetic retinopathy, hyperpituitarism, obesity, pituitary gigantism, precocious puberty, and pregnancy.

Decreased. Anorexia nervosa, cirrhosis, chronic illness, delayed puberty, diabetes mellitus, emotional deprivation syndrome, hepatoma, hypopituitarism, hypothyroidism, kwashiorkor, Laron dwarfs, liver disease, maternal deprivation syndrome, nutritional deficiency, and pituitary tumor.

Description. Insulin-like growth factor-I (IGF-I) is a small polypeptide produced primarily in the liver, transported in the plasma, and bound by carrier proteins. Acting via cell membrane receptors, IGF-I directly stimulates growth and proliferation of normal cells and mediates the level of growth hormone in the bloodstream. IGF-I affects glucose metabolism and is itself affected by growth hormone activity. IGF levels decrease with aging. Increased growth hormone in the bloodstream causes an increase in the level of IGF-I. Thus this test may be used when one is monitoring response to growth hormone treatment in growth hormone replacement therapy in adults or in pituitary dwarfism because levels are highest during growth spurts. IGF-1 is also used to evaluate the severity of acromegaly.

Professional Considerations
1. Consent form NOT required.
2. **Preparation:**
   A. Tube: Lavender topped.
   B. Specimens MAY be drawn during hemodialysis.
   C. See *Client and family teaching.*
3. **Procedure:**
   A. Draw a 2-mL blood sample.
4. **Postprocedure care:**
   A. Immediately separate and freeze serum. The specimen is stable for 30 days.
5. **Client and family teaching:**
   A. Fast from food and fluids from midnight before the test.
   B. Results may not be available for several days.
6. **Factors that affect results:**
   A. Decreased nutritional states.
   B. Results may be falsely elevated if the client received a radioactive scan within the previous 7 days.
7. **Other data:**
   A. Norms in pregnant women are higher than those in non pregnant women.
   B. IGF-I is now produced by recombinant DNA technology and may be useful in the treatment of acromegaly and certain types of dwarfism.
   C. IGF-II is similar in structure to IGF-I and is believed to be an important regulator of embryonic

and fetal growth. Its level remains fairly constant after an initial rise in the first year of life.

D. Recent studies of the interrelationship of IGF-I, insulin, and IGF-binding proteins indicate a possible correlation of increased bioavailability of IGF-I with increased risk of colon cancer.

E. The test was formerly known as somatomedin C.

INTERNATIONAL NORMALIZED RATIO, SERUM

(see Prothrombin time and International Normalized Ratio, Blood)

INTERNATIONAL SENSITIVITY INDEX

(see Prothrombin time and International Normalized Ratio, Blood)

INTRADUCTAL ULTRASONOGRAPHY, DIAGNOSTOC

(see Pancreas ultrasonography, Diagnostic)

INTRAOCULAR PRESSURE MEASUREMENT, DIAGNOSTIC

(see Tonometry test for glaucoma, Diagnostic)

INTRAVASCULAR COAGULATION SCREEN, BLOOD

Norm:

Fibrinogen

Adult	200-400 mg/dL
Newborn	125-300 mg/dL
Fibrin breakdown products	<10 µg/mL

Platelet Count

Adult	150,000-400,000/mm³
Newborn	84,000-478,000/mm³
Activated partial thromboplastin time (APTT)	25-35 seconds

Prothrombin Time

Adult	11-15 seconds
Newborn	2-35 seconds
Premature	3-5 seconds

Thrombin Time 16-23 seconds

Usage. Differentiation of acute disseminated intravascular coagulation (DIC) from chronic DIC.

Test	Acute DIC	Chronic DIC
D-Dimer	Increased	Increased
Fibrinogen	Decreased	Normal or increased
Fibrin breakdown	Positive	Positive
Platelet count	Decreased (or may appear normal if falling from a baseline high level)	Normal or increased
APTT	Increased	Normal
Prothrombin time	Increased	Normal
Thrombin time	Increased	Increased
Peripheral smear	Schistocytes present	

Description. Intravascular coagulation is a process whereby there are multiple fibrin thrombi with microinfarctions and tissue and organ necrosis. This is caused by activation of the clotting mechanism and depletion of clotting factors and platelets with a secondary fibrinolysis that results in bleeding.

In severe situations, the life-threatening condition of DIC can occur. DIC is triggered by systemic activation of the hemostasis system from release of tissue factor from endothelial cells or other circulating cells. The systemic activation eventually overcomes natural inhibitor mechanisms, allowing more coagulation to occur, which depletes the supply of fibrinogen and platelets. The end result is uncontrolled diffuse bleeding.

Professional Considerations

1. Consent form NOT required.
2. **Preparation:**
   A. Tubes: Three red topped, red/gray topped, or gold topped.
3. **Procedure:**
   A. Draw three 5-mL blood samples in the three tubes.
4. **Postprocedure care:**
   A. Place a pressure dressing on the venipuncture site. Monitor closely for bleeding.
5. **Client and family teaching:**
   A. Clients with disseminated intravascular coagulation (DIC) may be in acute crisis. Support the family; explain that there may be a need for blood product therapy.
6. **Factors that affect results:**
   A. Heparin increases clotting time.
7. **Other data:**
   A. DIC is eliminated only by eliminating the underlying cause. Short-term symptomatic support includes administration of cryoprecipitate, platelet concentrates, and fresh frozen plasma.

INTRAVASCULAR ULTRASONOGRAPHY, DIAGNOSTIC
(see Coronary intravascular ultrasonography, Diagnostic)

INTRAVENOUS CHOLANGIOGRAPHY

Norm. Even filling of the hepatic and biliary ducts. Complete filling of the gallbladder occurs. Negative for stones, stricture, or filling defects.

Usage. Alternative to oral cholecystography when client cannot tolerate oral iodopaque tablets or in clients with active intestinal inflammation; and detection of calculi (or their movement), strictures, or leaking anastamosis or anastamoses in the biliary ductal system.

Description. Intravenous cholangiography involves taking a series of radiographs of the gallbladder and hepatobiliary duct systems over several hours after the intravenous administration of a radiographic contrast medium. The contrast medium is allowed to circulate to the liver through the hepatic artery and empty into the biliary tree. Strictures or stones cause defects in the pattern of filling and can be visualized on the radiograph. Strictures occurring in the hepatobiliary ducts may be congenital or caused by ductal damage during exploratory or therapeutic biliary surgery or caused by benign or malignant tumor or inflammation. Intravenous cholangiography carries a diagnostic accuracy of 99% for detection of stones in the common bile duct; however, it has NOT been shown to provide incrementally superior information than other tests used to evaluate the hepatobiliary system (see *Professional Considerations, 7-A*).

Professional Considerations
1. Consent form IS required.

Risks
Hypotension, infection, nausea, respiratory failure, tachycardia, vomiting, allergic reaction to dye (itching, hives, rash, tight feeling in the throat, shortness of breath, bronchospasm, anaphylaxis, death), renal toxicity from contrast medium.

Contraindications
Respiratory failure; previous allergy to iodine, shellfish, or radiographic dye; renal insufficiency; during pregnancy (because of radioactive iodine crossing the blood-placental barrier).

2. **Preparation:**
   A. A laxative or cathartic may be administered 24 hours before the procedure.
   B. A cleansing or tap-water enema may be given the morning of the procedure.
   C. Establish intravenous access.

D. Have emergency equipment readily available.

E. See *Client and family teaching.*

3. **Procedure:**

A. The client is positioned supine on the scanning table.

B. A radiographic contrast medium is injected intravenously or infused by drip and allowed at least 30 minutes to circulate to the liver and become excreted into the bile ducts. Radiographs of the hepatic and bile ducts are taken at this time.

C. 2-3 hours are then allowed to pass to allow the gallbladder to fill with contrast medium. Radiographs may be taken of the gallbladder and biliary system at intervals for up to 8 hours after injection.

4. **Postprocedure care:**

A. Resume previous diet.

B. Assess for allergy to contrast medium for 24 hours.

C. Dysuria is not uncommon because the contrast medium is excreted in the urine.

5. **Client and family teaching:**

A. Fast from food and fluids overnight before the test.

B. Morning insulin may be withheld for diabetics because the test may take up to 8 hours.

C. A burning or flushing sensation may be experienced when the dye is injected.

D. Bring something to read, if desired, because the test may take several hours.

E. Blockage of the gallbladder can be caused by stones formed from natural bile salts and substances similar in nature to cholesterol. A low-fat diet is generally recommended for clients with gallbladder disease.

F. In women who are breast-feeding, formula should be substituted for breast milk for 1 or more days after the procedure.

6. **Factors that affect results:**

A. Hepatic failure with bilirubin >3.5 mg/dL (58 mmol/L, SI units) will interfere with gallbladder visualization. The dye must be processed in the liver before it passes into the gallbladder. The test will be canceled for a high bilirubin level.

7. **Other data:**

A. See also *Endoscopic retrograde cholangiopancreatography, Diagnostic,* and *Percutaneous transhepatic cholangiography, Diagnostic,* two tests that are used more commonly than intravenous cholangiography.

INTRAVENOUS PYELOGRAPHY (IVP, EXCRETORY UROGRAPHY), DIAGNOSTIC

Norm. Normal renal pelvis, ureters, and bladder. No obstruction or masses.

Usage. Berger's disease, glomerulonephritis, hydronephrosis, renal cell cancer, renal failure, renal hypertension, tubular necrosis, and Wilms' tumor. Examination of the superior ureters during pregnancy as compared with ultrasonography (see *Precautions*).

Description. An invasive test that uses contrast radiopaque dye to assess the ability of the kidneys to excrete dye in the urine. Radiographs are taken after dye injection to visualize the kidneys, ureters, and bladder to assess for obstruction, hematuria, stones, bladder injury, and renal artery occlusion of the renal pelvis. IVP is the first choice for evaluation for kidney stones, if non-contrast computed tomography is not available.

Professional Considerations

1. Consent form IS required.

Risks

Dysuria, nephrotoxicity, urinary tract infection, vasovagal response, allergic reaction to dye (itching, hives, rash, tight feeling in the throat, shortness of breath, bronchospasm, anaphylaxis, death), renal toxicity from contrast medium, weakness.

Contraindications

Dehydration, pregnancy (because of radioactive iodine crossing the blood-placental barrier), previous allergy to iodinated radiographic dye, renal insufficiency.

2. **Preparation:**

A. Bowel preparation of orally administered evacuation preparation 24 hours before the test and evacuation enema 8 hours before test.

B. Assess for high-risk clients: dehydration, elderly, severe diabetes mellitus, renal insufficiency, or multiple myeloma.

C. Have emergency equipment readily available.

3. **Procedure:**
   A. The client is placed in slight Trendelenburg position or supine.
   B. A venipuncture is performed, and dye is injected into a vein.
   C. Serial radiographs are taken periodically for the next 30 minutes.

4. **Postprocedure care:**
   A. The client should drink at least three 8-ounce glasses of liquid to flush the kidneys of the dye (when not contraindicated).
   B. Assess for signs of allergic reaction to the dye (listed above) for 24 hours.

5. **Client and family teaching:**
   A. It is normal to feel flushed and warm and to notice a salty taste soon after the dye is injected. This will last only a few moments.
   B. Stress the importance of drinking water after the test to flush dye from the body, prevent osmotic diuresis from the dye, and protect the kidneys.
   C. In women who are breast-feeding, formula should be substituted for breast milk for 1 or more days after the procedure.

6. **Factors that affect results:**
   A. Poor bowel evacuation or poor renal perfusion will decrease the uptake of dye, leading to poor radiograph quality.

7. **Other data:**
   A. Dosages of radiation range from 1047 to 1465 mR (milliroentgens).
   B. Magnetic resonance urography, although much more costly, is superior to renal ultrasonography in identifying pathology for clients with kidneys that do not opacify (such as those with renal transplants) during excretory urography.

INTRINSIC FACTOR ANTIBODY, BLOOD

Norm. Negative; none detected.

Positive. Graves' disease, insulin-dependent diabetes, megaloblastic anemia, and pernicious anemia.

Description. Intrinsic factor is produced by the parietal cells of the gastric mucosa and is required for the effective absorption of vitamin B_{12}. In some diseases, antibodies that bind the cobalamin–intrinsic factor complex are produced and prevent the complex from binding to receptors in the ileum.

Professional Considerations
1. Consent form NOT required.
2. **Preparation:**
   A. Tube: Red topped, red/gray topped, or gold topped.
   B. Do not collect a sample if vitamin B_{12} was injected or ingested by client within 48 hours before the test.
3. **Procedure:**
   A. Draw a 3-mL blood sample.
4. **Postprocedure care:**
   A. None.
5. **Client and family teaching:**
   A. If the test results show the presence of antibodies and a positive diagnosis is made of pernicious anemia, the client requires regular injections of vitamin B_{12} because of the body's loss of ability to produce the intrinsic factor secreted by the parietal cells in the stomach lining.
6. **Factors that affect results:**
   A. Reject if the client had a radioactive scan within 7 days before the test.
7. **Other data:**
   A. Causes of vitamin B_{12} deficiency include pancreatic insufficiency, parasitic infestations of the small intestine, regional enteritis, malnutrition, or transcobalamin protein abnormalities.

INULIN CLEARANCE TEST, DIAGNOSTIC

Norm:

Adults	90-130 mL/minute
>70 years	Decreased clearance up to 45% of adult value
Male	124 ± 25.8 mL/min
Female	119 ± 12.8 mL/min
Children	
<11 years	82-122 mL/minute
11-20 years	86-126 mL/minute

Usage. Assessment of glomerular filtration rate (GFR).

Increased. Diuresis.

Decreased. Decreased results occur when over 50% of renal nephrons are damaged, thus indicating impaired glomerular filtration; acute tubular necrosis, atherosclerosis (renal artery), congestive heart failure, decreased renal blood flow, dehydration, glomerulonephritis, malignancy (bilateral renal), nephrosclerosis, obstruction (renal artery), polycystic kidney disease, pyelonephritis (advanced bilateral chronic), renal lesions (bilateral), renal failure, shock (cardiogenic, hypovolemic), thrombosis (renal vein), tuberculosis (renal), and ureteral obstruction (bilateral). Drugs include aminoglycosides, amphotericin B, penicillins, and phenacetin.

Description. GFR is the standard measure of renal function and is critical for the management of renal diseases. The GFR in humans can be determined *exactly* by measurement of the clearance of an ideal filtration marker, such as inulin, which is a soluble dietary plant fiber that is freely filtered by the kidney and does not undergo metabolism, tubular secretion, or absorption. This method, however, is not suitable for routine clinical practice. The classic method of measuring inulin clearance in humans includes constant intravenous infusion of the compound and timed collections of urine. To avoid the need for timed urine collections, several alternative procedures have been devised. All these methods use only determination of inulin in plasma or serum. From these, the total body inulin clearance is obtained by means of pharmacokinetic calculations. To measure total body clearance, usually called "plasma clearance," inulin is given either as a constant intravenous infusion or as a bolus infusion. Both procedures overestimate GFR because of incomplete distribution of inulin during the study periods. The error may be minimized by means of model-independent pharmacokinetic calculations.

Professional Considerations
1. Consent form NOT required.

2. **Preparation:**
   A. Determination of systemic inulin clearance by the standard technique of constant intravenous infusion has long been accepted as a reliable method for measuring GFR without urine collection.
   B. Obtain alcohol wipes, a tourniquet, 5 needles, 5 syringes, 5 green-topped tubes, 5 clean specimen containers with lids, and a 500-mL bag of D_5W with Y tubing.
   C. Establish intravenous access, using 5% dextrose in water.
   D. Number each set of tubes and specimen containers 1, 2, 3, 4, and 5, and use them sequentially throughout the test.
   E. Obtain 25 mL of 10% inulin and 500 mL of 1.5% inulin along with an intravenous pump. Prepare the inulin by shaking the vial and heating it to promote crystal dissolution.
   F. Use this test cautiously in clients with cardiac disease because intravenous fluids given during the test may induce congestive heart failure.
   G. See *Client and family teaching.*
   H. Do NOT perform test or draw specimen during hemodialysis.
3. **Procedure:**
   A. Draw a 10-mL blood sample for inulin level, without hemolysis. Record the time of collection on each label.
   B. Infuse intravenously 25 mL of 10% inulin over 4 minutes.
   C. An hour later, begin an infusion of 1.5% inulin, 500 mL at 240 mL/hour.
   D. Draw a 10-mL blood sample for inulin level, without hemolysis, at 40, 60, 80, and 95 minutes after the initiation of the 1.5% inulin solution. Record the time of collection on each label.
   E. The test takes 2 hours.
4. **Postprocedure care:**
   A. Write the time and amount of each dose of inulin on the laboratory requisition.
   B. Each blood sample should be sent immediately to the laboratory after being collected.
   C. Resume previous diet.
5. **Client and family teaching:**
   A. Fast from food for 4 hours before the test, and refrain from exercise the morning of the test.

B. The test takes 2 hours to complete.
6. **Factors that affect results:**
   A. Hemolysis of blood will falsely decrease results.
   B. Failure to infuse intravenous inulin at the prescribed rate will decrease results.

7. **Other data:**
   A. The initial bolus of inulin should be administered within 1 hour of preparation.

IRF
(see Reticulocyte Count, Blood)

IRON (Fe), SERUM

Norm:

		SI UNITS
Adult female	40-150 µg/dL	7.2-26.9 µmol/L
Adult male	50-160 µg/dL	8.9-28.7 µmol/L
Newborn	100-250 µg/dL	17.9-44.8 µmol/L
Infant	40-100 µg/dL	7.2-17.9 µmol/L
Child	50-120 µg/dL	8.9-21.5 µmol/L

Increased. Acute hepatitis, aplastic anemia, blood transfusion, hemochromatosis, hemolytic anemia, hepatitis, lead poisoning, nephritis, pernicious anemia, polycythemia, sideroblastic anemia, thalassemia, and vitamin B_6 deficiency. Drugs include alcohol (wine, ethanol).

Decreased. Blood loss, burns, carcinoma, gastrectomy, infection, iron deficiency anemia, kwashiorkor, malabsorption, nephrosis, postoperative state, pregnancy, rheumatoid arthritis, schizophrenia (chronic), tetralogy of Fallot, and uremia.

Description. Iron is an inorganic ion, found mostly in hemoglobin, that acts as a carrier of oxygen from the lungs to the tissues and indirectly aids in the return of carbon dioxide to the lungs. Although the primary source of body iron is food, only a small portion of that consumed from the diet is absorbed. Iron is stored in the liver and reticuloendothelial tissue in the form of ferritin and hemosiderin and is released from storage as needed to meet the body's demands. Although iron levels are assumed to be highest in the morning due to a diurnal variation, studies have not shown that restricting specimen collection to the morning improves the reliability of the result.

Professional Considerations
1. Consent form NOT required.

2. **Preparation:**
   A. Tube: Red topped, red/gray topped, or gold topped.
   B. Screen client for use of herbal medicines or natural remedies.
   C. Document the date of the last blood transfusion on the laboratory requisition.
   D. Do NOT draw specimens during hemodialysis.
3. **Procedure:**
   A. If using Vacutainer and venipuncture for multiple samples, draw this sample first to avoid mixing heparin with the sample. Draw a 7-mL blood sample.
4. **Postprocedure care:**
   A. None.
5. **Client and family teaching:**
   A. The basic role of iron in hemoglobin formation is to allow blood to efficiently carry oxygen to the tissues. Foods rich in iron include red meats and some green, leafy vegetables.
6. **Factors that affect results:**
   A. Hemolysis of the specimens invalidates the results.
   B. Vitamin B_{12} ingested within 48 hours may increase the results.
   C. Herbs that interfere with iron absorption include St. John's wort and saw palmetto, which contain tannic acids.
7. **Other data:**
   A. Adenocarcinoma of the gastrointestinal tract may be detected by iron deficiency.

B. Increased serum iron concentrations of 300-500 mg/dL (53.7-89.6 mmol/L, SI units) can be the result of one ingested iron tablet.

C. Increased ferritin levels frequently accompany neoplastic activity.

D. See also *Iron and total iron-binding capacity/transferrin, Serum*.

IRON (Fe) AND TOTAL IRON-BINDING CAPACITY (TIBC)/TRANSFERRIN, SERUM

Norm:

		SI UNITS
Adult female	40-150 µg/dL	7.2-26.9 µmol/L
Adult male	50-160 µg/dL	8.9-28.7 µmol/L
Newborn	100-250 µg/dL	17.9-44.8 µmol/L
Infant	40-100 µg/dL	7.2-17.9 µmol/L
Child	50-120 µg/dL	8.9-21.5 µmol/L
TIBC		
Adult	250-400 µg/dL	44.8-71.6 µmol/L
Infant	100-400 µg/dL	17.9-71.6 µmol/L
Transferrin		
Adult	200-400 mg/dL	2-4.0 g/L
Maternal	305 mg/dL	3.0 g/L
(Term)		
Fetal	190 mg/dL	1.9 g/L
Newborn	130-275 mg/dL	1.3-2.8 g/L

Increased TIBC. Hepatitis, microcytic anemia, and pregnancy. Drugs include iron salts and oral contraceptives.

Decreased TIBC. Cirrhosis, dysmenorrhea, hemochromatosis, hemorrhage, hepatitis, hypothyroidism, kwashiorkor, microcytic anemia, myocardial infarction, neoplasm, nephrosis, pernicious anemia, thalassemia, and uremia. Drugs include ACTH, asparaginase, chloramphenicol, corticotropin, cortisone, dextran, steroids, and testosterone.

Description. This test differentiates anemia secondary to iron deficiency from other diseases associated with variations in cellular oxidation. Iron is an element necessary for many body processes, including the transport of oxygen to the tissues and for oxygen-carrying chromoproteins, hemoglobin, myoglobin, and enzymes such as xanthine oxidase and peroxidase. Transferrin is a plasma iron-transport protein, also called siderophilin, formed in the liver that has a half-life of 7-10 days. Transferrin is capable of binding more than its own weight in iron (that is, 1 g of transferrin can carry 1.43 g of iron).

In normal clients, iron saturation of transferrin is between 20% and 45%. Transferrin saturation by iron demonstrates a diurnal pattern, with a morning peak and an early evening trough. The formula for transferrin saturation by iron is:

$$(\text{Serum iron/TIBC}) \times 100 = \text{Transferrin saturation}$$

TIBC is the maximum amount of iron that can be bound to transferrin. It is useful in distinguishing anemia (increased value) from chronic inflammatory disorders (normal value). In this test, iron is added to the client's serum until all transferrin-binding sites are bound with iron. Then the excess iron is removed, and the total amount of remaining (bound) iron is measured, giving an assessment of the ability of the individual's transferrin to bind iron.

Professional Considerations

1. Consent form NOT required.
2. Preparation:
   A. Tube: Red topped, red/gray topped, or gold topped; and 20-gauge or larger needle.
   B. Document the date of the last blood transfusion on the requisition.

C. See *Client and family teaching.*
3. **Procedure:**
   A. Draw a 7-mL blood sample, without hemolysis.
4. **Postprocedure care:**
   A. None.
5. **Client and family teaching:**
   A. Fast 12 hours before sampling. Water is permitted.
   B. If the results indicate a low level of iron, eat foods rich in iron such as organ meats, eggs, and dried fruits.
6. **Factors that affect results:**
   A. Inflammatory states may decrease results below normal.
   B. Hemolysis may cause falsely elevated iron values.
7. **Other data:**
   A. A decrease in iron and an increase in TIBC are found in microcytic anemia.
   B. Serum transferrin may be calculated from TIBC using the formula "0.8 × TIBC − 43."
   C. See also *Soluble transferrin receptor assay, Serum.*

IRON STAIN, BONE MARROW, SPECIMEN
(see Bone marrow aspiration analysis, Specimen)

ISI
(see Prothrombin time and International Normalized Ratio, Blood)

ISOPROPYL ALCOHOL, BLOOD
(see Toxicology, Volatiles group by GLC, Blood or Urine

IVP
(see Intravenous pyelography, Diagnostic)

IVY BLEEDING TIME, DIAGNOSTIC
(see Bleeding time, Ivy, Blood; Aspirin tolerance test, Diagnostic)

KETONE, SEMIQUANTITATIVE, URINE
(see Ketone, Semiquantitative, Urine)

KETONE BODIES, BLOOD

Norm. Negative or 0.3-2.0 mg/dL (<0.17 mmol/L, SI units).

Panic Level. >20 mg/dL (>3.44 mmol/L, SI units).

Panic Level Symptoms and Treatment

Symptoms. Fruity breath, acidosis, ketonuria, depressed level of consciousness.

Treatment:
Note: Treatment choice(s) depend on client history and condition and episode history.
Blood glucose measurement every hour.
Insulin infusion.
Neurologic checks every hour.

Positive. After anesthesia, alcoholism, carbohydrate deficiency, diabetes mellitus, eclampsia, fasting, glycogen storage disease, high-fat (ketogenic) diet, hyperglycemia, isopropanol alcohol ingestion, ketoacidosis, pregnant diabetic, prolonged exercise, reducing diets, starvation, and von Gierke's disease. Drugs include: propranolol (poisoning).

Negative. Not applicable.

Description. Ketones are synthesized by the liver from fatty acids when a lack of glucose causes the body to use fat for energy. In a low-insulin state such as diabetes, fat and fatty acids are metabolized less efficiently than normal, resulting in a buildup of serum ketones. Ketone bodies consist of acetone, acetoacetic acid, and beta-hydroxybutyric acid. Beta-hydroxybutyric acid is the predominant type of ketone body occurring in diabetic ketoacidosis. Extremely elevated levels in the bloodstream can lead to coma. This test only measures acetone and acetoacetic acid and is used in conjunction with the *Beta-hydroxybutyrate, Blood* test to help differentiate coma caused by a hyperosmotic state (in which a negative test would be expected), from coma caused by ketoacidosis.

Professional Considerations
1. Consent form NOT required.

2. **Preparation:**
   A. Tube: Red topped, red/gray topped, or gold topped; or capillary tubes.
3. **Procedure:**
   A. Draw a 1-mL blood sample in a tube or collect the specimen in capillary tubes, filling them as completely as possible. Either central venous or peripheral blood is acceptable.
4. **Postprocedure care:**
   A. None.
5. **Client and family teaching:**
   A. Ketone bodies, a natural byproduct of metabolism, can be dangerously elevated in some diseases.
   B. Coma caused by diabetic ketoacidosis is usually reversible.
6. **Factors that affect results:**
   A. Hemolysis of the specimen invalidates the results.
   B. A low-carbohydrate or low-fat diet may cause elevated results.
   C. After 7 days of storage at −20° C, levels of acetoacetate are about 40% lower than at the time of specimen collection. After 40 days, levels are 100% lower. The degradation of acetoacetate can be slowed by storing at −80° C, resulting in 85% of the original acetoacetate still being present after 40 days.
   D. This test is not useful for monitoring response to treatment in DKA, because acetoacetate levels tend to remain stable, even with treatment. The *Beta-hydroxybutyrate, Blood* test should be used for treatment monitoring.
7. **Other data:**
   A. Elevated acetone with normal anion gap, bicarbonate, and plasma glucose is suggestive of rubbing alcohol (isopropanol) intoxication.
   B. Ketones appear in the urine before there is a significant increase in the blood.
   C. See also *Beta-hydroxybutyrate, Blood* and *Anion Gap, Blood.*

KETONE, SEMIQUANTITATIVE, URINE

Norm. Negative or Keto-Diastix negative.

Usage. Detection of ketones in the urine for carbohydrate deprivation, diabetes mellitus, diabetic ketoacidosis, or ketonuria.

Positive. Alcoholism, diabetes mellitus, convulsions, eclampsia, Fanconi syndrome, glycogen storage disease, ketogenic diet, ketoacidosis, and von Gierke's disease. Drugs include anesthesia, isopropyl alcohol (isopropanol), levodopa, and mesna.

Description. Ketone bodies consist of acetoacetic acid, beta-hydroxybutyric acid, and acetone and are by-products of fat and fatty acid metabolism. In a low-insulin state such as diabetes, fat and fatty acids are metabolized less efficiently than normal, resulting in a buildup of serum ketones. Elevated serum ketones are excreted through the kidneys into the urine. In this test, a dipstick is used for determining ketones in the urine. The reagent strip correlates only moderately well with quantitative acetoacetate in plasma and poorly with total blood ketones, but is a better screening test for diabetic ketoacidosis than the anion gap or serum bicarbonate. Semiquantitative results means testing several different dilutions of each urine specimen to obtain a better degree of differentiation of ketone body products that can be obtained from qualitative testing.

Professional Considerations
1. Consent form NOT required.
2. **Preparation:**
   A. Obtain a clean, plastic specimen container.
3. **Procedure:**
   A. Instruct the client to void and then to drink a glass of water.
   B. 30 minutes later, ask the client to void into the specimen container.
   C. Dip the stick into the urine for 5 seconds.
   D. Tap the edge of the stick against the container of urine to remove excess urine.
   E. After 15 seconds, compare the color of the ketone section (buff or purple) with the appropriate color chart. Report the results of ketones that are positive as either small, moderate, or large.
4. **Postprocedure care:**
   A. Send the specimen to the laboratory immediately. If the specimen cannot be tested immediately, refrigerate it. Cap the container tightly.

B. Testing must occur within 60 minutes of the specimen being obtained, for specimens kept at room temperature. Refrigerated urine may be tested later but must first be returned to room temperature.

5. **Client and family teaching:**

A. Assess over-the-counter medications for drugs that may cause false positives.

6. **Factors that affect results:**

A. Preservative in foods of 8-hydroxyquinoline may increase urine levels.

B. Drugs that may cause false-positive results include ascorbic acid, levodopa, phenazopyridine HCl (Pyridium), phthalein compounds given for liver or kidney tests, and valproic acid.

C. A low-carbohydrate or high-fat diet may cause elevated results.

7. **Other data:**

A. Ketones appear in the urine before serum elevations are seen.

B. Pentamidine therapy for AIDS may induce ketoacidosis in clients with diabetes mellitus.

C. Keto-Diastix assesses ketones only, not glucose.

D. Breath acetone testing is more practical than and as reliable as urine ketone testing when performing ongoing monitoring of ketone levels for clients receiving ketogenic diets for control of intractable seizures.

KETOSTIX, DIAGNOSTIC
(see Ketone, Semiquantitative, Urine)

KI-67 PROLIFERATION MARKER (MIB 1-3), SPECIMEN

Norm. Rated from low proliferation index to high proliferation index. Varies with tumor type.

Usage. Determination of the proliferation index (PI) of a specific tumor type to provide prognostic information in predicting the clinical outcome of certain tumors. The Ki-67 monoclonal antibody is used to determine the proliferation state of breast cancer, bone cancer, brain tumors, cervical cancer, colorectal cancer, endometrial cancer, liver tumors, lymphomas, plasma cell tumors, smooth muscle tumors, and soft-tissue tumors.

More studies are needed to determine the usefulness of Ki-67 as a predictor of tumor recurrence, as findings are mixed to date. Nonneoplastic conditions such as hemangiomas, inflammatory bowel disease, lupus nephritis, membranoproliferative glomerulonephritis, psoriasis, renal biopsy, and sarcoidosis also use the Ki-67 proliferation marker.

Description. Ki-67 is an IgG1-class, murine monoclonal antibody that reacts with a nuclear antigen expressed only by proliferating human cells. Expression of this antigen occurs during the late G1, S1, G2, and M phases of the cell cycle. The proliferation activity of a tumor tissue is determined by the growth fraction (number of cells in cell cycle) and the time taken to complete the cell cycle. A strong correlation exists between the proliferation rate of tumors and clinical outcome, and there is an association between a high proliferation rate and the degree of tumor aggressiveness. The Ki-67 immunostaining, along with histopathologic evaluation, has been shown to be beneficial in correlating the proliferation state of cancers such as breast, lymphatic, lung, and brain with clinical prognosis. Results of Ki-67 immunostaining as a prognostic factor vary with each tumor type using quantitative analysis. MIB 1-3 are newer antibodies that recognize the Ki-67 antigen in both fixed and frozen tissue, whereas the Ki-67 antibody requires a fresh, frozen sample.

Professional Considerations

1. Consent form IS required. See *Biopsy, Site-specific, Specimen,* for procedure-specific risks and complications.

2. **Preparation:**

A. The client is prepared for surgical biopsy or resection.

3. **Procedure:**

A. A fresh specimen, free of excess fat and blood and of at least 0.5-1.0 g, is obtained by surgical resection or needle biopsy.

B. The specimen is cut into small pieces and quick-frozen on dry ice, cryostat, or liquid nitrogen within 20 minutes of excision.

C. For Ki-67 immunostaining, do not place the specimen into formalin. Place the frozen specimen into a 60-mL solid-tumor biopsy bottle. The specimen must remain frozen ($-70°$ C).

K

D. For MIB-1 (Ki-67) the specimen may be prepared using a formalin-fixed paraffin block. Optimal fixation time is 12-24 hours, not to exceed 48 hours.

4. **Postprocedure care:**
   A. Apply a dry, sterile dressing to the biopsy or operative site.
   B. Assess the site for excessive bleeding, erythema, hematoma, or drainage.

5. **Client and family teaching:**
   A. Results will not be available for at least 2 days.

6. **Factors that affect results:**
   A. Thawed specimens will be rejected.
   B. Bronchial brushings are unacceptable because of tumor cell clumping and presence of mucus.
   C. The Ki-67 antigen is very sensitive to chemical denaturation and is destroyed in weak solutions of formalin.
   D. The Ki-67 antigen expression appears to be influenced by a cell's nutritional supply. Tissue taken from the central area of a large tumor may give an erroneously low value for the growth factor.

7. **Other data:**
   A. None.

KIDNEY BIOPSY, SPECIMEN

Norm. Interpretation required.

Usage. Alport syndrome, childhood idiopathic nephrotic syndrome, diabetic glomerulosclerosis, glomerulonephritis, Goodpasture syndrome, hematuria, Kimmelstiel-Wilson disease, nephrosis, nephrotic syndrome, renal failure, and toxemia.

Description. The surgical or percutaneous needle biopsy resulting in the aseptic removal of a small quantity of kidney tissue. This procedure is often performed under the guidance of ultrasound or computed tomography, but may also be an open (surgical) or a transjugular (transvenous) procedure. In the rare instance of pelvic kidney, a laparoscopy has been used to obtain the biopsy.

Professional Considerations
1. Consent form IS required.

Risks
Bleeding, infection, pneumothorax.

Contraindications
Percutaneous biopsy is contraindicated in uncooperative clients; in clients with bleeding diatheses, uncontrolled hypertension, or renal infection; or (usually) in clients with a solitary functional kidney. Mendelssohn and Cole (1995) recommend conditions under which clients with solitary functional kidneys might be considered candidates for kidney biopsy.

2. **Preparation:**
   A. Before the biopsy, an intravenous pyelography test or renal scan should be performed to document bilateral renal function.
   B. Obtain a biopsy tray, including a needle, sponges, lidocaine (Xylocaine), and slides or a sterile specimen jar.

3. **Procedure:**
   A. A renal biopsy can be performed percutaneously with a special needle or under direct visualization during surgery.

4. **Postprocedure care:**
   A. Send the specimen to the laboratory immediately.
   B. Monitor vital signs every 15 minutes × 4.
   C. Monitor for blood in the urine 8 hours after the biopsy.

5. **Client and family teaching:**
   A. This examination of renal tissue can provide valuable details in diagnosing kidney disease.
   B. Report any pain in the flank or abdomen after the procedure.

6. **Factors that affect results:**
   A. None found.

7. **Other data:**
   A. Indications for a renal biopsy are not clear-cut or universally agreed upon.
   B. A 1-year creatinine measurement has been shown to be as useful, and less risky, than kidney biopsy for prediction of long-term kidney function after kidney transplant.
   C. Histologic preparations using hematoxylin and eosin, periodic acid–Schiff, silver, or Trichrome (Masson) stains are also routinely performed on the tissue sample.
   D. Histologic preparations using hematoxylin and eosin, periodic

acid–Schiff, silver, or Trichrome (Masson) stains are also routinely performed on the tissue sample.

KIDNEY ECHOGRAPHY
(*see Kidney ultrasonography, Diagnostic*)

KIDNEY PROFILE, BLOOD
(*see SMA-7, Blood*)

KIDNEY SCAN, DIAGNOSTIC
(*see Renocystography, Diagnostic*)

KIDNEY STONE ANALYSIS, SPECIMEN

Norm. Interpretation required.

TYPE OF STONE	PREV- ALENCE	CHARAC- TERISTIC	CONDITION
Calcium compounds such as calcium oxalate and calcium phosphate	80%	Appear black, gray, or white	Chronic dehydration (failure to routinely drink adequate amounts of water throughout each day) Familial tendencies Hypercalcemia Hyperparathyroidism Hyperthyroidism Renal tubular acidosis Unknown cause (common) Vitamin D intoxication
Calcium oxalate			Intake of a diet high in oxalate-rich foods. Methoxyflurane anesthesia Vitamin B deficiency
Cystine	< 2%	Appear yellowish with flecks of shiny material	Renal tubular defects
Magnesium ammonium phosphate (struvite, staghorn stones)	5%-20%	Appearance similar to deer antlers	Urinary tract infection caused by *Proteus* type of bacteria
Uric acid	5%-10%	Difficult to visualize on an x-ray	Cancer Gout Lymphoproliferative disorders

K

Usage. Hematuria, kidney stone, and nephrolithiasis. Determination of the chemical composition of kidney stones gives an indication as to the underlying cause and helps guide future preventive treatment.

Description. Kidney stones (renal calculi) are formed in up to 20% of people from urine particulates such as calcium oxalate, magnesium ammonium phosphate, uric acid, and cystine. The occur- rence of kidney stones is higher in Caucasians than in African Americans, and in males than in females. Kidney stones can be diagnosed via computed tomography or an intravenous pyelogram. Kidney stones for analysis are either passed naturally through the ureters into the urine, or removed via surgery. In this procedure, infrared spectroscopy is used to examine the kidney stone(s) after the specimen has been washed free of tissue and blood to determine the composition. The spectra of the stone(s) is compared to the known spectra of chemical compounds. Knowing the composition helps understand the underlying causes, which are listed above. Factors that increase a person's risk for kidney stones include having a personal or family history of kidney stones, being a male aged 20-50, being on prolonged bed rest, spinal injury affecting the bladder, having frequent urinary tract infections, or having inflammatory bowel disease.

Professional Considerations
1. Consent form NOT required but IS required for the procedure used to obtain the specimen. See the individual procedure for risks and contraindications.
2. Preparation:
   A. Obtain a clean specimen container.
3. Procedure:
   A. Send the stone in a plastic or glass container to the laboratory immediately.
4. Postprocedure care:
   A. Encourage the intake of fluids.
   B. A mild analgesic may be prescribed for use as needed.
5. Client and family teaching:
   A. Strain the urine for further stones if they are needed for analysis.
   B. If the stone can be removed and the infection stopped, the client has a low probability of the condition returning.
   C. A low-oxalate diet may help prevent kidney stones formed from calcium oxalate. A low-oxalate diet includes avoiding soybean products, wheat germ, grapefruit juice, strawberries, bananas, orange juice, canned pineapples or tomatoes, kidney beans, beets, spinach, carrots, celery, onions, sweet and white potatoes, green and waxed beans, cauliflower, cucumber, squash, broccoli, eggplant, cabbage, cashews, peanut butter and other nuts, cola beverages, and tea.
6. Factors that affect results:
   A. Do not apply tape to stones because adhesives interfere with infrared spectroscopy.
7. Other data:
   A. Children commonly have stones from infection caused by calcium phosphate and magnesium ammonium phosphate

B. Large doses of vitamin B_6 may reduce the risk of kidney stone formation in women.
C. Helical computed tomography has been shown to be helpful in identifying the fragility of kidney stones, and thus potential susceptibility to shock wave lithotripsy. See *Computed tomography of the body, Diagnostic.*

KIDNEY ULTRASONOGRAPHY (KIDNEY ECHOGRAPHY, KIDNEY ULTRASOUND), DIAGNOSTIC

Norm. Bilateral kidneys are properly located and are of normal size and shape. The outer contour is smooth. Kidney is surrounded by echoes reflected from perirenal fat. Intense echoes are reflected by the renal sinus. Absence of calculi, cyst, hydronephrosis, obstruction, or tumor.

Usage. Alternative to renal dye imaging tests for clients with allergy to radiographic dyes Used for detection of hydronephrosis; diagnosis and localization of renal cysts, tumors, or calculi; evaluation of status after renal transplantation; and guidance for antegrade pyelography, biopsy, aspiration, or nephrostomy tube insertion. Although this procedure is inferior to intravenous pyelography when used alone, its advantages include the ability to detect some stones without the use of ionizing radiation. Disadvantages include risk of inaccurate measurement of calculus diameter, poor differentiation of true obstruction from non-obstructed dilatation, and inability to demonstrate the ureteral jet phenomenon at the uterovesical junction.

Description. Evaluation of the kidney structure by the creation of an oscilloscopic picture from the echoes of high-frequency sound waves passing over the flank area (acoustic imaging). The time required for the ultrasonic beam to be reflected back to the transducer from differing densities of tissue is converted by a computer to an electrical impulse displayed on an oscilloscopic screen to create a three-dimensional picture of the kidney. The kidney is imaged by use of the liver or spleen as an acoustic window. Renal cysts appear smooth, sonolucent, and spherical, with well-defined borders. In contrast, solid masses are of irregular shape with poorly defined borders and higher attenuation. Inflammatory cysts have thicker walls, less well-defined borders, and contain low-level echoes. Early hematomas look like cysts and become more echogenic over time. Hydronephrosis is demonstrated by a large extrarenal pelvis, with renal parenchyma not detectable. In multicystic disease, the kidney is of smaller than normal size, and the renal pelvis cannot be visualized. In polycystic disease, irregularly shaped cysts >1 mm diameter are present in variable shapes and sizes. Because this procedure cannot pinpoint obstruction, results that suggest the presence of hydronephrosis require additional confirmatory testing such as intravenous pyelography, computed tomography, or magnetic resonance urography.

Professional Considerations
1. Consent form NOT required.
2. **Preparation:**
   A. The client must be hydrated before the procedure.
   B. This test should be performed before intestinal barium tests or after the barium is cleared from the system.
   C. The client should disrobe below the waist or wear a gown.
   D. Obtain ultrasonic gel or paste.
3. **Procedure:**
   A. The client is positioned prone in bed or on a procedure table. Very young children are positioned supine.
   B. The flank area is covered with ultrasonic gel, and a lubricated transducer is passed slowly over the flank area at a variety of angles and at intervals about 1-2 cm apart.
   C. Photographs are taken of the oscilloscopic display.
4. **Postprocedure care:**
   A. Remove the lubricant from the skin.
   B. If a biopsy is performed, see *Biopsy, Site-specific, Specimen.*
   C. If an antegrade pyelography or a nephrostomy tube insertion is performed with this test, see *Antegrade pyelography, Diagnostic.*
5. **Client and family teaching:**
   A. The procedure is painless and carries no risks (if kidney ultra-

sonography is not performed with invasive procedures).
   B. This procedure takes about 30 minutes.
6. **Factors that affect results:**
   A. Dehydration interferes with adequate contrast between organs and body fluids.
   B. Intestinal barium obscures results by preventing proper transmission and deflection of the high-frequency sound waves.
   C. The more trunk fat present, the greater the attenuation (reduction in sound-wave amplitude and intensity), which interferes with the clarity of the picture. A lower frequency transducer should be used if a great deal of fat surrounds the kidney.
   D. Magnetic resonance urography, while much more costly, is superior to kidney ultrasonography in identifying pathology for clients with kidneys that do not opacify (such as those with renal transplants) during excretory urography.
   E. Proper hydration is essential for best detection. In clients who are not properly hydrated, up to 30% of obstructions and 25-65% of hydronephrosis may not be detected.
7. **Other data:**
   A. Further studies may include tomography or other radiographic imaging.
   B. See also *Antegrade pyelography, Diagnostic.*

KIDNEY ULTRASOUND
(*see Kidney ultrasonography, Diagnostic*)

KIDNEY-URETER-BLADDER, DIAGNOSTIC
(*see Flat-plate radiography of abdomen, Diagnostic*)

KIRSTEN, BLOOD
(*see K-ras, Blood*)

KLEIHAUER-BETKE STAIN, DIAGNOSTIC
(*see Betke-Kleihauer stain, Diagnostic*)

K

K-*ras* (KIRSTEN), BLOOD OR SPECIMEN

Norm. Negative for K-*ras* mutations.

Usage. Colorectal cancer, adenocarcinoma of the lung, endometrial carcinoma (up to 33%), pancreatic and bile duct carcinoma (>75%). Research is currently being conducted to determine its use in the detection, diagnosis, determination of response to therapy, and prognosis of colorectal cancer. It may be useful for the same reasons in pancreatic cancer.

Description. The K-*ras* oncogene is one of three members of the *ras* family of oncogenes, along with H-*ras* and N-*ras*. This oncogene resides on chromosome 12p12 and is involved in protein coding that modulates cellular proliferation and differentiation. Mutations of the K-*ras* gene occur early in tumorigenesis and are associated with >50% of colorectal adenocarcinomas and carcinomas. A strong correlation has been demonstrated between the presence of mutated K-*ras* gene in the colorectal tumor and the presence of the mutated K-*ras* gene in the blood. The mutant K-*ras* protein p21*ras* protein can be detected in the blood by use of a DNA-extraction method, such as a polymerase chain reaction (PCR)–based assay that utilizes sequence-specific primers to amplify the mutant DNA, thus detecting the tumor cells in blood. It can also be detected in tissue specimens using immunohistochemical methods. The K-*ras* oncogene has the potential to be a specific and sensitive marker for colorectal cancer.

Professional Considerations
1. Consent form is NOT required.
2. Preparation:
   A. Tubes with additives EDTA (lavender topped) or sodium citrate (blue topped). Heparinized tubes (green topped) have been used; however, there is some potential that heparin may inhibit the amplification assay. Confirm tube choice with the lab conducting the study. Clotted blood has been used. The mutated K-*ras* oncogene has been identified in serum and plasma samples.
3. Procedure:
   A. Amount of blood collected varies from 10 to 20 mL. Confirm amount of blood needed for the specimen with laboratory. A test

has been conducted on serum and plasma stored in frozen state after several years.
   B. Alternatively, tissue specimens may be obtained via biopsy. *See Biopsy, Site-specific, Specimen.*
4. Postprocedure care:
   A. If biopsy is used, see *Biopsy, Site-specific, Specimen.*
   B. None.
5. Client and family teaching:
   A. Results may not be available for several days if testing is performed at a distant site.
6. Factors that affect results:
   A. K-*ras* mutations are not present in all clients who have colorectal cancer. It is specific only in the 40%-50% of the colorectal cancers that are associated with K-*ras* mutations. The remaining 50%-60% of the colorectal cancers that are associated with other causes or markers will not be identified by the mutated K-*ras* gene (Anker et al, 1997).
   B. There have been incidents where clients with colorectal tumors containing the mutated K-ras gene did not have the K-ras gene identified in blood samples. These observations have been attributed to the possible genetic difference of metastatic lesions from the primary tumor, with the metastatic lesions being either lost or having never had the K-*ras* mutation.
   C. It has been speculated that the amount of circulating mutant K-*ras* gene could be increased after chemotherapy or surgery, increasing K-*ras* detection in the blood.
7. Other data:
   A. Generally, plasma or serum DNA mutations match the DNA mutations found in the primary tumor, leading to the assumption that the DNA mutations found in the blood are derived from the primary tumor.
   B. K-*ras*–mutated DNA associated with colorectal cancer has been found in colorectal tumors and in the feces of clients with colorectal cancer, holding implications for use in screening for colorectal cancer.

KUB (KIDNEY-URETERS-BLADDER), DIAGNOSTIC
(*see Flat-plate radiography of abdomen, Diagnostic*)

LABILE FACTOR, BLOOD
(see Factor V, Blood)

LA CROSSE VIRUS TITER, SERUM
(see California encephalitis virus titer, Serum)

LACTATE DEHYDROGENASE (LD), BLOOD

Norm:

		SI UNITS
Wróblewski Method	150-450 U/L	72-217 IU/L
30° C		
Adult		
≤60 years	45-90 U/L	45-90 U/L
>60 years	55-102 U/L	55-102 U/L
Newborn	160-500 U/L	160-500 U/L
Neonate	300-1500 U/L	300-1500 U/L
Infant	100-250 U/L	100-250 U/L
Child	60-170 U/L	60-170 U/L

Increased Total LD. Alcoholism, anemia (hemolytic, megaloblastic, pernicious), anoxia, burns (electric, thermal), cancer, cardiomyopathy, cerebrovascular accident, cirrhosis, congestive heart failure (with myocardial infarction), convulsions, delirium tremens, dysrhythmias (ventricular), folic acid anemia, hepatic neoplasm, hepatitis (acute, toxic), hypothyroidism, infectious mononucleosis, intracardiac prosthetic valves, jaundice (obstructive), lactic acidosis, leukemia (granulocytic, acute), lymphoma, malaria, megaloblastic anemia, mononucleosis (infectious), muscular dystrophy, myocardial infarction, myxedema, nephrectomy, nephritis, nephrotic syndrome, ovarian dysgerminoma, pain (muscle and bone), peritonitis, pernicious anemia, pheochromocytoma, *Pneumocystis carinii* pneumonia, polymyositis, pulmonary embolism, pulmonary infarction, renal cortical infarction, renal infection, renal malignancy, sickle cell anemia, shock, skeletal muscle necrosis, splenomegaly, sprue, toxic shock syndrome, trauma, tumors (malignant), and ulcerative colitis. Drugs include anesthetics, chlorpromazine hydrochloride, clofibrate, codeine, dicumarol, ethyl alcohol (ethanol), floxuridine, fluorides, imipramine, lithium carbonate, lorazepam, meperidine, methotrexate, metoprolol tartrate, mithramycin, morphine and other narcotic analgesics, niacin, nifedipine, nitrofurantoin, procainamide hydrochloride, propoxyphene, propranolol, quinidine, sufonamides, and thyroid hormone.

Decreased Total LD. Irradiation therapy. Drugs include oxalates.

Description. Lactate dehydrogenase (LD) is an intracellular enzyme found in almost all body tissues that is released after tissue damage. The highest concentrations are found in organs such as the heart, liver, kidneys, and skeletal muscle cells as well as the red blood cells. When body tissue is damaged from trauma, ischemia, or acid/base imbalance, LD is released into the bloodstream. The results of this test indicate that tissue damage has occurred but cannot pinpoint the specific location of damage. When total LD is elevated to at least 130 IU/L, the *Lactate dehydrogenase isoenzymes* test should be performed to narrow down the source of tissue damage.

Professional Considerations
1. Consent form NOT required.
2. Preparation:
   A. Tube: Red topped, red/gray topped, or gold topped.
   B. Do NOT draw during hemodialysis.
3. Procedure:
   A. Draw a 1-mL blood sample, without hemolysis.
4. Postprocedure care:
   A. None.
5. Client and family teaching:
   A. This test is used to look for compounds commonly found in the body after some type of damage to the tissue. If the results are elevated, another test is usually performed on the same blood speci-

L

men to help narrow down which type of tissue has been damaged.
6. Factors that affect results:
   A. Reject hemolyzed, frozen, or refrigerated samples. Hemolysis elevates the LD_1 isoenzyme, which will elevate total LD results.
   B. Heparin increases LD in one third of all clients being treated with heparin.
   C. In burn clients, plasma LD activity is higher than in serum, possibly due to leakage from ruptured platelets.
7. Other data:
   A. LD is recommended as a prognostic factor in colorectal carcinoma. Clients with an initially normal level versus those with an abnormal level had median survivals of 16 and 7 months, respectively. LD is also being studied for its use as a prognostic factor in myelodysplastic syndrome, with higher levels being associated with shorter survival
   B. See also *Lactate dehydrogenase isoenzymes, Blood.*

LACTATE DEHYDROGENASE (LD) ISOENZYMES, BLOOD

Norm:
LD_1 = 22-36% cardiac and RBC origin
LD_2 = 35-46% cardiac and RBC origin
LD_3 = 13-26% lung, lymph, skeletal, and spleen origin
LD_4 = 3-10% hepatic and skeletal muscle origin
LD_5 = 2-9% hepatic and skeletal muscle origin
$LD_2 > LD_1$
$LD_1:LD_2 \leq 1$
$LD_4 > LD_5$
$LD_5:LD_4 \leq 1:3$

Increased LD Total. Anemia (megaloblastic, hemolytic), cardiomyopathy, congestive heart failure, delirium tremens, hypothyroidism, inflammation, leukemia, muscle injury, myeloproliferative syndromes, myxedema, pulmonary infarction, and renal infarction. See *Lactate dehydrogenase, Blood.*

Increased LD_1. Folic acid anemia, hepatitis, megaloblastic anemia, myocardial infarction (rises 24 hours after injury, peaks at 72 hours, and returns to baseline level within 2

weeks), pernicious anemia, renal infarction, and testicular cancer.

Increased LD_2. Muscular dystrophy, pernicious anemia, and renal (cortex) infarction, rhabdomyolysis, tumor.

Increased LD_3. Advanced cancer, collagen disease, infection (viral), lymphocytosis, pancreatitis, pericarditis, platelet destruction, pulmonary embolism, pulmonary infarct with hepatic congestion, pulmonary pneumonia, and skeletal muscle injury.

Increased LD_4. Hepatitis, infectious mononucleosis, lymphoma, lymphocytic leukemia, and ovarian carcinoma, platelet destruction, pulmonary embolism, and skeletal muscle injury.

Increased LD_5. Alcoholism, cirrhosis, congestive heart failure, hepatitis, infectious mononucleosis, megaloblastic anemia, myocardial infarction, neonates, ovarian carcinoma, pulmonary infarct with hepatic congestion, and skeletal muscle injury.

Increased LD 1:2 Ratio. Inverted, or "flipped," in anemia (hemolytic, megaloblastic, pernicious, sickle cell [acute]), cardiac hypoxia, folic acid deficiency, hemolysis, megaloblastic anemia, myocardial infarction, renal infarction.

Increased LD 5:4 Ratio. Alcoholism.

Decreased. LD_1 is normally decreased in neonates.

Description. See *Lactate dehydrogenase, Blood.* This test is normally conducted when total LD levels are elevated. Electrophoresis is used to separate the five isoenzymes of lactate dehydrogenase (LD), an enzyme that catalyzes the reversible oxidation of lactic acid to pyruvic acid. LD isoenzymes help pinpoint whether tissue damage is of cardiac, red blood cell, hepatic, or skeletal muscle origin.

Professional Considerations
1. Consent form NOT required.
2. Preparation:
   A. Tube: Red topped, red/gray topped, or gold topped.
3. Procedure:
   A. Draw a 1-mL blood sample, without hemolysis. The test may also be performed on the original

specimen sent for total LD measurement.

4. Postprocedure care:
   A. Do not refrigerate or freeze the specimen.
5. Client and family teaching:
   A. This test is useful in diagnosing myocardial infarction, liver disease, tumors, and pulmonary embolus.
6. Factors that affect results:
   A. Reject hemolyzed specimens because this elevates LD_1.
7. Other data:
   A. Isoenzymes should not be measured if total LD is <130 IU/L.

LACTIC ACID, BLOOD

Norm:

		SI UNITS
Venous	0.5-2.2 mEq/L or 4.5-19.8 mg/dL	0.5-2.2 mmol/L
Arterial	0.5-1.6 mEq/L or 4.5-14.4 mg/dL	0.5-1.6 mmol/L

Increased:

TYPE A LACTIC ACIDOSIS	TYPE B LACTIC ACIDOSIS
Inadequate delivery of oxygen to the tissues	No evidence of inadequate delivery of oxygen to the tissues (Low tissue perfusion state may or may not be present)

Conditions causing poor tissue perfusion leading to hypoxia:

Left ventricular failure
Decreased cardiac output/cardiac arrest
Mesenteric ischemia
Shock

Reduced permeability of the vasculature

Reduced vascular tone
Decreased arterial oxygen
Hypoxemia
Severe anemia accompanied by poor perfusion
CO poisoning

Anaerobic muscular activity

Exercise (strenuous)
Seizures (grand mal)

B1 (caused by underlying disease or conditions)

Cholera
Cirrhosis
Diabetes mellitus
Hyperthermia
Malaria
Malignancy
Organ failure (liver, kidney)
Panic attack
Sepsis

B2 (caused by substances [e.g., drug and other substance toxicities])

Biguanides (e.g., phenformin), catecholamines, cocaine, cyanide, diethyl ether, ethanol, ethylene glycol, isoniazid, lactulose, methanol, nalidixic acid, niacin, nitroprusside, papaverine, paracetamol, paraldehyde, parenteral nutrition, salicylates, sorbitol, streptozotocin, theophylline, vitamin deficiency

B3 (caused by inborn errors of metabolism)

Congenital lactic acidosis
Enzyme deficiencies
D-lactic acid syndrome

From Cohen R, Woods H: *Clinical and biochemical aspects of lactic acidosis,* Oxford, 1976, Blackwell Scientific Publications.

Decreased. Hypothermia.

Description. Lactic acid is derived from carbohydrate metabolism and is used for muscle contraction when energy needs exceed oxygen supply (anaerobic metabolism). One fifth is oxidized through the citric acid cycle, and the rest is synthesized in the muscle to glycogen. Lactic acid is involved in the body's automatic compensatory systems that maintain acid base balance, increasing in response to compensate for respiratory alkalosis. Several classification schemes that diferentiate lactic acidosis are present in the literature.

Professional Considerations
1. Consent form NOT required.
2. Preparation:
   A. Tubes: Gray topped for the venous sample. Also obtain arterial puncture supplies and one heparinized tube.
   B. Draw the blood sample without a tourniquet if possible.
   C. Do NOT allow the client to clench and then unclench the hand before blood drawing.
3. Procedure:
   A. Obtain a 1-mL venous blood sample in a gray-topped tube containing a glycolytic inhibitor.
   B. Draw an arterial sample in a heparinized tube, place it on ice immediately, and transport it quickly to the laboratory. Note: Arterial samples are of little diagnostic value.
4. Postprocedure care:
   A. Assess the arterial puncture site after holding pressure for 5 minutes.
   B. Send the specimen to the laboratory immediately.
5. Client and family teaching:
   A. Pressure will be maintained on the area where the artery was accessed to avoid unnecessary bruising.
6. Factors that affect results:
   A. Reject specimens received more than 15 minutes after collection.
   B. Intravenous infusions may affect acid-base balance.
7. Other data:
   A. Lactic acidosis is accompanied by an increase in the anion gap.
   B. Lactic acidosis has been successfully treated with dichloroacetate.

LACTIC ACID, CEREBROSPINAL FLUID, SPECIMEN

(see Cerebrospinal fluid, Lactic acid, Specimen)

LACTIC DEHYDROGENASE (LDH), BLOOD

(see Lactate dehydrogenase, Blood)

LAPAROSCOPY (PERITONEOSCOPY), DIAGNOSTIC

Norm. Negative.

Usage. Ascites, biopsy, cholangiography, cirrhosis, dysmenorrhea, ectopic pregnancy, endometritis, fever of undetermined origin, gallbladder disease, identification of abdominal cavity adhesions, infertility, jaundice, lymphoma staging, malignancy staging, pancreatic disease, and pelvic inflammatory disease (PID). Used in conjunction with ultrasound to stage pancreatic cancer. Enables accurate staging of gastrointestinal malignancies and evaluation of liver disease; Provides a diagnostic route with access for therapeutic surgical interventions if abnormalities are identified. Also used therapeutically for surgical procedures, such as colectomy and nephrectomy.

Description. Direct inspection of the surfaces of the internal organs such as the liver, gallbladder, pancreas, fallopian tubes, ovaries, uterus, and lymph nodes by use of a fiberoptic telescope inserted transabdominally into the abdominal cavity. Diagnostic laparoscopy prevents unnecessary surgical laparotomies by providing direct visualization inside of the abdominal cavity with a minimally invasive procedure. Surgical procedures such as cholecystectomy, biopsy, or tubal ligation may be performed by means of laparoscopy. Use of electronic power morcellators is a newer method for removal of tissue that reduces the risk of postprocedure hernia by minimizing fascia damage, but carries with it higher risk for internal organ damage. Other advances in technology include 3-dimensional views and high-resolution digital images.

Professional Considerations
1. Consent form IS required.

Risks
Hemorrhage, infection, intestinal or organ puncture or damage, myocardial ischemia, peritonitis, respiratory acidosis, subcutaneous emphysema.

Contraindications
Advanced abdominal wall malignancy, anticoagulant therapy, bleeding disorders, chronic tuberculosis, intra-abdominal hemorrhage, multiple surgical adhesions, peritonitis, thrombocytopenia.

Precautions
Use with caution during pregnancy. "The occurrence of a miscarriage, premature labor or fetal death appears to be related to the underlying pathology, independent of the operative intervention" (Al-Fozan and Tulandi, 2002). The use of CO_2 insufflation has been associated with cardiorespiratory deterioration in clients with preexisting respiratory problems.

2. Preparation:
   A. Assess for allergies.
   B. Prepare the surgical site with a shave.
   C. Insert an indwelling urinary catheter.
   D. Administer a cleansing enema 4 hours before the procedure.
   E. The client should void just before the procedure.
   F. Bandage inguinal and umbilical hernias.
   G. See *Client and family teaching*.
3. Procedure:
   A. Anesthesia may be given. Regional anesthesia is associated with less postoperative side-effects and a shorter recovery period than is general anesthesia.
   B. A small surgical incision is made in the abdomen just below the umbilicus.
   C. Carbon dioxide is used to insufflate the abdominal cavity so that the organs are easily visualized.
   D. The laparoscope is inserted and visualization begins.
   E. Surgical specimens may be taken using electronic power morcellators
   F. The procedure takes about 30 minutes.

4. Postprocedure care:
   A. Assess the surgical incision area for signs of infection for 24 hours.
   B. Assess for signs and symptoms of hemorrhage as the major complication. Signs may include bleeding at the dressing site, increasing abdominal pain and firmness, and hypotension.
   C. Monitor vital signs every 30 minutes × 4 and PRN.
   D. Provide analgesia for incisional pain and for the pain caused by the carbon dioxide gas remaining in the peritoneal cavity.
5. Client and family teaching:
   A. Fast from food and fluids for 8-12 hours before the procedure.
   B. A common complaint after this procedure is shoulder, scapular, and general discomfort in the upper torso caused by referred pain from the carbon dioxide gas remaining in the abdomen. This pain can last for several days but should decrease in severity as each day passes. Pain medicine will be prescribed to help ease the pain.
   C. Avoid carbonated beverages for 1-2 days after the procedure because such beverages will add to the gas pains and may cause vomiting when added to the carbon dioxide left over from the procedure.
   D. Minimize physical activity for 3-7 days, as instructed by the physician.
   E. Notify the physician for increasing pain, redness, or drainage at the laparoscopy site.
6. Factors that affect results:
   A. Equipment should be in good working order.
7. Other data:
   A. Site-specific useful biopsy is a positive gain of this procedure.
   B. Nausea, puncture of the intestinal loop, infection, hemorrhage, and subcutaneous emphysema are possible complications of laparoscopy.

LASA
(see Lipid-associated sialic acid, Serum or Plasma)

LAXATIVE ABUSE TEST
(see Phenolphthalein test, Diagnostic)

LD, BLOOD
(see Lactate dehydrogenase, Blood)

LDH, BLOOD
(see Lactate dehydrogenase, Blood)

LE CELL TEST
(see Lupus test, Blood)

LE PREPARATION
(see Lupus test, Blood)

LE SLIDE CELL TEST
(see Lupus test, Blood)

LE TEST
(see Lupus test, Blood)

LEAD, BLOOD AND URINE

Norm:

		SI UNITS
Whole Blood		
Adult	<20 µg/dL	<1.0 µmol/L
Child	<10 µg/dL	<0.5 µmol/L
Industrial exposure	<60 µg/dL	<2.9 µmol/L
Lead encephalopathy in children*	>100 µg/dL	>4.8 µmol/L
Urine	0.08 mg/mL	0.39 mmol/L
	120 mg/24 hours	

*The Centers for Disease Control and Prevention defines lead toxicity in children as a blood level of ≥25 µg/dL combined with erythrocyte protoporphyrin ≥35 µg/dL.

Poisoning Level Symptoms and Treatment

Symptoms. Early signs of lead poisoning include anorexia, apathy or irritability, headache, dizziness, sleep disturbances, fatigue, anemia, weight loss, and abdominal "lead colic." Characteristic toxic effects include encephalopathy and peripheral neuropathy (wrist drop) and seizures. Elevated erythrocyte protoporphyrins in the blood is also suggestive of lead poisoning. Aminoaciduria, glycosuria, and Fanconi syndrome have been demonstrated in children exposed to lead.

Treatment:
Note: Treatment choice(s) depend on client history and condition and episode history.
Perform lavage of the stomach with magnesium sulfate or sodium sulfate.
Control seizures with diazepam (Valium).
Reduce cerebral edema with osmotic diuresis (mannitol) and corticosteroids.

Administer possible chelation therapy that includes several injections of calcium disodium EDTA and dimercaprol (see Lead mobilization test, 24-Hour urine).

Increased. Ataxia, metal poisoning, microcytic anemia from lead poisoning, and neuropathy; drinking from earthen teapots that contain lead. Herbal or natural remedies include the Chinese fungus Cordyceps sinensis.

Description. Lead is a heavy metal that is used in paint, leaded gasoline, insecticides, pottery glaze, and illicit liquor and is found in the fumes of old painted wood. It is an electropositive metal that has an affinity for the negatively charged sulfhydryl group and inhibits three enzymes in the body: delta-aminolevulinic acid dehydrase, coproporphyrinogen oxidase, and ferrochelatase. These enzymes are necessary for the production of heme, the iron-containing portion of hemoglobin. The majority of lead in the body is stored in the skeletal system and is thought to be released into the bloodstream in increasing amounts during periods of accelerated bone turnover and mineral loss. The acceptable levels for blood lead content have been gradually lowered over time as new information on lead's detrimental effects has become available. Lead measurements are performed on whole-blood specimens because whole-blood concentrations are 75 times higher than those of serum or plasma. Exposure of children to low levels of lead has been associated with reduced intellectual and neuropsychologic development. For this reason, many communities have in place routine screening for lead exposure of all schoolchildren. This test is the most appropriate test in screening for elevated lead levels in children and in workers in close contact with lead-containing substances.

Professional Considerations
1. Consent form NOT required.
2. **Preparation:**
   A. Tube: Lead-free, lavender topped or green topped for whole-blood sample. Samples MAY be drawn during hemodialysis.
   B. Obtain a 3-L, plastic, acid-washed urine collection container for the urine sample.
   C. Screen client for use of herbal medicines or natural remedies.
   D. See *Client and family teaching.*
3. **Procedure:**
   A. *Whole blood:* Draw a 3-mL blood sample.
   B. *Urine:* Collect all the urine voided in a 24-hour period in a 3-L plastic container that has been washed with 10% hydrochloric acid (HCl) solution.
4. **Postprocedure care:**
   A. *Urine:* Record starting and ending dates and times, as well as the total volume of urine, on the laboratory requisition.
5. **Client and family teaching:**
   A. Maintain on low-calcium diet for 3 days before collection of the 24-hour sample to mobilize lead from the bones and prevent false-positive results.
   B. Save all the urine voided in the container provided and avoid contaminating the urine with stool or toilet paper. If any urine is accidentally discarded, discard the entire specimen and restart the collection the next day.
   C. Avoid eating from old pottery bowls that may have been glazed with lead-base paint.
   D. Some herbal medicines contain high levels of lead, which can cause lead poisoning. Do not use these products without first consulting your physician.
6. **Factors that affect results:**
   A. Anticoagulant other than heparin is found in the tube.
   B. A high-calcium diet creates false-positive results in the urine test.
   C. A fungal remedy that may increase lead levels and induce lead poisoning as a result of its lead content is *Cordyceps sinensis* powder.
   D. There is some evidence that lactation increases the release of lead from bone storage into the bloodstream.
   E. It is thought that conditions of high bone turnover such as pregnancy, menopause and secondary hyperparathyroidism lead to increased release of lead into the bloodstream.
7. **Other data:**
   A. Fingerstick specimens are not recommended. If they are used, positive results should be confirmed with venous whole-blood testing to rule out contamination of the fingerstick specimen.
   B. Urine levels for lead toxicity may be normal when serum levels indicate lead toxicity.
   C. Urine uric acid levels and blood erythropoietin levels may be elevated in lead exposure.

LEAD MOBILIZATION TEST (CALCIUM DISODIUM EDTA MOBILIZATION TEST), 24-HOUR, URINE

Norm:

		SI UNITS
Normal Lead Level Before Mobilization Test		
Adult	<150 µg/day	<0.73 µmol/day
Child	<100 µg/day	<0.48 µmol/day

Continued

	SI UNITS

Normal Lead Level After Mobilization Test

Adult   <650 μg/day   <3.2 μmol/day

Child   <1 μg of Pb/mg of
CaNa$_2$-EDTA administered
over a 24-hour period

Lead Level in Clients With a Higher-Than-Normal Body Burden of Lead After Mobilization Test

Adult   >1000 μg/day   >4.9 μmol/day

Child   <1 μg of Pb/mg of
CaNa$_2$-EDTA administered
over 24-hour period

Usage. Diagnosis and treatment of lead poisoning. Used when blood lead levels are >100 mg/dL.

Description. Lead is an environmental trace metal of which the average client takes in 150-250 μg/day. Only a small fraction of that taken in is absorbed. Lead poisoning occurs when clients frequently come into contact with items or industries that contain large amounts of lead. Some examples are paint, batteries, gasoline, pottery, bullets, and printing materials and the mining, auto manufacturing, and welding industries. Lead affects many organs and tissues of the body, but most of it is stored in the bones. Symptoms of lead toxicity include gastrointestinal colic, vomiting, anorexia, anemia, and central nervous system abnormalities ranging from irritability, peripheral neuropathy, memory lapses, and impaired concentration to severe lead encephalopathy.

Calcium disodium EDTA (calcium disodium edetate, CaNa$_2$-EDTA, calcium versenate) is one of three substances known to bind to lead or form tight complexes with lead, resulting in removal of lead from the body tissues and excretion of lead through the kidneys. The complex forms when lead displaces calcium from the drug molecule. The test involves administering calcium disodium EDTA intravenously or intramuscularly and assessing the change in urinary lead excretion for 24 hours. Half-life of the drug is 20-60 minutes intravenously and 90 minutes intramuscularly. This test is currently the most reliable index of the body burden of lead.

Professional Considerations
1. Consent form NOT required.

Risks and Precautions
This procedure should be used with caution in clients with renal impairment.

Contraindications
Severe lead encephalopathy, pregnancy, anuria, or severe renal disease.

2. **Preparation:**
   A. Assess for adequate urinary output.
   B. Obtain a baseline 24-hour urine collection for lead level in a refrigerated, lead-free (polyethylene), 4-L container that has been rinsed with hydrochloric acid (HCl).
   C. Obtain a baseline urinalysis; a urine coproporphyrin level; blood urea nitrogen and serum creatinine, calcium, and phosphorus levels; and repeat daily throughout the test.
   D. Write the beginning time of the urine collection for the mobilization test on the laboratory requisition.
   E. Uncomfortable intramuscular injection site pain may be minimized by the addition of 1 mL of 1% procainamide to each milliliter of drug.

3. **Procedure:**
   A. Begin a 24-hour urine collection in a lead-free, 4-L container that has been washed with HCl.
   B. *Adults:* Perform the mobilization using one of the following three regimens:
      i. *Intravenous route:* Administer 1.0 g of CaNa$_2$-EDTA in 250-500 mL of 5% dextrose in water over 1-2 hours intra-

venously every 12 hours for no more than 5 days. Wait 2 full days before repeating the test, if necessary.

ii. *Intramuscular route:* Administer 2.0 g of CaNa$_2$-EDTA per day intramuscularly in divided doses (that is, 500 mg in each buttock, 12 hours apart).

iii. *Long-term mobilization:* Administer 1.0 g of CaNa$_2$-EDTA three times a week until the urine collection shows normal levels of lead excretion.

C. *Children:* Perform the mobilization using one of the following two regimens:

i. *For mildly to moderately increased lead levels:* Administer CaNa$_2$-EDTA 500-1000 mg/m^2/24 hours intramuscularly (preferred) or intravenously every 12 hours for 3-5 days. Do not exceed 50 mg/kg/24 hours. Wait 4 full days before repeating the test, if necessary.

ii. *For severe lead intoxication:* Administer CaNa$_2$-EDTA 50 mg/kg/24 hours or 1500 mg/m^2/24 hours intravenously or intramuscularly in divided doses. Do not exceed 70 mg/kg/24 hours.

D. Continue urine collection for 24 hours. Encourage the oral intake of fluids throughout the collection period except for clients with lead encephalopathy (because of the risk of increasing intracranial pressure).

4. **Postprocedure care:**

A. Write the ending time and total urine output on the laboratory requisition.

B. Transport the entire specimen to the lab. The lead measurement is performed in a lead-free laboratory space on an aliquot of the 24-hour specimen.

5. **Client and family teaching:**

A. Save all the urine voided in the container provided and avoid contaminating the urine with stool or toilet paper. If any urine is accidentally discarded, discard the entire specimen and restart the collection the next day.

B. Outline environmental sources of lead.

C. See also *Lead, Blood and Urine.*

6. **Factors that affect results:**

A. Clients who have reached the point of lead encephalopathy may not show clinical improvement after this procedure.

B. The higher the blood lead level, the greater the excretable amount of lead.

7. **Other data:**

A. Intake and output must be monitored during this test. Diminished urine output may result in symptoms of lead toxicity.

B. Other substances used to chelate lead include dimercaprol (British antilewisite [BAL]) and D-penicillamine.

C. Dimercaprol (BAL) may be combined with CaNa$_2$-EDTA for clients with extremely severe lead intoxication.

D. As blood lead is chelated and excreted in the urine, levels may rise again as stored bone lead is mobilized. The mobilization test may be repeated in this circumstance.

E. There is some evidence that lead mobilized from the bones after chelation becomes redistributed to body organs, especially the brain and liver.

F. CaNa$_2$-EDTA is reported to also chelate some other heavy metals.

LECITHIN/SPHINGOMYELIN RATIO
(see Amniocentesis and amniotic fluid analysis, Diagnostic)

LEEP
(see Colposcopy, Diagnostic and Pap smear, Diagnostic)

LEGIONELLA ANTIGEN (LEGIONELLA URINE ANTIGEN, LUA), URINE

Norm. Negative.

Usage. Provides rapid diagnosis for infection with *Legionella pneumophila.*

Description. Approximately 80% of clients with *Legionella* serogroup 1 infection will shed soluble *Legionella* antigens in their urine. Thus, this ELISA is the test of choice for rapid diagnosis of *Legionella* (serogroup 1) infection. Also see *Legionella pneumophila, Culture.*

Professional Considerations
1. Consent form IS required.
2. Preparation:
   A. Obtain a sterile specimen collection container.
3. Procedure:
   A. Collect a 10-mL mid-stream or catheter urine specimen.
4. Postprocedure care:
   A. None.
5. Client and family teaching:
   A. See *Legionella pneumophila, Culture.*
6. Factors that affect results:
   A. Sensitivity of this test for travel-associated *Legionella* infection is 95%, for community-acquired *Legionella* infection is 80%, and for nosocomial *Legionella* infection only 45% (Helbig et al, 2003).
7. Other data:
   A. See *Legionella pneumophila, Culture.*

LEGIONELLA PNEUMOPHILA, CULTURE

Norm. Negative. No growth. A positive culture may be grown in 2–7 days.

Positive. Legionnaires' disease.

Description. A gram-negative, non–acid fast bacillus that causes Legionnaires' disease, a form of lobar pneumonia, which causes symptoms of fever, headache, malaise, and diffuse alveolar damage. Concomitant symptoms of Legionnaires' disease may also include cardiac inflammation (endocarditis, pericarditis), pancreatitis, perirectal abscess, peritonitis, pyelonephritis, sinusitis, and wound infection. Two forms of this disease are a mild, self-limiting flulike syndrome of malaise and muscle aches and a more severe form in which pneumonia occurs. If untreated, *Legionella* is fatal in up to 25% of immunocompromised clients. Due to its ability to thrive in water, outbreaks of Legionnaires' disease have been attributed to community water supplies contaminated with *Legionella pneumophila.* In addition, strains have been found to persist for years in contamination of hospital water supplies. Symptoms develop 2–10 days after exposure to the organism. Clients at highest risk of developing this disease are smokers, those with preexisting pulmonary disease, and those who have received cytotoxic chemotherapy or cor-

ticosteroids. This test includes culture and direct fluorescent antibody (FA) smear of a fresh specimen, which may be obtained from a biopsy of the lung; pleural fluid; washings or brushings from the bronchi; transtracheal aspirates; blood; pus; or sputum.

Professional Considerations
1. Consent form NOT required for this test but IS required when bronchoscopy, lung biopsy, or lung aspiration is used to obtain the specimen. See the individual procedures for risks and contraindications.
2. Preparation:
   A. Obtain a sterile specimen container.
3. Procedure:
   A. The physician obtains a sterile specimen of tissue by bronchoscopy or biopsy or pleural fluid by aspiration. Sterile collections of sputum, blood, or pus may also be collected.
   B. Send the specimen to the laboratory immediately.
   C. Expectorated sputum will NOT have an FA smear.
4. Postprocedure care:
   A. Reports take 1–2 weeks.
   B. Do not freeze the specimen.
5. Client and family teaching:
   A. Undue pain or shortness of breath should be reported.
   B. Legionnaires' disease is treated by erythromycin (drug of choice) or rifampin if erythromycin does not eradicate the organism.
6. Factors that affect results:
   A. Contamination of the specimen will affect the results.
   B. The sensitivity of the sputum sample results is improved when the sample is treated with an acid wash before being cultured.
7. Other data:
   A. Lung biopsy provides the highest rate of identification (>90%), followed by sputum (80–90%). The specificity of blood testing is only ≤30%.
   B. A negative culture does not rule out the presence of *Legionella* because sensitivity of culturing methods may be 50%.
   C. Risk factors for Legionnaire's disease include cigarette smoking, immunosuppression, and status post–organ transplantation.

D. The most commonly used rapid diagnostic test for *Legionella* organism is *Legionella, Urine* test.

LEGIONELLA PNEUMOPHILA, DIRECT FA SMEAR, SPECIMEN

Norm. Negative.

Positive. Legionnaires' disease.

Description. See *Legionella pneumophila, Culture,* for a description of Legionnaires' disease. This test performs a direct fluorescent antibody microscopic examination of a specimen smear of lung tissue, pleural fluid, sputum, bronchial washing, or other body fluid. It provides rapid results (within 1-3 hours). The sensitivity of this test varies widely, from 24% to 80%, but has high specificity at >95%.

Professional Considerations
1. Consent form NOT required for the test but IS required for lung biopsy or lung aspiration by bronchial washing. See the individual procedure for risks and contraindications.
2. Preparation:
   A. Obtain the necessary sterile biopsy containers.
3. Procedure:
   A. Prepare for a lung biopsy, bronchial washing, pleural tap, or sterile sputum specimen.
4. Postprocedure care:
   A. Send the specimen to the laboratory in the sterile container immediately after collection.
5. Client and family teaching:
   A. Report undue pain or shortness of breath.
   B. Legionnaires' disease is treated by erythromycin (drug of choice) or rifampin if erythromycin does not eradicate the organism.
6. Factors that affect results:
   A. False-positive results are seen with tularemic pneumonia.
   B. False-negative results may occur if a saliva specimen, rather than a sputum specimen, is sampled.
7. Other data:
   A. There are several subgroups of *Legionella: L. bozemanii, L. dumoffii, L. gormanii, L. jordanis, L. longbeachae,* and *L. micdadei.*

B. The most commonly used rapid diagnostic test for *Legionella* organism is *Legionella, Urine* test.

LEGIONELLA URINE ANTIGEN
(see Legionella antigen, Urine)

LEGIONNAIRES' DISEASE ANTIBODIES, BLOOD

Norm. Negative or less than a fourfold change in titer between acute and convalescent samples.
A *fourfold rise in titer* >1:128 from the acute-to-convalescent sample provides evidence of recent infection.
A *single titer* ≥1:256 is evidence of infection at an undetermined time.

Positive. Legionnaires' disease.

Negative. Normal.

Description. See *Legionella pneumophila, Culture,* for a description of Legionnaires' disease. This test identifies specific antibodies produced after the body has been infected with the *Legionella* organism. In Legionnaires' disease, antibody titers rise and fall at a predictable rate. Levels are low the first week, rise steadily at weeks 2-4, peak during week 5 of the disease, and then drop slowly and remain elevated for many years.

Professional Considerations
1. Consent form NOT required.
2. Preparation:
   A. Tube: Red topped, red/gray topped, or gold topped.
3. Procedure:
   A. Draw a 10-mL blood sample.
4. Postprocedure care:
   A. Draw convalescent samples of blood 4-6 weeks after the onset of symptoms.
5. Client and family teaching:
   A. Legionnaires' disease is treated by erythromycin (drug of choice) or rifampin if erythromycin does not eradicate the organism.
6. Factors that affect results:
   A. Hemolysis of the specimen invalidates results.
   B. False-positive results may be caused when the client has tuberculosis.
   C. Clients with a past history of *Legionella pneumophila* infection can have elevated titers for several years.

D. 10%-20% of clients with *L. pneumophila* infection have false-negative results.

E. False-positive results may occur in clients infected with gram-negative organisms and non–*L. pneumophila* infections.

7. **Other data:**
    A. The most commonly used rapid diagnostic test for *Legionella* organism is *Legionella, Urine* test.

LEPTOSPIRA CULTURE, URINE

Norm. Negative; no *Leptospira* isolated.

Positive. Leptospirosis.

Description. *Leptospira* is a pathogenic spirochete causing human infection (leptospirosis). Common hosts include cattle, dogs, foxes, mice, opossums, rats, raccoons, and skunks. This is an occupational disease for veterinarians, animal caretakers, butchers, fish handlers, and dog wardens, who contract the disease through direct skin contact with the urine or tissue of infected animals. Symptoms are flulike but may be as severe as meningitis, renal insufficiency, and hemolytic anemia. The infection is not transmitted from human to human except in unusual circumstances. Isolation of *Leptospira* in culture may occur in as short as 6-14 days or in as long as 28 days. Serum *Leptospira* serodiagnosis for antibody identification should always be performed concomitantly with urine culture.

Professional Considerations
1. Consent form NOT required.
2. **Preparation:**
    A. Obtain a sterile urine specimen container.
    B. Alkalinization of the urine may reduce the chance of false-negative results.
3. **Procedure:**
    A. Collect a 50-mL midstream urine specimen in a sterile plastic container. See clean-catch collection instructions in the test *Body fluid, Routine, Culture.*
4. **Postprocedure care:**
    A. Transport the specimen to the laboratory within 1 hour.

5. **Client and family teaching:**
    A. The clean-catch urine technique must be used to decrease the risk of specimen contamination. See clean-catch collection instructions in the test *Body fluid, Routine, Culture.*
    B. Up to 4 weeks may be required for cultures to grow.
6. **Factors that affect results:**
    A. Repeat samples may be necessary if the sample is not tested immediately because acidic urine destroys *Leptospira* bacteria.
7. **Other data:**
    A. Serum should always be obtained for antibody studies when the urine culture is obtained.
    B. Leptospirosis is treated with penicillin or tetracycline.
    C. Urine results are normally available in 4-8 weeks.
    D. *Leptospira* cultures are difficult to grow and frequently give false-negative results when the specimen is not inoculated to medium within 30 minutes of its being obtained.

LEPTOSPIRA SERODIAGNOSIS, BLOOD

Norm. Negative.

Positive. Jaundice, leptospirosis (fourfold increase in titer between acute and convalescent specimens), meningitis, and renal failure (acute).

Description. See *Leptospira culture, Urine,* for a description of leptospirosis. This test is used to detect antibodies to *Leptospira* in the blood and can detect the antibodies when negative results are obtained from culture or dark-field examination for the *Leptospira* organism.

Professional Considerations
1. Consent form NOT required.
2. **Preparation:**
    A. Tube: Red topped, red/gray topped, or gold topped.
3. **Procedure:**
    A. Draw a 7-mL blood sample.
4. **Postprocedure care:**
    A. Draw a convalescent sample of blood 14-21 days later.
5. **Client and family teaching:**
    A. Leptospirosis cannot be ruled out just because cultures were nega-

tive. This test can identify antibodies to the organism, even when cultures are negative. It is important to return for convalescent sampling in 2-3 weeks.

6. Factors that affect results:
   A. Hemolysis of the specimen invalidates the results.
   B. A variety of rapid screening tests have demonstrated a low to high sensitivity during the first week of illness, when treatment decisions are crucial. Thus, choice of methods used for rapid detection should be literature-based.

7. Other data:
   A. None.

LEUCINE AMINOPEPTIDASE (LAP), BLOOD

Norm. Males: 80 to 200 U/mL
Females: 75 to 185 U/mL

Increased. Cancer of the liver, pancreas, or head and neck: cholelithiasis: cirrhosis; jaundice (obstructive); liver damage or dysfunction; pancreatitis, pregnancy (third trimester).

Description. Leucine aminopeptidase (LAP) is an enzyme present in liver cells, blood, bile, urine, and in the placenta. This test is helpful in the differential diagnosis of elevated alkaline phosphatase because the leucine aminopeptidase level is normal in clients with diseases of the bone. Because LAP is released into the bloodstream after liver damage and by liver tumors, it may serve as a marker for these conditions.

Professional Considerations
1. Consent form NOT required.
2. Preparation:
   A. Tube: Red topped, red/gray topped, or gold topped.
   B. See Client and family teaching.
3. Procedure:
   A. Draw a 7-mL blood sample.
4. Postprocedure care:
   A. None.
5. Client and family teaching:
   A. Fast, except for fluids, for 8 hours.
6. Factors that affect results:
   A. The last trimester of pregnancy increases the results.

7. **Other data:**
   A. Maternal serum placental LAP was shown in one study to decrease in women who subsequently experienced preterm labor.

LEUKOCYTE, BLOOD
(see Differential leukocyte count, Peripheral blood)

LEUKOCYTE ACID PHOSPHATASE, BLOOD
(see Tartrate-resistant acid phosphatase, Blood)

LEUKOCYTE ALKALINE PHOSPHATASE (LAP, NEUTROPHIL ALKALINE PHOSPHATASE, NAP), BLOOD

Norm. Score: 20-100 out of a maximum of 400. Score is based on a 0 to 4+ rating of 100 neutrophils.

Increased. Age ≤14 days, agnogenic myeloid metaplasia, aplastic anemia, burns, Down syndrome, Hodgkin's disease, immediately postoperatively, leukemia (acute lymphocytic or hairy cell), myelofibrosis with myeloid metaplasia, pregnancy and during lactation, polycythemia vera, stress, thrombocytopenia infection, tissue necrosis, trauma. Drugs include ACTH and oral contraceptives.

Decreased. Anemia (aplastic, pernicious), leukemia (acute monocytic, chronic granulocytic or chronic myelogenous), cirrhosis, collagen disease, congestive heart failure, diabetes mellitus, erythroleukemia, gout, hereditary hypophosphatemia, hypophosphatasia, idiopathic thrombocytopenic purpura, infectious mononucleosis (early), and paroxysmal nocturnal hemoglobinuria.

Description. Leukocyte alkaline phosphatase (LAP) is an enzyme present in neutrophilic granules from the metamyelocyte to the segmented stage and represents intracellular metabolism. Dye is added to a smear of blood, and a color reaction occurs, enabling the stained neutrophils to be identified by the appearance of red, blue, or

L

purple granules viewed in the cytoplasm of mature leukocytes. The neutrophils are given a rating of 0 to 4, based on the intensity of the color reaction. The score is the sum of the ratings for each neutrophil, with a total possible score of 400. This test helps differentiate chronic myelogenous leukemia, which produces low scores, from three other myeloproliferative diseases—polycythemia vera, myelofibrosis, and essential thrombocytopenia—which produce higher scores. It also is useful for differentiating polycythemia vera from secondary polycythemia, in which normal scores would be found.

Professional Considerations
1. Consent form NOT required.
2. **Preparation:**
   A. Preschedule the test with the laboratory.
   B. *For venous or arterial sample:* Tube: Green topped or black topped. Also obtain foil.
   C. *For capillary sample:* Obtain a lancet and 6 slides.
3. **Procedure:**
   A. Draw a 2-mL blood sample and wrap the tube in foil.
   B. Alternatively, obtain a peripheral fingerstick or earlobe capillary sample and smear it onto 6 slides.
4. **Postprocedure care:**
   A. Transport the specimen to the laboratory immediately. The slides must be fixed in formalin: methanol 1:9 for 30 seconds at 0°-5°C, washed in running water, and air dried within 30 minutes.
5. **Client and family teaching:**
   A. Fast for 6 hours before the test.
   B. Results are normally available within 4 hours.
6. **Factors that affect results:**
   A. Reject specimens collected in EDTA-anticoagulated (lavender-topped) tubes because EDTA inhibits the activity of LAP.
   B. Results are invalid if the client is neutropenic (that is, <1000/mm³ neutrophils).
7. **Other data:**
   A. Values are normal in myelomonocytic leukemia, lymphosarcoma, multiple myeloma, relative polycythemia, sickle cell crisis, and viral infections.

LEUKOCYTE CYTOCHEMISTRY (CYTOCHEMICAL STAIN), SPECIMEN

Norm. Requires interpretation.

Increased. Cushing's disease, diphtheria, Down syndrome, eclampsia, hemolytic anemia, hemorrhage, Hodgkin's disease, leukemia (acute lymphocytic), lobar pneumonia, leukocytosis (15,000-50,000/mL) associated with infection, lymphoma, malaria, meningitis, mercury poisoning, myeloid metaplasia, multiple myeloma, polycythemia vera, pregnancy, stress, syphilis, tissue necrosis, tuberculosis, tumors, and trauma. Drugs include ACTH and oral contraceptives.

Decreased. Anemia (aplastic), collagen disease, hereditary hypophosphatasia, idiopathic thrombocytopenic purpura, leukemia (acute and chronic myelocytic, acute monocytic), myelosclerosis, paroxysmal nocturnal hemoglobinuria, and pernicious anemia.

Description. A staining of blood smears and bone marrow that estimates alkaline phosphatase enzyme activity in neutrophilic granules. A newer microarray technique enables extensive immunophenotyping into distinctive patterns that differentiate chronic lymphocytic leukemia (CLL), hairy cell leukemia, mantle cell lymphoma, acute myeloid leukemia, and T-cell acute lymphoblastic leukemia.

Professional Considerations
1. Consent form IS required for bone marrow biopsy. See *Bone marrow biopsy aspiration analysis, Specimen,* for procedure risks and contraindications.
2. **Preparation:**
   A. Obtain a bone marrow biopsy tray, slides, a sterile container, an alcohol wipe, a tourniquet, a needle, a syringe, and a lavender-topped tube.
3. **Procedure:**
   A. Draw a 2-mL or capillary (preferred) blood sample.
   B. Obtain a bone marrow biopsy and place it in a sterile container.
4. **Postprocedure care:**
   A. Apply a pressure dressing to the bone marrow site and assess it for bleeding every 5 minutes × 3.

B. Transport the specimen to the laboratory immediately.

5. **Client and family teaching:**
   A. Bone marrow specimens are usually taken from the hip (iliac crest) or sternum. The procedure is transiently painful and has been described as extremely painful but only for a short time.

6. **Factors that affect results:**
   A. Tubes containing EDTA inhibit the activity of leukocyte alkaline phosphatase.

7. **Other data:**
   A. Normal levels found in kwashiorkor, leukemia (chronic lymphocytic, acute and chronic myelomonocytic), lymphosarcoma, and viral infections.
   B. See also *Bone marrow aspiration analysis, Specimen,* for care implications for the bone marrow biopsy procedure.

LEUKOCYTE DNA, SPECIMEN

Norm. DNA chain interpretation required.

Usage. Used in the establishment of genetic disorder, endocrinopathy, leukemias, myotonic dystrophies, prion encephalopathies, and cellular alterations such as tumors.

Description. DNA studies of all specimens use a technique called "polymerase chain reaction" (PCR) to amplify the quantity of DNA being studied. The polymerase chain reaction technique has diverse applications in detecting mutations and rare sequences of DNA. The discovery of heat-stable polymerase led to the invention of the PCR machine.

PCR has found its way into virtually all fields of biology, including medicine, evolutionary biology, and genetics.

Professional Considerations

1. Consent MAY BE required, depending on the procedure used to obtain the specimen.
2. **Preparation:**
   A. Contact the laboratory for specific collection regimens, depending on the specimen required.
3. **Procedure:**
   A. For blood samples, obtain a 7-mL sample in a citrate-anticoagulated or EDTA-anticoagulated tube.
   B. A reaction mixture consisting of specimen DNA, primers, DNA polymerase, nucleotides, and buffer containing magnesium is placed into the machine, which automatically runs through the cycles of heating and cooling. Generally 25-35 cycles are enough to amplify a single-copy genomic sequence by a factor of 10 million.
4. **Postprocedure care:**
   A. Care is specific to the procedure used to obtain the specimen. See each individual procedure for care implications.
5. **Client and family teaching:**
   A. Results may not be available for several days.
6. **Factors that affect results:**
   A. Anticoagulants mixed with samples invalidate the results.
7. **Other data:**
   A. This technique has the highest sensitivity of all molecular techniques up to now.

L-FORM, CULTURE
(*see Cell wall–defective bacteria, Culture*)

L

LIDOCAINE (XYLOCAINE), SERUM

Norm:

	TROUGH	SI UNITS
	1.5-6.0 µg/mL	6.4-25.6 µmol/L
Panic Level	6-8 µg/mL	25.6-34.2 µmol/L
Toxic Level	>8 µg/mL	>34.2 µmol/L

Panic Level Symptoms and Treatment

Symptoms. *Panic level:* Slurred speech, central nervous system depression, cardiovascular depression.
Toxic level: Coma, convulsions, decreased cardiac output, muscle twitching, obtundation.

Treatment:
Note: Treatment choice(s) depend on client history and condition and episode history.
Give continuous ECG monitoring for bradycardia, heart block, dysrhythmias, or cardiac arrest.
Support airway, breathing, and hemodynamic stability.
Monitor temperature every hour for hyperthermia. Use cool room or hypothermia, or both, as needed.
Take seizure precautions.
Hemodialysis will NOT remove lidocaine.

Increased. Convulsions and drug abuse. Drugs include anesthetics, cimetidine, norepinephrine, propranolol. Dysrhythmias.

Decreased. Dysrhythmias. Drugs include anesthetics, norepinephrine, phenobarbital, phenytoin, and propranolol.

Description. Lidocaine is a Class I antiarrhythmic and anesthetic drug used to treat ventricular tachycardia or defibrillation resistant to defibrillation. It is also used as a local anesthetic. Lidocaine suppresses automaticity of His-Purkinje system and elevates threshold of ventricle during diastole. Half-life is normally 70-140 minutes but in uremia is 77 minutes, in cirrhosis is 296 minutes, and in cardiac failure is 115 minutes. Because the half-life increases after 24-48 hours, the dose should be reduced after 24 hours when prolonged infusions are given. Lidocaine is metabolized in the liver and excreted in the urine. Steady-state levels are reached after 5-10 hours.

Professional Considerations
1. Consent form NOT required.
2. **Preparation:**
   A. Tube: Red topped, red/gray topped, or gold topped or lavender topped.
   B. Draw the first sample 12 hours after starting lidocaine.
   C. Specimens MAY be drawn during hemodialysis.
3. **Procedure:**
   A. Draw a 1-mL TROUGH blood sample. Obtain serial measurements at the same time each day.
4. **Postprocedure care:**
   A. Observe for signs of lidocaine toxicity.
5. **Client and family teaching:**
   A. Toxic symptoms normally resolve within 12-24 hours after cessation of lidocaine therapy.
6. **Factors that affect results:**
   A. Cardiopulmonary bypass surgery decreases serum levels.
   B. Do not collect in a serum separator tube because the separator gel may extract the lidocaine and cause falsely low results.
7. **Other data:**
   A. Action of drug begins 10-90 seconds after intravenous administration.

LIPASE, SERUM

Norm. <200 U/L with triolein; <160 U/L with olive oil.

		SI UNITS
Adults	13-141 U/L	0.22-2.40 µKat/L
20-60 years	31-186 U/L	0.53-3.16 µKat/L
>60 years	≤302 U/L	≤5.13 µKat/L
>90 years	26-267 U/L	0.44-4.54 µKat/L
Children	20-136 IU/L	0.34-2.30 µKat/L
Infants	9-105 IU/L	0.15-1.78 µKat/L

Increased. Cholecystitis, cirrhosis, duodenal ulcers, fat embolism, fructose malabsorption, gallstone colic, pain (abdominal), pancreatic carcinoma, pancreatic cholera, pancreatic trauma, pancreatitis, peritonitis, renal disease with impaired output, and strangulated bowel. Drugs include bethanechol, heparin, and narcotic analgesics.

Description. Lipase is a pancreatic enzyme that changes fats and triglycerides into fatty acids and glycerol. The pancreas is the only body organ that demonstrates significant lipase activity. In acute pancreatitis, serum lipase begins to increase in 2-6 hours, peaks at 12-30 hours, and remains elevated but slowly decreases for 2-4 days. Lipase rises and falls in tandem with amylase in acute pancreatitis but is a more specific marker than amylase for this condition.

Professional Considerations
1. Consent form NOT required.
2. **Preparation:**
   A. Tube: Red topped, red/gray topped, or gold topped.
3. **Procedure:**
   A. Draw a 1-mL blood sample.
4. **Postprocedure care:**
   A. None.
5. **Client and family teaching:**
   A. Results are normally available within 12 hours.
6. **Factors that affect results:**
   A. Endoscopic retrograde cholangiopancreatography procedure (ERCP) may increase lipase activity.
   B. Traumatic venipuncture can inhibit lipase activity.
   C. Baseline levels increase during pregnancy.
7. **Other data:**
   A. The sample is stable for several days at room temperature, longer if refrigerated or frozen.

LIPID-ASSOCIATED SIALIC ACID (LIPID-BOUND SIALIC ACID, LASA, LSA), SERUM OR PLASMA

Norm. *Serum:* <25 mg/dL
Plasma: <20 mg/dL

Increased. Cancer: Breast, brain, cervix uteri, colon, head and neck, leukemia, liver, lung, melanoma, metastatic, neuroblastoma, ovarian, pancreatic, renal, and uterine; hypertriglyceridemia, postmyocardial infarction (first 3 days).

Decreased. Response in therapy from high tumor burden to low tumor burden.

Description. Lipid-associated sialic acid (LASA) is a derivative of neuraminic acid, a widely distributed sugar that attaches itself to proteins and lipids. This lipid-associated tumor marker is found in the serum of clients with malignant disease and is associated with higher tumor burdens as opposed to low and moderate tumor burdens. Theoretically, LASA levels are believed to be increased in cancer because LASA has the ability to identify cells with altered surface properties, such as cancer cells, and bind to the surfaces, making the tumor cells more susceptible to metastasis and probable lysis by activated macrophages. LASA is also elevated after myocardial damage and is a constituent of total sialic acid, which is an independent cardiac risk factor.

Professional Considerations
1. Consent form NOT required.
2. **Preparation:**
   A. Tube: Lavender topped. Obtain ice.
3. **Procedure:**
   A. Draw a 5-mL blood sample.
4. **Postprocedure care:**
   A. Place the sample immediately on ice and deliver it to the laboratory for immediate spinning and freezing. The sample should be kept frozen until tested.
5. **Client and family teaching:**
   A. Results may take several days if the sample is sent off site to be tested.
6. **Factors that affect results:**
   A. None found.
7. **Other data:**
   A. No significant difference has been found in LASA levels between survivors and nonsurvivors of persons with a myocardial infarction.
   B. No significant difference has been found in LASA levels in persons with low and those with moderate tumor burdens from melanoma.
   C. The amount of sialic acid present on the surface of malignant cells has been correlated directly with the ability to metastasize.
   D. The research findings of Petrick et al (1994) suggest that sialic acid expression can change the binding of colorectal cancer cells. This binding is required for any cytotoxic effect to take place.

L

LIPID PROFILE, BLOOD

Norm. See individual test listings for age-specific norms, including norms for children.

		SI UNITS
Lipids, total	400-800 mg/dL	4.0-8.0 g/L
Triglycerides	10-190 mg/dL	0.2-4.8 mmol/L
HDL cholesterol		
Females	35-85 mg/dL	0.9-2.2 mmol/L
Males	30-65 mg/dL	0.8-1.7 mmol/L
LDL cholesterol	80-190 mg/dL	2.0-4.9 mmol/L
Total-to-HDL cholesterol ratio	Median=5	

CONDITION	TRIGLYC-ERIDES	TOTAL CHOLESTEROL	HDL	LDL
Alcoholism	Increase	Increase	Increase	Increase
Aortic aneurysm	Increase	Increase	Increase	Increase
Aortitis	Increase	Increase	Increase	Increase
Arteriosclerosis	Increase	Increase	Decrease	Increase
Diabetes mellitus	Increase	Increase	Increase	Increase
Glycogen storage	Increase	—	—	Increase
Hyperalimentation	Decrease	Decrease	Decrease	Decrease
Hypercholesterolemia	Increase	Increase	—	Increase
Hyperlipoproteinemia	Increase	Increase	Increase	Increase
Hypothyroid	Increase	—	Decrease	—
Malabsorption	Decrease	Decrease	Decrease	Decrease
Myxedema	Increase	Increase	Increase	Increase
Nephrotic syndrome	Increase	Increase	Increase	Increase
Pancreatitis	Increase	Increase	Increase	Increase

Description. Lipid profile is a battery of laboratory studies to help determine the risk factors in coronary artery disease. Blood lipids comprise cholesterol, triglycerides, and phospholipids. See individual test sections for further descriptions of the components of the *Lipid profile.*

TOTAL CHOLESTEROL–CORONARY HEART DISEASE RISK						
	Norm	Recommended mg/dL	Moderate Risk mg/dL	SI Units mmol/L	High Risk mg/dL	SI Units mmol/L
Adult	<200	<5.18	200-239	5.18-6.19	≥240	≥6.22
Child	<170	<4.40	170-199	4.40-5.15	≥200	≥5.18

HDL CHOLESTEROL–CORONARY HEART DISEASE RISK
High risk ≤35 mg/dL (≤0.91 mmol/L, SI Units)

TOTAL CHOLESTEROL–HIGH-DENSITY LIPOPROTEIN (mg/dL)			
Coronary Heart Disease Risk	Average Risk	2 × Average Risk	3 × Average Risk
Male	5.0	9.6	23.4
Female	4.4	7.1	11.0

LDL CHOLESTEROL–CORONARY HEART DISEASE RISK

	Norm	Recommended mg/dL	Moderate Risk mg/dL	SI Units mmol/L	High Risk mg/dL	SI Units mmol/L
Adult	<130	<3.37	130-159	3.37-4.12	≥160	≥4.14
Child	<110	<2.85	110-129	2.85-3.36	≥130	≥3.37

Professional Considerations

1. Consent form NOT required.
2. **Preparation:**
   A. Tubes: Two red topped, red/gray topped, or gold topped.
   B. See *Client and family teaching.*
3. **Procedure:**
   A. Draw two 7-mL blood samples.
4. **Postprocedure care:**
   A. None.
5. **Client and family teaching:**
   A. Maintain regular dietary habits for 2 weeks before the test.
   B. Fast from food and fluids for 12 hours before the test.
   C. Desirable levels and risk for coronary heart disease are shown in the table at bottom of p. 681.
6. **Factors that affect results:**
   A. Oral contraceptives may increase the levels of lipids in the serum.
   B. Herbal or natural remedy effects: Many studies have conflicting results concerning garlic's effect on lowering serum lipid level, but there are more studies showing this effect than there are studies showing equivocal results. Morcos (1997) showed an "11% decrease in cholesterol, a 34% decrease in triglyceride, and a 10% decrease in low-density lipoprotein (LDL) levels" in clients taking a combination of fish oil and garlic for 1 month. An herbal powder containing guar gum, *meshasringi (Gymnema sylvestre, mesha shringi,* Indian milkweed vine), *methi* (fenugreek leaves), and *tundika (Coccinia indica)* has been shown to reduce total cholesterol and LD levels but to have no effect on HDL and VLDL levels. Long-term treatment with Chinese herbal drugs *Cordyceps sinensis* (a fungus), *dai-saiko-to* (Chinese: *da⁴-chai²hu²-tang¹*, 'major *Bupleurum* prepara-

tion': mixture of *Pinellia, Scutellaria, Zizyphus,* ginseng, licorice, and ginger), and *saiko-ka-ryukotsu-boreito* (Chinese: $chai^2hu^2$-jia^1-$long^2gu^3$-mu^3li^4-$tang^1$, 'Bupleurum-with added-dragon bone-oyster-preparation', composed of *Bupleurum, Pinellia,* ginger, *Scutellaria, Zizyphus,* cinnamon, China root fungus [fu^2ling^2, hoelen, Poria cocos, P. sclerotium], Codonopsis, Chinese rhubarb, ginseng, oyster shell, and fossil bone for calcium) *has been shown to significantly increase HDL levels. Soy has been shown to reduce LDL,* triglycerides, and total cholesterol *as well as to increase HDL.* The Ayurvedic herb *amla* (emblic, *Phyllanthus emblica,* Indian gooseberry) was shown to reduce total and LDL cholesterol in an uncontrolled study. Lethicin has been known to be used to lower cholesterol.
   C. All levels except HDL are generally increased in obesity, whereas HDL levels are generally decreased.
7. **Other data:**
   A. Risk factors for heart disease include high-saturated-fat diet, cigarette smoking, hypertension, obesity, high salt intake, diabetes mellitus, and left ventricular hypertrophy.
   B. Risk for and incidence of coronary heart disease increase as the total-to-HDL cholesterol ratio increases.
   C. See also *Cholesterol, Blood.*

LIQUID ECSTASY

(see Gamma-hydroxybutyric acid, Blood or Urine)

LIQUID PAP TEST

(see Pap smear, Diagnostic)

L

LITHIUM, SERUM

Norm. Negative.

	THERAPEUTIC TROUGH LEVELS	SI UNITS
Treatment of acute mania	0.8-1.6 mEq/L	0.8-1.6 mmol/L
Ongoing prophylaxis	0.5-1.0 mEq/L	0.5-1.0 mmol/L
Panic level	>2.0 mEq/L	>2.0 mmol/L

Panic Level Symptoms and Treatment

Symptoms:

At levels = 1.5-2.5 mmol/L: Ataxia, coarse tremor, diarrhea, muscle weakness, sedation, and vomiting.

At levels = 2.5-4.0 mmol/L: Choreiform movements, confusion, convulsions, diminishing level of consciousness, increased deep tendon reflexes, muscle hypertonia, somnolence, stupor, T-wave flattening, renal toxicity accompanied by hypernatremia or hyponatremia.

At levels >4.0 mmol/L: Coma, death possible.

Treatment:

Note: Treatment choice(s) depend on client history and condition and episode history.

Perform gastric lavage.

Whole bowel irrigation and/or administration of sodium polystyrene sulfonate (Kayexalate) will decrease absorption of sustained-release lithium.

Administer intravenous normal saline or ½ normal saline to force diuresis and renal elimination of lithium.

Both hemodialysis and peritoneal dialysis WILL remove lithium. Some references indicate that dialysis should be considered in clients on chronic lithium therapy who are stable when lithium level is >4 mmol/L, or who are unstable when lithium level is >2.5 mmol/L, or when a change in mental status is present.

Usage. Drug abuse, manic-depressive psychosis, metal poisoning, and monitoring for therapeutic levels during lithium therapy.

Increased. Lithium overdose. Drugs include fluoxetine and thiazide diuretics.

Decreased. Herbal or natural remedies include psyllium (*Plantago psyllium, P. ovata*), fleawort (fleabane in Canada).

Description. Lithium is an alkali metal salt used mostly in the treatment of bipolar disorder (manic-depressive illness) and shows promise in the treatment of cluster migraine headaches. This drug is absorbed in the gastrointestinal tract, has a half-life of 17-36 hours and an onset of 5-10 days, and is excreted in the urine. Lithium alters the sodium transport in nerve and muscle cells, which assists in stabilizing mood.

Professional Considerations

1. Consent form NOT required.
2. Preparation:
   A. Tube: Green topped (not lithium-heparin).
   B. Do NOT draw during hemodialysis.
3. Procedure:
   A. Draw a 2-mL TROUGH blood sample 8-12 hours after the last dose.
4. Postprocedure care:
   A. Sodium, lithium, and fluid balance must be assessed weekly.
5. Client and family teaching:
   A. Periodic lithium levels are necessary to identify and prevent lithium toxicity symptoms. Teach symptoms from the list above.
   B. Clients with levels >2.5 mmol/L will require intensive care monitoring and intervention.
   C. For intentional overdose, refer the client and family for crisis intervention.
6. Factors that affect results:
   A. Reject the results if the specimen was collected in lithium-heparin.
7. Other data:
   A. The common side effects of lithium include elevated thyroid-stimulating hormone (TSH).

B. Levels correlate poorly with the appearance of toxic symptoms. Toxic symptoms may occur at normal lithium levels.

C. Higher lithium levels may be required in children than in adults to achieve therapeutic results.

LIVER BATTERY (PROFILE), SERUM

Norm:

Alanine Aminotransferase (ALT or Formerly SGPT)

Adult Female	4-35 U/L
Adult Male	7-46 U/L
Children	
<12 months	≤54 U/L
1-2 years	3-37 U/L
2-8 years	3-30 U/L
8-16 years	3-28 U/L

		SI UNITS
Alkaline Phosphatase (ALP)		
Adults (20-60 years)		
Bodansky	2-4 U/dL	10.7-21.5 IU/L
King-Armstrong	4-13 U/dL	25.0-92.3 IU/L
Bessey-Lowry-Brock	0.8-2.3 U/dL	13.3-38.3 IU/L
Elderly	Slightly higher	
Newborn	1-4 times adult values	
Children	Values remain high until epiphyses close	
Females		
2-10 years	100-350 U/L	
10-13 years	110-400 U/L	
Males		
2-13 years	100-350 U/L	
13-15 years	125-500 U/L	
Aspartate Aminotransferase		
Adult Females		
≤60 years	8-20 U/L	8-20 U/L
>60 years	10-20 U/L	10-20 U/L
Adult Males		
≤60 years	8-20 U/L	8-20 U/L
>60 years	11-26 U/L	11-26 U/L
Children		
Newborn	16-72 U/L	16-72 U/L
Infant	15-60 U/L	15-60 U/L
1 year	16-35 U/L	16-35 U/L
5 years	19-28 U/L	19-28 U/L
Bilirubin		
1 Month to Adult		
Premature Infant	<1.5 mg/dL	1.7-20.5 μmol/L
Cord	<2.8 mg/dL	<48 μmol/L
24 hours	1-6 mg/dL	17-103 μmol/L
48 hours	6-8 mg/dL	103-137 μmol/L
3-5 days	10-12 mg/dL	171-205 μmol/L

Continued

		SI UNITS
Full-term Infant		
Cord	<2.8 mg/dL	<48 μmol/L
24 hours	2-6 mg/dL	34-103 μmol/L
48 hours	6-7 mg/dL	103-120 μmol/L
3-5 days	4-6 mg/dL	68-103 μmol/L

Gamma-glutamyltransferase/Gamma-glutamyltranspeptidase (GGT/GGTP, Gamma-GT)

Adult Females	4-25 U	
	9-31 mU/mL	
	3.5-13 IU/L	
	3-33 U/L at 37° C	
Adult Males	7-40 U	
	12-38 mU/mL	
	4-23 IU/L	
	9-69 U/L at 37° C	
Children		
Cord blood	190-270 U/L at 37° C	
Premature infant	<140 U/L at 37° C	
1-3 days	56-233 U/L at 37° C	
4-21 days	0-130 U/L at 37° C	
3-12 weeks	4-120 U/L at 37° C	
3-6 months, female	5-35 U/L at 37° C	
3-6 months, male	5-65 U/L at 37° C	
>6 months, female	15-85 IU/L	
>6 months, male	5-55 IU/L	
1-15 years	0-23 U/L at 37° C	

Hepatitis B Surface Antigen
Negative

Lactate Dehydrogenase (LD/LDH)
Wróblewski Method 30° C

	150-450 U/L	72-217 IU/L
Adults		
≤60 years	45-90 U/L	45-90 U/L
>60 years	55-102 U/L	55-102 U/L
Children		
Newborn	160-500 U/L	160-500 U/L
Neonate	300-1500 U/L	300-1500 U/L
Infant	100-250 U/L	100-250 U/L
Child	60-170 U/L	60-170 U/L

Leucine Aminopeptidase (LAP)	12-33 IU/dL	<50 IU/L
5′-Nucleotidase (5′-NT or 5′-N)	0-17 U/L	2-15 IU/L
Bodansky units	0-1.6 U	0.3-3.2

Protein Electrophoresis

Norms are dependent on laboratory procedure. Percentage values are for the agarose method and represent the percentage of total protein:

Adult (Agarose Method)		
Total protein	6.4-8.3 g/dL	5.90-8.00
Albumin	58-74%	0.58-0.74
Alpha$_1$ globulin	2.0-3.5%	0.02-0.04
Alpha$_2$ globulin	5.4-10.6%	0.05-0.11
Beta globulin	7.0-14.0%	0.07-0.14
Gamma globulin	8.0-18.0%	0.08-0.18

		SI UNITS

Protein Electrophoresis—cont'd

Adult

Total protein	6.0-8.0 g/dL	60-80 g/L
Albumin	3.3-5.0 g/dL	35-50 g/L
Alpha$_1$ globulin	0.1-0.4 g/dL	1-4 g/L
Alpha$_2$ globulin	0.5-1 g/dL	5-10 g/L
Beta globulin	0.7-1.2 g/dL	7-12 g/L
Gamma globulin	0.8-1.6 g/dL	8-16 g/L

Premature infant

Total protein	4.4-6.3 g/dL	44-63 g/L
Albumin	3.0-4.2 g/dL	30-42 g/L
Alpha$_1$ globulin	0.11-0.5 g/dL	1.1-5 g/L
Alpha$_2$ globulin	0.3-0.7 g/dL	3-7 g/L
Beta globulin	0.3-1.2 g/dL	3-12 g/L
Gamma globulin	0.3-1.4 g/dL	3-14 g/L

Newborn

Total protein	4.6-7.4 g/dL	46-74 g/L
Albumin	3.5-5.4 g/dL	35-54 g/L
Alpha$_1$ globulin	0.1-0.3 g/dL	1-3 g/L
Alpha$_2$ globulin	0.3-0.5 g/dL	3-5 g/L
Beta globulin	0.2-0.6 g/dL	2-6 g/L
Gamma globulin	0.2-1.2 g/dL	2-12 g/L

Infant

Total protein	6.0-6.7 g/dL	60-67 g/L
Albumin	4.4-5.4 g/dL	44-54 g/L
Alpha$_1$ globulin	0.2-0.4 g/dL	2-4 g/L
Alpha$_2$ globulin	0.5-0.8 g/dL	5-8 g/L
Beta globulin	0.5-0.9 g/dL	5-9 g/L
Gamma globulin	0.3-0.8 g/dL	3-8 g/L

Child

Total protein	6.2-8.0 g/dL	62-80 g/L
Albumin	4.0-5.8 g/dL	40-58 g/L
Alpha$_1$ globulin	0.1-0.4 g/dL	1-4 g/L
Alpha$_2$ globulin	0.4-1.0 g/dL	4-10 g/L
Beta globulin	0.5-1.0 g/dL	5-10 g/L
Gamma globulin	0.3-1.0 g/dL	3-10 g/L

Prothrombin Time

Adult	10-15 seconds
Newborn	<17 seconds
Child	11-14 seconds

Usage. Work-up for liver disease, biliary disease; hepatoma; liver metastasis; chronic active hepatitis; cirrhosis, including biliary cirrhosis; hepatic complications associated with medications or TPN.

Increased. See individual test listing.

Decreased. See individual test listings.

Description. Liver battery includes testing for several blood levels that reflect hepatic function. In general, a liver battery includes the following: *Alanine aminotransferase, Serum; Alkaline phosphatase, Serum; Aspartate aminotransferase, Serum; Bilirubin, Serum; Gamma-glutamyl transpeptidase, Blood; Hepatitis B surface antigen, Blood; Lactate dehydrogenase, Blood; Leucine aminopeptidase, Blood; 5′-Nucleotidase, Blood; Protein, Electrophoresis, Serum; Prothrombin time, Blood.* See individual test listings for specific descriptions.

Professional Considerations
1. Consent form NOT required.
2. **Preparation:**
   A. Obtain foil or a paper bag.
   B. Tubes: 2 red topped, red/gray topped, or gold topped, *and* 1 blue topped.

3. **Procedure:**
   A. Completely fill all three tubes with blood. Cover one red topped, the red/gray topped, and the gold topped with foil, or place them in a paper bag to protect them from light.
4. **Postprocedure care:**
   A. Immediately spin the blue-topped tube, and then refrigerate it. The testing should be performed within 4 hours.
5. **Client and family teaching:**
   A. See individual test listings.
6. **Factors that affect results:**
   A. See individual test listings.
   B. Herbal or natural remedy. *Echinacea purpurea* may cause hepatotoxicity. The risk for this is increased when taken with other hepatotoxic drugs.
7. **Other data:**
   A. See individual test listings.
   B. Interpretation of LFTs is an art, not a science. There are no absolute rules regarding how mild, moderate, or severe liver damage is defined. When one is identifying abnormalities, the client's clinical condition and other diagnostic testing must be considered.
   C. Consider herbal medicines as contributors in otherwise unexplained hepatic injury.

LIVER BIOPSY (PERCUTANEOUS LIVER BIOPSY), DIAGNOSTIC

Norm. Normal liver cells and tissue. Negative for malignant or other abnormal cells and tissue.

Usage. Fine needle aspiration biopsy is the diagnostic procedure of choice for evaluation of liver lesions. Although primarily applied to malignant disease, it is also used in the evaluation of benign conditions. Almost all fine-needle aspiration biopsies of the liver utilize interventional radiology, primarily ultrasonography and computed tomography. This procedure is indicated for clients with unexplained hepatomegaly, unexplained jaundice, persistently elevated liver enzymes, and suspected liver disease. Used when the diagnosis or cause cannot be established by other means. Confirm diagnosis of amyloidosis, benign tumor, drug reaction, hemochromatosis, hepatic cirrhosis, hepatic cysts, hepatic encephalopathy, hepatitis, jaundice, liver abscess, liver cancer or metastasis, liver dysfunction, metabolic disorders, Reye syndrome, sarcoidosis, and schistosomiasis. Also indicated to assess client's response to therapy of chronic liver disease such as hepatitis C, monitor for hepatotoxicity of drug therapy, and evaluate liver transplant allografts.

Description. A liver biopsy is a safe, simple, and valuable method of diagnosing pathologic liver conditions. After the client is given local anesthetic, and while using an aseptic technique, a needle is inserted through the abdominal wall to the liver. Liver tissue is obtained by the needle biopsy for microscopic examination. Liver biopsy may be performed in conjunction with ultrasound or computed tomography guidance.

Professional Considerations
1. Consent form IS required.

Risks
Follow-up studies have indicated a very low rate of serious complications (0.06-0.32%) manifesting as pain, hemorrhage, bile peritonitis, liver cyst, penetration of abdominal viscera, and pneumothorax. Mortality is rare (0.006% to 0.1%). The estimated rate of needle-tract seeding is small in fine-needle aspiration of the liver. Only 3 cases reported.

Contraindications
Uncorrectable bleeding diathesis. Prothrombin time in the anticoagulant range (2-3 seconds over control values); platelet count less than 50,000/mm³; other bleeding disorders; anemia and inability to tolerate major blood loss associated with inadvertent puncture of an intrahepatic blood vessel; pronounced ascites; obstructive jaundice caused by a possible bile leakage; infection of the biliary tract; infection in the right pleural space or right upper quadrant of the abdomen; a hemangioma; or an inability to cooperate during procedure (such as remaining still and holding the breath during sustained exhalation). Sedatives are contraindicated in clients with central nervous system depression. See also *Computed tomography of the body, Diagnostic*, if CT will be used.

Precautions
See also *Computed tomography of the body, Diagnostic*, if CT will be used.

2. **Preparation:**
   A. Obtain a biopsy tray, sterile gloves, slides, sterile sponges, and tape for dressing.
   B. Ensure that all coagulation tests are normal.
   C. Administer any sedative medications as prescribed.
   D. A CT scan may need to be scheduled if the biopsy needle must to be inserted under CT guidance to obtain tissue from a specific area of the liver.
   E. See *Client and family teaching.*
3. **Procedure:**
   A. The area of the liver suspected of being abnormal is noted.
   B. The client is placed in the supine or left lateral position.
   C. The skin area used for puncture is anesthetized locally.
   D. The client is asked to exhale and hold the inhalation so that the liver descends and the possibility of a pneumothorax is decreased.
   E. The biopsy needle is inserted by the physician into the liver during the client's sustained exhalation, and a liver tissue is obtained.
   F. The needle is withdrawn from the liver.
   G. A pressure dressing is applied.
   H. The procedure takes approximately 30 minutes.
4. **Postprocedure care:**
   A. Touch-prints on glass slides may be made before fixation and may be submitted for cytologic evaluation.
   B. Needle rinses in 50% alcohol or saline may also provide helpful diagnostic material.
   C. Direct slides from needle aspirates may be made, and the slides may be fixed immediately in 95% alcohol.
   D. Tissue samples may be placed into a specimen bottle containing 10% formalin for fixation.
   E. Send the specimens to the pathology department.
   F. Assess vital signs frequently (every 15 minutes × 2) to determine evidence of hemorrhage (increased pulse and blood pressure) and peritonitis (increased temperature).
   G. Assess the biopsy site for bleeding.
   H. Place the client on the right side for 1-2 hours after the procedure. This position will compress the liver against the chest wall and will decrease the risk of hemorrhage or bile leak.
   I. Bed rest with 24-hour observation after the biopsy is usually prescribed. Some studies have found no increase in adverse outcomes when discharging clients with no complications one hour after fine needle aspiration liver biopsy.
5. **Client and family teaching:**
   A. Explain the purpose of the procedure.
   B. Fast from food and fluids after midnight on the day of the test.
   C. The procedure takes about 30 minutes. Local anesthetic is used to control pain.
6. **Factors that affect results:**
   A. False-negative results may occur, and localized liver disease may be missed, since a very small fragment of liver tissue, which is often partially destroyed, is taken in a random manner from a large organ. False-negative results may be attributable to (1) sampling error, since the detection rate of liver metastasis is approximately 60% with blind biopsy and about 85% using ultrasound guidance, and (2) degeneration or distortion, which has been caused by faulty preparation of the specimen.
   B. False-positive results may be attributable to incorrect interpretation of very reactive hepatocytes.
7. **Other data:**
   A. An experienced physician should perform the procedure.
   B. Specimens for histologic and cytologic examination may be obtained using ultrasound radiologic guidance and a tissue-core biopsy needle, such as the Menghini needle. Specimens for cytologic examination may be obtained only by use of a fine aspirate needle.
   C. Detection of portal vein tumor invasion in clients with hepatocellular carcinoma is important to determine therapy and prognosis. Fine-needle aspiration of a portal vein thrombus under ultrasonographic guidance helps to distinguish malignant from benign thrombus without resorting to laparotomy.
   D. See also *Hepatic function panel, Blood.*

L

LIVER ECHOGRAPHY
(*see Liver ultrasonography, Diagnostic*)

LIVER FUNCTION TESTS
(*see Liver battery, Diagnostic*)

LIVER ¹³¹I (ROSE BENGAL) SCAN, DIAGNOSTIC

Norm. Normal size, shape, and position of liver.

Usage. Cirrhosis, diffuse infiltrating processes affecting the liver (such as amyloidosis, sarcoidosis), granulomas, hepatomas, hepatic abscesses or cysts, jaundice, tuberculosis, and tumors. Also used as confirmatory test after other findings have been obtained.

Description. A nuclear medicine scan in which radioactive iodine is used to determine the uptake in the liver to outline and detect structural changes in the liver.

Professional Considerations
1. Consent form IS required.

Risks
Allergic reaction to dye (itching, hives, rash, tight feeling in the throat, shortness of breath, bronchospasm, anaphylaxis, death).

Contraindications
Previous allergy to iodine, shellfish, or radiographic contrast medium; renal insufficiency; during pregnancy (because of radioactive iodine crossing the blood-placental barrier) or breast-feeding.

2. Preparation:
   A. Have emergency equipment readily available.
3. Procedure:
   A. The client is transported to the nuclear medicine department. For inpatients, a nuclear medicine technologist may administer the radionuclide at the bedside.
   B. The client is injected intravenously with radioactive iodine 131.
   C. A gamma-ray detector is placed over the right upper quadrant of the client's abdomen 30 minutes after the client has been injected.
   D. The client is placed in lateral, prone, and supine positions, so that all the surfaces of the liver may be visualized.
   E. Scans are taken of the liver at intervals.
   F. The radionuclide image of the distribution of radioactive particles in the liver is recorded on either x-ray or Polaroid film.
4. Postprocedure care:
   A. Assess vital signs every 15 minutes × 2.
   B. Observe the client carefully for up to 60 minutes after the study for a possible (anaphylactic) reaction to the radionuclide.
   C. For 24 hours wear rubber gloves when discarding urine after the procedure. Wash the gloved hands with soap and water before removing the gloves. Wash the ungloved hands after the gloves have been removed.
5. Client and family teaching:
   A. No fasting or premedication is required.
   B. The IV injection of the radionuclide is the only discomfort associated with this procedure.
   C. You will not be exposed to large amounts of radiation, since only tracer doses of ¹³¹I are used.
   D. This procedure is performed by a trained technologist in approximately 1 hour. A physician trained in nuclear medicine interprets the results.
   E. Meticulously wash your hands with soap and water after each void for 24 hours after procedure.
   F. Family members must wear rubber gloves when discarding the client's urine for 24 hours after procedure, if family will be providing this care.
   G. Follow-up diagnostic tests (such as ultrasonography, CT scan, or biopsy) are needed to confirm the diagnosis.
6. Factors that affect results:
   A. Barium in the GI tract overlying the liver or spleen will produce defects on the scan, which may be mistaken for masses.
   B. False-negative results may occur in clients with space-occupying lesions (such as tumors, cysts, abscesses) smaller than 2 cm because the scan can demonstrate only filling defects greater than 2 cm in diameter.

C. False-positive results may occur in clients with cirrhosis. Because of the distortion of the client's liver parenchyma, the scan may be incorrectly interpreted as positive for filling defects.

7. **Other data:**

A. Health care professionals working in a nuclear medicine area must follow federal standards set by the Nuclear Regulatory Commission. These standards include precautions for handling the radioactive material and monitoring of potential radiation exposure.

B. If "cold spots" (areas that do not take up the radionuclide) appear, then cysts, abscesses, and tumors may be suspected.

C. The half-life of iodine 131 is 8 days.

LIVER SCAN, DIAGNOSTIC

(see Computed tomography of the body, Diagnostic; or Liver ^{131}I scan, Diagnostic)

LIVER/SPLEEN SCAN, DIAGNOSTIC

(see Hepatobiliary scan, Diagnostic)

LIVER ^{99m}TC SCAN OF BLOOD VESSELS, DIAGNOSTIC

(see Hepatobiliary scan, Diagnostic)

LIVER ULTRASONOGRAPHY (LIVER ECHOGRAPHY, LIVER ULTRASOUND), DIAGNOSTIC

Norm. Liver is of proper size, shape, and position and with a homogeneous soft echo pattern. Image indicates normal relationship to adjacent anatomic structures. Negative for intrahepatic duct dilatation, abscess, cyst, hematoma, or tumor.

Usage. Determine the cause of jaundice; differentiate between obstructive and nonobstructive jaundice; detect cirrhosis, hepatic abscess, cyst, hematoma, and tumors; differentiate cysts and abscesses from tumors; examine the shape and structure of intrahepatic ducts; visualize pleural effusion; evaluate hepatic hemodynamic flow balance;

evaluate ascites; and monitor hepatic metastasis response to cancer therapy. Used before and after placement of a TIPS. May be used before a liver biopsy or can help differentiate the constitution of abnormalities identified during hepatobiliary nuclear medicine scanning. It is useful with liver scanning to define the "cold spots." Serial scans may be used to determine the volume of the liver. Not reliable in detecting metastasis, especially when a client's liver is high and primarily under the rib cage. Alternative to hepatic dye imaging tests for clients with allergy to radiographic dyes.

Description. This noninvasive diagnostic technique provides an evaluation of the liver, intrahepatic duct structure, and ancillary areas of the gallbladder and diaphragm. It creates an oscilloscopic picture from the echoes of high-frequency sound waves, which pass over the right upper quadrant of the abdomen (acoustic imaging). A computer converts the time required for the ultrasonic beam to be reflected back to the transducer from differing densities of tissue to an electrical impulse. This impulse is displayed on an oscilloscopic screen to create a three-dimensional picture of the liver. Hepatitis and fatty liver may be indicated by hepatomegaly. Fatty infiltration also causes brighter-than-normal echoes, with decreased amount of vascular structures. Hepatic fibrosis is demonstrated by a smaller-than-normal liver size and inhomogeneity of the liver tissue. Cysts appear sonolucent with borders that are easily defined, and they have an echo-free nature. Abscesses may contain internal echoes. Malignant neoplasm (such as adenocarcinoma and other primary liver tumors) may appear as a diffusely distorted parenchymal area, where homogeneity of tissue would be expected. The image pattern, which is produced by malignant neoplasms, is called a "bull's-eye." This is attributable to the dense central echo pattern, which is surrounded by the less echo-producing halo.

Professional Considerations
1. Consent form NOT required.
2. **Preparation:**

A. This test should be performed before intestinal barium tests or after the barium is cleared from the system.

B. Obtain ultrasonic gel or paste.

C. See *Client and family teaching.*

3. **Procedure:**

    A. The client is positioned supine in bed or on a procedure table.

    B. The right upper quadrant of the abdomen is covered with ultrasonic gel, and a lubricated transducer is passed slowly over the area along the transverse plane at intervals 1 cm apart with the client in deep inspiration. This is followed by longitudinal scanning in 0.5- to 2-cm increments, moving from the umbilicus to the xiphoid process, with the transducer angled so that the sound waves pass under the rib cage. The client may be changed to a left lateral decubitus position to obtain lateral views of the liver by coronal scanning. If the client is dehydrated, he or she may be asked to expand the abdomen to enhance the smoothness of the anterior abdominal wall. The final views taken are right anterior oblique.

    C. Photographs are taken of the oscilloscopic display.

    D. The procedure takes less than 30 minutes.

4. **Postprocedure care:**

    A. Remove the lubricant from the skin.

5. **Client and family teaching:**

    A. Fast from food and fluids, and refrain from tobacco smoking overnight before the test.

    B. The procedure is painless and carries no risk.

    C. Wear a gown during the test.

6. **Factors that affect results:**

    A. Dehydration interferes with the adequate contrast between the organs and body fluids.

    B. Intestinal barium, gas, or food obscures results by preventing proper transmission and deflection of the high-frequency sound waves.

    C. Fatty liver causes scattering in the attenuation of the ultrasonic beam.

    D. The more abdominal fat present, the greater is the attenuation (reduction in sound-wave amplitude and intensity), which interferes with the clarity of the picture.

    E. Lung tissue may interfere with visualization of the liver dome in transverse views.

    F. Rib artifacts may obscure images of the right lobe of the liver.

7. **Other data:**

    A. See also *Gallbladder and biliary system ultrasonography, Diagnostic.*

LIVER ULTRASOUND
(see Liver ultrasonography, Diagnostic)

LORAZEPAM
(see Benzodiazepines, Plasma and Urine)

LOW-DENSITY LIPOPROTEIN (LDL) CHOLESTEROL, BLOOD

Norm:

AGE (years)	MALE mg/dL	MALE SI UNITS mmol/L	FEMALE mg/dL	FEMALE SI UNITS mmol/L
Adults				
20-24	66-147	1.71-3.81	57-159	1.48-4.12
25-29	70-165	1.81-4.27	71-164	1.84-4.25
30-34	78-185	2.02-4.79	70-156	1.81-4.04
35-39	81-189	2.10-4.90	75-172	1.94-4.45
40-44	87-186	2.25-4.82	74-174	1.92-4.51
45-49	97-202	2.51-5.23	79-186	2.05-4.82
50-54	89-197	2.31-5.10	88-201	2.28-5.21
55-59	88-203	2.28-5.26	89-210	2.31-5.44
60-64	83-210	2.15-5.44	100-224	2.59-5.80
65-69	98-210	2.54-5.44	92-221	2.38-5.72
>70	88-186	2.28-4.82	96-206	2.49-5.34

AGE	MALE		FEMALE	
(years)	mg/dL	SI UNITS mmol/L	mg/dL	SI UNITS mmol/L
Children				
Cord blood	20-56	0.52-1.45	21-58	0.54-1.50
5-9	63-129	1.63-3.34	68-140	1.76-3.63
10-14	64-133	1.66-3.44	68-136	1.76-3.52
15-19	62-130	1.61-3.37	59-137	1.53-3.55

LDL CHOLESTEROL LEVELS AND RECOMMENDATIONS

	Desirable Level	Level for Diet Therapy and Increased Exercise	Level for Drug Consideration
Without CHD and with fewer than 2 risk factors	<160 mg/dL	160-190 mg/dL	≥190 mg/dL*
Without CHD and with 2 or more risk factors	<130 mg/dL	100-160 mg/dL	≥160 mg/dL*
With CHD	≤100 mg/dL	100-130 mg/dL	≥130 mg/dL†

*In men <35 years of age and in premenopausal women with LDL cholesterol levels of 190 to 219 mg/dL, drug therapy should be delayed, except in high-risk clients (such as those with diabetes).
†In clients with CHD, with cholesterol levels of 100-129 mg/dL, the physician should exercise clinical judgment in deciding whether to initiate drug treatment.

Usage. Predict risk of coronary heart disease (CHD).

Increased. Acute myocardial infarction, anorexia nervosa, coronary arterial atherosclerosis, Cushing's disease, diabetes mellitus, diet high in cholesterol and saturated fats, dysglobulinemias, eclampsia, hepatic disease, type-II hyperlipoproteinemia, hyperlipidemia, hypothyroidism, Laënnec's cirrhosis, multiple myeloma, nephrotic syndrome, obesity (often), porphyria, pregnancy, and renal failure. Drugs include androgens, aspirin, catecholamines, diuretics, glucogenic corticosteroids, oral contraceptives, phenothiazines, and sulfonamides.

Decreased. Arteriosclerosis, abetalipoproteinemia, chronic obstructive lung disease, type-I hyperlipoproteinemia, hyperthyroidism, hypoalbuminemia, inflammatory joint disease, malabsorption, malnutrition, multiple myeloma, pulmonary disease, Reye syndrome, stress, and Tangier disease. Drugs include aspirin, cholestyramine, clofibrate, cortisone, estrogens, neomycin, nicotinic acid, probucol, tamoxifen and thyroxine. Herbs or natural remedies include garlic (aged extract taken on an ongoing basis); soy; and herbal powder containing guar gum, *meshasringi* (*Gymnema sylvestre, mesha shringi*, Indian milkweed vine), *methi* (fenugreek leaves), and *tundika* (*Coccinia indica*). The Ayurvedic herb *amla* (emblic, *Phyllanthus emblica*, Indian gooseberry) was shown to reduce total and LDL cholesterol in an uncontrolled study.

Description. Low-density lipoproteins (LDLs), the "bad lipids," carry the body's cholesterol in plasma from the liver to other parts of the body and deposit it in the peripheral tissues. LDL is associated with an increased risk of arteriosclerotic heart and peripheral vascular disease. High levels of oxidative LDLs are thought to be extremely atherogenic. Beta-lipoproteins, or LDLs, are moderately high in protein and cholesterol but low in triglycerides. LDL cholesterol is usually a calculation rather than a direct measurement. LDLs can be derived from the formula:

$$LDL = Cholesterol \times \frac{HDL + Triglycerides}{2}$$

Professional Considerations
1. Consent form NOT required.
2. **Preparation:**
   A. Tube: Red topped, red/gray topped, or gold topped.

B. Indicate on the laboratory requisition any drugs that may affect the test results.

C. See *Client and family teaching.*

3. **Procedure:**
   A. Draw a 2-mL blood sample.

4. **Postprocedure care:**
   A. None.

5. **Client and family teaching:**
   A. Fast from food for 14 hours before the test. Only water is permitted.
   B. Follow a regular diet for 2 weeks before the test.
   C. For elevated levels, provide information regarding appropriate body weight, diet, and acarus.
   D. If cholesterol is still elevated after life-style modifications, prescription medication may be an option to discuss with the physician.

6. **Factors that affect results:**
   A. Results are invalid if the client has undergone a radioactive scan within 7 days before this test.
   B. Consumption of alcoholic beverages within the previous 24 hours will affect the results.
   C. Test results could be elevated by a diet high in saturated fats and sugar (such as butter, cream, fatty meats, bacon, and candy).
   D. Binge eating can also alter lipoprotein values.

7. **Other data:**
   A. Calculation is not valid for specimens over 400 mg/dL or clients with type-III hyperlipoproteinemia.

LEIDEN MUTATION
(see *Factor V, Blood and Protein C, Blood*)

LOWER GI, DIAGNOSTIC
(see *Barium enema, Diagnostic*)

LP EXAMINATION
(see *Lumbar puncture, Diagnostic*)

L-PHASE, CULTURE
(see *Cell wall–defective bacteria, Culture*)

LSA
(see *Lipid-associated sialic acid, Serum or Plasma*)

LSD
(see *Lysergic acid diethylamide, Blood or Urine*)

L/S RATIO
(see *Amniocentesis and amniotic fluid analysis, Diagnostic*)

LUA
(see *Legionella antigen, Urine*)

LUMBAR PUNCTURE, DIAGNOSTIC

Norm. See *Cerebrospinal fluid, Glucose, Specimen; Cerebrospinal fluid, Immunoglobulin G, Immunoglobulin G ratios and immunoglobulin G index, Immunoglobulin G synthesis rate, Specimen; Cerebrospinal fluid, Lactic acid, Specimen; Cerebrospinal fluid, Myelin basic protein, oligoclonal bands, protein, and protein electrophoresis, Specimen; Cerebrospinal fluid, Routine analysis, Specimen; and Cerebrospinal fluid, Routine, Culture and cytology.*

Usage. To assist in the diagnosis of primary or metastatic brain or spinal cord neoplasm, cerebral hemorrhage, meningitis, encephalitis, degenerative brain disease, autoimmune diseases involving the central nervous system, neurosyphilis, and demyelinating disorders (such as multiple sclerosis, acute demyelinating polyneuropathy). Also, this procedure may be performed therapeutically to inject therapeutic or diagnostic agents, to administer spinal anesthetics, or to reduce/drain volume of CSF to a normal level in benign intracranial hypertension (pseudotumor cerebri, idiopathic intracranial hypertension). See individual test listings above for additional specific usage.

Description. An invasive sterile procedure that can be performed at the bedside. A needle is placed into the subarachnoid space of the spinal column. Cerebrospinal fluid (CSF) pressure is measured, and CSF is obtained for examination. The spinal fluid is analyzed to diagnose spinal cord and brain diseases. CSF protects the brain and spinal column from injury and transports products of neurosecretion and cellular metabolism. Under special circumstances, CSF may be obtained from a ventriculotomy or from cisternal or lateral cervical punctures.

Professional Considerations
1. Consent form IS required.

Risks
Bleeding-epidural hematoma, cerebral and spinal herniation, brain shift, cranial neuropathy, headache, hematoma (spinal subdural, or intracranial occipital), increased intracranial pressure, infection, low back pain, meningitis, nausea, nerve root irritation.

Contraindications
Degenerative joint disease affecting the spine; an agitated or uncooperative client; infection near the L2-S1 site, which could carry the infective process into the CSF and change cytologic results; coagulation defects, low back pain, or spinal deformities; brain shift (usually characterized by headache and vomiting; papilledema may or may not be present).
Note: Comatose clients with high intracranial pressure, but *without* brain shift may be candidates for lumbar puncture without prior CT when the need for the lumbar puncture diagnostic information is mandatory and urgent, such as in cases of suspected acute meningitis (van Crevel et al, 2002).

2. Preparation:
   A. See *Client and family teaching.*
   B. Obtain a lumbar puncture or a spinal tap sterile tray, sterile drapes, 1%-2% lidocaine (Xylocaine), and a dry, sterile dressing.
   C. If increased intracranial pressure is suspected, a computed tomographic scan of the brain should be performed to rule out this possibility before the lumbar puncture. Herniation of the brain may occur in such clients.
   D. Assess the client's vital signs. Perform a baseline neurologic assessment of the legs by assessing strength, sensation, and movement.
   E. Client should empty bowel and bladder before the procedure.
3. Procedure:
   A. Position the client in a lateral position with the knees drawn up to the abdomen, the chin placed

on the chest, and hands clasped around the knees.
   B. Assist the client in relaxing during the procedure by using soothing words and by instructing the client to breathe slowly and deeply with the mouth open. Give reassurance by using touch or holding the client's hand, unless this is opposed by the client.
   C. The puncture site is selected, usually in the lumbar sac at L3-L4 or at the L4-L5 site. A little bone at the L5-S1 interspace, the "surgeon's delight," facilitates selection of the puncture site.
   D. The site is thoroughly cleansed with an antiseptic solution.
   E. The surrounding area is draped carefully with sterile towels such that the towels do not obscure important landmarks.
   F. A local anesthetic (usually lidocaine) is injected into the L3-L4 or L4-L5 spinal column area, creating a burning sensation.
   G. A spinal needle, which contains an inner obturator (stylet), is placed through the skin and into the spinal canal. Postdural puncture headache may be decreased if the Sprotte atraumatic needle is used.
   H. The subarachnoid space is entered. The client may feel the entry (a "pop") of the needle through the dura mater. *Note:* In children a rule of thumb to use for mean insertion depth is 0.03 × height of child (cm).
   I. The obturator is removed, and CSF will be seen slowly dripping from the needle.
   J. The needle is attached to a sterile manometer.
   K. Ask the client to relax and straighten the legs. This will reduce the intra-abdominal pressure, which will cause an increase in CSF pressure.
   L. The opening CSF pressure is recorded.
   M. Three numbered sterile polypropylene CSF transfer tubes are filled sequentially, with a total of 3-12 mL of CSF.
   N. The Queckenstedt procedure is performed during a lumbar puncture if blockage in the CSF circulation in the spinal subarachnoid space is suspected. The jugular

L

vein is temporarily occluded manually by digital pressure or by a medium-sized blood pressure cuff inflated to approximately 20 mm Hg. The CSF pressure should increase to 15-40 cm H_2O within 10 seconds of jugular occlusion. No rise after 10 seconds is suggestive of a complete obstruction in the spinal canal. The pressure should return promptly to normal within 10 seconds of release of pressure. A sluggish rise or fall of CSF pressure is suggestive of partial blockage of CSF circulation.

O. The closing pressure of CSF is measured.

P. One may decrease a puncture headache by pointing the face of the bevel in the direction of the client's side, replacing the stylet, and rotating the needle 90 degrees before withdrawing the needle. Reinserting the stylet before removing the needle to reduce the incidence of post–lumbar puncture syndrome is recommended.

Q. The procedure takes 30 minutes.

4. Postprocedure care:
A. Discard the first specimen, which is likely to be contaminated with blood. Label all test tubes immediately with the proper number (1, 2, 3), the client's name, the date, and the room number. Colored or very cloudy spinal fluid requires additional mixing with 0.5 mL of sterile sodium citrate per 5 mL of CSF to prevent clotting.

B. Transport the specimens to the laboratory immediately. Analysis must be performed promptly on freshly collected specimens. Refrigerate the CSF or store the specimens for culture in a bacteriologic incubator when prompt analysis is not possible.

C. Apply a dry, sterile dressing to the lumbar puncture site.

D. Monitor vital signs and assess for changes in levl of consciousness, headache, and neurologic status every 15 minutes × 4, every 30 minutes × 4, and then hourly × 4.

E. Assess the client for numbness, tingling, and movement of the lower extremities; irritability; change in level of consciousness; nonreactive eye pupils; and ability to void.

F. Assess the puncture site for redness, swelling, drainage, and pain every 4 hours for 24 hours. Notify the physician of any unusual findings. Notify the physician immediately if there is a sign of leakage at the puncture site.

G. Encourage the client to drink increased amounts of fluid with a straw to replace CSF removed during the lumbar puncture, unless this is contraindicated.

H. Headache is common after lumbar puncture, usually beginning within 48 hours and may last up to 4 months, but it usually resolves within 1 week. The cause is thought to be related to CSF hypotension caused by spinal fluid leak. However, this is not proven. There is no correlation of amount of postprocedure bedrest with duration of headache; however, lying down typically reduces the severity of the symptoms. Treatment sometimes involves injection of a blood patch into the epidural space, as well as medication for pain.

5. Client and family teaching:
A. Explain the procedure, potential risks and benefits, and postprocedural care. Allay the client's fears, and allow him or her time to verbalize concerns.

B. There will be a burning sensation with the injection of local anesthetic, and transient pain or pressure may occur during the lumbar puncture.

C. No fasting or sedation is required.

D. Increase fluid intake to 6-8 glasses of water per day, unless contraindicated, to prevent and relieve possible headache.

E. Empty the bladder and bowels before the procedure.

F. You will have to lie on your side with your chin bent down onto your chest and to clasp your hands around your knees. The knees should be drawn up to but not compress the abdomen so that the back bows. (A sitting position, with the client straddling a straight-backed chair and flexing the head to the chest, can be used.)

G. It is important to lie very still throughout this procedure because movement may cause accidental injury.

H. Tell the client to refrain from holding his or her breath, straining, and talking during procedure.

I. Notify the physician or nurse if you are having severe back pain, numbness or tingling in the lower extremities, more than minor bleeding, headache that lasts more than 1 day, or a fever of higher than 101° F (38.3° C).

J. Headaches are common after this procedure. They usually resolve on their own within a week.

6. **Factors that affect results:**

A. Contamination of the specimen will cause inaccurate results. The first tube could be contaminated with blood from the spinal tap and should not be used for protein determination, cell count, or culture.

B. A traumatic spinal tap could cause blood to be present in the specimen, and this may be mistaken for a clinical problem.

C. Cloudy specimens may be caused by elevated white blood cells. Yellow specimens may be caused by elevated protein >100 mg/dL. Pink or red specimens may be caused by red blood cells. Turbid specimens may be caused by the presence of fungi.

D. Refrigeration will alter the test results if bacteriologic and fungal studies are done.

E. Certain drugs could cause a false increased CSF protein level, such as anesthetics, acetophenetidin (phenacetin), chlorpromazine (Thorazine), salicylates (aspirin), streptomycin, and sulfonamides.

F. CSF chloride level determination may be invalidated by IV fluid containing chloride.

G. Hyperglycemia could increase the CSF glucose level.

7. **Other data:**

A. Handle specimens cautiously to prevent self-contamination.

B. It is recommended that lumbar punctures continue to be performed in children with first febrile convulsions, especially if under 18 months of age.

C. The total amyloid beta peptide (Abeta) protein in CSF has not been found to be a useful marker for current diagnosis of Alzheimer's disease.

D. The role of routine lumbar puncture in the initial evaluation of symptom-free infants for congenital syphilis is not recommended because of the low yield of reactive VDRL in CSF and to the similar CSF leukocyte and protein values in the syphilis group and control group.

LUNG FUNCTION TEST
(see Pulmonary function test, Diagnostic)

LUNG SCAN, PERFUSION AND VENTILATION (V/Q SCAN), DIAGNOSTIC

Norm. Negative for emboli or thrombus.
Perfusion scan: Uniform uptake of particles within the entire lung vasculature
Ventilation scan: Equal gas distribution in the pulmonary airways

Usage. Diagnosis of pulmonary embolism or thrombosis; determination of the percentage of lungs functioning normally; assessment of pulmonary vasculature supply by providing an estimate of regional pulmonary blood flow and identifying areas of shunting and areas where capillaries are absent (that is, emphysema); and diagnosis of atelectasis, asthma, bronchitis, chronic obstructive pulmonary disease, inflammatory fibrosis, lung cancer or tumors, and pneumonia.

Description. This is a nuclear medicine procedure. There are three types of lung scans: (1) the perfusion scan, (2) the ventilation scan, and (3) the inhalation scan. In the perfusion scan, blood flow to the lungs is evaluated by use of a macroaggregated albumin (MAA) tagged with technetium (^{99m}Tc). This is injected intravenously. The radiolabeled particles become temporarily lodged in the pulmonary vasculature, since the diameter of these particles is larger than that of the pulmonary capillaries. A gamma-ray detector scans the client, and a scintillation camera records the distribution of particles within the pulmonary vascular supply. Although the lung perfusion scan is sensitive, it is not specific because a variety of pathologic conditions can cause the same abnormal results. Therefore, lung perfusion

L

scans should be performed with a lung ventilation scan. This scan determines the patency of the pulmonary airways and detects abnormalities in ventilation (such as pneumonia, pleural fluid, emphysema). Ventilation scans will show a normal wash-in and wash-out of radioactivity from the embolized lung area in embolic disorders. Conversely, the wash-in and wash-out will be abnormal in parenchymal disease (such as pneumonia). Finally, a normal inhalation scan looks much like a perfusion scan, except that the trachea and major airways are more visible.

Professional Considerations
1. Consent form IS required.

Risks
Allergic reaction to iodine 131 if use is planned (itching, hives, rash, tight feeling in the throat, shortness of breath, bronchospasm, anaphylaxis, death).

Contraindications
Lung perfusion scanning is contraindicated in clients with primary pulmonary hypertension or right-to-left heart shunts. During pregnancy or breastfeeding. Previous history of allergy to iodine, eggs, or shellfish if iodine 131 will be used.

Precautions
In pregnant or lactating women; Chang et al. (2002) conclude that pediatric risks are low when this procedure is performed during pregnancy.

2. **Preparation:**
   A. Have emergency equipment readily available.
   B. If iodine 131 is to be given (though this is rarely the case), give the client 10 drops of Lugol's solution several hours before the test. This will prevent iodine uptake by the thyroid gland.
   C. Sedation may be prescribed for very young children or those who are unable to lie still for the scan.
   D. Establish intravenous access.
   E. Breathing methods are reviewed with the client before injection and imaging.
   F. See *Client and family teaching*.
3. **Procedure:**
   A. Transport the client to the nuclear medicine department.

B. In a perfusion scan, a radionuclide-tagged MAA is injected slowly intravenously over several respiratory cycles. Half is injected while the client is sitting up, and the other half while lying down. The client is placed in the supine, prone, and various lateral positions on the nuclear medicine table under the camera. Scanning with a gamma-ray detector is begun immediately. The scintillation camera takes several single stationary images of the anterior, posterior, and lateral areas of the chest. Perfusion imaging lasts about 45 minutes.
C. In a ventilation scan, a client inhales a mixture of air and radioactive gas (xenon 133, krypton 85, krypton 81m, or ^{99m}Tc-diethylenetriaminepentaacetic acid [^{99m}Tc-DTPA]) through the mouthpiece of a face mask. The radioactive gas follows the same pathway as the air in normal breathing. A nuclear scan is performed at three phases: during the buildup of gas, after the client rebreathes from a bag and the radioactivity reaches a steady level, and after removal of the radioactive gas from the lungs. Ventilation imaging lasts about 30 minutes.
D. In an inhalation scan, droplets of radioactive material can be administered by a positive-pressure ventilator. The aerosol is then inhaled through the mouthpiece of a face mask.
4. **Postprocedure care:**
   A. Observe the client carefully for up to 60 minutes after the study for a possible (anaphylactic) reaction to the radionuclide.
   B. When urine is being discarded, rubber gloves should be worn for 24 hours after the procedure. Wash the gloved hands with soap and water before removing the gloves. Wash the ungloved hands after the gloves have been removed.
5. **Client and family teaching:**
   A. Peripheral venipuncture is the only discomfort associated with this test.
   B. A physician trained in diagnostic nuclear medicine interprets the results.

C. The total time for the procedure is approximately 2 hours.

D. No fasting or premedication is required.

E. The client will not be exposed to large amounts of radioactivity because only tracer doses of isotopes are used.

F. Remove jewelry around the chest area.

G. Meticulously wash your hands with soap and water after each void for 24 hours after procedure.

H. Family members must wear rubber gloves when discarding the client's urine for 24 hours after procedure if the family will be providing this care.

6. **Factors that affect results:**

A. Jewelry or metal objects in the x-ray field distort the results.

B. The client must lie motionless throughout the scan for the most accurate results.

C. Ventilation scans with ^{99m}Tc-DTPA require client cooperation with deep breathing and appropriate use of breathing equipment to prevent contamination with the radioactive gases.

D. The scan results of clients with pulmonary parenchymal disease (such as pneumonia, emphysema, pleural effusion, tumors) will appear to demonstrate perfusion defect and simulate pulmonary embolism.

E. False-positive scan results occur in vasculitis, mitral stenosis, and pulmonary hypertension and when tumors obstruct a pulmonary artery with airway involvement.

7. **Other data:**

A. In pulmonary emboli, perfusion is decreased, but ventilation is maintained. Diagnosis of pulmonary embolus cannot be made on the basis of a lung perfusion scan alone.

B. In pneumonia, ventilation is absent.

C. "Hot spots" are areas of normal blood flow. "Cold spots" are areas of low radioactivity uptake and indicate poor perfusion and emboli.

D. A chest radiograph should be obtained before or after a lung perfusion scan. Comparison of the perfusion scan with a chest radiograph can detect infiltrating disease.

E. The perfusion scan immediately follows the ventilation scan. However, ventilation scans using krypton can be performed before, during, or after perfusion scans.

F. Long-term anticoagulant therapy can be safely withheld in symptomatic clients (such as suspected pulmonary embolus) with a normal perfusion scan.

G. High-probability perfusion scans are usually diagnostic of pulmonary embolus.

H. Less client cooperation is needed during a ventilation scan with a krypton tracer. It can even be performed on a comatose client.

I. A pulmonary arteriogram is still necessary before an embolectomy can be attempted.

J. Health care professionals working in a nuclear medicine area must follow federal standards set by the Nuclear Regulatory Commission. These standards include precautions for handling the radioactive material and monitoring of potential radiation exposure.

K. Technetium half-life is 6 hours.

L. See also *Gas ventilation lung scan, Diagnostic.*

LUNG VOLUMES, DIAGNOSTIC
(see Pulmonary function test, Diagnostic)

LUPUS ANTICOAGULANT, BLOOD
(see Circulating anticoagulant, Blood)

LUPUS ERYTHEMATOSUS CELL TEST
(see Lupus test, Blood)

LUPUS PANEL, BLOOD

Norm:

		SI UNITS
Antinuclear antibody titer (ANA)	<1:20	
Anti-DNA titer	<1:10	
C3 complement, male	80-180 mg/dL	0.8-1.8 g/L
C3 complement, female	76-120 mg/dL	0.76-1.2 g/L
C4 complement, adult	15-45 mg/dL	0.15-0.45 g/L

Positive. Dermatomyositis, discoid lupus, infectious mononucleosis, lupoid hepatitis, myasthenia gravis, polyarteritis, rheumatoid arthritis, scleroderma, Sjögren syndrome, and systemic lupus erythematosus (SLE).

Negative. Normal finding; lack of SLE.

Description. Three distinct laboratory tests are used to verify the diagnosis of SLE. First, antinuclear antibody (ANA), which assesses tissue-antigen antibodies, is frequently used for diagnosing SLE. Antinuclear antibodies, which are gamma globulins, react with the nuclei of all organs of people or animals. These ANAs usually belong to more than one immunoglobulin class. Immunofluorescence detects ANAs and produces homogeneous and peripheral (RIM) staining patterns in clients with SLE. Second, anti-DNA, an antinuclear antibody, is almost always present in SLE and is present in lupus nephritis 95% of the time. Anti-DNA values may fluctuate according to the remission and exacerbation of the disease. Third, C3 and C4 complements are proteins that are activated into enzymes when IgG and IgM antibodies are combined with their specific antigens. These are measured during an acute or chronic inflammatory process. Both serum C3 and C4 complements will be decreased in clients with SLE.

Professional Considerations
1. Consent form NOT required.
2. **Preparation:**
   A. Tube: Red topped, red/gray topped, or gold topped.
3. **Procedure:**
   A. Draw a 5-mL blood sample.
4. **Postprocedure care:**
   A. None.
5. **Client and family teaching:**
   A. Signs and symptoms of SLE include fatigue, fever, rash (butterfly over the nose), leukopenia, and thrombocytopenia.
   B. If positive for SLE, have daily rest periods, which will help to decrease the symptoms.
   C. Lupus Foundation of America, Inc., 4 Research Place, Suite 180, Rockville, MD 10850-3226, (800) 558-0121.
6. **Factors that affect results**
   A. Hemolysis of the specimen invalidates the results.
   B. Several drugs may cause positive tests for ANAs. For example, clients who are receiving hydralazine or procainamide may demonstrate ANAs at increased titers, even though they do not exhibit any signs of SLE.
   C. Heat can destroy the complement components.
   D. The serum value of C3 may decrease if the sample is left standing for 1-2 hours at room temperature.
7. **Other data:**
   A. A positive (high) titer of ANAs does not necessarily indicate a disease process because ANAs are present in some apparently normal clients.
   B. Some clients with connective tissue disease or who may develop such a disease at a later time have developed a positive titer of ANAs.
   C. A negative test for total antinuclear antibody is strong evidence that the client does not have SLE.
   D. Anti-DNA titer correlates with systemic lupus erythematosus and the occurrence of glomerulonephritis.
   E. Other tests to confirm the diagnosis of SLE include (1) anti-SM, (2) CH_{50}, and (3) kidney or skin biopsy.

LUPUS TEST (LE TEST, LE CELL TEST, LE PREPARATION, LE SLIDE CELL TEST, LUPUS ERYTHEMATOSUS CELL TEST, LYMPHOCYTE ERYTHEMATOUS CELL TEST), BLOOD

Norm. Negative; no LE cells found.

Positive. Arthritis (rheumatoid), other rheumatic diseases, hepatitis, scleroderma, and systemic lupus erythematosus (SLE). Drugs include azulfidine (salicylazosulfapyridine), chlorpromazine, ethosuximide, hydralazine, isoniazid, methyldopa, penicillamine, phenytoin, practolol, primidone, procainamide, and thiouracils.

Description. This is a serologic test used to diagnose SLE and to monitor its treatment. Clients with SLE have antibodies against the components of nuclei within their own cells. One usually performs this test by traumatizing white blood cells and exposing the nuclear material within them. Then the nuclear material is incubated with the client's serum. Neutrophils in the affected client's serum will phagocytize the traumatized nuclear material. The phagocytized complex appears as a blue-staining, amorphous mass in the neutrophil's cytoplasm after the cells are stained with Wright's stain. When these neutrophils, which are now filled LE cells, are seen, the test is considered positive.

Professional Considerations
1. Consent form NOT required.
2. Preparation:
   A. Tube: Red topped, red/gray topped, or gold topped.
   B. Avoid heparin therapy for 2 days before the test.
3. Procedure:
   A. Draw a 5-mL blood sample.

B. List on the laboratory requisition any drugs that may affect results (from the list above, under "Positive," and from the list below, section 6).
4. Postprocedure care:
   A. None.
5. Client and family teaching:
   A. No fasting is required.
   B. Discuss the signs of potential infection at the venipuncture site with the client because clients with SLE are often immunocompromised.
6. Factors that affect results:
   A. Drugs that may cause false-negative results include heparin and steroids.
   B. Drugs that may cause false-positive results include acetazolamide, aminosalicylic acid, anticonvulsants (phenytoin [Dilantin], Mesantoin, Tridione), chlorprothixene, chlorothiazide, clofibrate, griseofulvin, isoniazid (INH), hydralazine (Apresoline), methyldopa (Aldomet), methysergide, oral contraceptives, penicillin, phenylbutazone, procainamide (Pronestyl), quinidine, reserpine, streptomycin, sulfonamides, and tetracyclines.
   C. This is a nonspecific test. False-positive results have been reported in those having rheumatoid arthritis, scleroderma, and drug-induced lupus, which were related to tetracycline, phenytoin, and oral contraceptives.
   D. Reject clotted specimens. Hemolysis of the blood sample could affect the results.
7. Other data:
   A. The LE test is positive in only 60%-80% of acutely ill cases.
   B. Use more sensitive tests, such as antinuclear antibodies or anti-DNA, to confirm SLE.

L

LUTEINIZING HORMONE, BLOOD

Norm. Ranges vary among laboratories.

		SI UNITS
Adult Females		
Follicular phase	5-30 mIU/mL	5-30 Arb units
Midcycle	75-150 mIU/mL	75-150 Arb units
Luteal phase	3-40 mIU/mL	3-40 Arb units
Postmenopausal	30-200 mIU/mL	30-200 Arb units

Continued

		SI UNITS
Adult Males	6-23 mIU/mL	6-23 Arb units
Female Children		
1-3 months	7.8-27 mIU/mL	7.8-27 Arb units
3-5 months	5.6-20.8 mIU/mL	5.6-20.8 Arb units
5-7 months	5.4-21.4 mIU/mL	5.4-21.4 Arb units
7-12 months	2.1-4.7 mIU/mL	2.1-4.7 Arb units
10-13 years	2-14 mIU/mL	2-14 Arb units
14-18 years	2-29 mIU/mL	2-29 Arb units
Male Children		
1-3 months	8.9-35.7 mIU/mL	8.9-35.7 Arb units
3-5 months	3.7-27.3 mIU/mL	3.7-27.3 Arb units
5-7 months	9.1-25.1 mIU/mL	9.1-25.1 Arb units
7-12 months	5.7-42.3 mIU/mL	5.7-42.3 Arb units
10-13 years	4-12 mIU/mL	4 12 Arb units
14-18 years	6-19 mIU/mL	6-19 Arb units

"Arb" means 'arbitrary.'

Usage. To evaluate infertility in women and men (high serum values of LH are related to gonadal dysfunction, and low values of LH are related to dysfunction or failure of the hypothalamus or pituitary gland); to evaluate hormonal therapy for inducing ovulation; and to evaluate endocrine problems related to precocious puberty in children.

Increased. Amenorrhea, anorchia (congenital absence of testicles), endocrine problems related to precocious puberty in children, hyperpituitarism, Klinefelter syndrome (in prepubertal boys)(such as sex chromosome disorder), liver disease, menopause, ovarian or testicular failure (primary gonadal dysfunction), Stein-Leventhal syndrome (polycystic ovarian disease), tumors (pituitary, testicular), and Turner's syndrome (ovarian dysgenesis). Drugs include anticonvulsants, clomiphene, naloxone, and spironolactone. Herbs or natural remedies include *Unkei-to*.

Decreased. Adrenal hyperplasia or tumor, amenorrhea (pituitary failure, secondary gonadal insufficiency), anorexia nervosa, anovulation, hypophysectomy, hypopituitarism, hypothalamic disorder, luteinizing hormone deficiency, malnutrition, pituitary disorder, prostate cancer and testicular failure (related to pituitary failure). Drugs include atrial natriuretic hormone (long-acting), digoxin, estrogen compounds, kaliuretic hormone, oral contraceptives, phenothiazines, proges-terone, stanozolol, testosterone, and vessel dilator hormone administration.

Description. Luteinizing hormone (LH), a glycoprotein is secreted by the anterior lobe of the pituitary gland in response to stimulation by the hypothalamic release of gonadotropic releasing hormone. LH plays a critical role in regulation of ovulatory and reproductive function. In women, LH initiates luteinization in the ovary, and together with follicle stimulating hormone (FSH) induces ovulation. A surge of LH in blood levels indicates that ovulation has occurred. In men, LH stimulates the secretion of androgens and increases the production of testosterone. Together with FSH, testosterone influences the development and maturation of spermatozoa. Luteinizing hormone levels peak at midcycle in women of childbearing age, surging when ovulation has occurred.

Professional Considerations
1. Consent form NOT required.
2. Preparation:
   A. Client may be asked to withhold estrogen-containing medications for 4 weeks before the test.
   B. Tube: Red topped, red/gray topped, or gold topped.
   C. For females, write date of the last menstrual period on the laboratory requisition. Note if the woman is menopausal. For all clients, write their age on the laboratory requisition.

D. Discuss with physician whether to withhold medications that could interfere with the test results.

3. **Procedure:**
   A. In men, one single sample is taken. In women, daily blood samples must be taken at the same time each day. A series of daily blood specimens can establish the presence or absence of a midcycle peak in women with anovulatory fertility problems. Alternatively, several samples may be taken in one day, 20-30 minutes apart. This because LH is released in a pulsatile manner with levels varying during the menstrual cycle.
   B. Draw a 1-mL blood sample without hemolysis.

4. **Postprocedure care:**
   A. None.

5. **Client and family teaching:**
   A. Encourage the client to express concerns related to infertility or other health problems to the nurse or the physician.
   B. Episodic fluctuations in LH can be great; thus multiple blood samples are more reliable than a single sample.

6. **Factors that affect results:**
   A. Hemolysis of the specimen invalidates the results.
   B. Results may be affected by the recent use of radioisotopes.
   C. Drugs that could increase or decrease plasma LH levels. (Refer to relevant sections above.)
   D. Women using oral contraceptives will have an absence of midcycle LH peak until the contraceptives are discontinued.
   E. Collection of the daily specimen at different times in the day may cause inaccurate results.
   F. Pulsatile secretion patterns may be disrupted in clients with seizure disorders.
   G. Radiology tests involving injection of a radioactive tracer within 7 days before the test can invalidate the results.

7. **Other data:**
   A. Follicle-stimulating hormone (FSH) level may be requested from the same specimen.
   B. Progesterone, not luteinizing hormone, concentrations at the time of ovum transfer is a significant variable associated with spontaneous abortion (miscarriage).

LUTEINIZING HORMONE, URINE

Norm:

Adult Female

Follicular phase	5-25 IU/24 hours
Midcycle	30-95 IU/24 hours
Luteal phase	2-24 IU/24 hours
Postmenopausal	40-100 IU/24 hours

Adult Male 5-25 IU/24 hours

Increased. See *Luteinizing hormone, Blood.*

Decreased. See *Luteinizing hormone, Blood.*

Description. See *Luteinizing hormone, Blood.* In addition, urine assays are used to monitor ovulatory cycles of clients undergoing in vitro fertilization.

Professional Considerations
1. Consent form NOT required.
2. **Preparation:**
   A. Obtain a specimen container for 24-hour urine collection. (The presence of a preservative eliminates the need for refrigeration.)
   B. Label the container with the client's name, test, date, and time. For females, write the date of last menstrual period on the laboratory requisition. Note if the woman is menopausal, and record her age.
3. **Procedure:**
   A. Discard the first morning urine specimen.

B. Save all the urine voided for 24 hours in the collection container. Include the urine voided at the end of the 24-hour period. For catheterized clients, keep the drainage bag on ice and empty the urine into the collection container hourly.

C. Refrigerate the urine if the 24-hour container does not contain a preservative.

4. **Postprocedure care:**
   A. Compare the urine quantity in the specimen container with the urinary output record for the test. If the specimen contains less urine than what was recorded as output, some urine may have been discarded, thus invalidating the test.
   B. Document the quantity of urine output for the collection period on the laboratory requisition.

5. **Client and family teaching:**
   A. Save all the urine voided in the 24-hour period and urinate before defecating to avoid loss of urine. If any urine is accidentally discarded, discard the entire specimen and restart the collection the next day.

6. **Factors that affect results:**
   A. Urine that is stored in a container without a preservative or urine that is not refrigerated will yield invalid results.

7. **Other data:**
   A. The 24-hour urine collection will minimize the episodic "peak-and-valley" secretion of LH that may occur with blood serum specimens.
   B. One or more blood samples of LH may also be evaluated.
   C. One-step test strip kits for detection of LH in urine are available for use at home.

LYME DISEASE ANTIBODY, BLOOD

Norm. Negative.
Indirect fluorescent antibody titer: ≤1:256.
ELISA: Nonreactive.
Western blot assay: 5 bands (confirmatory test).

Increased. Indicative of recent infection or past exposure to Lyme disease.

Description. Lyme disease was first named because of its close geographic clustering in Lyme, Connecticut, in 1975. Today, it is found mostly in the northeastern, upper midwestern, and western United States. This blood test identifies antibodies to the spirochete agent of Lyme disease, *Borrelia burgdorferi. B. burgdorferi* is carried by several tick vectors, primarily the deer tick, *Ixodes dammini* and is transmitted to humans through a tick bite. Lyme disease is an inflammatory disease involving multiple body systems and causing symptoms that mimic other diseases, beginning with a bull's eye rash and progressing to flulike symptoms and eventually to arthritis. If left untreated, Lyme disease can progress to symptoms as serious as encephalitis, cardiomegaly, and inflammation of the pericardium and sensory nerves. Until recently, indirect detection of Lyme disease via IgG and IgM antibody detection was the only method available for diagnosis. An initial enzyme-linked immunosorbent assay (ELISA) or indirect fluorescent antibody (IFA) test was followed by a Western blot confirmatory test. These methods are suitable for clients who have never had Lyme disease before. Levels of specific IgM antibodies peak during the third to sixth week after the onset of the disease and then gradually decline. Titers of specific IgG antibodies are usually low during the first several weeks of illness. The IgG antibodies will reach maximum levels months later and will often stay elevated for up to 20 years after the active disease has resolved. These methods are of limited use in certain clients; positive results will occur if the client has previously been vaccinated with the *B. burgdorferi* vaccine. Because 25% of those vaccinated fail to develop immunity, it is possible to become infected with Lyme disease even after vaccination. For previously vaccinated clients with current suspected Lyme disease, *the B. burgdorferi C6 Peptide Antibody Test, Serum* should be used.

Professional Considerations
1. Consent form NOT required.
2. **Preparation:**
   A. Tube: Red topped, red/gray topped, or gold topped.
   B. Ask the client if there has been any recent history of a tick bite.

C. Assess for a reddish, macular lesion at the site of the tick bite and elsewhere.
3. Procedure:
   A. Draw a 3-mL blood sample.
4. Postprocedure care:
   A. None.
5. Client and family teaching:
   A. No fasting or special preparation is required.
   B. Return as prescribed for serial specimen collection.
   C. A reddish, macular lesion usually occurs about 1 week after the tick bite.
   D. The primary disease occurs 4-20 days after the initial bite.
   E. The secondary disease develops after 3-24 weeks of infection.
   F. Wear clothing that covers the entire extremities when in areas infested by ticks and deer and when in the woods.
   G. See a doctor immediately if bitten by a tick or if a macular lesion results from a tick bite. Antibiotic therapy will usually be started.
6. Factors that affect results:
   A. False-positive results occur in 21% of clients with high rheumatoid factors.
   B. There is considerable cross-reactivity in clients with treponemal disease (syphilis).
   C. Reject specimens with low dilutions of serum.
   D. Due to the cross-reactivity of *B. burgdorferi* with other organisms, false positive results can occur if careful separation of the immune complexes from the serum is not done.
7. Other data:
   A. The organism may also be cultivated from cerebrospinal fluid or skin biopsy specimens.
   B. Serial serum samples are the preferred method of measurement.
   C. Seronegativity usually rules out the diagnosis of Lyme disease.
   D. The Lyme disease vaccine has been withdrawn from the market.

LYMPH NODE BIOPSY, SPECIMEN
(*see Biopsy, Site-specific, Specimen*)

LYMPHANGIOGRAPHY (LYMPHOGRAPHY, LYMPHANGIOGRAM), DIAGNOSTIC

Norm. Normal-sized vessels and nodes containing no filling defects.

Usage. Indicated in clients with edema of lower extremities with unknown cause, Hodgkin's disease, lymphadenopathy, lymphoma, prostate cancer, tumor metastatic to the lymphatic system. Used to stage clients with lymphoma, demonstrate the extent and level of lymphatic metastasis, and evaluate the effectiveness of chemotherapy or radiation therapy.

Description. Radiographic test of the lymphatic vessels and lymph nodes. A radiopaque iodine contrast oil, such as Ethiodol, is injected into the lymphatics of the foot or hand. The dye remains in the lymph nodes for 6 months to 1 year; thus repeat plain x-rays films can be performed for follow-up of disease progression or to determine the effectiveness of the cancer treatment.

Professional Considerations
1. Consent form IS required.

Risks
Allergic reaction to dye (itching, hives, rash, tight feeling in the throat, shortness of breath, bronchospasm, anaphylaxis, death); renal toxicity from contrast medium; lipid pneumonia (e.g., contrast dye causes micropulmonary emboli); lymphangiitis; infection or cellulitis.

Contraindications
Previous allergy to iodized oil, iodine preparations, contrast dye used in other x-ray tests, or shellfish are relative contraindications. If allergies exist, the radiologist may prescribe a diphenhydramine and steroid preparation, which may be given before the procedure. Then a hypoallergenic, nonionic contrast medium will be used during the test. Other contraindications: severe chronic lung diseases, pregnancy (because of radioactive iodine crossing the blood-placental barrier), pulmonary insufficiency, cardiac disease, and severe renal or hepatic disease.

L

2. **Preparation:**
   A. Have emergency equipment readily available.
   B. See *Client and family teaching.*
3. **Procedure:**
   A. In the radiology department, the client is positioned supine on the examination table.
   B. An oil-based dye is injected intradermally between each of the first three toes of each foot to outline the lymphatic vessels. (The stain can also be injected into the web of the skin between the fingers.)
   C. Under local anesthesia, a 1-2 inch incision is made in the dorsum of each foot (or hand) about 15-30 minutes later.
   D. The lymphatic vessel is identified. This will be easily visualized after the stain is taken up.
   E. A 30-gauge lymphangiographic needle with polyethylene tubing is carefully inserted into the identified lymphatic vessel. A low-rate infusion pump is used to administer an extremely low-pressure, slow injection (1-1.5 hours) of iodine contrast material.
   F. The flow of iodine dye is followed by fluoroscopy.
   G. When the contrast material reaches the level of the third and fourth lumbar vertebrae, the injection is stopped. This usually occurs in about $1\frac{1}{2}$ hours.
   H. Radiographs are then taken of the chest, abdomen, and pelvis. This will demonstrate the filling of the lymph nodes.
   I. The cannula is removed, and the incision is sutured closed after the injection of contrast is completed. The entire procedure takes about 3 hours.
   J. A second set of x-ray films is often made in 24-48 hours.
4. **Postprocedure care:**
   A. Elevate legs to prevent swelling for 24 hours if prescribed. Keep the client on bedrest for 24 hours or as prescribed.
   B. Assess for signs of oil embolism every 4 hours for 24 hours (such as dyspnea, pain, and hypotension).
   C. Observe injection and incision sites for evidence of cellulitis (such as redness, drainage, swelling, pain). Monitor temperature every 4 hours for 48 hours after the procedure.

D. The dressing is usually not changed for the first 48 hours.
   E. Allow the client to rest after the procedure.
   F. Monitor for complications, such as delayed wound healing or infection at the site of the incision or injection; edema of legs; allergic dermatitis; headache; sore mouth and throat; skin rashes; transient fever; lymphangitis; or oil embolism, which could occur if the contrast medium causes micropulmonary emboli and could produce lipid pneumonia.
5. **Client and family teaching:**
   A. No fasting or sedation is required.
   B. Discomfort may be felt when the stain is injected and when the feet are anesthetized.
   C. It is important to lie very still during the injection of the contrast dye. X-ray filming usually takes about 30 minutes.
   D. The dye will turn the urine and stool blue for 48 hours. Also, IV administration of the lymphatic stain or excessive infiltration of the stain may impart a transient bluish tint to the entire skin surface.
   E. Inspect the injection and incision sites for redness, swelling, and pain if the client will be returning home after the procedure.
   F. Sutures should be removed 7-10 days after the test.
6. **Factors that affect results:**
   A. Inability to cannulate lymphatic vessels.
7. **Other data:**
   A. To visualize axillary and supraclavicular nodes, injections are made in each hand.

LYMPHOCYTE, BLOOD
(see Differential leukocyte count, Peripheral blood)

LYMPHOCYTE ERYTHEMATOUS CELL TEST
(see Lupus test, Blood)

LYMPHOCYTE MARKER STUDIES
(see T- and B-lymphocyte subset assay, Blood)

LYMPHOCYTE SUBSET ENUMERATION, BLOOD
(see Acquired immunodeficiency syndrome evaluation battery, Diagnostic)

LYMPHOCYTE SUBSET TYPING
(see T- and B-lymphocyte subset assay, Blood)

LYMPHOCYTE (T & B) ASSAY
(see T- and B-lymphocyte subset assay, Blood)

LYMPHOGRANULOMA VENEREUM TITER (LGV), BLOOD

Norm. Negative; indirect fluorescent antibody titer ≤1:64.

Usage. *Chlamydia psittaci* infections and *Chlamydia trachomatis* infections, which are associated with lymphogranuloma venereum (LGV). In women, *Chlamydia* could cause pelvic inflammatory disease, endometriosis, or salpingitis. In men, *Chlamydia* could cause Reiter syndrome or epididymitis. Perihepatitis (Fitz-Hugh-Curtis syndrome) has also been linked to *Chlamydia.*

Description. Indirect fluorescent antibody test, which is useful in identifying *Chlamydia* antibodies. The bacterium *C. trachomatis* is associated with human diseases ranging from blinding trachoma to sexually acquired genital infections and the systemic disease LGV. LGV is a venereal infection caused by the L-1, L-2, or L-3 serotype of *C. trachomatis.* A primary lesion is followed by rapid swelling of regional lymph nodes.

Professional Considerations
1. Consent form NOT required.
2. Preparation:
   A. Tube: Red topped, red/gray topped, or gold topped.
3. Procedure:
   A. Draw a 7-mL blood sample.
   B. Draw a convalescent sample in 10-14 days.
4. Postprocedure care:
   A. None.

5. Client and family teaching:
   A. Return in 2 weeks to have a follow-up sample drawn.
6. Factors that affect results:
   A. Failure to collect a convalescent sample may indicate that the disease has not been fully treated.
7. Other data:
   A. A fourfold increase in titer indicates acute infection.
   B. Clients being evaluated for LGV should also be tested for syphilis.
   C. Diagnosis of *C. psittaci* should include a record of prior contact with sick birds (parrots) or employment in pet shops.
   D. Direct fluorescent test or ELISA on clinical specimens is now preferred over *Chlamydia* antibody titer.

LYMPHOGRAPHY
(see Lymphangiography, Diagnostic)

LYMPHS
(see Differential leukocyte count, Peripheral blood)

LSD (LYSERGIC ACID DIETHYLAMIDE), BLOOD OR URINE

Norm. Negative.

Positive. Drug abuse.

Description. A potent hallucinogen derived from ergot, a fungus that spoils rye grain. It is equally effective by the intravenous route as by the oral route, is metabolized in the liver and excreted in the bile, and affects both parasympathetic and sympathetic nervous systems. May produce hallucinations years after ingestion, without warning.

Professional Considerations
1. Consent form NOT required.
2. Preparation:
   A. Tube: Red topped, red/gray topped, or gold topped (for the blood sample).
   B. Obtain a sterile specimen container (for the urine sample).
3. Procedure:
   A. Draw a 7-mL blood sample or obtain 10 mL of urine.

4. Postprocedure care:
   A. Refrigerate or freeze specimen until testing.
5. Client and family teaching:
   A. This drug may cause delirium, delusions, and hallucinations.
   B. Clients who experience palinopsia (prolonged afterimages, visual perseveration) during LSD intoxication may continue to be symptomatic up to 3 years after they cease to ingest the drug.
   C. There is no systematic program of treatment for LSD ingestion. A quiet environment and diazepam may be effective in controlling the individual.
6. Factors that affect results:
   A. Levels may be decreased if stored at room temperature

B. The use of Stealth adulterant in the urine sample will cause negative results in a positive sample.
7. Other data:
   A. Signs of toxicity include hypertension, tachycardia, piloerection, and suicidal tendency. LSD-related violent behavior includes suicide, homicide, and accidental death

LYSOZYME, SERUM
(see Muramidase, Serum and Urine Muramidase, Serum and Urine and Urine)

MAGNESIUM, SERUM

Norm:

	NORMAL SERUM LEVELS	SI UNITS
Newborn	1.2-2.9 mEq/L	0.6-1.45 mmol/L
Child	1.6-2.6 mEq/L	0.8-1.3 mmol/L
Adult	1.3-2.5 mEq/L or 1.8-3.0 mg/dL	0.65-1.25 mmol/L
Panic level	<0.5 mEq/L or >3.0 mg/dL	<0.25 or >1.23 mmol/L
Toxic level	>12.0 mEq/L	>6 mmol/L

Panic Level Symptoms and Treatment

High Magnesium Symptoms. Lethargy, drowsiness, flushing, nausea, vomiting, slurred speech, hypotension, weak or absent deep tendon reflexes, electrocardiogram changes (such as prolonged PR and Q-T intervals, widened QRS, bradycardia), respiratory depression.

Treatment:
Note: Treatment choice(s) depend on client history and condition and episode history.
Administer magnesium salts intravenously (8-16 mmol of magnesium sulfate in 10-100 mL of D_5W over 10-15 minutes, followed by 40 mmol of magnesium sulfate in 500 mL of D_5W over 5 hours).

Reduce auditory, mechanical, and visual stimuli.
Monitor for respiratory depression and areflexia if intravenous magnesium sulfate is given.
Monitor for diarrhea and metabolic alkalosis if oral magnesium replacement is given.

Increased. Addison's disease, adrenalectomy, ataxia, dehydration (severe), diabetes (uncontrolled diabetes, diabetic acidosis before treatment, controlled diabetes in an older client), dysrhythmias, hypercalcemia, hypothyroidism, hypophosphatemia, kidney stone, leukemia (lymphocytic and myelocytic), mood disorders, nephrolithiasis, renal insufficiency or failure. Drugs include antacids containing magnesium (such as Maalox, Mylanta, Aludrox, DiaGel, Milk of Magnesia), calcium-containing medications, cathartics, Epsom salt gargle, ethacrynic acid, laxatives (such as Epsom salt, magnesium citrate), loop diuretics, and thyroid medications.

Decreased. Acute tubular necrosis (diuretic phase), alcoholism (chronic), aldosteronism, Bartter syndrome, bowel resection complications, convulsions, diabetic ketoacidosis, diarrhea (chronic), dysrhythmias, excessive lactation, excessive sweating, hepatitis, hepatic cirrhosis, hepatic insufficiency, hungry bone syndrome, hypokalemia, hypercalcemia, hyperthyroidism, hypoparathyroidism, intravenous solutions without magnesium, ketoacidosis, kwashiorkor (severe malnutrition), laxative abuse, magnesium-deficiency tetany syndrome, pancreatitis (chronic, acute), phosphate depletion, postoperatively, primary hyperaldosteronism, prolonged gastric drainage, reduced magnesium intake, reduced magnesium absorption (specific magnesium malabsorption, generalized malabsorption syndrome, excessive bowel resection, diffuse bowel disease or injury), renal disease (chronic), renal defect of magnesium resorption, renal transplantation, renal tubular acidosis, status post obstructive diuresis, stress states with catecholamine excess, tetany, toxemia of pregnancy, ulcerative colitis, volume expansion (extracellular fluid). Drugs include alcohol, amphotericin B, some antibiotics (neomycin, aminoglycosides), calcium gluconate, cisplatin, corticosteroids, cyclosporin A, diuretics (such as mercurial, ethacrynic acid), glucose, insulin, mannitol, and urea.

Description. Measurement of magnesium levels is used as an index to (1) metabolic activity in the body (such as carbohydrate metabolism, protein synthesis, nucleic acid synthesis, contraction of muscular tissue), and (2) renal function, since 95% of magnesium that is filtered through the glomerulus is reabsorbed in the tubules. Most of the body's magnesium, which is an electrolyte, is concentrated in the bone, cartilage, and the cell itself. In addition, magnesium is needed in the blood-clotting mechanism. Regulates neuromuscular irritability, acts as a cofactor that modifies the activity of many enzymes, and has a significant effect on the metabolism of calcium.

Professional Considerations
1. Consent form NOT required.
2. **Preparation:**
   A. Tube: Red topped, red/gray topped, or gold topped or green topped.
   B. Do NOT draw during hemodialysis.
   C. See *Client and family teaching.*
3. **Procedure:**
   A. Draw a 1-mL blood sample without hemolysis.
4. **Postprocedure care:**
   A. Separate serum from the red blood cells within 6 hours.
   B. If storage is necessary, refrigerate the specimen.
   C. Serum separated from the cells is stable for 2-3 days.
5. **Client and family teaching:**
   A. No special diet or fasting is required before sampling.
   B. Eat foods rich in magnesium (such as seafood, meats, green vegetables, whole grains, and nuts) if magnesium level is low.
   C. Avoid constant use of antacids or laxatives containing magnesium, if magnesium level is high. Check drug labels to identify magnesium-containing formulations.
6. **Factors that affect results:**
   A. Hemolysis of the specimen will create falsely elevated levels of magnesium.
   B. Glucuronic acid therapy will interfere with the color reaction in some laboratory methods and will produce falsely decreased results.
   C. Prolonged intravenous fluid therapy, hyperalimentation, exchange blood transfusions, or prolonged nasogastric suctioning may yield falsely decreased results.
   D. Prolonged use of magnesium products (such as antacids, laxatives), lithium compounds, or salicylate therapy will cause falsely increased levels, especially if renal damage is present.
   E. Hyperbilirubinemia interferes with serum magnesium, resulting in misleadingly low levels.
   F. High-phosphate diet suppresses both magnesium and calcium absorption.
   G. Levels may decrease from baseline in women taking oral contraceptives, and may increase from

M

baseline in women taking injectable contraceptives.
7. Other data:
A. Nutritional status is important to the interpretation of the test results.
B. If hypocalcemia is present, magnesium should also be measured. Magnesium deficiency may cause apparently unexplained hypocalcemia and hypokalemia.
C. Respiratory failure and death are possible when magnesium levels exceed 12 mEq/L. Magnesium level may be decreased after surgery for hyperparathyroidism.

MAGNESIUM, 24-HOUR URINE

Norm. Normal values vary with different test methods.
5-16 mEq/24 hours (2.5-8.0 μmol/24 hours)
12-199 mg/24 hours
7.3-12.2 mg/dL (random sample)

Increased. Alcoholism, Bartter syndrome, hypermagnesemia, and nephrolithiasis. Drugs include aldosterone, cisplatin, corticosteroids, diuretics (ethacrynic acid), and thiazides.

Decreased. Renal disease, kidney stones, magnesium deficit, osteoporosis, and syndrome of inappropriate antidiuretic hormone secretion (SIADHS).

Description. A 24-hour urine test useful in evaluation of renal disease and magnesium deficiency. In magnesium deficiency, urine magnesium decreases before serum magnesium. See also *Magnesium, Blood.*

Professional Considerations
1. Consent form NOT required.
2. Preparation:
A. Obtain a 3-L, acid-washed, metal-free urine collection container without preservatives.
3. Procedure:
A. Instruct the client to void and discard the initial specimen.
B. Collect all the urine voided in a 24-hour period in the above container. Maintain the specimen on wet ice throughout the collection period. Do not collect urine in a metal bedpan or urinal.
4. Postprocedure care:
A. Record total 24-hour urine volume and exact beginning and ending times of collection on the container and the laboratory requisition.
B. Send the specimen to the laboratory on wet ice.
5. Client and family teaching:
A. Save all the urine you void for 24 hours in the plastic container provided. If any urine is accidentally discarded, throw out the entire specimen and restart the collection the next day.
6. Factors that affect results:
A. Reject any urine specimen that has had contact with metal.
B. Increased blood alcohol level increases urine magnesium excretion.
7. Other data:
A. Urinary excretion of magnesium is diet-dependent.

MAGNETIC RESONANCE ANGIOGRAPHY (MRA), DIAGNOSTIC

Norm. Anatomy of normal vessels are well visualized, and blood flow is unobstructed.

Usage. Evaluate vascular structure; evaluate blood flow, especially in the venous system, for possible aneurysms, stenosis, thromboses, or blockages; determine tumor vascularity; assess for evidence of direct tumor involvement of vascular structures; evaluate clients with carotid stenosis preoperatively so that the carotid artery endarterectomy is performed with decreased complication; assist in diagnosis of cerebrovascular disease, cardiovascular disease, cerebral arteriovenous malformations, congenital heart disease, renal or hepatic vasculature disorder, trigeminal neuralgia; assess effectiveness of various therapeutic interventions related to vascular structure and blood flow.

Description. Magnetic resonance angiography (MRA) is a recently developed, noninvasive vascular imaging technique. This procedure is performed by use of the magnetic resonance imaging (MRI) scanner equipment, and MRA may be performed with MRI. MRA provides structural evaluation of arteries and veins and the image of blood flow. The two types of MRA are time of fight (TOF) and phase contrast (PC). TOF angiography uses a process described as "flow-related enhancement," which relies on the inflow of fully magnetized blood into the imaging plane. PC angiography directly measures flow by generating vascular images. These images detect changes in the phase of the blood's transverse magnetization as it moves along a magnetic field gradient. Therefore it relies on alterations in spin phase for image contrast. Both of these methods emphasize the signals in the structures, which contain blood flow, and reconstruct only those structures with flow. The computer subtracts images of other structures, which are of lesser interest, from the image. Both of these methods can obtain two- or three-dimensional images. MRA can be performed without injection of contrast medium or radiation exposure. However, some radiologists prefer using a contrast, such as gadolinium chelate or gadolium-DTPA, to enhance the visualization of venous flow.

Professional Considerations
1. Consent form IS required.

Risks
See *Risks, Magnetic resonance imaging, Diagnostic.*

Contraindications
See *Contraindications, Magnetic resonance imaging, Diagnostic.*

Precautions
See *Precautions, Magnetic resonance imaging, Diagnostic.*

2. Preparation:
   A. See *Preparation, Magnetic resonance imaging, Diagnostic.*
3. Procedure:
   A. See *Procedure, Magnetic resonance imaging, Diagnostic.*
4. Postprocedure care:
   A. If the client has been sedated for the procedure, make certain that he or she is fully awake before ambulating, and follow institutional protocol for postsedation monitoring.
5. Client and family teaching:
   A. This procedure may take 15-30 minutes to perform.
   B. See *Client and family teaching, Magnetic resonance imaging, Diagnostic.*
6. Factors that affect results:
   A. See *Factors that affect results, Magnetic resonance imaging, Diagnostic.*
   B. False-positive and false-negative results in cerebral aneurysm evaluation can be caused by vessel tortuosity and susceptibility artifacts (which occur at the interfaces of structures with different magnetic susceptibilities).
7. Other data:
   A. The same MRI scanner equipment, with different software and pulse sequences, is used to perform MRA.
   B. The results of MRA are beginning to guide medical management and determine the extent of surgical intervention.
   C. The use of MRA versus conventional angiography remains controversial. Gadolinium-enhanced MRA is more sensitive and specific, as well as less risky, than conventional arteriography for detection of renal artery stenosis. Risk for false results with MRA exist with cerebral aneurysms. MRA has been found to be as accurate as arteriography for carotid artery stenosis in large vessels, but not in smaller vessels such as the terminal carotid branch.

MAGNETIC RESONANCE CHOLANGIOPANCREATOG-RAPHY (MRCP), DIAGNOSTIC

M

Norm. Requires interpretation.

Usage. Used when more invasive procedures such as endoscopic retrograde cholangiopancreatography (ERCP) are contraindicated or have not been successful. Can detect choledocholithiasis, obstruction and dilation of the bile and pancreatic ducts due to malignancies, abnormal anatomy, or pancreatitis.

Used preoperatively to depict the anatomy of the ductal system before surgical drainage. Used postoperatively to evaluate the hepatobiliary system after gastrointestinal surgery. Superior to ERCP in visualizing dilated ducts proximal to an obstruction. The diffusion-weighted technique is particularly helpful in detecting early ischemic stroke, multiple sclerosis, and in differentiating neoplasm from brain abscess.

Description. Magnetic resonance cholangiopancreatography (MRCP) is a noninvasive, noncontrast procedure for evaluating the gallbladder, biliary tract, and pancreatic duct. MRCP is able to visualize extrahepatic bile ducts and central intrahepatic ducts. Because these structures contain fluid, they show up as bright images under magnetic resonance imaging. Because this procedure can be performed in about 10 minutes, can visualize the entire hepatobiliary system, and does not use risky contrast material, it is being used more often as a replacement for the traditional ERCP procedure. MRCP may be enhanced with the use of the breath-hold method, using intravenous gadolinium (Gd).

Professional Considerations
1. Consent form IS required.

Risks
See *Risks, Magnetic resonance imaging, Diagnostic.*

Contraindications
See *Contraindications, Magnetic resonance imaging, Diagnostic.*

Precautions
See *Precautions, Magnetic resonance imaging, Diagnostic.*

2. Preparation:
   A. See *Preparation, Magnetic resonance imaging, Diagnostic.*
3. Procedure:
   A. The client is positioned supine on the MRCP table and an antenna is coiled around the abdomen.
   B. *Non-contrast method:*
      i. A scout MRCP is performed to locate the biliary tract and pancreatic duct and then is used as a guide to acquire multiple images of the bile and pancreatic ducts.
      ii. A regular MRI of the abdomen may follow.
   C. *Breath-hold method:*
      i. An intravenous injection of 10 mL of gadolinium chelate is followed by fast-spoiled, gradient echo sequences acquired during breath-holding at 5, 10, and 15 minutes.
      ii. The collecting system is evaluated according to a scale of 0 to 3.
4. Postprocedure care:
   A. See *Postprocedure care, Magnetic resonance imaging, Diagnostic.*
5. Client and family teaching:
   A. MRCP is used to evaluate whether there are obstructions in the area of the gallbladder, liver, and pancreas.
   B. See *Client and family teaching, Magnetic resonance imaging, Diagnostic.*
6. Factors that affect results:
   A. See *Factors that affect results, Magnetic resonance imaging, Diagnostic.*
7. Other data:
   A. None.

MAGNETIC RESONANCE IMAGING (MRI), DIAGNOSTIC

Norm. Description of normal tissue, structure, and blood flow.

Usage. To detect abscesses, abnormalities in blood flow through coronary branches and through extremities, acute tubular necrosis, adenopathy, aortic and ventricular aneurysm, atrial and ventricular septal defects, avascular necrosis, blood clots, brain contusion, cancer and tumors (brain, bone, disk herniation, epidural hematoma on spine, extra-axial, head, intracardiac, hilar, mediastinal, neck, parenchymal, pericardiac, pituitary, pulmonary, renal, sarcoma, and spinal cord), cavernous hemangioma, cerebral infarction, congenital heart disease, cysts, dementia, demyelinating disease, edema, epilepsy, focal viral encephalitis, Gaucher's disease, glomerulonephritis, hemorrhage, hydronephrosis, hyperparathyroidism, infection, intervertebral disk abnormalities, knee abnormalities, Marfan syndrome, myocardial infarction (and afterward to detect scars, aneurysms, pseudoaneurysms, septal defects, mural thrombi and valvular regurgitations), multiple sclerosis, muscular disease, osteomyelitis, plaque formation, pulmonary atresia, renal transplants, renal vein thrombosis, seizures, shoulder abnormalities, skeletal abnormalities, soft-tissue infections, spinal cord compression or injuries, subarachnoid hemorrhage, subdural hematoma, temporomandibular joint abnormalities, tumor invasion (inferior vena cava and seminal vesicles), and tumor staging (cervix, large hydronephroma, prostate, urinary bladder, and uterus).

Description. MRI is a noninvasive diagnostic tool that enables health care professionals to visualize the body's tissues, structure, and blood flow. It uses a strong magnetic field, in conjunction with radio-frequency waves, to transmit signals from the body's cells to a computer. MRI actually stimulates the body to produce a signal of itself. The computer produces cross-sectional images of the body. The cell's nuclei react as tiny magnets in the presence of a strong external magnetic field (MRI). The signal density of the multiple body-plane images depends primarily on the tissue characteristics, pulse sequence, and timing parameters. Newer enhancements of MRI include the use of diffusion-weighted imaging, functional MRI, and fast MRI. In diffusion-weighted MRI, the intracellular and extracellular spaces are compared for the degree of diffusion of water molecules contained within them. Brighter areas indicate restricted diffusion, such as in ischemic cell damage or blockage by tumor. In functional MRI, successive images taken in rapid succession are compared for signal intensity and cerebral blood flow to help evaluate brain function in pathologic brain deterioration, psychiatric disorders, and can also be used to evaluate the auditory system. Fast MRI, which has become possible through software advances, allows shortened breath-holding timeframes, better resolution, completion in 30 minutes or less. Fast MRI is used for evaluation of fetal anatomy or pathology when ultrasound does not yield enough information, and is also showing promise for evaluation of heart failure and screening for metastases. In addition, the newest equipment called "Dual Mode Imaging" combines MRI with functional imaging modalities such as PET or SPECT for improved imaging results. (*See Dual Modality Imaging, Diagnostic.*) MRI is painless and has no known side effects. MRI is superior to computed tomography and ultrasound for its sensitivity in detection of changes in soft tissue. MRI is the standard in the diagnosis of most abnormalities of the brain and spine (except trauma). The ability of MRI to support the diagnosis of multiple sclerosis declines with increasing age of the client. MRI eliminates the need for many knee arthroscopies and has virtually replaced arthrography. Unlike computerized axial tomographic (CAT) scans, MRI can evaluate cerebral infarction within hours of the event. MRI virtually eliminates the need for myelography.

Professional Considerations

1. Consent form IS required. 1-2% of people refuse MRI because of claustrophobia.

Risks

Critical injury to the client could result from ferrous metal in the body (e.g., flecks of ferrous metal in eye could cause retinal hemorrhage).

Contraindications

Intraocular metal foreign bodies; heart valves manufactured before 1964 and middle ear prosthetics (these can be tested by obtainment of a duplicate, which is then placed into the bore, and if no torque is experienced, the test may be safely performed); nerve-stimulating devices may be a contraindication.

Precautions

Some older versions of aneurysm clips may not be ferromagnetic; verify this from manufacturer or hospital records. MRI uses non-ionizing radiation, and thus is considered the least risky of radiographic procedures during pregnancy and there is no evidence of teratogenic or developmental abnormalities associated with this procedure. However, the literature recommends that pregnant women should not be scanned unless absolutely necessary. Radiologists and operators must be informed of the presence of cardiac

M

pacemakers, implanted cardioverter-defibrillators and implanted venous access devices, and cochlear implants, though they are rarely a contraindication. Most stainless steel orthopedic implants and prosthetic devices are not ferromagnetic and are not affected by MRI. Clients with tattooed eyeliner may experience skin irritation or swelling around the eyes caused by the MRI's effects on ferrous pigments in the tattoo. Use of sedatives during this test is contraindicated in clients with central nervous system depression.

2. **Preparation:**
   A. See *Client and family teaching.*
   B. Screen the client for cardiac pacemaker, artificial heart valve, brain aneurysm clips or any type of surgical clip or staple, shunt, neurostimulation (TENS unit), implanted insulin pump, implanted venous access infusion devices, bone growth stimulator, internal electrodes, embolic spring coil, eye implant surgery (with staples), cochlear implant, hearing aid, foil or metallic medication patches, any orthopedic item(s) (such as pins, wires, rods, screws, clips, plates), artificial limb or joint, dental braces, any type of removable dental item, IUD, metallic eye makeup, metal fragments (in head, eye, skin), history of work in the machine tool industry, history of work with a metal lathe, or history of any accidents with metal or ferromagnetic objects (beebee [BB] guns, flecks of ferrous metal in eye). These items may be hazardous to the client's safety.
   C. Screen the accompanying adult for the above items if the client undergoing the procedure is a pediatric client.
   D. Remove any loose metal objects (such as hairpins, barrettes, watches, jewelry, pen clip, steel-toed shoes or clothing with metal snaps or zippers) because they can become projectile in the magnetic force.
   E. Inform the physician if the client is using an IV controller pump or computerized equipment because the magnets in the MRI can disrupt the function of the machine (such as IV flow).

   F. Elicit any problems with claustrophobia. Interventions to reduce claustrophobia include, as appropriate:
      i. Relaxation techniques or a sedative may be used.
      ii. Determine availability of an "open MRI."
      iii. Interact with client in an unhurried, relaxed manner.
      iv. Thorough explanation of the procedure, including methods to reduce anxiety, such as relaxation or controlled breathing techniques.
      v. Suggest that the client keep his or her eyes closed throughout the procedure.
      vi. Offer a cool cloth to be placed over the eyes.
      vii. Point out that the ends of the scanner are always open.
      viii. Offer to have client remove his or her shoes and be covered with a light sheet.
      ix. Keep room temperature cool. Use compressed air through a cannula positioned to blow past the client's face during the procedure.
      x. Arranging for family member to enter the scanner room to speak with the client between scans.
   G. If the client is very young or unable to follow directions, sedation may be indicated to complete the scan.
   H. Start an IV line, if contrast medium is to be given.
3. **Procedure:**
   A. The client is positioned on a padded table and moved into the cylinder-shaped scanner (such as a magnet bore).
   B. Contrast medium may be administered before the procedure if prescribed.
   C. The technologist will operate controls determining image-signal density, pulse sequence, and timing parameters.
   D. If blood flow is to be determined in an extremity, the arm or leg to be examined is placed into a cradlelike support. The technologist will mark reference sites to be imaged on the arm or leg. Then the extremity is moved into a flow cylinder.

E. The MR image is interpreted by a specially trained radiologist.

4. **Postprocedure care:**
   A. Continue the assessment of respiratory status after receiving sedation. If deep sedation was used, follow institutional protocol for postsedation monitoring. Typical monitoring includes continuous ECG monitoring and pulse oximetry, with continual assessments (every 5-15 minutes) of airway, vital signs, and neurologic status until the client is lying quietly awake, is breathing independently, and responds to commands spoken in a normal tone.
   B. Remove the IV line if one was inserted for injection of the contrast medium.

5. **Client and family teaching:**
   A. For pelvic or abdominal scans, do not eat or drink for 6 hours before the procedure.
   B. You will lie on a flat, narrow, padded surface and will be rolled into a cylinder-shaped scanner. The scanner will be around the area of the body that is being scanned.
   C. You will hear various noises from the test, including a muffled drumbeat sound. You may bring in earplugs for the test or use the earplugs that are available. In an open MRI machine, inform the client that there are no loud noises.
   D. You can communicate with MRI personnel, who will be in another room, by means of an intercom system.
   E. It is important to remain completely still during the scan.
   F. Remove jewelry, watches, hairpins, glasses, and any metal objects. The magnetic field can damage watches.
   G. Do not approach the MRI unit if you have a cardiac pacemaker.
   H. You will not be exposed to radiation during this procedure. The contrast medium that may be used is not an iodinated contrast.
   I. The procedure may take 45-90 minutes to scan the head or chest area and approximately 15 minutes to scan an arm or leg. In fast MRI, the procedure will take 30 minutes or less.

6. **Factors that affect results:**
   A. The image will be distorted by movement during the procedure.
   B. Metal, whether ferrous or nonferrous, may produce artifacts that degrade the images if the metal is in proximity to the area of the body that is being scanned.
   C. Because of the possibility of loss of data contained on magnetic recording media, MRI systems are normally contained within a restricted magnetic range, from 15 to 50 gauss.
   D. MRI does not use ionizing radiation; therefore there are none of the hazards found in x rays.

7. **Other data:**
   A. Intravenous gadolinium DTPA contrast, which is a commercially available contrast medium, may be necessary for some examinations at the discretion of the radiologist. This contrast is chemically unrelated to the iodinated contrast, which is used in conventional radiography.
   B. Magnetophosphenes (flickering lights in the visual field), which can occur with MRI, are completely reversible and have no known long-term health effects.
   C. MRI is more effective than CT in identifying white matter brain disease, such as multiple sclerosis.
   D. The Food and Drug Administration (FDA) has classified MRI devices into class II, which includes low-risk devices.

MAGNETIC RESONANCE NEUROGRAPHY (MRN, NEUROGRAPHY), DIAGNOSTIC

Norm. Description of normal nerve structure.

Usage. Helps diagnose and evaluate peripheral nerve tumors, carpal tunnel syndrome, ulnar nerve compression, thoracic outlet syndrome, brachial plexus injuries (including birth injuries), sciatica with no convincing spinal cause, any suspected nerve impingement, accidental injury to peripheral nerves, postirradiation neuritis, chronic nerve compression, and pain syndromes when an anatomic lesion is suspected. In the evaluation of clients with spinal problems, it can also be used as a follow-up or adjunct test to MRI, CT, and myelogram when there are ambiguous test results or if the client has clinical symptoms that are not confined to a single dermatome. MRN may also be useful in surgical planning to localize and determine the resectability of tumors through accurate depiction of the relation of the tumor to the nerve fascicles or presence of nerve laceration.

Description. MRN provides longitudinal and cross-sectional fascicular images of nerves. It is a noninvasive imaging technique that uses a magnetic resonance imaging (MRI) scanner that has been modified with a spin-echo pulse sequence combined with fat suppression and diffusion weighting to generate neurographic images. MRN images show the nerves as the most prominent feature, providing detail of the internal fascicular structure. The cross-sectional images can be viewed individually or reconstructed to provide fully isolated nerves and nerve structure (longitudinal views).

Professional Considerations
1. Consent form IS required.

Risks
See *Risks, Magnetic resonance imaging, Diagnostic.*

Contraindications
See *Contraindications, Magnetic resonance imaging, Diagnostic.*

Precautions
See *Precautions, Magnetic resonance imaging, Diagnostic.*

2. Preparation:
    A. See *Preparation, Magnetic resonance imaging, Diagnostic.*
3. Procedure:
    A. See *Procedure, Magnetic resonance imaging, Diagnostic.*
    B. Contrast medium is not used in this test.
4. Postprocedure care:
    A. See *Postprocedure, Magnetic resonance imaging, Diagnostic.*
5. Client and family teaching:
    A. See *Client and family teaching, Magnetic resonance imaging, Diagnostic.*

B. There is no contrast agent or injections involved.
C. The test takes about 30-40 minutes.
6. Factors that affect results:
    A. See *Factors that affect results, Magnetic resonance imaging, Diagnostic.*
    B. Variable sensitivity occurs in imaging very small nerves. Decreased sensitivity is associated with imaging small nerves that traverse multiple anatomic planes, such as those in the pelvis (that is, the ilioinguinal nerve).
    C. It is important that clinical evaluation correlate with abnormal findings of MRN. It has been reported that up to 60% of the population with no pain have been found to have a herniated disk, bone spurs, or narrowing of spinal canals. In a symptomatic client, these "commonly occurring" abnormalities may be inaccurately diagnosed as the cause of the symptoms when in actuality the pathologic condition is located at a more distal nerve site.
7. Other data:
    A. At this time, MRN cannot be accomplished by means of the "open" MRI machines. The magnet-field gradient required for MRN imaging cannot be maintained with the open MRI equipment.
    B. MRN is new and not widely available at present.

MAGNETIC RESONANCE SPECTROSCOPY (MRS), DIAGNOSTIC

Norm. Norms continue to be developed because this is a very new diagnostic modality. Qualitative and quantitative cellular biochemical data, such as steady-state cellular concentrations of metabolites, are visible with MRS.

Usage. Provide follow-up study and prognosis for clients with AIDS, cancer and tumors, diabetes mellitus, hepatic encephalopathy, intracranial mass, metabolic disorders, neurodegeneration, stroke, systemic lupus erythematosus (SLE); detect degeneration, inflammation, and necrosis in tissues;

and monitor and evaluate therapeutic interventions in conjunction with MRI. Evaluate biochemical basis for neuropsychiatric disorders and dementias. Future application may include detection of changes at the cellular level that precede morphologic changes detected with MRI or other radiologic imaging modalities.

Description. Magnetic resonance spectroscopy (MRS) is a recently developed noninvasive vascular imaging technique. This procedure is performed by use of the magnetic resonance imaging (MRI) scanner equipment and different software. Two types of MRS include the proton MRS and phosphorus-31 (^{31}P) MRS. The MRS describes the molecular state of water, the chemical environment of cells and tissues, and the qualitative and quantitative state of intermediary metabolism. It can produce specific metabolite profiles in various pathologic conditions.

Professional Considerations
1. Consent form IS required.

Risks
See *Risks, Magnetic resonance imaging, Diagnostic.*

Contraindications
See *Contraindications, Magnetic resonance imaging, Diagnostic.*

Precautions
See *Precautions, Magnetic resonance imaging, Diagnostic.*

2. Preparation:
   A. See *Preparation, Magnetic resonance imaging, Diagnostic.*
3. Procedure:
   A. See *Procedure, Magnetic resonance imaging, Diagnostic.*
   B. MRS always needs to be performed before contrast medium is added because a contrast medium may affect the expression of metabolites.
   C. To obtain the best image, the areas to be avoided in MRS include frontal and ethmoid sinuses, temporal bones, deep-in-posterior fossa, subcutaneous fat, and areas of high flow or hypervascular disorder.

4. Postprocedure care:
   A. See *Postprocedure care, Magnetic resonance imaging, Diagnostic.*
5. Client and family teaching:
   A. See *Client and family teaching, Magnetic resonance imaging, Diagnostic.*
6. Factors that affect results:
   A. See *Factors that affect results, Magnetic resonance imaging, Diagnostic.*
   B. Many factors influence the profile of the MR spectra, including magnetic-field uniformity, interclient variability, age, and developmental stage. Normal metabolite ratios change substantially during development, particularly from birth to 2 years of age. Quantification of metabolites is difficult as a result of the complexity of the spectra.
7. Other data:
   A. MRS may be performed with MRI.

MAGNETIC RESONANCE UROGRAPHY, DIAGNOSTIC

Norm. Requires interpretation.

Usage. Identification of urinary tract dilatation, particularly after transplantation; Detection of: neurogenic bladder dysfunction, ectopic ureters in children, Alternative to intravenous pyelography and computed tomography in renal-impaired clients for whom excretory urography is contraindicated, such as those with uremia and renal impairment or in those with no excretory function. Helpful during pregnancy and in those clients allergic to contrast medium, due to the noninvasive nature of the procedure. Other usage should be reserved for those clients in which less expensive testing has proven inconclusive.

Description. Magnetic Resonance Urography (MRU) is a costly but extremely accurate, noninvasive, and noncontrast method of identifying renal conditions which are not well identified with other technology such as computed tomography, pyelography and ultrasound. In MRU, urine appears white, and so the adequacy of the excretory route and obstructive impairments can be evaluated. The MRU may be enhanced with the use of the breath-hold method, using intravenous gadolinium (Gd).

M

Professional Considerations
1. Consent form IS required.

Risks
See *Risks, Magnetic resonance imaging, Diagnostic.*

Contraindications
See *Contraindications, Magnetic resonance imaging, Diagnostic.*

Precautions
See *Precautions, Magnetic resonance imaging, Diagnostic.*

2. **Preparation:**
   A. See *Preparation, Magnetic resonance imaging, Diagnostic.*
   B. Client must be well-hydrated prior to the procedure.
3. **Procedure:**
   A. The client is positioned supine on the MRU table and an antenna is coiled around the abdomen.
   B. *Non-contrast method:*
      A scout MRU is performed to locate the kidneys and ureters and then is used as a guide to acquire multiple images of the urinary system.
   C. *Breath-hold method:*
      An intravenous injection of 10 mL of gadolinium chelate is followed by fast-spoiled, gradient echo sequences acquired during breath-holding at 5, 10 and 15 minutes.
   D. The collecting system is evaluated according to a scale of 0 to 3.
4. **Postprocedure care:**
   A. See *Postprocedure care, Magnetic resonance imaging, Diagnostic.*
5. **Client and family teaching:**
   A. MRU is used to evaluate whether there are obstructions in the kidneys and ureters.
   B. See *Client and family teaching, Magnetic resonance imaging, Diagnostic.*
6. **Factors that affect results:**
   A. See *Factors that affect results, magnetic resonance imaging, Diagnostic.*
   B. Insufficient hydration will reduce the quality of the results.
7. **Other data:**
   A. MRU with contrast has been used to evaluate renal tumors and to evaluate the upper urinary tract in children.

MALARIA SMEAR, BLOOD

Norm. Negative.

Positive. Malaria (one of four *Plasmodium* species: P. *falciparum,* P. *vivax,* P. *malariae,* P. *ovale*) and trypanosomiasis.

Description. Malaria is a contact disease caused by a *Plasmodium.* The parasites, which are in the salivary glands of the anopheline mosquito, are introduced into the bloodstream of the human by means of mosquito bites. The parasites enter the cells of the liver, where they multiply without causing recognizable disease. A few days later, spores multiply asexually and fill red blood cells, destroying them and leading to fever and chills in the human. Malaria is most common in rural areas such as Central and South America, India, and Africa, but also exists in Eastern Europe. In the latter 1990's, over 1200 cases per year were reported in the United States and were attributed to acquisition of the disease when out of the country. Early detection via smear is essential so that treatment can be initiated and critical complications such as anemia, renal failure, pulmonary edema, disseminated intravascular coagulation, coma, and even death can be avoided. In this procedure, a thick and/or thin smear is collected. The thick smear only detects whether any of the *Plasmodium* species are present, whereas the thin smear is the only test that can pinpoint the specific *Plasmodium* species.

Professional Considerations
1. Consent form NOT required.
2. **Preparation:**
   A. Tube: Lavender topped.
   B. Obtain a lancet, 6 glass slides, Giemsa's stain, and methanol fixative.
   C. Monitor the client's temperature every 4 hours or as indicated.
   D. Report chills and fever to the physician.
   E. Obtaining specimens before fever spike is preferable.
   F. Include on the laboratory requisition any recent travel, including country and dates.
3. **Procedure:**
   A. Draw a 4-mL blood sample.
   B. Obtain fresh fingersticks (two or three each of thick and thin film on glass slides) stained with

Giemsa's stain. Both thick and thin smears may be collected on the same slide, if necessary. Fix thin smears with methanol.

4. **Postprocedure care:**
   A. None.
5. **Client and family teaching:**
   A. Inform the nurse when having chills.
6. **Factors that affect results:**
   A. Hemolysis of the specimen invalidates the results.
   B. The level of parasitemia varies from hour to hour (especially for *Plasmodium falciparum* infections).
7. **Other data:**
   A. Blood samples are usually drawn when fever and chills are present daily for 3 days at specified times, such as every 6 or 12 hours.
   B. The smear is considered positive if ≥2-30% of the red blood cells are infected.
   C. Blood should be examined several times a day for 2-3 days because results are seldom greater than 2% of the total cells.
   D. In *P. falciparum* malaria, severe parasitemia is 10% total infected cells and may reach levels of 20-30% or more.
   E. Clinical signs and symptoms may include myalgias, arthralgias, chills, fever of unknown origin, drenching sweat, fatigue, nausea, vomiting, abdominal pain, diarrhea, splenomegaly, hepatomegaly, and jaundice.
   F. American trypanosomiasis (Chagas' disease) and African trypanosomiasis (sleeping disease) are two diseases caused by trypanosomes, which are flagellated protozoans.
   G. A new nonradioactive DNA diagnostic procedure is available to detect malaria infection, which may aid in determining the diagnosis.

MAMMOGRAM
(see Mammography, Diagnostic)

MAMMOGRAPHY (MAMMOGRAM), DIAGNOSTIC

Norm. Radiographic image of normal breast tissue. Calcification, if present, is evenly distributed. Normal duct con-trast with gradual narrowing of branches of the ductal system is evident.

Positive. Benign or malignant masses in the breast tissue or nipple. Radiographic signs of breast cancer include asymmetric density; a poorly defined spiculated mass; fine, stippled clustered calcifications, which are seen as white specks on the x-ray film; and skin thickening. Malignant cancers are irregular and poorly defined and tend to be unilateral.

Negative. Normal finding.

Usage. Indicated to detect tumors that are clinically nonpalpable in women over 40 years of age as part of routine annual screening; to survey the opposite breast after mastectomy; to screen for breast cancer in clients at high risk (such as family history of breast cancer); to screen pendulous breasts, which are difficult to examine; to evaluate breasts when symptoms are present, such as skin changes, nipple or skin retraction, nipple discharge or erosion, breast pain, "lumpy" breast (such as multiple masses or nodules); to rule out breast cancer in a client with adenocarcinoma of undetermined site; to localize a mass before a biopsy is performed; to follow up after a previous breast biopsy; and to follow up after cancer treatment (such as surgery, radiation, chemotherapy) to determine its effectiveness. Used to diagnose benign breast masses, cysts, or abscesses; benign breast calcifications; breast cancer; fibrocystic breasts; intraductal papilloma of the breast; occult cancer (search in those with metastatic disease and unknown primary); suppurative mastitis; and Paget's disease of the breast.

Description. Mammography is a soft-tissue radiographic examination of the breast. Careful interpretation of these x-ray films can detect cancer, even before they become palpable lesions. The accuracy of breast cancer detection with mammography is approximately 85% and gives less than 10% false-positive diagnoses. It is believed that survival rates are improved with early detection of breast cancer. A "xeromammogram" provides the same information as a routine mammogram and has the same risks and benefits. However, xeromammograms are positive prints, unlike regular radiographs, which are negative prints. This

M

test has four views: oblique, lateral, craniocaudal, and chest wall. At least two views of each breast should be performed, one of which should be of the chest wall. Newer digital techniques are being developedthat are anticipated to improve diagnostic accuracy of mammography.

Professional Considerations
1. Consent form IS required.

Risks
The National Cancer Institute (United States) has estimated the risk of mammographically induced carcinogenesis to be 3.5 cancers per 1 million women per year per rad for Western women over 30 years of age at the time of exposure after a latent period of about 10 years.

Precautions
During pregnancy, risks of cumulative radiation exposure to the fetus from this and other previous or future imaging studies must be weighed against the benefits of the procedure. Although formal limits for client exposure are relative to this risk:benefit comparison, the United States Nuclear Regulatory Commission requires that the cumulative dose equivalent to an embryo/fetus from occupational exposure not exceed 0.5 rem (5 mSv). Radiation dosage to the fetus is proportional to the distance of the anatomy studied from the abdomen and decreases as pregnancy progresses. For pregnant clients, consult the Radiologist/Radiology Department to obtain estimated fetal radiation exposure from this procedure.

Contraindications
In clients who are pregnant because of the risk of fetal damage.

2. Preparation:
   A. Ask client to identify areas of lumps or thickening, if any.
   B. Ask the client if she is pregnant.
   C. Record client history of prior biopsies or breast surgeries or treatments.
   D. Be supportive. Allow time for questions and for verbalization of feelings.
   E. See *Client and family teaching*.
3. Procedure:
   A. The client is taken to the radiology department and stands or is

seated in front of the mammography machine.
   B. The breast(s) is (are) exposed, and one breast is placed on the x-ray plate.
   C. The x-ray cone is brought down on top of the breast to compress it gently between the broadened cone and the x-ray plate.
   D. The x-ray film is exposed. This creates the craniocaudal view.
   E. The x-ray plate is turned perpendicularly to the floor and then is placed laterally on the outer aspect of the breast.
   F. The broadened cone is brought in medially, and the breast is gently compressed. This is the lateral, or axillary, view.
   G. Occasionally a third view, the oblique view, is required. At least two views of each breast should be performed.
   H. This procedure is performed in 10-20 minutes by a radiologic technician.
   I. A hand-held scanner may be used by the radiologist to help detect early breast cancer that cannot be identified with conventional mammography.
4. Postprocedure care:
   A. Inform client that the radiographs must be interpreted by a radiologist.
   B. In the United States, the Mammography Quality Standards Act, phased in the 1990s, established standards for reporting of findings to the client within 5 days after the procedure if the findings may indicate malignancy and within 30 days after the procedure for findings not suggestive of malignancy.
5. Client and family teaching:
   A. The mammogram takes 10-20 minutes for both breasts to be x-rayed. Often the technologist or radiologist will palpate the breasts.
   B. Fasting is not required.
   C. Mammography is the single best method for detecting breast cancer in a curable stage.
   D. Some discomfort is experienced when the breast is compressed. Compression allows better visualization of the breast tissue. The breast will not be harmed in any

way, and discomfort is minimized if the test is scheduled during the week after your menstrual period ends.

E. Do not use any powder, deodorant, perfume, or ointments in the underarm area on the day of the test. Residue on the skin from these agents can obscure the visualization of the mammogram.

F. A minimal radiation dose will be used during the test.

G. Wear a blouse with a skirt or slacks, rather than a dress, since you will need to remove clothing from the upper half of the body.

H. If experiencing painful breasts, refrain from coffee, tea, cola, and chocolate 5-7 days before testing.

I. American Cancer Society mammography screening guidelines: screening mammogram by age 40; mammogram every 1 year if client is 40-49 years of age; mammogram annually at age 50 and older.

J. Call your doctor for results if you have not received a written or telephone test result within 10 days after the procedure.

K. Perform a monthly breast self-examination if 20 years of age or older and have a clinical breast examination by a health care provider at least every 3 years until age 40 and then every year. Breast self-examination should be performed after each menstrual period.

L. 80% of lumps found by a mammogram are benign.

6. Factors that affect results:

A. False-positive mammograms may result from calcifications of fibrocystic changes, calcification-like deposits in the skin secondary to tattoos, sebaceous gland secretions, and talcum powder. False-positive mammograms are more common in younger women.

B. False-negative results are possible. Up to 25% occur in women 40-49 years of age, and up to 10% occur in women 50-69 years of age.

C. Postoperative and postradiotherapy changes may be mistaken for carcinomas.

D. The principal cause of false-negative mammograms is dense parenchymal tissue because masses show up more clearly in fatty breasts.

E. Jewelry worn around the neck can preclude total visualization of the breast(s).

F. Breast-augmentation implants prevent total visualization of the breast(s).

7. Other data:

A. Magnification mammography is limited because of its higher radiation doses, but it can be useful in postoperative and postradiotherapy examinations, possibly preventing unnecessary biopsy.

B. Mammography immediately after stereotaxic breast biopsy is suboptimal for establishment of a new baseline view as a result of the frequent finding of hematoma.

C. According to one study, women undergoing mammography preferred to have their doctor call them with the result if the results were normal. If the results were abnormal, the subjects preferred to be told by their own physician in the office.

D. In one study (Lundstrom et al. 1999) an increase in mammographic density was much more common among women receiving continuous combination hormone replacement therapy.

MANTOUX SKIN TEST (PPD TEST, PURIFIED PROTEIN DERIVATIVE TEST, TB TEST, TUBERCULOSIS TEST), DIAGNOSTIC

Norm. Negative.

Positive. The appropriate criterion for defining a positive skin test reaction depends on the population being tested. For adults and children with HIV infection, close contacts of infectious cases, and those with fibrotic lesions on chest radiograph, a reaction of ≥5 mm is considered positive. For other at-risk adults and children, including infants and children younger than 4 years of age, a reaction of ≥10 mm is positive. Persons who are unlikely to be infected with *Mycobacterium tuberculosis* should generally not be skin tested. If a skin test is performed on a person without a defined risk factor for tuberculosis infection, ≥15 mm is positive.

M

Negative. Normal finding; lack of redness or induration of skin at site of skin test; zone of redness and induration <5 mm.

Usage. Screening is used to identify infected persons at high risk of disease who would benefit from preventive therapy and to find persons with clinical disease in need of treatment. As a screening tool, tuberculin skin testing is the standard method of identifying persons infected with M. tuberculosis. It is indicated for clients with signs suggestive of current tuberculosis (TB) disease (such as abnormality in mediastinum on radiograph) or symptoms (such as cough, hemoptysis, weight loss); recent contact with clients with confirmed or suspected cases of TB; clients with abnormal chest radiographs compatible with past TB; clients with medical conditions that increase the risk of TB (such as diabetes, immunosuppressive therapy, AIDS); groups at high risk for developing TB.

Description. An intradermal skin test to detect tuberculosis infection (active or dormant). Tuberculin, a protein fraction of tubercle bacilli, is injected intradermally in the human. A localized thickening with redness indicates an accumulation of small, sensitized lymphocytes, which occurs as a result of active or dormant tuberculosis. Clients at high risk for tuberculosis (HIV-infected persons, the very young and the very old, the malnourished, alcoholics, drug abusers, and the chronically ill) should be screened with the tuberculin skin test. Clients with human immunodeficiency virus infection are at increased risk for developing tuberculosis infection and should be screened with the tuberculin skin test. Other clients at high risk for becoming infected with Mycobacterium tuberculosis include the very young and the very old, those who are malnourished, alcohol and drug abusers, and the chronically ill.

Professional Considerations
1. Consent form IS required.

Risks
It is not known whether the test can cause fetal harm or affect reproductive capacity.

Contraindications
The test should be given to pregnant women only if clearly indicated. The test should not be given if the client has had a previous positive test.

2. **Preparation:**
   A. Assess for previous history of positive purified protein derivative (PPD) reaction. (The test should not be administered in this case.)
   B. Obtain a tuberculin syringe and PPD.
   C. Draw up PPD in a tuberculin syringe, following the manufacturer's directions. Use a ½-inch 26- or 27-gauge needle.

3. **Procedure:**
   A. Cleanse the injection site on the lower dorsal surface of the forearm with alcohol, and allow the area to dry.
   B. Stretch the skin taut.
   C. Inject intradermally 0.1 mL of a solution containing 0.5 tuberculin units of PPD. Injection should be made with a disposable needle and syringe just under the surface of the skin, with the needle bevel facing upward to provide a discrete, pale elevation of the skin (a wheal) 6 to 10 mm in diameter. Discard used needles and syringes in a puncture-resistant container (do not recap needles).

4. **Postprocedure care:**
   A. Mark the test area to locate it for reading.
   B. Read the test area 48-72 hours later. Examine the site, using good light. Inspect the skin for induration. Induration ≥5 mm diameter generally indicates infection. Rub lightly from the area of normal skin to the indurated area. Circle the induration with a pencil.
   C. An induration of >5 mm diameter should be interpreted as a positive reaction if the client has known contact with an individual with active tuberculosis or if there is a chest radiograph with findings consistent with tuberculosis. Isoniazid therapy is recommended to decrease the risk of developing the disease in positive reactors.
   D. A chest radiograph is necessary with all positive reactions.

E. Epinephrine hydrochloride solution (1:1000) should be readily available for use in the event of anaphylaxis.

5. **Client and family teaching:**
   A. The skin test does not distinguish between current disease and past infection.
   B. The skin test should not be administered to known tuberculin-positive reactors because of the possibility of severe reactions (vesiculation, ulceration, and necrosis).

6. **Factors that affect results:**
   A. Tuberculin must be stored as recommended by the manufacturer. Tuberculin solution should be stored between 2° and 8° C (35°-46° F). It should be exposed to light only when being withdrawn and administered. An open vial may be used only for 1 month.
   B. Subcutaneous rather than intradermal injection will nullify the test.
   C. Cross-reactions with nontuberculous mycobacteria may cause false-positive results.
   D. Serial testing may cause false-positive results.
   E. Vaccination with the *bacille* Calmette-Guérin (BCG) has a variable effect on the skin test reaction. However, a history of BCG vaccination should not alter interpretation of the skin test.
   F. False-negative reactions may occur in the following instances: bacterial infections, immunologic defects, immunosuppressive agents, live virus vaccinations (BCG, measles, mumps, polio, and rubella), malnutrition, old age, overwhelming tuberculosis, renal failure, and viral infections (chickenpox, measles, and mumps).
   G. False-negative results can occur, even in the presence of active TB, whenever sensitized T lymphocytes are temporarily depleted in the body.

7. **Other data:**
   A. None.

MAP-KINASE, SPECIMEN
(see Mitogen-activated protein kinase, Specimen)

MAPK, SPECIMEN
(see Mitogen-activated protein kinase, Specimen)

MAPROTILINE
(see Tricyclic antidepressants, Plasma or Serum)

MARIJUANA, BLOOD OR URINE
(see Cannabinoids, Qualitative, Blood or Urine)

MAXIMUM BACTERICIDAL DILUTION
(see Schlichter test)

MBD
(see Schlichter test)

MCA
(see Mucin-like carcinoma-associated antigen, Blood)

MCH, BLOOD
(see Blood indices, Blood)

MCHC, BLOOD
(see Blood indices, Blood)

MCV, BLOOD
(see Blood indices, Blood)

MEAN CORPUSCULAR HEMOGLOBIN, BLOOD
(see Blood indices, Blood)

MEAN CORPUSCULAR HEMOGLOBIN CONCENTRATION, BLOOD
(see Blood indices, Blood)

MEAN CORPUSCULAR VOLUME, BLOOD
(see Blood indices, Blood)

M

MEAN PLATELET VOLUME (MPV), BLOOD

Norm:

Preterm infants	7.5-9.5 fL
Term infants (0-1 month)	7.6-9.9 fL
1 month-48 months	6.3-8.9 fL
48 months-adult	7.0-9.0 fL

Usage. Evaluates platelet abnormalities; improves detection of platelet-related diseases when the platelet count is normal; determines the platelet changes associated with exercise and hyperthyroidism; predicts hypertensive crisis in pregnancy; predicts the presence of sepsis in neonates; and predicts hemorrhage in clients with rheumatoid arthritis, who are experiencing thrombocytopenia as a side effect of parental gold therapy. In screening clients with preexisting coronary artery disease, MPV over 11.6 fL was associated with an increased risk of subsequent myocardial infarction.

Increased. Acute poststreptococcal glomerulonephritis (APSGN), arterial disease (angina, atherosclerotic disease), coagulase-negative staphylococcal sepsis in neonates, cyanotic congenital heart disease, diabetes, hyperthyroidism, iron-deficiency anemia, ITP (idiopathic thrombocytopenic purpura), myeloproliferative disorders, myocardial infarction, pregnant women with preeclampsia, renal failure, rheumatic heart disease, smokers, splenomegaly, states of increased platelet production, and thrombocytopenia.

Decreased. Active inflammatory bowel disease, and in clients with rheumatoid arthritis who are receiving parental gold therapy.

Description. The MPV is an automated measurement of the average volume of platelets. It is the arithmetic mean volume of the platelet population derived from the platelet histogram on automated Coulter counters. Increased MPV may reflect either increased platelet activation or increased numbers of large, hyperaggregable platelets. Because the MPV increases during conditions of rapid platelet turnover, it can signify the release of larger, younger

platelets into the circulation. When the MPV is low, the platelets are generally smaller. The MPV is expressed in femtoliters (fL).

Professional Considerations
1. Consent form NOT required.
2. Preparation:
   A. Tube: Lavender topped.
3. Procedure:
   A. Leaving a tourniquet in place less than 1 minute, draw a 5-mL blood sample.
   B. Gently invert the tube two or three times.
4. Postprocedure care:
   A. Send the specimen to the laboratory within 1 hour.
5. Client and family teaching:
   A. Results are normally available within 4 hours.
6. Factors that affect results:
   A. When potassium EDTA is used as an anticoagulant, platelets demonstrate a progressive increase in mean platelet volume with storage, as measured by the Coulter counter. This increase is most noticeable within the first 2 hours but continues at a slower rate subsequently.
7. Other data:
   A. The mean platelet volume (MPV) is comparable to the mean corpuscular volume (MCV) of red blood cells.
   B. Younger platelets are larger than older platelets. Larger platelets are functionally and metabolically more active than smaller ones, contain more granules, and express more enzymatic activity in vitro.
   C. Increases in MPV can occur, even though thrombocytopenia has developed.
   D. The mean MPV may be normal in central thrombocytopenic diseases, such as aplastic anemia and acute leukemia.

MEAT FIBERS, STOOL

Norm. Negative.

Positive. Gastroenteritis, intestinal lymphoma, malabsorption syndrome, pancreatic insufficiency, severe ulcerative colitis, surgical removal of section of intestine, and Whipple's disease.

Description. Examination of stool for yield of meat fibers correlates with the amount of fat secretion in the stool. Meat fibers found in stool result from multiple abnormalities in absorption of nutrients. These include defects in the intestinal lumen that result in inadequate fat hydrolysis, inadequate proteolysis, altered bile salt metabolism, and defects in mucosal epithelial cells or intestinal lymphatics that affect absorbing surfaces and interfere with the transport of nutrients.

Professional Considerations
1. Consent form NOT required.
2. Preparation:
   A. Barium procedures or laxatives should be avoided for 1 week before specimen collection.
   B. Obtain an enema apparatus and warm saline, or a prepackaged enema, and a sterile plastic specimen container
   C. See *Client and family teaching.*
3. Procedure:
   A. Obtain a stool specimen by giving the client a warm saline enema or a prepackaged enema.
   B. Collect the stool specimen in a sterile plastic container.
4. Postprocedure care:
   A. None.
5. Client and family teaching:
   A. Include at least 3 ounces of red meat per day for 24-72 hours before the test.
   B. Results are normally available after 24 hours.
6. Factors that affect results:
   A. Reject specimens collected with enemas other than saline or Fleets (such as mineral oil, bismuth, or magnesium compounds).
7. Other data:
   A. Serum protein level should be determined because hypoproteinemia is the major clinical feature of protein-losing enteropathy.
   B. Biopsy of the intestinal mucosa is more useful than other diagnostic tests for definitive diagnosis of intestinal mucosal abnormalities.

MECKEL SCAN, DIAGNOSTIC

Norm. Negative; no increased uptake of radionuclide in the right lower quadrant of the abdomen.

Usage. Detection of Meckel's diverticulum, which contains ectopic gastric mucosa, in clients with abdominal pain or occult gastrointestinal bleeding.

Description. A nuclear medicine scan in which a radioisotope, ^{99m}Tc (technetium)-pertechnetate is injected intravenously. The radioisotope is concentrated in the normal gastric mucosa within the stomach and in the ectopic gastric mucosa in the Meckel's diverticulum. This is a very sensitive and specific test for this congenital abnormality.

Professional Considerations
1. Consent form IS required.

Risks
Hematoma, infection.

Contraindications
During pregnancy or breast-feeding.

2. Preparation:
   A. Assure the client that nuclear medicine personnel will remain within hearing range and will be able to see the client throughout the study.
   B. A histamine (H_2)-receptor antagonist (such as cimetidine orally every 6 hours for 24 hours) is usually administered for 1-2 days before the test. This drug inhibits acid secretion and allows for improved visualization of the Meckel's diverticulum.
   C. See *Client and family teaching.*
3. Procedure:
   A. In the nuclear medicine department, the client lies in a supine position.
   B. ^{99m}Tc-pertechnetate is administered intravenously 15 minutes before imaging.
   C. An anterior body-image view is obtained with a rectilinear scanner or scintillation (gamma) camera. Images are taken at 5-minute intervals for 1 hour.
   D. During the scan, the client may be asked to lie on the left side to increase the amount of radioisotope to the intestines.
   E. Total examining time is 60 minutes.
4. Postprocedure care:
   A. Observe the client carefully for up to 60 minutes after the study

M

for a possible (anaphylactic) reaction to the radionuclide.

B. Ask the client to void after the procedure, and a repeat image may be obtained.

C. Rubber gloves should be worn for 24 hours after the procedure when urine is being discarded. Wash the gloved hands with soap and water before removing the gloves. Wash the ungloved hands after the gloves are removed.

5. Client and family teaching:
A. It is necessary to lie still for 60 minutes for this scan. There is no pain associated with this test.
B. Refrain from eating or drinking anything for 6-12 hours before the test.
C. Void before the study to increase the visibility of the intestines.
D. Meticulously wash your hands with soap and water after each void for 24 hours after the procedure.
E. Family members must wear rubber gloves for 24 hours after the procedure when discarding the client's urine if the family will be providing this care.

6. Factors that affect results:
A. A positive scan is dependent on an adequate amount of gastric mucosa within Meckel's diverticulum. Only 25% of clients with Meckel's diverticulum will have sufficient ectopic gastric mucosa to produce a positive scan.
B. Meckel scan is unreliable for evaluation of gastrointestinal bleeding.
C. Other radionuclide studies performed within the previous 24 hours will interfere with this test.
D. A waiting period that is either too short or too long after the radionuclide injection will alter the results.
E. Premedication with pentagastrin and histamine (H_2)-receptor blocker (Zantac) may increase the sensitivity of the test.
F. Barium in the small or large bowel may mask the radionuclide concentration.

7. Other data:
A. Health care professionals working in a nuclear medicine area must follow federal standards set by the Nuclear Regulatory Commission. These standards include precautions for handling the radioactive material and monitoring of potential radiation exposure.
B. The half-life of technetium is 6 hours.

MEDIASTINOSCOPY, DIAGNOSTIC

Norm. Normal mediastinal structure and lymph nodes; no evidence of disease process.

Usage. To detect lymphoma (such as Hodgkin's disease), lung metastasis to mediastinal lymph nodes, granulomatous infection, mediastinal tuberculosis, sarcoidosis; to obtain biopsy specimen of mediastinal lymph nodes or intrathoracic lesions; to determine staging of bronchogenic carcinoma; and to evaluate tumor spread or intrathoracic diseases. Used when fine-needle aspiration biopsy of the thoracic structures has not yielded a diagnosis.

Description. Mediastinoscopy is a surgical endoscopic procedure that is performed with the client under general anesthesia. A small incision is made at the suprasternal notch, and a mediastinoscope is inserted into the mediastinum. The purpose of this procedure is to visualize the mediastinal structure and lymph nodes and to obtain biopsy sample of lymph nodes or other lesions. The lymph nodes in the mediastinum receive lymphatic drainage from the lungs. A mediastinoscopy is usually performed when radiographs, sputum cytologic evaluation, and lung scans (CT and nuclear) have not confirmed a diagnosis. Mediastinoscopy is an invasive procedure and is performed with the client under general anesthesia because of the pain and coughing that result from the manipulation of the trachea.

Professional Considerations
1. Consent form IS required.

Risks
Perforation of the trachea, esophagus, aorta, or other blood vessels; pneumothorax; laryngeal nerve damage; and infection.

Contraindications

Previous mediastinoscopy (caused by adhesions); clients who are not candidates for general anesthesia.

2. **Preparation:**
   A. See *Client and family teaching.*
   B. Complete preoperative checklist, and perform routine preoperative care, which is the same as with any other surgical procedure. Check if the client's blood needs to be typed and cross-matched.
   C. Measure and record baseline vital signs.
   D. Ask the client if he or she is allergic to any anesthetic medicine.
   E. Encourage the client and family members to express concerns about the procedure. Answer questions and refer those that you cannot answer to appropriate health care professionals.
   F. Administer preprocedural medication approximately 1 hour before the test, as prescribed.

3. **Procedure:**
   A. The client is transported to an operating room.
   B. General anesthesia is administered.
   C. A small incision is made in the suprasternal fossa.
   D. A mediastinoscope is passed through this neck incision, along the anterior course of the trachea, and into the superior mediastinum.
   E. The area is visualized. Photographs of specific areas and structures may be taken. Biopsies of the lymph nodes may also be performed.
   F. The mediastinoscope is withdrawn, and the incision is sutured closed.

4. **Postprocedure care:**
   A. Assess vital signs every 15 minutes × 2, then every 30 minutes × 2, then hourly × 4, and then every 4 hours until 24 hours after the procedure. Report changes in vital signs (such as increase in pulse rate or respiratory rate, decrease in blood pressure).
   B. Auscultate lung sounds, and assess for any respiratory abnormalities, such as dyspnea.
   C. Check for bright red blood or increased blood on the dressing. Observe the wound for symptoms of infection.
   D. Provide comfort measures as needed (such as position change, medication).
   E. Send biopsy specimens to the pathology laboratory immediately.

5. **Client and family teaching:**
   A. Refrain from eating or drinking for 8-12 hours before the procedure.
   B. Void before the surgical procedure.
   C. This procedure will take approximately 1 hour and is performed by a surgeon.
   D. You will be asleep during the procedure.

6. **Factors that affect results:**
   A. Phenytoin hypersensitivity may result in a "pseudolymphoma," causing false-positive cytologic results.

7. **Other data:**
   A. Thoracotomy is advisable in the instance of negative cytologic characteristics in lesions likely to be malignant.

MELANIN, URINE

Norm. Negative.

Positive. Malignant melanoma.

Description. Urine test to detect biochemical markers of melanoma progression. Melanin, which is the main pigment in the body, is synthesized by the melanocyte primarily in the skin and eyes. It is highly elevated in malignant melanoma. Both eumelanin (brown-black pigment) and pheomelanin (yellow-red pigment) are produced, with dihyroxyindole (DHI) and cysteinyl-dopa (CD) being the major precursors. Melanin metabolites are often released in the urine of clients with disseminated melanoma metastasis (melanuria). These metabolites include a pheomelanin metabolite, 5-S-CD, and a eumelanin metabolite, 6-hydroxy-5-methoxyindole-2-carboxylic acid (6H5MI2C). Melanogen, a colorless precursor of melanin, is also excreted in the urine of 25% of people with melanin-producing tumors.

Professional Considerations
1. Consent form NOT required.
2. Preparation:
   A. Obtain a sterile, plastic specimen container.
3. Procedure:
   A. Obtain a freshly voided urine specimen in a sterile, plastic container.
4. Postprocedure care:
   A. None.
5. Client and family teaching:
   A. Results are normally available within 24 hours.
6. Factors that affect results:
   A. Drugs that may cause false-positive results include salicylates.
7. Other data:
   A. The test is more frequently positive in people with hepatic metastasis.
   B. Urine exposed to room temperature for 24 hours will turn dark brown and later black as the melanogens oxidize to melanin.
   C. Plasma 6H5MI2C levels are usually high (>1.75 ng/mL) in clients with metastatic malignant melanoma, and it produces a more sensitive and reliable test than the melanin (5-S-CD) urine test.
   D. Elevated urine melanin in test results is a high-risk factor for metastatic malignant melanoma.

MELANOCYTE-STIMULATING HORMONE (MSH), URINE

Norm. Negative for melanin.

Positive. Addison's disease, hyperpituitarism, melanoma, and liver metastasis.

Description. Melanocyte-stimulating hormone (MSH) is part of the melanocortin system, which helps regulate the body's balance of energy via the hypothalamus. It is a hormone secreted by the anterior lobe of the pituitary gland that works in conjunction with leptin, leptin receptors, and neuropeptide Y to help control obesity. MSH secretion is closely linked to ACTH secretion, and experimental studies demonstrate body fact reduction after

treatment with exogenous MSH/ACTH. MSH also increases the amount of body melanin, the skin-darkening pigment that helps provide skin protection from damaging ultraviolet rays.

Professional Considerations
1. Consent form NOT required.
2. Preparation:
   A. Obtain a sterile, plastic specimen container.
3. Procedure:
   A. Obtain a freshly voided urine specimen in a sterile, plastic container.
4. Postprocedure care:
   A. None.
5. Client and family teaching:
   A. Results are normally available after 24 hours.
6. Factors that affect results:
   A. The secretion of MSH is increased when levels of circulating cortisol are low.
7. Other data:
   A. None.

MENDELIAN INHERITANCE IN GENETIC DISORDERS, DIAGNOSTIC

Norm. Negative for genetic disorders.

Usage. Used prospectively for genetic counseling to predict the probability that a future offspring will inherit a genetic disorder; used retrospectively to determine or confirm the presence of a mendelian disease.

Description. This procedure is an analysis of gene sequences on a person's DNA and RNA to detect the presence of genetic disorders in the family history or in a client himself. More than 4,000 mendelian diseases obey statistical laws and exist in a family. Examples are breast cancer, colon cancer, color blindness, congenital malformations, cystic fibrosis, hemophilia, Marfan syndrome, and sickle cell anemia. As genetic techniques improve, mendelian testing is becoming more commonly used for population-based screening, such as in screening newborns for phenylketonuria and other disorders. Screening carries with it legal and ethical dilemmas concerning confidentiality, privacy, discrimination, and interventions taken based on findings.

Professional Considerations
1. Consent form NOT required.
2. **Preparation:**
   A. Provide teaching.
3. **Procedure:**
   A. A family pedigree analysis is performed, including generational continuity of the disorder, sex relationship, and segregation (mendelian) ratio.
4. **Postprocedure care:**
   A. Genetic counseling and referral for follow-up study.
5. **Client and family teaching:**
   A. Inform the client about the reasons for genetic counseling.
6. **Factors that affect results:**
   A. Gene-mapping is most accurate in identifying simple genetic dis-orders, such as those caused by a single abnormal gene. Newer techniques are being developed to help identify genetic causes of more complicated diseases.
7. **Other data:**
   A. Other disorders can mimic mendelian disorders, such as chromosomal disorders, congenital infections, and mental retardation.
   B. The Online Mendelian Inheritance in Man (OMIM) databases, available via the worldwide web provide up-to-date information on gene mutation findings.

MEPHENYTOIN (MESANTOIN), BLOOD

Norm. Negative.

		SI UNITS
Mephenytoin Therapy		
Therapeutic level of mephenytoin	1-5 µg/mL or mg/L	4.6-23 µmol/L
Therapeutic level of mephenytoin and parent drug 5-phenyl-5-ethylhydantoin metabolite	25-40 µg/mL or mg/L	115-184 µmol/L
Panic level	>20 µg/mL or mg/L	>92 µmol/L
Normephenytoin	15-35 µg/mL or mg/L	69-161 µmol/L
Panic level	>50 µg/mL or mg/L	>230 µmol/L

Overdose Symptoms and Treatment

Symptoms. Ataxia, blood dyscrasias, coma, drowsiness, dysarthria, hypotension, nystagmus, and unresponsive pupils may be seen.

Treatment:
There is no specific treatment. Refer to a physician. Give general supportive care: lavage and maintenance of airway and blood pressure. Hemodialysis WILL remove mephenytoin and is utilized, especially with drug toxicity in children.

Increased. Overdose. Drugs include chloramphenicol and methsuximide.

Decreased. Convulsions, inadequate dosage, and noncompliance with therapeutic regimen.

Description. Mephenytoin (Mesantoin) is an anticonvulsant used to treat grand mal, tonic-clonic, psychomotor, temporal lobe, focal, and jacksonian seizures. It is metabolized in the liver and excreted in the urine.

Professional Considerations
1. Consent form NOT required.
2. **Preparation:**
   A. Tube: Red topped, red/gray topped, or gold topped.
   B. Do NOT draw during hemodialysis.
3. **Procedure:**
   A. Draw a 5-mL blood sample.
4. **Postprocedure care:**
   A. None.

5. **Client and family teaching:**
   A. Explain overdose symptoms and treatment (see above) as appropriate.
   B. Drug levels should be monitored routinely during therapy.

C. Refer clients with intentional overdose for crisis intervention.
6. **Factors that affect results:**
   A. Compliance with administration.
7. **Other data:**
   A. Trade name is Mesantoin.

MEPROBAMATE, BLOOD

Norm. Negative.

	SI UNITS
Meprobamate Therapy	
Therapeutic level	5-20 μg/mL or mg/L	23-92 μmol/L
Toxic level	>35 μg/mL or mg/L	>160 μmol/L
Panic level	>50 μg/mL or mg/L	>229 μmol/L
Lethal level	>200 μg/mL or mg/L	>916 μmol/L

Death has been reported with as little as 12 g, and survival with as much as 40 g.

Overdose Symptoms and Treatment

Symptoms. Drowsiness, lethargy, stupor, ataxia, hemolytic toxicity symptoms (fever, sore throat, bruising, bleeding), coma, shock, vasomotor and respiratory collapse, and death may occur.

Treatment:

Note: Treatment choice(s) depend on client history and condition and episode history.
Administer gastric lavage and supportive therapy as needed.
Both hemodialysis and peritoneal dialysis WILL remove meprobamate.
Osmotic diuresis with mannitol has also been effective.
Avoid dehydration.

Increased. Drug abuse and overdose.

Decreased. Noncompliance with therapeutic regimen.

Description. Meprobamate is a sedative-hypnotic used to treat anxiety disorders. A central nervous system depressant, metabolized in the liver, excreted in urine and feces. Meprobamate is a metabolite of carisoprodol (Soma), a muscle relaxant that some consider a suspect drug of abuse.

Professional Considerations
1. Consent form NOT required.
2. **Preparation:**
   A. Tube: Red topped, red/gray topped, or gold topped.
   B. Do NOT draw during hemodialysis.
3. **Procedure:**
   A. Draw 5-mL blood sample.
4. **Postprocedure care:**
   A. None.
5. **Client and family teaching:**
   A. Explain overdose symptoms and treatment (see above) as appropriate.
   B. For intentional overdose, refer for crisis intervention and counseling. Referrals to appropriate rehabilitation centers and therapeutic community programs should be offered to all clients who may be interested.
6. **Factors that affect results:**
   A. Onset of action is within 1 hour after oral dosage. Peak concentration is 2 hours from dosage, half-life is 6-17 hours, steady-state levels occur in 1.5-4.0 days.
7. **Other data:**
   A. An alternative method of determining meprobamate levels is by gas chromatography. This method is accurate and precise and is particularly suitable for toxicology studies.

MERCURY, BLOOD AND URINE

Norm:

		SI UNITS
Blood	<0.06 µg/mL or ≤60 ng/mL	≤0.3 nmol/L
Critical value	>0.6 µg/mL	>3 nmol/L
Panic value	>100 µg/mL	>500 nmol/L
Urine	≤10 µg/24 hours	≤0.05 µmol/day
Panic value	>50 µg/24 hours	>0.25 µmol/day

Panic Level Symptoms and Treatment

Symptoms. Symptoms appear when levels reach 600 µg/L (3 µmol/L, SI units) Signs of chronic poisoning include difficulty concentrating, short-term memory loss, irritability, fatigue, ataxia, muscle spasms, gingivitis, tremors, joint pain, and paresthesias.

Treatment:
Note: Treatment choice(s) depend on client history and condition and episode history.
Chelation with penicillamine. Monitor behavior and neurologic status closely.

Increased. Mercury poisoning.

Description. Mercury is the only metal that is liquid at ordinary temperatures. Mercury is primarily absorbed by inhalation but can also be absorbed through the skin and gastrointestinal tract. It is then distributed to the central nervous system and kidneys and excreted in the urine, having a half-life of up to 25 days. Mercury may exist in the body in three forms, elemental, inorganic, and organic. The more common sources of mercury poisoning are industrial inhalation of mercury vapors from paints and other materials and direct contact with mercury from broken thermometers or from dental fillings. This test is used to evaluate for mercury toxicity. Blood testing is best to evaluate methylmercury levels, and urine testing is best for evaluating inorganic mercury levels.

Professional Considerations
1. Consent form NOT required.

2. **Preparation:**
   A. For blood sample: Tube: Lavender topped, EDTA-tube.
   B. For urine specimen: Obtain a 3-L, acid-washed plastic specimen container without preservative.
   C. Assess the possible causes of mercury poisoning: occupational activities, hobbies (such as painting ceramics), target shooting, home renovation, and auto repair.
   D. Screen client for use of herbal preparations or "natural" remedies.
3. **Procedure:**
   A. *Blood:* Draw a 3-mL blood sample.
   B. *Urine:* Collect all the urine voided in a 24-hour period in a 3-L, acid-washed plastic container without preservative.
4. **Postprocedure care:**
   A. For increased levels, encourage fluids and monitor urine output because mercury is nephrotoxic.
5. **Client and family teaching:**
   A. *Urine:* Save all the urine voided in the 24-hour period and urinate before defecating to avoid loss of urine. If any urine is accidentally discarded, discard the entire specimen and restart the collection the next day.
   B. Some Chinese herbal medicines and remedies contain high levels of mercury. Do not use these preparations without first consulting your physician.
6. **Factors that affect results:**
   A. Drugs that may cause falsely low levels include iodine-containing medications.
7. **Other data:**
   A. Blood is the recommended specimen for measuring organic mercury.

M

B. Urine is the recommended specimen for measuring inorganic mercury and mercury secondary to dental amalgam fillings Hair is the recommended specimen for measurement of mercury levels secondary to seafood consumption. Saliva is not recommended as a substrate for mercury testing.

C. One study found high mercury levels to be associated with both male and female infertility and high seafood consumption by infertile clients with elevated blood mercury levels.

MESANTOIN, BLOOD
(see Mephenytoin, Blood)

METANEPHRINES, TOTAL, 24-HOUR URINE AND FREE, PLASMA

Norm:

PLASMA FREE METANEPHRINES	NORMAL	DIAGNOSTIC FOR PHEOCHROMOCYTOMA
Normetanephrine	<0.90 nmol/L	>1.5 pmol/L
Metanephrine	<0.50 nmol/L	>1.4 pmol/L

Diagnostic for Pheochromocytoma: (more than 4 and 2.5-fold above the upper reference limits) indicate a pheochromocytoma with 100% specificity.
Metanephrine >220 pg/mL

URINE METANEPHRINES	NORMAL	SI UNITS
Adults	<1.3 mg/24 hours	<5 μmol/day
	0.05-1.20 μg/mg of creatinine[2]	0.03-0.69 mmol/mol creatinine
Children		
<12 months	0.001-4.60 μg/mg of creatinine[2]	0.0006-2.64 mmol/mol creatinine
12-24 months	0.24-5.38 μg/mg of creatinine[2]	0.15-3.09 mmol/mol creatinine
24 months-5 years	0.35-2.99 μg/mg of creatinine[2]	0.21-1.72 mmol/mol creatinine
5-10 years	0.43-2.70 μg/mg of creatinine[2]	0.25-1.55 mmol/mol creatinine
10-15 years	0.001-1.87 μg/mg of creatinine[2]	0.0006-1.07 mmol/mol creatinine
15-18 years	0.001-0.67 μg/mg of creatinine[2]	0.0006-0.38 mmol/mol creatinine

Increased. Adrenal mass, brain tumors, chemodectomas, ganglioneuroblastoma, ganglioneuroma, hypertension with pheochromocytoma, malignant pheochromocytoma, metastasis (widespread), myasthenia gravis, neuroblastoma, pheochromocytoma, progressive muscular dystrophy, sepsis, and severe stress.

Description. This is a test to evaluate adrenomedullary function. Metanephrine testing is usually performed when a client with hypertension is suspected of having pheochromocytoma, which is a tumor of the chromaffin cells of the adrenal medulla. (Fewer than 1% of clients with hypertension have pheochromocytoma.) Metanephrines (such as normetanephrine and metanephrine) are one of the principle substances formed by the adrenal medulla, released into the bloodstream, and excreted into the urine. These substances contain a catechol nucleus and an amine group; therefore they are referred to as catecholamines.

The traditional method for testing has been a 24-hour urine test (sensitivity 89%-100%) because blood testing had too many interfering factors. The newest techniques for plasma testing provide an almost 100% sensitivity and specificity. Plasma metanephrine testing also provides the advantages of lower susceptibility to changing catecholamine levels due to posture changes, exercise or surgical stress, closer correlation with tumor size, less interference by medications, and insight into ongoing (long-term) production of catecholamines. Metanephrine testing is the best test for the diagnosis of pheochromocytoma because levels are unaffected by the many factors that affect catecholamine levels.

Professional Considerations

1. Consent form NOT required.
2. **Preparation:**
   A. *Plasma:* Obtain a lavender-topped tube and ice.
   B. *Urine:* Obtain a 3-L, plastic container with 20-25 mL of hydrochloric acid (HCl) preservative. Label the container with the client's name, the test, and the date.
   C. Discuss with the physician if any drugs are to be discontinued 3-7 days before the testing.
   D. See *Client and family teaching.*
3. **Procedure:**
   A. *Plasma test:* Obtain a 7-ml blood sample. Place specimen immediately on ice.
   B. *Urine:* Collect all the urine voided in a 24-hour period in a refrigerated, 3-L, plastic container to which 20-25 mL of HCl preservative has been added. For specimens collected from an indwelling urinary catheter, keep the drainage bag on ice, and empty urine into the refrigerated collection container hourly. Document urinary output throughout the collection period.
4. **Postprocedure care:**
   A. Write the beginning and ending times of collection and total urinary output (container quantity should match output record) on the laboratory requisition and on the specimen container.
   B. Send the urine specimen to the laboratory refrigerator after the 24-hour collection is completed. Metanephrines are stable for at least 1 week.

5. **Client and family teaching:**
   A. Save all the urine voided in the 24-hour period and urinate before defecating to avoid loss of urine. If any urine is accidentally discarded, discard the entire specimen and restart the collection the next day.
   B. Avoid caffeine, coffee, tea, cocoa products, bananas, vanilla products, aspirin, and phenothiazine-containing medications for 48 hours before collecting urine and during the urine collection.
   C. Encourage the client to rest, take in adequate food and fluids, and avoid stress during the test.
6. **Factors that affect results:**
   A. Drugs that may cause false-positive results include chlorpromazine, dopamine, guanethidine, hydralazine, hydrocortisone, imipramine, isoetharine, levodopa, monoamine oxidase (MAO) inhibitors, nalidixic acid, phenacetin, phenobarbital, phenylephrine, and tetracycline.
   B. Drugs that may cause false-negative results include clonidine, guanethidine, propranolol, reserpine, and theophylline.
   C. Dietary intake high in bananas may cause falsely increased results.
   D. Vigorous exercise may cause an increase in catecholamine levels.
   E. The 24-hour urine collection is problematic for practical reasons and for client compliance.
7. **Other data:**
   A. Urinary catecholamines and vanillylmandelic acid (VMA) are often measured with urine metanephrines.
   B. If a positive plasma result is followed by a negative result in repeat testing, pheochromocytoma can be ruled out. This is because metanephrines are continuously secreted by the tumor.

METHACHOLINE CHALLENGE TEST (BRONCHIAL CHALLENGE TEST), DIAGNOSTIC

Norm. Negative.

Usage. Diagnosis of asthma when the diagnosis cannot be made with

M

certainty from the history, physical examination, and conventional pulmonary function tests.

Description. The methacholine challenge test involves measurement of lung volumes before and after inhalation of methacholine chloride, a bronchial constrictor. This test is useful in demonstrating bronchial hyperreactivity (BHR), which is a defining characteristic of asthma. Clients with symptoms suggestive of asthma often have normal resting pulmonary function test results but are more sensitive to the bronchoconstrictive effects of methacholine than healthy people are.

Professional Considerations
1. Consent form NOT required.
2. Preparation:
   A. Obtain nebulizer and methacholine chloride.
3. Procedure:
   A. The client performs a forced vital capacity (FVC) test, and the forced expiratory volume (FEV) is measured.
   B. The client then inhales 3.12 mg of methacholine chloride from a nebulizer, waits 5 minutes, and performs the FVC and FEV test. A 20% reduction in the FEV is a positive response.
   C. If there is no response, the test is repeated with use of 6.25, 12.5, and 25 mg of methacholine,

respectively. Failure to achieve a 20% reduction in the FEV is considered a negative test.
4. Postprocedure care:
   A. Monitor respiratory status.
5. Client and family teaching:
   A. Symptoms suggestive of asthma include cough, chest tightness, and dyspnea.
6. Factors that affect results:
   A. Inability to follow directions and comply with instructions yields invalid results.
   B. Inhaled heparin may have an inhibitory role on methacholine bronchial challenge, possibly through a direct effect on smooth muscle.
7. Other data:
   A. This test has a positive predictive value of 60-88% and a negative predictive value of 100% to rule out asthma.
   B. Some experimental work is being done to evaluate the usefulness of a skin-prick test with methacholine in shortening the MCT. One study found that a negative skin-prick test reduced the chances of low-to-moderate risk clients having asthma by 10-20 fold.

METHANOL, BLOOD
(*see Toxicology, Volatiles group by GLC, Blood or Urine*)

METHAQUALONE, BLOOD

Norm. Negative.

		SI UNITS
Therapeutic level	2-3 µg/mL	8-12 µmol/L
Panic level	>8 µg/mL	>32 µmol/L
Toxic level	>10 µg/mL	>40 µmol/L

Panic Level Symptoms and Treatment

Symptoms. Pronounced drowsiness, confusion, dilated pupils, delirium, coma, restlessness, hyperexcitability, hypertonia, convulsions, shock, and cardiopulmonary failure may occur. Spontaneous vomiting with increased secretions may cause aspiration pneumonia or respiratory obstruction. Swelling, fluid retention, and abnormal bleeding may also occur. Death may occur from doses >5 g (20 mmol).

Treatment:

Note: Treatment choice(s) depend on client history and condition and episode history.
Maintain patent airway.
Support blood pressure.

Perform gastric lavage and evaluation of gastric contents by lavage after airway has been ensured.
Monitor neurologic, cardiac, and respiratory status closely.
Be prepared to mechanically ventilate and to treat bradycardia or cardiac arrest.
Analeptics are contraindicated.
Hemodialysis and peritoneal dialysis will NOT remove methaqualone. Hemoperfusion WILL remove methaqualone.

Usage. Drug abuse and therapeutic monitoring.

Description. Methaqualone (Quaalude) is a nonbarbiturate, sedative-hypnotic agent with unknown mechanism of action. It is absorbed from the gastrointestinal tract, metabolized in the liver, and excreted in the urine, bile, and feces. This drug has a high abuse potential. The minimum lethal dose of methaqualone is 5 g (20 mmol).

Professional Considerations
1. Consent form NOT required.
2. Preparation:
   A. Tube: Red topped, red/gray topped, or gold topped or lavender topped.
   B. If the client may also have taken diazepam or chlordiazepoxide, indicate so on the laboratory requisition.
   C. Specimens MAY be drawn during hemodialysis.

3. **Procedure:**
   A. Draw a 5-mL blood sample.
4. **Postprocedure care:**
   A. None.
5. **Client and family teaching:**
   A. Explain the procedure and the reason for drawing the specimen.
   B. Explain the overdose symptoms and treatment (see above), as appropriate.
   C. Withdrawal symptoms may not appear for 2-3 days, and convulsions may occur on the eighth or ninth day after cessation of the drug.
   D. For intentional overdose, refer client and family for crisis intervention.
   E. Referrals to appropriate rehabilitation centers and therapeutic community programs should be offered to all clients who may be interested.
6. Factors that affect results:
   A. The peak level of methaqualone is 2 hours after dose. Half-life is 33-38 hours, and steady-state levels occur in 7-8 days.
   B. Results are unreliable with concurrent administration of diazepam or chlordiazepoxide when the spectrophotometric method is used.
   C. Adulterants such as household chemicals, hand soap, and gluteraldehyde invalidate test results.
7. **Other data:**
   A. Monitor coagulation studies carefully if the client is taking an anticoagulant.
   B. Methaqualone can be detected in the urine for up to 7 days.

METHEMOGLOBIN, BLOOD

Norm:

% OF TOTAL HEMOGLOBIN		SI UNITS
≤2%	≤0.02 g/dL	≤3.1 µmol/L

Methemoglobinemia Signs and Symptoms

Normal pO_2 with decreased pCO_2
Decreased calculated oxygen saturation
Decreased HCO_3^-
>15% *methemoglobin:* Chocolate cyanosis (pale blue-gray skin, brownish lips, and mucous membranes).
>30% *methemoglobin:* Dizziness, fatigue, headache, tachycardia, weakness.
>45% *methemoglobin:* Signs of central nervous system (CNS) depression.

>55% *methemoglobin:* Acidemia, bradycardia, dysrhythmias, respiratory compromise.
>70% *methemoglobin:* Death may occur secondary to hypoxia. Fatal dose of nitroglycerin or sodium nitrite is reported to be 2 g.

Treatment:

Note: Treatment choice(s) depend on client history and condition and episode history.

Support symptoms: Protect airway, administer 100% oxygen, check neurologic status every hour.

Perform continuous pulse oximetry.

Do NOT induce emesis in clients with no gag reflex or with CNS depression or excitation.

Perform gastric lavage if it can be done soon after ingestion.

Draw arterial blood gas with measured oxygen saturation.

Methylene blue must be administered with caution when methemoglobin level is >30%. Methylene blue reverses the process of methemoglobin formation by reducing methemoglobin back to hemoglobin. This treatment should not be used in the presence of G6PD deficiency.

Give blood exchange transfusion(s).

Administer hyperbaric oxygen therapy.

Forced diuresis and urine alkalinization are NOT helpful.

Do NOT acidify urine.

Increased. Acquired or hereditary methemoglobinemia, carbon monoxide poisoning, ionizing radiation, sepsis or septic shock, smoking. Drugs include acetanilid, aniline dyes, benzene derivatives, benzocaine, Bromo-Seltzer, chlorates, chloroquine, dapsone, isoniazid, lidocaine, metoclopramide, nitrates, nitrites (including silver nitrate topical ointment), phenacetin, resorcinol, and sulfonamides.

Decreased. Pancreatitis.

Description. This test is used to help detect the adverse effects of drugs containing nitrates or nitrites, such as nitroglycerin. Methemoglobin is formed when the iron in the heme portion of deoxygenated hemoglobin is oxidized to a ferric form as a result of a hereditary deficiency of nicotinamide adenine dinucleotide-diaphorase or as a result of exposures to chemicals and drugs. In the ferric form, oxygen and iron cannot combine. This is a normal process, and it is balanced by the reduction of methemoglobin to hemoglobin. However, when a high concentration of methemoglobin is produced in the red blood cells (RBCs), the capacity of RBCs to combine with oxygen is reduced, and anoxia and cyanosis result. Methemoglobinemia occurs when greater than 1% of the blood hemoglobin has been oxidized to the ferric form and is a rare but potentially dangerous condition in which the oxygen-carrying capacity of blood is compromised. Infants are more susceptible to methemoglobinemia than adults because fetal hemoglobin is more easily converted to methemoglobin than is adult hemoglobin.

Professional Considerations
1. Consent form NOT required.
2. **Preparation:**
   A. Tube: Green topped. Also obtain ice.
3. **Procedure:**
   A. Draw a 2-mL venous blood sample.
4. **Postprocedure care:**
   A. Place the specimen on ice and deliver immediately to the laboratory. Specimens must be tested within 1 hour of collection.
5. **Client and family teaching:**
   A. Review with the client and family potential sources that may have caused methemoglobinemia and identify corrective measures for removal of the exposure.
6. **Factors that affect results:**
   A. The intestinal flora of nursing infants is capable of converting significant amounts of inorganic nitrate (such as well water) to the nitrite ion, which can produce serious toxicity.
   B. Amyl nitrite ingestion increases methemoglobinemia.
   C. Falsely elevated results occur when there is a delay of more than 1 hour after collection before the test is measured.
   D. Falsely low results may occur when the sample is not kept on ice until testing.

E. Symptoms will appear at lower than the above scale in clients who are anemic.

7. **Other data:**
   A. Clients suspected of having methemoglobinemia may experience symptoms of anoxia or cyanosis, without evidence of cardiovascular or pulmonary disease.
   B. Hidden sources of nitrates, which could cause methemoglobinemia, include spinach and Polish sausage, which is rich in nitrite and nitrate, and drinking well water, which contains nitrite.
   C. Nitrate can be absorbed from topical applications, such as silver nitrate (used to treat serious bums). It must be used sparingly when applied to infants to avoid serous conversion of nitrate to nitrite.
   D. Methemoglobin has been found to promote the growth of cancer cells in vitro testing for clients with solid tumors.
   E. Poisoning is reportable to public health authorities if secondary to occupational or environmental causes.
   F. See also *CO-oximeter profile, Blood.*

METHICILLIN-RESISTANT *STAPHYLOCOCCUS AUREUS* (MRSA), CULTURE

Norm. Negative.

Usage. Infections.

Description. MRSA is a strain of *Staphylococcus aureus* that is resistant to methicillin, the antibiotic most commonly used to treat staphylococcal infections. This organism is most commonly acquired in hospitals and is known for increasing length-of-stay in intensive care units. The mortality rate is high in clients with grafts infected with MRSA after vascular surgery. Rapid test kits are available that are less expensive, quicker to use, and highly sensitive and specific.

Professional Considerations
1. Consent form NOT required.
2. **Preparations:**
   A. Obtain a sterile cotton-tipped Culturette swab with sodium chloride medium.

3. **Procedure:**
   A. Culture a specific site, using a rotating motion for 10 seconds and using one swab per site.
   B. Place the swab in the sodium chloride medium.
4. **Postprocedure care:**
   A. Transport the sample to the laboratory within 8 hours.
5. **Client and family teaching:**
   A. Results are normally available within a few days.
6. **Factors that affect results:**
   A. Methicillin-resistant staphylococci are considered resistant to all cephalosporins and imipenem.
   B. Detection is enhanced by incubation at 30°-35° C and the use of sodium chloride medium.
7. **Other data:**
   A. Methicillin resistance occurs in up to 40% of isolated *Staphylococcus epidermidis* and is increasing as an isolate of *S. aureus* in hospitals and extended-care facilities.
   B. 0.3% triclosan (Bacti-Stat), used as a hand-washing soap, has eradicated MRSA outbreaks.
   C. One study (Itoh et al., 2000) found remission of MRSA in clients treated with the herb *hochu-ekki-to.*

METHOTREXATE (MTX), SERUM

Norm. Levels for therapeutic maintenance are variable.
   High dose MTX for cancer treatment: 10^{-6} M and 10^{-7} M at 24-72 hours after drug infused.

Panic Level. At 48 hours after high-dose MTX: 454 mg/mL or 1000 μmol/L.

Panic Level Symptoms and Treatment

Symptoms:

Increased severity of expected side effects, including stomatitis, nausea, vomiting, anorexia, diarrhea, infection, bleeding, bone marrow depression, gastrointestinal ulceration, and, with prolonged use, pneumonitis and serious hepatotoxicity. Drugs that increase toxicity include chloramphenicol, *para*-aminobenzoic acid, phenytoin, probenecid, salicylates, sulfonamides, and tetracycline.

M

Treatment:

Note: Treatment choice(s) depend on client history and condition and episode history.
Perform leucovorin calcium rescue.
Continued monitoring of blood levels is necessary.
Hemodialysis WILL but peritoneal dialysis will NOT remove methotrexate.

Usage. Monitor for therapeutic levels of methotrexate, which is used to treat cancer, cholangitis, rheumatoid arthritis, and sarcoidosis.

Description. A blood test for monitoring the serum levels of methotrexate. MTX is a protein-bound, folic acid antagonist and antimetabolite, and its action is specific in the cell cycle S-phase. It is used primarily in the treatment of cancer, including acute leukemias, but is also used for treatment of ectopic pregnancy. MTX interferes with normal biosynthesis of nucleic acids, which are necessary for synthesis of deoxyribonucleic acid (DNA) and ribonucleic acid (RNA). Intravenous methotrexate may be given in low doses (10-50 mg/m^2), medium doses (100-500 mg/m^2), or high doses (500 mg/m^2 or more). MTX is absorbed by the gastrointestinal tract and cleared by the kidneys, with a half-life of 1.5-15 hours and peak blood levels occurring 1-2 hours after dose.

Professional Considerations
1. Consent form NOT required
2. **Preparation:**
   A. Tube: Red topped, red/gray topped, or gold topped.
   B. Renal and hepatic function must be assessed before the administration of MTX.
   C. Do NOT draw specimens during hemodialysis.
3. **Procedure:**
   A. Draw a 1-mL blood sample.
4. **Postprocedure care:**
   A. Observe for symptoms of methotrexate toxicity.
5. **Client and family teaching:**
   A. Results are normally available within 24 hours.
6. **Factors that affect results:**
   A. Drugs that displace MTX from plasma proteins include chloral hydrate, phenytoin, salicylates, sulfonamides, and tetracyclines.
7. **Other data:**
   A. Leucovorin rescue is essential after high-dose MTX administration. It is generally administrated 24 hours after the first methotrexate dose began, and it is dosed every 6 hours for up to 12 doses.

p-METHOXYAMPHETAMINE
(*see Amphetamines, Blood*)

METHSUXIMIDE, SERUM

Norm. Negative.

		SI UNITS
Therapeutic range of metabolite *n*-desmethyl-methsuximide	10-40 µg/mL	53-212 µmol/L
Toxic level (of metabolite)	>40 µg/mL	>212 µmol/L
Panic level (of metabolite)	>150 µg/mL	>793 µmol/L

Panic Level Symptoms and Treatment

Symptoms. CNS symptoms (ataxia, confusion, dizziness, drowsiness, slurred speech, tremor, decreased level of consciousness) and GI symptoms (anorexia, abdominal pain, diarrhea, nausea, vomiting) are most common. Other symptoms include hypotension, severe depression, skin rash, periorbital edema, urinary frequency, vaginal bleeding, pancytopenia, hepatotoxicity, neuropathy.

Treatment:

Note: Treatment choice(s) depend on client history and condition and episode history.
Administer saline cathartic unless client has an ileus.
Administer sorbitol.

Perform gastric lavage if possible soon after ingestion.
Protect airway and support breathing.
Perform neurologic checks every hour.
Forced diuresis is not helpful.
Charcoal hemoperfusion may be helpful in removing the methsuximide metabolite in comatose clients. No information was found on the effectiveness of hemodialysis in removing methsuximide.

Increased. Overdosage ingestion.

Decreased. Convulsions and epilepsy. Drugs include valproic acid.

Description. Anticonvulsant for "absence seizures," also known as petit mal seizures, that depresses nerve transmission to the motor cortex, thereby decreasing paroxysmal spike-and-wave patterns. Methsuximide is also used to supplement other medications in clients with intractable seizures. Plasma half-life is 2-4 hours. Methsuximide is metabolized in the liver and excreted in urine.

Professional Considerations
1. Consent form NOT required.
2. **Preparation:**
   A. Tube: Red topped, red/gray topped, or gold topped.
   B. Do NOT draw specimens during hemodialysis.
3. **Procedure:**
   A. Draw a 7-mL blood sample before the next dose of medication.
4. **Postprocedure care:**
   A. None.
5. **Client and family teaching:**
   A. Explain overdose symptoms and treatment (see above) as appropriate.
   B. For an intentional overdose, refer the client and family for crisis intervention.
   C. Referrals to appropriate rehabilitation centers and therapeutic community programs should be offered to all clients who may be interested.
6. **Factors that affect results:**
   A. Obtaining specimens after medication has been ingested will cause increased results.
   B. Hepatic or renal dysfunction may cause increased results.

7. **Other data:**
   A. This drug may cause a positive albumin result in the urine and an elevated BUN.
   B. In pediatric clients, the C/D ratio (plasma concentration and dose per kilogram of weight) is less sensitive to both age and associated therapy.
   C. Methsuximide decreases valproic acid levels.

METHYLENEDIOXY-AMPHETAMINE, BLOOD
(see Amphetamines, Blood)

METHYLPHENIDATE, SERUM

Norm. Negative.
 Therapeutic level: 0.01-0.04 mg/mL (0.04-0.17 mmol/L, SI units).

Overdose Symptoms and Treatment

Symptoms. Agitation, hyperactive, talkative, sleepless for days, paranoia, hallucinations, violent behavior possible, confusion, dryness of mucous membranes, headache, mydriasis, hypertension, rapid and irregular pulse, sweating, vomiting, cerebral hemorrhage, seizures, convulsions, and coma.

Treatment:
Note: Treatment choice(s) depend on client history and condition and episode history.
Perform gastric lavage.
Perform forced diuresis.
Acid urine hastens excretion.
Administer cathartic.
Acidify urine.
Support symptoms.
Take precautions to prevent self-injury.
Treatments administered outside a health care facility should be used as directed by a poison control center.
No information on the effectiveness of dialysis is known.

Usage. Monitor levels of methylphenidate, which is used in the treatment of hyperkinetic disorders (such as ADHD, hyperactivity associated with minimal brain dysfunction), narcolepsy, mild depression, senile behavior, and children with perceptual problems; and methylphenidate also counteracts overdosage from depressant drugs.

Increased. Overdose and stimulant drug abuse.

Decreased. Subtherapeutic dose.

Description. Methylphenidate (Ritalin) is a central nervous system (CNS) stimulant and antidepressant that presumably activates brainstem and cortex arousal. Methylphenidate is well absorbed from the gastrointestinal tract and is distributed throughout the body. Its actions appear in about 1 hour after ingestion and last up to 6 hours. The drug is completely metabolized in the liver to inactive products that are excreted in urine.

Tolerance to the CNS and peripheral effects develops with continued use.

Professional Considerations
1. Consent form NOT required.
2. Preparation:
   A. Tube: Lavender topped.
   B. Do NOT draw specimens during hemodialysis.
3. Procedure:
   A. Draw a 7-mL blood sample.
4. Postprocedure care:
   A. None.
5. Client and family teaching:
   A. Counsel regarding proper dosing as needed.
   B. For intentional overdose, refer client and family for crisis intervention.
6. Factors that affect results:
   A. None found.
7. Other data:
   A. None.

METHYPRYLON, SERUM

Norm. Negative.

		SI UNITS
Therapeutic level	8-10 µg/mL	44-55 µmol/L
Panic level	>30 µg/mL	>164 µmol/L

Panic Level Symptoms and Treatment

Symptoms. Apnea, ataxia, bradycardia, central nervous system depression, confusion, hypotension, weakness, pulmonary edema, convulsions, shock, coma. Death has occurred after ingestion of 6 g.

Treatment:
Note: Treatment choice(s) depend on client history and condition and episode history.
Perform diuresis with IV fluids.
Give gastric lavage if possible soon after ingestion.
Give supportive therapy.
Hemodialysis, peritoneal dialysis, and hemoperfusion WILL remove methyprylon.

Usage. Monitoring for therapeutic drug level.

Description. Methyprylon is a sedative-hypnotic that induces sleep within 45

minutes by increasing the threshold of the arousal centers of the brain. Plasma half-life is 3-6 hours. It is conjugated in the liver and excreted in the urine. Addiction and physical dependence can occur.

Professional Considerations
1. Consent form NOT required.
2. Preparation:
   A. Tube: Red topped or red/gray topped or gold topped.
   B. Do NOT draw specimens during hemodialysis.
3. Procedure:
   A. Draw a 7-mL blood sample.
4. Postprocedure care:
   A. None.
5. Client and family teaching:
   A. Counsel regarding proper dosing as appropriate.
   B. For intentional overdose, refer client and family for crisis intervention.
   C. Referrals to appropriate rehabilitation centers and therapeutic community programs should be offered to all clients who may be interested.

6. **Factors that affect results:**
   A. Interferes with urine diagnostics for 17-KS and 17-OHCS.

7. **Other data:**
   A. The trade name is Noludar.

METYRAPONE (CORTISOL) TEST, SERUM

Norm:

		SI UNITS
11-Deoxycortisol	>7 µg/dL	>202 nmol/L
Cortisol	<3 µg/dL	<83 nmol/L

Increased. Adrenal carcinoma, Cushing syndrome, diabetic acidosis, fever, hepatic disease, hyperthyroidism, hypoalbuminemia, obesity, pain, pregnancy, renal disease, and stress. Drugs include estrogens, oral contraceptives, and spironolactone.

Decreased. Addison's disease, fungal invasion, hemorrhage, hepatic disease, hypopituitarism, hypothyroidism, low-birth-weight infants, respiratory distress syndrome, and tuberculosis. Drugs include amitriptyline, androgens, chlordiazepoxide, glucocorticoids, methysergide, oral contraceptives, phenobarbital, phenothiazines, phenytoin, progestins, rifampin, and steroids.

Description. The metyrapone test is a diagnostic test for secondary adrenal insufficiency. Metyrapone is an inhibitor of 11-betahydroxylase that prevents the conversion of 11-deoxycortisol to cortisol in the adrenal glands. The diminished level of cortisol stimulates the pituitary to produce adrenocorticotropic hormone (ACTH) in a negative-feedback mechanism. In normal individuals, more ACTH is produced.

Professional Considerations
1. Consent form NOT required.
2. **Preparation:**
   A. Tube: Red topped, red/gray topped, or gold topped or green topped. Also obtain ice.
   B. Metyrapone, 30 mg/kg (range 2-3 g), is given orally, usually with milk, at 11 PM.
   C. Assess for a history of heroin addiction or use and methadone maintenance because this test may induce a narcotic withdrawal-like syndrome.
3. **Procedure:**
   A. Draw a 1-mL blood sample at 8 AM the following morning.

4. **Postprocedure care:**
   A. Specimens should be placed on ice.
5. **Client and family teaching:**
   A. Return tomorrow at approximately 8 AM for a repeat blood draw.
6. **Factors that affect results:**
   A. Reject the specimen if the client had a radioactive scan within 7 days of the test.
   B. Specimens should be frozen if the test is not performed within 24 hours.
   C. Results are highly dependent on the time of day the specimen is obtained (circadian variation).
7. **Other data:**
   A. Do NOT perform this test if primary adrenal insufficiency is likely.
   B. Long-term treatment with metyrapone can cause hypertension.
   C. See also *Cortisol, Serum or Plasma; Metyrapone (cortisol), 24-Hour urine.*

METYRAPONE (CORTISOL), 24-HOUR URINE

Norm:
17-Hydroxycorticosteroids (17-OHCS):
   2-4 times base level.
17-Ketogenic steroids (17-KGS):
   2.5-3.0-fold rise but at least 10 mg/dL (35 µmol/day, SI units).
17-Ketosteroids (17-KS):
   >2 times base level.

Increased. Acute alcohol intoxication, Cushing syndrome, ectopic adrenocorticotropic hormone (ACTH) syndrome, hepatic disease, hyperthyroidism, obesity, and stress. Drugs include amphetamines, corticosteroids, morphine, phenothiazines, and reserpine.

Decreased. Addison's disease, adrenogenital syndrome, and pituitary insufficiency.

Description. Diagnostic test for secondary adrenal insufficiency. An inhibitor of 11-betahydroxylase that prevents the conversion of 11-deoxycortisol to cortisol. The diminished levels of cortisol stimulate the pituitary to produce more ACTH in a negative-feedback mechanism. In normal individuals, more ACTH is produced, which results in an increase in urinary hydroxysteroids and ketosteroids.

Professional Considerations
1. Consent form NOT required.
2. **Preparation:**
   A. Assess for history of heroin addiction and use or methadone maintenance because this test may cause narcotic withdrawal-like symptoms.
   B. Administer metyrapone to adults in doses of 750 mg every 4 hours × 6 doses. In the child, the dose is 300 mg/m^2.
   C. Begin administration at 11 PM.
3. **Procedure:**
   A. Begin a 24-hour urine collection at 8 AM the morning after the drug was ingested.
   B. Collection container must be acidified with either hydrochloric or acetic acid as a preservative.
4. **Postprocedure care:**
   A. Write the beginning and ending date and time, as well as total urine voided in the 24-hour period, on the laboratory requisition.
   B. Record the total dose and the time metyrapone was given on the laboratory requisition.
5. **Client and family teaching:**
   A. Minimize stress levels before urine collection.
   B. Save all the urine voided in the 24-hour period and urinate before defecating to avoid loss of urine. Keep the specimen on ice or refrigerate it during the collection period. If any urine is accidentally discarded, discard the entire specimen and restart the collection the next day.
6. **Factors that affect results:**
   A. Inaccurate collection of urine.
   B. When possible, hold all medications for several days before testing. Drugs that may interfere with results include estrogens, glucose, meprobamate, penicillin, and radiographic contrast materials.
   C. Obesity, pregnancy, and stress may affect results.
7. **Other data:**
   A. Hospitalization may be required to ensure accuracy of the 24-hour urine collection.
   B. Long-term treatment with metyrapone can cause hypertension.
   C. The 24-hour urine specimen reflects cumulative levels rather than circadian variation.
   D. See also *Cortisol, Urine; Metyrapone (cortisol) test, Serum; 17-OHCS, Urine; 17-KGS, Urine; 17-KS, Urine.*

MIB 1-3
(see Ki-67 proliferation marker, Specimen)

MIBG (IODINE-131-META-IODOBENZYLGUANIDINE) SCAN, DIAGNOSTIC

Norm. The adrenal glands will not be visualized. There is variable physiologic uptake by the bladder, colon, heart, spleen, and uterus.

Usage. Location and diagnosis of primary and metastatic pheochromocytoma, adrenal medullary hyperplasia, multiple endocrine neoplasia (MEN), Von Hippel-Lindau disease, Von Recklinghausen disease, neuroblastoma, paraganglioma, medullary carcinoma of thyroid, and other neuroendocrine tumors.

Description. A MIBG scan is a nuclear medicine scan of the whole body after injection of a radioactive tracer I-131 MIBG for the purpose of detecting areas of increased uptake by hyperactive endocrine tissue or tumor. MIBG is a catecholamine analog, similar to noradrenaline. Various organs and tumors take up the tracer at varying degrees. A series of scans is conducted at 24 and 48 hours following injection of radioisotope. The isotope is concentrated in hyperactive endocrine tissue, such as pheochromocytoma tissue, and appears on the scan as a "hot spot."

Professional Considerations

1. Consent form IS required.

Risks

Allergic reaction to tracer (itching, hives, rash, tight feeling in the throat, shortness of breath, anaphylaxis).

Contraindications

Previous allergy to MIBG or iodine solution (Lugol's solution or SSKI) or shellfish; pregnancy (because of radioactive iodine crossing the blood-placental barrier); breast-feeding; anuria; dialysis.

2. **Preparation:**
   A. See *Client and family teaching.*
   B. Assess client for history of allergy to iodine or shellfish.
   C. A prescribed dose of potassium iodide (SSKI) or Lugol's solution will be started 24 to 48 hours prior to the injection of the radioisotope to prevent uptake of radioisotope by the thyroid.
   D. Women of childbearing age should have a pregnancy test within 48 hours prior to the test.
   E. A bowel prep may be prescribed.
   F. Have emergency equipment readily available.
   G. Remove jewelry and metal objects before each scan.
3. **Procedure:**
   A. Position client in lying position and take baseline BP.
   B. Slowly inject radioisotope intravenously, over 1-2 minutes.
   C. Monitor BP during injection and 20 minutes following injection.
   D. A scan may be done 4, 24, 48, and possibly 72 hours following the injection of the isotope. For the scan, the client is positioned supine on the imaging table and the whole body is scanned using a gamma camera.
4. **Postprocedure care:**
   A. SSKI or Lugol's solution will be given throughout the test period and will continue for 4-7 days following the injection of MIBG.
   B. Check with institutional policy regarding special instructions for discarding urine for 24 hours following isotope injection.
5. **Client and family teaching:**
   A. Many prescribed and over-the-counter medications can interfere

with the results of this test. Be sure to inform physician of any medications that are being taken.
   B. Medications that may need to be discontinued up to 4-6 weeks prior to the test include labetalol, reserpine, loxapine, tricyclic antidepressants (doxepin, amitriptyline and derivatives, imipramine and derivatives, amoxapine), sympathomimetics (phenylephrine, phenylpropalamine, psuedoephedrine), calcium channel blockers, SSRI, catecholamine receptor agonists and antagonists, phenothiazines, butyrophenones (i.e., haloperidol), guanethidine, phenoxybenzamine.
   C. Inform the physician if pregnant, breastfeeding, or if young children are in the household.
   D. No fast is required for this test.
   E. You will need to lie still during the procedure. Young children may be need to be sedated.
   F. There is no discomfort associated with the scan.
   G. SSKI or Lugol's solution will be taken for 4-7 days, beginning 1-2 days before the injection of the radioisotope. This medication can be diluted in a glass of water or juice.
   H. Despite the use of thyroid blocking medication, the thyroid may be affected for a short period of time. Prolonged feelings of fatigue, temperature irregularities or changes in heart rate should be reported to the physician.
   I. The scan takes approximately 1-2 hours.
6. **Factors that affect results:**
   A. Many medications can impact the results of this test. Refer to *Client and family teaching.*
7. **Other data:**
   A. During the scan, the kidneys may be localized in relation to the adrenal glands by obtaining a correlative image of the kidneys using a renal tracer.
   B. MIBG is excreted by the kidneys. The half-life is 8 days.
   C. Health care professionals working in a nuclear medicine area must follow federal standards set by the Nuclear Regulatory Commission. These standards include precautions for handling

M

the radioactive material and monitoring of potential radiation exposure.

MICROALBUMIN, SPOT URINE
(see Albumin, Serum, Urine, and 24-Hour urine)

MICROFILARIAE, PERIPHERAL BLOOD

Norm. Negative or no parasite identified. An indirect hemagglutination titer of 1:128 as well as a bentonite flocculation titer of 1:5 are considered minimally significant titers.

Positive. Brugia, Dipetalonema, Loa loa, Mansonella, and Wuchereria.

Description. Filariae make up a large group of parasitic worms that produce an embryo known as a microfilaria (intermediate stage between egg and larva). These parasites invade the lymphatics, causing lymphedema and elephantiasis. Microfilaria are the smallest forms of filariae.

Professional Considerations
1. Consent form NOT required.
2. Preparation:
   A. Tube: Green topped.
   B. Include the client's recent travel history on the laboratory requisition.
3. Procedure:
   A. Draw a 4-mL blood sample.
   B. Repeat the test to obtain daytime and nighttime specimens.
4. Postprocedure care:
   A. Transport specimens to the laboratory immediately. Specimens should NOT be clotted.
5. Client and family teaching:
   A. Two specimens, drawn preferably 12 hours apart, are necessary.
6. Factors that affect results:
   A. One negative result does not rule out a parasitic infection.
   B. Circulating microfilariae may NOT be detected in blood for 6-12 months after transmission occurs.
7. Other data:
   A. Because Wuchereria and Brugia are nocturnal, the optimal blood sample time would be 10 pm to 2 am.

B. Because Loa loa is diurnal, the optimum time for the blood sample would be 12 PM (noon).

MICROHEMAGGLUTINATION TREPONEMA PALLIDUM (MHA-TP) TEST, SERUM

Norm. Titer <1:160 or nonreactive.

Usage. Serologic confirmation of syphilis when nontreponemal antibody tests (RPR or VDRL) are positive.

Description. Syphilis is a complex, sexually transmitted disease characterized by a wide range of symptoms that imitate other diseases and is caused by the organism Treponema pallidum. In this test, the client's serum is heat treated and mixed with T. pallidum–sensitized sheep red blood cells, incubated, and compared with a control. A positive result occurs when agglutination occurs in the test sample but not in the control. This test is less sensitive than the fluorescent treponemal antibody, absorbed double stain (FTA-Abs DS) test for primary syphilis. Positive results will occur in treponemal diseases of bejel, pinta, syphilis, or yaws.

Professional Considerations
1. Consent form NOT required.
2. Preparation:
   A. See Client and family teaching.
   B. Tube: Red topped.
3. Procedure:
   A. Draw a 1-mL blood sample.
4. Postprocedure care:
   A. Send the specimen to the laboratory and refrigerate them until tested.
5. Client and family teaching:
   A. Fast overnight before the test.
   B. The use of condoms significantly reduces the risk of sexually transmitted diseases.
   C. A referral for HIV testing may be indicated and should be discussed and offered to interested clients.
   D. If testing is positive:
      i. Notify all sexual contacts from the previous 90 days (if early stage) to be tested for syphilis.
      ii. Syphilis can be cured with antibiotics. These may

worsen the symptoms for the first 24 hours.

iii. Do not have sexual contact for 2 months and until after repeat testing has confirmed that the syphilis is cured. Use condoms after that for 2 years. Return for repeat testing every 3-4 months for the next 2 years to make sure the disease is cured.

iv. Do not become pregnant for 2 years because syphilis can be transmitted to the fetus.

v. If left untreated, syphilis can damage many body organs, including the brain, over several years.

6. **Factors that affect results:**
A. False-positive results may be attributable to autoimmune disorders, connective tissue diseases, infectious mononucleosis, leprosy, or systemic lupus erythematosus.

B. Testing errors may be associated with dusty or improper plates and pipetting errors.

7. **Other data:**
A. This test may remain positive indefinitely for clients previously infected with syphilis. Thus it is not useful for monitoring clinical response to treatment for syphilis.

B. Test results may become negative after treatment. Therefore, negative results do NOT necessarily exclude a past history of syphilis.

C. There is a significant correlation between the diagnosis of syphilis and seropositive HIV.

D. See also *FTA-Abs DS, Serum; RPR, Diagnostic; VDRL, Serum.*

MICROSOMAL ANTIBODY
(*see Thyroid Peroxidase Antibody, Blood*)

MIDAZOLAM
(*see Benzodiazepines, Plasma and Urine*)

MIF, BLOOD
(*see Migration inhibition factor, Blood*)

MILK PRECIPITINS, BLOOD

Norm. Negative.

Increased. IgA deficiency, celiac disease, infantile diarrhea, mongolism, pulmonary hemosiderosis, and Wiskoff-Aldrich syndrome.

Description. Milk precipitins are antibodies found occasionally in children who are sensitive to milk. This test involves adding blood to an agar gel and waiting for a specific antibody concentration to develop in a line formation. The distance of the precipitin line from the point of application of the blood is directly proportional to the concentration of antigens in the client's bloodstream.

Professional Considerations
1. Consent form NOT required.
2. **Preparation:**
A. Tube: Red topped, red/gray topped, or gold topped.
3. **Procedure:**
A. Draw a 7-mL blood sample.
4. **Postprocedure care:**
A. Results are normally available within 48 hours but may take several days if the test is performed off site.
5. **Client and family teaching:**
A. The test does not differentiate between sensitivity and allergy.
6. **Factors that affect results:**
A. Gross contamination.
B. A positive test does not necessarily mean that the child is allergic to milk because milk sensitivity may also produce a positive test.
7. **Other data:**
A. None.

MINI–MENTAL STATE EXAM (MMSE), DIAGNOSTIC

Norm: *Perfect score* (normal for clients with 12th grade or higher education and no cognitive impairment): 30 points.
Cognitive impairment: ≤24 points.

Usage. Detection and tracking of cognitive impairment.

Description. The Mini–Mental State Exam (MMSE) tests for cognitive impairment by evaluating orientation, registration, attention and calculation, recall and language. The MMSE has demonstrated an 85% specificity and 87% sensitivity for identifying cognitive impairment in hospitalized clients.

Professional Considerations

1. Consent form NOT required.
2. **Preparation:**
   A. Examination may be done at the client's bedside.
   B. Obtain copy of examination and a clipboard.
   C. Observe client's level of consciousness, educational level, visual impairments, and any physician limitations.
3. **Procedure:**
   A. Inform client that a series of questions will be asked. Instruct client to attempt to answer all the questions, even if they seem silly.
4. **Postprocedure care:**
   A. None.
5. **Client and family teaching:**
   A. Retesting should be done after 6 months if score is borderline (23-25 points).
6. **Factors that affect results:**
   A. Clients with less than a 4th-grade education do poorly on the reading and writing portions of this examination but may not be cognitively impaired.
   B. Medical conditions such as reduced vision ability, memory impairment, stroke, and diabetes have been associated with cognitive deterioration.
   C. Better self-care ability is related to better results on the simple processing items (registration, naming, repetition, commanding) and attention/ memory functions such as time/ place orientation, recall and attention.
7. **Other data:**
   A. None.

MIRALUMA

(see Scintimammography, Diagnostic)

MITOGEN-ACTIVATED PROTEIN KINASE (MAP KINASE, MAPK), SPECIMEN

Norm. Requires interpretation.

Usage. Prostate cancer, colon cancer, breast cancer. Use of MAPK in the detection, diagnosis, and determination of response to therapy for these conditions is in the research arena.

Description. MAP kinases act as transducers of extracellular signaling, by means of tyrosine kinase–growth factor regulators, to regulate a variety of transcription factors. MAP kinases are unique in that phosphorylation of both threonine and tyrosine residues are required for activation of the MAPK pathway cascade. One MAPK pathway is stimulated by serum growth factors that target extracellular regulated kinases (ERKs) resulting in cellular proliferation or differentiation. Another MAPK pathway is activated by stressors (that is, radiation or ultraviolet radiation) ultimately triggering apoptosis (organized cellular death). It is believed that various overexpressed or mutated oncogenes activate MAPK pathways and are responsible for stimulating tumor growth. Some of these oncogenes involved in the MAPK pathways include *ras, raf,* and *src*. MAPK activity is tested using immune complex assay. When compared to normal or noncancerous tissue, hyperexpression of MAP kinase is associated with carcinomas.

Professional Considerations

1. Consent form IS required for the procedure, that is, tumor resection or biopsy used to obtain the specimens used for this test. (See *Biopsy, Site-specific, Specimen,* for procedure-specific risks and contraindications.)
2. **Preparation:**
   A. See *Biopsy, Site-specific Specimen; Client and family teaching.*
   B. Obtain a sterile container and fixative or formalin.
   C. The requisition must include the operative diagnosis and the site of the specimen.

3. **Procedure:**
   A. The tissue sample is obtained with use of local or general anesthesia.
   B. Label the specimen with the client's name, age, sex, room number, and operative diagnosis; the source of the specimen; and the surgeon and other physicians desiring a copy of the pathology report
   C. A freshly frozen tissue sample may be used. See *Frozen tissue section, Diagnostic,* as appropriate.
4. **Postprocedure care:**
   A. Fresh tissue may be fixed in phosphate-buffered formalin. Confirm preferred tissue handling with physician.
   B. Deliver the specimen to the laboratory promptly.
   C. See *Biopsy, Site-specific, Specimen.*
5. **Client and family teaching:**
   A. See *Biopsy, Site-specific, Specimen.*
   B. Call the physician for signs of infection at the procedure site: increasing pain, redness, swelling, purulent drainage, for fever >101° F (38° C).
6. **Factors that affect results:**
   A. Poor sampling technique or contamination.
7. **Other data:**
   A. None.

MIXED LEUKOCYTE CULTURE (MIXED LYMPHOCYTE CULTURE), SPECIMEN

Norm. Requires interpretation.

Usage. Aplastic anemia, immunodeficiency (detection of T-lymphocyte abnormalities), transplants, and tuberculosis.

Description. Mixed leukocyte culture is performed to determine whether the mononuclear cells of a prospective tissue transplant recipient will react against a potential donor's leukocyte antigens. This histocompatibility test may be performed in two ways. In a one-way test, the potential donor sample is irradiated or treated with mitomycin C, which prevents the sample

from blast formation in reaction to mixture with the prospective recipient sample. This allows measurement of prospective recipient blast formation only. In a two-way test, blast formation of both samples is monitored by comparison of the amount of blast formation in the combined sample with that of each separate sample in combination with controls.

Professional Considerations
1. Consent form NOT required.
2. **Preparation:**
   A. Preschedule the test with the laboratory.
   B. Tube: 2 green-topped tubes.
3. **Procedure:**
   A. Draw a 7-mL blood sample from the prospective transplant donor. Label the tube "donor sample."
   B. Repeat the test for the prospective recipient. Label the tube "recipient sample."
4. **Postprocedure care:**
   A. Send the specimens to the laboratory within 2 hours.
   B. Specimens must be tested the same day.
5. **Client and family teaching:**
   A. Results are normally available in 7-10 days.
6. **Factors that affect results:**
   A. Reject any specimen that was not collected using a sterile procedure, not drawn in a heparinized tube, or has arrived in the laboratory more than 2 hours after collection.
   B. False-negative results may occur if the prospective recipient is severely immunocompromised.
7. **Other data:**
   A. May be helpful in predicting graft survival.
   B. This test should be repeated for several days.

MIXING STUDY (CIRCULATING ANTICOAGULANTS), PLASMA

Norm. Requires interpretation.

Usage. To determine if prolonged coagulation studies (prothrombin time

M

[PT], partial thromboplastin time [PTT], or activated partial thromboplastin time [APTT]) are resulting from circulating anticoagulants or factor deficiencies.

Description. The coagulation system involves numerous reactions (clotting cascade) that are initiated when bleeding occurs. The clotting cascade requires clotting proteins (factors I-XII, except factor IV), fibrinogen, lymphocytes, macrophage, neutrophils, platelets, and prothrombin. These substances are naturally circulating and awaiting activation. There are also naturally occurring anticoagulants that circulate and inhibit the clotting process. Examples of anticoagulants include antithrombin, antithromboplastin, and heparin. When prolonged clotting times are discovered (prolonged PT or PTT, or both), bleeding tendencies may arise. These prolonged studies may result from either factor deficiencies or circulating anticoagulants. To determine which problem is occurring, a MIXING study may be performed. A mixing study involves mixing the plasma sample from a specimen with a prolonged PT or PTT, or both, with a fresh plasma specimen having normal PT or PTT findings. Once the specimens are mixed a repeat PT and PTT study is performed to determine if a change or correction has occurred. If the cause of the prolonged coagulation study or studies is attributable to a circulating anticoagulant, the circulating anticoagulant will also alter the normal specimen it was mixed with and the PT or PTT will remain prolonged. If the problem is from a factor deficiency or from factor deficiencies, mixing the specimen with a normal specimen will correct the deficiency, resulting in a corrected or normal PT or PTT, or both. Disorders associated with factor deficiencies may include hemophilia (hemophilia A and B and von Willebrand's disease), hypoprothrombinemia, and disseminated intravascular coagulation. Identifying circulating anticoagulants, such as the lupus anticoagulant, may assist in the diagnosis of systemic lupus erythematosus (SLE) or identify clients with lymphoproliferative disorders and thrombotic tendencies.

Professional Considerations
1. Consent form NOT required.
2. **Preparation:**
   A. Preschedule this test with the laboratory.
   B. Tube: Four 5-mL blue-topped tubes.
   C. History of present or recent use of anticoagulant therapy or medications that may cause inhibitory effects must be documented on the laboratory requisition.
   D. See *Client and family teaching.*
3. **Procedure:**
   A. Venipuncture should be performed as nontraumatically as possible. The time the tourniquet is applied should be minimized.
   B. Draw 4 blood samples, completely filling each tube with 5 mL of blood.
   C. If multiple blood tests are to be drawn, the mixing-study specimens should be obtained LAST. If no other tests are to be drawn, discard at least 2 mL of blood before collecting the mixing-study specimens.
   D. If hematocrit is >55%, special collection tubes, without vacuum, must be used when the specimens are being obtained.
4. **Postprocedure care:**
   A. Promptly send the specimens to the laboratory. If the mixing study is not performed immediately, the specimens should be refrigerated. If testing is delayed >48 hours, the specimens should be double-spun and frozen.
   B. Specimens should be centrifuged for 10-15 minutes to produce platelet-poor plasma.
5. **Client and family teaching:**
   A. Fast for 8 hours before testing to minimize interference by lipemia.
   B. To minimize bleeding or injury, refrain from dental flossing or using a hard toothbrush. Do not receive intramuscular injections, aspirin, or nonsteroidal medications, and minimize activity that may produce physical injury when possible.
   C. Bleeding may not be unusual because of bleeding tendencies. An ice bag may be applied to the bruise, but excessive bruising should be reported to a physician.

6. Factors that affect results:
   A. Reject specimens if they are hemolyzed, their blood volume is insufficient, they are clotted, any processing error has occurred, or the specimens taken were from a heparinized intravenous line or arterial line site.
   B. Plasma not free of platelets (before freezing) or lipemia may affect results.
   C. Drugs that may affect results include antibiotics, chlorpromazine, phenytoin, procainamide, and quinidine.
7. Other data:
   A. Lupus anticoagulant is present in approximately 30% of clients with SLE and in those with lymphoproliferative disorders, recurrent abortions, and thrombotic phenomena.
   B. The more platelet-free the specimen, the greater is the sensitivity in identifying the lupus anticoagulant.
   C. Fresh normal plasma should be obtained from a specimen received no longer than 1 hour before the mixing study is performed.
   D. Acquired factor V inhibitors may occur transiently postoperatively or after blood transfusion.
   E. See also *Prothrombin time (PT), Serum; Activated partial thromboplastin time (APTT), Plasma.*

MJD GENE
(*see SCA2 Gene test, Diagnostic*)

MMSE
(*see Mini–Mental State Exam, Diagnostic*)

MONOCYTES, BLOOD
(*see Differential leukocyte count, Peripheral blood*)

MONOS, BLOOD
(*see Differential leukocyte count, Peripheral blood*)

MONOSPOT SCREEN (HETEROPHIL SCREEN), BLOOD

Norm. Negative.

Positive. Adenovirus, Burkitt's lymphoma, cytomegalovirus, Epstein Barr virus, herpes simplex virus, HIV, Hodgkin's disease, infectious mononucleosis, Izumi fever, leukemia, malaria, pancreatic cancer, rubella virus, rheumatoid arthritis, sarcoidosis, serum sickness, systemic lupus erythematosus, and viral or infectious hepatitis.

Negative. Normal finding or infection of bacterial cause.

Description. The monospot screen, a screening test that rapidly detects heterophil agglutinins, is performed on two slides, each containing serum and horse red cells, with one slide also containing guinea pig kidney and the other slide containing beef red cell stroma. Agglutination that occurs on only the slide with guinea pig kidney is diagnostic of infectious mononucleosis. Heterophil agglutinins can appear in serum approximately 6-10 days after contact. Detection may remain for up to 1 year and peaks between 4 and 8 weeks after exposure.

Professional Considerations
1. Consent form NOT required.
2. Preparation:
   A. Tube: Red topped, red/gray topped, or gold topped or lavender topped.
3. Procedure:
   A. Draw a 2-mL blood sample (red topped, red/gray topped, or gold topped) or a 3-mL blood sample (lavender topped).
4. Postprocedure care:
   A. Specimens should be refrigerated before being tested.
5. Client and family teaching:
   A. Results are normally available within 72 hours.
6. Factors that affect results:
   A. A hemolyzed or chylous sample invalidates the results.
   B. About 10% of adults (more for children) produce false-positive or false-negative results.

7. **Other data:**
   A. The monospot screen has a 99% specificity and an 86% sensitivity in helping to diagnose infectious mononucleosis.
   B. In the presence of infectious mononucleosis, 10%-25% atypical lymphocytes may be observed in the differential cell count.
   C. If mononucleosis is suspected based on clinical symptoms but the screening test is negative, more sensitive tests, such as heterophil antibody, cytomegalovirus, or *Toxoplasma* antibodies, should be considered.
   D. See also *Heterophil agglutinins, Blood.*

MORPHINE, BLOOD
(see *Toxicology, Drug screen, Blood*)

MORPHINE, URINE

Norm. Negative.

PANIC LEVELS		SI UNITS
Hydromorphone	>0.1 mg/dL	>0.2 μmol/L
Methadone	>0.2 mg/dL	>10 μmol/L
Morphine	>0.005 mg/dL	0.2 μmol/L

Panic Level Symptoms and Treatment

Symptoms. Bradycardia, itching, hypotension, bradypnea, hypoxia, muscle spasms, pinpoint (miotic) pupils, dilated pupils in mixed drug overdose or severe acidosis, coma.

Treatment:
Note: Treatment choice(s) depend on client history and condition and episode history.
Administer naloxone 0.4 to 2 mg IV every 2-3 minutes in adults.
Administer naloxone 0.01 mg/kg IV every 2-3 minutes in children.
Provide respiratory support.
Hemodialysis will NOT remove morphine.
Increased or Positive. Drug use or abuse (especially heroin).

Description. Morphine is a narcotic analgesic used for pain relief. It relieves anxiety and tension and causes sedation. It is habit forming and addictive. Overdose may cause bradycardia, hypotension, and severe respiratory and central nervous system depression.

Although morphine may be a potentially addictive or abused narcotic, two derivatives of morphine (heroin and codeine) are more commonly abused. Ninety percent of a morphine dose is excreted in the urine within 24 hours of administration, but levels may be detected for up to 7 days after heroin use.

Professional Considerations
1. Consent form NOT required unless the specimen is collected as legal evidence.
2. **Preparation:**
   A. Supervise the client when obtaining the sample if results may be used as medicolegal evidence.
   B. Obtain a sterile, preservative-free plastic or silanized (SiH$_4$)-glass specimen container.
   C. MAY be drawn during hemodialysis.
3. **Procedure:**
   A. Obtain a 25-mL random urine specimen.
4. **Postprocedure care:**
   A. If the results are to be used as legal evidence, the chain of possession must remain unbroken from the time the specimen is collected until court testimony.

5. Client and family teaching:
   A. For intentional overdose, refer client and family for crisis intervention.
   B. Referrals to appropriate rehabilitation centers and therapeutic community programs should be offered to all addicted clients who may be interested.
   C. Behavior and level of consciousness may be significantly altered under the influence of opiates.
   D. Signs and symptoms of withdrawal may include agitation, anorexia, anxiety, diaphoresis, disorientation, hallucinations, insomnia, seizures, and tremors.

6. Factors that affect results:
   A. Poppy seed ingestion may produce false-positive results with the immunoassay method for up to 60 hours after ingestion.
   B. Morphine, 10 mg intravenously, is detectable in the urine for up to 84 hours.
   C. One measurement method identified endogenous morphine excreted in the urine at the levels 0.71 pg/mL (2.5 fmol/mL, SI units)
   D. The use of Stealth adulterant in the urine sample will cause negative results in a positive sample.

7. Other data:
   A. Heroin is rapidly deacetylated to morphine in the human body.
   B. Hydromorphone is a semisynthetic phenanthrene derivative structurally similar to morphine. Hydromorphone has an 8-10 times more potent analgesic effect compared to morphine.
   C. Codeine is a phenanthrene derivative of opium made by methylation of morphine.
   D. Morphine levels can be measured in corpses for several days after death.
   E. See also *Toxicology, Drug screen, Urine.*

MOTILE SPERM, WET MOUNT, DIAGNOSTIC

Norm. Negative.

Usage. Reported sexual assault.

Description. Fresh vaginal specimen examined microscopically for presence of sperm.

Professional Considerations

1. Consent form or verbal consent IS usually required because specimens may be used as legal evidence.
2. Preparation:
   A. Obtain a speculum, a wooden Pap-smear stick, normal saline with a 60-mL syringe, a sterile specimen cup, and slides with frosted tips on which to label client information.
   B. See *Client and family teaching.*
3. Procedure:
   A. Have the specimen collection witnessed if the specimen may be used as legal evidence.
   B. Do NOT lubricate the speculum; this may inhibit sperm mobility.
   C. Obtain a vaginal specimen by vaginal wash with normal saline or a Pap-smear stick.
   D. Avoid cotton-tipped applicators.
4. Postprocedure care:
   A. Write the client's name, the date, exact time of collection, and specimen source on the laboratory requisition. Sign, and have the witness sign, the laboratory requisition.
   B. Transport the specimen to the laboratory immediately in a sealed plastic bag marked as legal evidence. All clients handling the specimen should sign and mark the time of receipt on the laboratory requisition.
5. Client and family teaching:
   A. The client may urinate before the procedure but should not wipe the vulva afterward; this may eliminate sperm.
   B. Survivors of sexual assault should be referred to appropriate crisis counseling agencies as well as for gynecologic follow-up study.
   C. Referral for HIV testing should be reviewed and offered to all sexual assault victims.
   D. Preventive treatment for chlamydiosis, gonorrhea, and syphilis should be provided to all survivors of sexual assault.
   E. The option of a postcoital contraceptive should be reviewed

M

with all survivors of sexual assault.

6. Factors that affect results:
   A. Avoid extreme temperature change or direct sunlight on slides when en route to the laboratory or a legal agency.
   B. Delayed delivery of the specimen or use of a condom may decrease the number of viable sperm.

7. Other data:
   A. The presence of sperm is not proof of rape because the definition of rape is a legal matter. Low levels do not exclude intercourse.
   B. Normal postcoital cervical mucosa reveal at least 10 motile sperm per high-power field.
   C. Federal and local laws, regulations, customs, and procedures must be known.

MPV

(see Mean platelet volume, Blood)

MRA

(see Magnetic resonance angiography, Diagnostic)

MRCP

(see Magnetic resonance cholangiopancreatography, Diagnostic)

MRI

(see Magnetic resonance imaging, Diagnostic)

MRN

(see Magnetic resonance neurography, Diagnostic)

MRSA

(see Methicillin-resistant Staphylococcus aureus, Culture)

MRU

(see Magnetic resonance urography, Diagnostic)

MSLT

(see Polysomnography, Diagnostic)

MUCIN CLOT TEST, SPECIMEN

Norm. Firm clot formation with surrounding fluid appearing clear.

Usage. Helps differentiate the types of joint diseases.

Description. The mucin clot test reflects the polymerization of synovial fluid hyaluronate and correlates with viscosity except in acute effusions. Test is normal with degenerative joint disease, rheumatic fever, and systemic lupus erythematosus. An abnormal test demonstrated by a friable clot and turbid surrounding fluid occurs in a wide variety of inflammatory joint diseases such as arthritis of acute bacterial, rheumatoid, septic, or tuberculous origin, and gout. The addition of acetic acid to synovial fluid causes a mucin clot that is graded good, fair, poor, or very poor. If normal, a firm clot forms surrounded by a clear solution. A soft clot formed in a slightly turbid solution is graded as fair. A friable clot formed in a turbid solution and shredding on agitation is graded as poor. No clot formation is graded as very poor.

Professional Considerations

1. Consent form IS required for synovial fluid aspiration. See *Biopsy, Site-specific, Specimen,* for procedure-specific risks and contraindications.
2. Preparation:
   A. Obtain a sterile aspiration tray.
   B. Tube: Lavender-topped or any sterile tube containing 20 mL of 5% acetic acid.
   C. A local anesthetic should be considered before aspiration of synovial fluid.
3. Procedure:
   A. Aspirate the synovial fluid into a sterile tube while using a sterile technique.
   B. Add 5 mL of fluid into 20 mL of 5% acetic acid. Normally a clot will form in 60 seconds.

4. **Postprocedure care:**
    A. Refrigerate specimens if not tested within 5 hours.
5. **Client and family teaching:**
    A. Monitor the site for bleeding, drainage, or inflammation for 24-48 hours.
    B. A mild analgesic may be required for pain control.
    C. Call the physician for signs of infection at the procedure site: increasing pain, redness, swelling, purulent drainage, or fever >101° F (38.3° C).
6. **Factors that affect results:**
    A. Lack of synovial fluid aspirate.
7. **Other data:**
    A. Results are nonspecific alone and are not diagnostic of a single pathologic entity.

MUCIN-LIKE CARCINOMA–ASSOCIATED ANTIGEN (MCA-AG), BLOOD

Norm. <11 U/mL

Increased. Breast cancer, cirrhosis of the liver, gastrointestinal cancer, hepatitis, lung cancer, mammary dysplasia, metastasis, and ovarian cancer.

Decreased. Not clinically significant.

Description. Mucinlike carcinoma-associated antigen (MCA) is a high-molecular-weight glycoprotein product of the MUC1 gene containing many side chains of carbohydrate. Small amounts of MCA are normally produced by epithelial cells that line the respiratory, gastrointestinal, and genitourinary tracts. Exocrine tissues such as mammary, salivary, and sweat glands will also produce small amounts of MCA. MCA can be useful as a serial marker for metastasis, in monitoring therapeutic responses to cancer treatment, in detecting relapse metastasis, in enhancing specificity of bone scintigraphy, and for tumor staging. Several cancer antigens are classified as "mucinlike," because they contain the same core MUC1 gene, with different variations of glycosylation. They include CA 15-5 commonly used for monitoring ovarian cancer, CA 19-9 used for monitoring gastrointestinal cancer, CA 50 used for monitoring lung and gastrointestinal cancers, CA 72-4 used for monitoring gastrointestinal and ovarian cancers, CA 125 used for monitoring breast and ovarian cancer, CA 549, newly identified as a marker for breast cancer, and carcinoma-associated mucin antigens (CA M) 28 and 29. CA M 28 and CA M 29 were found on one study to be superior to both CA 15-5 and CA 549 in detecting metastatic breast cancer disease. None of these markers are useful for detecting small tumor masses or early disease. See also, *CA 15-5, Blood and CA 549, Blood.*

Professional Considerations
1. Consent form NOT required.
2. **Preparation:**
    A. Tube: Red topped, red/gray topped, or gold topped for serum samples. Lavender topped for plasma samples.
3. **Procedure:**
    A. Draw a 0.5-mL blood sample.
4. **Postprocedure care:**
    A. If the specimen is not tested immediately, it can be refrigerated for up to 48 hours. If testing is delayed beyond 48 hours, the specimen should be frozen.
5. **Client and family teaching:**
    A. Results are normally available within 72 hours.
6. **Factors that affect results:**
    A. MCA is normally elevated in the second trimester of pregnancy and will steadily rise until the postpartum period. Thus in pregnant women, MCA is useful for monitoring breast cancer only in the early stages of pregnancy.
    B. When MCA is used to monitor therapeutic response to cancer treatment, it is necessary to consistently measure either serum or plasma samples; they should not be interchanged.
    C. Specimens should be rejected if 48 hours have passed since specimen collection and the specimen is not frozen.
7. **Other data:**
    A. Performance characteristics of testing have NOT been established.

B. Two thirds of all clients with breast or ovarian cancer have elevated MCA levels.

C. Single MCA levels are NOT helpful when one is screening women for breast cancer.

D. MCA has a 72% sensitivity in detecting reoccurrence of cancer in high-risk populations.

MUCOPOLYSACCHARIDES, QUALITATIVE, URINE

Norm. Negative.

Positive. Beta-glucuronidase syndrome, Hunter syndrome, Hurler syndrome, Maroteaux-Lamy syndrome, Morquio syndrome, Sanfilippo syndrome, and Scheie syndrome. Drugs include heparin.

Description. Mucopolysaccharidoses are a group of inherited, autosomal recessive diseases. These inborn errors of metabolism result in an increased excretion of urinary mucopolysaccharides because of a lysosomal enzyme deficiency of either alpha-l-iduronidase, sulfoiduronate sulfatase, chondroitin sulfate, or arylsulfatase B.

Professional Considerations

1. Consent form NOT required.
2. Preparation:
   A. Obtain a sterile specimen container.
3. Procedure:
   A. Obtain a 20-mL random urine specimen in a sterile container without preservative.
4. Postprocedure care:
   A. The specimen is stable for 1 week at 4° C.
5. Client and family teaching:
   A. Results are normally available within 72 hours.
6. Factors that affect results:
   A. Increased turbidity of urine causes positive results.
7. Other data:
   A. False-negative results can be as high as 32%.

MULTIGATED EQUILIBRIUM HEART SCAN (MUGA), DIAGNOSTIC
(see Heart scan, Diagnostic)

MULTIPLE SLEEP LATENCY TEST
(see Polysomnography, Diagnostic)

MUMPS ANTIBODY, BLOOD

Norm. Negative or titer <1:8.

Positive. Viral mumps. Recent infection with the virus is indicated by a fourfold rise in titer between the acute and convalescent specimens, with ratio of viral (V) to soluble (S) titer increasing.

Description. Mumps (infectious parotitis) is an acute, contagious, febrile disease that causes inflammation of the parotid glands and other salivary glands. Peak infection rates occur in the winter and spring months. Symptoms include fever, malaise, chills, headache, pain below the ear, and swelling of the parotid glands. In clients who have passed puberty, it may cause orchitis, oophoritis, and inflammation of many vital organs. Mumps virus contracted in the first trimester of pregnancy may be associated with a higher risk of congenital anomalies. Mumps is caused by the mumps paramyxovirus that is spread from client to client through droplet spray or direct contact with the saliva of an infected client. This test supports recent mumps virus infection or previous exposure to it. Besides mumps, this virus has been known to cause meningitis and encephalitis.

Professional Considerations

1. Consent form NOT required.
2. Preparation:
   A. Tube: Red topped, red/gray topped, or gold topped.
3. Procedure:
   A. Draw a 5-mL blood sample. Label the tube as the acute sample.
   B. Repeat the test in 7-14 days, and label the tube as the convalescent sample.
4. Postprocedure care:
   A. Place the specimens on ice.
5. Client and family teaching:
   A. Return in 1-2 weeks for drawing of a convalescent sample.
   B. If mumps is suspected, the client should be isolated for 9 days after parotid gland swelling appears, until the period of communica-

bility has passed. The incubation period is between 16 and 18 days.

C. Infection confers lifelong immunity.

D. There is no specific treatment for mumps after it has been acquired. Vaccination is available for clients who have not had the infection.

6. **Factors that affect results:**

A. Reject hemolyzed or chylous serum specimens.

B. Failure to collect a convalescent sample limits the value of the acute sample results.

7. **Other data:**

A. Increased hemagglutination-inhibition titer indicates either mumps or another parainfluenza virus.

MURAMIDASE (LYSOZYME), SERUM AND URINE

Norm:

SERUM			SI UNITS
Gel diffusion assay	0.4-1.3 mg/dL	4-13 µg/mL	4-13 mg/L
Nephelometric	0.36-0.78 mg/dL	3.6-7.8 µg/mL	3.6-7.8 mg/L
Radioimmunoassay	0.46 ± 0.08 mg/dL	4.6 ± 0.8 µg/mL	4.6 ± 0.8 mg/L
Turbidimetric	0.27-0.93 mg/dL	2.7-9.3 µg/mL	2.7-9.3 mg/L

URINE			
Random		<3 µg/mL	0-2.9 mg/L
24-Hour			1.3-3.6 mg/ 24 hours

Increased Serum and Urine Levels.

Glomerulonephritis, Hodgkin's disease, leukemia (acyte myelomonocytic, chronic myelomonocytic [CMML], chronic myelocytic [CML]), nephrosis, pleurisy (tuberculous type), pyelonephritis, renal insufficiency (severe), renal transplant rejection, urinary tract infection.

Increased Serum Levels.

Anemia (megaloblastic), Crohn's disease, infection (acute bacterial), sarcoidosis, ulcerative colitis, tuberculosis

Decreased. Neutropenia secondary to bone marrow hypoplasia.

Description. Muramidase (lysozyme) is an enzyme present in numerous body fluids (blood, saliva, sweat, tears, urine) and renal cells that is released into the bloodstream as a result of degradation of granulocytes and monocytes. Thus, it is a marker of mononuclear phagocytic cells. It normally functions in the process of gram-positive bacterial destruction. The proximal tubule of the kidney is the site of catabolism and reabsorption. Muramidase measurement may be used to differentiate lymphatic leukemia from myelogenous and monocytic leukemia, since muramidase is not produced when lymphocytes are degraded. Since levels drop when myelogenous and monocytic leukemia are successfully treated, muramidase can also provide an indicator of disease remission progress. The level of serum lysozyme has also been used as an indicator of central nervous system involvement associated with leukemia. Urine muramidase is excreted in renal tubular disease but not in glomerular disease. With normally functioning kidneys, serum levels must exceed three times the normal range before the enzyme will appear in the urine. However, in renal damage, serum levels may be normal in the presence of elevated urine levels.

Professional Considerations

1. Consent form NOT required.

M

2. **Preparation:**
   A. Tube: Red topped, red/gray topped, green-topped, or gold topped or lavender topped.
   B. Urine test should be prescheduled with the laboratory. Obtain a sterile, preservative-free plastic specimen container.
3. **Procedure:**
   A. Draw a 4-mL blood sample or collect a 5-mL random urine specimen.
4. **Postprocedure care:**
   A. Separate the serum and freeze it immediately in a plastic vial on dry ice.
   B. Freeze the urine specimen on dry ice if the specimen is not tested immediately.
5. **Client and family teaching:**
   A. Blood test results are normally available within 1 week. Urine results are normally available within 3 days.
6. **Factors that affect results:**
   A. Urine not maintained on ice after collection invalidates the results.
   B. Clients who are menstruating should be rescheduled for the urine test. Blood in the urine may produce falsely elevated results.
   C. Bacteria in the urine may produce falsely low results.
7. **Other data:**
   A. None.

MUSCLE BIOPSY, SPECIMEN

Norm. Interpretation by a pathologist is required.

Usage. Dermatomyositis, Duchenne's muscular dystrophy, muscular dystrophy, myalgia, polymyositis, neurogenic atrophy, pain (muscle and bone), trichinosis, and vasculitis.

Description. Microscopic examination of a piece of muscle for evaluation, diagnosis, or classification of muscular disease. The technique may be done via open muscle biopsy or via percutaneous fine needle aspiration muscle biopsy. The presence of hypercontracted fibers must be differentiated for cause. If accompanied by inflammation, hypercontracted fibers are indicative of

pathology. If no inflammation is present, hypercontracted fibers are attributed to strenuous exercise prior to the biopsy procedure.

Professional Considerations
1. Consent form IS required.

Risks
Bleeding, bruising, hematoma, infection.

Contraindications
Anticoagulant therapy, bleeding disorders, thrombocytopenia.

2. **Preparation:**
   A. Serum CK, 24-hour urine for creatine and serum creatinine, erythrocyte sedimentation rate (ESR), serum aldolase, and thyroid profile may be desirable before biopsy.
   B. Obtain a biopsy tray, sterile drapes, a sterile jar of sterile 0.9% saline, a sterile specimen container of formalin, and a sterile container of glutaraldehyde.
3. **Procedure:**
   A. Obtain a biopsy, using a sterile procedure. Biopsies for simple histologic examination may be obtained using thin needle aspiration. Fine needle aspiration may also be used for ocular muscle biopsy. To estimate capillary supply a sample sufficient to yield at least 50 muscle fibers is recommended.
   B. If histochemistry is desired, do not use epinephrine with lidocaine or procaine in securing the biopsy.
4. **Postprocedure care:**
   A. Place the biopsy in a sterile jar containing sterile saline. For histopathologic evaluation, place the specimen in formalin, and for electron microscopy, submit a small or minced specimen that is placed into glutaraldehyde.
   B. Label the container with the client's name, the room number, date, and site of specimen collection.
   C. The specimen should be delivered to the pathology department within 30 minutes. If the specimen cannot be delivered within

30 minutes, freeze it quickly, using liquid nitrogen.

D. Turnaround time is between 48 hours and 3 weeks.

5. **Client and family teaching:**
   A. Call a physician for signs of infection at the biopsy site over the next 24-48 hours: increasing pain, redness, swelling, purulent drainage, or for fever >101° F (38.3° C).
   B. Mild pain should be expected at the biopsy site. Severe pain should be reported to a physician.
   C. A mild analgesic may be required for pain control.
   D. Monitor for signs and symptoms of infection until the site is healed.

6. **Factors that affect results:**
   A. Use of wrong fixative.
   B. The specimen dries out.
   C. Unlabeled specimen container.
   D. Muscle that has been recently injected or undergone electromyographic studies may not be suitable for microscopic examination.

7. **Other data:**
   A. The quadriceps femoris is recommended for generalized diseases, and the gastrocnemius is suggested as a distal muscle for biopsy.
   B. The deltoid is not suitable for enzyme histochemistry.
   C. Tissue should be obtained from a relaxed, noncontracted isometric muscle.
   D. Optimally a specimen should be taken from a muscle with known disease that has NOT reached end-stage atrophy.
   E. Specimens for histologic examination are commonly stained with hematoxylin-eosin. This allows for the assessment of inflammatory processes.

MUSCLE PROFILE, SPECIMEN

(see Aldolase, Serum; Aspartate aminotransferase, Serum; Creatine kinase, Serum; Differential leukocyte count, Peripheral blood (eosinophils); Lactate dehydrogenase, Blood; Myoglobin, Serum; Thyroid test: Thyroxine (T₄) by RIA, Blood; Thyroid test: Thyroxine (T₄) free, Serum;

Thyroid test: Triiodothyronine (T₃) uptake, Blood; Thyroid test: Free thyroxine index, Serum)

MYCOBACTERIA, CEREBROSPINAL FLUID, CULTURE

(see Cerebrospinal fluid, Routine, Culture and cytology, Specimen)

MYCOPLASMA ENZYME IMMUNOASSAY, BLOOD

Norm. Current technology does not provide a recommended reference standard. There are inconsistencies in various test methodologies, laboratories, and manufacturers. Reference ranges are often determined by individual labs for each run.

Usage. Pneumonia, pertussis. Two M. *pneumoniae*–specific antibody levels, IgG and IgM, are typically used to evaluate the occurrence of current or past *M. pneumoniae* infection. The immune status of an individual can be determined with a single specimen. The use of paired samples, acute and convalescent, aids in the confirmation of the diagnosis of a recent or current infection. Testing should be done when clinical symptoms are present or exposure is suspected.

Description. *M. pneumoniae* is an aerobic bacteria, unique in that it does not have a cell wall. A *M. pneumoniae* infection may be asymptomatic or produce an upper respiratory tract disease or atypical pneumonia. *M. pneumoniae* is transmitted from an infected person in close contact with another person through respiratory droplets, and thus, is a common cause of community-acquired pneumonia. Signs and symptoms include nonproductive cough, sore throat, low-grade fever, malaise, middle-ear involvement, scattered rales and rhonchi, and cervical adenopathy. Extrapulmonary symptoms, such as gastrointestinal symptoms and skin rashes, may also occur. *M. pneumoniae* infection is difficult to differentiate from viral diseases by clinical symptoms alone. Differentiation of the organism is important because the typical

M

empirical treatment of respiratory infections with beta-lactam antibiotics is not effective with *M. pneumoniae.* This test involves an IgM enzyme immunoassay and is often carried out in conjunction with a polymerase chain reaction test on a nasopharyngeal sample. Together, these findings represent the most sensitive, specific and rapid diagnosis for *M. pneumoniae.*

Professional Considerations
1. Consent form NOT required.
2. **Preparation:**
   A. Tube: red topped, lavender topped, green topped, red/gray topped, or yellow topped.
   B. Obtain a specimen swab if a nasopharyngeal specimen will also be tested.
3. **Procedure:**
   A. Collect 6 mL of blood. (2-4 mL for children). Label sample clearly as "acute" or "convalescent." Acute samples should be collected as soon as possible after the onset of symptoms and not later than several days after onset. The second, or convalescent, sample should be collected 14 to 21 days after the acute specimen was collected.
   B. Obtain a nasopharyngeal specimen using the swab.
   C. Transport to laboratory immediately. Unacceptable samples include those that are severely lipemic, hemolyzed, or contaminated.
   D. Paired samples of acute and convalescent samples should be run together.
4. **Postprocedure care:**
   A. Stability of sample: after separation from clot; ambient (2°-8° C)—2 days, refrigerated (4° C)—2 weeks, frozen—1 year. Avoid repeated freeze-thaw cycles.
5. **Client and family teaching:**
   A. Results are normally available in 3-5 days.
6. **Factors that affect results:**
   A. A single positive serum result indicates prior exposure to *M. pneumoniae.* The antibody level in a single specimen does not typically indicate disease severity.
   B. *M. pneumoniae*–specific IgM antibodies become elevated 7 days after the onset of symptoms, and levels peak at 2-3 weeks. A single elevated IgM level is often used to support the diagnosis of a M. pneumoniae infection, however, low IgM levels can remain for years after an infection. The evaluation of paired sera, acute, and convalescent samples for an increasing IgM level is recommended if a more definitive diagnosis is necessary. The absence of *M. pneumoniae*–specific IgM antibody in the blood 10-20 days after the onset of symptoms has strong negative predictive value for the presence of a current *M. pneumoniae* infection.
   C. *M. pneumoniae*–specific IgG antibody levels increase 7-14 days after the onset of symptoms and can remain elevated for years. Use of paired IgG levels, acute and convalescent, or comparison of IgG levels to IgM levels is recommended for definitive diagnosis of acute *Mycoplasma* infection.
   D. False-positive results may occur in clients with *Ureaplasma, Mycoplasma hominis, Mycoplasma genitalium,* pancreatitis, bacterial meningitis, and other acute inflammatory disease. The incidence of *M. pneumoniae* IgG antibodies in the general population is high.
   E. False-negative results may occur if samples are drawn too early after the onset. Some individuals may never generate detectable antibody levels. Decreased production of specific IgM antibodies is associated with increased age and reinfection with *M. pneumoniae.*
7. **Other data:**
   A. *M. pneumoniae* infection can have a long incubation period, and reinfection may occur.
   B. Elevated cold agglutinins are associated with but not specific to *M. pneumoniae* infections. Other associated lab data include CBC (WB exceed 10,000/μL in approximately 30% of cases) and greatly elevated erythrocyte sedimentation rates. Culturing this bacteria is difficult, since the organism requires special growth media and incubation time is 5-20 days, which is 6-20 times slower than that of most bacteria.

C. *M. pneumoniae*–specific IgM and IgG antibodies play an important role in the ability of immunocompetent individuals to eliminate the infection in 10-14 days with the use of antimicrobial agents. Macrolides or tetracyclines are generally effective in reducing the duration of the illness.

D. See also *Mycoplasma titer, Blood.*

MYCOPLASMA TITER, BLOOD

Norm. Negative or complement fixation (CF) <1:64 and Seradyn Color Vue (SCV) agglutination <1:320.

Positive. Diarrhea and mycoplasmal pneumonia.

Description. *Mycoplasma* organisms are of the pleuropneumonia type that can pass through tiny bacteriologic filters, the smallest ranging from 125 to 250 nm. *Mycoplasma* bacteria are the smallest free-living organisms, characteristically have no cell wall, and are dependent for survival on a host, which is most commonly a child. The mechanisms by which *Mycoplasma* interact with the immune defenses of the host are elusive. Commonly causing upper respiratory tract infection in children, newer research is linking *M. pneumoniae*, along with *Chlamydia pneumoniae* as significant causative organisms in pneumonias of the lower respiratory tract in those under 5 years of age. There is no quick method for pinpointing the organism as a source of infection. Therefore, diagnosis and treatment are often based on clinical symptoms, with the *Mycoplasma* serologic titer, immunoassay or polymerase chain reaction.

Professional Considerations

1. Consent form NOT required.
2. Preparation:
   A. Tube: Red topped, red/gray topped, or gold topped.
3. Procedure:
   A. Draw a 3-mL blood sample.
4. Postprocedure care:
   A. Draw a convalescent sample of blood 10-14 days later.

5. Client and family teaching:
   A. Return in 10-14 days to have another blood sample drawn from the vein to obtain accurate results.
6. Factors that affect results:
   A. False-positive results may occur in clients with acute pancreatitis or streptococcal infection.
   B. A diet of green, leafy vegetables may produce false-positive results.
7. Other data:
   A. High titers are not significant for recent infection, since antibodies may persist >1 year and repeated infections occur.
   B. Mycoplasmal pneumonia is treated with tetracycline or erythromycin.
   C. Serologic confirmation is desirable, since *Mycoplasma* is difficult to culture. See *Mycoplasma enzyme immunoassay, Blood.*

MYELIN BASIC PROTEIN (MBP), SPECIMEN

(see *Cerebrospinal fluid, Myelin basic protein, oligoclonal bands, protein, and protein electrophoresis, Specimen*)

MYELOGRAM, DIAGNOSTIC

Norm. Normal cervical, lumbar, or thoracic myelogram. Normal spinal subarachnoid space with no obstructions.

Usage. Arachnoiditis, back pain, disk rupture, spinal problems, accidental injury, tumors of the spine, degenerative disease of the spine, nerve plexus lesions, cancer metastasis to the spine.

Description. Myelography is a radiographic study of the spinal cord and nerve roots by using contrast dye, contrast oil, or air injected by way of spinal needle into the spinal subarachnoid space. Myelography use is declining because magnetic resonance imaging (MRI) can usually match the findings of myelography with less risk to the client. Myelography is more often reserved for conditions that cannot be evaluated via MRI or CT, such as weight-bearing flexion and extension views, or walking views. Use of oil contrast has the disadvantage of tissue irritation and poor absorption by the subarachnoid spaces. Air contrast may be used instead of oil, but in this case, tomography is essential to improve visualization.

Professional Considerations

1. Consent form IS required.

Risks

Allergic reaction to dye (itching, hives, rash, tight feeling in the throat, shortness of breath, bronchospasm, anaphylaxis, death); contrast-induced renal failure, intramedullary cord injection. Multiple sclerosis may be worsened by this procedure.

Contraindications

Previous allergy to dye, iodine, or shellfish; renal insufficiency; bleeding abnormalities or clients receiving anticoagulants; increased intracranial pressure, low back pain, spinal deformities, or infections near the puncture site, pregnancy (because of radioactive iodine crossing the blood-placental barrier).

2. **Preparation:**
   A. Sedation or narcotic analgesia should be considered before this procedure.
   B. Shave the lumbar area if necessary.
   C. Obtain a lumbar puncture tray, sterile drapes, 1-2% lidocaine (Xylocaine), iodized Pantopaque oil or water-soluble iodine metrizamide contrast medium, antiseptic, and sterile gauze.
   D. If metrizamide is to be used as a contrast dye, discontinue the use of phenothiazines 48 hours before the procedure.
   E. Obtain baseline vital signs.
   F. Have emergency equipment readily available.
   G. If increased intracranial pressure is suspected, a CT of the rain should be performed before lumbar puncture to rule out this condition.
   H. See *Client and family teaching.*

3. **Procedure:**
   A. The client is positioned on the side with the knees drawn up toward the abdomen and the chin on the chest for the lumbar puncture.
   B. The lumbar puncture is verified by fluoroscopy.
   C. Spinal fluid is generally obtained for analysis.
   D. 5-15 mL of iodized Pantopaque oil dye or water-soluble iodine metrizamide contrast is injected into the subarachnoid space in the lumbar area or into the cisterna magna.
   E. The client is tilted to maneuver oil up and down the spine.
   F. Radiographic films are taken.
   G. Oil is removed by aspiration after the procedure.

4. **Postprocedure care:**
   A. Cleanse the puncture site with antiseptic and cover with a dry, sterile dressing.
   B. See *Lumbar puncture, Diagnostic.*
   C. Do not administer phenothiazines for nausea or vomiting if water-soluble contrast was used.
   D. Results are normally available within 48 hours.

5. **Client and family teaching:**
   A. The client should fast from food and fluids for 4-8 hours before the procedure.
   B. The procedure takes 1 hour.
   C. Review activity limitations.
   D. Drink 6-8 glasses of water or other fluids each day for 2 days (when not contraindicated) to hasten removal of any contrast medium.
   E. Potential side effects or complications include arachnoiditis, headache, nausea and vomiting, seizures, spinal infection, subarachnoid bleeding, and tingling at the puncture site.
   F. Observe the puncture site for bleeding, hematoma, or swelling for 24-48 hours after the procedure.
   G. A mild analgesic may be required for pain control.
   H. Monitor the lumbar puncture site for signs and symptoms of infection until the site is healed.

6. **Factors that affect results:**
   A. Conditions such as convulsions, pain, stiffness of the neck, and stupor may interfere with the procedure.
   B. Severe kyphosis or scoliosis may prohibit completion of this procedure.
7. **Other data:**
   A. Dye usage affects preparation and postprocedure care.

MYOGLOBIN, QUALITATIVE, URINE

Norm. Negative or <20 ng/mL.

Positive. Acute alcohol intoxication with delirium tremens, acute or chronic muscular disease, barbiturate toxicity, burns (severe), diabetic acidosis, glycogen and lipid storage diseases, hyperthermia, hypothermia, hypokalemia, hypophosphatemia, muscular dystrophy, myocardial infarction, poisoning, polymyositis, renal failure, rhabdomyolysis, surgical procedure, trauma, and viral or bacterial infection. Herbs or natural remedies include licorice (*Glycyrrhiza glabra*), which can cause an intoxication.

Description. Myoglobin is a heme-containing, oxygen-binding, low-molecular-weight protein similar to hemoglobin that is exclusive to striated and nonstriated skeletal or cardiac muscle. It serves as a short-term oxygen store, carrying the muscle from one contraction to the next. It is released into the interstitial fluid as early as 3 hours after any muscle injury including a myocardial infarct and remains detected in the urine for up to 7 days later.

Professional Considerations
1. Consent form NOT required.
2. **Preparation:**
   A. Obtain a sterile specimen container.
3. **Procedure:**
   A. Collect a 10-mL random urine specimen in a sterile plastic container without preservatives.
   B. Collection time should be early morning when possible.

4. **Postprocedure care:**
   A. Specimens should be refrigerated.
5. **Client and family teaching:**
   A. Results are normally available within 72 hours.
6. **Factors that affect results:**
   A. False-negative results are likely if the test is used for screening.
   B. The presence of hypochlorite or microbial peroxidase or other oxidizing contaminants may cause false-positive results.
   C. Clients should not receive isotopes 7 days before testing.
   D. High concentrations of vitamin C decrease the sensitivity of this test.
7. **Other data:**
   A. Because myoglobin is excreted by the kidney, renal function should be assessed.
   B. Serum levels are preferred to urine levels when one is obtaining myoglobin values.
   C. See also *Myoglobin, Serum.*

MYOGLOBIN, SERUM

Norm. RIA <85 ng/mL (or 5-70 µg/L, SI units).

Usage. In combination with other tests, helps diagnose myocardial ischemia; serial values are used to monitor for reinfarct, success of thrombolytic treatment, and myocardial injury during open-heart surgery.

Increased. Acute alcohol intoxication with delirium tremens, after cardioversion (possible increase), after open-heart surgery, angina (possible increase), burns (severe), congestive heart failure (possible increase), dermatomyositis, dysrhythmias (possible increase), glycogen and lipid storage diseases, hyperthermia, hypothermia, muscular dystrophy, myocardial infarction (increased levels are detected 2-3 hours after injury, peak at 6-9 hours, and return to baseline level within 36 hours), polymyositis, renal failure, rhabdomyolysis, shock, skeletal muscle injury or extreme skeletal muscle exertion, surgical procedure, systemic lupus erythematosus (SLE), trauma, and viral or bacterial infection. Drugs include ethyl alcohol (ethanol)

M

(heavy use). Herbs or natural remedies include licorice (*Glycyrrhiza glabra*), which can cause intoxication.

Description. Myoglobin is a heme-containing, oxygen-binding protein similar to hemoglobin that is exclusive to striated and nonstriated skeletal or cardiac muscle. It serves as a short-term oxygen store, carrying the muscle from one contraction to the next. It is released into the interstitial fluid with elevated serum levels detected as early as 30-60 minutes after a myocardial infarct or damage to any muscle tissue. Serum myoglobin is generally detected earlier than traditional cardiac enzymes (total creatinine kinase [CK] or isoenzyme creatinine kinase–MB [CK-MB]). Because myoglobin is contained in both skeletal and cardiac muscle, it is not used alone to diagnose myocardial infarction. Tests used in combination with myoglobin for this purpose include troponin, CK-MB, with or without carbonic anhydrase III (a marker for skeletal muscle damage). Myoglobin characteristics are being studied for their use in post-MI risk stratification. One study found that levels above the MI detection threshold (>110 μg/L) independently predictive of an increased mortality rate at 6 months. Another study found that when the 12-hour post-MI myoglobin level is lower than 240 ng/mL, clients had a high 30-day survival rate.

Professional Considerations
1. Consent form NOT required.
2. **Preparation:**
   A. Tube: Red topped, red/gray topped, or gold topped.
3. **Procedure:**
   A. Draw a 2-mL blood sample.
4. **Postprocedure care:**
   A. Specimens should be refrigerated.
   B. Specimens may be frozen and stored for up to 2 years.
5. **Client and family teaching:**
   A. Results are normally available within 48 hours.
6. **Factors that affect results:**
   A. Hemolysis of the specimen invalidates the results.
   B. False-negative results are likely if the test is used for screening.

C. Clients should have no isotopes 7 days before testing.
D. Serum levels must be obtained within 2-12 hours of the onset of symptoms of a myocardial infarct to be useful in assessing myocardial injury.
E. Normal levels may be higher in men compared to women but increase in both sexes with age.
F. Hypertriglyceridemia or postprandial specimens may affect the results.
G. Serum myoglobin has been found to increase proportionally with the size of muscle damage.
7. **Other data:**
   A. Serum myoglobin may lack specificity in the diagnosis of myocardial infarct. Elevated levels are also observed after angina, chest trauma, cocaine use, electrical accidents, exercise, intramuscular injection, muscular injury of any type, and renal failure. Within 8 hours of symptoms, myoglobin specificity is 97.9% for acute MI, as opposed to CK-MB, which has 100% specificity.
   B. Increased levels should be correlated with client signs and symptoms.
   C. Myoglobin can be measured by a variety of approaches, including fluorometric measurement, latex agglutination, and nephelometric and turbidimetric assay. Each approach has its own reference range.
   D. IM injections, bicycle exercise, and cardiac catheterization should NOT increase levels.
   E. See also *Myoglobin, Qualitative, Urine.*

MYOGLOBIN, URINE
(*see Myoglobin, Qualitative, Urine*)

MYSOLINE
(*see Primidone, Serum*)

NAP
(*see Leukocyte alkaline phosphatase, Blood*)

NARCOTICS DRUG SCREEN, URINE
(see Toxicology, Drug screen, Urine)

NASOPHARYNGEAL CULTURE, SWAB, DIAGNOSTIC
(see Culture, Routine, Specimen)

NASAL CULTURE, SWAB, DIAGNOSTIC
(see Culture, Routine, Specimen)

NATRIURETIC PEPTIDES, ATRIAL (ANP, ATRIAL NATRIURETIC HORMONE, ATRIAL NATRIURETIC FACTOR), BRAIN (BNP, B-TYPE), C-TYPE (CNP), PLASMA

Norm:

	IMMUNOFLUORESCENCE ASSAY	SI UNITS
ANP		
Adults	20-77 pg/mL	20-77 ng/L
Children		
10-15 years	>55 pg/mL	>55 ng/L
Infants		
3 days	165-185 pg/mL	165-185 ng/L
1 week	165-185 pg/mL	165-185 ng/L
10 days	98-122 pg/mL	98-122 ng/L
30-60 days	52-72 pg/mL	52-72 ng/L
BNP		
Male		
<45 years	<25 pg/mL	<25 ng/L
45-54 years	<4 pg/mL	<4 ng/L
55-64 years	<73 pg/mL	<73 ng/L
65-74 years	<64 pg/mL	<64 ng/L
≥75 years	<79 pg/mL	<79 ng/L
Female		
<45 years	<48 pg/mL	<48 pg/mL
45-54 years	<73	
55-64 years	<82	
65-74 years	<96	
≥75 years	<181	
CNP	Norms not established. Consult reference range provided with test results.	

Usage. Helps distinguish heart failure from other causes of dyspnea; Under investigation for usefulness in assessing prognosis for long-term survival of clients with heart failure and acute myocardial infarction.

Increased ANP. Atrial fibrillation, congestive heart failure (acute), cardiovascular disease accompanied by increased preload, dysrhythmia (parox-ysmal atrial tachycardia), hyperthyroidism, lactate-induced panic attacks, left ventricular enlargement, myocardial ischemia, myotonic dystrophy, pacemaker (atrial), sleep apnea, small cell lung cancer, subarachnoid hemorrhage, ventricular pacing.

Increased BNP. Congestive heart failure (acute), cardiovascular disease accompanied by increased preload, hyperthyroidism, lactate induced panic attacks, left ventricular enlargement, myocardial ischemia, myotonic dystrophy, pacemaker (atrial), sleep apnea, small cell lung cancer, subarachnoid hemorrhage, ventricular pacing.

Increased CNP. Has been found to increase in response to local inflammation.

Decreased ANP. Congestive heart failure (chronic). Drugs include prazosin, urapidil, and xipamide.

Decreased BNP. BNP has been found to return to normal levels after successful treatment of volume overload.

Decreased CNP. Not established.

Description. Natriuretic peptides are substances produced by the body that function in regulation of fluid balance through feedback mechanisms from and to the renin-angiotensin-aldosterone system. *Atrial natriuretic peptide* (ANP) is released by cardiac cells in the atria of the heart and *Brain or B-type natriuretic peptide* (BNP) is released by cardiac cells in the ventricles of the heart. Both ANP and BNP are secreted in response to the stimulation of the heart's volume receptors by the stretch from increased blood volume. ANP is also released in response to atrial fibrillation and supraventricular tachycardia. ANP and BNP reduce renal reabsorption of sodium, thus having diuretic and antihypertensive effects. They also reduces blood pressure by blocking the secretion of aldosterone and renin and inhibiting the action of angiotensin II. The net effect is reduced preload, afterload, blood volume, and a reduction in systemic hypertension. Measurement of ANP and BNP helps identify a subnormal levels as a cause of chronic congestive heart failure. *C-type natriuretic peptide* (CNP) is produced in the brain, by most of the major endocrine glands, and locally from endothelial tissue and from macrophages and is not considered to be a cardiac peptide. CNP is thought to contribute to local neuroendocrine regulation.

Professional Considerations
1. Consent form NOT required.

2. **Preparation:**
   A. Tube: Lavender topped. Also obtain ice.
   B. For dialysis clients, collect the sample AFTER dialysis and on the same day of the week as prior samples.
3. **Procedure:**
   A. Draw a 5-mL blood sample.
4. **Postprocedure care:**
   A. Place the specimen immediately on ice and deliver it to the laboratory for immediate spinning.
5. **Client and family teaching:**
   A. Results are normally available within 24 hours.
6. **Factors that affect results:**
   A. Results are invalidated if the sample is not kept on ice until it is spun and frozen.
7. **Other data:**
   A. Secretion of ANH and vasopressin by small cell lung cancer may be a contributing factor to hyponatremia.
   B. Natriuretic peptides are relatively new in medical knowledge. ANP was first identified in 1984 and BNP was not identified until 1988.
   C. Recombinant natriuretic peptides such as nesitiride (Natrecor) are being used for treatment of acute decompensated congestive heart failure.

NEEDLE ASPIRATION, DIAGNOSTIC

Norm. Nonmalignant, or negative.

Usage. Essential to diagnosing malignancies and benign growths. Also used to evaluate tissue for reaction to hormones; these results assist in selecting appropriate therapy for cancer.

Description. Surgical procedure in which a sample of body tissue or fluid is removed transcutaneously through a needle and then examined microscopically for abnormal cells or tested in a hormone receptor assay. This procedure can be performed on an ambulatory surgery basis under local anesthesia and can help prevent unnecessary surgery.

Professional Considerations
1. Consent form IS required.

Risks

Infection at needle aspiration site.

Contraindications

Cutaneous infection at site.

2. **Preparation:**
   A. Obtain 1%-2% lidocaine (Xylocaine) for local anesthesia, a cutting needle, a sterile cup with normal saline, and a heparinized tube.
3. **Procedure:**
   A. Position the client supine.
   B. Under local anesthesia, a cutting needle such as the Cope's or Vim-Silverman is inserted into the suspected area, and a core of tissue is removed and placed into normal saline, or fluid is aspirated and placed into a heparinized tube.
4. **Postprocedure care:**
   A. Apply a dry, sterile dressing to the site.
   B. Label the specimens and transport them to the laboratory promptly.
   C. Assess vital signs every 15 minutes × 2.
   D. Monitor the site every 2 hours × 3 for bleeding, inflammation, or drainage.
   E. Results are normally available in 48-72 hours.
5. **Client and family teaching:**
   A. Monitor for drainage and inflammation for 24-48 hours.
   B. A mild analgesic may be required for pain control.
   C. Call the physician for signs of infection at the procedure site: increasing pain, redness, swelling, purulent drainage, or for fever >101° F (38.3° C).
6. **Factors that affect results:**
   A. Failure to obtain adequate sample(s) or a sample from a nonsuspect site or to properly prepare the smear can result in a false negative finding.
7. **Other data:**
   A. Permanent microscopic sections are preferred to frozen sections because permanent sections have more clarity.
   B. A negative result does not always exclude the diagnosis of cancer.

NEISSERIA GONORRHOEAE SMEAR, SPECIMEN

Norm. Negative.

Positive. Gonorrhea.

Description. *Neisseria gonorrhoeae* is a pyogenic, gram-negative, oxidase-positive cocci that is an obligate parasite of humans. *N. gonorrhoeae* inhabits the mucous membranes of the genital tract, causing gonorrhea. Symptoms include dysuria, fever, pharyngitis, peripheral skin lesions, proctitis, and purulent urethral discharge. It may also cause inflammation of any of the mucous membranes of the body. Females are often asymptomatic. Left untreated, gonorrhea leads to skin lesions, arthritis, meningitis, and reproductive problems. *N. gonorrhoeae* is most often found in the urethra of males and the endocervical canal of females. This test is performed using nucleic acid amplification, a method with improved sensitivity over and higher cost than older methods. It is often performed in conjunction with testing for *Chlamydia trachomatis*, another sexually transmitted organism.

Professional Considerations
1. Consent form NOT required.
2. **Preparation:**
   A. Determine the potential infected area(s): anus, cervix, conjunctivae, endocervix, skin lesion, throat, and urethra.
   B. Wait 1 hour after urination to collect urethral specimens.
   C. Obtain a wooden scraper or swab and a glass slide with frosted edges.
3. **Procedure:**
   A. Obtain a sterile microbiologic smear. With a swab, swab the potential infected area for 10 seconds.
   B. Apply to a glass slide and allow to air dry.
   C. Label the slide.
4. **Postprocedure care:**
   A. Place the air-dried slide in a sterile container and send it to the laboratory.
   B. Results are normally available immediately or within 24 hours.
5. **Client and family teaching:**
   A. The client should be referred for medical follow-up examination

N

after the treatment is concluded. Repeat cultures or smears may be necessary to assess response to treatment.

B. The use of condoms significantly reduces the risk of sexually transmitted diseases.

C. Gonorrhea infection is treatable with antibiotics.

D. If results are positive, provide the client with the appropriate information on sexually transmitted diseases.

   i. Notify all sexual partners from the previous 90 days to be tested for gonorrhea infection.

   ii. Do not have sexual relations until the physician confirms that the infection is gone.

   iii. Referral for HIV testing should be reviewed and offered to all clients.

E. Do not use feminine hygiene sprays or douche during treatment.

F. Wear underpants and pantyhose that have a cotton lining in the crotch.

G. Take showers instead of tub baths until the infection is gone.

6. **Factors that affect results:**

A. False-positive results occur in 50% of endocervical specimens because normal flora have similar morphologic appearance.

B. Insufficient specimen volume.

7. **Other data:**

A. DNA probe assay (Gen-Probe, San Diego) is an alternative test that can be used to diagnose *N. gonorrhoeae*.

B. A culture is necessary to confirm diagnosis.

C. See also *Genitals, Neisseria gonorrhoeae, Culture.*

NEPHROTOMOGRAPHY, DIAGNOSTIC

Norm. Normal kidney size, shape, and position.

Usage. Adrenal tumor, carcinoma of the kidney, nephrolithiasis, polycystic kidney disease (diagnostic when used in conjunction with ultrasound), and renal laceration.

Description. Radiographic examination of a single plane of renal tissue. It is a routine procedure performed during urography. Delineates renal borders and aids in distinguishing cystic from solid lesions. Precisely locating the kidneys, however, can be difficult. Nephrotomography may be performed with excretory urography (intravenous pyelography). Delineates renal borders and aids in distinguishing cystic from solid lesions. The use of this test for detection of nephrolithiasis is decreasing as the newer technique of three-dimensional spiral computed tomography equals the accuracy of nephrotomography for this purpose.

Professional Considerations
1. Consent form IS required.

Risks
Radiation exposure, allergic reaction to contrast media (itching, hives, rash, tight feeling in the throat, shortness of breath, bronchospasm, anaphylaxis, death), contrast-induced renal failure.

Contraindications
Pregnancy, previous allergy to dye, iodine, or shellfish, pregnancy (because of radioactive iodine crossing the blood-placental barrier), renal insufficiency.

2. **Preparation:**

A. Have emergency equipment readily available.

B. Residual barium from prior studies should be completely cleared from the gastrointestinal tract before this test is performed.

C. See *Client and family teaching.*

3. **Procedure:**

A. A plain film of the kidneys is taken.

B. Contrast medium is injected intravenously, the first half in 5 minutes (rapid phase) and the next half in 10 minutes (slow phase).

C. Serial tomograms are initiated as soon as the slow phase begins.

D. The procedure takes 1 hour.

4. **Postprocedure care:**

A. Monitor vital signs and urinary output every 4 hours for 24 hours.

5. Client and family teaching:
   A. Fast from food and fluids for 8 hours before the procedure.
   B. Be alert for an allergic reaction to the dye for 24 hours (itching, hives, shortness of breath, hypotension). Call the physician immediately if these symptoms occur or go to the nearest emergency room.
6. Factors that affect results:
   A. Residual barium interferes with visualization.
7. Other data:
   A. Perform this procedure with caution on individuals who have severe cardiovascular disease, multiple myeloma, asthma, pheochromocytoma, or myasthenia gravis.
   B. This test is routinely performed with an intravenous pyelogram (IVP).
   C. See also *Intravenous pyelography (IVP, Excretory urography), Diagnostic.*

NERVE BIOPSY, DIAGNOSTIC

Norm. Negative.

Usage. Amyloid infiltration, demyelination, hypertrophic polyneuropathy, inflammation axonal degeneration, lepromatous leprosy lesions, metachromatic leukodystrophy, peripheral neuropathy, sarcoidosis, and vasculitis.

Description. Removal of peripheral nerve tissue for electromicroscopic, biochemical, histochemical, or virologic examination to establish a diagnosis for neuropathies when radiologic evaluation and direct inspection have been inconclusive. Findings must be used in conjunction with clinical history and assessment findings for the most accurate diagnosis.

Professional Considerations
1. Consent form IS required.

Risks
Bruising, infection.

Contraindications
Anticoagulant therapy, bleeding disorders, thrombocytopenia.

2. Preparation:
   A. Prepare for local anesthesia and obtain biopsy instruments and a 3 × 5-inch index card.
   B. Consult laboratory personnel for special handling of the specimen if electron microscopic examination is required.
3. Procedure:
   A. Place a 1.5-cm portion of nerve on cardboard with the firmness of a 3 × 5-inch index card and then straighten and slightly stretch it.
   B. Allow the specimen to adhere to the cardboard for 1 minute.
   C. Keep the handling of specimens to a minimum.
   D. Submerge the specimen in 0.05 mol/L phosphate-buffered glutaraldehyde.
4. Postprocedure care:
   A. Transport specimens to the laboratory immediately.
5. Client and family teaching:
   A. Monitor for drainage and inflammation for 24-48 hours.
   B. A mild analgesic may be required for pain control.
   C. Call the physician for signs of infection at the procedure site: increasing pain, redness, swelling, purulent drainage, or for fever >101° F (38.3° C).
6. Factors that affect results:
   A. Drying out of samples invalidates the results.
7. Other data:
   A. The nerve where the biopsy specimen was taken will not regenerate.
   B. The most common nerve used for biopsy is the superficial peroneal sensory nerve.

NERVE CONDUCTION STUDIES, DIAGNOSTIC

Norm. Maximum conduction velocity = 40-80 msec for those 3 years of age and older. Distal latency <4 msec and amplitude 13.2 mV. Values decreased by half for infants and elderly. Equipment and technique vary; thus laboratories establish their own norms.

N

Usage. Carpal tunnel syndrome, peripheral entrapment neuropathies, tarsal tunnel syndrome, and thoracic outlet syndrome.

Description. Percutaneous stimulation of peripheral, sensory, or mixed sensory motor nerve fibers. Recording of muscle and sensory action potentials distinguishes between disease processes that cause both segmental demyelinative lesions and axonal losses.

Professional Considerations
1. Consent form IS required.

Risks
Pain at needle-electrode sites.

Contraindications
Nicotine-patch drug users.

2. Preparation:
   A. Shave the area for better conduction if needed.
3. Procedure:
   A. An electrode is applied to the specific nerve area.
   B. Electrical current is passed through and read distally to determine nerve conduction time.
4. Postprocedure care:
   A. Assess the skin area for irritation.
5. Client and family teaching:
   A. Results are normally available within 48 hours.
6. Factors that affect results:
   A. Poor conduction of electrodes due to use of outdated electrodes, improper site preparation, or movement during the procedure.
   B. Lower amplitudes are demonstrated in obese clients than in thin clients.
7. Other data:
   A. Professional interpretation must follow the results of the study.
   B. Supplements electromyographic studies.

NEUROGRAPHY

(see Magnetic resonance neurography, Diagnostic)

NEURON-SPECIFIC ENOLASE (NSE), SERUM

Norm.   0-12.5 ng/mL
Cord blood: 4.8-19.4 µg/L
Method:
  Serum RIA   0-9 ng/mL
  Serum EIA   1-6 ng/mL

Increased. Brain cell distress (e.g., secondary to seizure, tumor, cerebral edema, traumatic brain injury), medullary carcinoma of the thyroid, neuroblastoma (marker) that is metastatic, pancreatic islet cell tumor, small cell carcinoma of the lung, and uremia.

Decreased. Not applicable.

Description. Neuron-specific enolase (NSE) is an isoenzyme of a glycolytic enzyme found in neuronal and neuroendocrine cells of the central and peripheral nervous system. NSE is produced by adult T-cell leukemia and other tumor cells and is a sensitive tumor marker used to monitor response to therapy or detect neuroendocrine cell destruction disease progression because there is a strong correlation between disease state and concentration. NSE levels correlate with outcome in neuroblastoma.

Professional Considerations
1. Consent form NOT required.
2. Preparation:
   A. Tube: Red topped, red/gray topped, or gold topped. Also obtain ice.
3. Procedure:
   A. Collect a 2-mL blood sample. Place the specimen in a container of ice.
4. Postprocedure care:
   A. Send the specimen to the laboratory immediately. Serum must be separated and refrigerated within 45 minutes of collection. The specimen should be frozen at −70° C if not tested the same day.
5. Client and family teaching:
   A. Results may not be available for as long as 7 days.
6. Factors that affect results:
   A. Serum is not separated after collection.

7. Other data:

A. This test is not useful in screening for early stages of neoplasms.

B. Clients with NSE over 15 ng/mL are likely to have metastatic small cell lung cancer.

NEUT, BLOOD

(see Differential leukocyte count, Peripheral blood)

NEUTROPHIL ALKALINE PHOSPHATASE

(see Leukocyte alkaline phosphatase, Blood)

NEUTROPHILS, BLOOD

(see Differential leukocyte count, Peripheral blood)

NH₃, BLOOD

(see Ammonia, Blood and Urine)

NIPPLE DISCHARGE CYTOLOGY, SPECIMEN

(see Cytologic study of nipple discharge, Diagnostic)

NITRITE, BACTERIA SCREEN, URINE

Norm. <0.1 mg/dL, <100,000 organisms/mL, or negative.

Usage. Cystitis, differentiation between acute bacterial infections and viral or tuberculosis (TB) infections, dysuria, pyelonephritis, shigellosis, and urinary tract infection.

Description. Humans normally oxidize ingested nitrite and excrete it as nitrate. The presence of nitrite in urine indicates a urinary tract infection caused by organisms that reduce nitrate back to nitrite.

Professional Considerations
1. Consent form NOT required.

2. Preparation:

A. Cleanse the urethral orifice with a sterile wipe.

B. Obtain a sterile plastic container.

3. Procedure:

A. Collect a first morning void of 12 mL of urine, or a specimen collected at least 4 hours after the client last voided, in a sterile plastic container.

4. Postprocedure care:

A. Refrigerate the sample within 2 hours.

5. Client and family teaching:

A. Results are normally available within 72 hours.

6. Factors that affect results:

A. Incidence of false-positive results is 12%-34% as a result of age less than 2 months, Candida albicans and Nocardia infections, echovirus, hemophilia A, Hodgkin's disease, lymphoma, malaria, and parasitic infections.

B. Incidence of false-negatives is 5%-9% as a result of agammaglobulinemia, diabetes mellitus, localized infection, sickle cell anemia, and systemic lupus erythematosus.

C. Drugs that may cause false-positive results include oral contraceptives and phenazopyridine.

D. Drugs that may cause false-negative results include antibiotics, anti-inflammatories (corticosteroids and phenylbutazone), and ascorbic acid concentration >25 mg/dL in specimens containing <0.03 mg/dL of nitrite ions.

E. Diuresis, delay of several hours without refrigeration of specimen, and contamination in obtaining specimen invalidate the results.

F. Dipsticks stored in ambient humidity may produce false-negative results.

G. Another degree of color development on the reagent test strip is NOT proportional to the number of bacteria present.

H. Bacteria infections are less likely to be detected when the urine output is high.

N

I. An increased urine specific gravity will decrease the sensitivity of this test.
7. Other data:
   A. Urinary tract infections may be caused from organisms that will not produce a positive nitrite test
   B. If nitrites are positive on the dipstick or are negative but the client is symptomatic, a urine culture should be performed.

NITROBLUE TETRAZOLIUM TEST (NBT), DIAGNOSTIC

Norm. 2%-8% segmented neutrophils reduce the dye.

Increased. Ulcerative colitis.

Usage. Chronic granulomatous disease in childhood.

Description. This demanding test uses different reagents to differentiate bacterial from nonbacterial infections. Nitroblue tetrazolium is a yellow compound that turns blue when reduced by an increase in the hexose monophosphate shunt generated by phagocytic activity. In granulomatous disease, neutrophil phagocytic activity is absent, thus resulting in absence of blue dye formation. This test is often replaced by the formazan test, which depends on the reduction of nitroblue tetrazolium to insoluble formazan. The formazan test is simpler to perform and more cost effective.

Professional Considerations
1. Consent form NOT required.
2. Preparation:
   A. Preschedule this test with the laboratory.
   B. Tube: Green topped (heparinized) tube.
3. Procedure:
   A. Draw a 4-mL blood sample.
4. Postprocedure care:
   A. Write the collection time on the laboratory requisition.
   B. Transport the specimen to the laboratory immediately.

5. Client and family teaching:
   A. Results are normally available in 72 hours.
6. Factors that affect results:
   A. Reject clotted specimens or specimens received more than 1 hour after collection.
   B. False-negative results may occur in clients with solid cancerous nonlymphomatous tumors.
   C. Specificity is poor because many secondary diseases cause false-positive results.
   D. Diets high in fats may affect the results.
7. Other data:
   A. Neutrophils reduce the dye to dark blue-black on phagocytosis.
   B. Unreliable in differentiating bacterial from viral infections.

NITROGLYCERIN SCAN
(*see Heart scan, Diagnostic*)

NOCARDIA CULTURE, ALL SITES, SPECIMEN

Norm. Negative.

Positive. Human immunodeficiency virus, immunodeficiency, leukemia, lymphoma, lymphoreticular malignancy, pulmonary alveolar proteinosis, tuberculosis, and wounds. Drugs include corticosteroids and chemotherapeutic agents.

Description. Microscopic examination to detect gram-positive filamentous branching bacteria that may segment into reproductive bacillary fragments. *Nocardia* is found in soil, grass, grain, straw, and decaying matter. The human infections produced are primary skin lesions (rare), lung (60%-80%), and brain (20%-40%). Increasingly, *Nocardia* is being recognized as a primary pathogen for organ transplant clients.

Professional Considerations
1. Consent form NOT required.
2. Preparation:
   A. Preschedule the test with the laboratory.
   B. Obtain a sterile Culturette or a sterile plastic container.

3. Procedure:
   A. Obtain a sterile culture from a suspected site.
4. Postprocedure care:
   A. Send the specimen to the laboratory within 1 hour.
5. Client and family teaching:
   A. Results are normally available from 72 hours to 30 days.
6. Factors that affect results:
   A. A contaminated culture invalidates the results.
7. Other data:
   A. *Nocardia* grows on various media but may take 3-30 days or more to appear.
   B. *Nocardia* is extremely difficult to culture. A modified acid-fast stain is helpful in the diagnosis of *Nocardia*.
   C. *Nocardia* infections are uncommon, with approximately 500-1000 reported cases annually in the United States.
   D. Respiratory symptoms appear first because the lung is the most common portal of entry.
   E. Brain abscess is the most fatal complication of *Nocardia*.
   F. Sulfonamides or minocycline is the treatment of choice.

NOCTURNAL PENILE TUMESCENCE TESTING
(see Polysomnography, Diagnostic)

NON–STRESS TESTING (NST), DIAGNOSTIC
(see Fetal monitoring, External, Non–stress testing [NST], Diagnostic)

NOREPINEPHRINE, SERUM
(see Catecholamines, Plasma)

NORPACE, SERUM
(see Disopyramide, Serum)

NORTRIPTYLINE, BLOOD
(see Tricyclic antidepressants, Plasma or Serum)

NOSE, ROUTINE, CULTURE
(see Culture, Routine, Specimen)

NST (NON–STRESS TESTING), DIAGNOSTIC
(see Fetal monitoring, External, Non–stress testing [NST], Diagnostic)

5'-NUCLEOTIDASE, SERUM

Norm. 2-15 IU/L, 0-17 U/L, 0-1.6 U, or 0.3-3.2 Bodansky units.

Increased. Alcoholism, cirrhosis, drug-induced cholestasis, extrahepatic obstruction, granulomatous infiltrative disease, liver dysfunction, liver failure, liver metastasis, Rheumatoid arthritis inflammation, sickle cell anemia, and surgery. Drugs include acetaminophen, aspirin, narcotics, phenothiazines, and phenytoin.

Decreased. Hepatitis.

Description. A plasma membrane enzyme that is an isozyme of alkaline phosphatase that is found in hepatic parenchyma and bile ductal cells. This test aids differential diagnosis between bone and liver cancer because 5'-nucleotidase is rarely elevated in bone cancer. When coupled with elevated alkaline phosphatase, the levels are indicative of liver metastasis.

Professional Considerations
1. Consent form NOT required.
2. Preparation:
   A. Tube: Red topped, red/gray topped, or gold topped or blue topped.
3. Procedure:
   A. Draw a 2-mL blood sample.
4. Postprocedure care:
   A. The sample remains stable for 5 days at room temperature, 1 week when refrigerated, and 1 month when frozen.
5. Client and family teaching:
   A. Results are normally available within 72 hours.
6. Factors that affect results:
   A. Contaminated sample and hemolysis.

N

7. **Other data:**
   A. Liver enzyme studies should be evaluated with results.

O₂ SAT, BLOOD
(*see Blood gases, Arterial, Blood*)

O-BANDING, CSF OR PLASMA

Norm. Negative.

Usage. Burkitt's lymphoma, cryptococcal meningitis, multiple sclerosis, neurosyphilis, polyneuropathy, rubella panencephalitis of progressive nature, and subacute sclerosing panencephalitis.

Description. Serum electrophoresis to diagnose inflammatory and autoimmune central nervous system (CNS) diseases that produce quantitative changes in oligoclonal proteins in the serum. O-banding can also be performed on cerebrospinal fluid (CSF) by electrophoresis. Two or more definite bands with no counterparts is considered positive identification.

Professional Considerations
1. Consent form NOT required.
2. **Preparation:**
   A. Tube: Red topped, red/gray topped, or gold topped.
   B. See also *Lumbar puncture, Diagnostic.*
3. **Procedure:**
   A. If both plasma and CSF are being evaluated, they should be drawn at approximately the same time.
   B. Draw a 1-mL blood sample and/or a 5-mL CSF sample.
4. **Postprocedure care:**
   A. Plasma or CSF specimens should be frozen if testing is delayed.
   B. See *Lumbar puncture, Diagnostic.*
5. **Client and family teaching:**
   A. Results are normally available within 72 hours.
   B. See also *Lumbar puncture, Diagnostic.*
6. **Factors that affect results:**
   A. Unlabeled specimens.
7. **Other data:**
   A. These bands are not seen in vascular disease, brain tumors, or other nonimmunologic brain disorders.

B. O-banding is not a significant prognostic factor in heart transplant recipients, HIV infections, or multiple sclerosis.
C. This test has a 90% sensitivity level.

OBSTETRIC ULTRASONOGRAPHY (OBSTETRIC ECHOGRAM, OBSTETRIC ULTRASOUND), DIAGNOSTIC

Norm. Fetus(es) and sac are of normal size for gestational date. No fetal abnormality detected.

Usage. Evaluate amniotic fluid volume, fetal age, position, size, or viability for proper timing of induced or cesarean delivery; fetal abnormality detection; and multiple gestation determination. Helps diagnose abruptio placentae, ectopic tubal pregnancy, endometriosis, fetal death, molar pregnancy, ovarian size, ovarian torsion, pelvic inflammatory disease, placenta previa, uterine size or rupture; and provides guidance for amniocentesis, cervical cerclage placement, fetoscopy, or intrauterine procedures. Tumor detection, localization, characterization, staging; can identify Down syndrome structural markers (duodenal atresia, cardiac abnormalities, brachycephaly, mild ventriculomegaly, macroglossia, abnormal facies, nuchal edema, echogenic or hyperechoic bowel, pyelectasis, and shortening of the limbs), indicating the need for genetic karyotyping.

Description. Evaluation of size, status, and location of fetus, fetal sac, and pelvic organs by the creation of an oscilloscopic picture from the echoes of high-frequency sound waves passing over the pregnant abdomen (acoustic imaging). The time required for the ultrasonic beam to be reflected back to the transducer from differing densities of tissue is converted by a computer to an electrical impulse displayed on an oscilloscopic screen to create a three-dimensional picture of the pelvic contents. Two-dimensional ultrasound has been found to be superior to the three-dimensional technology for evaluation of both healthy and malformed fetuses.

Professional Considerations

1. Consent form IS required. Although the procedure does not pose physical risks, informed consent information should include the diagnostic accuracy of this procedure for detecting fetal abnormalities.
2. Preparation:
   A. This test should be performed before intestinal barium tests or else after the barium is cleared from the system.
   B. The client should disrobe below the waist or wear a gown.
   C. Obtain water-soluble gel, a transducer for the ultrasound machine, a camera and videotape, with or without an oscilloscope.
   D. See *Client and family teaching*.
3. Procedure:
   A. The client is positioned supine.
   B. The pelvic and abdominal areas are coated with water-soluble gel.
   C. A lubricated transducer is passed slowly and firmly over the abdominal and pelvic area at a variety of angles.
   D. Photographs are taken of the images transmitted to the oscilloscopic screen.
   E. The procedure should take approximately 30-60 minutes.
4. Postprocedure care:
   A. Wipe the gel off the abdominal and pelvic area.
   B. Instruct the client to empty her bladder immediately.
5. Client and family teaching:
   A. The client should drink 1 quart of water 1 hour before the procedure because a full bladder is needed to define pelvic organs by serving as an acoustic window for transmission of the sound waves. The full bladder also properly positions the uterus so that it is perpendicular to the transducer. Do not void until the test is completed.
   B. Lying supine may cause shortness of breath. This may be relieved by elevation of the upper body or by lying on either side.
6. Factors that affect results:
   A. Miscalculation of the conception date.
   B. Dehydration interferes with adequate contrast between the organs and body fluids.
   C. Intestinal barium or gas obscures the results by preventing the proper transmission and deflection of the high-frequency sound waves.
   D. Although a full bladder is recommended, during the first trimester, one that is overfilled may compress the uterus, making it difficult to obtain adequate pictures of the early embryonic and extra-embryonic structures.
7. Other data:
   A. An abnormal echo pattern may indicate a multiple pregnancy.
   B. This procedure has a 98% accuracy rate for identifying the placental site.
   C. In the first trimester of pregnancy, a transvaginal approach to ultrasonography may be preferred. This method requires an empty bladder and the passage of a small transducer gently into the vagina. This process eliminates the interference of transverse abdominal tissue, allowing for more detailed visualization.
   D. A chaperone should be present during transvaginal ultrasonography.

OBSTETRIC ULTRASOUND

(see Obstetric ultrasonography, Diagnostic)

OC

(see Osteocalcin, Plasma or serum)

OCA 125 ANTIGEN, SERUM

(see CA 125, Blood)

OCCULT BLOOD, GASTRIC CONTENTS, DIAGNOSTIC

(see Gastric analysis, Specimen)

OCCULT BLOOD, STOOL

Norm. Negative.

Positive. Alcohol abuse, colon cancer, Crohn's disease, diverticulitis, esophageal varices, gastric ulcer, gastritis, gastrointestinal bleeding, hemorrhage, intussusception, pancreatic carcinoma, peptic ulcer, stress ulcers, tumors, and ulcerative colitis. Drugs include aspirin, boric acid, bromides, colchicine, indomethacin, iodine, iron preparations, potassium preparations, reserpine, salicylates, steroids, and thiazide diuretics.

Description. Rapid method for qualitative detection of red blood cells in stool, based on pseudoperoxidase reaction between hemoglobin, the developer (hydrogen peroxide and denatured ethyl alcohol), and guaiac. The methodology used is testing of a sample of stool. Specimens obtained via digital rectal exam are considered unsuitable for fecal occult blood testing due a risk of false-negative results. Occult blood detection has long been used to screen for colorectal cancer, the second highest cause of cancer deaths. However, this method is underused due to public expectation of discomfort. Newer methods of screening include detection of molecular markers, such as the K-*ras* oncogene mutation, which holds promise for becoming a more sensitive and specific test than fecal occult blood testing for screening for colorectal cancer. See *K-ras, Blood or specimen.*

Professional Considerations
1. Consent form NOT required.
2. Preparation:
   A. See *Client and family teaching.*
   B. Obtain a guaiac-impregnated card for occult blood testing and a wooden applicator.
   C. Check the developer and the slides for expiration dates.
3. Procedure:
   A. Obtain a stool sample.
   B. Open the front flap of the guaiac-impregnated slide.
   C. Using the applicator provided, apply a thin smear of stool in each box. Use a separate sample from a different part of the stool specimen for each smear.
   D. Close the slide cover.
   E. Open the flap on the back of the slide.
   F. Apply two drops of developer to each box and to the quality control monitor.
   G. Read the results after 30 seconds and within 2 minutes. Any trace

of blue color is positive for occult blood.
   H. Repeat for three consecutive bowel movements.
   I. Test stools within 48 hours of collection.
4. Postprocedure care:
   A. Assess the rectal area for irritation.
5. Client and family teaching:
   A. Follow a meat-free, high-residue diet for 24-48 hours before the test. The diet should also be free of vegetables with high peroxidase activity (including bananas, beets, broccoli, cantaloupe, cauliflower, grapes, horseradish, mushrooms, parsnips, and turnips).
   B. The client may perform this test at home following the same procedure stated above. Slides should be mailed to the physician's office or to the laboratory as instructed.
   C. Factors that may interfere with results should be reviewed with the client and avoided before testing.
6. Factors that affect results:
   A. Specimens will be positive if contaminated by menstrual or hemorrhoidal blood or povidone-iodine solution.
   B. Diets rich in meats, green leafy vegetables, poultry, and fish may produce false-positive results. Drugs include alcohol, anti-inflammatory agents, ascorbic acid (vitamin C), ETOH, and nonsteroidal agents.
   C. Ascorbic acid (vitamin C) may also produce false-negative results.
   D. Inadequate stool on the slide may produce false-negative results.
   E. False-positives occur in about 10% of tests.
7. Other data:
   A. None.

OCCULT BLOOD, URINE

Norm. Negative, <5000-10,000 RBC/mL or 2-3 RBCs per high-power field.

Positive. Bladder cancer, benign familial hematuria, benign prostatic hypertrophy, burns, cystitis, dysuria, glomerulonephritis, Goodpasture syndrome, heavy exercise, hematuria, hemophilia, nephrolithiasis, thrombocytopenia, transfusion reaction, trauma, and urinary tract infection. Drugs include heparin, salicylates, and warfarin.

Description. Screening by dipstick or examination of urine sediment for asymptomatic hematuria, which may be associated with a serious urologic disease, or the presence of active bleeding with a hematologic disorder.

Professional Considerations
1. Consent form NOT required.
2. Preparation:
   A. Obtain a plastic specimen container and a centrifuge tube. If testing is to be performed immediately, obtain reagent strips with the manufacturer's instructions.
3. Procedure:
   A. Cleanse the genital area with soap and water.
   B. Collect a 10-mL random urine specimen in a centrifuge tube and send the tube to the laboratory, or collect a specimen in a clean plastic cup for dipstick usage as directed by the manufacturer.
4. Postprocedure care:
   A. Perform a dipstick reading according to the manufacturer's directions immediately, or send the specimen to the laboratory within 2 hours.
   B. Write the collection time on the laboratory requisition.
5. Client and family teaching:
   A. Results are normally available within 24 hours.
6. Factors that affect results:
   A. Reject specimens received more than 2 hours after collection because leaving a specimen standing destroys red blood cells.
   B. The presence of urinary bacteria may cause false-positive results, as large amounts of ascorbic acid or formaldehyde in urine will.
   C. False-positives may also be caused by contact of the specimen with povidone-iodine solution, bleach, menstrual blood, or hemorrhoidal blood.

D. Failure to mix the sample, resulting in no RBCs in supernatant and high levels of nitrite, may cause false-negative results.
E. Vitamin C may cause false-negative results, and ethyl alcohol (ethanol) may cause false-positive results.
F. Do NOT use a reagent strip to test urine if the client is receiving tetracycline (Panmycin), oxytetracycline (Terramycin), bromides, or copper because these create false-positive results.
7. Other data:
   A. Sensitivity of reagent strips decreases with age and if urine contains high protein or high specific gravity readings.
   B. Reagent strips are more sensitive to free hemoglobin than to intact red blood cells.

OCT (OXYTOCIN CHALLENGE TEST), DIAGNOSTIC
(see Fetal monitoring, External, Contraction stress test [CST] and Oxytocin challenge test [OCT], Diagnostic)

OCTREOTIDE SCAN (SOMATOSTATIN-RECEPTOR SCINTIGRAPHY), DIAGNOSTIC

Norm. Physiological tracer uptake demonstrates normal size, shape and position of liver, spleen, bladder and kidney.

Usage. Location and diagnosis of primary and metastatic cancers arising from the neuroendocrine system that express somatostatin receptors such as carcinoid tumors, gastrinomas of pancreas and duodenum, thymoma, thymic carcinoma, pheochromocytoma, pituitary adenomas (growth hormone, TSH tumors), islet cell tumors (insulinoma, glucagonoma), neuroblastoma, small cell carcinoma of the lung, paragangliomas, medullary carcinoma of thyroid, meningioma, astrocytoma, lymphoma, astrocytoma, lymphoma, Merkel cell tumor, and breast cancer; staging of Hodgkin's disease; may help in the client selection for clinical trials using somatostatin analogs in the treatment of neuroendocrine cancers.

Description. An Octreotide scan is a nuclear medicine scan of the whole body after injection of a radioactive tracer [In-111-DTPA-D-Phe] or [I-123-Thy3] Octreotide for the purpose of detecting areas of increased uptake by somatostatin-receptor tumors. The Octreotide tracer is a somatostatin analog. Various organs and tumors uptake the tracer at varying degrees. The tracer radiation is emitted as gamma rays and is detected by gamma cameras. A series of images are taken from various angles around the client and compiled by single photon emission computed tomography (SPECT). Cross-sectional and three-dimensional imaging can be accomplished. A series of scans are conducted at 4 and 24 hours following injection of radioisotope. Additional scans may be done.

Professional Considerations
1. Consent form IS required.

Risks
Octreotide may produce severe hypoglycemia in clients with insulinomas. An intravenous line is recommended for clients with suspected insulinomas for the administration of glucose solution as needed.

Contraindications
Women who are breast-feeding.

Precautions
During pregnancy, risks of cumulative radiation exposure to the fetus from this and other previous or future imaging studies must be weighed against the benefits of the procedure. Although formal limits for client exposure are relative to this risk:benefit comparison, the United States Nuclear Regulatory Commission requires that the cumulative dose equivalent to an embryo/fetus from occupational exposure not exceed 0.5 rem (5 mSv). Radiation dosage to the fetus is proportional to the distance of the anatomy studied from the abdomen and decreases as pregnancy progresses. For pregnant clients, consult the radiologist/radiology department to obtain estimated fetal radiation exposure from this procedure.

2. **Preparation:**
   A. See *Client and family teaching.*
   B. Octreotide acetate therapy should be discontinued 24-48 hours prior to scan, while monitoring client for signs of withdrawal.
   C. Jewelry and metal objects should be removed before scanning.
   D. A bowel prep such as Golytely (Colyte) or MagCitrate (magnesium citrate) may be recommended for the evening of the injection, prior to the 24-hour scan.
   E. The client should be well hydrated.
3. **Procedure:**
   A. Intravenous radioactive tracer is administered 3½-4 hour prior to the first scan.
   B. The client should drink two glasses of water immediately following the injection and continue to increase fluid intake for the next 2 days.
   C. The client is placed in a supine position and the whole body is scanned with a gamma camera.
   D. A bowel prep such as Golytely (Colyte) or MagCitrate (magnesium citrate)may be recommended for the evening of day 1.
   E. Repeat scan will be done 24 hours later.
   F. Repeat scans may be done on days 3 and 4.
4. **Postprocedure care:**
   A. Continue to maintain hydration throughout test period.
5. **Client and family teaching:**
   A. Fasting is NOT required for this test.
   B. You may feel a warm sensation when the radioisotope is injected into your vein.
   C. The level of radiation exposure to is low and not associated with any significant risks.
   D. You will need to lie still on a hard table during the procedure.
   E. Each scan takes 1-2 hours and is painless.
   F. Drink plenty of fluids during the 2 days following the injection of the isotope.
6. **Factors that affect results:**
   A. Reduced sensitivity of Octreotide imaging may occur in clients receiving therapeutic doses of octreotide acetate (Sandostatin) therapy.

7. **Other data:**
   A. The radioisotope tracer is primarily excreted by the kidney. Studies have not been conducted in clients with poor renal function. It is not known if Octreotide can be removed by dialysis.
   B. The physical half-life of [In-111-DTPA-D-Phe] Octreotide is 2.8 days.
   C. The scan is often used to identify tumors unrevealed by CT or MRI scans.
   D. Uptake of the Octreotide tracer may indicate the client is a candidate for Octreotide injections to treat the cancer.
   E. Health care professionals working in a nuclear medicine area must follow federal standards set by the Nuclear Regulatory Commission. These standards include precautions for handling the radioactive material and monitoring of potential radiation exposure.

OCULAR CYTOLOGY, SPECIMEN

Norm. Negative.

Usage. Adenovirus infection, *Chlamydia,* conjunctivitis, dry eye conditions, Kaposi's sarcoma, keratitis, and metastatic cancer from the breast or melanoma.

Description. An ocular smear or cellulose acetate filter paper impression is histologically evaluated for the presence of polymorphs or other inflammatory cells. Mapping of the ocular surface can be done from the impression specimen, providing information about changes in the surface cells of the eye, mucus production, and tear function. This test commonly includes staining by either Papanicolaou or Giemsa stain.

Professional Considerations
1. Consent form IS required for the fine needle aspiration technique.

Risks of Fine Needle Aspiration Technique
Infection, unilateral blindness.

Contraindications of Fine Needle Aspiration Technique.
Central retinal artery occlusion.

2. **Preparation:**
   A. For fine needle aspiration, obtain a sterile fine-needle aspiration tray, a sterile plastic container, and a sterile 2 × 2-inch gauze or sterile cotton-tipped applicator approved for microbiologic use and two glass slides and spray the fixative.
   B. For the impression technique, obtain 5-mm-thick half-circular cellulose acetate filter paper.
3. **Procedure:**
   A. *Needle aspiration technique:* A fine-needle biopsy specimen is taken from the eye or by a cotton-tipped application, or a scraping is obtained. Place the smears on two clean glass slides, and immediately fix one slide with the spray and let the other slide air-dry.
   B. *Impression technique:* Place filter paper in the upper and lower quadrants around the limbus, and press lightly against the surface. Remove filter paper and place in a sterile container. Topical anesthesia is not used.
4. **Postprocedure care:**
   A. Assess the aspiration area every 5 minutes × 4 for bleeding, edema, or redness.
   B. Results are normally available in 24 hours.
5. **Client and family teaching:**
   A. Monitor ocular site for inflammation or redness for 24-48 hours.
   B. A mild analgesic may be required for pain control.
   C. Monitor ocular site for signs and symptoms of infection until the site is healed.
6. **Factors that affect results:**
   A. A contaminated sample of the aspirate invalidates results.
7. **Other data:**
   A. None.

OCULOPLETHYSMOGRAPHY (OPG), DIAGNOSTIC

Norm. Negative, or all pulses should occur simultaneously.

Usage. Ataxia, status after carotid endarterectomy, syncope, and transient ischemic attacks.

Description. Noninvasive test that measures ocular artery pressure by comparing pulse arrival times in the eyes with the ears, which reflects the adequacy of cerebrovascular blood flow in the carotid arteries.

Professional Considerations
1. Consent form IS required.

Risks
Corneal abrasion.

Contraindications
Clients who have had eye surgery within 2-6 months, cataract, conjunctivitis, diabetes mellitus, uncontrolled glaucoma, enucleation, history of retinal detachment or lens implantation, or in those who are hypersensitive to local anesthetic or uncooperative and combative clients.

2. Preparation:
   A. Obtain anesthetic eye drops, an eyecup, and photoelectric cells.
3. Procedure:
   A. Instill the anesthetic eye drops and apply the eyecup to the corneas with light suction (40-50 mm Hg).
   B. Apply the photoelectric cells to earlobes.
   C. Record the cyclic changes in volume on a graphic machine.
4. Postprocedure care:
   A. Observe for ocular pain or photophobia, which may indicate corneal abrasion.
5. Client and family teaching:
   A. Do not rub the eyes or insert contact lenses for 30 minutes after the test.
   B. Anesthetic eye drops may cause slight temporary burning.
   C. It is not unusual to experience blurred vision for a short period after this procedure.
   D. Continued blurred vision or pain should be reported to the physician.
   E. The procedure takes a few minutes.
6. Factors that affect results:
   A. Constant blinking, nystagmus, or poor cooperation prevent accurate measurement.

7. Other data:
   A. A 20-msec or greater delay in the pulse wave in the ophthalmic artery is abnormal, signifying stenosis.
   B. Delayed arrival of the ocular pulse is associated with ipsilateral carotid stenosis.
   C. This test does NOT distinguish between a completely occluded internal carotid artery and one that is nearly occluded.
   D. This procedure is extremely useful for evaluating deep orbital circulation.
   E. See also *Carotid phonoangiography and oculopneumoplethysmography (OPPG), Diagnostic.*

OCULOPNEUMOPLETHYSMOGRAPHY (OPPG), DIAGNOSTIC

Norm. Difference between ophthalmic artery pressures should be <5 mm Hg. Ophthalmic artery pressure divided by the higher brachial systolic pressure should be >0.67.

Usage. Ataxia, carotid bruits of asymptomatic origin, carotid endarterectomy monitoring, carotid occlusive disease, syncope, and transient ischemic attacks.

Description. A vacuum applied to the sclera allows adjustment of intraocular pressure and a recording of ocular pressure waveform. Ophthalmic artery pressures are compared with the higher brachial pressure and with each other.

Professional Considerations
1. Consent form IS required.

Risks
Corneal abrasion, erythema, hematoma (scleras).

Contraindications
Anticoagulant therapy, conjunctivitis, enucleation, retinal detachment or history, uncontrolled glaucoma, eye surgery within the previous 2-6 months, increased intracranial pressure.

2. Preparation:
   A. Obtain anesthetic eye drops such as 0.5% proparacaine, an eyecup, suction vacuum apparatus, a plethysmograph, a sphygmomanometer, and a stethoscope.

3. Procedure:
   A. Instill the anesthetic eye drops.
   B. Attach the eyecup to the scleras of the eyes.
   C. Apply a vacuum of 300 mm Hg to each eye so that the pulse disappears. Then gradually release the suction until the pulse returns.
   D. Take both brachial pressures.
   E. The higher systolic brachial pressure is compared with the ophthalmic artery pressures.
4. Postprocedure care:
   A. Observe for ocular pain or photophobia, which may indicate corneal abrasion.
5. Client and family teaching:
   A. Transient loss of vision when suction is applied is not unusual.
   B. Anesthetic eye drops may cause slight temporary burning.
   C. Do not rub the eyes or insert contact lenses for 2 hours after the test.
   D. Continued pain should be reported to the physician.
6. Factors that affect results:
   A. Constant blinking, hypertension, nystagmus, and poor cooperation prevent accurate measurement.
   B. Results may be difficult to interpret if the client has a history of hypertension.
   C. Cardiac dysrhythmias may alter the results.
7. Other data:
   A. This method is more accurate than oculoplethysmography.
   B. See also *Oculoplethysmography (OPG), Diagnostic.*

OKT-3 CELLS, OKT-4 CELLS, OKT-8 CELLS

(*see Acquired immunodeficiency syndrome evaluation battery, Diagnostic*)

OLIGOCLONAL BANDS, CEREBROSPINAL FLUID, SPECIMEN

(*see Cerebrospinal fluid, Myelin basic protein, oligoclonal bands, protein, and protein electrophoresis, Specimen*)

OLIGOCLONAL BANDS, DIAGNOSTIC

(*see O-Banding, Serum*)

OMT, SPECIMEN

(*see Oral mucosal transudate, Specimen*)

ONCOFETAL FIBRONECTIN

(*see Fetal fibronectin, Specimen*)

ONE-STEP, DIAGNOSTIC

(*see Glucose monitoring machines, Diagnostic*)

ONE TOUCH, DIAGNOSTIC

(*see Glucose monitoring machines, Diagnostic*)

OPHTHALMODYNAMOMETRY, DIAGNOSTIC

Norm. No difference in pressure of both eyes.

Usage. Carotid occlusive disease, extracranial vascular disease, and transient ischemic attacks.

Description. Compares the retinal artery pressures in both eyes in the supine and upright positions. A decrease in retinal arterial pressure with a normal brachial pressure when the client moves from a supine position to an upright position indicates carotid occlusive disease.

Professional Considerations
1. Consent form NOT required.

Risks
Corneal abrasion.

Contraindications
In thrombocytopenia and for clients receiving anticoagulants.

2. Preparation:
   A. Obtain an ophthalmoscope, a blood pressure cuff, a stethoscope, and a sphygmomanometer.
3. Procedure:
   A. The ophthalmoscope is pressed gradually against the eye to measure arterial systolic pressure and

diastolic pressures in supine and upright positions.

B. Brachial blood pressures are also measured in the arm.

4. **Postprocedure care:**
   A. Assess for ocular photophobia or pain, which may indicate corneal abrasion.

5. **Client and family teaching:**
   A. Results are normally available within 24 hours, with interpretation to follow.

6. **Factors that affect results:**
   A. Constant blinking, nystagmus, and poor cooperation.

7. **Other data:**
   A. The oculoplethysmography test is the preferred test when one is evaluating carotid arteries when compared to the ophthalmodynamometry test.
   B. A 20% difference in diastolic pressure between eyes is suggestive of insufficient carotid artery flow on the side with the lower finding.
   C. See also *Oculoplethysmography (OPG), Diagnostic.*

OPN
(see Osteopontin, Serum)

ORAL CAVITY CYTOLOGY, SPECIMEN

Norm. Negative.

Usage. Cancers of the tongue, gum, or mouth; *Candida albicans*; herpesvirus infection; human immunodeficiency virus; Klinefelter syndrome; pemphigus; trisomy 13, 18, and 21; and Turner syndrome.

Description. Microscopic examination of cells scraped from the oral cavity surface.

Professional Considerations
1. Consent form NOT required.
2. **Preparation:**
   A. Obtain a glass of water, a spatula or tongue blade, a glass slide, a specimen container of 95% ethyl alcohol (ethanol) or spray fixative, and a light source.

B. Label the slide with the client's name and the specimen source.
3. **Procedure:**
   A. The client should rinse the mouth vigorously with water several times before the scraping is performed.
   B. The lesion or oral surface is scraped with a spatula or tongue blade.
   C. Smear the scraping on a labeled glass slide and fix it immediately in 95% alcohol or spray fixative.

4. **Postprocedure care:**
   A. The requisition should include age, physical findings, history of smoking, dentures, skin lesions, and reverse smoking; and history of chemotherapy, immunotherapy, or radiation therapy.

5. **Client and family teaching:**
   A. Results are normally available in 24-48 hours.

6. **Factors that affect results:**
   A. Failure to fix specimens invalidates the results.

7. **Other data:**
   A. Occasional diagnosis of palatal salivary gland neoplasm occurs.
   B. *Candida albicans* can spread to the esophagus and down to the intestines.

ORAL GLUCOSE SCREENING
(see Glucose challenge test, Diagnostic)

ORAL MUCOSAL TRANSUDATE (OMT, HIV ORAL TEST), SPECIMEN

Norm. Negative AIDS battery, nonreactive.
Antibody detection: Negative for HIV antibodies.

Usage. Used in combination with a modified ELISA and salivary Western blot assay. Offers clinical and outreach advantage to health care personnel who provide counseling and testing. It is an excellent alternative for clients with poor venous access or who are unwilling to donate a blood sample.

Description. Oral mucosal transudate is a serous fluid that derives from transudation at the gingival crevice. The OMT method detects the presence of HIV antibodies using a micro–enzyme-linked immunosorbent assay similar to the ELISA. Samples collected are place in a nontoxic stabilizing preservative that prevents bacterial growth and degradation of IgG by bacteria protease. Modifications in collection technology and immunosorbent assays have improved the detection of HIV-1 antibodies in oral specimens. The EpiScreen HIV-1 Oral Specimen Collection device is currently the only FDA-approved oral HIV antibody test and is restricted to testing with the oral fluid Vironstika HIV-1 Microelissa System. (Organon Teknika Corporation, Durham, N.C.) The salivary Western blot is an in vitro qualitative assay developed specifically for oral mucosal transudate (Epitope, Inc.). The OraSure Specimen Collection Device (Epitope, Inc.) is an FDA-approved device that looks similar to a toothbrush with a padded end that is used for collection of oral specimens for HIV testing. Oral mucosal specimens follow the algorithm recommended for blood samples by the Centers for Disease Control and Prevention.

Professional Considerations

1. Consent form IS required.
2. **Preparation:**
   A. Only properly trained personnel may test using the oral specimen kits according to the manufacturer's directions.
   B. Wear gloves and have timer available.
3. **Procedure:**
   A. OMT: A fiber pad is treated with a hypotonic salt solution. The client rubs the pad between the lower gum and cheek several times and then holds the pad in place for a minimum of 2 minutes to a maximum of 5 minutes. The OraSure Specimen Collection Device may also be used to collect the sample.
   B. The time must be verified by the collector. The client immediately places the pad in the provided container. Follow further the manufacturer's instructions.

4. **Postprocedure care:**
   A. Dispose of the equipment in the room.
   B. Specimen may be stored at room temperature.
5. **Client and family teaching:**
   A. Each client is given the pamphlet provided with the kit and is explained the purpose of the test, the procedure for collection, and the alternative of giving a blood specimen.
   B. The test might leave a slightly salty taste in your mouth.
   C. Results may not be available for several days.
   D. If the results are positive, it is recommended to follow with serum samples for ELISA and serum for Western blot or immunofluorescence assays.
   E. Assess client understanding of safe sex practices and provide counseling as needed.
6. **Factors that affect results:**
   A. False-positive ELISA results may be seen in pregnant women in the first trimester because of immunoglobulin reaction and sloughing of epithelial tissue.
   B. False-positive ELISA results have been documented in clients with anticoagulation therapy, an oral pathologic condition, autoimmune disease other than AIDS, and with monoclonal or polyclonal gammopathy.
   C. False-negative results may occur as a result of the absence of antibodies to HIV-1 in the early phase of the infection.
7. **Other data:**
   A. OMT testing is not intended for use in clients under 13 years of age.
   B. This test is not designed to screen blood donors.

ORNITHINE CARBAMOYLTRANSFERASE (OCT), BLOOD

Norm. 0-500 sigma units/mL, or 0-16 U/L.

Increased. Acute viral hepatitis, cholecystitis, cirrhosis, enteritis, hepatic necrosis, hepatotoxicity caused by drugs or alcoholism (rare), infectious mononucleosis, liver dysfunction, obstructive jaundice, metastatic liver carcinoma, and prolonged exercise. Drugs include all hepatotoxic drugs, heavy alcohol, and oral contraceptives.

Decreased. Congenital hyperammonemia. Drugs include mercuric salts, *p*-chloromercuribenzoate, and 2,3-dimercaptopropanol.

Description. Ornithine carbamoyltransferase (OCT) is an enzyme found in the liver and to a lesser extent in the intestinal mucosa that is involved in urea metabolism of the Krebs' cycle. An elevation specifically and sensitively indicates liver cell disease. Insufficient production of OCT is an inherited X-linked dominant genetic defect that leads to neurological damage. The exact occurrence of the inherited X-linked genetic defect is unknown but has been estimated to be 1:80,000, with males more affected.

Professional Considerations
1. Consent form NOT required.
2. Preparation:
   A. Tube: Red topped, red/gray topped, or gold topped.
3. Procedure:
   A. Draw a 7-mL blood sample.
4. Postprocedure care:
   A. None.
5. Client and family teaching:
   A. Results are normally available within 72 hours to 1 week.
6. Factors that affect results:
   A. Hemolysis of the specimen invalidates the results.
7. Other data:
   A. The test is more sensitive than AST (SGOT) or ALT (SGPT) in assessing liver function.
   B. The test does not distinguish between hepatic and biliary diseases.

OSMOLALITY, CALCULATED TEST (OSMOLAR GAP), BLOOD

Norm:

		SI UNITS
Serum osmolality	280-300 mOsm/kg H_2O	280-300 mmol/kg H_2O
Critical low	≤230 mOsm/kg H_2O	≤230 mmol/kg H_2O
Critical high	≥375 mOsm/kg H_2O	≥375 mmol/kg H_2O
Osmolar gap	<10 mOsm/kg H_2O	<10 mmol/kg H_2O

Increased. Alcoholism, azotemia, burns, convulsions, dehydration, diabetes insipidus, diarrhea, hyperaldosteronism, hyperlipidemia, hyperproteinemia, presence of hyperosmolar substances such as ethyl alcohol (ethanol) or methanol or lactic acid, syndrome of inappropriate antidiuretic hormone secretion (SIADHS), and uremia. Drugs include mannitol.

Decreased. Hyponatremia and overhydration.

Description. Osmolality refers to a solution's concentration of solute particles per kilogram of solvent and is expressed in mOsm/kg. In the laboratory, it is measured by an osmometer. However, it is possible to calculate serum osmolality using serum measurements of sodium, glucose, and urea (BUN) according to the formula(s) listed under "Procedure," below. The osmolar gap is the difference between the laboratory serum osmolarity value and the calculated osmolar value. Assessing this gap is most important in the diagnosis of ethyl alcohol (ethanol) or methanol poisoning.

Professional Considerations
1. Consent form NOT required.
2. Preparation:
   A. None, other than locating the results of serum sodium, glucose, and BUN levels.

3. **Procedure:**
    A. Calculate osmolality as follows:

    $(1.86 \times Sodium) + (Glucose/18) + (BUN/2.8)$

    B. Rounded formula:

    $(2 \times Sodium) + (Glucose/18) + (BUN/2.8)$

    C. Dr. Weisberg's formula:

    $(2 \times Sodium) + (Glucose/20) + (BUN/3)$

    D. Calculated osmolar gap =

    $$\frac{1.86\, Na^+ + Glucose + BUN}{182.8}$$

4. **Postprocedure care:**
    A. Calculated osmolality may be compared to laboratory-measured osmolality.
5. **Client and family teaching:**
    A. Results are normally available within 72 hours.
6. **Factors that affect results:**
    A. Hemolysis of specimens used to obtain sodium, glucose, and BUN values invalidates results.
    B. Herbal or natural remedy goldenseal (*Hydrastis canadensis*) causes increased renal water loss, whereas sodium is spared. This may increase osmolality.
    C. Na^+ concentration may decrease by 1 mEq/L for every 4.6 g/L of plasma lipids, causing pseudohyponatremia.
    D. Na^+ concentration may decrease by 1.6 mEq/L for every 100 mg/dL increase in plasma glucose because of an osmotic shift of water into the bloodstream.
7. **Other data:**
    A. A difference between measured and calculated serum osmolality (osmolar gap) of >10 mOsm/kg of H_2O may indicate pseudohyponatremia. Causes of an osmolar gap may include the following:
        i. A decrease in serum water content (as by displacement because of severe hyperlipidemia).
        ii. Hyperproteinemia, as occurs in macroglobulinemia and multiple myeloma.
        iii. The presence of low-molecular-weight solutes such as ethyl alcohol (ethanol), methanol, ethylene glycol, isopropanol, or mannitol in the blood.
        iv. In diabetics when hyperglycemia is present.
        v. In clients with chronic renal failure when dialysis is needed.
    B. Abnormal calculated results should be confirmed by a serum osmolality test.
    C. See also *Osmolality, Serum*.

OSMOLALITY, SERUM

Norm:

		SI UNITS
Adult	280-300 mOsm/kg H_2O	280-300 mmol/kg H_2O
Child	270-290 mOsm/kg H_2O	270-290 mmol/kg H_2O
Panic levels	<240 mOsm/kg H_2O	<240 mmol/kg H_2O
	>320 mOsm/kg H_2O	>320 mmol/kg H_2O

Panic Level Symptoms and Treatment

Symptoms. Poor skin turgor or interstitial edema, listlessness, acidosis by decreased pH, shock, seizures, coma, cardiopulmonar arrest. Respiratory arrest may occur when value exceeds 360 mOsm/kg.

Treatment:
Note: Treatment choice(s) depend on client history and condition and episode history.

Assess electrolytes.
Administer IV fluids in specific osmotic concentrations to shift fluid into or out of the intravascular space as appropriate.
Add corrected electrolytes as needed.
Monitor for side effects of fluid and electrolyte imbalance.
Possibly conduct cardiac monitoring, depending on electrolyte values.
Perform neurologic checks every 1-4 hours.

Treatment—cont'd

Implement seizure precautions (the client is at risk for intracerebral edema or brain cell dehydration, depending on the relative serum osmolality in comparison with intracellular osmolality).
Treat gastrointestinal symptoms supportively.
Identify and correct cause.

Increased. Acidosis, advanced liver disease, alcoholism, burns, dehydration (associated with diabetes insipidus because too much antidiuretic hormone causes the kidney to excrete large amounts of water), diabetic ketoacidosis, hyperbilirubinemia, hypercalcemia, hyperglycemia, hyperglycemic hyperosmolar nonketotic coma, hypernatremia, high-protein diet, hypovolemic shock, methanol poisoning, nephrogenic diabetes insipidus.

Decreased. Acute renal failure; Addison's disease; hyponatremia; overhydration; syndrome of inappropriate antidiuretic hormone secretion (SIADHS), which is often associated with cancers (especially oat cell of the lung) or medications such as chemotherapy, oral agents for diabetes mellitus and tricyclic antidepressants, and narcotics; and disorders of the posterior pituitary.

Description. Osmolality is a measure of the concentration of particles in the serum per kilogram of water. Osmolarity is nearly the same but measures said concentration per liter of water. Used to assess the fluid state of the client and determine the cause of fluid and electrolyte imbalances, particularly in endocrine disorders. The normally functioning osmoregulation system maintains the serum osmolality (the concentration of the blood) within a tight normal range. Receptors in the hypothalamus adjust the level of antidiuretic hormone from the posterior pituitary, which affects the free water excreted from the kidney. Disorders of the hypothalamus, the posterior area of the pituitary, or the kidney may alter serum osmolality. Dehydration from any cause increases osmolality. Overhydration decreases serum osmolality.

Either is dangerous to the client. Urine osmolarity is usually obtained with serum osmolality because the comparison gives the true picture of the fluid-balance state. The set of serum electrolytes (especially sodium and glucose) will also be assessed.

Professional Considerations
1. Consent form NOT required.
2. Preparation:
    A. Tube: Red topped, red/gray topped, or gold topped.
    B. Do NOT draw samples during hemodialysis.
3. Procedure:
    A. Draw a 1-mL blood sample.
4. Postprocedure care:
    A. Measure the intake and output every hour until the results are within normal limits.
5. Client and family teaching:
    A. Results are normally available within 4 hours.
    B. Clients with adrenocortical insufficiency should consult a physician about the continuation of steroid therapy.
6. Factors that affect results:
    A. The specimen is stable for only 10 hours if refrigerated.
    B. The use of mineralocorticoids, osmotic diuretics, insulin, or mannitol may increase values because of the effect on fluid balance.
    C. Hemolysis of specimens invalidates the results.
    D. Lipemic serum may alter the results.
    E. Herbs or natural remedies: $che^1qian^2zi^3$ ('cart-before-seeds', seeds of *Plantago major*, var. *asiatica*, ribgrass), fu^2ling^2 (*hoelen, Poria cocos, P. sclerotium*, China root fungus), goldenseal (*Hydrastis canadensis*), ze^2xie^4 ('marsh-purge', *Alisma orientale*, water plantain), and zhu^1ling^2 ('pig-fungus', *Polyporus umbellatus*, pore fungus) increase osmolality because of their aquaretic (orally absorbable, nonpeptidergic competitive ADH antagonistic) or diuretic effects.
7. Other data:
    A. See *Osmolality, Calculated tests, Blood*, for information on "Osmolar gap."

OSMOLALITY, URINE

Norm. See range below; the concentration of the urine has a wide range as the body adjusts to varying fluid intake and requirements.

		SI UNITS
13 months–adult	200-1200 mOsm/kg H_2O	200-1200 mmol/kg H_2O
0-12 months	50-600 mOsm/kg H_2O	50-600 mmol/kg H_2O

The comparison of urine osmolality to serum osmolality is important for determining the significance of the urine osmolality.

Increased. Acidosis; Addison's disease; congestive heart failure; high-protein diet; hyperglycemia; hypernatremia; hypovolemia; intracellular dehydration; renal disease; shock; and syndrome of inappropriate antidiuretic hormone secretion (SIADHS), in which the serum osmolality will be decreased.

Decreased. Aldosterone insufficiency, diabetic ketoacidosis, diabetes insipidus (levels <200 mOsm/kg H_2O), diuretic therapy, hypokalemia, hyponatremia, nephrogenic diabetes insipidus, overhydration with intravenous D_5W, psychogenic polydipsia, renal disease that affects the kidneys' ability to concentrate urine. Drugs include lithium (long-term treatment).

Description. Measure of the number of osmotically active particles in a given urine volume, which reflects the kidney's concentrating ability. Normal fluid balance is achieved by the action of the posterior pituitary (ADH secretion) and properly functioning kidneys. Fine adjustments are made continuously to maintain normal fluid and electrolyte balance. The kidney is able to adjust the urine concentration over a wide range to maintain a normal serum concentration, or osmolality. Normally, when the client becomes even slightly dehydrated, the urine will become more highly concentrated. Therefore, if there is high fluid intake, the urine will become more dilute in ridding the body of the excess fluid.

Professional Considerations
1. Consent form NOT required.
2. Preparation:
   A. The collection may be random, or the client may be required to fast from food and fluids from midnight before the collection the next day.
   B. Obtain a sterile, plastic specimen container.
3. Procedure:
   A. Collect a 10-mL random or morning urine specimen in a sterile, plastic container without preservatives.
4. Postprocedure care:
   A. Send the specimen to the laboratory for immediate processing.
   B. Intake and output (I&O) until the results are normal.
5. Client and family teaching:
   A. Results are normally available within 24 hours.
   B. Clients with adrenocortical insufficiency should consult a physician about the continuation of steroid therapy.
6. Factors that affect results:
   A. Anesthetics, antibiotics, carbamazepine, chlorpropamide, detergent, dextran, diuretics, glucose, mannitol, and radiographic contrast agents affect the urine volume and therefore cause abnormal results.
   B. Herbs or natural remedies: che[1]qian[2] zi[3] ('cart-before-seeds', seeds of *Plantago major*, var. *asiatica*, ribgrass), *fu[2]ling[2]* (*hoelen, Poria cocos, P. sclerotium*, China root fungus), goldenseal (*Hydrastis canadensis*), *ze[2]xie[4]* ('marsh-purge', *Alisma orientale*, water plantain), and *zhu[1]ling[2]* ('pig-fungus', *Polyporus umbellatus*, pore fungus) increase urine osmolality because of their aquaretic (orally absorbable, non-peptidergic competitive ADH antagonistic) or diuretic effects.
7. Other data:
   A. Urine osmolality is considered a better measurement than specific gravity to assess for the state of hydration.

B. Wakefield et al (2002) found positive associations between the color of urine and urine specific gravity and urine osmolality and the BUN/creatinine ratio when searching for a low-cost method for monitoring dehydration status in an elderly population.

OSMOLAR GAP, BLOOD
(*see Osmolality, Calculated tests, Blood*)

O'SULLIVAN TEST, DIAGNOSTIC
(*see Glucose challenge test, Diagnostic*)

OSTEOCALCIN (Oc, BONE GLA PROTEIN, BGP), PLASMA OR SERUM

Norm. *Note:* No standardized reference norms exist for this marker. Reference ranges below are provided for guidance only. Refer to individual lab reference norms provided with test results.

Adult males:	1.1-10.8 ng/mL
Adult females (premenopausal):	0.7-6.4 ng/mL

Usage. The identification of women at risk of developing osteoporosis; monitoring bone metabolism in clients with growth hormone deficiency, hypothyroidism, hyperthyroidism, and chronic renal failure and in women during perimenopause and postmenopause, during hormone replacement therapy and treatment of premenopausal women with LH-RH agonists, monitoring glucocorticoid-induced suppression of bone turnover, monitoring renal osteodystrophy therapy.

Increased. Hyperparathyroidism, rapid bone growth in children (peak levels occur between ages of 10-16), postmenopausal females, low estrogen production, low calcium intake, low physical activity, osteomalacia, Paget's disease, hyperthyroidism (decreases with treatment), fractures (for up to 1 year), renal failure with dialysis (if assay includes measurements of Oc fragments). Drugs include 1,25-dihydroxy-vitamin D, calcitrol.

Decreased. Hypoparathyroidism, multiple myeloma, hypercalcaemia associated with malignancy, liver cirrhosis. Drugs include glucocorticoids, heparin, warfarin, tamoxifen, postmenopausal hormone replacement therapy.

Description. Osteocalcin is a gamma-carboxylated protein of bone matrix that is used as a serum marker of bone turnover because it is specifically produced by the osteoblast. Oc is an integral part of bone formation process; however, a small amount of Oc does enter the circulation. The circulating levels of Oc are a specific indicator of recent bone turnover.

Professional Considerations
1. Consent form NOT required.
2. **Preparation:**
   A. Tube: 3 or 7 mL, confirm type of collection tube with laboratory.
   B. Fasting is not generally required.
3. **Procedure:**
   A. Draw a 2-5 mL blood sample. Avoid hemolysis.
   B. If serial samples are drawn, collect the samples at the same time of day.
4. **Postprocedure care:**
   A. Send specimen immediately to the laboratory. Refrigerate the specimen immediately if not taken immediately to the laboratory.
5. **Client and family teaching:**
   A. The results are usually available in 3-5 days.
6. **Factors that affect results:**
   A. The tube additive, EDTA may invalidate the results, depending on the analytical method used. Confirm correct sample collection tube with lab.
   B. The serum samples are relatively instable, especially when at room temperature
   C. With RIA, very high osteocalcin levels (>5000 ng/mL) may exceed the highest standard concentration and appear as low values due to the "hook" effect. If this

occurs, the test should be repeated with a diluted sample.

D. Because of the variety of evaluation methods available for measuring osteocalcin levels, there can be significant difference in the normal range between labs.

E. Diurnal variations in Oc levels have been reported, peaking in early morning (4:00 AM).

F. Menstrual cycle phase: highest level occurs during luteal phase.

G. Serum osteocalcin has a short half-life and is easily fragmented. Some assays detect only intact Oc, while others also detect Oc fragments. Since Oc is sensitive to in vitro degradation, assays that measure only intact Oc may provide lower values and assays that detect fragments may provide higher Oc values.

7. **Other data:**

A. Vitamin K (phylloquinone) is required for the carboxylation of Oc, which is essential for the synthesis of mature Oc. Low serum concentrations of vitamin K are associated with increased levels of undercarboxylated Oc. Undercarboxylated Oc can be measured by some assays, providing information regarding bone quality.

OSTEOGRAM, DIAGNOSTIC

(*see Radiography of the skull, chest and cervical spine, Diagnostic*)

OSTEOPONTIN (OPN), SERUM

Norm. There are no universal standards established. Use the reference values provided by laboratory that provides the test results.

Usage. Malignant ovarian cancer, breast cancer, prostrate, lung cancer, colon cancer. Research is currently being conducted to determine the use of OPN in the detection, diagnosis, monitoring, and/or staging of these and other cancers. Research has indicated that OPN may be useful in determining the prognosis and guiding therapy in clients with head and neck squamous cell carcinoma.

Increased. Malignant ovarian cancer, breast cancer, lung cancer, prostate cancer, gastric cancer, colon cancer, granulomas, hepatocellular carcinoma, sarcoidosis, atherosclerosis.

Description. Osteopontin is an acidic glycoprotein, synthesized by preosteoblasts, osteoblasts and osteocytes and is incorporated into bone. It is also found in many other areas of the body, including the brain, kidney, placenta. It is a chemotactic factor for macrophages and T cells. An overexpression of OPN has been associated with tumorigenesis and metastasis in several cancers. OPN level is measured with ELISA.

Professional Considerations

1. Consent form NOT required.
2. **Preparation:**
   A. See *Client and family teaching.*
   B. Clarify type of collection tube needed with institutional lab.
3. **Procedure:**
   A. Clarify amount of blood required with institutional lab.
   B. Transport specimen to the laboratory immediately.
4. **Postprocedure care:**
   A. None.
5. **Client and family teaching:**
   A. Fasting is NOT required for this test.
   B. The use of OPN as a tumor biomarker is currently under research.
6. **Factors that affect results:**
   A. Research has indicated that inflammatory and noninflammatory disease processes may reflect an overexpression of OPN, decreasing the specificity of the OPN as a tumor marker.
7. **Other data:**
   A. The use of this test as a tumor biomarker is in the research phase.

OTOSCOPY, VIDEO, DIAGNOSTIC

Norm. Normal structure, absence of inflammation, infection, growths or obstruction.

Usage. Anatomy and physiology of the ear canal, visualization of the tympanic membrane. Any trauma causing bleeding may be diagnosed as well as vascular tumors of the middle ear. Using pneumatic video-otoscopy, the mobility of the tympanic membrane is observed. Video recordings can be made during surgery.

Description. This technique combines the standard methods of ENT endoscopy with a small, hand-held, video camera for viewing and recording the examination and ENT procedure. It can be used with the ears, nose, or larynx. The advantage of the video is in the visual record of the anatomy and physiology, which can be carefully studied at a later time without further discomfort to the client adding to the increased means of physician consultation and as an excellent teaching tool. The recording is stored as part of the client record.

Professional Considerations
1. Consent form IS required.

Risks
Infection.

Contraindications
Sedatives are contraindicated in clients with central nervous system depression.

2. **Preparation:**
   A. Obtain a video camera; a light source; a video cassette recorder; a video printer; a monitor and an enhancer; and film.
   B. Obtain an endoscope: Hopkins 4.0 mm for adults and Hopkins 2.7 mm for children.
   C. Anesthetic spray and sedation as prescribed. Monitor respiratory status closely throughout the procedure if sedation is given.
   D. Obtain instruments to remove wax and superficial hairs from the ear.
   E. See *Client and family teaching.*
3. **Procedure:**
   A. Wax and hair are removed.
   B. A topical anesthetic is applied to the canal.
   C. Sedatives may be given intravenously.
   D. The client is placed in an upright or supine position, and the endoscope is inserted.
   E. The video recording may begin at the time of insertion.
4. **Postprocedure care:**
   A. Continue the assessment of the respiratory status. If deep seda-

tion was used, follow institutional protocol for postsedation monitoring. Typical monitoring includes continuous ECG monitoring and pulse oximetry, with continual assessments (every 5-15 minutes) of airway, vital signs, and neurologic status until the client is lying quietly awake, is breathing independently, and responds to commands spoken in a normal tone.
   B. Assess for postoperative complications, including bleeding and pain.
5. **Client and family teaching:**
   A. The procedure should take less than 1 hour.
   B. Hold very still during the procedure.
6. **Factors that affect results:**
   A. The client must be able to sit still for an extended length of time.
7. **Other data:**
   A. Videos are also used in rhinoscopy and laryngoscopy.

OVA AND PARASITES (O & P), STOOL
(see Parasite screen, Stool)

OVARIAN CANCER ANTIGEN-125, SERUM
(see CA 125, Blood)

OXALATE, 24-HOUR URINE

Norm. 8-40 mg/24 hours (92-456 mmol/24 hours, SI units).

Increased. Celiac disease, cirrhosis, Crohn's disease, ethylene glycol poisoning, diabetes mellitus, hyperoxaluria (primary), kidney stone, nephrolithiasis, pancreatic insufficiency, sarcoidosis, vitamin B_6 deficiency. Drugs include megadoses of ascorbic acid and calcium. Also ingestion of certain foods—see *Client and family teaching* below.

Decreased. Gastrointestinal disease or surgery that affects absorption; renal failure.

Description. Oxalate is an end product of metabolism that is excreted through the urine. It may accumulate in the soft and connective tissues of the kidneys and bladder and cause renal calculi and chronic inflammation and fibrosis.

Professional Considerations
1. Consent form NOT required.
2. **Preparation:**
   A. Obtain a 3-L plastic container to which 30 mL of 6 N hydrochloric acid (HCl) has been added.
   B. See *Client and family teaching.*
3. **Procedure:**
   A. Collect all the urine voided in a 24-hour period in a refrigerated, 3-L plastic container to which 30 mL of 6 N HCl has been added. For specimens collected from an indwelling urinary catheter, keep the drainage bag on ice and empty the urine into the collection container hourly. Document the quantity of the urinary output throughout the collection period. Not all laboratories require refrigeration.
4. **Postprocedure care:**
   A. Write the beginning and ending dates and times as well as the total 24-hour urine output on the collection container and the laboratory requisition.
   B. Transport the specimen to the laboratory and refrigerate it until testing.
5. **Client and family teaching:**
   A. For 48 hours before testing, maintain a diet that avoids increasing oxalate by avoiding soybean products, wheat germ, grapefruit juice, strawberries, rhubarb, bananas, orange juice, canned pineapples or tomatoes, kidney beans, beets, spinach, carrots, tomatoes, celery, onions, sweet and white potatoes, green and waxed beans, cauliflower, cucumber, squash, broccoli, eggplant, cabbage, spinach, cashews, chocolate, cocoa, gelatin, peanut butter and other nuts, cola beverages, and tea.
   B. Urinate before defecating, and avoid contaminating the urine with the stool or toilet tissue. If any urine is accidentally discarded, discard the entire specimen and restart the collection the next day.

C. A high-calcium diet may promote the development of kidney stones. Consult a dietitian.
D. Results are normally available within 24 hours.
6. **Factors that affect results:**
   A. Failure to include all urine voided in the 24-hour period invalidates the results.
   B. Ascorbic acid may interfere with the testing process. It does not affect the level of oxalate excretion.
   C. Certain foods need to be avoided because they raise oxalate levels (see section 5A above).
7. **Other data:**
   A. Studies show that stone formation is not age specific or gender specific.
   B. Grapefruit juice ingestion has been found to increase urinary oxalate excretion.

OXAZEPAM
(see Benzodiazepines, Plasma and Urine)

OXIMETRY (PULSE OXIMETRY, SpO₂), DIAGNOSTIC

Norm. Adult arterial blood saturation is 94%-100%; newborn arterial blood saturation, 40%-92%, is dependent on lung development.

Usage. Any clinical situation in which adequate oxygenation is potentially compromised. Particularly helpful when used between arterial blood gas (ABG) determinations, to reduce both the number of blood draws and costs when the accuracy and correlation is known to the clinicians. *Advantages:* quick, noninvasive, and continuous, and can detect variations in saturation that may not be noted with ABGs. *Disadvantage:* provides only one of the determinants of the ABG and may be of only limited value when single readings are obtained. Must be carefully correlated with the clinical situation (see 6-h). Conditions when it is used include acute myocardial infarction, acute respiratory distress syndrome (ARDS), anesthesia monitoring, asthma, cerebrovascular accident, chronic obstructive pulmonary disease, congenital heart defects, congestive heart failure, cor pulmonale, cystic fibrosis, emphysema, head trauma, intraoperatively, lung cancer, oxygen therapy, postoperatively, premature infant monitoring, pulmonary edema, pulmonary emboli, sickle cell anemia, tuberculosis, ventilator dependence, and weaning from mechanical ventilation

Description. Pulse oximetry involves the spectrophotometric estimate of functional oxygen saturation on hemoglobin. This is a noninvasive measurement of oxygen saturation (see *Arterial blood gases*), a percentage representing the ratio of arterial hemoglobin saturated with oxygen. Measurement is performed by means of a spectrophotometer probe connected to the adult's finger, temporal area, or bridge of the nose, or to an infant's foot or toe. The probe emits red and infrared light that passes through the body part directed at a photodetector that determines the amplitude of the transmitted light and isolates the blood's pulsatile flow. This enables calculation of SpO_2 through measurement of light absorption based on known amounts absorbed by saturated and reduced hemoglobin. Newest pulse oximetry equipment is available with motion-resistant capabilities, which improves consistency and accuracy of readings through reduction of motion artifact. The type of technology used in these is called "3-wavelength reflectance."

Professional Considerations
1. Consent form NOT required.
2. Preparation:
   A. Cleanse the area with water and dry it before attaching the probe.
   B. For clients with impaired tissue perfusion, use a nasal probe or a temporal probe. If a finger probe must be used, apply a warm pack around the hand and the extremity for 10 minutes before the probe application. The newest equipment uses centrally-placed forehead censors which deliver improved sensitivity and rapid detection of hypoxemia.
3. Procedure:
   A. The skin should be clean and dry before placement. Attach the probe to the toe or foot for

infants; the finger, temporal area, or bridge of the nose for adults; and the bridge of the nose for obese clients. Nasal probes should be placed over cartilage for best results.
   B. Activate the pulse oximeter and set low and high alarm limits according to the manufacturer's instructions.
   C. Note SpO_2 after allowing at least 30 seconds for the reading to stabilize.
   D. For continuous or periodic oximetry, observe for downward trends in SpO_2. Generally, decreased SpO_2 below 90%-92% must be addressed by thorough assessment of the client and clinical status.
4. Postprocedure care:
   A. Remove the probe. Clean nondisposable probes according to the manufacturer's instructions.
   B. Wash the area with soap and water.
5. Client and family teaching:
   A. Results are normally available immediately.
   B. Alarms are normally set to sound for a trend downward in values. Keeping the probe covered with a cloth improves signal clarity.
   C. In cases of lung disease, discuss smoking cessation programs and strategies if applicable.
6. Factors that affect results:
   A. Hyperbilirubinemia, hypotension, hypothermia, use of vasopressor medications, impaired tissue perfusion, or cold extremities may result in no reading or a falsely low reading, necessitating use of ABG SpO_2. Desaturation by pulse oximetry may be used as a sign of severe hypotension requiring evaluation.
   B. Failure to place the probe properly may result in no reading or a falsely low or high reading.
   C. Very bright light surrounding the probe may make obtaining a reading difficult. If so, cover the probe with a sheet or other opaque material.
   D. Falsely elevated results may occur in the presence of dyshemoglobins (carboxyhemoglobin, >3%; methemoglobin, 1.5 g/dL; sulfhemoglobin, 0.5 g/dL),

necessitating periodic validation with ABG SaO$_2$.

E. Falsely decreased results may be caused by hyperbilirubinemia >20 mg%, necessitating periodic validation with ABG SaO$_2$.

F. Unreliable results may occur with the injection of radiographic dyes, necessitating periodic validation with ABG SaO$_2$.

G. Results may not be accurate in clients with rapid oxygen desaturation, low perfusion states, or hypothermia.

H. Clients who are anemic may have misleadingly high saturation of hemoglobin and still be hypoxemic because of decreased oxygen-carrying capacity.

I. Interarterial injection of Patent Blue lowers the pulse oximeter reading.

7. **Other data:**

A. Accurate between SaO$_2$ levels of 85% and 100%.

B. Some pulse oximeters give slightly false higher readings in dark-skinned clients, but use after validation with ABG is not affected.

C. In healthy volunteers, significant delays in the detection of acute hypoxemia by pulse oximetry occur when pulse oximeters are placed at the toe as compared with probes at either the ear or the hand.

D. Richmond et al. (2002) found routine pulse oximetry useful in screening asymptomatic newborns for postductal saturation as a means of identifying those in whom further examinations revealed congenital heart defects.

OXYGEN SATURATION (O$_2$ Sat, SO$_2$, SaO$_2$), BLOOD
(see Blood gases, Arterial, Blood; Blood gases, Venous, Blood; Blood gases, Capillary, Blood; Oxyhemoglobin dissociation curve, Diagnostic)

OXYHEMOGLOBIN DISSOCIATION CURVE (P-50), DIAGNOSTIC
(see Blood gases, Arterial, Blood)

OXYTOCIN CHALLENGE TEST (OCT), DIAGNOSTIC
(see Fetal monitoring, External, Contraction stress test [CST] and Oxytocin challenge test [OCT], Diagnostic)

P-50
(see Blood gases, Arterial, Blood)

PA
(see Transthyretin, Serum)

p-ANCA
(see Anti-neutrophil cytoplasmic antibody screen, Serum)

PANCREAS ULTRASONOGRAPHY (PANCREAS ECHOGRAM, PANCREAS ULTRASOUND), DIAGNOSTIC

Norm. The pancreas is properly located and positioned and is of normal size and shape, with a regular border, and homogeneous pattern that is of finer texture than that of the peritoneum, more intense than area soft tissue, and less intense than the liver. Major supporting arteries and veins as well as the pancreatic duct are visible and normal.

Usage. Aids diagnosis of pancreatic inflammation, pseudocyst, or tumor; guidance for needle biopsy of pancreas; and ongoing monitoring of pancreatic carcinoma response to therapy (that is, change in the size of a tumor). Work-up of abdominal pain, particularly in clients with alcoholism, blunt abdominal trauma, gallbladder stones, and known hyperlipidemia because they are more prone to pancreatitis. The Endoscopic/Intraductal method using miniprobes with or without fine needle aspiration is used experimentally to identify intraductal papillary-mucinous tumor and cystic lesions of the pancreas *(see Endoscopic Ultrasonography, Diagnostic)*.

Description. Evaluation of pancreatic structure by the creation of an oscilloscopic picture from the echoes of high-frequency sound waves passing over the epigastric area (acoustic imaging). A variation of the technique involves moving the probe intraductally via endoscopic ultrasonography (see *Endoscopic Ultrasonography, Diagnostic*). The time required for the ultrasonic beam to be reflected back to the transducer from differing densities of tissue is converted by a computer to an electrical impulse displayed on an oscilloscopic screen to create a three-dimensional picture of the pancreas. An advantage of this test is that it can help diagnose acute pancreatitis retrospectively. In acute pancreatitis, the pancreas appears larger than normal and is less echogenic than the liver is. The edema may cause compression of the inferior vena cava, and the pancreatic duct may appear enlarged. In chronic pancreatitis, calculi, shadows, strictures, or stenoses may be viewed in the pancreatic duct as well as calcified areas in the body of the pancreas. An abscess may appear as an irregular-shaped, highly echogenic structure with thick walls. Adenocarcinoma may cause the gland to appear enlarged, with an irregular border and absence of normal parenchymal echo pattern. True cysts may be differentiated from pseudocysts by their spherical, sonolucent appearance. Pseudocysts are nonspherical and may contain scattered echoes caused by debris contained within them.

Professional Considerations

1. Consent form NOT required.
2. **Preparation:**
   A. See *Client and family teaching*.
   B. This test should be performed before intestinal barium tests, or after the barium is cleared from the system.
   C. If the pancreas alone will be studied, a full stomach improves visualization of the posterior portion of the pancreas. The client should drink 500-1000 mL of tomato or orange juice or a cellulose to distend the stomach. Alternatively, glucagon (1 mg) or a cellulose suspension may be administered intravenously, with 500 mL of water ingested a few minutes later to reduce stomach peristalsis. This causes the stomach to function as a fluid-filled window

for scanning for up to 60 minutes.
   D. The client should wear a gown.
   E. Obtain ultrasonic gel or paste.
3. **Procedure:**
   A. The client is positioned supine in bed or on a procedure table.
   B. The area of the abdomen overlying the pancreas is covered with conductive gel, and a lubricated transducer is passed slowly and repeatedly over the pancreas. Scanning begins with transverse views taken at 1-cm intervals with the client in full inspiration. Scanning is started at the level of the xiphoid process and proceeds until the presence of intestinal gas hinders the view. The client may then be changed to a rising position, which moves gastric air to the fundus and distends the abdominal veins to provide landmarks for identifying the pancreas. This is followed by sagittal scanning, which alternates moving from midline to the right and then midline to the left, at 1-cm intervals. The client may be asked to suspend breathing on inhalation or exhalation to reduce motion artifact.
   C. Photographs of the oscilloscopic display are taken.
4. **Postprocedure care:**
   A. Remove the gel from the skin.
   B. If a biopsy is performed, see *Biopsy, Site-specific, Specimen*.
5. **Client and family teaching:**
   A. This transabdominal procedure is painless and carries no risks.
   B. If the biliary system will also be examined, a fast from food and fluids for 8 hours before the test is required.
   C. Oral ingestion of fluids before the procedure is for stomach distension that aids in the visualization of the pancreas.
   D. It is important to lie still during the procedure. You may be asked to stop breathing for a few seconds during the procedure.
   E. The procedure takes less than 60 minutes, and results are normally available within 48 hours.
6. **Factors that affect results:**
   A. Dehydration interferes with adequate contrast between the organs and body fluids. Dehydration may

cause the duodenum to be mistaken for the pancreas.
B. Intestinal barium, gas, or food obscures the results by preventing proper transmission and deflection of the high-frequency sound waves.
C. The more abdominal fat present, the greater is the attenuation (reduction in sound-wave amplitude and intensity), which interferes with the clarity of the picture. Abdominal muscles and cartilage may have the same effect, necessitating repositioning of the client.
D. The stomach may interfere with views of the pancreatic anatomy in transverse scans.
E. If the left lobe of the liver is very small (<2 cm), it will function poorly as an acoustic window.
7. Other data:
A. Severe dehydration, especially when combined with obesity, has the potential to impair visualization of the pancreas and the surrounding area.
B. See also *Endoscopic Ultrasonography, Diagnostic.*

PANCREATIC SECRETORY TRYPSIN INHIBITOR (PSTI) SERUM (TATI)

Norm. 16.6 ± 0.7 ng/mL.

Increased. Crohn's disease, pancreatitis, and with severe infection of the GI tract or with cell destruction in the mucosal layers of the GI tract. Considered a marker for malignant pancreatic endocrine tumors. The related TATI tumor-associated trypsin inhibitor is considered a marker for certain cancers such as lung and ovarian. Levels may increase with rejection of transplanted pancreas. It is considered a marker for threatened organ rejection. Drugs: misoprostol (Cytotec).

Decreased. None.

Description. PSTI is a potent protease inhibitor found in the pancreas, the mucus-secreting cells of the gastrointestinal tract, and in the breasts, lungs, and kidneys. It is believed to be involved in healing after injury because it inhibits the proteolytic breakdown of mucus. It may also be capable of promoting growth activity. Newer studies suggest than PSTI gene alteration may be a associated with the risk of developing chronic pancreatitis. PSTI is absorbed into the bloodstream and therefore can be measured by immunoradioassay. Absorbed PSTI is excreted in the urine. This test is performed by radioimmunoassay.

Professional Considerations
1. Consent form NOT required.
2. Preparation:
A. Tube: Red topped, red/gray topped, or gold topped.
B. No fasting required.
3. Procedure:
A. Draw 5 mL of blood.
4. Postprocedure care:
A. No special handling of the specimen is known.
5. Client and family teaching:
A. Results will not be available for up to 5 days.
6. Factors that affect results:
A. Radioisotope testing within the previous week invalidates the results.
B. Hemolysis of blood samples invalidates the results.
C. Oral contraceptives and steroids have a possibility of interfering with test results.
7. Other data:
A. None.

PAP
(see Prostatic acid phosphatase by RIA, Blood)

Pap SMEAR, DIAGNOSTIC

Norm. Results are reported according to the Bethseda System in a descriptive statement regarding the adequacy of the sample, followed by a descriptive diagnosis. Abnormalities are described as either benign, low-grade squamous, high-grade squamous, glandular, or severe dysplasia with carcinoma in situ.

Abnormal. Terms used to describe abnormal cells include the following:

TERMINOLOGY	MEANING	MAY ALSO BE CALLED
Atypical squamous cells of undetermined significance (ASCUS)	May indicate the need for further diagnostic evaluation	
Dysplasia, mild, moderate or severe	Appearance of cells is abnormal; no invasion of healthy tissue; cells may develop into early cervical cancer SIL, CIN 3	Mild: low-grade SIL, CIN 1 Moderate: high-grade SIL, CIN 2 Severe: high-grade
Squamous intraepithelial lesion (SIL), low grade or high grade	Abnormal appearance of cervical surface cells, which appear thin and flat	
Cervical intraepithelial neoplasia (CIN)	Presence of abnormal cell growth in the cervical surface cells; may be further described with number 1 to 3 to indicate how much of the cervix contains abnormal cells	
Carcinoma in situ	Presence of preinvasive cancer cells on the surface of the cervix	High-grade SIL, CIN 3

Previous Terminology:

Class I   Normal
Class II   Probably normal
Class III   Doubtful (may be malignant)
Class IV   Probably malignant
Class V   Malignant

Positive. Abnormal cells indicative of endocrine disorders, cancer (uterine), endometriosis, lymphogranuloma venereum, tumors (cervical), and vaginal adenosis or inflammation that could lead to cancer.

Negative. Normal cervical cells.

Usage. This test is primarily used in the early detection of cervical and vaginal carcinomas and scrapings from the uterus. The *smear technique* can also used to detect cancerous cells of the breast (aspiration of mammary gland tissue), lung (bronchial brushing and washing from bronchoscopy or coughed-up sputum), stomach (aspirated gastric secretions), and renal system (urine sediment). It is indicated as routine screening and for work-up of disorders of reproduction function.

Description. The Pap smear, the most widely-used cancer-screening tool, is a cytologic examination of desquamated epithelial tissue to differentiate normal from anaplastic cells. Both a traditional slide method and a newer liquid method are described here. In the traditional method, one prepares the smears by scraping or aspirating cells from the tissue to be examined (that is, the cervix) and fixing them on glass slides, using ether and 95% ethyl alcohol (ethanol) solution. Slides are then dried, stained, and examined under a microscope by a pathologist or cytotechnologist. In the newer liquid Pap method, the tissue scrapings are placed in liquid to remove mucus and debris, which can interfere with the view through the microscope. Many studies have found that most human cervical cancers harbor types of high-risk human papillomavirus (HPV). For this reason, studies are being conducted to evaluate whether circulating HPV DNA in the plasma can serve as a marker for cervical cancer. (See *Human papillomavirus in situ hybridization, Specimen.*)

Professional Considerations
1. Consent form NOT required.
2. Preparation:
   A. See *Client and family teaching.*
   B. Interview the client; record age, date of last menstrual period, prior history of abnormal Pap smear results, and pregnancy status.
   C. Obtain a glass slide, a sterile Ayre spatula, a tongue blade, a pipette, a sterile cotton swab, sterile gloves, ether/95% alcohol solution (1:1), spray fixative, a graphite pencil, and a speculum. Using the graphite pencil, label the frosted ends of the slide with the client's name and the collection site. For liquid procedure, obtain ThinPrep.
   D. The client should disrobe below the waist.
   E. Position the client recumbent on a gynecologic examination table in the lithotomy position and drape for comfort and privacy.
3. Procedure:
   A. *Liquid Pap Method:* Follow the steps below, substituting transfer of the specimen to the ThinPrep Pap container, instead of to a slide.
   B. Note: Fixative must be applied to the slide before any drying of the specimen occurs. If a two-step specimen is taken, fixative should be applied after each step. Remove excess mucus by placing a 2 × 2-inch gauze pad over the cervix and gently peeling it away after a few seconds.
   C. *Endocervical Smear:*
      i. Aspirate endocervical secretions from the cervical os as through a pipette. Spread the secretions onto a glass slide. Dip or spray the slide with the prepared fixative and dry it.
      OR
      ii. Insert a sterile spatula into the cervical os and rotate it 360 degrees, using one continuous motion. Smear the scrapings onto a glass slide, using a single continuous stroke to avoid traumatizing

the cells. Fix immediately as described above.
      OR
      iii. Lightly brush the cervical os circumference and secretions 90 to 180 degrees with a tapered synthetic fiber brush. Gently roll the brushings onto the slide and immediately fix as described above.
      OR
      iv. Insert a sterile cotton swab into the cervical os and rotate it 360 degrees. Leave the swab in place for 10-20 seconds. Remove the swab and smear onto a glass slide. Fix it immediately as described above.
      v. *Ectocervical Scraping:* Using a wooden tongue blade or the blunt side of a wooden Ayre spatula inserted into the cervical os, rotate or scrape the entire surface at the squamo-columnar junction. Remove the tongue blade and smear onto a glass slide. Fix immediately as described above.
   D. *Cervical Scraping:* Insert the pointed edge of a wooden Ayre spatula into the cervical os and rotate the spatula 360 degrees. Spread the cervical scrapings on a glass slide, fix it with an ether/95% ethyl alcohol solution, and dry the slide. A Cervex-Brush sampling device may be used, and it is recommended to be rotated a full 180 degrees to improve the sampling for abnormal cervical cells.
   E. *Vaginal Pool:* Using the blunt side of a wooden Ayre spatula, scrape the vaginal floor behind the cervix. Spread the vaginal pool secretions on a glass slide, spray or soak them in fixative, and dry the slide. Vaginal fluid is obtained for suspected endometrial cancer or for a hormonal evaluation.
   F. *Vulva Smear:* Using the blunt side of a wooden Ayre spatula, directly scrape the vulvar lesion. Spread the scraping on a glass slide and fix it immediately with spray fixative.
4. Postprocedure care:
   A. Write the client's age; the reason for the study; the date of the last menstrual period; any chemotherapy or hormonal medications; and history, including any previous

abnormal Pap smears, and treatment for cancer or abnormal vaginal bleeding on the laboratory requisition.
B. Send the slides to the cytology laboratory.

5. **Client and family teaching:**
   A. For clients of childbearing age, test should be done 10-20 days after the first day of the last menstrual period.
   B. Do NOT douche for 18-72 hours before the procedure.
   C. It is customary practice for the client to be informed of the results, either positive or negative. The method of information exchange needs to be arranged with the client's physician.

D. Results are normally available within 1 week.
E. Further testing may be needed, including a repeat Pap, endometrial biopsy, or colposcopy. This decision will be made when the results of the test are received.
F. Pap smears should be performed at the earlier of either yearly after 21 years of age or 3 years after becoming sexually active. If the client is sexually active, has a family history of cervical or uterine cancer, has venereal disease, or has a mother who took diethylstilbestrol during pregnancy, a Pap smear should be performed before 18 years of age and yearly thereafter.

YEARS	REGULAR (TRADITIONAL) Pap	LIQUID-BASED Pap (ThinPrep BY QUEST DIAGNOSTICS)
<21	Begin annual screenings at three years after becoming sexually active	Same
21-30	Annually	Every 2-3 years
30-70	If the last three tests were normal, decrease frequency to every 2-3 years	Every 2-3 years
70	Consider discontinuation of screening if the last three tests were normal AND if there were no abnormal results in the last 10 years	Same
After subtotal hysterectomy	Same as above	Same as above
After total hysterectomy due to invasive cervical disease	Every 3 months × 2 years, then every 6 months.	
After total hysterectomy not necessitated by cancer or precancerous conditions	Not needed unless client has risk factors for cervical cancer	Same

6. **Factors that affect results:**
   A. Smears that dry before fixative is applied cannot be properly interpreted.
   B. Do not lubricate the speculum; such lubrication distorts cells.
   C. Use of formalin as a fixative invalidates the results.
   D. Water or lubricant on the specimen can distort the cells.

E. A smear taken any time other than in the midmenstrual cycle can result in abnormal findings. The best time for a cervical cytology study is 5-6 days after menses.
F. Inadequate specimens may require retesting.
G. Tetracycline or digitalis preparations can affect the look of squamous epithelium.

H. Blood, mucus, or pus on the slide makes accurate specimen interpretation difficult.

I. Cells that are damaged from excessive manipulation during collection may be interpreted as atypical.

7. **Other data:**

A. False-positive Pap smear results requiring a repeat in 6-12 weeks, as is standard, may be avoided if a culture for *Chlamydia* and *Neisseria gonorrhoeae* and wet-mount slides are examined at the time of the examination.

B. False-negative results can be minimized by obtaining double scrapings and smear cultures.

C. See also *Papanicolaou smear, Ultrafast,* and *Fine-needle aspiration, Diagnostic.*

D. Precancerous cervical cells often take up to 5 years to become cancerous. The American Cancer Society revised its recommendations for frequency of cervical cancer screening via Pap smear to reflect studies that have shown that less frequent testing only slightly increases the risk of missing precancerous conditions, but reduces the likelihood of detecting and subsequently overtreating benign cervical conditions.

E. Many studies have found that most human cervical cancers harbor the high-risk human papillomavirus (HPV) types. For this reason, studies are being conducted to evaluate whether circulating HPV DNA in the plasma can serve as a marker for cervical cancer.

Consensus Guidelines of the American Society for Colposcopy and Cervical Pathology (ASCCP) Recommend Follow-up for Abnormal Pap Smears

Finding	Recommended Follow-Up
Atypical squamous cells (ASC) of undetermined significance (ASCUS)	Two repeat cytology tests OR Immediate colposcopy with loop electrosurgical excision procedure (LEEP) (see *Colposcopy, Diagnostic*) OR DNA testing for high-risk types of human papillomavirus (preferred choice, if method used for Pap testing was liquid-based cytology). See *Human papillomavirus in situ hybridization, Diagnostic.*
Finding cannot exclude high-grade squamous intraepithelial lesion (HSIL; ASC-H)	Immediate colposcopy with loop electrosurgical excision procedure (LEEP)
Low-grade squamous intraepithelial lesion or atypical glandular cells	Immediate colposcopy with loop electrosurgical excision procedure (LEEP)

Pap SMEAR, ULTRAFAST (UFP) AND FINE-NEEDLE ASPIRATION, DIAGNOSTIC

Norm. Normal cell and structure for the area biopsied. Absence of tumor cells or abnormalities of the cell nucleus.

Usage. Adenocarcinoma, of various organs; squamous cell carcinoma; neuroendocrine carcinomas; clear cell–type renal cell carcinoma; schwannoma; lymphoid hyperplasia, with small round lymphocytes, small cleaved lymphocytes, large noncleaved lymphocytes, and histocytes (macrophages). Breast-tissue lesions, thyroid lesions, Hürthle cell carcinoma, and colloid nodule with hemorrhagic degeneration.

Description. This procedure involves fine-needle aspiration for cytologic evaluation and may be performed intraoperatively or during a colposcopic examination (see *Colposcopy, Diagnostic*). The ultrafast technique is particularly useful when a quick result is important. The method is particularly advantageous for looking at the cell nucleus because it provides the cytologist or histologist with a clear, stained view of the cell and organelles.

Professional Considerations

1. Consent form IS required for all fine-needle aspiration biopsy procedures. For specimens taken during surgery, the client gives consent for the surgical procedure.
2. Preparation:
   A. Obtain clear glass slides, a syringe, and 18-gauge needles; Choplin jars; normal saline, and 95% ethyl alcohol for storage and transport to the laboratory.
   B. Notify the laboratory for on-site processing, staining, handling, and consultative interpretation of the specimen.
3. Procedure:
   A. Depends on the body site and location of the area for biopsy. Some clients will be prepared for surgery and taken to an operating room.
   B. Ambulatory care and ward procedures may require local anesthesia.
   C. The skin is prepared for the procedure.
   D. Needle aspiration of the tissue is obtained; sometimes special procedures such as fluoroscopy or isolation of a nodule are required. The specimen is taken with a sterile technique, and smears are made on the clear microscope slides. It is air-dried and processed for 30 seconds in normal saline and then in 95%

ethyl alcohol and sent immediately to the laboratory for processing or the cytologist at the procedure handles the specimen. The developers suggest that fine-needle aspirations for cytology follow this procedure: (1) prepare several clear glass slides and air-dry; (2) stain and process the ultrafast slide; (3) save the other slides for laboratory use for other methods such as Diff-Quik Stain, which has other advantages for final diagnosis.
4. Postprocedure care:
   A. The specimen is carefully labeled and transported immediately to the cytology laboratory.
   B. Apply a dry, sterile dressing over the site.
   C. Monitor for bleeding at the site.
   D. Give postsurgical care as appropriate.
5. Client and family teaching:
   A. Call the physician for signs of infection at the procedure site: increasing pain, redness, swelling, purulent drainage, or for fever >101° F (38.3° C).
   B. Results are normally available within 24 hours.
6. Factors that affect results:
   A. Inappropriate processing.
7. Other data:
   A. Total turn-around time for these specimens may be as little as 30 minutes.
   B. See also *Pap smear, Diagnostic*.

PARACENTESIS (PERITONEAL FLUID ANALYSIS), DIAGNOSTIC

Norm:

Appearance	Clear, serous, light yellow
Amount	<50 mL
Protein	<4.1 g/dL
Glucose	70-100 mg/dL (equals serum)
Amylase	140-400 U/L (equals serum)
Ammonia	<50 mg/dL
Alkaline phosphatase	
Adult female	45-250 U/L
Adult male	90-240 U/L
Red blood cells	Negative
White blood cells	<300/mL
Culture	Negative
Cytologic result	No malignant cells
CEA and CA 125	Negative
Fungus	Negative

Usage. Used diagnostically to remove and examine small amounts of fluid for undiagnosed causes of abdominal effusion. May be used to instill and remove saline lavage to examine for the presence of blood if blunt trauma to the chest and abdomen is suspected.

Abnormal Appearance
Bloody: Trauma (or traumatic tap).
Turbid (cloudy): Infection, pancreatitis, intestinal perforation, and cirrhosis.
Milky: Chylous ascites.

Increased Protein. Cancer, tuberculosis, peritoneal carcinomatosis, and peritonitis.

Increased Amylase. Pancreatitis and intestinal strangulation, necrosis (intestinal), pancreatic pseudocyst, pancreatic trauma.

Increased Alkaline Phosphatase. Intestinal strangulation and ruptured intestine.

Increased Red Blood Cells. Intra-abdominal trauma, neoplasm, and tuberculosis.

Increased White Blood Cells. Infection and chylous ascites, cirrhosis, and peritonitis. Granulocyte count of >250 cells/mL is diagnostic for infection.

Increased CEA and CA 125. Malignancy. *Note:* an elevated CA125 without elevation in CEA indicates primary malignancy is ovarian or endometrial.

Decreased Glucose Below Serum Level. Malignancy or TB peritonitis.

Description. Paracentesis is the trans-abdominal removal of fluid from the peritoneal cavity for analysis of electrolytes, red blood cells, white blood cells, bacterial and viral cultures, and cytology studies. The procedure may be done in conjunction with endoscopic ultrasound guidance, particularly when used to reach small areas of effusion. Paracentesis may also be used therapeutically to remove ascitic fluid when the accumulation is large and disabling (e.g., interferes with venous return, normal breathing, appetite, and activities of daily living) such as in ascites attributable to hepatic encephalopathy or other causes.

Professional Considerations
1. Consent form IS required.

Risks
Abdominal wall infection, hemorrhage, perforated bowel, increased peritonitis.

Contraindications
This procedure should be used with caution during pregnancy and in clients with coagulation abnormalities or bleeding tendencies.

2. **Preparation:**
   A. Have the client urinate or empty the bladder by catheterization. This will help prevent accidental bladder trauma.
   B. Measure abdominal girth, weight, and baseline vital signs. Monitor vital signs every 10-15 minutes during the procedure.
   C. Obtain povidone-iodine solution, sterile gauze sponges, 1%-2% lidocaine (Xylocaine), 10- and 30-mL syringes, 22- and 24-gauge needles, sterile gloves, sterile drapes, a trochar with a cannula, a sterile vacuum collection bottle, plastic tubing, a scalpel, a suture, a needle holder, and tape.

3. **Procedure:**
   A. Position the client sitting on the edge of a bed or examination table with the back supported and the feet resting on a stool. The procedure may also be performed with the client lying prone.
   B. Cleanse the client's abdomen with povidone-iodine solution and allow it to dry; then cover the areas surrounding the site with a sterile drape.
   C. Numb the area with 1%-2% lidocaine (Xylocaine), first using a 22-gauge needle locally and then changing to a 24-gauge needle and anesthetizing the area deeper.
   D. A scalpel is used to make a stab wound into the peritoneal cavity midway between the umbilicus and the symphysis pubis. Alternatively the insertion may be through the iliac fossa, through the flank, or in each abdominal quadrant. The trochar-cannula is threaded through the incision. An audible sound may be heard when the needle pierces the peritoneum. The trochar is removed, and plastic tubing is attached to the cannula; the other end of the tubing is placed in the collection receptacle (usually a 500- to 1000-mL vacuum bottle). The fluid is slowly drained from the

abdominal cavity. The client may need to be repositioned to improve drainage.

E. Do not drain more than 5L at a time. If hypovolemia occurs as a result of rapid drainage, raise the bottle to slow the drainage rate or clamp the drainage tube. To reduce risk of infection, do not leave drain in place longer than 6 hours.

F. When the fluid collection is complete, remove the cannula, and suture the incision if necessary.

4. **Postprocedure care:**
   A. Apply a dry, sterile dressing to the site.
   B. Observe the site for bleeding or drainage.
   C. Measure abdominal girth and weight.
   D. Monitor vital signs for evidence of hemodynamic changes every 30 minutes for 2 hours, every hour for 4 hours, and then every 4 hours for 24 hours.
   E. Write any recent antibiotic therapy on the laboratory requisition. Send the samples to the laboratory for analysis immediately.
   F. Document in the client's record the time of the procedure; the name of the physician; the color, consistency, and amount of fluid withdrawn; and the client's response to the procedure.
   G. Monitor daily sequential multiple analyzer (SMA7) blood work.
   H. Observe for hematuria caused by bladder trauma. If this is suspected at the time of the procedure, a BUN and creatinine value obtained on the paracentesis fluid should be sent to confirm the condition.

5. **Client and family teaching:**
   A. Notify the physician immediately if you notice bloody, pink, or red urine.
   B. Results are normally available within 72 hours.

6. **Factors that affect results:**
   A. Inadvertent internal organ injury, including female organs, may contaminate the sample with bile, blood, urine, or feces or with bacterial flora.
   B. Delay in analysis may cause inaccurate results.
   C. Care must be taken to ensure a sterile technique, especially in handling specimens for culture and Gram stain.

7. **Other data:**
   A. Frequently, salt-poor albumin or mannitolum is infused for 24 hours after paracentesis for clients with ascites and poor nutrition, which increase the third spacing of fluid into this cavity.
   B. Transient initial bloody fluid may result from a traumatic tap.

PARACENTESIS, FLUID ANALYSIS, SPECIMEN
(see Paracentesis, Diagnostic)

PARASITE SCREEN, BLOOD

Norm. Negative. Acute parasitic infection is strongly indicated when titers increase fourfold (for most organisms) between acute and convalescent sera.

Usage. Nonspecific detection of parasitic infection.

Positive. Chagas' disease, small protozoa of malaria (*Plasmodium falciparum, P. malariae, P. ovale,* and *P. vivax*), cysticercosis, *Babesia, Echinococcus, Entamoeba histolytica, Fasciola hepatica,* filariasis (*Wuchereria bancrofti*), *Giardia,* kala-azar (leishmaniasis), *Paragonimus, Strongyloides, Taenia solium, T. saginata,* toxoplasmosis (*Toxoplasma gondii*), trichinosis, trypanosomiasis (*Trypanosoma brucei* and *T. brucei rhodesiense*), and VLM (*Ascaris* and *Toxocara*).

Description. Parasites are organisms that must live in or on a host to survive and often require different hosts at different stages of development. Parasitic infections in humans may be acquired from the fecal-oral route, contaminated food, animals, and some arthropods. Some parasites survive on the host by changing antigenic characteristics or becoming coated with host immunoglobulins, so that they are no longer recognized as foreign by the immune system. The most accurate method of diagnosing a blood-borne parasitic infection is to identify the actual parasite in a Giemsa-stained thick or thin film of blood. This is not always easy, however, because the amount of blood-borne parasites present at any given time may vary depending on the parasitic stages and cycles. The parasite screen is used when the presence of the actual parasite cannot be established. This screen involves several laboratory procedures that help to detect the presence of parasite antigen-antibody complexes in a sample of blood. Three of the methods typically used to identify parasitic infection are complement fixation, hemagglutination inhibition, and immunodiffusion. Results are reported in titers as the highest dilution of serum that tests positive for parasitic antibodies.

Professional Considerations
1. Consent form NOT required.
2. **Preparation:**
   A. Tube: Red topped, red/gray topped, or gold topped or pink topped, or Corvac tube.
3. **Procedure:**
   A. Parasite screen the fresh blood for filariae and trypanosomes, which should be collected between 2200 (10 PM) and 2400 (12 AM) hours.
   B. Draw a 5-mL blood sample.
   C. Avoid causing hemolysis.
   D. An acute sample should be drawn as soon as possible after a parasitic infection is suspected.
   E. Draw a convalescent sample in 2-4 weeks.
4. **Postprocedure care:**
   A. None.
5. **Client and family teaching:**
   A. Return in 2-4 weeks to have a follow-up sample drawn.
   B. Avoid donating blood until the results are known.
6. **Factors that affect results:**
   A. Hemolysis of the specimen may cause false-negative results.
   B. A single test has little significance unless the results are extremely high.
   C. For several of the parasites, false-negative results may be caused by the presence of antibodies from past infection.
7. **Other data:**
   A. Even with positive results, diagnosis of a parasitic infection cannot be confirmed without recovery of the parasite.

PARASITE SCREEN (OVA AND PARASITES), STOOL

Norm. Negative. No parasite, ova, or larvae identified.

Usage. Diagnosis of parasitic infestation of the intestinal tract.

Positive. *Ancylostoma duodenale* (hookworm), *Ascaris lumbricoides* (roundworm), *Balantidium coli, Blastocystis hominis, Capillaria philippinensis, Chilomastix mesnili, Clonorchis sinensis, Cryptosporidium* spp., *Dientamoeba fragilis, Diphyllobothrium latum* (fish tapeworm), *Dipylidium caninum* (tapeworm), *Endolimax nana, Entamoeba histolytica, E. hartmanni, E. polecki, Enterobius vermicularis* (pinworm), *Enteromonas hominis, Escherichia coli, Fasciola hepatica, Fasciolopsis buski, Giardia lamblia,* helminths and protozoa, *Heterophyes, Hymenolepis diminuta* (tapeworm), *Hymenolepis nana* (dwarf tapeworm), *Iodamoeba bütschlii, Isospora belli, Metagonimus yokogawai, Necator americanus* (hookworm), *Opisthorchis sinensis, Paragonimus westermani* (long fluke), *Retortamonas intestinalis, Sarcocystis* spp., *Schistosoma mansoni* (blood fluke ova), *Strongyloides stercoralis* (threadworm), *Taenia saginata* (beef tapeworm), *T. solium* (pork tapeworm), *Trichinella spiralis, Trichomonas hominis, Trichostrongylus* spp., and *Trichuris trichiura* (whipworm).

Description. Microscopic examination of stool to detect parasites at various stages of development from ova through mature or motile forms. A parasite screen is performed on a stool sample when a parasitic infection is suspected as evidenced (usually) by diarrhea of unknown origin. A parasite is an organism that survives at the expense of a host organism. Frequently, protozoa, amebas, and worms infect the gastrointestinal tract from contaminated food and water sources. Parasites, larvae, or ova may not be continuously present in fecal specimens; thus, at least three samples, spaced 2-3 days apart, or as prescribed, are taken. For a screen the laboratory will need to know travel information and will likely perform screens based on the parasites usually found in that location. Laboratory preparations for each parasite to be identified may vary.

Professional Considerations
1. Consent form NOT required.
2. **Preparation:**
   A. Question the client carefully about any recent travel and about hygiene practices.
   B. Clarify whether a preservative is needed by contacting the laboratory that will be performing the

test. If a preservative is to be used, stools for ova and parasite examination should be preserved in 5% formalin or polyvinyl alcohol solutions. Specimens should be diluted in a 3:1 stool-to-preservative ratio.

C. Obtain a clean plastic, waxed cardboard, or glass container and a tongue blade; or obtain clear cellophane tape, a tongue blade, a glass slide, and a clean container. If protozoa, amebas, or flagella are suspected, the specimen must be taken "stat" to the laboratory for examination.

D. See *Client and family teaching.*

3. Procedure:
   A. *Stool collection:* Collect three random stool samples, each 2-3 days apart. The specimens should be collected in a plastic, waxed cardboard, or glass container with a tight-fitting lid. The client should defecate directly into the container or into a clean, sterile bedpan. If a bedpan is used, lift 2 tablespoons of stool into the container with a wooden tongue blade, being cautious not to contaminate the outside of the container. Apply the lid tightly.
   B. *Collection of pinworm or tapeworm eggs:* Collect the specimen between 2200 (10 PM) and 2300 (11 PM) hours or early in the morning before bath or bowel movement. Wrap clear cellulose tape around the end of a tongue blade and firmly press it against three or four separate portions of the perianal area, close to the anus. Do not insert the tongue blade into the anus. Remove the tape and, using a cotton ball, press it lightly onto a glass slide with the gummed side against the glass. Place the slide in a clean container for transport to the laboratory.
   C. *Collection of tapeworm:* If tapeworm is suspected, send the entire stool so that the head of the tapeworm can be identified.

4. Postprocedure care:
   A. Write the collection time, travel history, and suspected diagnosis on the laboratory requisition.
   B. Send the specimen to the laboratory within 1 hour of collection. Unformed stools should have a preservative added.
   C. Several specimens are usually prescribed: 3 is a standard number.

5. Client and family teaching:
   A. Collect the stool specimen according to the procedure described above and avoid contaminating it with urine.
   B. Cook food properly, boil water, and wash hands thoroughly if contamination is suspected.
   C. Have water analyzed, especially well water.
   D. With diarrhea, avoid milk, milk products, greasy foods, and spicy foods. Drink clear fluids with electrolytes.

6. Factors that affect results:
   A. Fresh, room-temperature stool samples provide the best specimens. Do not incubate, refrigerate, or freeze the specimens.
   B. Reject specimens contaminated with urine, toilet paper, diapers, or toilet water.
   C. Mineral oil or magnesium antacids, MOM, kaolin, antimalarial drugs, or bismuth may interfere with accuracy.
   D. Specimens obtained by means of saline or phosphosoda enemas are acceptable. Often the first stool after the enema is discarded, and the subsequent stools are examined.
   E. Stool samples should be collected during laboratory hours so that they can be promptly examined.
   F. Antimicrobial or antiamebic therapy within 5-10 days before specimen collection may cause false-negative results.
   G. Residual barium from recent gastrointestinal studies may interfere with microscopic examination. Wait 1 week after barium procedures or laxative administration before collecting stool samples.
   H. Drugs and other substances that interfere with microscopic examination of fecal samples include antacids, antibiotics, barium, bismuth, castor oil, enemas, iron, magnesia, Metamucil, and tetracyclines.

7. Other data:
   A. Use with caution when handling the sample because some parasitic infections are very contagious.
   B. One negative result does not rule out a parasitic infection.
   C. A 24-hour stool collection may be requested to obtain an estimated egg count in known parasitic infestation.

D. Information about travel is of utmost importance to the laboratory in detecting the suspected parasite because different techniques are used to analyze stool when one is looking for specific parasites or ova.

PARATHYROID HORMONE (PTH), BLOOD

Norm. *Note:* norms vary by test method use. Check laboratory-specific norms.

		SI UNITS
Serum	11-54 pg/mL	11-54 ng/L
Cord	≤3 pg/mL	≤3 ng/L
2-20 years	9-52 pg/mL	9-52 ng/L
Adults	10-65 pg/mL	10-65 ng/L
Plasma	1.0-5.0 pmol/L	

Midmolecule and C-terminal

Serum		
1-16 years	51-217 pg/mL	51-217 ng/L
Adults	50-330 pg/mL	50-330 ng/L
Plasma	50 μLEq/mL	<50 mLEq/L

N-terminal

Serum		
2-13 years	14-21 pg/mL	14-21 ng/L
Adults	8-24 pg/mL	8-24 ng/L
Plasma	<6.1 pmol/L	

Usage. Primarily in the evaluation of abnormal calcium states to assist with the diagnosis of hyperparathyroid or hypothyroid disease. An ionized calcium is usually drawn with the parathyroid hormone (PTH) sample. Levels are also followed in chronic renal clients to identify the development of hyperthyroid function caused by phosphate retention and to monitor clients treated for same.

Increased. As a response to low serum calcium levels caused by calcium malabsorption, chronic renal failure, dietary vitamin D deficiency, osteomalacia, and renal dialysis. Also, ectopic production of PTH, lactation, primary hyperparathyroidism, parathyroid adenoma, parathyroid carcinoma, parathyroid hyperplasia, pregnancy, pseudohypoparathyroidism (sometimes), renal hypercalciuria, rickets (vitamin D dependent, vitamin D deficient), secondary hyperparathyroidism, and squamous cell carcinoma (kidney, lung, ovary, pancreas). PTH levels increase with the aging process.

Decreased. As a response to high calcium levels, autoimmune disease or cancer, Graves' disease, hypomagnesemia, hypoparathyroidism, parathyroidectomy (transient decrease), sarcoidosis, and vitamin A and D intoxication. Drugs include thiazide diuretics.

Description. Parathyroid hormone (PTH) is measured by radioassay using competitive protein-binding agents to identify and measure several molecular forms of PTH: intact and midmolecule fragments. N-terminal fragments and C-terminal fragments may be tested in some laboratories. Intact PTH is secreted by the parathyroid gland and is metabolized by the liver and kidneys into N-terminal fragments and C-terminal fragments. The intact and N-terminal fragments are helpful in identifying acute conditions, whereas C-terminal fragments indicate chronic disturbances of PTH metabolism. Parathyroid hormone is directly responsible for the plasma regulation of calcium and phosphorus. When the body's normal autoregulatory mechanism senses a decrease in serum calcium, the parathyroid gland is stimulated to secrete PTH. The elevated serum PTH triggers the release of calcium from bone and stimulates the renal tubules to increase reabsorption of calcium ions in the distal convoluted tubules and to decrease reabsorption of phosphorus in the proximal convoluted tubules. When the serum calcium concentration again becomes adequate, the parathyroid gland decreases PTH secretion. In the presence of primary parathyroid tumor or hyperplasia, the PTH-calcium autoregulation fails. As PTH secretion increases, so does the serum calcium level, ultimately resulting in a hypercalcemic condition that can be life threatening. Assessment of radioassayed PTH is helpful in differentiating parathyroid causes from nonparathyroid causes of hypercalcemia. Other causes of hypercalcemia generally display normal to slightly high or low PTH secretion. Thus PTH should always be evaluated in conjunction with serum ionized calcium levels.

Professional Considerations
1. Consent form NOT required.
2. Preparation:
   A. Tube: Red topped, red/gray topped, or gold topped or lavender topped; and ice.
   B. A morning fasting sample is recommended because there is a diurnal variation in PTH levels.
   C. Do NOT draw during hemodialysis.
   D. See *Client and family teaching.*
3. Procedure:
   A. Completely fill the red-topped, red/gray-topped, or gold-topped tube with blood.
   B. Some laboratories require that the sample be packed in ice.
   C. Some laboratories request 7 mL of blood in a lavender-topped tube as well.
4. Postprocedure care:
   A. Send the specimen to the laboratory immediately.
   B. Resume previous diet.
   C. Assess for signs of hypercalcemia: lethargy, headache, thirst, increased urinary output, decreased muscle tone, nausea, thirst, and flank pain.
   D. Assess for signs of hypocalcemia: lethargy, nausea, cramps, dysrhythmias, shallow breathing, tetany, and Chvostek's and Trousseau's signs.
5. Client and family teaching:
   A. Fast overnight before sampling.
   B. A change in diet may be needed, based on results. A diet either low or high in calcium may be indicated. Consider consulting a dietitian.
   C. Calcium is important to your body. It helps with blood clotting, bone strength, and heart contraction.

6. **Factors that affect results:**
   A. Reject lipemic specimens or specimens not received on ice.
   B. Ingestion of milk before the test may cause falsely low values.
   C. Radioisotope testing within the last 7 days may alter the results.
7. **Other data:**
   A. A neck venipuncture PTH level should be compared to a peripheral venipuncture PTH level if the test is performed to rule out parathyroid adenoma. The neck vein technique may help to confirm the diagnosis of hyperparathyroidism if the PTH level is much higher than that from a peripheral site.

PARATHYROID HORMONE RADIOIMMUNOASSAY, DIAGNOSTIC
(*see Parathyroid hormone, Blood*)

PARIETAL CELL ANTIBODY, BLOOD

Norm. Negative, none detected, or titer <1:120

Abnormal. Weakly positive, titer 1:120-1:140

Positive. Titer >1:180

Usage. Aids in differential diagnosis of autoimmune gastritis and pernicious anemia. Not so widely accepted as in the past for the diagnosis of pernicious anemia.

Positive. Autoimmune atrophic gastritis or pernicious anemia and thyroiditis. Parietal cell antibodies are also found in (but are not diagnostic of) Addison's disease, gastric ulcer, juvenile diabetes mellitus, iron deficiency anemia, myasthenia gravis, and Sjögren syndrome.

Description. Parietal cells are located among the epithelial cells of the stomach and secrete hydrochloric acid (HCl), which is essential for protein breakdown. Many adults who suffer from alterations in gastric acid stimulation (such as pernicious anemia) have an autoimmune response with circulating parietal cell antibodies or other antibodies. Parietal cell antibodies are present in 20-30% of people who have other autoimmune disorders. They are occasionally present in people who have gastric cancer or ulcers and are also found in up to 2% of normal children and 20% of older adults, particularly the siblings of clients with pernicious anemia. Some researchers believe that there may be a genetic component to pernicious anemia or gastric ulcer with parietal cell antibody activity. The antibodies can be detected with indirect immunofluorescence.

Professional Considerations

1. Consent form NOT required.
2. Preparation:
   A. Tube: Red topped, red/gray topped, or gold topped.
3. Procedure:
   A. Draw a 10-mL blood sample.
4. Postprocedure care:
   A. None.
5. Client and family teaching:
   A. Results are normally available within 72 hours.
6. Factors that affect results:
   A. One study found that the levels increased with increasing severity of atrophic gastritis in clients positive for *Helicobacter pylori*.
7. Other data:
   A. It has not been shown that parietal cell antibodies affect a person's ability to absorb B vitamins.

PAROXETINE
(see Selective serotonin reuptake inhibitors, Blood)

PARTIAL THROMBOPLASTIN TIME (PTT), PLASMA
(see Activated partial thromboplastin time and partial thromboplastin time, Plasma)

PAS
(see Periodic Acid–Schiff stain, Specimen)

PCG, DIAGNOSTIC
(see Phonocardiography, Diagnostic)

PCHE, PLASMA
(see Pseudocholinesterase, Plasma)

PCO, BLOOD
(see Carbon dioxide, Partial pressure, Blood and arterial blood gases)

PCP, URINE
(see Phencyclidine, Qualitative, Urine)

PELVIC ECHOGRAM
(see Gynecologic ultrasonography, Diagnostic)

PELVIC ULTRASONOGRAPHY
(see Gynecologic ultrasonography, Diagnostic)

PELVIMETRY AND PELVICEPHALOGRAPHY, DIAGNOSTIC

Norms:

Pelvic Inlet (Anteroposterior Diameters)	
Diagonal conjugate	12.5 cm
Obstetric conjugate	11.0 cm
True conjugate	11.5 cm

Pelvic Cavity (Midpelvis)	
Midplane	12.75 cm
Anteroposterior diameter	11.5-12.0 cm
Posterior sagittal diameter	4.5-5.0 cm
Transverse	10.5 cm

Pelvic Outlet	
Anteroposterior diameter	9.5 cm
Obstetric anteroposterior diameter	11.5 cm
Transverse diameter	8.0 cm
Suprapubic angle	85-90 degrees

Usage. Evaluation of pelvic adequacy for vaginal delivery when any of the following conditions are present: labor has been dysfunctional or slow; fetal positioning is breech, the fetal head fails to engage, or other abnormal positioning in labor occurs, especially in primigravidas, when maternal pelvic adequacy is questioned; history of pelvic fracture or injury or congenital deformity or disease, such as rickets, polio, or hip dysplasia, may affect the bony pelvis or hips. Examination of very small women or those with kyphoscoliosis or dwarfism. May be indicated when the physician is considering oxytocin administration. It is not the pelvic measurements alone but the pelvic measurements in relation to the size of the fetal head that are important to ensure safe delivery for these indicators. Pelvimetry measurements may be used when previous deliveries have been difficult or have produced large infants or in previous deliveries with an unplanned forceps delivery or nonelective cesarean section before another pregnancy. The radiographic tests are not performed as often as they were a decade ago.

Description. Pelvimetry is measurement of the internal dimensions of the bony pelvis, usually to determine the adequacy and shape of the maternal pelvis in relationship to fetal size and positioning for or during vaginal delivery. Estimates of pelvic measurements may be performed digitally during the physical examination by an obstetrician, nurse midwife, or trained obstetrical nurse (see *Pelvic measurements*). Other methods for more specific measurements of the pelvic outlet capacity and the fetal head size may be performed by radiography, CT scan, or MRI. Ultrasound pelvimetry is not considered accurate at this time. Pelvicephalography is a measurement of the fetal head diameters by a radiologic measurement. It is performed with special methods used to correct for radiographic distortion and magnification. Pelvimetry by radiography, ultrasonography, or computed tomography requires a physician's prescription.

Precautions

During pregnancy, risks of cumulative radiation exposure to the fetus from this and other previous or future imaging studies must be weighed against the benefits of the procedure. Although formal limits for client exposure are relative to this risk:benefit comparison, the United States Nuclear Regulatory Commission requires that the cumulative dose equivalent to an embryo/fetus from occupational exposure not exceed 0.5 rem (5 mSv). Radiation dosage to the fetus is proportional to the distance of the anatomy studied from the abdomen and decreases as pregnancy progresses. For pregnant clients, consult the radiologist/radiology department to obtain estimated fetal radiation exposure from this procedure.

Professional Considerations

1. Consent form NOT required.
2. **Preparation:**
   A. Prepare the client for transport to the appropriate radiology department.
3. **Procedure:**
   A. *Radiographic pelvimetry* is completed in the x-ray department. The client is positioned carefully for an erect lateral view of the pelvis and a supine AP view of the pelvis. It is important that exact measurement of the woman's position and distance from the film at the time of radiography be taken for a correction factor used in the computation of pelvic measurements. The disadvantages include radiation hazards to the fetus and the fact that radiography alone is no longer considered reliable as a tool to diagnose problems with labor and delivery.
   B. *Computed tomograph pelvimetry* is considered more accurate and easier to perform. There is less x-ray exposure to the fetus and less chance of distortion if the woman is positioned correctly on the table. Three views are taken: anterior, lateral, and axial. Electronic calipers are used to take the numerical pelvic measurements. CT is particularly useful in women with a history of pelvic fractures and before delivery for any situation except those in which a cesarean section is already planned.
   C. *Ultrasonography* is not yet clinically helpful. A radiograph is also required, and a fetal pelvic index that estimates proportion or disproportion for vaginal delivery must be computed.
   D. *MRI* is considered quite accurate and allows for imagery of the complete fetus as well as the mother's pelvis and pelvic measurements. The MRI has the advantage of evaluation of the soft tissues of the pelvic region as reasons for dystocia and uses NO radiation to the fetus. MRI is costly and difficult to access in emergency situations.
   E. *Cephalopelvic proportion:* Use of the above radiographic techniques late in the pregnancy or during a difficult labor to assess the mother's pelvic dimensions as relates specifically to the size of the fetal head and position.

F. Knowledge of the course of normal labor and delivery and full understanding of the correction factors for radiographic pelvimetry are essential.

G. For digital examination, the lengths of the first two fingers on either hand of the examiner are measured in centimeters. These fingers should be used for obtaining all measurements.

4. **Postprocedure care:**
   A. Assist the woman to a position of comfort.
   B. Assess the parents' readiness for new roles; include information on feeding, supplies, safety, and referral agencies.

5. **Client and family teaching:**
   A. The procedure takes 15 minutes.
   B. The client must remove clothes and put on a gown.
   C. Explain the relationship of the results to the type of delivery—vaginal versus cesarean.

6. **Factors that affect results:**
   A. None.

7. **Other data:**
   A. Emotional support is more likely needed during this test than at other times during pregnancy.

PELVIMETRY, DIAGNOSTIC (PELVIC EXAMINATION, DIGITAL)

Norm. *Pelvic inlet:* 11.0 cm.
Pelvic outlet: 8.0 cm.

Usage. Evaluation of the pelvic adequacy for vaginal delivery. Clinical, noninvasive estimations of the important pelvic measurements in pregnancy. If there have been pelvic injuries, known bony abnormalities, or a previous difficult labor, a radiograph or a CT scan is needed to fully assess the adequacy for vaginal delivery.

Description. Digital pelvimetry may be performed by the physician or nurse midwife during pregnancy or nearing delivery to estimate the adequacy of the woman's pelvic measurements for vaginal delivery. Any abnormality noted with this method is confirmed by other methods, and pelvicephalography is utilized to fully assess the prospects of normal delivery.

Professional Considerations
1. Consent form NOT required.
2. **Preparation:**
   A. Obtain rubber gloves, lubricant, and a ruler or Thom's pelvimeters.
   B. Position the woman on the examination table in the dorsal lithotomy position with her feet supported in stirrups.
3. **Procedure:**
   A. The lengths of the first two fingers on either hand of the examiner are measured in centimeters. These fingers should be used for obtaining all measurements.
   B. *Pelvic inlet measurement:* The examiner inserts these fingers into the vagina, using the middle finger to locate the lower border of the symphysis pubis and the sacral promontory. To measure the diagonal conjugate, the other hand is used to indicate where the pubis makes contact with the proximal part of the hand. This distance is calculated in centimeters. The obstetric conjugate is calculated by subtraction of 1.5 cm from the length of the diagonal conjugate. The true conjugate is calculated by subtraction of 1.0 cm from the diagonal conjugate. Since the obstetric conjugate is the narrowest anteroposterior diameter through which the fetus must travel, radiographic examination for accurate measurement is helpful. To measure the obstetric conjugate on radiographic film, locate the inner point of the symphysis and measure back to the sacral promontory. This distance should be approximately 11.0 cm.
   C. *Pelvic capacity measurement:* The sagittal posterior diameter is the only midpelvis diameter that can be palpated. The fingers are inserted into the vagina, locating the sacrospinous ligament. This ligament is traced by palpation from the ischial spines to the sacrum. The sacrospinous ligament is usually three fingerbreadths long, or 4-5 cm. The capacity of the midpelvis, particularly the midplane, will give the examiner an idea of how labor will progress, if at all.
   D. *Pelvic outlet measurement:* The pelvic outlet is the area in which

the fetal head crowns and extends for delivery. The pelvic outlet measurements can be obtained by palpation. The most important diameter is the obstetric antero-posterior outlet diameter. The flexibility and mobility of this diameter are usually assessed by palpation of the coccyx. With the finger inserted into the rectum while the thumb externally grasps the coccyx, the examiner attempts to move the coccyx downward. An immobile coccyx indicates a decreased outlet diameter. The anteroposterior outlet diameter is obtained by insertion of two fingers into the vagina and locating the tip of the sacrum and externally locating the symphysis pubis with the other hand. The distance between the fingers is marked. The suprapubic angle is estimated by placement of the thumbs, side by side, at the symphysis border. The fingers are then separated from the thumbs and placed flat against the thighs. The angle at which the fingers are able to separate from the thumbs is the suprapubic angle. If the suprapubic angle is narrow, minimal finger-thumb separation will occur. Another way to measure the suprapubic angle is to insert one finger into the vagina, locating the internal margin while the other hand externally palpates the top of the symphysis pubis. An imaginary line is drawn between the two points and assessments of the depth and bend of the symphysis pubis are made. From these calculations, an estimate of the angle is made. Preferably the symphysis pubis is short and continues inward, allowing for an adequate obstetric conjugate. If it were bony and elongated, the fetus might have difficulty extending the head during delivery. The transverse outlet diameter is measured with the fist on Thom's pelvimetry position between the ischial tuberosities. Pelvimetry outlet measurements are important in the assessment of the potential for fetal head injuries and perineal tearing during the final stages of labor.

4. **Postprocedure care:**
   A. Assist the woman to a position of comfort.
5. **Client and family teaching:**
   A. The procedure takes 15 minutes.
   B. Explain the implications of the findings in relation to the type of delivery anticipated.
6. **Factors that affect results:**
   A. The accuracy of the results depends on the skill and performance technique of the examiner.
7. **Other data:**
   A. Outlet dystocia is a narrowing of the pubic arch and may make it difficult for the fetus to extend its head, resulting in the need for a forceps delivery.

PEMPHIGUS ANTIBODIES, BLOOD

Norm. Negative.

Usage. Confirmation of diagnosis and management of pemphigus and pemphigoid. Diagnosis is usually made by clinical findings and biopsy with findings of a histologic picture of disruption of the epidermal intercellular connections (which is called "acantholysis") and microscopic deposits of IgG.

Description. Pemphigus and pemphigoid are autoimmune blistering diseases of the skin and mucus membranes. Its cause is unknown, and it occurs in middle-aged or older adults. Initial lesions are located in the mouth or on the scalp. After the blisters break, secondary infections may occur in the raw, eroded areas. Before the discovery of steroid therapy, the disease was fatal in 95% of cases. Pemphigus is an autoimmune disease, with cause unknown, in which the autoantibodies cause a separation of the epidermal cells, especially after even mild trauma to a specific area. The circulating IgG antibodies can be detected by indirect immunofluorescence.

Professional Considerations
1. Consent form NOT required.
2. **Preparation:**
   A. Tube: Red topped, red/gray topped, or gold topped.
3. **Procedure:**
   A. Draw a 3-mL blood sample.

4. Postprocedure care:
   A. None.
5. Client and family teaching:
   A. Pemphigus is treatable with immunosuppressive and steroid drugs. These drugs can cause side effects that include slow healing, weight redistribution, and psychoses. It is important to watch for signs of these changes and tell the doctor about them.
   B. Bed rest and attention to nutrition are important.
   C. Anesthetic mouth rinses may reduce oral pain, especially before eating.
   D. Secondary infection and fluid and electrolyte losses are the most common complications and causes of mortality.
6. Factors that affect results:
   A. False-positive results may occur in the presence of lupus, burns, or drug reactions.
7. Other data:
   A. In pemphigoid, antibody titer levels may provide a correlate for disease activity and may be used to follow management or predict a relapse.
   B. Pemphigus may be drug induced by penicillamine or captopril.

PENICILLIN SKIN TEST, DIAGNOSTIC

Norm. Absence of immediate wheal and flare.

Usage. Determination of hypersensitivity to penicillin after previous history of allergic sensitivity.

Description. After a period of time, many people stop expressing IgE sensitivity to beta-lactam antibiotics (that is, penicillin), particularly if the reaction occurred during childhood or while the drug was taken orally. This test is used for individuals with a previous history of hypersensitivity to penicillin and who require the drug to treat a particular infection. By injecting small amounts of PrePen (Kremer-Urban), benzylpenicilloyl polylysine, or benzylpenicillin G intradermally and examining for evidence of an enlarged wheal with erythema, one can identify many individuals at risk for developing anaphylaxis.

Professional Considerations
1. Consent form NOT required.

Risks
Allergic reaction to intradermal injection (itching, hives, rash, tight feeling in the throat, shortness of breath, bronchospasm, anaphylaxis, death).

Contraindications
Previous anaphylactic reaction to penicillin.

2. Preparation:
   A. Withhold antihistamines for 24-48 hours before the test.
   B. *Emergency readiness:* The test should be completed in an area where appropriately trained ACLS personnel and emergency medical equipment are available because of the possibility of anaphylactic reaction.
   C. Obtain 0.9% saline for the injection, PrePen or benzylpenicillin G, alcohol, tuberculin syringes, and 25-gauge $\frac{1}{2}$-inch needles for intradermal injection.
3. Procedure:
   A. Initially prick or scratch the skin on a distal extremity with PrePen or benzylpenicillin G.
   B. Wait 15 minutes to examine the area for evidence of wheal and flare.
   C. If these are not evident, proceed with one of the following procedures:
      i. *PrePen test:* Inject 0.02-0.04 mL of PrePen reagent intradermally to make a 3-mm bleb on the form. At the same time, inject the same amount of 0.9% saline intradermally near the same area, making the same-sized bleb for use as a control site. After 15-20 minutes, examine the forearm for wheals. Measure the wheals, if present, in millimeters. A positive result will be >5 mm in diameter, with or without a surrounding erythematous area.
      ii. *Benzylpenicillin G test:* Inject a small bleb of benzylpenicillin G, 100 U/mL, intradermally in the forearm. At the same time, inject the same amount of 0.9% saline intradermally

near the same area, making the same-sized bleb for use as a control site. If no reaction occurs after 15-30 minutes, repeat the procedure, using benzylpenicillin G, 1000 U/mL. If no reaction occurs after 15-30 minutes, repeat the procedure using benzylpenicillin G, 10,000 U/mL. A 0.9% saline control should be administered with each successive dose. After 15-20 minutes, examine the forearm for wheals. Measure the wheals, if present, in millimeters. A positive result will be >5 mm in diameter, with or without a surrounding erythematous area.
iii. If the procedure is to be repeated using several strengths of penicillin, start with the lowest concentration.
4. **Postprocedure care:**
   A. Keep the area uncovered and open to air.
5. **Client and family teaching:**
   A. Call the physician immediately if symptoms of a delayed allergic reaction (listed above, under *Risks*) occur, and seek immediate medical attention if any difficulty in swallowing or breathing occurs.
   B. The penicillin skin test allows assessment only for immediate or accelerated hypersensitivity reactions. There is no test to assess for risk of delayed reactions.
   C. Clients with a positive skin test to penicillin are also generally reactive to first-generation cephalosporins.
6. **Factors that affect results:**
   A. Recent administration of antihistamines may cause false-negative results.
7. **Other data:**
   A. A positive skin test indicates a 67%-73% risk of immediate to accelerated reaction to penicillin therapy.
   B. 2%-6% of clients with negative penicillin skin test results have anaphylactic reactions with the administration of penicillin.
   C. Repeat skin testing should be performed before reinitiation of penicillin therapy if the initial test was negative and the first course of the drug has been completed.

D. It is not necessary to withhold corticosteroids before penicillin skin testing.
E. Clients with a negative skin test should still be given penicillin cautiously; IV administration may quickly resensitize the client to the drug.

PENICILLINASE TEST (BETA-LACTAMASE PRODUCTION TEST), DIAGNOSTIC

Norm. Negative for penicillinase.

Usage. Client on antibiotic therapy for bacterial infections, especially *Haemophilus influenzae*, *Staphylococcus aureus*, and *Moraxella (Branhamella) catarrhalis*. To test for bacterial strains that may be resistant to the penicillin type of antibiotics.

Description. Penicillin and some cephalosporin antibiotics work by attaching to a receptor in the cell membrane of bacteria and inhibiting bacteria cell synthesis. When the receptor/penicillin bond is broken, the bacteria is destroyed. Penicillin's bonding ring is a beta-lactam ring. Certain strains of bacteria may have penicillinase (also called beta-lactamase), an enzyme that destroys the beta-lactam ring of penicillin, making it ineffective against the bacteria. When certain strains of bacteria, including *Staphylococcus*, *Neisseria gonorrhoeae*, *Haemophilus influenzae*, and others produce penicillinase, drugs such as penicillins and first- and second-generation cephalosporins are rendered ineffective against them. This test is performed to detect the presence of penicillinase on isolates of body substances when penicillin treatment shows no improvement in clinical condition. If test results are positive, the treatment is changed to a penicillinase-resistant penicillin or a cephalosporin such as Augmentin, Unasyn, or Timentin.

Professional Considerations
1. Consent form NOT required.
2. **Preparation:**
   A. For sputum samples, obtain a suction catheter and tubing, a sputum trap, and a suction source.

B. For wounds or abscesses, obtain a sterile needle, a syringe, and a red-topped tube.

C. For urine, obtain a straight catheter and a sterile container; or a syringe, a needle, and alcohol wipes; or a clean-catch urine collection kit.

3. **Procedure:**

A. Using a sterile technique, collect at least a 1-mL sample of the particular body substance to be tested.

B. For sputum, collect the sample directly into a sputum trap by suction.

C. For wounds or abscesses, aspirate 1 mL through a needle into a syringe and inject it into a red-topped tube.

D. For urine, obtain the sample by straight catheterization by aspirating through the collection port of an indwelling urinary catheter or by a voided clean-catch technique. See clean-catch collection instructions in the test *Body fluid, Routine, Culture.*

4. **Postprocedure care:**

A. Write the specimen source, collection time, and recent antibiotic therapy on the laboratory requisition.

B. Send specimens to the laboratory immediately.

5. **Client and family teaching:**

A. Deep coughs are necessary to produce sputum rather than saliva, To produce the proper specimen, take in several breaths without fully exhaling each. Then expel sputum with a "cascade cough."

B. The necessity of the test is associated with the choice of antibiotic to treat the infectious organism.

C. Results are normally available within 48 hours.

6. **Factors that affect results:**

A. Do not contaminate the specimen with surrounding tissue.

7. **Other data:**

A. This test is not routinely performed before penicillin therapy is initiated.

B. Recent development of a fluorescent developer for use in the laboratory has increased the sensitivity of the test.

PEPSINOGEN I (PEPSINOGEN A, PGI) AND PEPSINOGEN II (PGII), BLOOD

Norm:

		SI UNITS
Pepsinogen I		
Adults	124-142 ng/mL	124-142 µg/L
Women at delivery	116-138 ng/mL	116-138 µg/L
Cord blood	24-28 ng/mL	24-28 µg/L
Children		
<12 months	72-82 ng/mL	72-82 µg/L
12 months to <2 years	90-106 ng/mL	90-106 µg/L
3-6 years	80-104 ng/mL	80-104 µg/L
7-10 years	77-103 ng/mL	77-103 µg/L
11-14 years	96-118 ng/mL	96-118 µg/L
Premature infants	20-24 ng/mL	20-24 µg/L
Pepsinogen II	3-19 ng/mL	3-19 mg/L
PGI:PGII Ratio	4:1	
Atrophic gastritis	<2.5	

Increased Pepsinogen I. Diseases or situations in which gastric acid is increased: duodenal ulcer (30%-50% of clients with duodenal ulcer have increased pepsinogen levels); gastrinomas; gastritis, acute and chronic; hyper- gastrinemia; and hypertrophic gastropathy. It is associated with chronic renal failure, *Helicobacter pylori* infection, and Zollinger-Ellison syndrome. May be inherited autosomal dominant trait. Drugs include omeprazole.

Increased Pepsinogen II. Acute and chronic superficial gastritis and duodenal ulcers, *H. pylori* infection and Zollinger-Ellison syndrome. Drugs include omeprazole.

Decreased Pepsinogen I. Diseases or conditions in which there is a decrease in the mass of chief cells: Addison's disease, atrophic gastritis, gastric cancer, hypopituitarism, myxedema, pernicious anemia, and after vagotomy. Absence of pepsinogen I is seen with achlorhydria with pernicious anemia. Drugs include gastric inhibitory polypeptides (GIP), anticholinergics, and histamine (H₂)-antagonists.

Decreased Pepsinogen II. Addison's disease, gastric neoplasia, gastric resection, gastritis, myxedema, status postgastrectomy.

Usage. Pepsinogen levels, especially pepsinogen II, are useful to help diagnose atrophic gastritis and as a clinical monitor to assess the efficacy of the treatment of gastric ulcer disease.

Description. The term *pepsinogen I* (PGI) encompasses five of the eight fractions of pepsinogen found in the bloodstream. Pepsinogen I (PGI) is an inactive precursor of the proteolytic enzyme pepsin and is produced by the chief cells of the gastric glands. Pepsinogen secretion is stimulated by the vagus nerve as well as hormonal activity of gastrin, secretin, and cholecystokinin. When the pH of the stomach is acidic, pepsinogen I is converted to pepsin, which acts on amino acids in the first step of protein digestion. Activated pepsin is capable of converting additional pepsinogen(s) to active enzymes. The remaining related pepsinogens are collectively termed, "*pepsinogen II.*" Pepsinogens group II are related to the pepsinogen I group but are found in Brunner's gland and pyloric glands in the gastric antrum and proximal portion of the duodenum. The PGI:PGII ratio decreases linearly with the severity of atrophic gastritis, and decreased ratio has been associated with an increased risk of gastric cancer. A small amount of pepsinogen (1%) is absorbed into the bloodstream and can be assayed

Professional Considerations
1. Consent form NOT required.

2. **Preparation:**
   A. Preschedule this test with the laboratory. The sample should be a fasting morning specimen.
   B. Tube: Red topped, red/gray topped, or gold topped.
   C. See *Client and family teaching.*
3. **Procedure:**
   A. Draw a 10-mL blood sample.
   B. Send the sample to the laboratory for evaluation or storage (frozen) immediately.
4. **Postprocedure care:**
   A. Begin meals as prescribed.
5. **Client and family teaching:**
   A. Fast overnight before the test.
   B. High pepsinogen is considered a risk factor for duodenal ulcer. High serum pepsinogen II level is a risk factor for developing gastric ulcers.
   C. High pepsinogen I levels and low pepsinogen I:II ratios are associated with *H. pylori* infection, which is now associated with ulcer disease.
   D. Results are normally available within 48 hours.
6. **Factors that affect results:**
   A. Impaired renal function causes elevated results.
   B. Pepsinogen levels may increase with age.
   C. There is a diurnal pattern to pepsinogen II secretion; failure to obtain an early-morning specimen may affect the interpretation of results.
7. **Other data:**
   A. Endoscopy is considered of more use in diagnosing gastric and duodenal abnormalities than the pepsinogen I level is.
   B. A diagnosis of chronic atrophic gastritis is recommended if PGI is less than 70 ng/mL and PGI:PGII ratio is less than 3.0.
   C. In pernicious anemia, Pepsinogen I is decreased, while Pepsinogen II is normal.
   D. See also *Pepsinogen I antibody, Blood.*

PEPSINOGEN I ANTIBODY, BLOOD

Norm. Negative.

Usage. Method of detection of autoantibodies of pepsinogen I in the serum.

Positive. Pernicious anemia (some gastric lesions and some duodenal lesions).

Description. One performs this test by using the enzyme-linked immunosorbent assay to detect the occurrence of autoantibodies against pepsinogen. Pepsinogen I antibody has been shown to be a major chief cell antigen. Its presence may indicate the presence of a gastric or duodenal lesion that destroys the mucosa of the surrounding area. This destruction is believed to trigger the production of autoantibodies against the pepsinogen cell contents not recognized as self by the immune system.

Professional Considerations
1. Consent form NOT required.
2. Preparation:
   A. Tube: Red topped, red/gray topped, or gold topped.
3. Procedure:
   A. Draw a 7-mL blood sample.
4. Postprocedure care:
   A. None.
5. Client and family teaching:
   A. Results are normally available within 48 hours.
6. Factors that affect results:
   A. Renal failure may enhance positive results.
7. Other data:
   A. This test may serve as a subclinical marker of clients with ulcer tendencies.
   B. See also *Pepsinogen I and pepsinogen II, Blood.*

PEPTAVLON STIMULATION TEST
(*see Gastric acid analysis test, Diagnostic*)

PERCUTANEOUS LIVER BIOPSY
(*see Liver biopsy, Diagnostic*)

PERCUTANEOUS TRANSHEPATIC CHOLANGIOGRAPHY (PTHC, PTC), DIAGNOSTIC

Norm. Normal diameter and filling of the cystic, hepatic, and common bile ducts. Normal-shaped gallbladder; no masses or irregular borders.

Usage. Identification and determination of obstructive jaundice. The procedure may also be completed as part of a work-up for continued pain after cholecystectomy.

Description. Fluoroscopic examination of the biliary ducts using an iodine-based contrast dye, performed in the radiology department by a radiologist under IV sedation or local anesthesia. This allows visualization of all the bile ducts and biliary flow. These ducts will appear dilated if there is an obstruction. Biliary obstruction causes that can be identified may be filling defects, spasms of the sphincter of Oddi, strictures, tumors, and stones, particularly those located in the common bile duct. This test may be performed in conjunction with magnetic resonance imaging or computed tomography.

Professional Considerations
1. Consent form IS required.

Risks
Allergic reaction to dye (itching, hives, rash, tight feeling in the throat, shortness of breath, bronchospasm, anaphylaxis, death); bleeding, extravasation of contrast dye into the peritoneal cavity, peritonitis, renal toxicity from contrast medium, septicemia, and subcapsular injection.

Contraindications
Previous allergy to iodine, shellfish, or radiographic dye; massive ascites or uncontrolled coagulopathies; pregnancy (because of radioactive iodine crossing the blood-placental barrier), renal insufficiency; sedatives are contraindicated in clients with central nervous system depression.

Relative Contraindication
Client may be premedicated with diphenhydramine to prevent reaction.

2. Preparation:
   A. See *Client and family teaching.*
   B. Notify the physician and the radiologist of any known or possible allergy to determine if premedication will be prescribed.
   C. Obtain baseline prothrombin time, clotting time, and platelet counts. Notify the physician and the radiologist of any abnormalities. Transfusion to normalize coagulation may be prescribed just before the study.

D. A sedative may be prescribed, especially for children. Monitor the respiratory status continually if sedation is given.

E. Obtain a surgical scrub and povidone-iodine solution, 2% lidocaine (Xylocaine), a 23-gauge flexible needle, sterile gloves and drapes, and contrast medium.

F. Have emergency equipment readily available.

G. When this procedure uses the small, flexible needle, surgical backup is no longer considered necessary. If a large-bore needle is used, this procedure should have surgical backup.

3. **Procedure:**

A. The client is secured in a supine position on the fluoroscopy tilt table.

B. The upper right quadrant of the abdomen is cleansed with surgical scrub solution and prepared with povidone-iodine solution. The entire abdomen is covered with sterile drapes.

C. The skin is anesthetized with 2% lidocaine.

D. By means of a long, flexible, 23-gauge needle, the liver is punctured, and the needle is advanced under fluoroscopy until bile is aspirated from the duct. A small amount of contrast dye is injected, and placement is visualized by fluoroscopy. Once the needle is located in the biliary tract, the remaining contrast dye is injected. If the bile ducts appear dilated, the contrast material will be diluted to allow for full visualization to the biliary tract without additional contrast-medium dose.

E. Fluoroscopy is used to observe the flow of contrast medium through the ducts into the small intestine. It may be necessary to gently rotate the scanning table vertically and horizontally, or the client may be asked to change to a side-lying position. Erect or decubitus films may be required to visualize the complete system.

4. **Postprocedure care:**

A. Apply a dry, sterile dressing to the injection site.

B. Assess the injection site for bleeding, swelling, or tenderness every hour × 4 and then every 8 hours until 24 hours after the procedure.

C. Continue postsedation assessment of the respiratory status. If deep sedation was used, follow institutional protocol for postsedation monitoring. Typical monitoring includes continuous ECG monitoring and pulse oximetry, with continual assessments (every 5-15 minutes) of airway, vital signs, and neurologic status until the client is lying quietly awake, is breathing independently, and responds to commands spoken in a normal tone.

D. Maintain bed rest for several hours as prescribed. A right-side lying position may be prescribed.

E. Resume previous diet.

F. Analgesics may be prescribed for pain.

G. Observe for signs of septicemia, peritonitis, hemorrhage, and tension pneumothorax.

H. Antibiotics may be continued for 2-3 days.

5. **Client and family teaching:**

A. Fast from food and fluids for 8-12 hours before the procedure.

B. A mild laxative such as magnesium citrate may be prescribed the night before the procedure.

C. Antibiotics may be prescribed during the 24-48 hours before the procedure.

D. Transient pain may be experienced during the injection of the dye.

E. It is important to lie still for the study to avoid injury to internal organs. Sedation may be used to help you lie still.

F. There should be a responsible adult available to take you home and care for you for 24 hours.

G. Surgical intervention may be required if obstruction is diagnosed.

H. The procedure takes up to 1 hour.

6. **Factors that affect results:**

A. Gas overlying the biliary ducts or obesity can interfere with radiograph clarity.

B. Barium, from previous studies, may interfere with the fluoroscopy.

7. **Other data:**

A. None.

PERFUSION LUNG SCAN, DIAGNOSTIC

(see Lung scan, Perfusion and ventilation, Diagnostic)

PERICARDIOCENTESIS, DIAGNOSTIC

Norm:

FEATURE	FINDINGS
Normal	
Quantity of fluid	10-50 mL
Appearance	Clear, straw-colored
Bacteria	Absent
Glucose	Approximates blood glucose level
Erythrocytes	Absent
Leukocytes	Absent
Abnormal	
Blood streaks	Tuberculosis or tumors
Turbid	Infection, pericarditis, or malignancy
Grossly bloody	Traumatic tap, cardiac rupture, or bleeding disorders
Blood obtained on pericardiocentesis	If it clots, this indicates entering the heart. If it does not clot, it is from the pericardium.
Milky	Lymphatic drained into the pericardium, chylopericardium
Chemistry	
Low glucose compared to serum levels	Bacterial infection or malignancy
CEA levels	Tumor—correlate with cytology studies

Usage. Effusion (pericardial), emergency treatment for pericardial tamponade, and removal of pericardial fluid for diagnostic testing.

Description. Pericardiocentesis is the aspiration of fluid surrounding the heart and contained within the pericardial sac. The procedure involves the transthoracic insertion of a needle through the intercostal space into the pericardium and may be done with guidance from transesophageal echocardiography, when the effusions are small and harder to locate. Excess fluid may accumulate because of pericarditis, after cardiac surgery, heart transplant rejection, cardiac trauma, myocardial rupture, acute rheumatic fever, metabolic diseases (fluid will likely be clear), or tumor. If the amount is greater than 50 mL or accumulates rapidly, it may result in restricted ventricular filling and stroke volume, which progresses to elevated venous blood pressure, tachycardia, and, eventually, cardiac tamponade. Other less common causes of pericardial effusion are blunt chest trauma in children, sarcoidosis and other connective tissue disorders, and AIDS. Cases of chylopericardium after aortic valve surgery or coronary artery bypass grafting have been recorded.

Professional Considerations

1. Consent form IS required unless the procedure is performed as an emergency.

Risks

Air embolism, cardiac arrest, cardiac tamponade, coronary artery laceration, dysrhythmias, gastric puncture, hemorrhage, hemothorax, hepatic puncture, hydropneumothorax, infection, laceration of coronary artery, peritoneal puncture, pneumothorax, puncture of cardiac chamber, vasovagal arrest, ventricular fibrillation, and ventricular perforation.

Contraindications

Anticoagulant therapy, bleeding disorders, thrombocytopenia.

2. Preparation:
   A. Obtain baseline vital signs and neurologic check, and monitor closely throughout the procedure. The procedure will likely be performed in the cardiac

catheterization laboratory or an intensive care unit.

B. Have an emergency cart, a defibrillator, and a 12-lead ECG machine at the bedside, with appropriate personnel trained in ACLS.

C. Establish intravenous access.

D. Obtain 1%-2% lidocaine (Xylocaine), sterile gloves, povidone-iodine solution, and a sterile pericardiocentesis tray. The tray should include a short-beveled, 14- to 18-gauge, 4- to 5-inch cardiac needle or Cath-Over Needle (spinal needle); a 25-gauge needle; a 35- to 50-mL syringe; a three-way stopcock; red-topped, green-topped, and lavender topped tubes; sterile gauze; a Kelly clamp; ground wire; and an alligator clip.

E. Perform continuous ECG monitoring before, during, and after the procedure. Observe for development of potentially life-threatening dysrhythmias.

F. See *Client and family teaching.*

3. Procedure:

A. Position the client semirecumbent with the head of the bed elevated between 30 and 60 degrees.

B. Cleanse the skin of the chest from the xiphoid process to the left costal margin with povidone-iodine solution.

C. The subxiphoid insertion site is injected with 1%-2% lidocaine.

D. A sterile alligator clip is used to attach the ECG lead V to the aspiration needle, or an echocardiogram is utilized to guide the needle insertion. In emergency situations, in cardiac arrest, the needle insertion is performed "blind."

E. An open three-way stopcock with a 50-mL syringe attached is connected to the cardiac needle. The needle is then inserted into the subxiphoid area, between the xiphoid and the costal margin.

F. The ECG (grounded) is used to monitor and to guide the needle insertion as follows: The appearance of an acute increase in the QRS complex indicates pericardial penetration. Epicardial ventricular contact by the needle is indicated by elevation of the ST segment and ventricular ectopy, and atrial contact by the needle is indicated by elevation of the PR segment. An abnormally shaped QRS complex may indicate myocardial perforation. Echocardiography is increasingly used, especially in the nonemergency situation to guide pericardiocentesis.

G. When the pericardium is penetrated, pericardial fluid should appear in the syringe. Grossly bloody aspirate will occur if a cardiac chamber is perforated. At this point, a Kelly clamp applied to the needle at the point of insertion stabilizes the position. The remainder of the pericardial fluid is aspirated.

H. The Kelly clamp and syringe are then removed, and a gauze pad is applied with pressure to the site for 3-5 minutes.

I. The pericardial fluid is measured and injected into the red-topped, green-topped, and lavender-topped tubes.

4. Postprocedure care:

A. Label the specimen tubes with the site and time of collection. Write the diagnosis and any recent antibiotic therapy on the laboratory requisition. Send the specimens to the laboratory.

B. The client is usually maintained in the intensive care unit to monitor continuous ECG for 24 hours after the procedure.

C. Assess vital signs every 15 minutes × 4, then every 30-60 minutes for 2 hours, and then every 4 hours for 24 hours if the client is hemodynamically stable.

D. Monitor for symptoms of cardiac tamponade for at least 24 hours. Beck's triad, the classic symptoms of cardiac tamponade, includes neck vein distention, hypotension, and heart sounds that are muffled and distant. The narrowing of pulse pressure (when the systolic and diastolic blood pressure numbers begin to go toward one another) may also be a sign of cardiac tamponade.

5. Client and family teaching:

A. Inform the client and family about the procedure and the seriousness of the condition. They should, if possible, understand the procedure and the need for ICU care before consent.

B. It is important to lie motionless throughout the procedure.

C. Assure that the client and family fully understand the condition related to the pericardiocentesis.

D. Signs and symptoms to report to the physician include chest pain, shortness of breath, and dizziness or light-headedness.

E. The catheter may be left in place if there is a need for further fluid drainage.

F. The family should be approached on CPR readiness and given resources on how to learn CPR.

6. Factors that affect results:
   A. Prepericardiocentesis echocardiographic localization of the effusion helps to minimize the chance of complications from the procedure.

7. Other data:
   A. None.

PERIODIC ACID–SCHIFF STAIN (PAS), SPECIMEN

Norm. No abnormal findings.

Usage. Limited clinical use includes the following:

1. Whole blood or bone marrow indicative for leukemia diagnosis, though phenotyping for the markers of the various forms of leukemia are more accurate and more widely used.

2. PAS may also be used to identify a fungus infection. The polysaccharide cell walls of fungus are stained by PAS so that a fungal infection is suspected when exudate, body fluids, or tissue homogenates are stained with PAS and the cell walls or portions of the cell wall identified. The test is nonspecific for the type of fungus.

Description. The agent stains glycogen, whole blood, and bone marrow specimens, and gives a pattern when positive that is indicative for several forms of leukemia. PAS does not stain normal lymphocytes, myeloblasts normoblasts, or megakaryoblasts. It stains granulocytes, platelets, megakaryocytes, fungus, and some bacteria.

Professional Considerations

1. Consent form NOT required for whole-blood specimens or for swabs of most body fluids and exudates. Consent IS required for bone marrow aspiration. Consent IS required for tissue sampling for PAS for fungus or for sampling of exudates, which requires an invasive procedure. See individual procedures for risks and contraindications.

2. Preparation:
   A. Obtain a sterile swab approved for microbiologic use, a glass slide, and a sterile container. Obtain sterile saline if the conjunctivae will be swabbed.
   B. Determine the specimen source and equipment required for the specimen.

3. Procedure:
   A. Obtain 10 mL of whole blood in a nonheparinized tube.
   B. See *Bone marrow aspiration analysis, Diagnostic,* if the test is to be performed on bone marrow.

4. Postprocedure care:
   A. Write the specimen source, the collection time, and the client's diagnosis on the laboratory requisition.
   B. Send the specimen to the laboratory within 2 hours.

5. Client and family teaching:
   A. Results are normally available within 5 days.
   B. This test does not identify specific fungi, nor can it distinguish between ALL and AML.

6. Factors that affect results:
   A. Contamination of specimens invalidates the results.

7. Other data:
   A. The smears of blood or bone marrow of clients with acute lymphatic leukemia show coarse granules or blocks of PAS-positive material in 67% of cases.
   B. The smears of blood or bone marrow of clients with acute monocytic leukemia have PAS-positive discrete granules.
   C. The "hairy" appearance of cells in hairy cell leukemia indicates PAS positivity.
   D. PAS cannot be used to distinguish between acute lymphatic leukemia and acute myeloid leukemia, nor can it be used to determine benign or malignant lymphatic disorders.

E. PAS does not identify the type of fungal infection, only that fungal infection is present.

PERITONEAL FLUID ANALYSIS, SPECIMEN
(see Paracentesis, Diagnostic)

PERITONEOSCOPY, DIAGNOSTIC
(see Laparoscopy, Diagnostic)

PERSANTINE-SESTAMIBI STRESS TEST AND SCAN, DIAGNOSTIC
(see Heart scan, Diagnostic)

PET SCAN
(see Positron emission tomography, Diagnostic)

PET/CT
(see Dual modality imaging, Diagnostic)

PFT
(see Pulmonary function test, Diagnostic)

pH, BLOOD
(see Blood gases, Arterial, Blood; Blood gases, Capillary, Blood; Blood gases, Venous, Blood)

pH, STOOL

Norm:

Adult	7.0-7.5
Newborn	5.0-7.0
Bottle-fed infant	Neutral to slightly alkaline pH of 7.0-8.0
Breast-fed infant	Slightly acidic

Increased. Colitis, protein breakdown, and villous adenoma.

Decreased. Breast-fed infants, celiac disease, disaccharidase deficiency, diabetes mellitus, lactose intolerance, malabsorption (carbohydrates, fats), malnutrition, nontropical sprue (adult celiac disease), and tropical sprue. Drugs include antibiotics.

Description. pH of stool is used to screen clients with gastrointestinal tract disorders for malabsorption of carbohydrates and fats and disaccharide intolerance. Stools with pH >6.0 are indicative of disaccharide intolerance, whereas those <6.0 indicate malabsorption of sugars and fats.

Professional Considerations
1. Consent form NOT required.
2. **Preparation:**
   A. The client should not have undergone barium procedures or taken laxatives for 1 week before specimen collection.
   B. Obtain a bedpan, a stool specimen container with a lid, a tongue blade, and pH paper.
3. **Procedure:**
   A. Collect a random stool specimen in a bedpan or collection container. Mix the specimen with water to make a suspension. Test it with commercially prepared pH paper as directed.
4. **Postprocedure care:**
   A. Refrigerate the specimen if the test cannot be performed promptly.
5. **Client and family teaching:**
   A. Results are normally available within 24 hours.
   B. Do not contaminate the stool with urine or other secretions or with toilet paper.
6. **Factors that affect results:**
   A. Reject specimens mixed with urine, toilet paper, or toilet water.
7. **Other data:**
   A. Acidic stools will have a sickly sweet odor in both adults and children.
   B. Stool pH may be one factor related to the development of cancers of the gastrointestinal tract.

pH, URINE

Norm. Normal values have a wide range because the renal system acts as a buffer for the body and adjustments in urine pH provide homeostasis. Urine pH should be evaluated with other data and client information.

Adult

Early-morning specimen	pH 5-6
Random	4.5-8.0 as the body adjusts acid base
Average	5-6
Newborn	5.0-7.0

Increased. As a response to alkali overdose, a diet high in vegetables and fruits (especially citrus) and after meals. Also occurs with metabolic alkalosis without potassium loss, Fanconi syndrome, prolonged gastric suction or vomiting, hyperaldosteronism, hypokalemia, renal insufficiency, respiratory alkalosis, and urinary tract infection with *Proteus* or *Pseudomonas*. Drugs include acetazolamide, aldosterone, amiloride, amphotericin B, carbenoxolone, epinephrine, mafenide acetate, niacinamide, phenacetin, potassium citrate, and sodium bicarbonate. Increased pH levels may be associated with renal calculi.

Decreased. Diets high in meat protein and cranberries or starvation diets; achlorhydria, alkaptonuria, diabetes, or other metabolic acidosis; severe diarrhea caused by potassium depletion; methanol poisoning; phenylketonuria; respiratory acidosis; and renal tuberculosis. Drugs include acid phosphate, ascorbic acid, ammonium chloride, corticotropin, diazoxide, hippuric acid, methiomine, mandelate, and methenamine. Herbal or natural remedies include cranberry juice.

Description. Measurement of free hydrogen-ion excretion in urine. Urine pH is reflective of plasma pH and is an indicator of renal tubular function. Playing a role in acid-base balance, normally functioning kidneys will excrete excess hydrogen ions in the urine.

Professional Considerations

1. Consent form NOT required.
2. **Preparation:**
   A. Early-morning voids are preferred for urine pH testing.
   B. Obtain a clean specimen container with a lid.
3. **Procedure:**
   A. Have the client urinate into a 50- to 100-mL collection container. A fresh specimen may be taken from a urinary drainage bag.
   B. pH results should be read immediately. If urine is to be tested with a commercially prepared test reagent, follow the manufacturer's directions.
4. **Postprocedure care:**
   A. Cover the container tightly and send the specimen to the laboratory if it is not tested immediately with a commercially prepared test reagent.
5. **Client and family teaching:**
   A. Notify the nurse immediately after you have collected the sample.
   B. Results are normally available within 24 hours.
6. **Factors that affect results:**
   A. Urine pH testing must be performed on a freshly collected specimen. Urine left to stand will falsely raise the pH.
   B. Urine with glucose may have falsely low pH caused by bacterial activity.
   C. Bacterial infections can alter the pH in either direction.
7. **Other data:**
   A. Urine pH is related to diet and may be one factor in the development of renal stones.

PHENCYCLIDINE (PCP, ANGEL DUST), QUALITATIVE, URINE

Norm. Negative.

Nonfatal level	0.2 μg/L
Fatal level	1-5 μg/L

Overdose Symptoms and Treatment

Symptoms of phencyclidine use:

Stage I. Psychiatric signs: drunken or euphoric with possible ataxia, muscle spasms, fever, tachycardia, flushing, small pupils, diaphoresis, salivation, nausea, and vomiting.
Stage II. Stupor, convulsions especially after stimulation, hallucinations, and progressive increases in

heart rate, fever, and blood pressure. CNS stimulation or depression may occur.
Stage III. Increases in heart rate and metabolism progress to cardiac and respiratory failure.

Treatment:
Note: Treatment choice(s) depend on client history and condition and episode history.
Provide respiratory support if needed.
Administer a cathartic such as sorbitol, followed by gastric lavage and suction for oral ingestion.
Administer benzodiazapines or haloperidol for severe agitation.
Treat seizures as needed.
Give IV nutrition and fluid and electrolyte support as needed.
Acidification of urine will increase the rate of phencyclidine excretion.
If rhabdomyolysis occurs, IV fluids, mannitol, and diuretics are required.
Close observation of electrolytes, respiratory, and circulatory status until the client returns to baseline level.
Chronic abusers may become increasingly psychotic after the drug wears off.
Drug counseling and psychiatric counseling are advised.

Usage. Screening for drug abuse or PCP toxicity, and psychosis or coma (unexplained), which may be related to PCP use. Metabolites of abused drugs are excreted and can be detected in the urine for several days after ingestion. PCP is just one of the drugs tested for in urine toxicology screening as recommended by the National Institute of Drug Abuse (NIDA) for new-job physicals, criminals, and after industrial accidents.

Description. Phencyclidine is a highly addictive, illegal, hallucinative drug designed for use as an anesthetic and a veterinary tranquilizer. It causes euphoria by accelerating the metabolism of the body. Phencyclidine is available in powder or capsule form and can be smoked, snuffed, injected, or swal-

lowed. It is excreted by the kidneys and is detectable in the urine for 7 days. The effects of PCP can be observed at concentrations as low as 12 ng/mL.

Professional Considerations
1. Consent form NOT required.
2. **Preparation:**
   A. Obtain a clean plastic container.
3. **Procedure:**
   A. Obtain a 100- to 125-mL random urine sample in a clean plastic container. A fresh specimen may be taken from a urinary drainage bag.
4. **Postprocedure care:**
   A. Send the specimen to the laboratory. For screening for known drug abusers: Special care MUST be taken in obtaining the specimen and in specimen handling to avoid falsification of results. Documentation of observed collection and handling may be required.
5. **Client and family teaching:**
   A. Obtain a past and recent history of drug abuse.
   B. For intentional overdose, refer client and family for crisis intervention.
   C. Referrals to appropriate rehabilitation centers and therapeutic community programs should be offered to all addicted clients who may be interested.
6. **Factors that affect results:**
   A. Peak serum concentrations occur within 15 minutes after smoking phencyclidine. Half-life is 11 hours.
   B. Drugs that may cause false-positive results include ketamine hydrochloride.
7. **Other data:**
   A. Qualitative urine testing identifies the presence of phencyclidine but does not indicate toxic levels.
   B. PCP can be detected in blood samples stored at 4° C or −20° C for up to 3 years.

PHENDIMETRAZINE
(see Amphetamines, Blood)

PHENMETRAZINE, BLOOD
(see Amphetamines, Blood)

PHENOBARBITAL, PLASMA OR SERUM

Norm. Negative. Therapeutic levels are relative. For control of seizures, the clinical picture is important.

		SI UNITS
Therapeutic Levels		
Adults	15-40 µg/mL	65-173 µmol/L
Infants	15-30 µg/mL	65-129 µmol/L
Children	15-30 µg/mL	65-129 µmol/L
Toxic Level	>40 µg/mL	>172 µmol/L
Panic Levels		
Coma with reflexes	65-117 µg/mL	280-504 µmol/L
Coma without reflexes	>90 µg/mL	>430 µmol/L

Panic Level Symptoms and Treatment

Symptoms. Cold, clammy skin; ataxia; CNS depression; hypothermia; hypotension; cyanosis; Cheyne-Stokes respirations; tachycardia; coma. Toxicity may cause severe renal impairment.

Treatment:

Note: Treatment choice(s) depend on client history and condition and episode history.

Perform gastric lavage, followed by a slurry of multiple-dose activated charcoal (MDAC) with cathartic.

Urine alkalinization is no longer recommended, as MDAC has been found to be more effective alone than in combination with urinary alkalinization.

Protect the patient's airway.

The client may require intubation and mechanical ventilation, especially during gastric lavage if the gag reflex has been affected by the barbiturates.

Monitor closely for hypotension.

Hemodialysis, peritoneal dialysis, and hemoperfusion all WILL remove phenobarbital. Charcoal hemoperfusion is very effective in removing phenobarbital.

Usage. Suspected drug toxicity or abuse in clients with symptoms of lethargy, dizziness, ataxia, and diplopia. Monitoring therapeutic levels of phenobarbital especially for seizure disorders during puberty, after weight gain or loss, and if renal failure develops.

Increased. Drug (barbiturate) abuse and renal failure in clients treated with phenobarbital. Drugs that can increase levels for clients taking phenobarbital include monoamine oxidase (MAO) inhibitors, sodium valproate, and valproic acid.

Decreased. (Below therapeutic range.) Inadequate therapy, noncompliance, and malabsorption (oral doses).

Description. A long acting, schedule-IV barbiturate most commonly used for its anticonvulsant effect and occasionally used as a sedative. It is widely distributed throughout the body and metabolized by the liver, and 50% is excreted unchanged in the urine. The half-life is normally 50-120 hours in adults and 40-70 hours in children. Allowance of time for steady-state levels after changes in dosage should be considered, with monitoring of therapeutic blood levels. For rapid detection, the fluorescence polarization assay method can be used.

Professional Considerations

1. Consent form NOT required.
2. Preparation:
   A. Tube: Red topped, red/gray topped, or gold topped or black topped.
   B. Do NOT draw specimens during hemodialysis.
3. Procedure:
   A. Draw a 1-mL blood sample.
4. Postprocedure care:
   A. None.
5. Client and family teaching:
   A. Discuss the schedule and dose of taking medication.

B. Results are normally available within 24 hours.

C. Return for serum reevaluation within 7 days for long-term phenobarbital therapy.

D. If activated charcoal was given for elevated levels, the client should drink 4-6 glasses of water each day for 2 days to prevent constipation. Activated charcoal will cause stools to be black for a few days.

E. Consult physician before taking any herbal or natural remedies or medicines because some may lower seizure threshold when taken with anticonvulsants.

6. Factors that affect results:
   A. Draw the specimen within 1 hour before the next dose for ongoing monitoring.
   B. Remeasure the phenobarbital level 7 days after dosage change for long-term therapy.

7. Other data:
   A. Mephobarbital is metabolized to phenobarbital.
   B. Peak levels occur 6-18 hours after dose.
   C. Herbal or natural remedy concomitant ingestion of evening primrose (family Onagraceae) oil and borage (*Borago officinalis*) may lower seizure threshold.

PHENOLPHTHALEIN TEST (LAXATIVE ABUSE TEST), DIAGNOSTIC

Norm. Negative.

Usage. Anorexia nervosa (laxative use for weight loss), chronic self-prescribed laxative use, and unexplained diarrhea.

Description. The phenolphthalein test is a toxicologic screening for evidence of recent laxative use. Phenolphthalein is the active ingredient of many over-the-counter laxative preparations. It causes stool evacuation by enhancing fluid and electrolyte accumulation in the intestines. After ingestion, phenolphthalein is excreted in both the feces and the urine and is detectable for up to 32 hours. It may also have laxative effects for up to 4 days and cause fluid and electrolyte abnormalities. This test is performed on an aliquot of a 24-hour urine sample to detect the presence of phenolphthalein by thin-layer chromatography.

Professional Considerations

1. Consent form NOT required.
2. **Preparation:**
   A. Preschedule this test with the laboratory.
   B. Obtain a clean, 3-L container without preservative.
   C. Write the beginning time of collection on the laboratory requisition.
3. **Procedure:**
   A. Discard the first morning-urine specimen.
   B. Begin to time a 24-hour urine collection.
   C. Save all the urine voided for 24 hours in a refrigerated, clean, 3-L container. Document the quantity of urine output during the specimen collection period. Include the urine voided at the end of the 24-hour period. For catheterized clients, keep the drainage bag on ice and empty the urine into the collection container hourly.
4. **Postprocedure care:**
   A. Compare the urine quantity in the specimen container with the urinary output record for the test. If the specimen contains less urine than what was recorded as output, some of the sample may have been discarded, thus invalidating the test.
   B. Document the quantity of urine output and the ending time for the 24-hour collection period on the laboratory requisition.
   C. Send the entire 24-hour urine specimen to the laboratory for testing. The test is performed on a 20-mL aliquot of the 24-hour specimen.
5. **Client and family teaching:**
   A. Save all the urine voided in the 24-hour period and urinate before defecating to avoid loss of urine. If any urine is accidentally discarded, discard the entire specimen and restart the collection the next day.
   B. Results are normally available within 24 hours.
   C. Discuss psychologic and rehabilitation services if laxative abuse is determined.

6. **Factors that affect results:**
   A. Repeating the collection on consecutive days for a total of three 24-hour specimens increases the likelihood of detecting laxative abuse.
7. **Other data:**
   A. Methods are available to test for a wide range of laxative ingredients in urine.

B. Complications of laxative abuse may include diarrhea, abdominal pain, hypokalemia, hypermagnesemia, cathartic colon, and the development of ammonium urate renal calculi.

PHENOTHIAZINES, BLOOD

Norm. Negative.

QUANTITATIVE TESTS		SI UNITS
Chlorpromazine (Thorazine)		
Adults	50-300 ng/mL	157-942 nmol /L
Children	40-80 ng/mL	126-251 nmol/L
Panic level	>750 ng/mL	>2355 nmol/L
Fluphenazine (Prolixin)	0.2-4.9 ng/mL	0.4-8.4 nmol/L
Prochlorperazine (Compazine)	<0.5 µg/mL	
Panic level	>1.0 µg/mL	
Thioridazine (Mellaril)	1.0-1.5 µg/mL	2.7-4.1 µmol/L
Panic level	>10 µg/mL	>27 µmol/L
Trifluoperazine (Stelazine)	<500 ng/mL	<1040 nmol/L
Panic level	>1000 ng/mL	>2080 nmol/L

Overdose Symptoms and Treatment

Symptoms. Extrapyramidal symptoms, central nervous system (CNS) depression, respiratory depression. Sodium-channel blockade manifesting as early prolonged QRS interval, rightward axis of 40 msec, presence of an R-wave in aV_R lead and an S-wave in leads I and aV_L. CNS and respiratory depressive effects are worse when alcohol or antihypertensives are concomitantly ingested.

Treatment:
Note: Treatment choice(s) depend on client history and condition and episode history.
Monitor for CNS and cardiac depression.
ECG monitoring.
Perform gastric lavage for oral doses or a saline cathartic for oral spansules.
Do not induce vomiting.

Hemodialysis and peritoneal dialysis will NOT remove chlorpromazine. No information was found on prochlorperazine, thioridazine, and trifluoperazine regarding dialysis effect on blood levels.

Increased. Phenothiazine abuse and phenothiazine overdose. Drugs that may increase levels above therapeutic for clients on various phenothiazines include monoamine oxidase (MAO) inhibitors.

Decreased. Inadequate therapy. Drugs include antacids, antidiarrheals, anticholinergics, barbiturates, CNS depressants, and lithium carbonate. Thorazine absorption from the gut is pH dependent, and so H_2 antagonists may decrease steady-state levels for client on thorazine therapy.

Description. A group of drugs with antipsychotic, antihistaminic, antipruritic, and antiemetic effects that act centrally on the reticular activating system and peripherally with anticholinergic and alpha-adrenergic blocking effects. Phenothiazines are widely distributed in body tissues, metabolized by the liver, and excreted by the kidney, with a half-life of 20-40 hours. Correlation of therapeutic effectiveness with blood levels is poor. This test is mainly used to determine whether or not the phenothiazine is being taken or for the diagnosis of possible overdose. Fatalities from large doses are rare.

Professional Considerations
1. Consent form NOT required.
2. **Preparation:**
   A. Tube: Red topped, red/gray topped, or gold topped.
   B. Chlorpromazine levels MAY be drawn during hemodialysis.
3. **Procedure:**
   A. Draw a 7-mL blood sample.
4. **Postprocedure care:**
   A. Send the specimen to the laboratory immediately and refrigerate it until tested.

5. **Client and family teaching:**
   A. Evaluate the need for psychologic and rehabilitation support if an overdose is involved. Referrals to appropriate rehabilitation centers and therapeutic community programs should be offered to all addicted clients who are interested.
6. **Factors that affect results:**
   A. For therapeutic monitoring, draw samples within 1 hour before the next dose and at least 3 hours after the last dose.
7. **Other data:**
   A. Newer phenothiazines include trifluopromazine (Vesprin), perphenazine (Trilafon), fluphenazine (Prolixin), and mesoridazine (Serentil).

PHENTERMINE, BLOOD
(see Amphetamines, Blood)

PHENYLALANINE, BLOOD

Norm:

		SI UNITS
Infant	<4 mg/dL	<272 µmol/L
Newborn	1.2-3.4 mg/dL	73-206 µmol/L
Premature or low birth weight	2.0-7.5 mg/dL	121-454 µmol/L
Adult	0.8-1.8 mg/dL	48-109 µmol/L
Adult—monitored for diet compliance	1.3-3.4 mg/dL	78-204 µmol/L

Positive Test (Increased Result). Phenylketonuria (PKU) is diagnosed and confirmed by:
1. Greater than 4 mg/dL serum phenylalanine.
2. Associated with low tyrosine less than 0.6 mg/dL.
3. Urinary excretion of phenylpyruvic acid.

Description. PKU is caused by an autosomal recessive gene. The infant (client) lacks the ability to produce the enzyme phenylalanine hydroxylase, which converts phenylalanine to tyrosine. The resulting buildup of phenylalanine leads to severe mental retardation. The carrier rate for PKU is 2% in the United States. This test is performed when either a urine screening or Guthrie test screening for PKU has been positive or as the PKU screening test in newborns.

Professional Considerations
1. Consent form NOT required.
2. **Preparation:**
   A. Mark the birth date and the date of initiation of feedings on the laboratory requisition.
   B. Tube: Green topped.
3. **Procedure:**
   A. Draw a 0.5-mL blood sample. Do not use cord blood.
4. **Postprocedure care:**
   A. None.

5. Client and family teaching:
   A. Refer parents with PKU infants for genetic counseling.
   B. Clients with PKU may be monitored for serum phenylalanine levels for life. The client must follow a low-protein diet, which is effective treatment but not a cure.
   C. Level of mental capacity has been shown to be related to serum levels. Range is 1.3-3.4 mg/dL for best control.
   D. Results are normally available within 48 hours.
6. Factors that affect results:
   A. False-negative results may occur with other tests for PKU before the third day of feeding, but the serum phenylalanine test for PKU has the advantage that it is usually accurate in the first 24 hours of life, especially in breast-fed babies because colostrum has a high protein content.
   B. Phenylalanine clearance has been shown to be delayed in elderly males.
   C. Do not use cord blood.
   D. Fasting in not needed even for monitoring of older PKU clients.
   E. The presence of antibodies in the sample make results uninterpretable.
7. Other data:
   A. Diagnosis of PKU may be made with concomitant urine testing and a plasma level >2 mg/dL (121 mol/L, SI units) on consecutive tests.
   B. Male infants with PKU increase levels of phenylalanine at a faster rate than affected females do.
   C. See also *Guthrie test for phenylketonuria, Diagnostic (Filter paper test)*.

PHENYLPROPANOLAMINE
(see *Amphetamines, Blood*)

PHENYTOIN, SERUM

Norm:

	TROUGH	SI UNITS
Therapeutic range	10-20 µg/mL	40-79 µmol/L
Toxic level	45-112 µg/mL	177-442 µmol/L
Panic level	>60 µg/mL	>237 µmol/L

Panic Level Symptoms and Treatment

Symptoms. Double vision, nystagmus, lethargy. Central nervous system depression: drowsiness, confusion, slurred speech, coma, and respiratory depression.

Treatment:
Note: Treatment choice(s) depend on client history and condition and episode history.
Support airway and brathing.
   Administer oxygen as needed.
ECG monitoring (for levels over 75 µg/mL), although the risk for arrhythmias is minimal.
Phenytoin levels every 4 hours.
Activated charcoal (multiple dose) every 2-6 hours as needed.
Administer IV fluids and vasopressor, as needed for hypotension.
Saline cathartic.
The use of sorbitol cathartic has NOT been shown to increase clearance values of phenytoin.
Hemodialysis and peritoneal dialysis will NOT remove phenytoin. One study found that direct hemoperfusion WILL remove phenytoin at a rate of about 20% per session.

Increased. Phenytoin abuse, phenytoin overdose, and renal disease in clients on maintenance phenytoin (Dilantin). Drugs that may increase phenytoin levels for clients on chronic treatment include allopurinol, amiodarone, anticoagulants (oral), benzodiazepines, chloramphenicol, chlordiazepoxide, cimetidine, diazepam, H_2 antagonists, disulfiram, estrogens, ethyl alcohol (acute intake), ethosuximide, fluoxetine, isoniazid, methsuximide, methylphenidate, phenacemide, phenothiazines, phenylbutazone, propoxyphene, salicylates, sulfonamides, thiazides, trazodone, tolbutamide, trimethoprim, and vinblastine sulfate.

Decreased. Inadequate phenytoin therapy; noncompliance. Drugs that may alter (speed up) metabolism of phenytoin leading to lower serum levels for clients receiving Dilantin include carbamazepine, diazoxide, ethyl alcohol (chronic intake), folic acid, loxapine, methotrexate, sulfonylureas, theophylline, reserpine, sucralfate, and calcium-containing medications. Herbs include the Ayurvedic preparation *shankhapushpi* (often misspelled *shankapulshpi,* from Sanskrit *shankhapushpi,* feminine form of 'conch-flower', that is, [1] *Canscora decussata,* of the Gentianaceae family and containing iridoids and possible cyanogens and saponins/sapogenins, or [2] *Convolvulus microphyllus* [synonym *Convolvulus pluricaulis*], bindweed, containing various alkaloids). Enteral tube feedings may decrease absorption of oral phenytoin. Drugs that may *either increase or decrease* levels: phenobarbital, sodium valproate, and valproic acid.

Description. A hydantoin-derivative anticonvulsant also used as an antidysrhythmic. Phenytoin is widely distributed throughout the body, metabolized by the liver, and excreted in bile and urine, with a half-life of approximately 22 hours for oral administration. Five or 6 days of therapy are required to reach steady-state levels in adults, and 2-5 days are necessary in children. For rapid detection, the fluorescence polarization assay method can be used.

Professional Considerations
1. Consent form NOT required.
2. Preparation:
   A. Tube: Red topped, red/gray topped, or gold topped.
   B. Specimens MAY be drawn during hemodialysis.
   C. Screen client for the use of herbal preparations or medicines or "natural" remedies.
3. Procedure:
   A. Draw a 1-mL TROUGH blood sample. Obtain serial specimens at the same time each day.
4. Postprocedure care:
   A. None.

5. Client and family teaching:
   A. Explore the reasons for inappropriate ingestion of phenytoin if appropriate.
   B. If activated charcoal was given for elevated levels, the client should drink four to six glasses of water each day for 2 days to prevent constipation. The activated charcoal will cause stools to be black for a few days.
   C. Consult physician before taking any herbal or natural remedies or medicines because some may lower seizure threshold when taken with anticonvulsants.
   D. For intentional overdose, refer client and family for crisis intervention.
   E. Referrals to appropriate rehabilitation centers and therapeutic community programs should be offered to all clients who may be interested.
6. Factors that affect results:
   A. Tube feedings should be held before and up to 2 hours after oral phenytoin administration.
   B. Peak levels should be drawn 3-9 hours after oral administration of phenytoin. Trough levels should be drawn just before the administration of the next dose.
   C. Five days should be allowed before measurement of phenytoin level after a change in dose.
   D. Postmortem levels are not stable and were found to drop significantly in one study.
   E. Levels may be significantly lower in clients with acquired immunodeficiency syndrome. It is believed that this may be a result of the hypoalbuminemic state that accompanies this condition.
   F. An herbal or natural remedy used to control seizures, *shankhapushpi* (see above) has been shown to decrease phenytoin concentrations in rats when given in multiple coadministered doses.
   G. Hypoalbuminemia and concurrent valproic acid administration may increase free phenytoin levels. Clients with both conditions are at risk for exceeding the therapeutic range, even at normal dosages.
7. Other data:
   A. Susceptibility to side effects and toxic effects, including Stevens-

Johnson syndrome, may be increased in clients with head injuries or those with intracranial lesions, especially if irradiation is used as a treatment modality.

B. Herbal or natural remedy: Concomitant ingestion of evening primrose (family Onagraceae) oil and borage (*Borago officinalis*) may lower seizure threshold.

PHLEBOGRAPHY
(*see Venography, Diagnostic*)

PHONOCARDIOGRAPHY (PCG), DIAGNOSTIC

Norm. Normal S_1 and S_2 appear as spikes above the baseline on phonocardiograph paper. Absence of abnormal heart sounds as recorded by the phonocardiogram.

Usage. Aids diagnosis of cardiac valve abnormalities, hypertrophic cardiomyopathy, and left ventricular failure. May be performed and retained for reference as part of the client's permanent record as a visual representation of the intensity and loudness of murmurs and other abnormal heart sounds. Excellent teaching tool because it allows the learner to visualize the different heart sounds.

Description. A pictorial recording of the cardiac sounds heard on auscultation. A phonocardiogram uses microphones to transduce and amplify the sound into electrical impulses that are graphically recorded as a waveform by a high-speed recording apparatus. Generally, PCG is performed simultaneously with an electrocardiograph (ECG); The S_1, S_2, and any additional sounds, including S_3, S_4, murmurs, and clicks, are recorded. By comparing the ECG and PCG, one can locate normal and abnormal heart sounds and cardiac events and time them during the cardiac cycle. Phonocardiography with the addition of echocardiography is becoming a valuable noninvasive diagnostic tool. Newer phonocardiography technology may soon be available to noninvasively study coronary artery flow as well as estimate great vessel pressures, provide more reliable diagnosis, and stratify the severity of cardiac value dysfunction.

Professional Considerations
1. Consent form NOT required.
2. **Preparation:**
   A. Obtain electrodes and alcohol.
   B. Clip the hair from the electrode sites before placement.
3. **Procedure:**
   A. The client is positioned supine. The electrode sites should be cleansed with alcohol and lightly scraped with the edge of an electrode before placement.
   B. After the heart apex and base are located with a stethoscope, a microphone is strapped (or secured with suction cups) in place over each site.
   C. Both an ECG and PCG are recorded simultaneously for four complete cardiac cycles of sinus rhythm. For dysrhythmias, 7 to 10 cardiac cycles are recorded. The procedure is repeated with the client changed to upright and left-lateral oblique positions. The client may be asked to change his or her breathing patterns (that is, hold breath or perform deep inspiration and expiration).
4. **Postprocedure care:**
   A. Remove the electrodes and the residual electrode gel.
5. **Client and family teaching:**
   A. Cooperation is imperative throughout the procedure.
   B. Phonocardiography is noninvasive and takes about 30 minutes.
6. **Factors that affect results:**
   A. Failure to obtain secure electrode placement causes an artifact in the electrocardiographic recording.
   B. Careful calibration is needed for the results to be diagnostic and generalizable.
7. **Other data:**
   A. Phonocardiography with esophageal echocardiography provides a valuable permanent and comparable record of cardiac valve murmurs. The progress of the disease process can be followed using serial recordings.

PHOSPHOLIPIDS, SERUM

Norm:

Males > females except during pregnancy

All	180–320 mg/dL
Adult ≤65 years	125–275 mg/dL

Adult >65 years	196-366 mg/dL
Birth	75-170 mg/dL
Infant	100-275 mg/dL
Child	180-295 mg/dL

Usage. Evaluation of fat metabolism. Less used today because there are other specific tests for the plasma phospholipids. Levels are increased or decreased in the diseases listed below with more specific diagnostic tests available for most. Amniotic fluid levels of phospholipids reflect the surfactant level and give an indication of fetal lung maturity.

Increased. Diabetes mellitus, biliary cirrhosis, cholestasis, LCAT deficiency, hypothyroidism, ETOH cirrhosis, obstructive jaundice, and nephrotic syndrome with breast cancer, and chronic pancreatitis. Drugs include estrogens, epinephrine, and some phenothiazine.

Decreased. Primary hypolipoproteinemia, Tangiers disease, abetalipoproteinemia, and a dietary restriction of fat intake. Drugs include antilipemic agents such as clofibrate.

Description. Phospholipids also known as "compound lipids," are the largest and most soluble of the lipid elements of the blood Phospholipids which contain phosphorus, fatty acids, and nitrogen are needed for lipid transport and are essential components in cellular membranes. Serum phospholipid determinations may be monitored when disorders in lipid metabolism are suspected; however, cholesterol levels are more often prescribed and evaluated for this purpose.

Professional Considerations
1. Consent form NOT required.
2. **Preparation:**
   A. Tube: Red topped, red/gray topped, or gold topped.
   B. See *Client and family teaching.*
3. **Procedure:**
   A. Draw a 5-mL fasting blood sample in the morning before any medications are administered.
4. **Postprocedure care:**
   A. Note any medications taken on the laboratory requisition.
   B. Specimens should be taken to the laboratory immediately.
5. **Client and family teaching:**
   A. Do NOT drink alcohol for 24-48 hours before sampling.
   B. Consume a low- to moderate-fat evening meal on the day before the test.
   C. Fast from midnight before sampling.
6. **Factors that affect results:**
   A. Hemolysis of the specimen invalidates results.
   B. Recent intravenous injection of radiographic dye invalidates results.
   C. Significant weight changes within 2 weeks before the test invalidate results.
7. **Other data:**
   A. This test is not included in a routine assay of a "lipid profile."

PHOSPHOLIPID ANTIBODIES
(*see Antiphospholipid antibodies, Serum*)

PHOSPHORUS (INORGANIC PHOSPHATE), SERUM

Norm:

		SI UNITS
Adults ≤60 Years	2.7-4.5 mg/dL	0.87-1.45 mmol/L
Females >60 Years	2.8-4.1 mg/dL	0.90-1.30 mmol/L
Males >60 Years	2.3-3.7 mg/dL	0.74-1.20 mmol/L
Children and Infants		
Cord blood	3.7-8.1 mg/dL	1.20-2.62 mmol/L
Premature infant	5.4-10.9 mg/dL	1.74-3.52 mmol/L
Newborn	4.5-9 mg/dL	1.45-2.91 mmol/L
Infant (10 days-24 months)	4.5-6.7 mg/dL	1.45-2.16 mmol/L
Child (24 months-12 years)	4.5-5.5 mg/dL	1.45-1.78 mmol/L

Increased. >4.7 mg/dL or 1.3 mmol/L fasting: acromegaly, acute or chronic renal disease, bone tumors or metastases, diabetic ketoacidosis, healing bone fractures, hyperthyroidism, hypoparathyroidism, lactic and respiratory acidosis, leukemia (myelogenous), magnesium deficiency, malignant hyperpyrexia after anesthesia, massive blood transfusions, metastatic bone tumors, milk-alkali (Burnett) syndrome, multiple blood transfusions, multiple myeloma, portal cirrhosis, Paget's disease, pseudohypoparathyroidism, pulmonary embolism, sarcoidosis, sickle cell, renal failure, sarcoidosis, secondary hypoparathyroidism, uremia, vitamin D toxicity. Drugs include androgens, beta-adrenergic blockers, chemotherapy, diphosphates, ethyl alcohol (ethanol), furosemide (Lasix), growth hormone, hydrochlorothiazide, methicillin, parathormone, phenytoin, phosphate enemas or infusions, phosphate laxative abuse, steroids, and tetracycline (nephrotoxicity). Herbal or natural remedies include products containing aristolochic acids (*Akebia* spp., *Aristolochia* spp., *Asarum* spp., birthwort, *Bragantia* spp., *Clematis* spp., *Cocculus* spp., *Diploclisia* spp., Dutchman's pipe, *Fang chi, Fang ji, Fang chi, Guang fang ji, Kan-Mokutsu, Menispernum* spp., *Mokutsu, Mu tong, Sinomenium* spp., and *Stephania* spp.).

Decreased. <0.8 mg/dL, panic <0.3 mg/dL: acute alcoholism, burns (diuretic phase), Crohn's disease (caused by vomiting and diarrhea), diabetic ketoacidosis, dialysis, Fanconi syndrome (renal tubular defects), gout, hyperalimentation (without phosphorus supplement), hypercalcemia (severe), hyperinsulinism, hyperparathyroidism, hypokalemia, hypomagnesemia, hypothermia, hypovolemia, malabsorption, malnutrition, nasogastric suction, osteomalacia, respiratory alkalosis, rickets (primary or familial hypophosphatemia), salicylate poisoning, septicemia (gram-negative bacterial), sprue, vitamin D deficiency. Drugs include albuterol, acetazolamide, amino acids, anticonvulsants, anesthetic agents, antacids (aluminum-containing and phosphate-binding), carbamazepine, calcitonin, diuretics, epinephrine, estrogens, glucagon, glu-

cocorticoids, glucose IV, insulin, isoniazid, oral contraceptives, phenytoin, RenaGel (phosphate binder).

Description. The majority (85%) of phosphorus is stored in the bones in organic compounds. The remainder exists inorganically as phosphate anions within the soft tissue cells of the body and in the bloodstream. Phosphate functions in urinary acid-base buffering, energy storage and release, and metabolism of carbohydrates and lipids. Phosphorus is absorbed in the small intestine with the help of vitamin D and phosphorus levels in the blood, along with calcium levels, are regulated by parathyroid hormone, calcitonin, vitamin D, and the renal phosphate excretion rate. An inverse relationship of calcium and phosphorus blood levels exists.

Professional Considerations
1. Consent form NOT required.
2. Preparation:
   A. The client must fast for 8-12 hours.
   B. Tube: Red topped, red/gray topped, or gold topped.
   C. Do NOT draw samples during hemodialysis.
   D. See *Client and family teaching*.
3. Procedure:
   A. Draw a 1-mL blood sample.
4. Postprocedure care:
   A. Send the specimen to the laboratory for immediate spinning.
5. Client and family teaching:
   A. Foods high in phosphorus include beans, chicken, eggs, fish, milk, and milk products.
   B. Avoid excessive antacid intake and laxatives or enemas containing sodium phosphate.
   C. For low phosphorus levels, avoid other persons with infections because phosphorus interferes with the functioning of the white blood cells.
6. Factors that affect results:
   A. Hemolysis of the specimen causes falsely elevated results.
   B. Serum levels vary throughout the day and are lowest in the morning.
   C. Eating before the test may falsely lower the phosphate level.
   D. Hemodialysis will reduce phosphate levels.

E. Drugs that cause falsely decreased results include citrates, mannitol, oxalates, tartrate, and phenothiazines.

F. Levels may decrease from baseline in women taking oral contraceptives, and may increase from baseline in women taking injectable contraceptives.

7. Other data:
A. Calcium levels should also be prescribed to aid interpretation of results.
B. Hyperphosphatemia is related to LOW calcium levels and associated symptoms: tetany, dysrhythmias, and seizures.

C. Hypophosphatemia is associated with muscle weakness, difficult-to-wean chronic ventilator clients, encephalopathy, poor platelet function, decreased cardiac contractility, and paresthesias.

D. A 24-hour urine test for phosphate may be helpful in the workup of low phosphate levels.

PHOSPHORUS, URINE

Norm:

		SI UNITS
Adults	0.4-1.3 g/24 hours	13-42 mmol/day
Restricted diet	<1.0 g/24 hours	<32 mmol/day

Note: Restricted diet contains 0.9-1.5 g (29-48 mmol) of phosphorus and 10 mg (0.25 mmol) of calcium per day.

Increased. Bone fractures (transiently), Fanconi syndrome (renal tubular damage), familial hypophosphatemia, hyperparathyroidism, nonrenal acidosis (because phosphate excretion is a buffering mechanism), paraplegia, vitamin D–resistant rickets, and vitamin D toxicity. Drugs include acetazolamide, asparagine, bicarbonate, bismuth salts, calcitonin, corticosteroids, dihydrotachysterol, diuretics, hydrochlorothiazide, metolazone, phosphates (increased intake), PTH, valine, and vitamin D. Herbal or natural remedies include products containing aristolochic acids (*Akebia* spp., *Aristolochia* spp., *Asarum* spp., birthwort, *Bragantia* spp., *Clematis* spp., *Cocculus* spp., *Diploclisia* spp., Dutchman's pipe, *Fang chi, Fang ji, Fang chi, Guang fang ji, Kan-Mokutsu, Menispernum* spp., *Mokutsu, Mu tong, Sinomenium* spp., and *Stephania* spp.)

Decreased. Hypoparathyroidism or parathyroidectomy, pseudohypoparathyroidism. Drugs include aluminum-containing antacids; alanine in the obese fasting client; RenaGel, a phosphate binder, decreased urinary phosphate excretion in rats.

Description. See *Phosphorus, Serum.*

Professional Considerations
1. Consent form NOT required.
2. **Preparation:**
   A. Obtain a clean, detergent-free, 3-L urine container to which acetic acid wash has been added.
   B. Write the beginning time of collection on the laboratory requisition.
3. **Procedure:**
   A. Discard the first morning-urine specimen.
   B. Save all the urine voided for 24 hours in a clean, refrigerated, 3-L container. Document the quantity of urine output during the specimen-collection period. Include urine voided at the end of the 24-hour period. For catheterized clients, keep the drainage bag on ice and empty the urine into the collection container hourly.
4. **Postprocedure care:**
   A. Compare the urine quantity in the specimen container with the urinary output record for the test. If the specimen contains less urine than what was recorded as output, some of the sample may

have been discarded, invalidating the test.

B. Document the quantity of urine output and the ending time on the laboratory requisition.

C. HCl acid is added in the laboratory on arrival for preservation.

5. **Client and family teaching:**
A. Save all the urine voided in the 24-hour period and urinate before defecating to avoid loss of urine and to avoid contaminating the urine with stool. If any urine is accidentally discarded, discard the entire specimen and restart the collection.

6. **Factors that affect results:**
A. All urine voided for the 24-hour period must be included to avoid a falsely low result.

7. **Other data:**
A. Because phosphorus levels vary throughout the day, this test is most informative if performed on a 24-hour urine sample.

B. Poor creatinine clearance will invalidate the results.

PINWORM, CULTURE
(see Parasite screen, Stool)

PIR
(see Pulse volume recording of peripheral vasculature, Diagnostic)

PKU
(see Phenylalanine, Blood)

PLASMA FREE METANEPHRINES
(see Metanephrines, Total, 24-Hour urine, and Free, Plasma)

PLASMA RENIN ACTIVITY
(see Renin activity, Plasma)

PLASMINOGEN ASSAY, BLOOD

Norm. 20 mg/dL, 2.5-5.2 U/mL or 3.8-8.4 CTA (Council on Thrombolytic Agents) U/mL.

Increased. Anxiety, congenital defect in the release of plasminogen inhibitors, deep-vein thrombosis, infancy, infection, inflammation, malignancy, myocardial infarction, pregnancy, stress, and surgery. Drugs include oral contraceptives.

Decreased. Cirrhosis, congenital defect in the release of plasminogen activators, disseminated intravascular coagulation, fibrinolysis, hyaline membrane disease, hypofibrinogenemia (acquired), liver disease, nephrosis, surgery (coronary artery bypass graft, postoperatively), and thrombosis. Drugs include atelplase, l-asparaginase, streptokinase, and urokinase.

Description. Plasminogen is a beta globulin protein found in fibrin clots of blood vessels, soft tissue, and any body cavity lined with endothelial cells. When healing or cellular repair has occurred, endothelial cell enzymes trigger the conversion of plasminogen to the fibrinolytic enzyme plasmin, and lysis of the fibrin clot begins. Plasminogen has a biologic half-life of 2 days. Plasminogen assays are used in the evaluation of fibrinolysis and increased fibrin-fibrinogen degradation products and in the diagnosis of the source of hypofibrinogenemia.

Professional Considerations
1. Consent form NOT required.
2. **Preparation:**
A. Clarify with the laboratory whether this test must be prescheduled for processing.
B. Tube: Blue topped.
C. Do not use plasma collected in the presence of fluoride, EDTA, or heparin.
D. Specimens without lipidemia or hemolysis are preferred.
E. Specimens MAY be drawn during hemodialysis.
3. **Procedure:**
A. Draw and discard a 2-mL blood sample and discard the syringe, leaving the needle in place. Perform venipuncture and withdraw 2 mL of blood into a syringe or vacuum tube. Remove the syringe or tube, leaving the needle in place. Attach a second syringe, and draw a sample quantity of 2.4 mL for a 2.7-mL tube and 4.0 mL for a 4.5-mL tube. Immediately place the specimens in a container of ice.

4. Postprocedure care:
   A. Write the collection time on the laboratory requisition.
   B. Send the specimens to the laboratory and refrigerate them if not processed within 8 hours.
5. Client and family teaching:
   A. If results are elevated, the client may need to change from oral contraceptives to other forms of birth control.
6. Factors that affect results:
   A. Reject hemolyzed or clotted specimens.
7. Other data:
   A. Clients with decreased plasminogen concentration may be prone to developing recurrent thromboses.
   B. Plasminogen concentrations are decreased with acquired or secondary hypofibrinogenemia and remain normal when congenital causes exist.

PLATELET ADHESION TEST, DIAGNOSTIC

Norm. Glass bead retention: 50%-95% (most commonly, 90%-95%).

Increased. Aging, atherosclerosis, burns, carcinoma, diabetes mellitus, exertion, homocystinuria, hypercoagulability, hyperlipemia, infection (acute), multiple sclerosis, pregnancy, surgery, thrombosis, and trauma. Drugs include oral contraceptives.

Decreased. Afibrinogenemia, anemia (severe), azotemia, Bernard-Soulier syndrome, Chediak-Higashi syndrome, congenital heart disease, Glanzmann's thrombasthenia, glycogen storage disease, macroglobulinemia, multiple myeloma, myeloid metaplasia, myeloproliferative disorders, plasma cell dyscrasia, platelet release defect, storage pool disease, thrombasthenia, thrombocytopathy, uremia, and von Willebrand's disease. Drugs include vitamin E and dietary fish oil supplementation. Herbs or natural remedies include garlic (aged extract taken on an ongoing basis).

Description. This test evaluates the ability of platelets to adhere to foreign bodies during blood clotting by running blood through a collection of glass beads and counting the number of platelets adhering to the beads.

Professional Considerations
1. Consent form NOT required.
2. Preparation:
   A. Preschedule this test with the laboratory.
   B. Tube: Red topped, red/gray topped, or gold topped.
   C. Specimens MAY be drawn during hemodialysis.
   D. Screen client for the use of herbal preparations or medicines or "natural" remedies.
   E. See *Client and family teaching.*
3. Procedure:
   A. Draw a 10-mL blood specimen.
4. Postprocedure care:
   A. None.
5. Client and family teaching:
   A. Do not take drugs that inhibit platelet adhesion within 10 days before the test.
   B. Do not take drugs that decrease platelet levels within 10 days before the test (see *Platelet count, Blood*).
   C. Fast for 8 hours before this test.
   D. If results are elevated, the client may need to change from oral contraceptives to other forms of birth control.
6. Factors that affect results:
   A. Reject clotted specimens or specimens with an extremely low platelet count.
   B. Platelet adhesiveness is increased during the spring season.
   C. Platelet adhesiveness is highest during the afternoon hours.
7. Other data:
   A. This test is difficult to standardize.

PLATELET AGGREGATION, BLOOD; PLATELET AGGREGATION, HYPERCOAGULABLE STATE, BLOOD

Norm. 60%-100% or according to specific laboratory.
   Hypercoagulable state: Normal values are reported in descriptive terms of rate of spontaneous platelet aggregation of samples as compared to rate of platelet aggregation of control, evaluation of a

second wave of aggregation with adenosine diphosphate (ADP) reagent, and platelet response to serial dilutions of epinephrine.

Increased. Atheromatosis, cholangiocarcinoma, diabetes mellitus, hypercoagulability, hyperlipemia, polycythemia vera, smoking. Drugs include thiopental.

Decreased. Afibrinogenemia, anemia (sideroblastic), Bernard-Soulier syndrome (ristocetin test), beta-thalassemia major, Chediak-Higashi syndrome, cirrhosis, Glanzmann's thrombasthenia (ADP, epinephrine, and collagen test), gray platelet syndrome (ADP, epinephrine, thrombin, collagen tests), Hermansky-Pudlak syndrome, homocystinuria, idiopathic thrombocytopenic purpura (ADP, collagen, epinephrine), macroglobulinemia, myeloid metaplasia, plasma cell dyscrasia, platelet release defects (ADP, second phase; epinephrine, second phase; and collagen tests), preleukemia, scurvy, storage pool disease (ADP, second phase; epinephrine, second phase; and collagen tests), snakebite, thrombasthenia (ADP, epinephrine, collagen), thrombocythemia (hemorrhagic), uremia, von Gierke's disease, von Willebrand's disease (ristocetin test), and Wiskott-Aldrich syndrome. Drugs include alphaprodine, antibiotics, anticoagulants, antihistamines, aspirin, azlocillin, carbenicillin indanyl sodium, carvedilol, cephalothin sodium, chlordiazepoxide, chloroquine hydrochloride, chloroquine phosphate, clofibrate, cocaine hydrochloride, corticosteroids, cyproheptadine hydrochloride, dextran, dextropropoxyphene, diazepam, diphenhydramine hydrochloride, dipyridamole, eptifibatide, flufenamic acid, furosemide, gentamicin sulfate, guaifenesin, heparin calcium, heparin sodium, ibufenac, ibuprofen, iloprost (aerosolized), imipramine, indomethacin, interferon alpha 2b, ketamine, marijuana, mefenamic acid, naproxen sodium, nebivolol, nitric oxide, nitrofurantoin, nortriptyline hydrochloride, oxyphenbutazone, penicillin G benzathine, penicillin G potassium, penicillin G procaine, phenothiazines, phenylbutazone, promethazine hydrochloride, propranolol, pyrimidine compounds, sibrafiban, statin drugs, sulfinpyrazone, theophylline, ticlopidine hydrochloride, tricyclic antidepressants, vitamin E, volatile general anesthetics (methoxyflurane, halothane, nitrous oxide), and zomepirac. Herbs or natural remedies include *Cordyceps sinensis*, dan¹shen¹ ('red-ginseng', *Salvia miltiorrhiza*), feverfew, *Ganoderma lucidum* (a bracket fungus), garlic (aged extract taken on an ongoing basis), Ligustrazine isolated from Chuangxiong, Pycnogenol, tetramethylpyrazine (at high concentrations of 1.0 mmol). Other: Red wine is thought to exert cardioprotective effects through inhibition of platelet aggregation polyphenol resveratrol, one of its constituents.

Description. The platelet aggregation test assesses the ability of platelets to adhere to each other by mixture of the client's platelets in solution with substances that induce aggregation and measurement of the amount of light that passes through the solution after clumping has occurred. Substances that induce aggregation include ADP, epinephrine, ristocetin, collagen, arachidonic acid, and thrombin. The platelet aggregation test for a hypercoagulable state is a modification on the standard platelet aggregation test. This test assesses the ability of platelets to adhere to each other in the following ways. First, the rate and amount of spontaneous platelet aggregation of the sample is compared to a known normal control sample. Second, the platelet-aggregating reagent, ADP, is added to the client's sample, which is then observed for evidence of a second wave of aggregation. Third, serial dilutions of epinephrine, another platelet-aggregating reagent, are added to the sample and the sample is studied for an enhanced platelet response.

Professional Considerations
1. Consent form NOT required.
2. Preparation:
    A. Preschedule this test with the laboratory.
    B. Tube: Blue topped.
    C. Do NOT draw specimens during hemodialysis.
    D. Screen client for the use of herbal preparations or medicines or "natural" remedies.
    E. See *Client and family teaching.*

3. **Procedure:**
   A. Draw a 10-mL blood sample.
   B. Traumatic venipuncture may cause contamination, thereby increasing aggregation.
4. **Postprocedure care:**
   A. Write the specimen collection time on the laboratory requisition.
   B. Deliver the specimen to the laboratory immediately. Do not refrigerate it. Testing should be performed within 2 hours after collection. Keep the specimen stable at room temperature for 1-3 hours.
5. **Client and family teaching:**
   A. Do not take drugs that inhibit platelet aggregation within the previous 10 days unless the test is being used to evaluate the drug effect on platelet function.
   B. Do not eat or drink caffeine-containing products within 12 hours.
6. **Factors that affect results:**
   A. Reject hemolyzed or clotted specimens or specimens received more than 2 hours after collection.
   B. Platelet count <100,000/mm^3 causes inaccurate results.
   C. A delay in testing may cause a loss of platelet ability to aggregate.
   D. Lipemia may interfere with accurate measurement.
   E. There is some evidence that red wine inhibits platelet aggregation.
   F. Females have greater aggregability than males. The reason is hypothesized to be related to sex-related differences in testosterone levels.
7. **Other data:**
   A. Von Willebrand's disease may be ruled out by a normal response to ristocetin aggregating agent. Platelet aggregation inhibition caused by ingestion of aspirin may be ruled out by an inhibited response to arachidonic acid aggregating agent. Gray platelet syndrome may be ruled out when aggregation occurs with ristocetin but not with other aggregating agents.

PLATELET ANTIBODY, BLOOD

Norm. Negative or <1000 molecules of IgG per platelet.

Positive. Thrombocytopenia caused by platelet autoantibodies causing idiopathic thrombocytopenic purpura (ITP), posttransfusion purpura, platelet refractoriness, isoimmune purpura, drug-induced (quinidine, quinine, furosemide, sulfonamides), or caused by platelet isoantibodies after receipt of multiple transfusions.

Description. The platelet antibody test is performed to detect the presence of platelet autoantibodies and platelet isoantibodies (alloantibodies). Platelet autoantibodies are IgG immunoglobulins of autoimmune origin and are present in all cases of ITP. A quantitative antiglobulin consumption test or other methods may be used to detect platelet autoantibodies. Platelet isoantibodies develop in clients when they become sensitized to platelet antigens of transfused blood. This results in destruction of both donor and native platelets and shortened survival time of platelets in the transfusion recipient. A complement fixation test (or other methods) may be used to detect platelet isoantibodies.

Professional Considerations
1. Consent form NOT required.
2. **Preparation:**
   A. Preschedule this test with the laboratory.
   B. Tubes: Two blue topped.
   C. Do NOT draw during hemodialysis.
3. **Procedure:**
   A. Completely fill two sodium citrate-anticoagulated, blue-topped tubes with a blood sample.
   B. If testing will be delayed, collect the sample into tubes containing acid citrate dextrose obtained from the laboratory.
4. **Postprocedure care:**
   A. Send the specimens to the laboratory. Plasma should be separated from the red cells and frozen in a plastic tube at −25° C.
   B. For specimens collected into acid citrate dextrose, store the sample as collected at 4° C.
   C. Specimens may be frozen up to 3 years.
5. **Client and family teaching:**
   A. If thrombocytopenia is present, avoid rough physical activity and bumping into furniture. Use a

stool softener and avoid straining to have a bowel movement. Use a soft toothbrush and watch for and report signs of bleeding: bruising, petechiae, blood in the stool/urine/sputum, bleeding from invasive lines, bleeding gums, abnormal or excessive vaginal bleeding.

6. **Factors that affect results:**
   A. Reject hemolyzed or clotted specimens.
7. **Other data:**
   A. Samples with mean fluorescence greater than 2 standard deviations above the mean of the negative control sample are considered positive.

PLATELET (THROMBOCYTE) COUNT, BLOOD

Norm:

PLATELETS (PLT)		SI UNITS
Adults	150,000-400,000/μL	150-400 × 10⁹/L
Critical low	<30,000/μL	<30 × 10⁹/L
Critical high	>1,000,000/μL	>1000 × 10⁹/L
Children		
Cord	100,000-290,000/μL	100-290 × 10⁹/L
Premature	100,000-300,000/μL	100-300 × 10⁹/L
Newborn	100,000-300,000/μL	100-300 × 10⁹/L
Neonate	150,000-390,000/μL	100-390 × 10⁹/L
3 months	260,000/μL	260 × 10⁹/L
Infant	200,000-473,000/μL	200-473 × 10⁹/L
1-10 years	150,000-450,000/μL	150-450 × 10⁹/L
Critical low	<20,000/μL	<20 × 10⁹/L
Critical high	>1,000,000/μL	>1000 × 10⁹/L

Increased. After splenectomy, anemia (hemolytic, iron-deficiency, postmenorrhagic, sickle cell), asphyxia, asplenism, carcinoma, cirrhosis, collagen disease, cryoglobulinemia, exercise, fractures, heart disease, hemorrhage (acute), idiopathic thrombocythemia, infection (acute), inflammation, leukemia (chronic granulocytic, chronic myelogenous), malignancy, multiple myeloma, myelofibrosis, myeloproliferative disease, polycythemia vera, postoperatively, post partum, pregnancy (more in twin than single pregnancies), pseudothrombocytosis, reticulocytosis, rheumatoid arthritis, surgery, and tuberculosis. Drugs include epinephrine, epinephrine bitartrate, epinephrine borate, epinephrine hydrochloride, and oral contraceptives.

Decreased. After splenectomy (2 months), anemia (aplastic, megaloblastic, pernicious), aplastic or hypoplastic bone marrow, autoimmune disorders, Bernard-Soulier syndrome, blood transfusion (incompatible, large amounts), burns (severe), carcinoma (metastatic), cirrhosis, clostridial infection, collagen diseases, defibrination syndrome, diphtheria, disseminated intravascular coagulation, extracorporeal circulation, Gaucher's disease, hemorrhage, hemolytic disease of the newborn, heparin therapy, histoplasmosis, hypersplenism, idiopathic thrombocytopenic purpura, lymphoproliferative disease, infections (acute), irradiation, leukemia (acute granulocytic, acute lymphocytic, monocytic), malaria, May-Hegglin anomaly, megakaryocytic hypoplasia, menstruation, multiple myeloma, myelofibrosis, radiation, regular plateletpheresis donors, septicemia, typhoid fever, uremia, and Wiskott-Aldrich syndrome. Drugs include acetazolamide, acetohexamide, amidopyrine, aminosalicylic acid, amphotericin B, ampicillin, antimony, antimony potassium tartrate, antineoplastics, arsenicals, aspirin, aurothioglucose, barbiturates, brompheniramine maleate, carbamazepine, chloramphenicol, chlorpropamide, chloroquine hydrochloride, chloroquine phosphate, chlorothiazide, colchicine, diazoxide, digitoxin, ethacrynate sodium, ethacrynic acid, ethoxzolamide, furosemide, gold sodium thiomalate, hydroxychloroquine sulfate, indomethacin, iothiouracil, isoniazid, mefenamic acid, meprobamate, methazolamide, methimazole, methyldopa, methyldopate hydrochloride, oral hypoglycemics, organic insecticides (some), oxyphenbutazone, oxytetracycline, oxytetracycline calcium, oxytetracycline hydrochloride, penicillamine, penicillins, phenylbutazone, phenytoin, phenytoin sodium, pyrimethamine, quinidine gluconate, quinidine polygalacturonate, quinidine sulfate, quinine sulfate, rifampin, salicylates, streptomycin sulfate, sulfonamides, thiazides, tolbutamide, tricyclic antidepressants, and vaccines. Herbal or natural remedies include the Chinese bracket fungus *Ganoderma lucidum.*

Description. Platelets are nonnucleated, disk-shaped cells that function in hemostatic plug formation, clot retraction, and coagulation factor activation. They are produced by the bone marrow from megakaryocytes released into the bloodstream to function in hemostasis.

Professional Considerations
1. Consent form NOT required.
2. **Preparation:**
   A. Tube: Lavender topped.
   B. Do NOT draw specimens during hemodialysis.
3. **Procedure:**
   A. Leave a tourniquet in place less than 1 minute.
   B. Draw a 5-mL blood sample.
   C. Gently invert the tube two or three times.
4. **Postprocedure care:**
   A. Send the specimen to the laboratory within 1 hour.
   B. Closely monitor the site for bleeding with clients with known thrombocytopenia.
5. **Client and family teaching:**
   A. If thrombocytopenia is present, avoid rough physical activity and bumping into furniture. Use a stool softener and avoid straining to have a bowel movement. Use a soft toothbrush and watch for and report signs of bleeding: bruising, petechiae, blood in the stool/urine/sputum, bleeding from invasive lines, bleeding gums, abnormal or excessive vaginal bleeding.
6. **Factors that affect results:**
   A. Reject hemolyzed specimens or specimens received more than 1 hour after collection.
   B. High altitudes, chronic cold weather, and exercise increase platelet counts.
7. **Other data:**
   A. The serum sample is stable at room temperature for 10 hours, may be refrigerated for up to 18 hours, and should not be frozen.
   B. Feverfew is an herb or natural remedy that may inhibit platelet activity and increase bleeding.

PLETHYSMOGRAPHY, DIAGNOSTIC
(see Pulse volume recorder testing of peripheral vasculature, Diagnostic)

p-METHOXYAMPHETAMINE
(see Amphetamines, Blood)

PNEUMOCYSTIS IMMUNOFLUORESCENT ASSAY, SERUM

Norm. Antibodies <1:16. No organisms observed.

Usage. Diagnosis of *Pneumocystis* pneumonia associated with acquired immunodeficiency syndrome (AIDS), immunosuppressed cancers, and organ transplants.

Description. *Pneumocystis carinii* are protozoan bacteria that produce an inflammatory infection within the lungs known as *Pneumocystis* pneumonia. This type of pneumonia does not generally develop in humans unless they are immunocompromised by steroid therapy or cell-mediated immunodeficiencies. The alveolar exudate produced by *Pneumocystis* is a proteinaceous material pervaded with cysts and trophozoites. The antigens present in the bacterial cell walls produce antibodies that circulate in the blood. These antibodies can be examined under a microscope when stained with immunofluorescent dyes and examined under ultraviolet radiation.

Professional Considerations
1. Consent form NOT required.
2. Preparation:
   A. Tube: Red-topped or pink-topped or Corvac tube.
   B. Specimens MAY be drawn during hemodialysis.
3. Procedure:
   A. Draw a 10-mL blood sample.
4. Postprocedure care:
   A. Handle the specimen with caution because of potential cross-infection.
5. Client and family teaching:
   A. Results are normally available within 24 hours.
6. Factors that affect results:
   A. Immunofluorescent antibody titers are elevated in only about 30% of clients with *Pneumocystis*.
   B. Serum antibody or antigen detection is not reliable for definitive diagnosis of *P. carinii*.
7. Other data:
   A. A diagnostic bronchoscopy for tissue brushings should be performed if the serum specimen is positive for *P. carinii*.

PNEUMOTONOMETRY
(*see Tonometry test for glaucoma, Diagnostic*)

POLIOMYELITIS 1, 2, 3 TITER, BLOOD

Norm. <1.8 is normal. A fourfold increase in the antibody titer between the acute and convalescent blood specimens is diagnostic for poliomyelitis. Presence of a high IgM titer may also indicate recent infection.

Usage. Identification and diagnosis of the enterovirus poliovirus and differentiation of the serotype (1 = Brunhilde, 2 = Lansing, 3 = Leon).

Description. Poliomyelitis is an extremely contagious systemic infection resulting in necrotic and inflammatory lesions of the motor and autonomic neurons of the brain and spinal cord. Poliomyelitis usually manifests as a systemic viremia with headache, fever, vomiting, and back and neck pain progressing in severity to a prominent paralysis and possibly death. The virus is transmitted by ingestion of contaminated water or food. The virus incubates and replicates in the lymphoid tissue of the tonsils, Peyer's patches, pharynx, and alimentary tract. Enteroviruses (polioviruses) are excreted in the feces and can remain active outside of the human cells for months. The incubation period for poliomyelitis is 5-35 days, with acute symptoms occurring 7-12 days after exposure. Both acute and convalescent blood samples are tested to detect a rise in titer levels. Antigen-neutralization tests quantitate titers and serotype the virus from centrifuged serum. Type I, Brunhilde poliovirus, is associated with paralysis, chronic cardiomyopathy, diabetes, fetal malformation, myocarditis, and pericarditis. Orally administered vaccines available since the 1950s have decreased the incidence of this disease worldwide. A global poliomyelitis eradication initiative that began in 1998 has reduced the cases worldwide by over 99%. Polio is considered endemic in only 10 countries, as of 2001.

Professional Considerations
1. Consent form NOT required.
2. Preparation:
   A. Tube: Red topped, red/gray topped, or gold topped.
   B. Specimens MAY be drawn during hemodialysis.
3. Procedure:
   A. Draw an 8- to 10-mL (adults) or a 3- to 4-mL (pediatric) blood sample.
4. Postprocedure care:
   A. None.
5. Client and family teaching:
   A. Strict isolation precautions may be instituted if serum titers indicate infection secondary to the extreme contagiousness.
6. Factors that affect results:
   A. In 50% of people with poliomyelitis, the serum titers have already peaked before testing.
7. Other data:
   A. Use extreme caution when handling or transporting samples and wash hands well after handling a sample.
   B. Poliovirus is human specific.

POLYSOMNOGRAPHY (PSG, CARDIOPULMONARY SLEEP STUDY, CPAP TITRATION STUDY, MULTIPLE SLEEP LATENCY TEST, MSLT, SLEEP APNEA STUDY, SLEEP OXIMETRY, SLEEP STUDY), DIAGNOSTIC

Norm. No abnormal patterns of sleep or breathing.

Usage. Obstructive sleep apnea, CPAP titration study (treatment for obstructive sleep apnea), narcolepsy, periodic movement syndrome, disorders of arousal (sleepwalking, night terrors), rapid eye movement (REM) behavioral disorder, dissociative disorders, nocturnal seizures, nocturnal reflux, nocturnal pain syndromes, erectile dysfunction, restless legs syndrome. Rarely: insomnias, depression, and sleep-wake disorders.

Description. Polysomnography (PSG) is a procedure that takes recordings of the electric potentials generated by the cerebral cortex of the brain during sleep. Electrical potentials demonstrated on PSG are of six types: (1) those generated by eye movements, (2) surface electrical potentials generated by chin muscle activity, (3) surface electrical potentials generated by the heart, (4) surface electrical potentials generated by the muscles in the leg (anterior tibalis), (5) nasal and oral airflow (each separately or combined), and (6) respiratory effort of chest and abdomen by piezoelectric or inductance belts. In special instances additional sensors are placed either on the head or abdomen or to measure penile erections. This study can be coordinated with a multiple sleep latency test when an evaluation of excessive daytime sleepiness (that is, narcolepsy) is desired. The use of computerized digital monitoring provides objectivity in scoring of sleep-related events.

Professional Considerations

1. Consent form is NOT required.
2. **Preparation:**
   A. See *Client and family teaching.*
   B. Document the client's current medications, and his or her height and weight.
   C. Verify with the physician whether certain medications should be withheld before the test.
   D. Review and complete the pretest questionnaire with the client.
3. **Procedure:**
   A. Sensor placement:
      i. The client sits on a bed or chair and electrodes are placed on the scalp (see the EEG description), about the eyes, and under the chin.
      ii. The airflow monitors are placed near the mouth and nose, and the respiratory belts are placed about the chest and abdomen.
      iii. Electrodes are placed on the chest to measure the ECG and on the legs to measure movements. For *nocturnal penile tumescence testing,* a mercury strain gauge will be placed at the base and tip of the penile shaft.
      iv. Other sensors, such as a pH probe, are placed as necessary.
   B. The client is asked to follow several commands to ensure that the sensors are functioning properly. This includes eye blinking, looking right, looking left, breath holding, right and left leg movements. This is known as "biocalibration."
   C. The client then sleeps, and the PSG recordings are taken. A technician is continuously monitoring the recordings and client to detect lead detachment. For nocturnal penile tumescence testing, pressure is placed on the head of the penis with a pressure plate to determine at what pressure the penis will buckle.
   D. Recordings:
      i. The data obtained from a polysomnogram include the amount of sleep during the test, the amount of each stage of sleep, any events occurring during sleep, the number of arousals, the number of respiratory events, and the degree of desaturation.
      ii. Apneas are defined as a complete cessation of breathing, whereas hypopneas are a partial cessation of breathing. These are usually reported as the number of respiratory events (apneas plus hypopneas) for an hour. This is

known as the RDI, respiratory distress index, or the AHI, apnea hypopnea index.

E. *CPAP titration studies:*
   i. CPAP (continuous positive air pressure) is a treatment for obstructive sleep apnea and is essentially an air splint. Room air is blown through a mask covering the nose. The air pressure opens the posterior area of the pharynx eliminating the obstruction and snoring.
   ii. The air pressure is titrated throughout the night, usually being slowly increased until both the obstructive respiratory events and the snoring are eliminated.
   iii. Occasionally a bi-level machine that provides separate inspiratory and expiratory pressures is used.

F. *"Split-night" studies:*
   i. In these studies the first half of the night is used to confirm the existence of significant sleep-disordered breathing. The second half of the night is used to titrate CPAP. The use of "split-night" studies is still controversial. Not all laboratories will perform them.

G. *The multiple sleep latency test (MSLT):*
   i. The MSLT measures the degree of daytime sleepiness.
   ii. Usually only the brain waves (EEG), eye movements (EOG), chin muscle activity (EMG), and heart activity (ECG) are measured during the (MSLT).
   iii. The MSLT consists in five naps taken throughout the day, each 2 hours apart.
   iv. The client is given up to 20 minutes to fall asleep on each nap. If the client falls asleep, he or she is given 15 minutes to sleep.
   v. Two results are obtained: The first is the average time to fall asleep on the five naps known as the "mean sleep latency." The second is the number of naps on which REM is seen known as "sleep-onset REMs."

4. **Postprocedure care:**
   A. The various sensors are removed, and the conductive medium is removed from the scalp.
   B. Every sleep lab should have facilities available for a client's morning toilet.

5. **Client and family teaching:**
   A. Often a pretest questionnaire is filled out the night of this study or mailed to the client before the study.
   B. You will sleep all night in the sleep lab, and a videotape will be taken of you while you sleep. If the PSG will be followed by a multiple sleep latency test, you will spend the day in the sleep laboratory.
   C. You will have wires and sensors attached to you, which are needed to perform the sleep study. The wires and sensors receive signals from your brain waves, muscle movement, heart, and breathing patterns that help evaluate your sleep patterns.
   D. For clients who will have a CPAP titration study: A CPAP mask might be used for part or all of the test to determine whether it will help reduce sleep apnea. This mask fits very snugly over your nose and mouth. It delivers air into your lungs under pressure, and so it might be uncomfortable until you get used to it. You will be able to select the mask that is most comfortable for you.
   E. You will be able to perform normal daily activities after the test.
   F. Your test results will be sent to your referring physician, who will explain the results to you.

6. **Factors that affect results:**
   A. The use of caffeine or other stimulants before the test.
   B. The client's normal sleep-wake cycle.
   C. The client's information before the study and comfort sleeping in an unusual situation.
   D. Nocturnal penile tumescence testing results may be inconclusive due to the client's anxiety, embarrassment, or startle response during testing, as well as sleep disorders that cause a reduction in the amount of REM-type of sleep Most penile nocturnal erections occur during REM sleep.

E. CPAP titration studies: A client success in using CPAP is highly dependent on the skill of the sleep technician. The degree of client education about CPAP before the study of CPAP is a factor that can affect how well the client is able to tolerate the CPAP mask while sleeping. The technicians should be aware of the presence of any claustrophobia or difficulties the client might have by having things on the face.

7. **Other data:**
   A. Even moderate weight reduction reduces the incidence of sleep-disordered breathing in obese clients with obstructive sleep apnea.

PORPHYRINS, QUANTITATIVE, BLOOD

Norm:

		SI UNITS
Total erythrocyte porphyrins	<31 µg/dL	
ALA	<1 mg/dL	
Coproporphyrin	0.5-2.3 mg/dL	
Protoporphyrin	4-52 mg/dL	0.07-0.93 µmol/L
Uroporphyrin	Negative to trace	Negative to trace

Increased ALA. Chemical toxicity, cirrhosis (alcoholic), lead poisoning, and porphyrias.

Increased Coproporphyrin. Anemia (hemolytic, pernicious, sideroblastic), cirrhosis (alcoholic), coproporphyria (erythropoietic), erythroid hyperplasia, exercise (extreme), fever, hemochromatosis, Hodgkin's disease, lead poisoning, leukemia, myocardial infarction (acute), poliomyelitis (acute), porphyria (congenital erythropoietic), protoporphyria (erythropoietic), thyrotoxicosis, and vitamin deficiencies.

Increased Protoporphyrin. Anemia (hemolytic, sideroblastic), carbon tetrachloride and benzene toxicity, erythropoiesis, infection, iron deficiency, lead poisoning, protoporphyria (erythropoietic), and thalassemia.

Increased Uroporphyrin. Cirrhosis, lead poisoning, and porphyria (acute, intermittent, congenital erythropoietic).

Decreased ALA. Not applicable.

Decreased Coproporphyrin. Not applicable.

Decreased Protoporphyrin. Anemia (megaloblastic).

Decreased Uroporphyrin. Not applicable.

Description. Porphyrins are compounds necessary for heme synthesis in hemoglobin metabolism. ALA (delta-aminolevulinic acid) is the basic building block of porphyrins and is involved in the synthesis of coproporphyrin and protoporphyrin. Coproporphyrin is the main porphyrin found in urine, whereas protoporphyrin is the main porphyrin found in erythrocytes. When iron is added to protoporphyrin, the final heme molecule is formed. As the hemoglobin is eventually broken down, these products used for heme synthesis again appear in the blood, urine, and stool as hemoglobin-breakdown products. Clients with one of the congenital or acquired diseases classified as the "porphyrias" secrete and excrete increased amounts of these compounds. The diseases are characterized by neurologic abnormalities, acute abdominal pain, acute cutaneous pain, photosensitivity, or psychiatric disturbances. This test is used most frequently with the measurement of urine porphyrin levels to differentiate the cause and type of porphyria occurring.

Professional Considerations
1. Consent form NOT required.
2. **Preparation:**
   A. Tube: Green topped, lavender topped, or black topped.
   B. Do NOT draw specimen during hemodialysis.
   C. See *Client and family teaching.*

3. **Procedure:**
   A. Draw a 3-mL blood sample without hemolysis.
4. **Postprocedure care:**
   A. None.
5. **Client and family teaching:**
   A. Do not drink alcohol for 24 hours before testing.
   B. Clients with positive test results should avoid ethyl alcohol (ethanol), barbiturates, and anticonvulsants that might cause an acute attack of neurologic or psychotic porphyria (elevated ALA).
   C. Clients with positive test results should avoid sunlight.
   D. Genetic counseling may be necessary for the inherited form of porphyria.
6. **Factors that affect results:**
   A. Hemolysis of the specimen invalidates the results.
   B. Increased levels may occur during menstruation or pregnancy.
7. **Other data:**
   A. See also *Protophorphyrin, Free erythrocyte, Blood; Coproporphyrin, Urine.*

POSITRACE IMAGING, DIAGNOSTIC
(*see Dual modality imaging, Diagnostic*)

POSITRON EMISSION TOMOGRAPHY (PET), DIAGNOSTIC

Norm. Requires interpretation according to the type of study being performed.

Usage. Enables noninvasive regional tissue physiology study of metabolic changes in body tissues. Comparison of cerebral blood flow and energy metabolism; evaluation for leakage of the blood-brain barrier; study of brain pharmacology; evaluation of brain hemodynamics in cerebrovascular disease; localization of seizure foci in clients with focal seizures; evaluation of regional myocardial blood flow, metabolism and thus viability; study of the distribution of pulmonary edema; and study of solid tumor proliferation, blood flow, glucose, and oxygen utilization alone and in response to therapy; diagnosing, staging, and restaging of cancer (lung, colorectal, lymphoma,

melanoma, head and neck, and esophageal.).

Description. Positron emission tomography (PET) is a noninvasive radiographic method for studying blood flow and metabolic changes occurring in specific organs or regions of the body tissues. It involves the injection or inhalation of gamma ray-emitting, biologically compatible radioisotopes and the creation of images of radioisotope distribution in the body. As the radioisotopes disintegrate, they emit positrons, which are positively charged particles similar to electrons. As the positrons are captured by electrons, both are destroyed, resulting in the emission of two photons, which travel outward in opposite directions. The photons are detected simultaneously by the PET camera, an event known as a "coincidence." The summation of these coincidences allows for the creation of a continuous map of the metabolic activity of the body. A computer then creates pictures of cross-sections of the body area studied, which show brighter areas according to the amount of radioisotope present.

Some examples of radioisotopes include oxygen 15, nitrogen 13, carbon 11, and fluorine 18, which are labeled onto substances such as water, carbon dioxide, or glucose. Because the radioisotopes are biologically compatible, they take the place of the body's chemical elements (such as oxygen, nitrogen, or fluorine), and the resulting scan gives a true representation of the physiologic function of the body processes. The choice of radioisotope and material to be labeled is based on the body function to be studied. For example, blood flow is studied using ^{15}O-labeled HO, glucose metabolism is studied using ^{18}F-labeled glucose, tissue perfusion is studied using ^{13}N-labeled NH, and anaerobic metabolism is studied using ^{11}C-labeled acetate. Some conditions in which the use of PET has been studied include Alzheimer's disease, asthma, brain tumors, cerebral atrophy, cerebrovascular disorders, chronic obstructive pulmonary disease, coronary artery disease, epilepsy, head trauma, Huntington's disease, myocardial infarction, obsessive compulsive disorder, pulmonary edema, schizophrenia, and unstable angina.

The newest equipment called "Dual Mode Imaging" combines PET with structural imaging modalities such as Ultrafast CT or MRI for improved imaging results. See *Dual Modality Imaging, Diagnostic.*

Professional Considerations
1. Consent form MAY be required.

Risks
Hematoma, infection.

Precautions
During pregnancy, risks of cumulative radiation exposure to the fetus from this and other previous or future imaging studies must be weighed against the benefits of the procedure. Although formal limits for client exposure are relative to this risk:benefit comparison, the United States Nuclear Regulatory Commission requires that the cumulative dose equivalent to an embryo/fetus from occupational exposure not exceed 0.5 rem (5 mSv). Radiation dosage to the fetus is proportional to the distance of the anatomy studied from the abdomen and decreases as pregnancy progresses. For pregnant clients, consult the radiologist/radiology department to obtain estimated fetal radiation exposure from this procedure.

2. **Preparation:**
   A. A premedication may be prescribed to be given before transport to the nuclear medicine department.
   B. Diuretics should be withheld before the study unless an indwelling urinary catheter is present or will be inserted.
   C. If pelvic imaging is to be performed, an indwelling urinary catheter should be inserted.
   D. The client should have a meal before the procedure. Diabetics should be given their morning insulin before the procedure.
   E. If abdominal imaging is indicated, a bowel preparation may be prescribed.
   F. See *Client and family teaching.*
3. **Procedure:**
   A. The client is placed in a supine position on the scanning table, with an arm supported in extension.
   B. Intravenous access is established.
   C. A heparin flush solution is slowly infused.
   D. An arterial line may be inserted for some procedures.

E. For brain scans, a polymer clay (Polyform)-molded face mask is placed over the temporal level of the face and secured to the headrest to immobilize the client's head. The mask is marked with a reference point to ensure exact repeat positioning for any necessary future PET studies.
F. The scanning table is moved into position within the lumen of the positron emission scanner.
G. Once the client is positioned he or she must remain motionless throughout the study.
H. Some studies are conducted by having the client inhale the radioisotope. Others use intravenous injection.
I. An example of the steps involved in one type of scan follows.
J. *Cardiac PET:*
   i. ^{15}O-labeled HO is injected intravenously, and a 15-minute test scan is conducted to verify proper positioning.
   ii. A 30-minute transmission scan is then performed to correct for the attenuation of the chest and lungs.
   iii. ^{13}N-labeled NH is injected intravenously and allowed to equilibrate for 3 minutes. Then a PET study is performed for approximately 30 minutes to study cardiac tissue perfusion.
   iv. Finally, glucose metabolism of the heart is studied. If the client is a diabetic, with a glucose level >150 mg/dL, insulin may be given before this step. If the client has a low blood glucose level, either orally administered glucose or intravenous 50% dextrose in water will be given. Fluorodeoxyglucose (FDG) is injected intravenously to study glucose metabolism of the heart. After waiting 30 minutes for the FDG to circulate, one performs a 30-minute PET study.
4. **Postprocedure care:**
   A. The arterial line, if inserted for the PET study, is discontinued, and the site should be monitored for the development of hematoma.

5. Client and family teaching:
   A. You must remain motionless in an enclosed space for 1-3 hours.
   B. Wear comfortable clothing to the test.
   C. You may bring a cassette tape to listen to during the study.
   D. Do not drink large quantities of fluid or caffeine-containing beverages within 2 hours before the study unless you have been informed that an indwelling catheter will be inserted.
   E. Have a meal before the procedure.
   F. You may need a bowel preparation if abdominal imaging is indicated.
   G. Lactating women should not breast-feed for at least 20 hours after the scan.
6. Factors that affect results:
   A. Hypoglycemia may alter the results of PET of glucose metabolism.

   B. Movement more than about 1 cm may blur the resulting pictures. The ability of the client to remain motionless in an enclosed space affects whether an accurate study can be obtained.
   C. Insulin-dependent diabetics must have insulin administered the day of the study if glucose metabolism will be a focus of PET.
   D. Anxiety in the client that causes tension in the neck area can cause increased uptake of the fluorine type of isotope, which can be misinterpreted as metastases.
7. Other data:
   A. PET takes 1-3 hours. The half-life of the specific radioisotope used affects the length of the study.
   B. Claustrophobia may occur during the procedure.

POTASSIUM, SERUM

Norm:

		SI UNITS
Adult	3.5-5.3 mEq/L	3.5-5.3 mmol/L
Panic values	<2.5 mEq/L or >6.6 mEq/L	<2.5 mmol/L or >6.6 mmol/L
Premature Infant		
Cord blood	5.0-10.2 mEq/L	5.0-10.2 mmol/L
2 days	3.0-6.0 mEq/L	3.0-6.0 mmol/L
Full-term Newborn		
Cord blood	5.6-12.0 mEq/L	5.6-12.0 mmol/L
Newborn	3.7-5.0 mEq/L	3.7-5.0 mmol/L
Infant	4.1-5.3 mEq/L	4.1-5.3 mmol/L
Newborn, panic value	<2.5 mEq/L or >8.1 mEq/L	<2.5 mmol/L or >8.1 mmol/L
Child	3.4-4.7 mEq/L	3.4-4.7 mmol/L

Panic Level Symptoms and Treatment

Note: Treatment choice(s) depend on client history and condition and episode history.

Hyperkalemia Symptoms. Irritability, diarrhea, cramps, oliguria, difficulty speaking, cardiac dysrhythmias including peaked T-waves and progressing to refractory ventricular fibrillation with tachycardia.

Hyperkalemia Treatment:

Provide continuous ECG monitoring.
Administer sodium polystyrene sulfonate (Kayexalate).
Administer intravenous insulin and dextrose.
Administer sodium bicarbonate.
Administer calcium chloride or gluconate.
Both hemodialysis and peritoneal dialysis WILL remove potassium.

Hypokalemia Symptoms. Malaise, thirst, polyurea, anorexia, weak pulse, low blood pressure, vomiting, decreased reflexes, ECG changes, including depressed T-waves and ventricular ectopy.

Hypokalemia Treatment. Potassium replacement.

Increased. Acidosis, Addison's disease, adrenocortical insufficiency, anemia (hemolytic), anxiety, asthma, burns, dialysis (hemodialysis or peritoneal), diet (excessive potassium intake), dysrhythmia, hemolysis, hypoventilation, increased osmolality, infection (acute), ketoacidosis, leukocytosis, malignant hyperthermia (early), massive rapid red blood cell transfusion, metabolic acidosis, muscle necrosis, near-drowning, obstruction (intestinal), ostomies, pneumonia, pseudohypoaldosteronism, renal failure, renal hypertension, sepsis, shock, status epilepticus, syndrome of inappropriate antidiuretic hormone secretion (SIADHS), thrombocytosis, tissue trauma, uremia, and Waterhouse-Friderichsen syndrome. Drugs include aldosterone antagonists, amiloride, aminocaproic acid, antineoplastic agents, captopril, cyclophosphamide, digoxin, ephedrine, ephedrine sulfate, epinephrine, estrogens, heparin calcium, heparin sodium, histamine, ibuprofen, indomethacin, isoniazid, lithium, mannitol, methicillin, methicillin sodium, nonsteroidal anti-inflammatory agents, potassium bicarbonate, potassium chloride, potassium citrate, potassium gluconate, potassium salts of penicillin, phenformin, propranolol, salt substitutes, spironolactone, succinylcholine, tetracyclines, timolol maleate, triamterene and tromethamine.

Decreased. After sigmoidoscopy, acute tubular necrosis (diuretic phase), alcoholism, aldosteronism (primary), alkalosis, anorexia, barium intoxication, Bartter syndrome, bradycardia, cancer (colon), cerebral palsy, cholera, cirrhosis (chronic), congestive heart failure, Crohn's disease, Cushing's disease, dehydration, diabetes insipidus, diabetes mellitus, diarrhea, dumping syndrome, dysrhythmias, Fanconi syndrome, fever, fistulas, folic acid deficiency, hyperaldos-teronism, hyperalimentation, hypercorticoadrenalism, hypertension, hypomagnesemia, hypothermia, hypovolemia, hysterectomy, kwashiorkor, ketoacidosis, laxative abuse, lymphoma, malabsorption, malignant hyperthermia (late-stage), metabolic alkalosis, nephritis, organic brain syndrome, ostomies, pancreatitis (acute), paralytic ileus, pseudoaldosteronism, pyelonephritis (chronic), pyloric obstruction, renal tubular acidosis, salicylate intoxication, salt-losing nephropathy, sweating, suction (gastric), surgery (postoperatively), starvation, stress, toxic shock syndrome, ureterosigmoidostomy, villous adenoma, vipoma, vomiting, and Zollinger-Ellison syndrome (with diarrhea). Drugs include acetazolamide, albuterol, ammonium chloride, amphotericin, aspirin, bisacodyl, bronchodilators, carbenicillin, carbenoxolone, chlorthalidone, corticosteroids, corticotropin, EDTA, diuretics, ethacrynic acid, furosemide, gamma-hydroxybutyrate (GHB), gentamicin sulfate, glucose, insulin, mercurial diuretics, penicillin G, piperacillin, salicylates, sodium bicarbonate, sodium chloride, succinylcholine chloride (in children), thiazides, thiopental, ticarcillin, and trimethaphan camsylate. Herbs or natural remedies include aloe (long-term use), licorice (*Glycyrrhiza glabra*), which can cause intoxication, and products containing aristolochic acids (*Akebia* spp., *Aristolochia* spp., *Asarum* spp., birthwort, *Bragantia* spp., *Clematis* spp., *Cocculus* spp., *Diploclisia* spp., Dutchman's pipe, *Fang chi, Fang ji, Fang chi, Guang fang ji, Kan-Mokutsu, Menispernum* spp., *Mokutsu, Mu tong, Sinomenium* spp., and *Stephania* spp.).

Description. Potassium (K^+) is the major intracellular cation. The body obtains potassium through dietary ingestion, and the kidneys either preserve or excrete it depending on cellular need. Potassium is responsible for the regulation of cellular water balance, electrical conduction in muscle cells, and acid-based homeostasis. Although the majority of potassium is stored and used within tissue cells, serum potassium analysis can be helpful in evaluating electrolyte balance. Serum potassium levels are used in the evaluation of clients with cardiac dysrhythmias, renal dysfunction, mental confusion, gastrointestinal distress, and intravenous replacement therapy.

Professional Considerations
1. Consent form NOT required.
2. **Preparation:**
   A. Tube: Red topped, red/gray topped, or gold topped or green topped.
   B. Do NOT draw specimens during hemodialysis.
3. **Procedure:**
   A. Draw the specimen without using a tourniquet.
   B. Using a 20-gauge or larger needle, draw a 1-mL blood sample.
   C. Do not aspirate strongly or push the plunger into the vacuum tube too forcefully.
   D. Avoid hemolysis.
4. **Postprocedure care:**
   A. Write the collection time on the laboratory requisition.
   B. Note on the laboratory requisition if the client is receiving potassium by pill, liquid, or intravenously.
   C. Send the specimen to the chemistry laboratory for spinning within 1 hour of collection.
   D. Serum and plasma must be separated from the red cells, or elevated results may occur.
5. **Client and family teaching:**
   A. The client must follow the prescribed dosage of potassium.
   B. Foods high in potassium are apricots, bananas, meats, potatoes, prunes, and tomatoes.
6. **Factors that affect results:**
   A. Reject hemolyzed specimens or specimens received more than 1 hour after collection.
   B. Use of a tourniquet and pumping the hand before obtaining a venous sample can increase the laboratory value by up to 20%.
   C. Do NOT draw the specimen from a site where an intravenous infusion exists.
   D. Clients with elevated white blood counts and platelet counts may have falsely elevated serum potassium levels.
   E. Incomplete separation of the serum from the clot may cause falsely elevated results.
   F. Acidemia causes potassium to move from cells into the extracellular fluid in exchange for hydrogen ions moving intracellularly.
   G. Values are 0.2-0.4 mEq/L higher in samples collected in the afternoon and early evening.
7. **Other data:**
   A. For elevated potassium levels, an arterial blood gas should be evaluated for acidemia.
   B. Green et al, (2002) found a higher risk for stroke in clients with low potassium intake (<2.5 g/day) and in clients on diuretics with lower potassium levels (<4.1mEq/L or <4.1 mmol/L).

POTASSIUM, URINE

Norm:

		SI UNITS
Adult	25-123 mEq/24 hours (intake-dependent)	25-123 mmol/day
Child	17-57 mEq/24 hours	17-57 mmol/day

Increased. Alkalosis, Cushing's disease, dehydration, diabetic ketoacidosis, diet (excessive potassium intake), fever, head trauma, hyperaldosteronism, hypokalemia, renal tubular acidosis, renal failure (chronic), salicylate intoxication, and starvation. Drugs include acetazolamide, ammonium chloride, amphotericin, fosinopril, glucocorticoids, loop diuretics, mercurial diuretics, penicillin, potassium, and thiazide diuretics.

Decreased. Addison's disease, diarrhea, hyperkalemia, hypomagnesemia, malabsorption syndrome, nephrotic syndrome, potassium deficiency, renal failure (acute), and syndrome of inappropriate antidiuretic hormone secretion (SIADHS). Drugs include laxatives, epinephrine, levarterenol, and general anesthetic agents.

Description. Potassium (K^+) is the major intracellular cation. The body obtains potassium through dietary ingestion, and the kidneys either preserve or excrete it, depending on cellular need. Potassium is responsible for the regulation of cellular water balance, electrical conduction in muscle cells, and acid-base homeostasis. A 24-hour urine collection is obtained to determine excreted potassium levels. Urine potassium levels are helpful in the assessment of endocrine abnormalities and renal tubular function.

Professional Considerations
1. Consent form NOT required.
2. Preparation:
   A. Obtain a 3-L container without preservatives, or a pediatric urine collection device/bag and tape.
   B. Write the beginning time of the collection on the laboratory requisition.
   C. Note diuretic or glucocorticoid therapy on the laboratory requisition.
3. Procedure:
   A. Discard the first morning urine specimen.
   B. Save all urine voided for 24 hours in a refrigerated, clean, 3-L container without preservatives. Document the quantity of urine output during the specimen collection period. Include urine voided at the end of the 24-hour period. For catheterized clients, keep the drainage bag on ice and empty urine into the collection container hourly.
   C. *Pediatric/infant specimen collection:*
      i. Place the child in a supine position with the knees flexed and the hips externally rotated and abducted.
      ii. Cleanse, rinse, and thoroughly dry the perineal area.
      iii. To prevent the child from removing the collection device/bag, a diaper may be placed over the genital area.
      iv. *Females:* Tape the pediatric collection device/bag to the perineum. Starting at the area between the anus and vagina, apply the device/bag in an anterior direction.
      v. *Males:* Place the pediatric collection device/bag over the penis and scrotum and tape it to the perineal area.
4. Postprocedure care:
   A. Compare the urine quantity in the specimen container with the urinary output record for the test. If the specimen contains less urine than what was recorded as output, some of the sample may have been discarded, invalidating the test.
   B. Document the quantity of urine and the collection ending time on the laboratory requisition.
   C. Send the specimen to the laboratory and refrigerate it.
5. Client and family teaching:
   A. Save all the urine voided in the 24-hour period and urinate before defecating to avoid loss of urine. If any urine is accidentally discarded, discard the entire specimen and restart the collection the next day.
6. Factors that affect results:
   A. All urine voided for the 24-hour period must be included to avoid a falsely low result.
7. Other data:
   A. Urine potassium levels exhibit a diurnal variation, with higher levels occurring at night.

PPD
(see Mantoux skin test, Diagnostic)

PRA
(see Renin activity, Plasma)

PRAZEPAM
(see Benzodiazepines, Plasma and Urine)

PREALBUMIN
(see Transthyretin, Serum)

PRECIPITIN TEST AGAINST HUMAN SPERM AND BLOOD, VAGINAL SWAB

Norm. Negative.

Usage. Used to identify the presence of semen or blood of human origin from vaginal secretions after sexual assault or rape.

Description. Human semen contains specific antibodies that are unique to the species. When vaginal secretions containing semen or blood are mixed with antisera solution, an antigen-antibody reaction or linkage will occur if the source is human sperm. The reaction is the result of the antigen binding to the antibody and forming an insoluble precipitate. One can perform this test by mixing the vaginal aspirate with antisera solution in a test tube or capillary tube. If an antigen-antibody reaction occurs, the cells will clump and fall to the bottom of the test tube, an indication that semen or blood present in the sample is from a human source. The result of the semen precipitation test is recorded as permanent evidence that coital relations occurred. Vaginal aspirations can also be tested for hemagglutination of ABO blood typing.

Professional Considerations
1. Consent form NOT required.
2. **Preparation:**
   A. Obtain a rape examination tray.
   B. Use a speculum rinsed with 0.9% saline for examination and specimen collection.
3. **Procedure:**
   A. The collection of specimens is governed by the laws of each state.
   B. Follow the directions in the "sex evidence kit" according to the requirements of the state.
4. **Postprocedure care:**
   A. Follow directions in the "sex evidence kit" for the proper chain of command of evidence.

B. The specimen is generally given to the police and forwarded to the proper authorities for evidence testing.
5. **Client and family teaching:**
   A. Vaginal douching or bathing decreases the likelihood of obtaining positive results.
   B. Survivors of sexual assault should be referred to appropriate crisis counseling agencies as well as for gynecologic follow-up examination.
   C. Referral for HIV testing should be reviewed and offered to all sexual assault victims.
   D. Preventive treatment for chlamydiosis, gonorrhea, and syphilis should be provided to all survivors of sexual assault.
   E. The option of postcoital contraceptive should be reviewed with all survivors of sexual assault.
6. **Factors that affect results:**
   A. The laboratory must receive vaginal washing immediately, or else the specimen should be frozen.
7. **Other data:**
   A. No universal threshold exists for evidence of intercourse or rape. A decrease in acid phosphatase after intercourse varies from hours to 4 days.

PREGNANCY TEST (HCG) ROUTINE, SERUM AND QUALITATIVE, URINE

Norm. *Note:* Norms are greatly dependent on test method used.

		SI UNITS
HCG, Serum		
Males	<3.0 mIU/mL	<3.0 IU/L
Females		
Nonpregnant	<3.0 mIU/mL	<3.0 IU/L
Pregnancy, first 6 weeks	Values double about every 2 days.	
10 weeks of gestation	100,000 mIU/mL	
≥14 weeks of gestation	Levels trend downward	
HCG, Qualitative, Urine	Negative	

Increased. Breast cancer, bronchogenic carcinoma, choriocarcinoma, embryonal carcinoma, gastric carcinoma, hepatocarcinoma, hydatidiform mole, malignant melanoma, multiple myeloma, pancreatic cancer, pregnancy, seminoma, teratoma, and trophoblastic tumor.

Decreased. Abortion (threatened, actual) and ectopic pregnancy.

Description. Human chorionic gonadotropin (HCG) is a hormone uniquely secreted by the placenta of a fertilized ovum implanted in the uterine wall. HCG production begins 8-10 days after conception or during day 21-23 of the cycle. It reaches peak concentration at 8-12 weeks of gestation and then gradually decreases until returning to normal within 3-4 days after normal full-term delivery. This test can be most accurately performed 2 days after missed menses up to 3 weeks.

Serum testing is performed by incubation of serum with antihuman chorionic gonadotropin (anti-HCG). If HCG is present in the sample, it combines with the anti-HCG antibodies and inactivates them. When these inactivated antibodies are exposed to the indicator, which is red or latex cells coated with HCG, clumping of the cells does not occur, resulting in a positive pregnancy test. If clumping does occur, the test is negative.

Professional Considerations
1. Consent form NOT required.
2. **Preparation:**
   A. Tube: Red topped, red/gray topped, or gold topped for serum test.
   B. Obtain random urine collection container for urine test.
   C. Serum specimens MAY be drawn during hemodialysis.
   D. See *Client and family teaching.*

3. **Procedure:**
   A. Draw a 1-mL blood sample for serum test.
   B. Obtain a 4-mL random urine specimen.
4. **Postprocedure care:**
   A. None.
5. **Client and family teaching:**
   A. May help differentiate actual pregnancy from an ectopic pregnancy in conduction with an ultrasonogram.
   B. Avoid medications such as anticonvulsants, antiparkinsonian agents, hypnotics, and tranquilizers, which may cause a false-positive result in the serum test
6. **Factors that affect results:**
   A. False-positive results may be caused by incorrect performance or handling of the test, excessive production of luteinizing hormone (LH) of the pituitary gland, absence of gonadal hormones in menopausal women, HCG-producing tumors or tubo-ovarian abscess.
   B. False-negative results may result when test is performed very early in pregnancy.
7. **Other data:**
   A. Although not usually present in healthy males or nonpregnant females, elevated levels of HCG may be detected in these clients with certain malignant tumors.
   B. See also *Human chorionic gonadotropin, Beta subunit, Serum.*

PREGNANETRIOL, URINE

Norm:

		SI UNITS
Adult female	0.5-2.0 mg/24 hours	1.5-5.9 mmol/day
Adult male	0.4-2.4 mg/24 hours	1.2-7.1 mmol/day
Child		
<6 years	<0.2 mg/24 hours	<0.6 mmol/day
7-16 years	0.3-1.1 mg/24 hours	0.9-3.3 mmol/day

Increased. Adrenogenital syndrome, congenital adrenocortical hyperplasia, hirsutism, Stein-Leventhal syndrome, 21-hydroxylase deficiency, tumor (ovarian, adrenal cortex), and virilization.

Description. Pregnanetriol, a metabolite of 17-hydroxyprogesterone, is involved in the synthesis of adrenal cor-

ticoids and is normally excreted in the urine in only small amounts. Increased urinary excretion is caused by a deficiency in the enzyme that converts 17-hydroxyprogesterone to cortisol. The decreased cortisol production results in increased adrenocorticotropic hormone (ACTH), which leads to increased serum hydroxyprogesterone.

This in turn stimulates the release of adrenal androgens. As the increased amounts of hydroxyprogesterone are metabolized, urine pregnanetriol levels increase. This test is most commonly abnormal in adrenogenital syndrome, which results in symptoms of hypertension, craving for salt, premature physical development of sexual characteristics in males, failure to thrive in infants, and pseudohermaphroditism (females with male genitalia).

Professional Considerations

1. Consent form NOT required.
2. Preparation:
   A. Obtain a clean, 3-L container without preservative or to which acetic acid preservative has been added.
   B. For pediatric/infant specimens, obtain a pediatric urine collection device/bag and tape.
   C. See *Client and family teaching.*
3. Procedure:
   A. Discard the first morning-urine specimen.
   B. Save all the urine voided for 24 hours in a refrigerated, clean, 3-L container without preservative or to which acetic acid preservative has been added. Document the quantity of urine output during the specimen collection period. Include urine voided at the end of the 24-hour period. For catheterized clients, keep the drainage bag on ice and empty the urine into the collection container hourly.
   C. *Pediatric/infant specimen collection:*
      i. Place the child in a supine position with the knees flexed and the hips externally rotated and abducted.
      ii. Cleanse, rinse, and thoroughly dry the perineal area.
      iii. To prevent the child from removing the collection device/bag, a diaper may be placed over the genital area.
      iv. *Females:* Tape the pediatric collection device/bag to the perineum. Starting at the area between the anus and vagina, apply the device/bag in an anterior direction.

v. *Males:* Place the pediatric collection device/bag over the penis and scrotum and tape it to the perineal area.
4. Postprocedure care:
   A. Compare the urine quantity in the specimen container with the urinary output record for the test. If the specimen contains less urine than what was recorded as output, some of the sample may have been discarded, invalidating the test.
   B. Document the urine quantity on the laboratory requisition.
5. Client and family teaching:
   A. Save all the urine voided in the 24-hour period and urinate before defecating to avoid loss of urine. If any urine is accidentally discarded, discard the entire specimen and restart the collection the next day.
   B. Avoid muscular exercise before or during the specimen collection period.
6. Factors that affect results:
   A. All the urine voided for the 24-hour period must be included to avoid a falsely low result.
   B. Results are invalid if the specimen was not refrigerated throughout the collection period.
   C. Exercise during the collection period causes increased androgen release.
7. Other data:
   A. In 21-hydroxylase deficiency, there is also an increase in serum 17-hydroxyprogesterone and urinary 17-ketosteroids.

PREKALLIKREIN, PLASMA
(see Factor, Fletcher plasma)

PRENATAL SCREEN, DIAGNOSTIC
(see ABO group and Rh type, Blood; Coombs' test, Indirect, Serum)

PRIMIDONE (MYSOLINE), SERUM

Norm. Negative.

	TROUGH	SI UNITS
Therapeutic Levels		
Adults	5-12 µg/mL	23-55 µmol/L
Children <5 years	7-10 µg/mL	32-46 µmol/L
Panic level	>24 µg/mL	>110 µmol/L

Panic Level Symptoms and Treatment

Symptoms. Decreased level of consciousness, ataxia, anemia.

Treatment:
Note: Treatment choice(s) depend on client history and condition and episode history. Discontinue primidone.
Protect airway.
Support hemodynamics.
Hemodialysis WILL remove primidone.
Treat anemia with folic acid or vitamin B_{12}.
Drugs that may speed the conversion of primidone to its metabolite phenobarbital include phenytoin and phenytoin sodium.

Usage. Monitoring the effectiveness of primidone therapy and prevention of primidone toxicity.

Increased. Drugs include carbamazepine, isoniazid, monoamine oxidase (MOA) inhibitors, phenobarbital, and sodium valproate.

Decreased. Subtherapeutic treatment. Drugs include acetazolamide and methsuximide.

Description. Primidone is an anticonvulsant used in the treatment of temporal lobe epilepsy and other grand mal seizures that are resistant to other anticonvulsants. When metabolized by the liver, it breaks down into phenobarbital and phenylethylmalonamide. These two metabolites have a synergistic ability to raise the seizure threshold. The metabolites of primidone are excreted by the kidneys. Half-life is 4-12 hours in adults and 4-6 hours in children. Peak time varies from 0.5-0.9 hours. Steady-state levels are reached after 16-60 hours in adults and after 20-30 hours in children. For rapid detection, the fluorescence polarization assay method can be used.

Professional Considerations
1. Consent form NOT required.
2. **Preparation:**
   A. Tube: Red topped or green topped
   B. Do NOT draw during hemodialysis.
3. **Procedure:**
   A. Draw a 5-mL blood TROUGH sample. Obtain serial specimens at the same time each day.
4. **Postprocedure:**
   A. Monitor for panic level symptoms (see above).
   B. Monitor for convulsions if the drug is discontinued.
5. **Client and family teaching:**
   A. Take medication as prescribed and report any adverse side effects such as sedation, dizziness, nausea, vomiting, nystagmus, and loss of libido.
   B. For accidental overdose, teach the client and family early warning symptoms of overdose (see above).
   C. For intentional overdose, refer the client and family for crisis intervention.
6. **Factors that affect results:**
   A. Reject hemolyzed or lipemic specimens to avoid falsely elevated results.
   B. Peak levels occur 2-4 hours after the oral dose.
7. **Other data:**
   A. Data indicate there is no evidence of good seizure control with levels of above 10 mg/mL.

PROACCELERIN, BLOOD
(see Factor V, Blood)

PROCAINAMIDE, SERUM

Norm. Negative.

	TROUGH	SI UNITS
Procainamide	4.9-12 µg/mL	20.7-50.8 µmol/L
Toxic level	12-20 µg/mL	50.8-84.6 µmol/L
Panic level	>20 µg/mL	>84.6 µmol/L
Procainamide + NAPA	<30 µg/mL	<126.7 µmol/L
Toxic level	>30 µg/mL	>126.7 µmol/L

Toxic Level Symptoms and Treatment. Toxic symptoms occur in 10% of people with levels >12 µg/mL. Serious toxicity occurs in 40% of people with levels over 16 µg/mL.

Symptoms. Sodium-channel blockade manifesting as early prolonged QRS interval, rightward axis of 40 msec, presence of an R-wave in aV_R lead and an S-wave in leads I and aV_L. Torsades de pointes, nausea, vomiting, hepatic disturbances, agranulocytosis.

Treatment:

Note: Treatment choice(s) depend on client history and condition and episode history.
Protect airway.
Support hemodynamic stability.
Force emesis.
Perform gastric lavage.
Administer infusion of a molar sodium lactate solution.
Hemodialysis WILL but peritoneal dialysis will NOT remove procainamide.

Increased Procainamide. Hepatic dysfunction. Drugs include amiodarone.

Increased Procainamide and NAPA. Renal dysfunction. Drugs include quinidine.

Decreased. NAPA: Hepatic dysfunction.

Description. Procainamide is an antidysrhythmic used in the treatment of atrial and ventricular dysrhythmias. It is most commonly administered as an oral or intravenous drug and metabolized by the liver. 25% of procainamide is metabolized to N-acetylprocainamide (NAPA) by the liver; 60% of the dose is excreted via the kidneys, with a half-life of 3-4 hours. Procainamide's primary metabolite is NAPA, which has similar antidysrhythmic properties and a half-life of approximately 6 hours but is not metabolized by the liver. The differences in the half-lives result in slightly high NAPA levels until both reach stabilization approximately 18 hours after initiation of therapy. At this time, a 1:1 ratio exists between procainamide and NAPA. An increase or decrease in the ratio between them can alter the therapeutic effectiveness or result in toxicity. Therefore, when procainamide is assayed, NAPA levels should be monitored simultaneously. Steady-state levels of procainamide are reached after 11-20 hours. Steady-state levels of NAPA are reached after 22-40 hours.

Professional Considerations

1. Consent form NOT required.
2. **Preparation:**
   A. Tube: Red topped, red/gray topped, or gold topped.
   B. Do NOT draw specimens during hemodialysis.
3. **Procedure:**
   A. Draw a 1-mL TROUGH blood sample. Obtain serial measurements at the same time each day.
4. **Postprocedure care:**
   A. Monitor for panic level symptoms (see above).
5. **Factors that affect results:**
   A. Reject hemolyzed or lipemic specimens.
6. **Client and family teaching:**
   A. Take medication as prescribed.
   B. Report side effects such as anorexia, nausea, and vomiting.
   C. For intentional overdose, refer client and family for crisis intervention.
7. **Other data:**
   A. For the initial evaluation, draw a trough level just before the next dose of procainamide and draw a peak level 75-90 minutes after oral administration or immedi-

ately after the loading dose and at 2, 6, 12, and 24 hours for intravenous administration.

B. For continuous therapeutic drug monitoring, three normal-range levels within one dosing interval are required initially. Then only trough levels are required unless toxicity is suspected.

PROCHLORPERAZINE
(see Phenothiazines, Blood)

PROCONVERTIN, BLOOD
(see Factor VII, Blood)

PROCTOSCOPY, DIAGNOSTIC

Norm. The rectal lining is continuous, reddish, and free of lesions, abscesses, inflammation, ulcerations, and polyps. The anal lining appears grayish tan and smooth.

Usage. Melena or bleeding from the anorectal area, persistent diarrhea, changes in bowel habits, passage of pus and mucus, suspected chronic inflammatory bowel disease, bacteriologic and histologic studies, surveillance of known rectal disease or after rectal surgery, rectal pain, screening for suspected polyps or tumors, foreign-body removal, or adjunct to barium enema.

Description. A proctoscopy is the endoscopic, direct visual examination of the lining of the rectum and anal canal using a rigid, lighted proctoscope. Specimens for biopsy, cytologic evaluation, or culture may be taken during the procedure. Proctoscopy is usually performed with flexible sigmoidoscopy for clients demonstrating unexplained anemia, unexplained diarrhea, or the presence of blood in the stool.

Professional Considerations
1. Consent form IS required.

Risks
Bowel perforation, hemorrhage, peritonitis.

Contraindications
Severe necrotizing enterocolitis, toxic megacolon, painful anal lesions, or severe cardiac dysrhythmias.

2. Preparation:
   A. A tap-water, hypertonic phosphate, or saline enema may be prescribed. Clients with ulcerative colitis or acute diarrhea can be examined without an enema.
   B. Obtain drapes, gloves, 1%-2% lidocaine (Xylocaine), a proctoscope with an obturator, and a light source. If a biopsy is to be performed, obtain a specimen container of 10% formalin. If cytology slides are to be prepared, obtain cytology slides and a Coplin jar of 95% ethyl alcohol (ethanol). If cultures are to be performed, obtain sterile swabs with culture tube.
   C. See Client and family teaching.
3. Procedure:
   A. The client is placed in a left-lateral or knee-to-chest position and draped for comfort and privacy.
   B. The physician inserts a lubricated finger through the anus to assess for patency and the presence of obstruction.
   C. After patency is determined, the lubricated proctoscope with obturator is inserted fully into the rectum through the anus, and the obturator is removed.
   D. After a light is inserted, the physician carefully inspects the interior lining of the rectum and anal canal as the proctoscope is slowly withdrawn.
   E. If biopsy specimens are taken, the site may be anesthetized first with 1%-2% lidocaine or another local anesthetic.
   F. Any liquid drainage is removed with suction during the procedure.
4. Postprocedure care:
   A. Send the specimens to the laboratory immediately.
   B. The client should lie flat for 10-15 minutes before leaving.
   C. Monitor for signs of fatigue, abdominal pain or distention, fever, hypotension, or rectal bleeding.
   D. Bloody stools are normal for 1-2 days after a rectal biopsy.
   E. No enemas or barium studies for 1 week after rectal biopsy secondary to the increased risk of perforation.

5. **Client and family teaching:**
   A. Client may be asked to follow a clear liquid diet for 2 days or fast for 8 hours.
   B. Try to defecate before the procedure.
   C. An urge to defecate may be felt during the procedure, and slow, controlled deep breathing may help to diminish this feeling.

6. **Factors that affect results:**
   A. Residual barium from prior testing will impair visualization.
   B. The presence of stool in the rectum impairs visualization.

7. **Other data:**
   A. Complications of proctoscopy include rectal perforation, minimal bleeding from lacerations, transient abdominal discomfort, and cardiac dysrhythmias.

PROGESTERONE RECEPTOR ASSAY, SPECIMEN

Norm. Negative.

		SI UNITS
Negative	<5 fmol/mg protein	<5 nmol/kg protein
Positive	>10 fmol/mg protein	>10 nmol/kg protein

Usage. Determination of the likelihood of carcinoma to respond to hormone or antihormone therapy, monitoring the responsiveness of tumors to hormonal or antihormonal therapy, and determination of the need for oophorectomy.

Positive. Breast cancer, hormonal therapy, meningioma, and metastasis.

Negative. Normal finding. Normal results may be obtained in the presence of a benign and nonresponsive tumor.

Description. Progesterone receptors are located primarily in mammary gland tissue but are also present in the corpus luteum, prostate, uterus, vaginal epithelium, and placenta. Progesterone receptors transfer and bind steroid molecules into cell nuclei to exert hormonal function. This test is usually performed with an estrogen receptor assay and involves testing an excised or biopsied tumor for the degree of responsiveness (positivity) of the progesterone receptors in the tissue. In some clients with carcinoma, the degree of progesterone receptor positivity correlates to the amount of cellular subtype differentiation and is a measure of potential tumor responsiveness to hormonal or antihormonal therapy. Clients with positive tests are more likely to respond to these types of therapy than those with negative results. In monitoring tumor response to therapy, the best prognosis can be expected in clients whose progesterone receptor assay results remain positive. In clients who have negative tests after positive initial tests, the prognosis is poor. Clients who remain negative have the poorest outcome.

Professional Considerations

1. Consent form NOT required for this test but IS required for the procedure used to obtain the specimen tested. See individual procedure for risks and contraindications.
2. **Preparation:**
   A. The client is prepared for a surgical biopsy or resection.
   B. Arrange for a person to be standing by to transport the iced specimen to the pathology laboratory immediately after excision.
   C. Obtain a waxed cardboard specimen container without preservatives. Do not place it into formalin.
3. **Procedure:**
   A. A fresh tissue specimen of at least 150 mg and preferably 1 g (1 mL) is obtained by means of needle biopsy or resection and placed into a container free of formalin.
   B. The specimen is transported to the pathology laboratory immediately.
4. **Postprocedure care:**
   A. Apply a dry, sterile dressing to the biopsy or operative site.
   B. Specimens must be stored at temperatures lower than $-70°$ C. Spec-

imens transported to another institution must be packed in dry ice.
5. Client and family teaching:
   A. Results of the test may dictate the type of anticipated therapy.
6. Factors that affect results:
   A. Reject specimens not stored at temperatures lower than −70° C or those contaminated with formalin.
   B. Reject specimens not transported to the pathology laboratory immediately because a delay of even 15 minutes results in degradation of receptor sites.
   C. The presence of massive tumor necrosis or tumors with low cellular composition lowers the assay result.
7. Other data:
   A. The estrogen receptor assay should also be performed on all specimens.
   B. Progesterone receptors are found in up to 75% of estrogen receptor-positive mammary cancers.
   C. Estrogen and progesterone positive tumors have a 75% response rate to endocrine therapy, whereas estrogen and progesterone negative tumors have a 5%-10% response rate.

PROGESTERONE, SERUM

Norm:

		SI UNITS
Female		
Follicular phase	0.2-0.6 ng/mL	<2 nmol/L
Luteal phase	6-30 ng/mL	19-95 nmol/L
Midluteal phase	5.7-28.1 ng/mL	18-89 nmol/L
Oral contraceptives	0.1-0.3 ng/mL	<2 nmol/L
Postmenopause	0-0.2 ng/mL	<2 nmol/L
Pregnancy		
1-12 weeks	9-47 ng/mL	28-149 nmol/L
13-24 weeks	16.8-146 ng/mL	53-464 nmol/L
25 weeks to term	55-255 ng/mL	175-811 nmol/L
Male	0.1-0.3 ng/mL	<2 nmol/L
Child (Prepubertal)	7-52 ng/mL	0.2-1.7 nmol/L

Usage. Assessment of corpus luteum formation and placental function, and assistance in determining the day of ovulation.

Increased. Adrenal hyperplasia (congenital, males), corpus luteum cyst, lipid ovarian tumors, molar pregnancy, ovarian chorionepithelioma, ovarian neoplasms, placental tissue (retained after parturition), precocious puberty, and theca lutein cyst. Drugs include adrenocortical hormones, estrogens, and progesterones (oral or vaginal application).

Decreased. Adrenogenital syndrome, amenorrhea, anovular menstruation, fetal abnormality or death, luteal deficiency, menstrual abnormalities, ovarian failure, panhypopituitarism, placental failure or insufficiency, preeclampsia, Stein-Leventhal syndrome, threatened abortion, toxemia of pregnancy, Turner syndrome, and primary and secondary hypogonadism. Drugs include ampicillin, ethinyl estradiol.

Description. Progesterone is a steroid sex hormone secreted by the corpus luteum during the latter half of the menstrual cycle in nonpregnant women, by the placenta in large amounts of pregnant women, and by the adrenal cortex in men. Progesterone causes secretory changes in the mucosa of the fallopian tubes and assists in nourishing the fertilized ovum as it travels through the tubes to the uterus. It prepares the endometrium for implantation of the fertilized ovum, stimulates growth of the breasts and proliferation of the vaginal epithelium, and decreases myometrial excitability and uterine contractions.

Professional Considerations

1. Consent form NOT required.
2. **Preparation:**
   A. Tube: Red topped or green topped.
   B. Specimens MAY be drawn during hemodialysis.
3. **Procedure:**
   A. Draw a 7-mL blood sample.
4. **Postprocedure care:**
   A. Record the first day of the last menstrual cycle or the week of gestation on the laboratory requisition.
5. **Client and family teaching:**
   A. Results are normally available within 24 hours.
6. **Factors that affect results:**
   A. The sample may be refrigerated for 4 days or frozen up to 1 year and is stable at room temperature for 7 days.
7. **Other data:**
   A. Serial testing is recommended.
   B. For diagnosis of a short luteal phase, correlation with endometrial biopsy is recommended.
   C. Levels are higher with twin pregnancies than with single pregnancies.
   D. Topical progesterone was shown in one study to increase salivary progesterone levels, but not serum levels.

PROLACTIN (HUMAN PROLACTIN, HPRL), SERUM

Norm. Prolactin levels do not differ between males and females before the onset of puberty.

		SI UNITS
Adult Female, Nonlactating	<23 ng/mL	<23 ng/dL
Follicular phase	<28 ng/mL	<28 ng/dL
Luteal phase	5-40 ng/mL	5-40 ng/dL
Postmenopause	<12 ng/mL	<12 ng/dL
Pregnancy		
Trimester 1	<80 ng/mL	<80 ng/dL
Trimester 2	<160 ng/mL	<160 ng/dL
Trimester 3	<400 ng/mL	<400 ng/dL
Adult Male	<20 ng/mL	<20 ng/dL
Pituitary Tumor	>100 ng/mL	>100 ng/dL
Newborn	>10 times adult levels	

**Prolactin Levels in Response to TRH Stimulation Test
(Used for Differentiation of Prolactinoma from Other Causes of Hyperprolactinemia)**

	Baseline Value	Peak after Injection of 400 µg of TRH Intravenously
Adult Female	4.0-25 µg/L Median: 10.0 µg/L	Median: 51 µg/L Relative increase: >250%
Adult Male	0.5-19.0 µg/L Median: 8.5 µg/L	Median: 41 µg/L Relative increase: >250%

Increased. Serum level >300 ng/mL is assumed to be pathognomonic of a pituitary tumor.

Other conditions in which increases may be found: Acromegaly, Addison's disease, amenorrhea, anorexia nervosa, breast stimulation, bronchogenic carcinoma, Chiari-Frommel syndrome, coitus, del Castillo syndrome, ectopic tumors, endometriosis, erectile dysfunction, exercise, Forbes-Albright syndrome, galactorrhea, HIV infection (20% of males with stable HIV), hyperestrogen states, hyperpituitarism, hypothalamic disorders, hypothyroidism (primary), hysterectomy, idiopathic causes (such as early microadenoma that are undetectable by radiology), impotence, lactation, multiple myeloma (advanced), Nelson syndrome, neurogenic causes, pituitary tumors, polycystic ovaries, pregnancy, renal failure (chronic), sleep, stress, and systemic lupus erythematosus. Drugs include amitriptyline, amoxapine, amphetamines, benzamides, chlorprothixene, desipramine, doxepin, droperidol, estrogens, gamma-hydroxybutyrate (GHB), haloperidol, imipramine, isoniazid, maprotiline, meprobamate, methyldopa, metoclopramide, nortriptyline, opiates, oral contraceptives, phenothiazines, procainamide hydrochloride, protriptyline, reserpine, thioridazine, thiothixene, thyrotropin, Triavil (perphenazine and amitriptyline HCl), and trimipramine maleate.

Decreased. Gynecomastia, hirsutism, osteoporosis, and pituitary necrosis or infarction. Drugs include apomorphine hydrochloride, clonidine, bromocriptine mesylate, dihydroergotamine mesylate, dopamine, ergonovine maleate, ergotamine tartrate, ergoloid mesylate, lergotrile, levodopa, and lisuride hydrogen maleate. Herbal or natural remedies include Licorice and St. John's wort. In addition, chaste tree (*Vitex agnus-castus*) berry has been shown to reduce prolactin levels in a study of women with hyperprolactinemia.

Description. Prolactin is a peptide hormone produced by the anterior pituitary gland that promotes growth of breast tissue and is essential for the initiation and maintenance of milk production. Also called the lactogenic hormone, luteotropic hormone, LTH, and mammotropin. It is identical to luteotropin.

Professional Considerations
1. Consent form NOT required.

2. **Preparation:**
   A. Tube: Red topped, red/gray topped, or gold topped.
   B. Specimens MAY be drawn during hemodialysis.
   C. Screen client for the use of herbal preparations or "natural" remedies.
   D. See *Client and family teaching.*
3. **Procedure:**
   A. Draw a 5-mL blood sample without trauma.
   B. Samples should be drawn in the morning.
4. **Postprocedure care:**
   A. Samples remain stable for 4 days at room temperature and then must be frozen if analysis is delayed.
5. **Client and family teaching:**
   A. Fast for 12 hours before testing.
6. **Factors that affect results:**
   A. Hemolysis of the specimen invalidates the results.
7. **Other data:**
   A. Differentiation between a pituitary tumor and other prolactin disorders can be done by means of the thyrotropin-releasing hormone (TRH) stimulation test. Prolactin levels in clients with pituitary tumors do not increase.
   B. Men with elevated prolactin levels generally have low serum testosterone. Symptoms will not reverse unless prolactin is reduced.
   C. Hankinson et al, (1999) found that women with prolactin levels in the highest 25% were twice as likely to develop breast cancer as those with prolactin levels in the lowest 25%.

PROLIFERATION MARKER MIB 1-3
(*see Ki-67 proliferation marker, Specimen*)

PROPOXYPHENE, BLOOD

Norm. Negative.

PROPOXYPHENE THERAPY		SI UNITS
Therapeutic levels	0.1-0.4 µg/mL	0.3-1.2 µmol/L
Panic level	>0.5 µg/mL	>1.5 µmol/L

Usage. Suspected drug abuse, drug overdose, or suicide.

Panic Level Symptoms and Treatment

Symptoms. Coma; respiratory depression; circulatory collapse; pulmonary edema; dysrhythmias, including heart block, trigeminy, and prolongation of the QRS complex; sodium-channel blockade manifesting as early prolonged QRS interval, rightward axis of 40 msec, presence of an R-wave in the aV_R lead and an S-wave in leads I and aV_L; and nephrogenic diabetes insipidus. Overdosage may be fatal in as little as 1 hour after ingestion.

Treatment:

Note: Treatment choice(s) depend on client history and condition and episode history.
Supportive therapy, including maintenance of airway and hemodynamic stability; opiate antagonists; and forced emesis.
Hemodialysis and peritoneal dialysis will NOT remove propoxyphene.

Description. Propoxyphene is a schedule-IV, nonnarcotic analgesic structurally related to methadone. It is one half to two thirds as potent as codeine. Propoxyphene is metabolized in the liver and excreted in the urine, with a half-life of 30-36 hours.

Professional Considerations

1. Consent form NOT required.
2. Preparation:
   A. Tube: Red topped, red/gray topped, or gold topped or black topped.
   B. Specimens MAY be drawn during hemodialysis.
3. Procedure:
   A. Broad-spectrum drug screening: Draw a 20-mL blood sample.
4. Postprocedure care:
   A. None.
5. Client and family teaching:
   A. Take medication as prescribed to avoid an overdose.
   B. Report any adverse side effects to the physician.
   C. For intentional overdose, refer client and family for crisis intervention.
   D. Referrals to appropriate rehabilitation centers and therapeutic community programs should be offered to all clients who may be interested.
6. Factors that affect results:
   A. Peak serum levels occur in 2-5 hours for propoxyphene hydrochloride and in 3-4 hours for propoxyphene napsylate.
   B. Metabolism and excretion are delayed with hepatic and renal dysfunction.
7. Other data:
   A. A 100-mL urine sample, collected without preservatives, should be obtained at the time of the serum sample.

PROPRANOLOL, BLOOD

Norm. Negative.

PROPRANOLOL THERAPY		SI UNITS
Therapeutic level	50-100 ng/mL	193-386 nmol/L
Panic level	>500 ng/mL	>1930 nmol/L

Panic Level Symptoms and Treatment

Symptoms. Coma; respiratory depression; circulatory collapse; pulmonary edema; dysrhythmias, including heart block, trigeminy and widening of the QRS complex, sodium-channel blockade manifesting as early prolonged QRS interval, rightward axis of 40 msec, presence of an R-wave in the aV_R lead and an S-wave in leads I and aV_L; and nephrogenic diabetes insipidus. Overdosage may be fatal in as little as 1 hour after ingestion.

Treatment:

Note: Treatment choice(s) depend on client history and condition and episode history.
Supportive therapy, including maintenance of airway and hemodynamic stability;

opiate antagonists; gastric lavage; and forced emesis. Hemodialysis and peritoneal dialysis will NOT remove propoxyphene.

Increased. Propranolol overdosage. Drugs include flecainide, methimazole, and propylthiouracil.

Description. Propranolol hydrochloride is a beta-adrenergic blocking drug classified as a type II cardiac antidysrhythmic. It competes with epinephrine and norepinephrine for beta-adrenergic receptors, resulting in inhibition of myocardial beta-adrenergic stimulation. Cardiac effects include reduced irritability and heart rate because the automaticity of the SA node, AV node, and intraventricular conduction velocity is depressed. Large doses depress cardiac function. Propranolol may also cause hypoglycemia without warning in diabetics. Propranolol is bound to plasma proteins, metabolized in the liver, and excreted in the urine, with a half-life of 2-6 hours. Steady-state levels are reached after 10-30 hours.

Professional Considerations
1. Consent form NOT required.
2. Preparation:
   A. Tube: Red topped, red/gray topped, or gold topped.
   B. Specimens MAY be drawn during hemodialysis.
3. Procedure:
   A. Draw a 7-mL blood sample in a syringe.
B. After removing the stopper, inject the specimen promptly into the tube (plasma propranolol binding is reduced when blood passes through the stopper of a vacuum tube).
C. Replace the stopper.
D. Collect the specimen before the next dose (trough) if drawing to evaluate therapeutic value.
4. Postprocedure care:
   A. Monitor the client for evidence of increasing congestive heart failure.
5. Client and family teaching:
   A. Take mediation as prescribed to prevent overdose.
   B. Report any side effects to the physician.
   C. Take your pulse daily and notify the physician if it falls below the level your physician specifies.
   D. For intentional overdose, refer client and family for crisis intervention.
6. Factors that affect results:
   A. Smoking decreases plasma concentration of propranolol.
   B. Peak propranolol levels occur 1-2 hours after oral administration.
   C. Propranolol metabolism and excretion are delayed with hepatic and renal dysfunction.
7. Other data:
   A. When you are obtaining serial levels, the same time interval between drug dosing and specimen collection should be maintained.

PROSTASIN, SERUM

Norm. Interpretation required. Preliminary studies report:

	MEAN	RANGE
Normal	7.5 µg/mL	6.6 µg/mL-8.3 µg/mL
Ovarian cancer subjects	13.7 µg/mL	10.5 µg/mL-16.9 µg/mL

Increased. Ovarian cancer.

Decreased. May decrease after surgery for ovarian cancer.

Description. Prostasin is a trypsin-like serine proteinase normally secreted by the prostate gland. Prostasin is expressed at lower levels in other body tissues, including kidneys, liver, pancreas, salivary gland, lung, bronchus, and colon but its functions in these tissues has not been determined. Preliminary studies have suggested that prostasin is released from ovarian cancer cells, migrates to the bloodstream, and may be a novel marker for the early diagnosis and management of ovarian cancer. Whether prostasin levels will be elevated in clients with other cancers has not been determined.

Professional Considerations

1. Consent form NOT required.
2. **Preparation:**
   A. Tube: Red topped, red/gray or gold topped.
3. **Procedure**
   A. Draw a 1-ml blood sample.
   B. Specimen may remain at room temperature for up to 7 days but must be refrigerated if assay not performed within 7 days.
4. **Postprocedure care**
   A. None.
5. **Client and family teaching.**
   A. This test may be used as a marker for early ovarian cancer.
   B. Results should be available within 3 working days.
6. **Factors that affect results:**
   A. Serum levels may decrease postoperatively after surgery for ovarian cancer
7. **Other data:**
   A. Combining serum prostasin levels and CA125 levels as a marker for ovarian cancer reveals a sensitivity of 94% (compared with a sensitivity of 64.9% for CA125 and of 51.4% for prostasin).

PROSTATE ULTRASONOGRAPHY (PROSTATE ECHOGRAM, PROSTATE ULTRASOUND), DIAGNOSTIC

Norm. The prostate gland is round and about 3 cm in diameter. Prostatic tissue is homogeneous and causes only a slight bladder wall indentation.

Usage. Adjunct to digital examination of the prostate, diagnosis and staging of and screening for prostate cancer, evaluation of the size and shape of the prostate gland, monitoring response to treatment in prostate disease, and providing guidance for transrectal biopsy of the prostate gland or for positioning of clients for radiation of the prostate gland.

Description. Evaluation of the prostate gland by the creation of an oscilloscopic picture from the echoes of high-frequency sound waves passing through the anterior rectal wall or through the urethra over the pelvic area (acoustic imaging, endosonography). The time required for the ultrasonic beam to be reflected back to the transducer from differing densities of tissue is converted by a computer to an electrical impulse displayed on an oscilloscopic screen to create a three-dimensional picture of the pelvic contents. Because of the risk of sepsis and trauma from transurethral ultrasonography, the transrectal route is preferred. For staging prostate cancer, transrectal ultrasonography costs less than magnetic resonance imaging, with comparable or superior accuracy. This technique may help detect prostate lesions before they become large enough to palpate. Ultrasound techniques are still inferior to prostate biopsy in sensitivity for diagnosing prostate cancer.

Professional Considerations

1. Consent form IS required.

Risks

Transurethral route: Sepsis and trauma. *Transrectal route:* Hematuria, Infection, Urinary retention. *Note:* Complications are more frequent in clients who receive a preprocedure enema.

Contraindications

Nonprostate disease. *Transurethral route:* Bleeding disorders, thrombocytopenia.

2. **Preparation:**
   A. This test should be performed before intestinal barium tests, or after the barium is cleared from the system.
   B. Obtain ultrasonic gel or paste.
   C. For transrectal ultrasonography, a hypertonic enema of sodium phosphate or a bisacodyl suppository may be prescribed.
   D. The client must disrobe below the waist or wear a gown.
   E. See *Client and family teaching.*
3. **Procedure:**
   A. An injection of lidocaine or inhalation of a nitrous oxide/air mixture may be used to manage procedure-associated pain.
   B. The client is positioned supine, and a short transabdominal ultrasonogram may be performed to evaluate for kidney distention.
   C. A suprapubic examination of the prostate is performed, and the rectum is examined digitally for obstruction.
   D. The client is assisted to a knee-elbow, lateral decubitus, or rising position.
   E. The probe is covered with an air-free, sterile, transparent cover or

condom. The condom is then coated with sterile lubricant, and the probe is slowly inserted into the rectum.

F. After the probe is inserted into the rectum, the condom may be inflated with 20-60 mL of deaerated water, depending on the practitioner's preference.

G. The probe is angled anteriorly, and ultrasonography of the prostate is performed.

H. Photographs of the oscilloscopic display are taken. Doppler ultrasonography may be used to further define abnormalities in vascular supply and differentiate vascular differences in the prostate tissue.

I. A biopsy of the prostate lesions may be performed during ultrasonography.

4. Postprocedure care:
   A. Remove the gel from the skin.

B. Sterilize the endosonography probes by soaking them in glutaraldehyde solution for 10 minutes.

5. Client and family teaching:
   A. An enema may be prescribed before the procedure.
   B. Drink normal amounts of fluids for 24 hours before the procedure.
   C. Clients under age 60 experience more discomfort than older men during the procedure. Both local and topical anesthesia may be used to reduce discomfort.

6. Factors that affect results:
   A. Dehydration interferes with adequate contrast between organs and body fluids.
   B. Lower intestinal barium obscures results by preventing proper transmission and deflection of the high-frequency sound waves.

7. Other data:
   A. Allow at least 6 weeks between procedures if biopsies are taken.

PROSTATE-SPECIFIC ANTIGEN (PSA), SERUM

Norm:

	Total PSA*	**Complexed (bound to alpha-chymotrypsin)**	**PSA Density**
Male (Normal levels increase with age, secondary to increasing prostate size)			
0-49 years	<2.5 ng/mL or µg/L	<3.75 µg/mL	<0.15
Black	<2.0 ng/mL or µg/L		
Asian	<2.0 ng/mL or µg/L		
Caucasian	<2.5 ng/mL or µg/L		
50-59 years	<3.5 ng/mL or µg/L	<3.75 µg/mL	<0.15
Black	<4.0 ng/mL or µg/L		
Asian	<3.0 ng/mL or µg/L		
Caucasian	<3.5 ng/mL or µg/L		
60-69 years	<5.5 ng/mL or µg/L	<3.75 µg/mL	<0.15
Black	<4.5 ng/mL or µg/L		
Asian	<4.0 ng/mL or µg/L		
Caucasian	<4.6 ng/mL or µg/L		
>69 years	<6.5 ng/mL or µg/L	<3.75 µg/mL	<0.15
Black	<5.5 ng/mL or µg/L		
Asian	<5.0 ng/mL or µg/L		
Caucasian	<6.5 ng/mL or µg/L		
Female	0.5 ng/mL or µg/L		

*Vashi AR, Oesterling JE: Percent free prostate-specific antigen: entering a new era in the detection of prostate cancer, *Mayo Clin Proc* 72:337-344, 1997.

Usage. Assists in the identification, differentiation, classification, staging, and localization of tumor; monitoring preoperatively, postoperative therapeutic interventions or cytotoxic drug therapy; and assists in assessment of tumor response to treatment protocols. Can serve as a marker for the success of total prostatectomy for prostate cancer.

Probability of Prostate Cancer*

PSA

0-2 ng/mL	1%
2-4 ng/mL	15%
4-10 ng/mL	25%
>10 ng/mL	>50%

% Free PSA:Total PSA Ratio
= free-PSA/total PSA × 100

0-10%	56%
10-15%	28%
15-20%	20%
20-25%	16%
>25%	8%

*Findings in combination with a negative digital rectal examination.

Increased. Benign prostatic hypertrophy (levels up to 10 ng/mL), cirrhosis, impotence, osteoporosis, prostate cancer or infarct, prostatic needle biopsy, prostatitis, pulmonary embolism, renal osteopathy, transurethral resection (TUR), urethral instrumentation, and urinary retention. Herbal or natural remedies include *Dendranthema morifolium Tzvel, Ganoderma lucidum Karst, Isatis indigotica Fort, Panax pseudo-ginseng,* and *Rabdosia rubescens Hara.*

Decreased. Drugs include finasteride (decreases levels by 50%). Herbal or natural remedies include *Glycyrrhiza uralensis Fisch, Scutellaria baicalensis Georgi,* and *Serenoa repens.*

Description. Prostate-specific antigen (PSA) is a glycoprotein produced by the prostate gland that liquefies clotted semen. PSA was previously believed to be exclusive to the prostate epithelium, but is now known to exist in normal and cancerous breast tissue, as well as some female body fluids. *Total PSA* is comprised of free and complexed PSA. The percent of free PSA is lower in men with prostate cancer than in men free of the disease because tumor catabolic activity and accelerated metabolic rate in prostate carcinoma elevate the serum value of PSA without proportionately elevating the free PSA. The *free PSA* test includes measuring both free and total PSA, then calculating a ratio and has been recommended in men with a negative digital rectal exam accompanied by an elevated total PSA level. It can help provide guidance to select those

that need prostate biopsies, particularly when PSA levels are between 4 and 10 ng/mL. More recently, testing for *complexed PSA* alone has been found in one large study to be more sensitive than free or total PSA in detecting prostate cancer. However, subsequent studies have not reproduced the same findings. Currently being investigated is *PSA fractionation,* in which subforms of PSA, called "Intact" PSA and "Nicked" PSA have been identified and may be helpful in more specifically differentiating between benign and malignant disease of the prostate. In one study, the ratio of intact to free PSA was higher in malignant than in benign cancer. *PSA density* is a division of the total PSA level by the prostate size in cubic centimeters and provides insight into whether the amount of PSA produced is out of proportion to the size of the prostate gland. *PSA velocity* (PSAV) is a term used by some to describe changes over time in the PSA levels. Overall, PSA is a reliable immunocytochemical marker used in the detection of prostate cancer. The majority of PSA elevation is attributed to benign prostatic hypertrophy, which normally raises PSA no higher than 10 ng/mL, and also produces higher free-to-total ratios. Although 70% of those with elevated values are prostate-cancer free, when higher than 50 ng/mL, PSA is 98.5% accurate in predicting that a prostate biopsy will be positive for cancer. Only about 45% of clients with prostate cancer have PSA values over 10 ng/mL. PSA is smaller than the prostatic acid phosphatase molecule, more stable, and does not demonstrate diurnal variations. It is measured using an immunoreactive antibody assay.

Professional Considerations
1. Consent form NOT required.
2. **Preparation:**
   A. Draw sample BEFORE performing digital rectal examination.
   B. Tube: Red topped, red/gray topped, or gold topped.
   C. Specimens MAY be drawn during hemodialysis.
   D. See *Client and family teaching.*
3. **Procedure:**
   A. Draw a 1-mL blood sample.
4. **Postprocedure care:**
   A. The sample is stable at room temperature for 24 hours and may be refrigerated.
5. **Client and family teaching:**
   A. Fast for 8 hours.

B. Do not have the test drawn less than 24 hours after a rectal or prostate examination.

6. **Factors that affect results:**
   A. Falsely elevated results may be associated with blood drawn 1 to 24 hours after a rectal examination.
   B. Levels can rise and remain elevated up to 50 times higher than baseline value for several weeks after prostate procedures, such as transurethral resection of prostate needle biopsy.
   C. Approximately 25% of men with benign prostatic hypertrophy have an elevated PSA.
   D. Up to one third of clients with localized prostate cancer have false-negative values.

E. Levels can normally vary 20% from one day to the next.

7. **Other data:**
   A. Although this test aids in the diagnosis of malignant states, some benign diseases can also demonstrate antigen marker abnormalities.
   B. Adult levels are reached at approximately 15 years.
   C. A routine PSA with an annual rectal examination is recommended for men older than 50 years.
   D. In the study of women with breast cancer, one study found a 30% decrease in the risk of relapse or of death in clients with PSA-positive disease as compared to those with disease that was PSA negative.

PROSTATIC ACID PHOSPHATASE (PAP), BLOOD

Norm. Values are dependent on laboratory method.

		SI UNITS
Fishman-Lerner	0-0.7 U/dL	
Bessey, Lowry, and Brock (BLB)		
Female	0.02-0.55 U at 37° C	0.3-9.2 U/L
Male	0.15-0.65 U at 37° C	2.5-10.8 U/L
Bodansky	0-3 U/dL	0-16.1 U/L
King-Armstrong	0-3 U/dL	0-5.3 U/L
RIA	2.5-3.7 ng/mL	

Increased. Hyperparathyroidism, metastatic bone cancer (elevated in 75%-80%), metastatic prostatic carcinoma (elevated in 50%-75%), multiple myeloma, non-metastatic prostatic carcinoma (10%-25%), osteogenesis imperfecta, Paget's disease, and prostatic infarct.

Decreased. Down syndrome. Drugs include estrogen therapy for prostatic carcinoma and ethyl alcohol (ethanol).

Description. Prostatic acid phosphatase, an isoenzyme of acid phosphatase, is a lysosomal enzyme that hydrolyzes phosphate esters. It is found in the prostate, erythrocytes, kidneys, liver, and spleen. Prostatic acid phosphatase is a prostate-specific epithelium differentiation antigen that regulates the growth of the prostate; thus prostate tissue has a concentration of acid phosphatase 100 times higher than that of other tissues. Serum activity of the prostatic isoenzyme is greatly increased in metastatic cancer of the prostate in which the tumor has extended beyond the capsule surrounding the prostate gland. Therefore this test is used as both a marker for and a monitor of the disease course.

Professional Considerations
1. Consent form NOT required.
2. **Preparation:**
   A. Draw sample BEFORE performing digital rectal examination.
   B. Tube: Red topped, red/gray topped, or gold topped or lavender topped.
   C. Specimens MAY be drawn during hemodialysis.
3. **Procedure:**
   A. Draw an early-morning, 5-mL blood sample.
4. **Postprocedure care:**
   A. Transport the specimen to the laboratory immediately. Serum specimens deteriorate rapidly at room temperature.
5. **Client and family teaching:**
   A. Wait at least 24 hours after prostatic massage, extensive prostate

palpation, or a transurethral resection before the blood test.

B. This test may be drawn in conjunction with the prostate-specific antigen test.

6. **Factors that affect results:**
   A. PAP levels exhibit a diurnal variation, with the highest levels occurring during the early morning.
   B. Recent administration of clofibrate invalidates the results.
   C. Falsely elevated results may be associated with blood drawn 1 to 24 hours after a rectal examination.
   D. False-positive results have been reported in hemolyzed serum samples.
   E. False-negative results have been reported in serum specimens contaminated with fluoride, oxalate, or phosphate.

7. **Other data:**
   A. Refrigerated specimens or specimens frozen with 0.01 mL of 20%

acetic acid per milliliter of serum can remain stable for up to 1 week.

B. With the increased reliability of prostate-specific antigen (PSA), screening serum PAP testing may become more limited in value for prostate carcinoma.

PROTEIN, CEREBROSPINAL FLUID, SPECIMEN
(see Cerebrospinal fluid, Myelin basic protein, oligoclonal bands, protein, and protein electrophoresis, Specimen)

PROTEIN ELECTROPHORESIS, CEREBROSPINAL FLUID, SPECIMEN
(see Cerebrospinal fluid, Myelin basic protein, oligoclonal bands, protein, and protein electrophoresis, Specimen)

PROTEIN ELECTROPHORESIS, SERUM

Norm. Norms are dependent on laboratory procedure. Percentage values represent the percentage of total protein for the agarose method:

		SI UNITS
Adult Percentage		
Total protein	100%	5.90-8.00
Albumin	58-74%	0.58-0.74
Alpha$_1$ globulin	2.0-3.5%	0.02-0.04
Alpha$_2$ globulin	5.4-10.6%	0.05-0.11
Beta globulin	7.0-14.0%	0.07-0.14
Gamma globulin	8.0-18.0%	0.08-0.18
Adult Quantitative		
Total protein	6.0-8.0 g/dL	60-80 g/L
Albumin	3.3-5.0 g/dL	35-50 g/L
Alpha$_1$ globulin	0.1-0.4 g/dL	1-4 g/L
Alpha$_2$ globulin	0.5-1.0 g/dL	5-10 g/L
Beta globulin	0.7-1.2 g/dL	7-12 g/L
Gamma globulin	0.8-1.6 g/dL	8-16 g/L
Premature infant		
Total protein	4.4-6.3 g/dL	44-63 g/L
Albumin	3.0-4.2 g/dL	30-42 g/L
Alpha$_1$ globulin	0.11-0.5 g/dL	1.1-5 g/L
Alpha$_2$ globulin	0.3-0.7 g/dL	3-7 g/L
Beta globulin	0.3-1.2 g/dL	3-12 g/L
Gamma globulin	0.3-1.4 g/dL	3-14 g/L
Newborn		
Total protein	4.6-7.4 g/dL	46-74 g/L
Albumin	3.5-5.4 g/dL	35-54 g/L
Alpha$_1$ globulin	0.1-0.3 g/dL	1-3 g/L

Continued

		SI UNITS
Newborn—cont'd		
Alpha$_2$ globulin	0.3-0.5 g/dL	3-5 g/L
Beta globulin	0.2-0.6 g/dL	2-6 g/L
Gamma globulin	0.2-1.2 g/dL	2-12 g/L
Infant		
Total protein	6.0-6.7 g/dL	60-67 g/L
Albumin	4.4-5.4 g/dL	44-54 g/L
Alpha$_1$ globulin	0.2-0.4 g/dL	2-4 g/L
Alpha$_2$ globulin	0.5-0.8 g/dL	5-8 g/L
Beta globulin	0.5-0.9 g/dL	5-9 g/L
Gamma globulin	0.3-0.8 g/dL	3-8 g/L
Child		
Total protein	6.2-8.0 g/dL	62-80 g/L
Albumin	4.0-5.8 g/dL	40-58 g/L
Alpha$_1$ globulin	0.1-0.4 g/dL	1-4 g/L
Alpha$_2$ globulin	0.4-1.0 g/dL	4-10 g/L
Beta globulin	0.5-1.0 g/dL	5-10 g/L
Gamma globulin	0.3-1.0 g/dL	3-10 g/L

Usage. Assists in the diagnosis of blood dyscrasias, dysproteinemias, gastrointestinal disorders, hepatic disease, hypergammaglobulinemias, hypogammaglobulinemias, inflammatory states, neoplasms, and renal disease.

Increased Total Protein. Macroglobulinemia, multiple myeloma, and sarcoidosis.

Increased Prealbumin Zone Intensity. Alcoholism.

Increased Albumin Zone Mobility. Acute pancreatitis. Drugs include aspirin and penicillins.

Increased Albumin-Alpha$_1$ Globulin Interzone Intensity. Alcoholism (chronic), females during puberty, and pregnancy.

Increased Alpha Globulin Zone Intensity. Acute-phase response in inflammation (alpha$_1$, alpha haptoglobin), acute rheumatic fever (alpha$_2$), aged (alpha$_2$), analbuminemia (alpha$_2$), chronic glomerulonephritis (alpha$_2$), cirrhosis (increased alpha$_1$ with normal or only slightly elevated alpha$_2$), diabetes mellitus (alpha$_2$), dysproteinemia (familial idiopathic), glomerular protein loss (alpha$_2$-macroglobulin), hepatic damage, hepatic metastasis (increased alpha$_1$ with normal alpha$_2$), Hodgkin's disease (alpha$_1$, alpha$_2$), hypoalbuminemia, infancy (alpha$_2$ zone dominated by macroglobulin), infection (acute), meningitis (alpha$_2$), metastatic carcinomatosis (alpha$_1$, alpha$_2$), myocardial infarction, myxedema, nephrosis (alpha$_2$), nephrotic syndrome (alpha$_2$), osteomyelitis (alpha$_2$), peptic ulcer disease (alpha$_1$, alpha$_2$), pneumonia (alpha$_2$), polyarteritis nodosa (alpha$_2$), pregnancy (increased alpha$_1$, with normal alpha$_2$), protein-losing enteropathy (alpha$_1$, alpha$_2$), rheumatoid arthritis (alpha$_2$), sarcoidosis (alpha$_2$), stress (alpha$_1$, alpha$_2$), systemic lupus erythematosus (alpha$_2$), and ulcerative colitis (alpha$_1$, alpha$_2$). Drugs that increase alpha$_1$ with little change in alpha$_2$ include estrogens.

Increased Alpha$_2$-Beta$_1$ Interzone Intensity. Hypercholesterolemia (type II), nephrotic syndrome, and pregnancy.

Increased Beta Globulin Zone Intensity. Acute-phase response (beta$_2$), analbuminemia, diabetes mellitus (poorly controlled), dysproteinemia (familial idiopathic), glomerular protein loss, hepatitis (viral), hypercholesterolemia, hyperlipemia, iron-deficiency anemia (beta$_1$) jaundice (obstructive), macroglobulinemia, nephrotic syndrome, pregnancy (beta$_1$), rheumatoid arthritis, and sarcoidosis. Drugs that increase beta$_1$ globulin include estrogens and oral contraceptives.

Increased Gamma Globulin Zone Intensity. Acute viral hepatitis (sometimes), amyloidosis, analbuminemia, carcinoma (advanced), chronic aggressive hepatitis (appearance of oligoclonal bands), chronic hepatic disease (IgM), chronic lymphatic leukemia (IgM paraprotein), chronic viral infections (appearance of oligoclonal bands), cirrhosis (IgA), cryoglobulinemia, cystic fibrosis (IgG, IgA), Hashimoto's disease, hepatic disease, Hodgkin's disease, hypergammaglobulinemia, hypersensitivity reaction, infection (severe), juvenile rheumatoid arthritis (IgG, IgA, IgM), Laënnec's cirrhosis, leukemia (myelogenous, monocytic), lymphosarcoma (IgM paraprotein), macroglobulinemia, multiple myeloma, respiratory infection (IgA), rheumatoid arthritis (IgA, IgM), sarcoidosis, scleroderma (sometimes), skin disease (IgA), Sjögren syndrome (IgG), systemic lupus erythematosus (active) (IgM), and Waldenström's macroglobulinemia (IgM paraprotein).

Decreased Total Protein. Analbuminemia, cholecystitis (acute), chronic glomerulonephritis, Hodgkin's disease, hypertension (essential with congestive heart failure), hypogammaglobulinemia, leukemia (myelogenous, monocytic), nephrosis, peptic ulcer disease, and ulcerative colitis.

Decreased Prealbumin Zone Intensity. Acute-phase response (day 1) and cirrhosis.

Decreased Albumin Zone Intensity. Acute rheumatic fever, analbuminemia, carcinomatosis (metastatic), cholecystitis (acute), diabetes mellitus, gastrointestinal protein loss (inflammatory or neoplastic disease), glomerular protein loss, glomerulonephritis (chronic), hepatic disease, hepatitis (acute viral), Hodgkin's disease, hyperthyroidism, hypertension (essential with congestive heart failure), Laënnec's cirrhosis, leukemia (lymphatic, myelogenous, monocytic), lymphoma, macroglobulinemia, malnutrition, meningitis, multiple myeloma, nephrosis, nephrotic syndrome, osteomyelitis, peptic ulcer disease, pneumonia, polyarteritis nodosa, protein-losing enteropathy, pyrexia, rheumatoid arthritis, sarcoidosis, stress, systemic lupus erythematosus, and ulcerative colitis. Drugs include corticosteroids.

Decreased Albumin-Alpha₁ Interzone Intensity. Cirrhosis, hepatitis (acute), and inflammation (severe).

Decreased Alpha Globulin Zone Intensity. Acute viral hepatitis (alpha₁, alpha₂), congenital hypohaptoglobinemia (alpha₂ haptoglobin), hepatic disease, intravascular hemolysis (hemolytic anemia, hepatic metastases, cirrhosis, and splenomegaly cause decreased alpha₂ haptoglobin), malabsorption, pulmonary emphysema (alpha₁), scleroderma, starvation, and steatorrhea.

Decreased Alpha₂-Beta₁ Interzone Intensity. Diabetes mellitus, inflammation, and pancreatitis.

Decreased Beta Globulin Zone Intensity. Autoimmune disease, carcinomatosis (metastatic), hepatic disease (beta₁), immune complex disease (beta₂), leukemia (lymphatic, monocytic, myelogenous), lymphoma, malabsorption, malnutrition (beta₁), nephrosis, scleroderma, starvation, steatorrhea, systemic lupus erythematosus, and ulcerative colitis.

Decreased Gamma Globulin Zone Intensity. Acute viral hepatitis (sometimes), agammaglobulinemia, glomerular protein loss, hypogammaglobulinemia, leukemia (lymphatic), lymphoma, nephrosis, nephrotic syndrome, malabsorption, protein-losing enteropathy, scleroderma (sometimes), starvation, steatorrhea, and ulcerative colitis.

Description. Protein electrophoresis is the most frequent measurement of the primary blood proteins, albumin, and globulins (alpha₁, alpha₂, beta, and gamma). Under the influence of an electrical field, at a pH of 8.6, the proteins separate by electrical charge, molecular size, and shape. Plotted on treated paper, the serum proteins form five homogeneous bands of the relative protein values in percentages. These percentages, when multiplied by the total protein concentration, reflect the absolute value of each protein. High-resolution electrophoresis allows the detection of additional bands or zones. Immunoelectrophoresis may be performed to identify the nature of suspicious bands or to monitor the progress of gammopathies, disturbances in immunoglobulin synthesis. The most rapid form of unknown band identification combines high-resolution electrophoresis with immunoprecipitation.

Certain protein-electrophoresis band patterns are characteristic of specific disease states.

Professional Considerations

1. Consent form NOT required.
2. Preparation:
   A. Tube: Red topped, red/gray topped, or gold topped.
   B. Specimens MAY be drawn during hemodialysis.
3. Procedure:
   A. Draw a 1-mL blood sample, without trauma.
4. Postprocedure care:
   A. None.
5. Client and family teaching:
   A. Immunoelectrophoresis may take up to 3 days for results.
   B. Medications that interfere with serum protein levels may be prescribed to be withheld.
6. Factors that affect results:
   A. Falsely elevated total protein levels may occur with the use of contrast dyes.
   B. Hemolysis of the specimen invalidates the results.
   C. Electrophoresis may be performed on serum or plasma. The alpha-beta interzone is absent in heparinized plasma.
   D. At least a 30% drop in albumin is required before changes can be detected by electrophoresis.
   E. Aged serum samples may cause decreased beta globulin and increased beta globulin density.
   F. Protein electrophoresis is unreliable for diagnosis of IgA deficiency.
   G. Recent dialysis distorts protein values.
7. Other data:
   A. None.

PROTEIN ELECTROPHORESIS, URINE

Norm. Interpretation of urine electrophoretic patterns is required. Normal urine electrophoretograms show individual variance and show a globulin pattern that is generally diffuse. Distinct bands may not be identifiable. The dominant protein, albumin, rapidly migrates to the anode, producing a spike in the pattern. Normally there is only a trace amount of alpha$_1$ globulin and alpha$_2$ globulin. The beta globulin and gamma globulins are negligible to absent. In contrast to serum electrophoresis, urine electrophoresis does not contain beta-lipoproteins and beta globulin.

	Total Protein	SI Units
Albumin	37.9%	0.379
Alpha$_1$ globulin	27.3%	0.273
Alpha$_2$ globulin	19.5%	0.195
Beta globulin	8.8%	0.088
Gamma globulin	3.3%	0.033

Usage. Detection of albumin, Bence Jones proteins, hemoglobin, myoclonal gammopathies, myoglobin, renal disease, and systemic lupus erythematosus.

Interpretation of Abnormals. Proteinuria associated with increased glomerular permeability exhibits an electrophoretic pattern that is dominated by albumin, with moderate beta globulin, some alpha globulin, trace alpha$_1$ globulin, and trace gamma$_1$ globulin. Basement-membrane glomerular capillary damage occurs with amyloidosis, congestive heart failure, glomerulosclerosis (diabetic), inflammation, increased venous pressure, nonrenal infectious disease, or renal vein thrombosis. Glomerular dysfunction may occur with idiopathic nephrotic syndrome, membranous glomerulonephritis, immune complex disorders such as poststreptococcal glomerulonephritis, and systemic lupus erythematosus. These conditions produce proteinuria. Proteinuria can result from chyluria, increased circulating proteins, increased glomerular permeability, or renal tubular dysfunction.

Prerenal conditions include hemoglobinuria, inflammatory syndrome, monocytic leukemia, myoglobinuria, and paraproteinemias. Prerenal electrophoretic patterns vary, based on the specific low-molecular-weight excess protein present in serum. These circulating proteins may be normal or abnormal. Their excess results in the excretion of proteins in the presence of normal glomerular function.

Hemoglobinuria or intravascular hemolysis produces an electrophoretic pattern that is dominated by beta globulin, with some albumin, trace alpha$_1$ globulin, trace alpha$_2$ globulin, and negligible to absent gamma$_1$ globulin.

Inflammatory syndromes include acute infection, burns, cancer, collagen diseases, hyperthyroidism, and pregnancy. This electrophoretic pattern consists of moderate alpha$_1$ globulin, some albumin, some alpha$_2$ globulin, and negligible to absent beta$_1$ globulin and gamma$_1$ globulin.

Monocytic and monomyelocytic leukemia result in a cationic peak or dominant migration to the cathode, moderate albumin, trace alpha$_1$ globulin, trace alpha$_2$ globulin, and negligible to absent beta$_1$ globulin and gamma$_1$ globulin.

Myoglobinuria associated with crushing injuries or electrocution demonstrates a pattern of dominant to absent gamma$_1$ globulin, some albumin, trace alpha$_1$ globulin, trace alpha$_2$ globulin, and negligible to absent beta$_1$ globulin.

Paraproteinemias such as multiple myeloma with Bence Jones proteinuria produce moderate to absent beta$_1$ globulin and gamma$_1$ globulin, with some albumin, trace alpha$_1$ globulin, and alpha$_2$ globulin.

Inflammatory conditions (such as chronic osteomyelitis), increased glomerular permeability, and tubular dysfunction (such as chronic renal failure) produce a pattern that is dominated by albumin, with moderate alpha$_1$ globulin elevation, some alpha$_2$ globulin, trace beta$_1$ globulin, and negligible to absent gamma$_1$ globulin.

Renal tubular disorders include acute renal tubular failure, Balkan neuropathy, cadmium poisoning (chronic), cystinosis, Fanconi syndrome, galactosemia, hypokalemia (chronic, severe), intoxication (phenacetin or vitamin D), medullary cystic disease, monoclonal gammopathy, oculocerebral renal syndrome, polycystic kidney disease, pyelonephritis (chronic), renal transplantation, renal tubular acidosis, sarcoidosis, and Wilson's disease. The electrophoretic pattern is dominated by beta$_1$ globulin, with some alpha$_2$ globulin, some gamma$_1$ globulin, trace albumin, trace alpha$_1$ globulin, and a trace cationic migration or peak.

Retroperitoneal lymphatic injury from inflammation, obstruction, or trauma can result in aberrant communication of the retroperitoneal lymph vessels, chyle ducts of the intestine, and urinary tract. This condition causes chyluria. The electrophoretic pattern noted in chyluria is one dominated by albumin, with moderate gamma$_1$ globulin, some alpha$_2$ globulin, some beta$_1$ globulins, and trace alpha$_1$ globulin.

Upright or orthostatic position–dependent proteinuria is characterized by dominant albumin, moderate beta$_1$ globulin, some alpha$_1$ globulin, trace alpha$_2$ globulin, and trace gamma$_1$ globulin. The recumbent position reflects a normal electrophoretic pattern. Activity-related proteinuria demonstrates a pattern that is more accentuated than normal but not so elevated as orthostatic proteinuria. An exercise pattern produces moderate albumin, some alpha$_1$ globulin and alpha$_2$ globulin, trace beta$_1$ globulin, and trace gamma$_1$ globulin.

Description. Normally the urine is free of protein or contains only trace amounts of albumin and globulin because the glomeruli prevent the passage of proteins from the plasma to the glomerular filtrate. Protein electrophoresis is a quantitative measurement of proteins, which under the influence of an electrical field, at a pH of 8.6, separate by charge, size, and shape. The separation produces homogeneous bands that are plotted on treated paper. Protein electrophoresis detects the presence of free light chains and other proteins associated with myoclonal gammopathies. The normally round and broad curves form a "church spire," or sharp peak. The immunoelectrophoretic technique is able to demonstrate a large number of components that are identical to the serum electrophoretic patterns. It is used to identify light-chain, Bence Jones, and kappa-, lambda-, and heavy-chain proteins. The test helps detect specific abnormalities by identifying patterns of protein characteristic of different disease states. The meaning of the results of urine electrophoresis is best interpreted when the test is run simultaneously with a serum sample for electrophoresis.

Professional Considerations
1. Consent form NOT required.

2. **Preparation:**
   A. Obtain a clean 50-mL container for a random urine collection or a 3-L container without preservatives or to which toluene or acetic acid has been added. For pediatric/infant specimen collection, also obtain a pediatric urine collection device/bag and tape.
   B. Write the beginning time of the 24-hour collection on the laboratory requisition.
   C. See *Client and family teaching.*
3. **Procedure:**
   A. *Random sample:* Obtain a 25-mL fresh, first morning-voided urine sample in a clean container. A fresh specimen may be taken from a urinary drainage bag.
   B. *24-Hour sample:* Discard the first morning-urine specimen. Save all urine voided for 24 hours in a refrigerated, clean 3-L container without preservatives or to which toluene or acetic acid preservative has been added. Document the quantity of urine output during the specimen collection period. Include the urine voided at the end of the 24-hour period. For catheterized clients, keep entire drainage bag on ice and empty the urine into the collection container hourly.
   C. *Pediatric/infant specimen collection:* Empty the urine into the refrigerated collection container after each void.
      i. The child is placed in a supine position with the knees flexed and the hips externally rotated and abducted.
      ii. Cleanse, rinse, and thoroughly dry the perineal area.
      iii. To prevent the child from removing the collection device/bag, a diaper may be placed over the genital area.
      iv. *Females:* Tape the pediatric collection device/bag to the perineum. Starting at the area between the anus and vagina, apply the device/bag in an anterior direction.
      v. *Males:* Place the pediatric collection device/bag over the penis and scrotum and tape it to the perineal area.

4. **Postprocedure care:**
   A. Compare the urine quantity in the specimen container with the urinary output record for the test. If the specimen contains less urine than what was recorded as output, some of the sample may have been discarded, invalidating the test.
   B. Document the urine quantity on the laboratory requisition.
5. **Client and family teaching:**
   A. For 24-hour urine collection for home collection: Save all urine voided in the 24-hour period and urinate before defecating to avoid loss of urine. If any urine is accidentally discarded, discard the entire specimen and restart the collection the next day.
   B. Avoid drugs that may cause proteinuria (listed below) for specific lengths of time before the test as specified by the physician.
6. **Factors that affect results:**
   A. Contamination of the specimen with stool invalidates the results. The test must be repeated or restarted.
   B. Drugs that cause proteinuria include amikacin sulfate, amphotericin B, aurothioglucose, bacitracin, gentamicin sulfate, gold sodium thiomalate, kanamycin, neomycin sulfate, netilmycin sulfate, penicillins, phenylbutazone, polymyxin B, streptomycin sulfate, sulfonamides, tobramycin sulfate, and trimethadione.
7. **Other data:**
   A. Urine protein electrophoresis results should be evaluated with consideration given to serum protein electrophoresis patterns.

PROTEIN, QUANTITATIVE, URINE
(*see Protein, Urine*)

PROTEIN, SEMIQUANTITATIVE, URINE
(*see Protein, Urine*)

PROTEIN, TOTAL, SERUM

Norm:

		SI UNITS
Adults	6.0-8.0 g/dL	60-80 g/L
Children	4.3-7.6 g/dL	43-76 g/L
Premature	4.6-7.4 g/dL	46-74 g/L
Newborn	6.0-6.7 g/dL	60-67 g/L
Infant	6.2-8.0 g/dL	62-80 g/L

Increased. Amyloidosis, Addison's disease, autoimmune collagen disorders, chronic infection, Crohn's disease, dehydration (relative increase), diarrhea, Franklin's disease, hemolysis, liver disease, macroglobulinemia, multiple myeloma, protozoal diseases (kala-azar), renal disease, sarcoidosis, vomiting, and wound drainage. Drugs include clofibrate, corticosteroids, corticotropin, dextran, heparin calcium, heparin sodium, insulin, levothyroxine sodium/T, radiographic contrast dye, somatotropin, sulfobromophthalein (Bromsulphalein), thyrotropin, and tolbutamide.

Decreased. Acute cholecystitis, analbuminemia, burns, chronic glomerulonephritis, cirrhosis, congestive heart failure, Crohn's disease, diarrhea, edema, essential hypertension, exfoliative dermatitis, frequent plasma donation, hemorrhage, hepatic disease (severe), Hodgkin's disease, hyperalimentation, hyperthyroidism, hypoalbuminemia, hypogammaglobulinemia, infectious hepatitis, kwashiorkor, leukemia (monocytic, myelogenous), malabsorption, malnutrition, nephrosis, nephrotic syndrome, peptic ulcer, pregnancy, protein-losing enteropathies, sprue, ulcerative colitis, and water intoxication. Drugs include ammonium ion, dextran, excessive intravenous fluids containing glucose, oral contraceptives, pyrazinamide, and salicylates.

Description. Total serum protein reflects the total amount of albumin and globulins in the serum. The serum proteins that are synthesized in the liver and reticuloendothelial system constitute over 100 different substances and are grouped as albumin and globulins. Serum proteins are essential to the reg-

ulation of colloid osmotic pressure, and comprise coagulation factors for hemostasis, enzymes, hormones, tissue growth and repair, and pH buffers. They produce antibodies, transport blood components (bilirubin, calcium, lipids, metals, oxygen, steroids, thyroid hormones, and vitamins) and are the preservers of chromosomes.

Professional Considerations
1. Consent form NOT required.
2. **Preparation:**
   A. Tube: Red topped, red/gray topped, or gold topped.
   B. Medications that interfere with serum protein levels may be withheld.
   C. Do NOT draw specimens during hemodialysis.
   D. See *Client and family teaching.*
3. **Procedure:**
   A. Draw a 1-mL blood sample without trauma.
   B. Avoid prolonged application of a tourniquet, which can cause an increase in protein concentrations.
   C. Obtain the sample away from IV solution, which can lower protein levels through local dilution.
4. **Postprocedure care:**
   A. Samples may be refrigerated for up to 1 week.
5. **Client and family teaching:**
   A. Do not ingest a high-fat diet for 8 hours before the test.
   B. Medications that interfere with serum protein levels may be prescribed to be withheld before the test.
6. **Factors that affect results:**
   A. Reject hemolyzed or lipemic specimens.
   B. Falsely elevated total protein levels occur for up to 48 hours after

the use of sulfobromophthalein contrast dye.

C. Recent dialysis distorts protein values.

D. Hyperglycemia may cause total protein concentration to appear to be greater than actual.

E. Serum total protein for bedridden clients is lower by approximately 0.3 g/dL than expected for the same age.

7. **Other data:**

A. See also *Protein electrophoresis, Blood.*

B. The significance of the total protein is difficult to interpret without knowledge of the level of the individual fractions (albumin/ globulin) obtained through electrophoresis.

PROTEIN, URINE

Norm. Negative; no detectable protein.

SEMIQUANTITATIVE NORMS		SI UNITS
Normal	<20 mg/%	<0.2 g/L
Reagent Strip/Stick		
Negative	0-5 mg/dL	0-0.05 g/L
Trace	5-20 mg/dL	0.05-0.2 g/L
1+	30 mg/dL	0.3 g/L
2+	100 mg/dL	1.0 g/L
3+	300 mg/dL	3.0 g/L
4+	1000 mg/dL	10.0 g/L

QUANTITATIVE NORMS		SI UNITS
Adults	30-150 mg/24 hours	0.03-0.15 g/day
Children <10 years	<100 mg/24 hours	<0.10 g/day

Newborn: Increased protein in urine for 3 days after delivery.

Increased or Positive

Nonrenal disease. Abdominal tumor, aging, anemia (severe), ascites, bacterial toxins (acute streptococcal, diphtheria, pneumonia, scarlet and typhoid fever), cardiac disease, central nervous system lesion, convulsive disorders, fever, hepatic disease (jaundice), hypersensitivity reaction, hyperthyroidism, infection (acute), ingestion of or overexposure to certain substances (arsenic, carbon tetrachloride, ether, lead, mercury, mustard, opiates, phenol, propylene glycol, sulfosalicylic acid, turpentine), intestinal obstruction, leukemia (chronic lymphocytic), subacute bacterial endocarditis, toxemia, and trauma.

Transient proteinuria. Dehydration, diet (excessive protein), emotional stress, exposure to cold, exercise (strenuous), fever, orthostatic hypotension, proteinuria, posthemorrhage, and sodium depletion. Drugs include epinephrine bitartrate, epinephrine borate, epinephrine hydrochloride, and levarterenol bitartrate.

Prerenal disease. Amyloidosis, Bence Jones proteinuria associated with myeloma, congestive heart failure, convulsions, exercise, leukemia (myelocytic), orthostatic hypotension, proteinuria, and Waldenström's macroglobulinemia.

Renal disease. Collagen diseases, cryoglobulinemia, Henoch-Schönlein purpura, hypertension (malignant, renovascular), and thrombotic thrombocytopenic purpura.

Glomerular disease. Amyloidosis, diabetic glomerulosclerosis and nephropathy, glomerulonephritis and lesion, Goodpasture syndrome, high molecular weight proteinuria, membranous nephropathy, polycystic disease, pyelonephritis (chronic), renal vein thrombosis, and systemic lupus erythematosus.

Interstitial disease. Bacterial pyelonephritis, deposition of calcium, uric acid, or urate, and idiosyncratic pharmacologic reactions to the following drugs: methicillin sodium, phenytoin, phenytoin sodium, phenindione, and sulfonamides.

Tubular disease. Acute tubular necrosis, Bartter syndrome, beta-microglobulinemia, Bright's disease, Butler-Albright syndrome, Fanconi syndrome, galactosemia, heavy metal poisoning (cadmium, lead, mercury), Kimmelstiel-Wilson syndrome, nephrotic syndrome, and renal tubular acidosis.

Postrenal disease. Cystitis (severe), tumor metastasis of the bone, and tumor (urinary bladder, renal pelvis). Drugs that cause proteinuria include amikacin sulfate, amphotericin B, aurothioglucose, bacitracin, gentamicin sulfate, gold sodium thiomalate, netilmicin sulfate, neomycin sulfate, penicillins, phenylbutazone, polymyxin B, streptomycin sulfate, sulfonamides, and trimethadione.

Decreased. Not applicable.

Description. The semiquantitative urine test is a random screening test for urinary protein and is part of the routine urinalysis. The reagent-strip color indicators and use of sulfosalicylic acid in the laboratory are two methods used to confirm the presence of urinary protein. A small amount of protein in the urine is regarded as normal and consists of albumin and low-molecular-weight plasma proteins (beta-microglobulin, globulins, haptoglobulin, light chains, and Tamm-Horsfall glycoprotein). Protein in the urine is a key indicator of renal disorder.

Quantitation of urinary protein is indicated when a random urine sample is positive for more than a trace of protein. Normally, only low-molecular-weight proteins are small enough to pass through the glomerular membrane into the glomerular filtrate, and most of these are reabsorbed by the renal tubules. Proteinuria is a key indicator of renal disorder and can

result from glomerular leakage, tubular impairment, breakdown of renal tissue, or excessive concentrations of low-molecular-weight proteins. Transient proteinuria may result from nonpathologic states such as physical or emotional stress and body position. Protein substances are excreted at different rates and at varying times in a 24-hour period; thus the 24-hour timed quantitative urine test for protein provides the most accurate reflection of kidney function.

Professional Considerations
1. Consent form NOT required.
2. **Preparation:**
   A. *Semiquantitative test:*
      i. Obtain a clean, dry plastic container or a pediatric urine-collection device and a container of reagent strips.
   B. *Quantitative test:*
      i. Obtain a clean, 3-L container that is free of preservative. For pediatric/infant collections, also obtain tape and a pediatric urine-collection device/bag.
      ii. Write the beginning time of the 24-hour collection on the laboratory requisition.
3. **Procedure:**
   A. *Semiquantitative test:*
      i. An early-morning specimen or the first voided specimen of the day after the client stands upright is preferred.
      ii. Instruct the client to void into a clean, dry container. The specimen may be transferred to a plastic container.
      iii. Specimens may be tested immediately or sent to the laboratory for testing.
      iv. To test the sample immediately, dip the reagent strip into the urine and remove any excess urine by gently tapping the strip on the side of the collection container. The strip should then be held at a horizontal plane to prevent mixing of any other chemicals on the strip. Immediately and carefully compare the color of the test pad on the reagent strip to the color chart provided on the container from

which it was taken. Record the result according to the negative to 4+ range of approximate milligrams per deciliter (mg/dL) of protein.

B. *Quantitative test:*

i. Early morning is the preferred time to begin a 24-hour collection.

ii. Discard the first morning urine specimen.

iii. Save all the urine voided for 24 hours in a refrigerated, clean, 3-L container that is free of preservatives. Document the quantity of urine output during the specimen collection period. Include the urine voided at the end of the 24-hour period. For catheterized clients, keep the drainage bag on ice and empty the urine into the refrigerated collection container hourly.

iv. Pediatric/infant specimen collection:

a. Empty the collection bag into the refrigerated collection container after each void.

b. The child is placed in a supine position with the knees flexed and the hips externally rotated and abducted.

c. Cleanse, rinse, and thoroughly dry the perineal area.

d. To prevent the child from removing the collection device/bag, a diaper may be placed over the genital area.

e. *Females:* Tape the pediatric collection device/bag to the perineum. Starting at the area between the anus and vagina, apply the device/bag in an anterior direction.

f. *Males:* Place the pediatric collection device/bag over the penis and scrotum and tape it to the perineal area.

4. **Postprocedure care:**

A. *Semiquantitative test:*

i. To be most accurate, specimens sent to the laboratory must be transported within 2 hours of the collection of the sulfosalicylic acid precipitation of the protein. Specimens must be refrigerated.

B. *Quantitative test:*

i. Compare the urine quantity in the specimen container with the urinary output record for the test. If the specimen contains less urine than what was recorded as output, some of the sample may have been discarded, thus invalidating the test.

ii. Document the urine quantity and ending time on the laboratory requisition.

5. **Client and family teaching.**

A. Save all the urine voided in a 24-hour period; urinate before defecating to avoid loss of urine; and avoid contamination of the specimen with stool, toilet tissue, or prostatic or vaginal secretions. If any urine is accidentally discarded, discard the entire specimen and restart the collection the next day.

B. Parents may be taught a pediatric collection technique for specimens collected on infants at home.

6. **Factors that affect results:**

A. Drugs that may cause false-positive semiquantitative results include acetazolamide, aminosalicylic acid, cephaloridine, chlorpromazine, penicillins, phenazopyridine, promazine hydrochloride, radiographic contrast media, sodium bicarbonate, sulfisoxazole, sulfonamides, thymol, and tolbutamide.

B. Drugs that may cause falsely elevated quantitative results include acetazolamide, aminosalicylic acid, aspirin, barbiturates, cephalosporins, corticosteroids, iodine, iodine contrast medium, mercurial diuretics, penicillins, sodium bicarbonate, sulfonamides, tolbutamide, and tolmetin sodium.

C. First-voided urine samples are the most accurate for semiquantitative measurement because they are the most uniformly concentrated, are the most acidic pH, and are most likely to exhibit abnormalities.

D. False-positive semiquantitative results can occur with incorrect matching of the reagent strip to the color chart and with prolonged exposure of the strip or stick to the urine.

E. False-positive results have been reported with gross hematuria.

F. Reject specimens contaminated with blood, heavy mucus, purulent drainage, stool, prostatic or vaginal secretions, or toilet tissue.

G. The presence of many white blood cells can alter the results.

H. False-negative results have been reported with very dilute urine, highly buffered alkaline urine, urine high in sodium, and urea-splitting infectious organisms of the urinary tract.

I. Reject quantitative specimens in which the last void before the testing period was not discarded.

J. All urine voided for the 24-hour period must be included to avoid a falsely low quantitative result.

K. Increased protein concentrations are found during the daytime and after exercise.

L. The reagent strip is most sensitive to albumin and less sensitive to globulins.

M. The reagent strip method will not detect Bence Jones protein, globulins, mucoproteins, or myeloma protein.

N. Semiquantitative testing with a regent strip will show a trace positive reaction at a protein concentration of 100-200 mg/L.

7. **Other data:**

A. The creatinine clearance test is often prescribed with the quantitative urine protein test.

B. Bence Jones protein may be present if the reagent strip method is negative and the sulfosalicylic acid test is positive. An electrophoresis and immunoelectrophoresis search for light chains is indicated because Bence Jones proteins are associated with amyloidosis, chronic lymphocytic leukemia, hyperparathyroidism, macroglobulinemia, malignant lymphoma, metastatic bone tumor, multiple myeloma, and osteomalacia.

C. See also *Protein electrophoresis, Urine.*

PROTEIN C (AUTOPROTHROMBIN IIA), BLOOD

Norm:

PROTEIN C	RANGE
Normal level of protein C	58%-148%
Critical value	<50%
Heterozygous protein C deficiency	20%-74%
Homozygous protein C deficiency	As low as 0%

ACTIVATED PROTEIN C RESISTANCE TEST	
APC-APTT/APTT Ratio	>2.0
Resistance to activated Protein C	≤2.0 with confirmatory DNA testing to identify Factor V Leiden mutation

Usage. Helps diagnose cause of thrombosis. Protein C:Protein S ratio is helpful in identifying carriers of congenital protein C deficiency.

Description. Activated protein C is a plasma, vitamin K–dependent glycoprotein that counters coagulation activity by inhibiting factors V and XIII. Protein C was first identified in the early 1980s. Sixty percent of protein C is bound to complement protein, and its activity is enhanced by cofactor protein S. Protein C deficiency may be congenital or acquired. *Congenital protein C deficiency* is an inherited, autosomal dominant thrombophilia present in 3%-5% of clients with venous thrombosis. Congenital deficiency may be exhibited either as reduced protein C levels or as resistance to protein C despite normal levels. Clients with homozygous deficiencies usually die as a result of thrombosis during their first year of life, which is often preceded by neonatal purpura fulminans. Those with heterozygous deficiency often have venous thromboembolisms, such as deep vein thrombosis or pulmonary embolism, at a young age. *Acquired protein C deficiency* is seen in acute respiratory distress syndrome, disseminated intravascular coagulation, hemolytic-uremic syndrome, hepatic disease, infection, postoperative states, vitamin K deficiency, and clients receiving warfarin sodium (Coumadin). Protein C deficiency is responsible for a much greater proportion of venous thromboses than arterial thromboses. The *Factor V Leiden mutation,* newly identified in the 1990s, is a thrombotic molecular defect in Factor V making it resistant to anticoagulant activation by protein C. It is a significant cause of deep vein thrombosis, as the mutation is thought to be present in 5% of the population. The Leiden mutation is identified by performing an activated protein C resistance test (APTT with and without commercially-available activated protein C) and confirming an abnormal result with DNA evaluation for the Leiden mutation.

Professional Considerations
1. Consent form NOT required.
2. **Preparation:**
    A. Tube: 4.5-mL blue topped. Also obtain ice.

    B. Indicate on the laboratory requisition if the activated protein C resistance testing is needed.
3. **Procedure:**
    A. Withdraw 2 mL of blood into a syringe or vacuum tube. Remove the syringe or tube, leaving the needle in place. Attach a second syringe, and draw a 2.4-mL sample in a 2.7-mL tube or a 4.0-mL sample in a 4.5-mL tube. Place the specimens immediately into a container of ice.
    B. Gently tilt the tube five or six times to mix.
4. **Postprocedure care:**
    A. Place the specimens on ice immediately.
    B. For clients with coagulopathy, hold pressure over the sampling site for at least 5 minutes and observe the site closely for development of a hematoma.
    C. Write the collection time on the laboratory requisition.
    D. Transport the specimens to the laboratory immediately, discard the ice, and refrigerate the specimens.
5. **Client and family teaching:**
    A. For results showing congenital deficiency, refer client or parents for genetic counseling as appropriate.
6. **Factors that affect results:**
    A. Reject hemolyzed or clotted specimens, specimens not completely mixed, tubes partially filled with blood, specimens not refrigerated, specimens diluted or contaminated with heparin, or specimens received more than 2 hours after collection.
    B. Specimen results are invalidated if client is receiving a recently adjusted (within previous week) dose of warfarin.
7. **Other data:**
    A. Protein C deficiency is treated with ongoing anticoagulation with or without protein C or factor IX concentrates. There is no treatment for Factor V Leiden mutation.

PROTEIN S, TOTAL AND FREE, BLOOD

Norm:

	TOTAL	FREE	% FREE AS A PERCENTAGE OF HEALTHY CONTROL
Protein S	74-112 U/dL	27-63 U/dL	68-140%
Critical low			<50%

Usage. Helps diagnose cause of thrombosis. Protein C:Protein S ratio is helpful in identifying carriers of congenital protein C deficiency.

Description. Protein S is a plasma, vitamin K–dependent glycoprotein manufactured in the liver that functions in the coagulation pathway. It exists in free form (active) and bound to a complement protein (inactive). Protein S functions as a cofactor to protein C, which inactivates Factors Va and VIIIa. Deficiencies of protein S may be of two types. *Congenital protein S deficiency* is an autosomal dominant disorder responsible for about 5% of thromboses, in which the client has a higher-than-normal risk of thrombosis at a young age. *Acquired protein S deficiencies* are seen in pregnancy, disseminated intravascular coagulation, hepatic disease, and clients receiving warfarin. Protein S deficiency is responsible for a much greater proportion of venous thromboses than arterial thromboses.

Professional Considerations
1. Consent form NOT required.
2. Preparation:
   A. Tube: 4.5-mL blue topped. Also obtain ice.
3. Procedure:
   A. Withdraw 3 mL of blood into a syringe or vacuum tube. Remove the syringe or tube, leaving the needle in place. Attach a second syringe, and draw a 2.4-mL sample in a 2.7-mL tube or a 4.0-mL sample in a 4.5-mL tube. Place the specimens immediately into a container of ice.
   B. Gently tilt the tube five or six times to mix.
4. Postprocedure care:
   A. Place the specimens on ice immediately.
   B. For clients with coagulopathy, hold pressure over the sampling site for at least 5 minutes and observe the site closely for development of a hematoma.
   C. Write the collection time on the laboratory requisition.
   D. Transport the specimens to the laboratory immediately, discard the ice, and refrigerate the specimens.
5. Client and family teaching:
   A. For results showing congenital deficiency, refer client or parents for genetic counseling as appropriate.
6. Factors that affect results:
   A. Reject hemolyzed or clotted specimens, specimens not completely mixed, tubes partially filled with blood, specimens not refrigerated, specimens diluted or contaminated with heparin, or specimens received more than 2 hours after collection.
   B. Specimen results are invalidated if client is receiving a recently adjusted (within previous week) dose of warfarin.
7. Other data:
   A. Once discovered, protein S deficiency is treated with ongoing anticoagulation.

PROTHROMBIN TIME (PT) AND INTERNATIONAL NORMALIZED RATIO (INR), BLOOD

Normal PT. Each laboratory establishes a normal value, or control, based on the method and reagents used to perform the test. A value within ±2 seconds of the control set by each laboratory is considered within a normal range

	PROTHROMBIN TIME
Adult	10-15 seconds
Newborn	<17 seconds
Child	11-14 seconds
Panic value	>40 seconds
Nonanticoagulated condition	>20 seconds
Anticoagulated condition	>3 times the control

Normal International Normalized Ratio (INR).

Coumadin therapy. There are, in general, two therapeutic ranges for clients receiving warfarin sodium (Coumadin):

Standard (Low-Intensity) Therapy	High-Dose (High-Intensity) Therapy
≤2.5 INR to minimize risk of bleeding during endoscopic procedures. 2.0 INR (range 1.6-2.5) for stroke prevention in clients over 75 years of age who have atrial fibrillation. 2.5 INR (range 2.0-3.0) for stroke prevention in clients up to 75 years of age who have atrial fibrillation. 2.0-3.0 INR is appropriate for management of deep vein thrombosis, prevention of systemic embolism, and mitral or aortic prosthetic tissue valves.	2.5-3.5 INR is appropriate for management of client's status after recent acute myocardial infarction, or clients with bi-leaflet or tilting-disk mechanical heart valves, or for evaluation of client's status after left-sided prosthetic valve thrombosis and recurrent systemic embolism; and for prophylaxis in high-risk surgery.

Panic Level Symptoms and Treatment

Symptoms. Bleeding from venipuncture, arterial, or intravenous catheter sites; ecchymoses; hematoma; hematuria; blood in stool; ecchymosis; or hallmark signs of intracerebral, gastrointestinal, or retroperitoneal bleeding.

Treatment:

Note: Treatment choice(s) depend on client history and condition and episode history.
Discontinue or reduce rate of IV anticoagulant.

Maintain patent airway.
Apply pressure for 10 minutes or more to bleeding line or venipuncture sites.
Observe and intervene for hemodynamic stability.
For active bleeding, consider administration of whole blood, fresh frozen plasma or prothrombin complex concentrate.
Administer vitamin K. Crowther et al, (2002) found that the oral route of administration is faster than the subcutaneous route in reducing the INR.

Route	Coagulation Factors Increase	Bleeding Control Occurs	INR Becomes Normal	Risks
IV (Aqua-MEPHYTON) (route not recommended unless other routes are not feasible)	1-2 hours	3-8 hours	12-14 hours	Anaphylaxis
Subcutaneous (Aqua-MEPHYTON)	Progressive Increase	Progressive length	24-48 hours	Hemorrhage at injection site
Intramuscular (Aqua-MEPHYTON)			24-48 hours	Hemorrhage at injection site
Oral (Mephyton)	6-12 hours		24-48 hours	Considered safest and preferred method of administration

Increased PT. Afibrinogenemia, alcoholism, biliary obstruction, cancer, celiac disease, circulating anticoagulants, cirrhosis, colitis, collagen disease, congestive heart failure, diarrhea (chronic), disseminated intravascular coagulation (DIC), dysfibrinogenemia, factor deficiency (I, II, V, VII, X), fever, fibrinogen degradation products (FDP), fistula, hemorrhagic disease of the newborn, hepatic disease (abscess, biopsy, failure, jaundice, infectious hepatitis), hypernephroma of kidney, hyperthyroidism, hypervitaminosis A, hypofibrinogenemia (<100 mg/dL), idiopathic familial hypoprothrombinemia, idiopathic myelofibrosis, increased fibrinolytic activity, jaundice (hemolytic, hepatocellular, obstructive), leukemia (acute), malabsorption, malnutrition, obstetric complications, pancreatic carcinoma, pancreatitis (chronic), polycythemia vera, premature infants, prolonged hot weather, prothrombin deficiency, Reye syndrome, snakebite, sprue, steatorrhea, toxic shock syndrome, vitamin K deficiency, and vomiting. Drugs include alcohol, allopurinol, aminosalicylic acid, amiodarone hydrochloride, anabolic steroids, antibiotics, bromelains, chenodiol, chloral hydrate, chlorpropamide, chymotrypsin, cimetidine, clofibrate, dextran, dextrothyroxine, diazoxide, diflunisal, disulfiram, diuretics, ethacrynic acid, fenoprofen, fluoroquinolone antibiotics, fluoxetine, glucagon,

hepatotoxic drugs, ibuprofen, indomethacin, influenzavirus vaccine, mefenamic acid, methyldopa, methylphenidate, metronidazole, miconazole, monoamine oxidase inhibitors, nalidixic acid, naproxen, narcotics (prolonged), pentoxifylline, phenylbutazone, phenytoin sodium, propafenone, pyrazolones, quinidine, quinine, ranitidine, salicylates, sulfinpyrazone, sulfonamides (long-acting), sulindac, tamoxifen, thyroid drugs, tolbutamide, trimethoprim-sulfamethoxazole, and warfarin sodium (underdosage).

Increased INR. Excess oral anticoagulant. INR is also increased by conditions that increase PT. Herbs or natural remedies include *dan[1]shen[1]* ('red-ginseng', *Salvia miltiorrhiza*), *dang[1]gui[1]* (variants: *tangkuei, dong quai, Angelica sinensis*) (in clients receiving warfarin concurrently), feverfew, garlic, *Ginkgo biloba*, ginseng, and ginger.

Decreased PT. Arterial occlusion, deep vein thrombosis, edema, hereditary coumarin resistance, hyperlipemia, hyperthyroidism, hypothyroidism, multiple myeloma, myocardial infarction, peripheral vascular disease, pulmonary embolism, spinal cord injury, thromboembolism (acute), and transplant rejection. Drugs include adrenocortical steroids, alcohol, aminoglutethimide, antacids, antihistamines, barbiturates, carbamazepine, chloral hydrate, chlordiazepoxide, cholestyramine, diuretics, ethchlorvynol, glutethimide, griseofulvin, haloperidol, meprobamate, nafcillin, oral contraceptives, paraldehyde, primidone, ranitidine, rifampin, sucralfate, trazodone, vitamin C, and warfarin sodium (underdosage).

Decreased INR. Insufficient oral anticoagulant. INR is also decreased by conditions and drugs that decrease PT.

Description. Prothrombin is a vitamin K-dependent glycoprotein produced by the liver that is necessary for firm fibrin clot formation. It converts to thrombin in the clotting-cascade process and should not appear in the serum after clot formation. Prothrombin time (PT) measures the amount of time taken for clot formation after reagent tissue thromboplastin (brain tissue extract) and calcium are added to citrated plasma. PT is used to monitor response to warfarin therapy or to screen for dysfunction involving the extrinsic system resulting from liver disease, vitamin K deficiency, factor deficiency, or DIC. The most accurate PT values are reported as the number of seconds taken for the client's plasma to form a clot, along with the number of seconds taken for a laboratory control sample to clot. Very small PT fluctuations can have profound physiologic effects.

The PT is usually not prolonged until Factors (II, V, VII, X) are decreased or less than 50% of normal or the fibrinogen is decreased to less than 80-100 mg/dL.

Because individual responses to same-dose warfarin anticoagulant therapy vary, the efficacy and safety of management are dependent on maintaining the anticoagulant effect within a defined therapeutic range. The INR improves the usability of the PT test in monitoring response to anticoagulation therapy. Since 1977, the World Health Organization has advocated that all PT results be reported as an INR, which is the PT ratio that would result if the sample was tested with WHO international standard reference thromboplastin reagent. The standardization guidelines of the World Health Organization (WHO) state that freshly prepared specimens from 20 normal individuals and 60 patients receiving coumarin must be used to calibrate the International Sensitivity Index (ISI). An International Sensitivity Index (ISI) number is assigned to each thromboplastin reagent that is used in mathematically calculating the INR to correct for varying thromboplastin sensitivities: The INR is calculated when the observed PT ratio is raised to the power of the ISI specific to the particular thromboplastin reagent used, or:

$$INR = \frac{(\text{Client's PT in seconds})^{ISI}}{\text{Mean normal PT in seconds}}$$

CIRCUMSTANCES	RECOMMENDED INR FREQUENCY
5 mg loading dose* of Coumadin	Baseline prior After 24 hours of therapy, then 2-4 times per week until steady levels are obtained.
Ongoing Coumadin therapy	Every 4-6 weeks. Lidstone et al (2002) found it safe to extend intervals between INR testing to 14 weeks in clients with a wide INR target range of 3-4.5.

*The literature contains several studies that demonstrate that using 5 mg instead of 10 mg loading doses of Coumadin is as effective in reaching a therapeutic INR between 2.0 and 3.0 by day 4-5, but poses less incidence of overanticoagulation.

Professional Considerations
1. Consent form NOT required.
2. **Preparation:**
   A. Baseline PT should be drawn before anticoagulant therapy is started.
   B. Tube: 2.7-mL or 4.5-mL blue-topped tube and a control tube and a waste tube or syringe.

C. Do NOT draw specimens during hemodialysis.
D. Screen client for the use of herbal preparations or medicines or "natural" remedies. See 6-H and 6-I.
E. See *Client and family teaching.*

3. **Procedure:**
   A. Perform venipuncture and withdraw 2 mL of blood into a syringe or vacuum tube. Remove the syringe or tube, leaving the needle in place.
   B. Attach a second syringe and completely fill a blue-topped tube with a blood sample collected without trauma. The sample quantity should be 2.4 mL for a 2.7-mL tube and 4.0 mL for a 4.5-mL tube.
   C. A 9:1 ratio of blood to citrate is critical.
   D. Gently tilt the tube several times to thoroughly mix the specimen.

4. **Postprocedure care:**
   A. Write the specimen collection time on the laboratory requisition.
   B. Send the specimen to the laboratory immediately. Results take about 1 hour, if the test is performed immediately.
   C. The specimen should be refrigerated until testing. Testing should be performed within 12-18 hours.
   D. In the presence of a coagulation defect, the venipuncture site should have digital direct pressure to the site for 3-5 minutes after the needle is removed. The venipuncture site should be observed for bleeding or excessive ecchymosis.

5. **Client and family teaching:**
   A. Abstain from coffee and alcohol for 24 hours before the test.
   B. Follow normal dietary patterns for vitamin K–containing foods during the 24 hours before the test.
   C. Oral anticoagulant medication should be taken at the same time daily. Regular PT checks may be required for clients on long-term anticoagulant medication.
   D. Report any unusual bleeding.
   E. Women of childbearing age should be advised to avoid pregnancy during oral anticoagulation because warfarin is teratogenic and can cause fetal death. Heparin, which does not cross the placenta, should be used if pregnancy is desired.
   F. Warfarin enters breast milk. Women should not breast-feed when taking warfarin.
   G. Many herbs can interfere with Coumadin's effects. For this reason, do not take any herbal preparations or natural remedies without receiving your doctor's approval.
   H. It is important to keep taking the same brand of warfarin, if prescribed, because changing brands can alter the anticoagulation effect and INR.

6. **Factors that affect results:**
   A. Reject specimens if:
      i. Hemolyzed.
      ii. Lipemic.
      iii. Received more than 3 hours after collection.
      iv. Specimens in which collection tubes are incompletely filled
      v. Not promptly transported to the laboratory
      vi. Not refrigerated
   B. Concurrent therapy with heparin can lengthen PT for up to 5 hours after dosing. To minimize this influence, blood for PT determinations should be drawn 5 hours after IV heparin and 24 hours after subcutaneous heparin injection. Concurrent therapy with warfarin and fluoxetine can cause a slightly increased PT and delayed normalization.
   C. The problem of loss of accuracy of the INR system can be resolved by the use of sensitive thromboplastins with ISI values close to 1.0 (WHO reagent ISI = 1.0). However, even without this sensitivity, the INR system has been shown to be more accurate than reporting the results as a PT ratio.
   D. The use of automated clot detectors requires the use of sensitive thromboplastins or calibration of each new batch of thromboplastins with lyophilized plasmas with certified INR values obtained by the manual method to obtain valid and reliable results. ("True" INR values were obtained by the manual method.)
   E. It is recommended that reagents insensitive to heparin be used to avoid obtaining falsely elevated INRs when a client is receiving heparin and Coumadin concurrently. Innovin and Thromboplastin C Plus meet this criterion.
   F. Herbs or natural remedies that have a synergistic effect with warfarin to prolong bleeding include *dan¹shen¹(Salvia miltiorrhiza)*, *dang¹gui¹* (variants: *tangkuei, dong quai, Angelica sinensis*), *chuan¹xiong¹* (*ch'uanhsiung, Ligusticum chuanxiong* or *L. wallichi, Cnidium*, or *Conioselinum universitatum*), papaya

(*Carica papaya*), *tao²ren²* (*Prunus persica* and *P. davidiana*, semen Persicae, peach seed), *hong²hua¹* (safflower, *Carthamus tinctorius*), and *shui³zhi⁴* (leech, *Hirudo* and *Whitmania*).

G. Antibiotic therapy, mineral oil, and clofibrate can affect the PT.

H. Diets excessively high in green leafy vegetables can increase the absorption of vitamin K, which shortens the PT.

I. Intake of alcohol within 48 hours prior to the test can falsely decrease the INR.

J. Intake of the herb coffee (*Coffea*) within 48 hours prior to the test can falsely decrease the INR.

K. A minimum of 100 g/dL of fibrinogen must be present for the PT to be accurate.

L. The PT is affected by many pharmacologic agents, including those that alter protein-binding patterns, those that inhibit the formation of intestinal microorganisms, and those that are precursors of enzyme production.

M. Contamination of the specimen with tissue thromboplastin may alter the results. This is the reason for the double-draw technique.

7. **Other data:**

A. PT/INR should be measured frequently: daily × 5 when treatment is initiated, twice a week the following 1-2 weeks, once a week for the next 1-2 months, and every 2-4 weeks thereafter. Also, PT/INR should be performed whenever a drug that interacts with warfarin is added to or deleted from the regimen (see *Prothrombin time, Blood*).

B. The INR system is invalid in clients with liver disease (different reagents do not give the same INR for the same sample) but is no less valid than the PT in this client population.

C. The PT should be evaluated daily and used as a basis for dose adjustments during initial anticoagulation therapy.

D. A time interval of 16-48 hours may occur before warfarin affects the PT value.

E. A PT >30 seconds places the client at risk for hemorrhage.

F. Oral anticoagulation therapy usually maintains the prothrombin time at 1.5-2 times the laboratory control value. Clients with cardiac disease may be maintained at 2-2.5 times the laboratory control value.

G. Home testing kits are now available for clients on warfarin therapy.

H. Portable bedside INR testing is not recommended for anticoagulated clients.

PROTOPORPHYRIN, FREE ERYTHROCYTE, BLOOD

Norm:

		SI UNITS
Piomelli Method		
Adult female	19-52 mg/dL	0.34-0.92 µmol/L
Adult male	11-45 mg/dL	0.20-0.80 µmol/L
Hematofluorometer		
Adult female	<40 mg/dL	0.71 µmol/L
Adult male	<30 mg/dL	0.53 µmol/L
Panic level	>190 mg/dL	>3.38 µmol/L
Erythrocyte Precursor		
Protoporphyrin	4-52 mg/dL	0.07-0.92 µmol/L

Increased. Erythropoiesis, erythropoietic protoporphyria (>2200 mg/dL), hemolytic anemia (>50 mg/dL), infection (>50 mg/dL), iron deficiency (>200 mg/dL), lead poisoning (>200 mg/dL), protoporphyria, sideroachrestic anemia (acquired) (>50 mg/dL), and thalassemia.

Decreased. Megaloblastic anemia (<30 mg/dL).

Description. Protoporphyrin is a derivative of porphin that combines with iron to form the heme portion of hemoglobin and constitutes the predominant porphyrin in red blood cells

(RBCs). After hemoglobin breakdown, protoporphyrin is converted into bilirubin, combines with albumin, and remains unconjugated in the circulation. In conditions interfering with heme synthesis, increased amounts of protoporphyrin can be detected in erythrocytes, urine, and stool. Protoporphyria is an autosomal dominant disorder in which increased amounts of protoporphyrin are secreted and excreted. It is believed to be caused by an enzyme deficiency and is detected by the identification of increased concentrations of protoporphyrin in RBCs. Protoporphyria causes photosensitivity and may lead to cirrhosis and cholelithiasis because of protoporphyrin deposition. The free erythrocyte protoporphyrin (FEP) test measures the concentration of protoporphyrin in RBCs.

Professional Considerations
1. Consent form NOT required.
2. Preparation:
    A. Write the current hematocrit value on the laboratory requisition.
    B. If this test is being used for evaluation of lead intoxication, a blood sample for lead measurement should also be obtained.
    C. Tube: Green topped, lavender topped, or black topped.
    D. Do NOT draw specimens during hemodialysis.
3. Procedure:
    A. Draw a 3-mL blood sample, without hemolysis.
    B. Capillary tube samples from pediatric heel sticks are acceptable. (See notation regarding infant testing in item 6 below.)
4. Postprocedure care:
    A. Protect specimens from light.
5. Client and family teaching:
    A. Because protoporphyria is a hereditary disease, genetic counseling may be advised.
    B. Inform the client of lead poisoning detection and prevention.
6. Factors that affect results:
    A. Hemolysis of the specimen invalidates the results.
    B. This test is considered to be unreliable in infants less than 6 months of age.
7. Other data:
    A. This test can be used to screen for elevated lead in chil-

dren after iron deficiency is ruled out.
    B. See also *Porphyrins, Quantitative, Blood; Coproporphyrin, Urine.*

PROTRIPTYLINE
(see Tricyclic antidepressants, Plasma or Serum)

PSA, SERUM
(see Prostate-specific antigen, Serum)

PSA DENSITY, SERUM
(see Prostate-specific antigen, Serum)

PSA FRACTIONATION, SERUM
(see Prostate-specific antigen, Serum)

PSA VELOCITY, SERUM
(see Prostate-specific antigen, Serum)

PSAV, SERUM
(see Prostate-specific antigen, Serum)

P-SELECTIN, PLASMA

Norm. sP-selectin: 0.6-10 ng/mL.

Usage. Being developed for use in helping to identify a myocardial origin of chest pain symptoms earlier than other markers available. Also being tested for its use as a first trimester marker for risk for preeclampsia.

Increased. Acute coronary syndromes, acute lung injury, arthritis (rheumatoid), connective tissue diseases, coronary spasm, Graves' disease, inflammatory bowel disease (active), surgical trauma, thrombosis.

Description. P-selectin is a glycoprotein that exists in two forms, a soluble protein (sP-selectin) and bound to platelets and endothelial cells and is thought to help modulate platelet-leukocyte-endothelial activity during acute coronary syndromes. P-selectin is thought to be a marker for platelet activation because it exists only on platelets that have undergone the release action, is involved with leukocytes on endothelial tissue, and levels increase within minutes of triggers. Levels of both the soluble and bound forms of P-selectin have been found to be elevated in clients with acute coronary syndromes, and so it is possible that P-selectin levels may serve as a coronary marker in the future. The P-selectin profile measures both soluble and bound forms of the glycoprotein via enzyme immunoassay. While the sensitivity of this test is over 90%, the specificity for chest pain is currently only about 55%. This is because many other non-cardiac causes of chest pain also involve inflammatory processes that trigger rises in P-selectin.

Professional Considerations
1. Consent form NOT required.
2. **Preparation:**
    A. Tube: 2.7-mL or 4.5-mL blue-topped tube and a control tube and a waste tube or syringe.
    B. Do NOT draw specimens during hemodialysis.
3. **Procedure:**
    A. Perform venipuncture and withdraw 2 mL of blood into a syringe or vacuum tube. Remove the syringe or tube, leaving the needle in place.

B. Attach a second syringe and completely fill a blue-topped tube with a blood sample collected without trauma. The sample quantity should be 2.4 mL for a 2.7-mL tube and 4.0 mL for a 4.5-mL tube.
C. A 9:1 ratio of blood to citrate is critical.
D. Gently tilt the tube several times to thoroughly mix the specimen.
4. **Postprocedure care:**
    A. Write the specimen collection time on the laboratory requisition.
    B. Send the specimen to the laboratory immediately.
5. **Client and family teaching:**
    A. None.
6. **Factors that affect results:**
    A. Lower levels on serial measurements may indicate depletion.
    B. Aspirin has been found experimentally to decrease levels more than warfarin.
    C. One study found that drinking 5 cups of black tea per day lowered levels of plasma P-selectin.
7. **Other data:**
    A. Heparin does not affect P-selectin levels.

PSEUDOCHOLINESTERASE (CHOLINESTERASE, CHOLINESTERASE II, CHS, PCHE), PLASMA

Norm. Norms vary, depending on the laboratory substrate test method.

		SI UNITS
RID method	0.5-1.5 mg/dL	5-15 mg/L
DuPont ACA method	7-19 U/mL	7-19 kU/L
Other methods	3.0-8.0 U/mL	
	8-18 IU/L	
	0.5-1.3 pH U/hour	
Female	204-500 IU/dL	
Male	274-532 IU/dL	
Dibucaine inhibition	81-87%	0.81-0.87
Fluoride inhibition	44-54%	0.44-0.54

Increased. Diabetes mellitus, hyperthyroidism, insecticide exposure of organic phosphates, and nephrotic syndrome.

Decreased. Acute burns, anemia (severe pernicious, aplastic), carcinomatosis, cirrhosis, congenital deficiency, congestive heart failure (causing liver disease), dermatomyositis, hepatic carcinoma (metastatic), hepatitis (infectious), hypoproteinemia, infections (acute), infectious mononucleosis, insecticide exposure (carbamate, organophosphate), jaundice (obstructive), malnutrition, metastasis, muscular dystrophy, myocardial infarction, organophosphate insecticide poisoning

(DFP, parathion, sarin, triocresyl phosphate), parenchymatous liver disease, recent plasmapheresis, shock, skin diseases, succinylcholine hypersensitivity, tuberculosis, and uremia. Drugs include estrogens, morphine sulfate, neostigmine bromide, neostigmine methylsulfate, oral contraceptives, physostigmine sulfate, physostigmine salicylate, pyridostigmine bromide, and phospholine iodine.

Description. Pseudocholinesterase (PCHE) is a nonspecific cholinesterase that hydrolyzes noncholine esters as well as acetylcholine. It exists in several forms and serves to inactivate acetylcholine. PCHE is synthesized by the liver and found in plasma and is well distributed throughout the body. This enzyme's activity is inhibited reversibly by carbamate insecticides and irreversibly by organophosphate insecticides. Clients with an inherited PCHE deficiency exhibit an increased sensitivity to the effects of succinylcholine, which is normally inactivated by PCHE. Inherited deficiencies can be detected by the identification of abnormal genotypes of PCHE through dibucaine and fluoride inhibition tests. Although normal forms of PCHE are inhibited by these substances, the abnormal forms are not.

Professional Considerations
1. Consent form NOT required.
2. **Preparation:**
   A. Tube: Red topped or green topped.
   B. Specimens MAY be drawn during hemodialysis.
   C. See *Client and family teaching.*
3. **Procedure:**
   A. Draw a 5-mL blood sample, without trauma.
4. **Postprocedure care:**
   A. If the test purpose is to screen for organophosphate insecticide poisoning, the sample should be transported to the laboratory for immediate spinning and refrigeration. For other purposes, serum samples remain stable at room temperature for up to 1 week, refrigerated for 2 weeks, and frozen for up to 3 months.
5. **Client and family teaching:**
   A. Ten percent of the population may carry the gene for an uncommon form of PCHE.

B. Elevated results may indicate exposure to organophosphates, and the source would need to be identified.
C. If the test is to be using inhibition by dibucaine with fluoride, the client should not have taken muscle relaxants or anticholinergic drugs within 24 hours.
6. **Factors that affect results:**
   A. Hemolysis of the specimen causes falsely elevated results.
   B. Pregnancy decreases values by 30%.
   C. Exposure of the sample to chemicals such as fluoride, citrate, and borate will cause falsely decreased results.
7. **Other data:**
   A. A 20% drop in PCHE activity between baseline value and subsequent samples indicates overexposure to organophosphate insecticides.
   B. PCHE (pseudocholinesterase) is not to be confused with acetylcholinesterase (true cholinesterase, cholinesterase I, AcCHS).
   C. PCHE levels are an earlier indicator of organophosphate exposure than acetylcholinesterase levels are.
   D. One study suggested use of PCHE as an indicator of recovery progress after acute burns. In clients studied, PCHE decreased during the first 24 hours were correlated with burn severity and mortality. Levels did not return to normal for several days.

PSITTACOSIS TITER, BLOOD

Norm. *Chlamydia* antibody IgG test. Titer ≤1:640. Low titers may be found in psittacosis. A fourfold elevation indicates recent infection.

Usage. Screening for antibodies indicating infection with *Chlamydia psittaci.*

Description. Psittacosis (parrot fever, ornithosis) is a viral infectious disease caused by *C. psittaci. Chlamydia* transmission to humans is believed to be through inhalation of the aerosols of dried droppings and exudates from parrots, birds, and domestic fowl. Person-to-person transmission is rare. Symptoms of psittacosis include mild respiratory symptoms along with fever, headache, muscle aches, and chills. Because laboratory recovery of *C. psittaci* is often difficult, diagnosis is made after a significant rise in the titer of antibodies directed at the psittacosis-lymphogranuloma group of *Chlamydia* is detected.

Professional Considerations
1. Consent form NOT required.
2. **Preparation:**
   A. Tube: Red topped, red/gray topped, or gold topped.
   B. Specimens MAY be drawn during hemodialysis.
3. **Procedure:**
   A. Draw a 10-mL blood sample, without hemolysis.
   B. Paired samples, an acute-phase specimen, and a convalescent-phase specimen, 2-3 weeks apart, should be obtained.
4. **Postprocedure care:**
   A. None.
5. **Client and family teaching:**
   A. The disease is transmitted through inhalation near bird feces.
   B. If a cough is present in the acute stage, psittacosis is communicable. The client must be placed on respiratory isolation, with close contacts wearing masks for protection. All bodily discharges must be disinfected.
6. **Factors that affect results:**
   A. Other infections such as brucellosis and Q fever can cause false-positive results.
7. **Other data:**
   A. Titer levels collected in the latter course of the infection provide more conclusive evidence of the disease.
   B. Albuminuria is common, whereas sputum culture and smear show normal flora. Cold agglutination is negative.
   C. In many countries, psittacosis is a reportable disease.
   D. Tetracyclines are used for the treatment of psittacosis.
   E. For diagnosis of psittacosis, prior contact with sick birds or employment in poultry business or a pet shop should be documented.

PTC
(see Percutaneous transhepatic cholangiography, Diagnostic)

PTH
(see Parathyroid hormone, Blood)

PTHC
(see Percutaneous transhepatic cholangiography, Diagnostic)

PTT
(see Activated partial thromboplastin time and partial thromboplastin time, Plasma)

PULMONARY ANGIOGRAM (PULMONARY ANGIOGRAPHY, PULMONARY ARTERIOGRAPHY), DIAGNOSTIC

Norm. Radiopaque iodine contrast material should circulate symmetrically and without interruption through the pulmonary circulatory system.

Usage. Visualization of the size and shape of the pulmonary artery, its branches, and the pulmonary vascular bed; measurements of pressures within these structures, cardiac output, and pulmonary vascular resistance determinations; assessment of pulmonary vascular perfusion defects, including aneurysms, blood vessel displacement, stenosis, thrombi, and vascular filling defects; definitive diagnostic test for pulmonary thromboembolism, in the symptomatic client and in clients at risk on anticoagulation therapy and when lung scans are normal or inconclusive; definitive test for lung torsion; and evaluation of the pulmonary circulatory system preoperatively in clients with congenital heart disease.

Description. Pulmonary angiography is an invasive roentgenographic, fluoroscopic procedure after injection of iodine radiopaque contrast material via a catheter inserted through an antecubital or femoral vein into the pulmonary artery or one of its branches. Recurrence rates of pulmonary embolism are low if a normal result is found.

Professional Considerations
1. Consent form IS required.

Risks
Acute pulmonary hypertension, acute renal failure (related to the presence of contrast material), arterial occlusion, dysrhythmias, embolism, hemorrhage, infection, allergic reaction to dye (itching, hives, rash, tight feeling in the throat, shortness of breath, bronchospasm, anaphylaxis, death), perforation of pulmonary artery or myocardium, renal toxicity from contrast medium, venous occlusion, ventricular dysrhythmias.

Contraindications
Previous allergy to iodine, radiographic dye, or shellfish; pregnancy (because of radioactive iodine crossing the blood-placental barrier); renal insufficiency. Sedatives are contraindicated in clients with central nervous system depression.

2. **Preparation:**
   A. Recent coagulation times, platelet count, and renal function should be noted.
   B. A mild sedative may be prescribed.
   C. Establish intravenous access for use in the event of a hypersensitivity or dysrhythmic complication.
   D. Obtain electrocardiographic patches, surgical scrub solution, povidone-iodine solution, sterile drapes, 1-2% lidocaine (Xylocaine), radiopaque contrast material, a pulmonary artery catheter, and a pulmonary angiography tray. The amount of contrast dye used is based on the client's body weight.
   E. Have an emergency cart readily available.
   F. See *Client and family teaching*.
3. **Procedure:**
   A. The client is placed in the supine position. Electrodes are connected to a cardiac monitor.
   B. The femoral or antecubital vein site is cleansed with surgical scrub solution, followed by povidone-iodine solution, and covered with sterile drapes.
   C. After a local anesthetic is injected over the site, a needle puncture is made into the vein, a guidewire is placed through the needle, and a long catheter is introduced over

the wire through the antecubital or femoral vein and advanced into the pulmonary vasculature. Pressures are measured as the catheter passes through the right atrium, right ventricle, and into the pulmonary artery.
   D. As the contrast material is injected, rapid, serial roentgenographic images or films record the circulation of the dye through the pulmonary vasculature.
   E. Monitor the client throughout the procedure for cardiac dysrhythmias or a hypersensitivity reaction to the contrast material.
   F. The catheter is removed, and a pressure dressing is applied over the insertion site.
4. **Postprocedure care:**
   A. Monitor the catheter-insertion site for bleeding, inflammation, or hematoma formation.
   B. Assess vital signs according to institutional protocol (usually every 15 minutes × 4 and then every 4 hours × 4).
   C. Although hypersensitivity reactions usually occur during the first 30 minutes after injection of radiopaque iodine, a delayed reaction is possible.
   D. Resume previous diet.
   E. No blood pressures should be taken from the extremity used for injection for 24 hours.
5. **Client and family teaching:**
   A. Fast for 8 hours before the procedure.
   B. For 5 minutes after the injection of the contrast material, an urge to cough, flushing, nausea, or salty taste may occur.
   C. The client must lie motionless during the procedure.
6. **Factors that affect results:**
   A. The client must be able to lie motionless during the procedure.
7. **Other data:**
   A. Small peripheral emboli may not be visible with angiography, but these rarely produce symptoms or result in the usual outcomes of embolism.

PULMONARY ARTERIOGRAPHY, DIAGNOSTIC
(see Pulmonary angiogram, Diagnostic)

PULMONARY ARTERY CATHETERIZATION, DIAGNOSTIC

Norm:

ADULT PRESSURES

Right atrial (RA) pressure	3-11 mm Hg
Central venous pressure (CVP)	2-6 mm Hg
	(2.7-12 cm H_2O)
Right ventricular systolic pressure (RVSP)	20-30 mm Hg
Right ventricular end-diastolic pressure (RVEDP)	<5 mm Hg
Pulmonary artery systolic (PAS) pressure	20-30 mm Hg
Pulmonary artery end-diastolic pressure (PAEDP)	8-15 mm Hg
Pulmonary artery mean (PAM) pressure	<20 mm Hg
Pulmonary artery wedge pressure (PAWP)	4-12 mm Hg
or pulmonary capillary wedge pressure (PCWP)	
Cardiac output (CO)	5-8 L/minute
Cardiac index	2.5-3.5 L/minute/m^2
Pulmonary vascular resistance	80-240 dyne/second/cm^{-5}
Systemic vascular resistance	800-1300 dyne/second/cm^{-5}

Usage. Assessment, diagnosis, and evaluation of the effects of therapy on right and left ventricular function; measurement of cardiac output and cardiac and pulmonary pressures; access to central venous blood and mixed venous blood samples; monitoring of mixed venous oxygen saturation (SvO$_2$); temporary atrial, ventricular, or atrioventricular sequential pacing by means of a thermodilution pulmonary arterial pacing catheter; and preoperative, intraoperative, and postoperative uses, including monitoring of high-risk clients (those with a history of angina, cardiopulmonary disease, or potential fluid shifts during surgery), elderly clients, and high or low cardiac output states, and in situations when hypotensive anesthesia is used. Indications for pulmonary artery catheterization include acute myocardial infarction, angina (severe), burns (severe), cardiomyopathy, congestive heart failure, cardiac tamponade, intraoperative cardiac collapse, failure to respond to appropriate resuscitative measures, fluid-related hypotension and hypovolemia, intravascular control problems, noncardiogenic pulmonary edema, pulmonary congestive states, pulmonary edema, pulmonary failure, pulmonary hypertension, renal disease, right and left ventricular failure, shock states (cardiogenic, hypovolemic, septic, traumatic with concomitant heart failure), tissue perfusion (altered), and titration of chronotropic, inotropic, or vasoactive pharmacologic agents.

Description. Pulmonary artery (PA) catheterization is an invasive procedure using a radiopaque polyvinyl chloride, flow-directed, balloon-tipped catheter containing fluid-filled proximal, distal, and thermistor lumens and a balloon inflation lumen with a valve. Proper placement of the catheter in the PA, in the lower one third of the lung (zone 3), where venous pressures are greater than alveolar pressure, allows for measurement of CVP, PAS, PAEDP, PAM, and PAWP pressures. Intermittent occlusion of the PA branch by inflation of the balloon tip with air or carbon dioxide (never fluid) temporarily impedes blood flow from the right side of the heart to the lungs. The mitral valve opens during diastole, permitting the distal part of the catheter to record pressure that is reflected backward through the left atrium and pulmonary capillary bed. Identical pressures in the left ventricle, left atrium, and pulmonary vasculature momentarily occur during diastole and are captured as the PAWP when the balloon is inflated.

Professional Considerations
1. Consent form MAY be required.

Risks
Air embolism, arterial occlusion, dysrhythmias, hemothorax, infection, per-

foration of the pulmonary vasculature or myocardium, pneumothorax, pulmonary embolus or thrombus, ventricular tachycardia, cardiac valvular damage, complete heart block in clients with pre-existing left bundle branch block.

Contraindications
History of latex allergy (for catheters containing latex or latex balloons).

2. **Preparation:**
   A. Cardiac assessment for history of complete left bundle branch block is indicated before insertion of a PA catheter because there is slight risk for developing a right bundle branch block during catheter insertion, resulting in complete heart block. Standby external transcutaneous pacemaker, insertion of temporary pacemaker, or use of a pacing thermodilution PA catheter can be used for those at risk for this complication.
   B. Assemble and prepare monitoring equipment according to institutional protocol. This includes the following:
      i. Program the monitor for PA pressure display.
      ii. Prepare a transducer with high-pressure tubing for hemodynamic monitoring and a pressure bag of normal saline or heparin flush solution according to institutional protocol.
      iii. Balance the transducer at the phlebostatic axis (the level of the client's right atrium, the fourth intercostal space at the midaxillary line).
   C. Have an emergency cart on standby. Have lidocaine (100 mg) for intravenous use at the bedside in the event of sustained ventricular tachycardia caused by catheter irritation of the right ventricle.
   D. Obtain povidone-iodine solution, sterile drapes, 1%-2% lidocaine (Xylocaine), introducer (sheath, Cordis) trays, a pulmonary artery catheter tray, and 0.9% saline or heparin flush solution.
   E. The physician(s) performing the procedure should wear the fol-

lowing: a sterile gown, a sterile mask, a cap, and sterile gloves.
   F. The procedure may be performed at the bedside or under fluoroscopy.

3. **Procedure:**
   A. The PA catheter may be inserted percutaneously into the external or internal jugular veins, femoral or subclavian veins, and the antecubital fossa veins by venous cutdown.
   B. The client is placed in the supine position. For subclavian or internal jugular insertions, the head of the bed is lowered slightly into a shallow Trendelenburg position. The flat supine position is preferred; however, if not tolerated by the client, a low semi-Fowler's position is acceptable, provided that the same position is maintained throughout the procedure.
   C. Electrocardiographic monitoring is performed throughout the procedure.
   D. After the site is cleansed with povidone-iodine solution and allowed to dry, it is covered with sterile drapes.
   E. A protective sleeve is placed over the PA catheter, and the catheter is flushed with sterile 0.9% saline or heparin flush solution (heparin 100 U/mL of 0.9% saline). The balloon at the distal end of the PA catheter is tested for proper inflation and integrity by injection of 1-1.5 mL of air into the PA distal injection port.
   F. The PA distal port is connected to the transducer tubing and a paper printout of the PA tracing is started and run continuously throughout the catheter insertion.
   G. The site is anesthetized with 1%-2% lidocaine. For subclavian or internal jugular (IJ) insertions, the Seldinger technique is used as follows. The vessel is cannulated with a 22- or 25-gauge needle (IJ insertions only; subclavian insertions omit this step). A large-bore needle is inserted over the small needle, and the small needle is removed. A guidewire is inserted through the large-bore needle, and that needle is removed. The introducer is then inserted

over the guidewire, and the guidewire is removed. The introducer is then secured into place.

H. The PA catheter is inserted through the introducer and directed into the right atrium and through the tricuspid valve into the right ventricle. As the catheter traverses the right ventricle, the balloon at the distal portion of the catheter is inflated to permit normal cardiac blood flow to carry (float) the catheter through the pulmonic valve into the PA. Inflation of the balloon and flow-direction minimize the potential of catheter-induced ventricular dysrhythmias and irritability. However, the risk for ventricular tachycardia is greatest while the PA catheter tip is passing through the right ventricle. If ventricular tachycardia occurs, the catheter should be either advanced through the pulmonary valve or withdrawn into the right atrium. Lidocaine and emergency measures are seldom needed because the removal of the catheter as a ventricular irritant is usually sufficient to stop the tachycardia.

I. As the catheter is slowly inserted, placement and progress are assessed by observation of the monitor for the waveform and pressure changes characteristic of the different chambers and vessels of the cardiac and pulmonary anatomy. When the waveform changes from a PA waveform to a PAWP waveform, the balloon is allowed to deflate, and the catheter is secured into this position. The syringes of flush solution are removed, and the ports are either connected to a continuous flush solution or capped, according to the policy of the institution.

4. **Postprocedure care:**
   A. Apply an occlusive sterile dressing to the PA catheter-insertion site.
   B. Obtain a chest radiograph for verification of the catheter placement if fluoroscopy has not been used.
   C. PA pressures should be monitored continuously. The waveform should be frequently observed for progression of the catheter tip into a wedge position.

5. **Client and family teaching:**
   A. If the access is subclavian or jugular, the head will be covered with a sterile drape during the procedure.
   B. Activity may be limited during the time a PA catheter is in place.

6. **Factors that affect results:**
   A. The mechanical factors that invalidate pressure measurements include the following:
      i. *Air bubbles* in pressure tubing system or transducer cause dampening of the waveform.
      ii. *Kinking of pressure tubing* causes dampening of the waveform.
      iii. *Improper tubing length:* Tubing should not exceed 48 inches in length from the client to the transducer.
      iv. *Loose connections* interfere with the high-pressure pathway along the tubing and may cause waveform artifact and false readings.
      v. *Stopcocks* between the transducer and the PA distal port distort PA pressures slightly, but effects increase with an increased number of stopcocks. For this reason, use no more than one stopcock for ports through which pressures are monitored.
      vi. *Blood return* in the transducer tubing. The continual flush–counteracting pressure should be maintained at 300 mm Hg.
      vii. *Catheter artifact* (catheter whip, catheter fling) results from excessive catheter movement during cardiac contraction when the distal tip of the catheter is too close to the pulmonary valve.
      viii. *Catheter displacement* may result from backward recoil into the right ventricle as evidenced by large RV waveforms. It may also result from forward migration into a wedged position.
      ix. *Migration of the catheter against the vessel wall* may cause a dampened waveform and affect pressure readings.

Repositioning the client or asking the client to cough may help to return the tip to a floating position. The catheter should never be flushed if a spontaneous wedge position is suspected.

x. *A flush solution rate* affects pressure readings. Clot formation near the distal port as a result of too slow a flush rate dampens the waveform and causes falsely low readings. Falsely high readings may result from a flush rate >3-6 mL/hour.

xi. *Incorrect transducer* position below the phlebostatic axis causes falsely low pressure readings. A transducer higher than the phlebostatic axis causes falsely high pressure readings. Each 1 cm difference alters the reading by 1 mm Hg.

xii. *Malfunction of equipment,* which may include the amplifier, the oscilloscope, the recording devices, or the transducer.

xiii. *Positive-pressure mechanical ventilation* (PEEP) elevates pressures slightly. Formulas are available to compensate for this effect. PEEP should never be discontinued to obtain pressure readings because the discontinuation has been shown to be deleterious to the client's condition.

xiv. *Overinflation of the balloon* results in inflation larger than what is necessary for the vessel size, recognized by a drifting up or down of the PAWP waveform. Overinflation may cause rupture of the pulmonary capillary. Air should be injected into the balloon very slowly while one continuously watched for a waveform change to a wedge position. Proper placement of the PA catheter is indicated when a PAWP waveform is obtained with 0.8-1.2 cc of air. At no time should more than 1.5 cc of air be injected into the balloon. Assessment or adjustment of PA catheter placement by a physician is indicated if a PAWP waveform cannot be obtained with ≥1.5 cc of air.

xv. *A ruptured balloon* is indicated when one feels no resistance to air injection into the balloon port, along with an absence of a PAWP waveform or by the presence of blood in the PA distal (balloon) port. Balloon rupture may result from a manufacturing defect or from balloon weakening after many inflations. Manual deflation may accelerate balloon weakening. If a ruptured balloon is suspected, no more air should be injected, and a physician should immediately assess the client.

xvi. *Respiratory variation* as a result of inspiration and expiration cannot be accounted for by digital averaging. The most accurate readings of pressures are calculated manually from paper recordings of the waveforms at end expiration.

xvii. *Retrograde injection* during cardiac output measurement is indicated when a backflow of blood or fluid is detected in the introducer or protective sleeve of the catheter. This is an indication that the catheter injectate opening is located within the lumen of the introducer, rather than in the right atrium. Retrograde injection results in inadequate thermodilution and falsely high cardiac output values.

B. Physiologic conditions that alter pressure measurements of the different chambers and vessels include the following:

   i. *RA/CVP:* Cardiac tamponade, fluid overload, pulmonary disease, pulmonary hypertension, right heart failure, tricuspid regurgitation, and tricuspid stenosis.

   ii. *RV:* Chronic congestive heart failure, constrictive pericarditis, pericardial effusion, pulmonary hypertension, pulmonary valvular stenosis, right ventricular failure, and ventricular septal defects.

iii. *PAS/PAD:* Chronic obstructive pulmonary disease, increased pulmonary blood flow, left-to-right shunts secondary to atrial or ventricular septal defects, mitral stenosis, pulmonary edema, pulmonary embolus, and pulmonary hypertension.
iv. *PAWP/PCWP:* Cardiac insufficiency, cardiac tamponade, left ventricular failure, mitral regurgitation, and mitral stenosis.

7. **Other data:**
   A. Transducers should be balanced every 2-4 hours with position and ventilator changes and before each measurement of PA catheter parameters.
   B. PA catheter balloons should never be manually deflated. The air should be allowed to flow back into the syringe spontaneously.
   C. The flexible PA catheter includes two-lumen, three-lumen, four-lumen thermodilutional, and five-lumen catheters of varying lengths. Sizes include 5, 6, 7, and 7.5 Fr, with markings at 10-cm increments along the outer surface.
   D. Although the information obtained from the pulmonary artery catheter can help diagnose certain conditions, a meta-analysis routine perioperative use in vascular surgery and a study of use of continuous SvO_2 monitoring during cardiac surgery have not been consistently shown to reduce morbidity and mortality.
   E. Later generations of catheter development include the capability for atrial, ventricular, or AV sequential pacing; continuous mixed venous oxygen saturation (SvO_2); continuous cardiac output; using fiberoptic oximetry; and additional lumens or ports for fluid infusions.

PULMONARY FUNCTION TESTS (PFT), DIAGNOSTIC

Norm. The observed values are reported as percentages of normal with use of prediction equations calculated according to age, height, sex, race, and weight. Results are considered abnormal if they are less than predicted 80% of the calculated values. For spirometry measurement, forced vital capacity, forced expiratory volumes, and peak expiratory flow rates are at predicted value for age, race, sex, and height.

VOLUME	AVERAGE RESULTS FOR ADULTS
Tidal volume (V_T)	500 cc
Expiratory reserve volume (ERV)	1500 cc
Residual volume (RV)	1500 cc
Inspiratory reserve volume (IRV)	2000 cc
Diffusion capacity carbon monoxide	25 mL/min/mm Hg
Spirometry Norms	
Forced vital capacity (FVC)	>80% of predicted volume
Forced expiratory volume (FEV_1)	>80% of predicted volume
FEV_1/FVC ratio	>80%
Elderly clients	70-80%
Forced expiratory flow (FEF) 25-75	>50%

Usage. Diagnosis and monitoring the progress of pulmonary dysfunction (asthma, bronchitis, bronchiolitis obliterans, emphysema, and myasthenia gravis); quantify the severity of known lung disease; evaluate the effectiveness of medications (bronchodilators); determination of whether a functional abnormality is obstructive or restrictive; identification of clients at high risk for postoperative pulmonary complications; evaluation of the risk of pulmonary resection; used in conjunction with a cardiopulmonary exercise stress test for evaluation of functional ability; serial measurements used to evaluate response to treatment in cardiopulmonary vascular disease.

MEASUREMENT	INCREASED	DECREASED
Total Lung Capacity (TLC) = (V_T + ERV + RV + IRV) (total volume of lungs when maximally inflated is divided into four volumes)	Overdistention of the lungs associated with obstructive disease	Restrictive disease
Tidal Volume (V_T) (volume of air inhaled and exhaled in normal quiet breathing)	May indicate bronchiolar obstruction with hyperinflation or emphysema	May indicate fatigue, restrictive parenchymal lung disease, atelectasis, cancer, edema, pulmonary congestion, pneumothorax or thoracic tumor; decreased V_T necessitates further testing
Inspiratory Reserve Volume (IRV) (maximum volume that can be inhaled after a normal quiet inhalation)	n/a	Decreased IRV as an isolated value does not indicate disease
Expiratory Reserve Volume (ERV) (maximum volume that can be exhaled after a normal quiet exhalation)	n/a	May occur with obesity, pregnancy, or thoracoplasty
Residual Volume (RV) (volume remaining in the lungs after maximal exhalation)	Increased RV above 35% of the TLC indicates obstructive disease; RV is also increased with aging	n/a
Forced Expiratory Volume (FEV) (volume expired during specified time intervals [0.5 and 1 second]).	Restrictive disease	Decreased FEV_1 after the administration of beta-blockers may indicate the presence of bronchospasm and contraindicate the continued use of the specific pharmacologic therapy involved
Forced Expiratory Volume I (FEV_1) (air volume forcefully exhaled in 1 second)	Restrictive disease	Decreased FEV_1 as percentage of the vital capacity (FEV_1/FVC) indicates obstructive disease 65%-80% of predicted = mild disease 50%-65% of predicted = moderate disease <50% of predicted = severe disease

Continued

MEASUREMENT	INCREASED	DECREASED
Functional Residual Capacity (FRC) = (ERV + RV) (amount of volume in the lungs after normal exhalation)	Overdistention of the lungs associated with chronic obstructive pulmonary disease Pulmonary cysts	Acute respiratory distress syndrome (ARDS) Heart failure Kyphoscoliosis Muscular weakness Pulmonary granulomatosis Restrictive diseases and mixed obstructive and restrictive diseases
Inspiratory Capacity (IC) = (IRV + V_T) (maximum volume that can be inhaled after a normal quiet exhalation); useful in evaluating time-liness of weaning from mechanical ventilation	n/a	Restrictive disease
Vital Capacity (VC) = (IRV + V_T + ERV) (total volume that can be exhaled after maximum inspiration) **Forced Vital Capacity (FVC)** (total volume exhaled forcefully and rapidly after maximum inhalation)	Increased or normal VC and FVC with decreased flow rates indicate an obstructive defect (airway diseases)	Decreased VC with normal or increased flow rates indicates restrictive defect (diaphragmatic impairment; drug overdose, head injury, limited thoracic expansion, and neuromuscular disease) With concurrent heart disease, may indicate pulmonary congestion, pleural effusion, cardiomegaly or muscular weakness
Thoracic Gas Volume (TGV) (total volume of the lungs including nonventilated and ventilated airways)	Indicates air trapping caused by obstructive disease and requires special equipment to monitor	n/a
Minute Volume (MV) = (Respiratory Rate × V_T) (total amount of gas breathed during 1 minute)	Air embolism Bronchospasm Burns Hyperthyroidism Hypovolemia Metabolic or respiratory acidosis PEEP causing increased Intrathoracic pressure Pulmonary embolism Pulmonary parenchymal disease Sepsis Shallow breathing Shock	n/a

MEASUREMENT	INCREASED	DECREASED
Maximum Voluntary Ventilation (MVV) (maximum volume of gas breathed during rapid, forced breathing in 1 minute under testing conditions)	n/a	Obstructive disease
Maximum Breathing Capacity (MBC) (the largest volume of air that can be inhaled and exhaled in 1 minute)	n/a	Obstructive disease
Peak Expiratory Flow Rate (PEFR) (peak flow rate during expiration)	n/a	Asthma
FEV_1/FVC (ratio of FEV_1 to FVC, expressed as a percentage)	n/a	Obstructive airway disease Obstruction
Forced Expiratory Flow (FEF 25-75) (the average forced expiratory flow during the midportion [25%-75%] of the forced vital capacity); useful in clients with small airways, such as children	n/a	Obstructive airway disease

Description. Pulmonary function tests (PFTs) are several different tests used to evaluate lung mechanics, gas exchange, and acid-base disturbance through spirometric measurements, lung volumes, and arterial blood gases. Spirometry testing is included in pulmonary function testing. A spirometer is an instrument that measures lung capacity, volume, and flow rates. The instrument consists of a bell suspended in a container of water. The bell rises and falls in response to the client's breathing. The movement of the bell is recorded on a kymograph or electrical potentiometer. The pattern of the air flow on the graph must be interpreted to identify artifact and abnormalities, such as cough and upper airway obstruction. Full PFTs include measuring the amount of air that can be maximally exhaled after a maximum inspiration and the time required for that expiration and determining the ability of the alveolar capillary membrane to transport oxygen into the blood and carbon dioxide from the blood into the expired air.

Professional Considerations
1. Consent form NOT required.

Risks
Pneumothorax, increased intracranial or intraocular pressure, syncope, dizziness, chest pain, paroxysmal coughing, bronchospasm, oxygen desaturation, hypertension, strain on recent abdominal or thoracic incisions, aneurysm rupture.

Contraindications
Relative contraindications include hemoptysis of unknown origin, pneumothorax, unstable cardiovascular status, recent cardiac event or pulmonary embolus, recent eye surgery, concurrent nausea or vomiting, recent thoracic or abdominal surgery, thoracic, abdominal or cerebral aneurysm.

2. Preparation:
   A. Assess medication record for recent analgesic that may depress respiratory function.

B. Bronchodilators and intermittent positive-pressure breathing therapy may be withheld before the tests.

C. The client should void and then loosen any restrictive clothing.

D. Record the client's age, sex, and race on the test requisition.

E. Carefully measure and record weight and height.

F. Assess baseline vital signs.

G. See *Client and family teaching*.

3. **Procedure:**

A. Position the client sitting with both feet flat on the floor or standing with something to lean on and a chair behind him or her for use if dizziness occurs.

B. Connect the mouthpiece to the spirometer (even in the handled version) and place mouthpiece in the client's mouth.

C. Place the clip over the nose so that only breathing through the mouth is possible.

D. Instruct the client to breathe through a mouthpiece. Up to 8 efforts per measurement period may be needed to obtain results that are reproducible three times.

E. Criteria for acceptable test:
   i. Extrapolated volume of 95% of the FVC or 150 mL, whichever is greater.
   ii. No false starts.
   iii. Rapid start-to-rise time.
   iv. No cough.
   v. Exhalation time of at least 6 seconds.
   vi. The two largest FEV and FEV_1 vary by no more than 0.200 L.
   vii. MVV 12-15 seconds.

F. The two highest MVVs are within 10% of each other.

G. If the test is ordered to include a bronchodilator, administer bronchodilator and wait 15 minutes before repeating the procedure.

4. **Postprocedure care:**

A. Assess vital signs every 5 minutes until they return to baseline value.

B. Resume normal diet and any bronchodilators or intermittent positive-pressure breathing therapy.

C. Results are normally available within 30 minutes. Consideration of client's clinical condition is necessary when one is interpreting results.

D. Flush out air at least 5 times in a volume-displacement spirometer to reduce risk of airborne spread of infection to future clients.

E. Dispose of or disinfect any portions of the test equipment that come into contact with the client.

5. **Client and family teaching:**

A. Withhold short-acting bronchodilator medication for 5 hours before the test or as ordered by physician. Long-acting bronchodilators will be withheld for a longer period of time. If you experience difficult breathing, you should use your bronchodilator.

B. Refrain from smoking or eating a heavy meal for 4-6 hours.

C. Dentures should not be removed.

D. Take a maximal inhalation, hold it, and then maximally and forcibly exhale. A modified technique with an initial forced exhalation followed by a relaxed exhalation continued for as long as possible may be used.

E. After a short rest period, the procedure is repeated two more times.

F. The procedure takes about 20 minutes.

6. **Factors that affect results:**

A. The client's ability to voluntarily and actively participate is essential to complete the indicated tests.

B. An inadequate seal around the mouthpiece invalidates the results.

C. An ineffective nose clip causes unreliable results.

D. Gastric distention, hypoxia, metabolic disturbances, narcotic analgesia, pregnancy, and sedatives may alter the results. Fatigue as a result of repeated efforts may also alter the results.

E. Daily monitoring and calibration is required to ensure accuracy and reproducibility of spirometry results.

F. In one study, obstruction of PFTs included use of tobacco, CAP or hay fever history, age, and male sex.

G. Bronchodilators administered before the tests may obscure true pulmonary function.

H. Herbs or natural remedy effects: In one study, people who received 200 mg of ginseng twice each day for 3 months demonstrated improved FVC, FEV$_1$, and PEFR as well as arterial blood oxygen and walking distance.
7. **Other data:**
   A. Pulmonary function tests are normally performed in a pulmonary laboratory.
   B. See also *Lung scan, Perfusion; Ventilation, Diagnostic; Diffusing capacity carbon monoxide (DLCO).*

PULMONARY SCINTIPHOTOGRAPHY
(see Lung scan, Perfusion and ventilation, Diagnostic)

PULSATILITY INDEX RATIO
(see Pulse volume recording of peripheral vasculature, Diagnostic)

PULSE OXIMETRY
(see Oximetry, Diagnostic)

PULSE VOLUME RECORDER TESTING OF PERIPHERAL VASCULATURE, DIAGNOSTIC

Norm. The waveform recording demonstrates rapid upstroke or an anacrotic limb, a sharp peak, a brisk decline or catacrotic limb, and a clearly discernible visual diastolic wave. Bilateral consistent augmentation of the pulse amplitude from proximal-to-distal measurement sites is present throughout the waveform recordings.

Usage. Assists in the diagnosis, location, and monitoring of the progression of arterial vascular lesions and arterial narrowing; preoperative, intraoperative, and postoperative evaluations; aids in the determination of the need for arterial angiography; differentiation of aortoiliac and superficial femoral artery occlusion and neuropathies; assists in the evaluation of the severity of arterial occlusions and the detection of arterial pressure changes in distal extremity vessels that cannot be measured by a Doppler probe; helps evaluate penile blood flow and intercavernous pressure; TFI method used to monitor venous grafts at risk for failing.

Description. *Pulse volume recording* measures pressure changes of arterial vessels and displays the pressure changes as waveforms. Pressure changes are recorded by a transducer during blood pressure cuff inflation and deflation. Segmental air plethysmography records the pulse waveform tracings onto graph paper. These pressure recordings supplement segmental limb pressure studies and are a sensitive indicator of arterial vascular occlusive disease of the distal vessels of the feet and toes. Recordings may be taken before or after segmental limb-pressure measurements. Arterial narrowing distal to a vascular lesion produces a loss of the diastolic wave, a prolonged catacrotic limb (prolonged downstroke tracing), rounding of the normally sharp peak, and a decrease in the slope of the anacrotic limb (vertical ascending limb). Progression of arterial occlusive disease results in a broadened, flattened, lengthened, and dampened waveform with depression in the amplitude of the diastolic wave. A *transfer function index* (TFI) or *pulsatility index ratio* (PIR) may be generated by the equipment to demonstrate abnormalities in perfusion via color coding. A variation of the pulse volume recording procedure is *pulse volume plethysmography,* in which a water-filled cuff is placed around the penis and an assessment of continuous blood flow and intercavernous pressure is taken.

Professional Considerations
1. Consent form NOT required.
2. **Preparation:**
   A. Remove clothing from each extremity.
3. **Procedure:**
   A. Traditional pulse volume recording:
      i. The client is placed in the prone position.
      ii. Blood-pressure cuffs that have a length of 80% of the limb circumference and a width of 40% of the limb circumference and a pneumatic inflatable bladder that is 20% wider than the limb diameter are selected.

iii. The pressure cuffs are placed bilaterally 2.5 cm above the antecubital crease of the arm, just above the wrist, as high as possible on the thigh, just below the knee, and just above the malleolus of the ankle.

iv. Transmetatarsal and penile pressure recordings may be obtained.

v. Pulse volume recordings are measured at brachial, radial, ulnar, femoral, popliteal, dorsalis pedis, and posterior tibial levels of each resting extremity.

vi. Pressure changes are recorded by a transducer during cuff inflation and deflation.

vii. Cuff inflation is measured by standard mercury-gravity or aneroid manometer.

viii. Cuff deflation is measured by stethoscope, plethysmography, or the Doppler velocity detector, which is the most convenient and sensitive measurement device.

ix. A segmental air plethysmography records the pulse-waveform tracings onto graph paper.

x. The same procedure is used for pediatrics.

B. Pulse volume plethysmography of penile blood flow:

i. The procedure may be performed to measure natural variations in blood flow while the client sleeps, or during visual sexual stimulation or during artificial erection.

ii. A cuff filled with water is placed around the penis and connected to a three-way tap. One of the taps is covered with a latex membrane, which displaces in response to penile blood flow. Another tap is connected to a pressure bag positioned 30 cm above the penis. A second cuff is placed around the base of the penis.

iii. As variations in blood flow occur, the displacement of the latex membrane is recorded by a photoplethysmograph. Artificial variations in blood

flow may be induced by compression of the penis artery via the base cuff.

iv. Findings are used by the equipment to determine a *pulsatility index ratio* (PIR), which is a ratio of total vascular resistance in the penis divided by functional impedance at the current heart rate. The PIR, along with the transfer function index display a color coded screen that represents differing perfusion between adjacent cuff segments.

4. Postprocedure care:
A. Remove cuffs.

5. Client and family teaching:
A. The procedure takes 30 minutes, unless performed during sleep.
B. Results are available immediately.

6. Factors that affect results:
A. Improper size, inflation, or loose cuff application causes inaccurate results.
B. False-negative results have been reported in clients with a short segmental occlusion of the superficial femoral artery in which they have developed large femoral collateral circulation. The pulse-volume recording produced a very depressed thigh tracing without discernible augmentation over the occluded site while circulation to the extremity was maintained.

7. Other data:
A. Pulse-volume recording of peripheral vascular pulses reports 97% accuracy for detecting superficial femoral artery occlusion.

PURE TONE AUDIOMETRY, DIAGNOSTIC
(*see Audiometry test, Diagnostic*)

PYELOGRAPHY, ANTEGRADE, DIAGNOSTIC
(*see Antegrade pyelography, Diagnostic*)

PYELOGRAPHY, RETROGRADE, DIAGNOSTIC
(*see Retrograde pyelography, Diagnostic*)

PYP SCAN
(see Heart scan, Diagnostic)

4-PYRIDOXIC ACID
(see Vitamin B$_6$, Urine)

PYRIDOXAL
(see Vitamin B$_6$, Plasma)

PYRIDOXINE
(see Vitamin B$_6$, Plasma)

PYRIDOXAMINE
(see Vitamin B$_6$, Plasma)

Q

QUINIDINE, SERUM

Norm. *Note:* Quinidine takes 2 days to reach steady-state.

	TROUGH	SI UNITS
Therapeutic level	2-5 µg/mL	6.16–15.41 µmol/L
Toxic level	>6 µg/mL	>18.49 µmol/L
Lethal level	>30 µg/mL	>92.46 µmol/L

Panic Level Symptoms and Treatment. 65% of people with levels over 14 µg/mL (for the double extraction test methodology) have toxic symptoms.

Symptoms. Asthmatic or angioneurotic phenomena, Ataxia, cinchonism (headache, dizziness, hearing loss, ringing in the ears), respiratory depression, vomiting, diarrhea, severe hypotension, syncope, anuria, cardiac dysrhythmia (asystole, heart block, widening of QRS and QT interval, sodium-channel blockade manifesting as early prolonged QRS interval, rightward axis of 40 msec, presence of an R-wave in the aV$_R$ lead and an S-wave in leads I and aV$_L$, paradoxical tachycardia, ventricular tachycardia), embolism, hallucinations, paresthesia, irritability.

Treatment:
Note: Treatment choice(s) depend on client history and condition and episode history.
Maintain airway and hemodynamic stability.
Provide transcutaneous or transvenous temporary pacemaker.
Acidify urine.
Perform gastric lavage.
Implement forced emesis.
Administer infusion of a sodium molar lactate.
Treat respiratory depression with caffeine, ephedrine, oxygen, or mechanical ventilation.
Administer epinephrine and/or antiasthmatics for angioneurotic or asthmatic symptoms phenomena.
Consider administration of nitrates and methacholine for toxic amaurosis (residual visual impairment).
Transfusion, if warranted due to severe hemoglobinuria.
Both hemodialysis and peritoneal dialysis WILL remove quinidine in small amounts.

Increased. Impaired hepatic function, impaired renal function, and urine alkalinity. Drugs include acetazolamide, amiodarone, antacids, carbonic anhydrase inhibitors, cimetidine, magnesium hydroxide, nifedipine, propranolol, sodium bicarbonate, thiazide diuretics, and verapamil.

Decreased. Urine acidity. Drugs include ascorbic acid, barbiturates, nifedipine, phenobarbital, phenytoin, phenytoin sodium, primidone, and rifampin.

Description. Quinidine is class 1A antidysrhythmic that exerts a depressant effect on myocardial excitability, conduction velocity, and contractility. It causes decreased sodium, potassium, and calcium influx across the cell membrane, resulting in a prolongation of the myocardial refractory period. In larger doses, the ventricular response rate is increased through anticholinergic inhibition of vagal stimulation of the AV node. Quinidine is metabolized by the liver and excreted unchanged in the urine, with a half-life of 4-10 hours. Steady-state levels are reached after 20-35 hours. Toxicity may result in prolongation of the QRS complex >25% from baseline value, hypotension, and cardiac standstill. Because 70%-80% of quinidine is bound to plasma protein and plasma binding varies among individuals, it is recommended that the *unbound* portion of quinidine be measured and doses be adjusted in conjunction with serial measurements. This is of particular importance during pregnancy, when changes in protein-binding occur.

Professional Considerations

1. Consent form NOT required.
2. **Preparation:**
   A. Tube: royal blue topped. Do NOT use a serum separator tube.
   B. Do NOT draw specimens during hemodialysis.
3. **Procedure:**
   A. Draw a 3-mL TROUGH blood sample. Obtain serial measurements at the same time each day.
4. **Postprocedure care:**
   A. None.
5. **Client and family teaching:**
   A. Take medication as prescribed.
   B. Report any side effects, such as nausea, vomiting, and dizziness.
   C. Check pulse every day when taking quinidine. The client should notify the physician when panic level symptoms (see p. 941) are noted.
6. **Factors that affect results:**
   A. When obtaining serial samples, the same time interval between drug dosing and sample collection should be observed.
   B. Peak quinidine levels occur 1.5-2 hours after oral administration.
   C. Acidification of the urine increases excretion of quinidine. Alkalinization of the urine decreases excretion of this drug.
   D. If the radioimmunoassay is used for testing, instead of high-performance liquid chromatography (HPLC), values may be overestimated due to the cross-reactivity of dihydroquinone, an impurity present in up to 15% of quinidine preparations.
7. **Other data:**
   A. Coadministration of quinidine with digoxin increases the risk of digoxin toxicity.
   B. Quinidine may cause an increase in bleeding tendencies secondary to inhibition of hepatic production of vitamin K-dependent clotting factors.

RABIES, BLOOD
(see Animals and rabies, Serum)

RADIOALLERGOSORBENT TEST, SERUM
(see Allergin-specific IgE antibody, Serum)

RADIOGRAPHIC ABSORPTIOMETRY, DIAGNOSTIC
(see Bone densitometry, Diagnostic)

RADIOGRAPHY, DIAGNOSTIC
(see Bone radiography, Diagnostic; Cardiac radiography, Diagnostic; Chest radiography, Diagnostic; Esophageal radiography; Eye radiography, Diagnostic; Flat-plate radiography of abdomen, Diagnostic; Radiography of skull, chest, and cervical spine, Diagnostic; Sinus radiography, Diagnostic)

RADIOGRAPHY OF SKULL, CHEST, AND CERVICAL SPINE, DIAGNOSTIC

Norm. Negative for fracture or dislocation.

Usage. Trauma and determination of location and extent of suspected skull fracture or cervical spine damage.

Description. This procedure involves radiographic examination of the skull, chest, and cervical spine to detect skull and spinal injuries resulting from accidents or physically induced. Fractures of the skull are classified by location and type. Types of skull fractures may be penetrating, depressed, bending, lin-

R

ear, or diastatic (involving the skull suture area or areas). The orbits are examined for the presence of free air, which indicates a fractured sinus area. Radiography of the chest and cervical spine identifies the seven cervical spine segments as well as the C7-T1 area and relationship. Definite indications for cervical spine radiographs include neck pain or a tender cervical area. Other indications may include decreased level of consciousness, paresthesias, decreased sensation, weakness, muscle spasm near the cervical area, or decreased anal tone.

Professional Considerations
1. Consent form NOT required.

Precautions
During pregnancy, risks of cumulative radiation exposure to the fetus from this and other previous or future imaging studies must be weighed against the benefits of the procedure. Although formal limits for client exposure are relative to this risk:benefit comparison, the United States Nuclear Regulatory Commission requires that the cumulative dose equivalent to an embryo/fetus from occupational exposure not exceed 0.5 rem (5 mSv). Radiation dosage to the fetus is proportional to the distance of the anatomy studied from the abdomen and decreases as pregnancy progresses. For pregnant clients, consult the radiologist/radiology department to obtain estimated fetal radiation exposure from this procedure.

2. **Preparation:**
   A. Move the client only the minimal amount necessary to obtain the different radiographic views.
   B. Maintain strict body alignment throughout transport and transfer of the client. If uncooperative or combative, the client may need to be intubated, paralyzed, and mechanically ventilated to maintain alignment.
3. **Procedure:**
   A. *Skull radiography:* Conventional plain-film radiography of the skull is performed, including the following views: posteroanterior, anteroposterior in Towne's projection, two lateral views, posteroanterior Waters's, and lateral views designed to highlight the facial area.

   B. *Chest and cervical spine radiography:* Conventional plain-film radiography of the cervical spine is performed, including the following views: anteroposterior, lateral, both obliques, and one that shows the ondontoid process. Risks versus benefits must be considered before flexion and extension views are taken.
4. **Postprocedure care:**
   A. Maintain strict body alignment until radiograph results are known.
   B. Perform postsedation or paralytic monitoring per institutional protocol if either was used.
5. **Client and family teaching:**
   A. Results are normally available within 24 hours or immediately in case of emergency.
   B. Body alignment should be maintained until results are known.
6. **Factors that affect results:**
   A. Linear skull fractures may not be detected if their location is not on the side of the skull closest to the film. They must be distinguished from vascular grooves of the skull.
   B. Skull suture area (diastatic) fractures are difficult to detect without a great deal of experience in radiographic interpretation.
   C. Skull radiograph interpretation should take into consideration clinical findings from scalp and soft-tissue examination.
7. **Other data:**
   A. Nuclear medicine studies can help pinpoint fractures near the base of the skull that are not demonstrable by conventional radiography.
   B. Computed tomography of the spine may be needed to detect spinal fractures not demonstrable by conventional radiography.
   C. Because as many as half of spinal injuries occur below the cervical area, radiographs of the lower spine should also be taken.

RADIONUCLIDE BREAST IMAGING, DIAGNOSTIC
(*see Scintimammography, Diagnostic*)

RADIONUCLIDE VENOGRAPHY
(*see Venography, Diagnostic*)

RAJI CELL ASSAY, BLOOD

Norm:

Normal	<13 μg AHG Eq/mL
Borderline	13-25 μg AHG Eq/mL
Abnormal	≥26 μg AHG Eq/mL

Usage. Detection of immune complexes in the following: autoimmune disorders; celiac disease; cirrhosis; Crohn's disease; cryoglobulinemia; dermatitis herpetiformis; disseminated malignancy; drug reactions; microbial, parasitic, and viral infections; and sickle cell anemia.

Description. Complement receptors for IgG are found on the Raji cells, which are lymphoblastoid cells that contain receptors for complement, particularly C3b. Raji cells are derived from Burkitt's lymphoma and are used to recognize and bind protein-bound immune complexes that contain C3b. Results are reported in the quantity of precipitated immune complexes. Detection of circulating immune complexes is used to help determine the mechanisms of autoimmune diseases.

Professional Considerations

1. Consent form NOT required.
2. **Preparation:**
   A. Preschedule this test with the laboratory.
   B. Tube: Chilled green topped.
   C. Specimens MAY be drawn during hemodialysis.
3. **Procedure:**
   A. Draw a 5-mL blood sample.
   B. Heelstick is acceptable, collected in a Microtainer.
   C. Place the tube in a container of ice and water.
4. **Postprocedure care:**
   A. Transport the specimen to the laboratory immediately.
5. **Client and family teaching:**
   A. The test is used to help diagnose autoimmune diseases.
6. **Factors that affect results:**
   A. Results may be unreliable if the client has undergone a recent scan involving the injection of radioactive dye.
7. **Other data:**
   A. AHG measurement stands for aggregated human gamma globulin equivalents.
   B. See also *Immune complex assay, Blood.*

RAPID PLASMA REAGIN (RPR) TEST, BLOOD

Norm. Negative, nonreactive sample.

Positive. Borderline, reactive, and weakly reactive are considered positive results for the syphilis antibody. A reactive result is suggestive of contraction of syphilis, but diagnosis must be confirmed by medical examination and history.

Negative. RPR nonreactive results may be reported in clients who are treated before the appearance of the primary chancre (in the primary phase), those treated after the appearance of the primary chancre but before the appearance of the reagin, and those treated in the secondary phase of the disease. This test can be substituted for the Venereal Disease Research Laboratory (VDRL) test. Seronegative results occur with alcohol ingestion before the test and during inactive or latent-phase syphilis.

Description. Syphilis is a complex sexually transmitted disease characterized by a wide range of symptoms that imitate other diseases. It is caused by the organism *Treponema pallidum.* The RPR test is a macroscopic agglutination screening test for the presence of reagin, the antibody specific for the treponemal spirochete. In this test, an antigen (cardiolipin phospholipid derived from beef heart) to reagin is used to detect an agglutination reaction, indicating a positive test result. The RPR test is most useful during the secondary stage of syphilis, at the peak of reagin antibody presence in the blood. This test is inexpensive and widely used for mass testing for syphilis. However, its sensitivity in primary syphilis is fairly poor, and many biologic false-positive results are possible.

Professional Considerations

1. Consent form NOT required.
2. **Preparation:**
   A. Tube: Red topped, red/gray topped, or gold topped.
   B. See *Client and family teaching.*
   C. Specimens MAY be drawn during hemodialysis.
3. **Procedure:**
   A. Draw a 7-mL blood sample.
   B. Heelstick is acceptable, collected in a Microtainer.

4. **Postprocedure care:**
   A. State law may require completion of a confidential department of health form when a specimen is reported as reactive.
5. **Client and family teaching:**
   A. Do not drink alcohol for 24 hours before the test.
   B. Assess the client's understanding of safe sexual practices.
   C. If testing is positive and a syphilis diagnosis is confirmed:
      i. Notify all sexual contacts from the last 90 days (if early stage) to be tested for syphilis.
      ii. Syphilis can be cured with antibiotics. These may worsen the symptoms for the first 24 hours.
      iii. Do not have sex for 2 months and until after repeat testing has confirmed that the syphilis is cured. Use condoms after that for 2 years. Return for repeat testing every 3-4 months for the next 2 years to make sure the disease is cured.
      iv. Do not become pregnant for 2 years because syphilis can be transmitted to the fetus.
      v. If left untreated, syphilis can damage many body organs, including the brain, over several years.
6. **Factors that affect results:**
   A. Alcohol ingestion within the previous 24 hours produces transient nonreactive results.
   B. Hemolysis of the specimen invalidates the results.
   C. Serum samples should be drawn before meals because chyme alters the reaction.
   D. Refrigeration destroys *Treponema* spirochetes in 72 hours.
   E. Conditions that may cause false-positive results include active immunization in children, antinuclear antibodies, antiphospholipid antibody syndromes, blood loss (with multiple transfusions), chancroid, chickenpox, cirrhosis, the common cold, diabetes mellitus, fever (relapsing), hepatitis (infectious), HIV, hypergammaglobulinemia, leprosy, leptospirosis (Weil's disease), Lyme disease, lymphogranuloma venereum, lymphoma, infection (chronic), malaria, measles, mononucleosis (infectious), *Mycoplasma* pneumonia, nonsyphilitic treponemal diseases (bejel, pinta, yaws), periarteritis nodosa, pneumococcal pneumonia, pneumonia, pregnancy, rat-bite fever, rheumatic fever, rheumatic heart disease, rheumatoid arthritis, scarlet fever, scleroderma, senescence, subacute bacterial endocarditis, systemic lupus erythematosus, tuberculosis (advanced pulmonary), treponematosis, trypanosomiasis, tuberculosis, typhus fever, and vaccinia.
7. **Other data:**
   A. Results may be nonreactive while infectious organisms are present in the bloodstream because immunologic response is not detectable for 14-21 days after contraction of the spirochetes.
   B. The greatest risk for transmission of syphilis occurs in freshly drawn blood products that must be administered immediately (platelets) or those not refrigerated for 72 hours before infusion.
   C. Negative results in the presence of definite clinical signs of syphilis or suspected biologic false-positive tests necessitate the *fluorescent treponemal antibody absorption test.*
   D. Test has been found to be highly sensitive and specific, even if antigen is improperly stored at temperature of 36°C.

RAST TEST, SERUM
(*see Allergin-specific IgE, Serum*)

RAYNAUD'S COLD STIMULATION TEST, DIAGNOSTIC

Norm. Within 15 minutes, digital temperature returns to prebath temperature. Recovery time >20 minutes indicates Raynaud syndrome.

Usage. Detection of Raynaud syndrome after occlusive disease of the peripheral arteries is ruled out.

Description. This test records digital temperature changes after submersion of the digits in an ice-water bath. Raynaud syndrome is an idiopathic, vasospastic disorder of small cutaneous arteries and arterioles of the extremities characterized by intense paroxysmal bilateral pallor and cyanosis of the fingers or toes with or without local gangrene. The attacks may occur in response to exposure of the affected extremities to cold temperature. Idiopathic or primary occurrence of this syndrome is referred to as "Raynaud's disease." "Raynaud's phenomenon" is the term used when accompanied by paresthesia and caused by underlying disease processes such as connective tissue disorders.

Professional Considerations
1. Consent form NOT required.

Risks
Increased infection in open wounds on fingers.

Contraindications
Gangrenous digits, or open or infected wounds on the hands.

2. **Preparation:**
   A. All jewelry should be removed from the fingers and wrists.
3. **Procedure:**
   A. Digital temperatures are measured by thermistors attached to each digit.
   B. The hands are then submerged in an ice-water bath for 20 seconds.
   C. Serial temperature recordings are taken beginning immediately after the hands are removed from the bath and continue every 5 minutes for 20 minutes.
4. **Postprocedure care:**
   A. None.
5. **Client and family teaching:**
   A. Avoid exposing the hands to extreme cold.
   B. Smoking greatly increases difficulties in clients with peripheral circulatory problems.
6. **Factors that affect results:**
   A. Excessively cold or warm ambient temperature can alter the physiologic response.
7. **Other data:**
   A. Laser Doppler flowmetery is being studied for its usefulness as an adjunctive diagnostic tool for Raynaud's conditions.

RBC, BLOOD
(*see Red blood cell, Blood*)

RDI
(*see Polysomnography, Diagnostic*)

RECOMBIGEN LATEX AGGLUTINATION ASSAY
(*see Acquired immunodeficiency syndrome evaluation battery, Diagnostic*)

RECTAL CULTURE, SWAB, DIAGNOSTIC

Norm. Negative for pathogenic organisms.

Usage. Screening for causes of bacterial diarrhea such as *Campylobacter, Chlamydia, Neisseria gonorrhoeae, Salmonella,* and *Shigella;* and detection of aerobic and anaerobic intestinal flora.

Description. The rectal swab culture is a screening test for pathogenic organisms of the rectum.

Professional Considerations
1. Consent form NOT required.
2. **Preparation:**
   A. Obtain a sterile culture swab, a closed sterile container, and drapes.
   B. The client should disrobe below the waist.
3. **Procedure:**
   A. Drape the client in the left lateral position with the knees and hips flexed.
   B. Gently insert a sterile, cotton-tipped swab at least 2.5-3 cm into the rectum. Rotate the swab from side to side and leave it in place for a few seconds to allow absorption of rectal flora.
   C. If the swab is being obtained for *N. gonorrhoeae* culture, the swab must be discarded and the procedure repeated if fecal material contaminates the swab.
   D. Place the swab in a sterile container and cover it tightly. If a Culturette is used, insert the swab into the medium compartment of the culture tube and crush the distal end to release the ampule of medium.
4. **Postprocedure care:**
   A. Label the specimen with the site and collection time.

5. **Client and family teaching:**
   A. The test is used to determine the potential bacterial cause of diarrhea.
6. **Factors that affect results:**
   A. Swabs should be sent to the laboratory immediately.
   B. Refrigerate specimens not tested immediately.
   C. There is a high false-negative rate when testing for vancomycin-resistant enterococcus (VRE) in stool.
7. **Other data:**
   A. The rectal culture is not used to determine carrier state.

RECTAL MANOMETRY, DIAGNOSTIC
(see Rectal motility test, Diagnostic)

RECTAL MOTILITY TEST (RECTAL MANOMETRY), DIAGNOSTIC

Norm. *Adult:* 40-120 mm Hg. Distention of the rectum produces relaxation of the internal sphincter and contraction of the external sphincter.

Usage. Assists in the diagnosis of colonic dilatation, constipation, diarrhea, external sphincter disorders (hypothyroidism, myasthenia gravis, myotonic dystrophy, polymyositis), Hirschsprung's disease, incontinence, and internal sphincter disorders (scleroderma); detection of anal achalasia; and evaluation of intrinsic ganglionic innervation of the internal sphincter of the rectum.

Increased. Crohn's disease. Decreased anal squeeze pressure, and/or rectal motility and/or rectal sensation: Hyperglycemia, irritable bowel syndrome, post anorectal repair or microscopic surgery, post-irradiation of the prostate, multiple sclerosis, proctalgia fugax, severe idiopathic chronic constipation, and ulcerative colitis.

Description. This test measures the pressures within the rectum and provides an evaluation of the strength and function of the internal and external anal sphincters. The anal canal length is 5 cm, with a functional length of 3-5 cm. Functional length is determined by the extent of pressure generated by the involuntary internal and voluntary external anal sphincter muscles within the anal canal. Increasing rectal distention from filling produces progressive increasing electromechanical activity in the surrounding tissue accompanied by increasing proximal pressure and decreasing distal pressure along the rectal canal until the contents are expelled. This test is a more sensitive indicator of short segments of anal achalasia than barium enema. A small, thin, flexible balloon catheter with four sensing ports is introduced into the proximal portion of the rectum. The catheter is connected to three pressure transducers. Pressure readings of the rectum and sphincter are measured and recorded onto a graph or computer.

Professional Considerations
1. Consent form NOT required.
2. **Preparation:**
   A. The client should disrobe below the waist.
   B. If a large amount of stool is present, a Fleet enema is given, and the examination is performed 1 hour after rectal evacuation.
3. **Procedure:**
   A. *Adults:*
      i. The client is placed in the left lateral position.
      ii. A small, thin, flexible balloon catheter with four sensing ports is introduced into the proximal portion of the rectum.
      iii. The catheter is inserted 8-10 cm above the mucocutaneous level, with the balloon portion in the proximal portion of the rectum and the sensing ports in the anal canal.
      iv. The catheter is connected to three pressure transducers.
      v. The rectum is distended with an inflated balloon for 7-12 seconds until resistance to balloon distention is demonstrated by passive movement of a syringe. Usually, 30-50 cc of air is required and is dependent on the client's age, the balloon size, and rectal dilatation capacity.
      vi. The amount of air required for the client to feel resistance is recorded as the internal anal sphincter response.

vii. Air is withdrawn in 5- to 10-cc amounts until distention is no longer felt. This smallest volume reflects the threshold of rectal sensation. Most people have relaxation of the internal sphincter with a distention volume of 15 cc.

viii. The client is asked to squeeze the external sphincter tightly for 2 seconds and then relax.

ix. Anal canal pressures are measured at eight points, in 0.5- to 1.0-cm increments, with the highest resting and voluntary squeeze pressures recorded at each point.

x. Pressure readings of the rectum and sphincters are recorded onto graph paper, or images are configured on a computer.

xi. The catheter is removed.

B. *Children:*

i. The procedure as above is consistent with the following changes: The catheter is inserted 5 cm above the mucocutaneous level, and the child may be sedated to prevent unnecessary movements and crying.

C. *Infants:* A cleansing enema is not given.

4. **Postprocedure care:**
   A. Cleanse the anal area.

5. **Client and family teaching:**
   A. Once home, call your doctor if rectal bleeding or discharge occurs.

6. **Factors that affect results:**
   A. Rectal stool decreases pressure readings.
   B. Insufficient rectal distention results in decreased pressure readings.
   C. Improper placement of the anal balloon or equipment malfunction.

7. **Other data:**
   A. Rectal manometry has not been demonstrated to be reliable in the newborn.
   B. To avoid bacterial growth, store the equipment tubing dry. To detect bacterial growth, perform regular water quality testing.

RECTOSPHINCTERIC MANOMETRY, DIAGNOSTIC
(*see Rectal motility test, Diagnostic*)

RED BLOOD CELL (RBC), BLOOD

Norm:

		SI UNITS
Adult female	4-5.5 million/μL	$4\text{-}5.5 \times 10^{12}/L$
Pregnant	3-5.0 million/μL	$3\text{-}5.0 \times 10^{12}/L$
Adult male	4.5-6.2 million/μL	$4.5\text{-}6.2 \times 10^{12}/L$
Infant	3.8-6.1 million/μL	$3.8\text{-}6.1 \times 10^{12}/L$
1-2 years	3.6-5.5 million/μL	$3.6\text{-}5.5 \times 10^{12}/L$
6-15 years	4.7-4.8 million/μL	$4.7\text{-}4.8 \times 10^{12}/L$

Increased. Anoxia, burns (severe), cardiovascular disease, cerebellar hemangioblastoma, Cushing's disease, dehydration (severe), diarrhea, erythema, erythropoietin production increase, hemorrhage, hemoconcentration (exercise, fright, stress), hepatic carcinoma, hereditary spherocytosis, high-oxygen-affinity hemoglobinopathy, hypernephroma, poisoning, polycythemia vera, pulmonary disease and fibrosis, renal cyst, shock, sickle cell disease, surgery, thalassemia, and trauma. Drugs include gentamicin sulfate, methyldopa, and methyldopate hydrochloride.

Decreased. Addison's disease, anemias (aplastic, hemolytic, hemorrhagic, iron deficiency, pernicious, pure red cell), bone marrow suppression, cirrhosis, fatty liver, fluid overload, Gaucher's disease, hemorrhage, hemodilution, hemolysis, Hodgkin's disease, hydremia in pregnancy, hypothyroidism, idiopathic steatorrhea, infection (chronic), leukemia (chronic myelogenous), malaria, multiple myeloma, myxoma of left atrium of the heart, rheumatic fever, systemic lupus erythematosus, subacute bacterial endocarditis, and vitamin deficiency (B_6, B_{12}, folic acid). Drugs include acetaminophen, aminosalicylic acid, ampicillin, antineoplastics, carbamazepine, chloramphenicol, chloroquine hydrochloride or phosphate, haloperidol, hydralazine hydrochloride, hydroxychloroquine sulfate, indomethacin, isoniazid, mefenamic acid, methsuximide, methyldopa, methyldopate hydrochloride, nitrofurantoin, novobiocin sodium, penicillamide, phenobarbital, phenylbutazone, phenytoin, phytonadione, rifampin, spectinomycin hydrochloride, tetracyclines, thiazide diuretics, thiocyanates, tolbutamide, tripelennamine hydrochloride, valproic acid, and vitamin A. Herbs or natural remedies that potentiate anemia include American mandrake or mayapple (*Podophyllum peltatum*), European mistletoe (*Viscum album*), pennyroyal (*Hedeoma pulegioides*), *Rauwolfia serpentina,* Indian squill (*Urginea indica*), squill (*Urginea maritima*).

Description. Red blood cells constitute the majority of peripheral blood cells. They are formed by red bone marrow, have a life span of about 120 days, and are removed from the blood by the liver, spleen, and bone marrow. Red blood cells function in hemoglobin transport, which results in delivery of oxygen to the body tissues. Red blood cell development is characterized by passage through several characteristic stages, beginning with erythroblasts, which are immature, nucleated red blood cells.

Professional Considerations

1. Consent form NOT required.
2. **Preparation:**
   A. Tube: Lavender topped.
   B. Draw the sample from an extremity that does not have intravenous fluids infusing.
   C. Do NOT draw specimens during hemodialysis.
3. **Procedure:**
   A. Draw a 4-mL blood sample.
   B. Heelstick is acceptable, collected in a Microtainer.
4. **Postprocedure care:**
   A. Invert the tube 10 times to mix the contents.

   B. The sample is stable at room temperature for 10 hours and refrigerated for 18 hours.
5. **Client and family teaching:**
   A. This test evaluates the body's ability to produce red blood cells in sufficient numbers.
6. **Factors that affect results:**
   A. False low values occur in the presence of cold agglutinins.
   B. Traumatic venipuncture and hemolysis invalidate the results.
7. **Other data:**
   A. Red blood cell indices are useful in further differentiating conditions.

RED BLOOD CELL ENZYME DEFICIENCY SCREEN, BLOOD

Norm. Red blood cell enzyme is present.

Usage. Assists in the differential diagnosis of chronic nonspherocytic hemolytic anemias.

Description. Erythrocytes contain many enzymes that are involved in numerous metabolic activities. Any of the red blood cell enzymes may be congenitally deficient or become deficient because of acquired abnormalities. Either type of deficiency falls under the category of nonspherocytic anemia. The red blood cell enzyme deficiency screen is a battery of tests that assists in the differential diagnosis of chronic nonspherocytic hemolytic anemias.

Glucose-6-phosphate dehydrogenase (G6PD) is an enzyme present in red blood cells that plays an important role in the hexose monophosphate shunt. The majority of those affected by G6PD deficiency remain asymptomatic, and few exhibit chronic hemolytic anemia. After exposure to certain drugs, deficiency of this enzyme may result in hemolytic anemia. This trait is carried on the X chromosome, is expressed in the hemizygous male and the homozygous female, and is one of the most common red blood cell deficiencies, with over 50 variants of this sex-linked disorder.

Glutathione reductase (GR) is a red blood cell enzyme that is a catalyst in the reduction of NADPH to glutathione in the hexose monophosphate shunt. Exposure to certain drugs may cause a deficiency of this enzyme, resulting in hemolytic anemia.

Pyruvate kinase (PK) is a red blood cell glycolytic enzyme of the Embden-Meyerhof pathway and, when deficient, is the second most frequent cause (after G6PD deficiency) of congenital, homozygous, nonspherocytic hemolytic anemia.

2,3-Diphosphoglycerate (2,3-DPG) is the most abundant intracellular organic phosphate in red blood cells. It is a by-product of the glycolytic pathway in the Rapoport-Luebering shunt. 2,3-DPG controls oxygen transport to the tissues and binds to specific amino acid sites on proteins. In the presence of decreased levels of hemoglobin (anemia), 2,3-DPG acts on the beta chains of the deoxyhemoglobin to decrease oxygen affinity or release oxygen to the tissues. Increased production of 2,3-DPG causes the oxyhemoglobin dissociation curve to "shift to the right." Conversely, deficiency of this enzyme or conditions that increase oxygen affinity results in defects in the unloading of oxygen to the tissues.

Professional Considerations
1. Consent form NOT required.
2. **Preparation:**
   A. Tube: Lavender topped, red topped, red/gray topped, or gold topped; or capillary tube.
   B. Specimens MAY be drawn during hemodialysis.
3. **Procedure:**
   A. Draw a 7-mL blood sample without trauma.
   B. Fingerstick samples should be collected into 7 microhematocrit tubes, three fourths full and gently rotated 7 times to ensure complete mixing of the sample and anticoagulant.
   C. For 2,3-DPG, draw a 3-mL blood sample.
4. **Postprocedure care:**
   A. None.
5. **Client and family teaching:**
   A. This test evaluates and helps differentiate the different anemias.
6. **Factors that affect results:**
   A. Reject hemolyzed or clotted specimens.
   B. High altitudes increase 2,3-DPG results.

C. Banked or stored blood decreases 2,3-DPG results.
D. False-normal G6PD results may occur in black clients if the sample is collected during a hemolytic episode.
7. **Other data:**
   A. Phenotyping of RBC enzymes has been applied to paternity testing.

RED BLOOD CELL COUNT, SERUM
(see Red blood cell, Blood)

RED BLOOD CELL MASS, BLOOD
Norm:

Female: 24.24 ± 2.59 mL/kg (standard deviation)
Male: 28.27 ± 4.11 mL/kg (standard deviation)

Increased. Addison's disease, burns, carboxyhemoglobinemia, cerebellar hemangioblastoma, Cushing's disease, dehydration, emphysema, hepatoma, high altitude, increased erythropoietin production, left-to-right shunt (because of cardiovascular disease), lung disease (producing hypoxia), methemoglobinemia, myeloproliferative syndrome, pickwickian syndrome, polycythemia vera, renal cell adenocarcinoma, renal cyst, secondary polycythemia, smokers, stress states, and uterine myoma.

Decreased. Addison's disease, anemias, blood loss (acute), carcinoma, edema (severe), hemorrhage, infection (chronic), inflammation (chronic), myxedema, panhypopituitarism, radiation, renal failure (chronic), and starvation.

Description. Red blood cell mass is a direct measurement of the total number of red blood cells in the systemic circulation and is expressed in relation to body weight as milliliters per kiloliter (mL/kg). Red blood cell mass reflects the equilibrium between the rate that the bone marrow produces and releases erythrocytes and the rate of peripheral erythrocyte destruction. This test assists in differential diagnosis of absolute and relative polycythemia, anemia, erythrocytosis, and Gaisböck syndrome.

Professional Considerations
1. Consent form NOT required.

Risks
Hematoma, infection.

Contraindications
During pregnancy or breast-feeding.

2. **Preparation:**
   A. Tube: Two green topped.
   B. Do NOT draw speciment during hemodialysis.
3. **Procedure:**
   A. Draw an 8-mL blood sample.
   B. The sample is mixed with a radioactive isotope (^{51}Cr-, ^{131}I-, or ^{125}I-labeled albumin) and is reinjected into the client after 15 minutes.
   C. Draw an 8-mL blood sample 15 minutes after reinjection.
4. **Postprocedure care:**
   A. Observe the client carefully for up to 60 minutes after the study for a possible (anaphylactic) reaction to the radionuclide.
   B. When urine is being discarded, rubber gloves should be worn for 24 hours after the procedure. Wash the gloved hands with soap and water before removing the gloves. Wash the ungloved hands after gloves are removed.

5. **Client and family teaching:**
   A. This test is a measurement of the body's ability to produce RBCs.
   B. Instruct the client to meticulously wash the hands with soap and water after each void for 24 hours.
6. **Factors that affect results:**
   A. Active bleeding, edematous extremities, or intravenous infusions during measurement may alter the results.
   B. Recent scans involving the administration of radioactive isotopes will obscure the results.
7. **Other data:**
   A. Total blood volume and plasma volume are obtained at the time of this test.
   B. Health care professionals working in a nuclear medicine area must follow federal standards set by the Nuclear Regulatory Commission. These standards include precautions for handling the radioactive material and monitoring of potential radiation exposure.
   C. Iodine-131 half-life is 8 days. Iodine-125 half-life is 60 days. Chromium-51 half-life is 27.8 days.

RED BLOOD CELL MORPHOLOGY, BLOOD

Norm. Microscopic interpretation is required.

Color	Uniformly normochromic
Size	6-8 μm, only slight size variation
Shape	Round, biconcave disk
Stained appearance	Mature erythrocytes stain uniformly and contain a normal concentration of hemoglobin with an area of central pallor
Nucleus	Absent
Nuclear remnants	Absent
Cellular inclusions	Absent
Acanthocytes	Absent
Crescent bodies	Absent
Drepanocytes	Absent
Echinocytes	Absent
Leptocytes	Absent
Poikilocytes	Absent
Schizocytes	Absent
Spherocytes	Absent
Stomatocytes	Absent
Cabot rings	Absent
Heinz bodies	Absent
Siderocytes	Absent

CLASSIFICATION OF VARIATION FROM NORMAL		
ABNORMAL RBCS/HPF	**SCORE**	**INTERPRETATION**
3-6	1+	Slight
7-10	2+	Moderate
11-20	3+	Significant
>20	4+	Pronounced

Usage. Detection of blood dyscrasias; and differentiation of anemias, leukemia, and thalassemia.

DESCRIPTION OF ABNORMALITIES OF RBC COLOR	POSSIBLE CAUSES OF ABNORMAL RBC COLOR
Anisochromia is demonstrated by variable staining intensities indicating unequal hemoglobin content because of multiple populations of red blood cells (RBCs).	*Anisochromatism:* Iron-deficiency anemia treated with transfused blood
Hyperchromia is demonstrated by the presence of cells having a smaller than normal area of central pallor, causing the cells to take on excessive staining and demonstrate higher-than-normal pigmentation. Increased amounts of these cells are called "hyperchromatism."	*Hyperchromatism:* Dehydration, increased bone marrow iron stores, inflammation (chronic), and in the presence of spherocytes that have increased cell wall thickness
Hypochromia is demonstrated by the presence of cells having a larger-than-normal area of central pallor, causing the cells to stain weakly and appear to have less than normal pigmentation. Increased amounts of these cells are called "hypochromatism."	*Hypochromatism:* Anemia (iron deficiency) and decreased hemoglobin concentration
Polychromatophils are cells that are stainable with many types of stains, such as stains with both an acid and a base component. They are demonstrated by a bluish pink tinge caused by the presence of both hemoglobin stained by acid and cytoplasmic ribonucleic acid (RNA) stained by the basic component. Both the larger-than-normal cell size and the presence of cytoplasmic RNA indicate that polychromatophils are reticulocytes (newly made red blood cells). Increased amounts of polychromatophils are called "polychromatosis" and occur in accelerated RBC production.	*Polychromatosis:* Hemorrhage, hemolysis, reticulocytosis, and therapy for iron-deficiency anemia or pernicious anemia
Acanthocytes are cells with irregular, thorny, spiculated membrane surface projections containing bulbous, rounded ends. They result from an irreversible defect in the lipid content of the RBC membrane. The presence of acanthocytes is called "acanthocytosis."	*Acanthocytosis:* Abetalipoproteinemia (most common cause), alcoholic cirrhosis, hemolytic anemia (induced by pyruvate kinase deficiency), hepatic disease, status after splenectomy, and retinitis pigmentosa. Drugs include heparin calcium and heparin sodium.

DESCRIPTION OF ABNORMALITIES OF RBC SHAPE	POSSIBLE CAUSES OF ABNORMAL RBC SHAPE
Crescent bodies (achromocytes) are cells with a faint quarter-moon shape caused by RBC rupture.	*Achromocytosis:* Any condition that increases the fragility of red blood cells (that is, sickle cell anemia, reduced oxygen supply).
Drepanocytes or *sickle cells,* are cells formed in the shape of a sickle with a point at one end. The presence of these cells is called "drepanocytosis."	*Drepanocytosis:* Anemia (hemolytic, sickle cell) and hemoglobin SC disease.
Echinocytes, burr cells, or *crenated* RBCs, have a cell surface with 10-30 uniformly distributed, blunt spicules. Echinocytes may be commonly attributable to pH changes caused by faulty drying during smear preparation, but certain physiologic conditions, including a reversible defect in the lipid content of the RBC membrane, have been associated with their presence. The presence of these cells is called "echinocytosis."	*Echinocytosis:* Bile acid abnormalities, blood loss (acute), burns (extensive), carcinoma of the stomach, disseminated intravascular coagulation (DID), gastric ulcers (bleeding), increased free fatty acids, microangiopathic hemolytic anemia, pyruvate kinase deficiency, renal failure, thrombotic thrombocytopenic purpura, and uremia. Drugs include barbiturates, heparin calcium, heparin sodium, and salicylates.
Elliptocytes, or *ovalocytes,* have a cigar shape, which distinguishes them from the more oval shape of the ovalocytes. They are normal constituents of mature RBCs. Higher-than-normal amounts of these cells are called "elliptocytosis."	*Elliptocytosis:* Anemias (iron deficiency, pernicious, sickle cell), hereditary elliptocytosis, leukemia, megaloblastic hematopoiesis, and thalassemia
Leptocytes, or *target cells,* have an increased ratio of surface to volume, often because of a shape that looks like a cup, bell, or hat. They have a colorless center and are thinner and lighter staining than normal RBCs because of abnormally low amounts of hemoglobin. When they are stained, the depth of the "cup" collapses, causing a bull's-eye appearance. The presence of leptocytes is termed "leptocytosis."	*Leptocytosis:* Anemia (iron deficiency, sickle cell), cellular dehydration, cirrhosis, hemoglobin C disease, hemoglobin SC disease, hepatitis, jaundice (obstructive), status after splenectomy, and thalassemia.
Poikilocytes occur in varying shapes, ranging from slightly irregular to dumbbell-like, pear shaped, or teardrop shaped. Defective bone marrow production causes poikilocytosis, a general term used to describe the presence of cells demonstrating variation from the normal shape of the RBC.	*Poikilocytosis:* Anemia (iron deficiency, hemolytic, megaloblastic, pernicious), myelofibrosis, myeloid metaplasia, and thalassemia
Schizocytes, or *schistocytes,* are RBCs with adhesions of spiral and triangular red blood cell fragments because of hemolysis, hemoglobinopathies, or erythrocytic mechanical damage from fibrin strands. The presence of these cells is called "schizocytosis."	*Schizocytosis* or *schistocytosis:* Anemia (acute hemolytic, microangiopathic hemolytic), burns (severe), disseminated intravascular coagulation (DIC), prosthetic heart valves, pyruvate kinase deficiency, renal graft rejection, uremic-hemolytic syndrome, valve prosthesis, and valvular stenosis.

Continued

DESCRIPTION OF ABNORMALITIES OF RBC SHAPE	POSSIBLE CAUSES OF ABNORMAL RBC SHAPE—cont'd
Spherocytes are cells that are globelike rather than biconcave, with an abnormally small dimple. They are thicker than normal, with many fine needle-like projections. Spherocytes lack an area of central pallor (as a result of an increased mean corpuscular hemoglobin concentration) and have a smaller surface area relative to their size. Spherocytes are caused by mechanical fibrin strand damage to circulating RBCs. The presence of spherocytes is called "spherocytosis."	*Spherocytosis:* ABO hemolytic disease of the newborn, accelerated reticuloendothelial red blood cell destruction, anemia (hemolytic), status after blood transfusion, hereditary spherocytosis, and thermal injury of the cell membrane.
Stomatocytes are cup-shaped RBCs with an abnormal area of central pallor that may be oval or rectangular, elongated, or slit like. These cells are produced by antibodies or hydrocytosis. The presence of these cells is called "stomatocytosis."	*Stomatocytosis:* Alcoholism, cirrhosis, erythrocyte sodium pump defect, hepatic disease (obstructive), hereditary spherocytosis, hereditary stomatocytosis, and Rh_{null} (Rh_0) cells.

DESCRIPTION OF ABNORMALITIES OF RBC SIZE	POSSIBLE CAUSES OF ABNORMALITIES OF RBC SIZE
Anisocytosis is a general term that describes any variation in the size of the RBC.	*Anisocytosis:* Anemias (iron deficiency, pernicious), folic acid deficiency, status after blood transfusion of normal cells into an abnormal red blood cell population, leukemia, newborns, and reticulocytosis.
Macrocytes are large erythrocytes having a diameter >8 μm, a mean corpuscular volume <95 m, and higher-than-normal hemoglobin content. They are usually increased because of stress erythropoiesis. Increased amounts of macrocytes are called "macrocytosis."	*Macrocytosis:* Alcoholic lever disease, anemia (hemolytic, pernicious), folic acid deficiency, hepatic disease, hyperthyroidism, idiopathic steatorrhea, newborns, reticulocytosis, status after hemorrhagic states, and thalassemia.
Microcytes have a RBC diameter <6 μm, a mean corpuscular volume <80 μm, and a mean corpuscular hemoglobin concentration <27%. Increased amounts of microcytes are called "microcytosis."	*Microcytosis:* Anemia (from chronic hemorrhage, iron deficiency), hemoglobinopathies, hereditary spherocytosis, and thalassemia.

DESCRIPTION OF ABNORMALITIES OF RBC CONTENT OR STRUCTURE	POSSIBLE CAUSES OF ABNORMAL RBC CONTENT OR STRUCTURE
Agglutination: Clumping together of RBCs is an immune mechanism caused by antibody formation.	*Agglutination:* Invading antigen(s).

DESCRIPTION OF ABNORMALITIES OF RBC CONTENT OR STRUCTURE	POSSIBLE CAUSES OF ABNORMAL RBC CONTENT OR STRUCTURE

Basophilic stippling is demonstrated by the presence of minute basophilic granules that cause a bluish-to-purple color when reticulocytes are stained. They are caused by ribosomal aggregation that occurs as smears are prepared. Small amounts of basophilic stippling normally occur as the smears are dried. Increased amounts occur in conditions in which RNA has aggregated in the cells.

Increased basophilic stippling: Alcoholism, anemia (megaloblastic, sickle cell), heavy metal intoxication (bismuth, lead, mercury, and silver), hemorrhage (gastrointestinal), leukemia, and thalassemia.

Cabot's rings are cells containing mitotic spindle remnants appearing as fine, threadlike filaments of bluish purple color in the shape of a single ring or a double ring (figure-eight shape).

Presence of Cabot's rings: Anemia (severe, pernicious), lead poisoning, myelofibrosis, and myeloid metaplasia.

Heinz bodies are denatured particles of hemoglobin attached to the RBC membrane that appear when stained with cresyl blue or new methylene blue. Heinz bodies usually indicate abnormal erythrocyte stability because of hemolytic conditions or hemoglobinopathies.

Presence of Heinz bodies: Alphathalassemia, anemia (hemolytic), glucose-6-phosphate dehydrogenase deficiency, hemoglobinopathies, methemoglobinemia, and status after splenectomy. Drugs include analgesics, antipyretics, chlorates, phenacetin, phenothiazines, phenylacetamide, phenylhydrazine, phenylamine, primaquine phosphate, resorcinol, and sulfapyridine.

Howell-Jolly bodies are nuclear fragments contained in red cells that stain purple or violet. They are normally present in immature RBCs and in mature erythrocytes before they pass through the splenic circulation. In conditions causing increased RBC production, erythrocytes contain higher-than-normal amounts of these bodies.

Presence of Howell-Jolly bodies: Anemia (hemolytic, megaloblastic), leukemia, splenic absence (congenital or surgical removal), and splenic atrophy.

Platelets on red blood cells appear as a halo that resists staining and can be easily confused with RBC inclusion bodies.

n/a

Rouleaux formation is demonstrated by a cellular configuration in stacks or rolls. Increased rouleaux formation may be caused by increased fibrinogen or globulins in the blood. Rouleaux formation is decreased by the presence of abnormally shaped RBCs, which inhibits adherence of the cells in a stacked shape. Rouleaux formation may also result from a delay in slide preparation.

Increased rouleaux formation: Hyperfibrinogenemia, macroglobulinemia, and multiple myeloma.
Decreased rouleaux formation: Hereditary spherocytosis.

Continued

DESCRIPTION OF ABNORMALITIES OF RBC CONTENT OR STRUCTURE—cont'd	POSSIBLE CAUSES OF ABNORMAL RBC CONTENT OR STRUCTURE—cont'd
Siderocytes, or *Pappenheimer* bodies, are cells with mitochondrial concentrations of ferritin (nonhemoglobin iron) deposits. These cells stain as purple bluish granules only in the presence of iron stains such as Prussian-blue reactions. Pappenheimer bodies are noniron basophilic granules contained in the iron-protein matrix and stain positive for iron in the presence of noniron stains. Ferritin is normally absent in RBCs. During hemoglobin formation in the premature infant and newborn, siderocyte free-iron granules commonly occur in developing normoblasts and reticulocytes. The presence of siderocytes is called "siderocytosis."	*Siderocytosis* or *Pappenheimer bodies:* Anemia (chronic hemolytic, congenital spherocytic, dyserythropoietic, megaloblastic, pernicious, refractory, sideroblastic), burns (severe), hemochromatosis, infection, lead poisoning, status post splenectomy, and thalassemia.

Description. Red blood cells (RBCs) constitute the majority of peripheral blood cells and function in hemoglobin transport, which results in delivery of oxygen to the body tissues. RBC development is characterized by passage through several characteristic stages, beginning with erythroblasts, which are immature, nucleated RBCs. RBC morphology is the examination of red blood cells under a microscope, comparing the actual appearance with calculated values for each indice of color, size, shape, developmental stage, and structure or content.

Professional Considerations

1. Consent form NOT required.
2. Preparation:
   A. Tube: Lavender topped.
   B. Specimens MAY be drawn during hemodialysis.
3. Procedure:
   A. Draw a 7-mL blood sample.
   B. Heelstick is acceptable, collected in a Microtainer.
4. Postprocedure care:
   A. None.
5. Client and family teaching:
   A. This test evaluates the structure of the RBCs.
6. Factors that affect results:
   A. Automated methods of counting and sizing of the RBCs should not be used in the presence of red cell agglutination. Instead, hand counts must be performed.

7. Other data:
   A. RBC morphology stained smear is usually carried out at the same time as the differential white blood cell count.

RED BLOOD CELL SIZE DISTRIBUTION WIDTH (RDW), BLOOD

Norm. 13.4%-14.6%. Microscopic electronic interpretation is required.

Increased. Alcoholic liver disease, celiac disease, iron deficiency. See *Red blood cell (RBC), Blood; Red blood cell morphology, Blood.*

Decreased. Defects in iron reutilization, renal failure See *Red blood cell (RBC), Blood; Red blood cell morphology, Blood.*

Description. Red blood cell volume distribution width, or RDW, is a coefficient of variation (CV) in red blood cell volume. This is derived from anisocytosis. RDW becomes abnormal earlier in iron deficiency than in any other blood cell parameters. RDW may be a useful tool in differential diagnosis of microcytic and macrocytic anemias. It may also be used in monitoring for improved absorption of nutrients in response to a gluten-free diet in celiac disease. It should be remembered that RDW is a CV, and it should be correlated with other erythrocytic indices for most accurate diagnoses. (See *Red blood cell morphology, Blood.*)

Professional Considerations
1. Consent form NOT required.
2. Preparation:
   A. Tube: Lavender topped.
   B. Specimens MAY be drawn during hemodialysis.
3. Procedure:
   A. Draw a 5-mL blood sample.
4. Postprocedure care:
   A. None.
5. Client and family teaching:
   A. This test will evaluate iron intake and utilization in the body.
6. Factors that affect results:
   A. RDW is obtained by electronic evaluation (anisocytosis).
   B. See *Reticulocyte count, Blood; Hematocrit, Blood.*
7. Other data:
   A. See *Reticulocyte count, Blood; Hematocrit, Blood.*

RED BLOOD CELL SURVIVAL, BLOOD
(see ^{51}Cr *[chromium]-red blood cell survival, Blood*)

REDUCING SUBSTANCES, STOOL

Norm:

Normal	<2 mg/g of stool
Borderline	2-5 mg/g of stool
Abnormal	>5 mg/g of stool

Increased. Disaccharidase deficiencies, infant diarrhea (some forms), intestinal mucosal defects, and metabolic disorders.

Decreased. Beta-lipoprotein deficiency, blind loop syndrome, celiac disease, cystic fibrosis of the pancreas, *Giardia* infestation, and malnutrition (severe). Drugs include colchicine, neomycin sulfate, and oral contraceptives.

Description. The presence of reducing substances in the stool demonstrates the inability of intestinal border enzymes to absorb disaccharide carbohydrates, especially sucrase and lactase. These unabsorbed sugars are reduced by metal ions, such as copper contained in the frequently used Clinitest reduction tablet.

Professional Considerations
1. Consent form NOT required.
2. Preparation:
   A. Obtain a clean, dry plastic specimen container.
3. Procedure:
   A. Collect at least 1 g of stool in a clean, dry, plastic specimen container with a lid.
4. Postprocedure care:
   A. Send the specimen to the laboratory immediately.
   B. Freeze the specimen if not tested immediately.
5. Client and family teaching:
   A. This test measures the digestive tract's ability to absorb disaccharides.
   B. Urinate before defecating to avoid contaminating the stool sample with urine.
6. Factors that affect results:
   A. False-low results because of bacterial fermentation may occur when analysis is delayed in nonfrozen specimens.
   B. Reject specimens that have been placed on an absorbent surface (diaper, cardboard).
7. Other data:
   A. The weight and pH of the specimen are usually obtained and included in the results.

REFRACTION VISION TEST, DIAGNOSTIC

Norm. Emmetropia or no refractive error.

Refractive power of the human eye, without accommodation:	58 diopters
Refractive power of the structures of the eye:	
Cornea	44 diopters
Aqueous humor	44 diopters
Lens	10-14 diopters

Note: The vitreous humor has little refractive power and primarily transmits light.

Usage. Assists in the evaluation of visual acuity; diagnosis of ametropias (refractive errors), including astigmatism, hyperopia (farsightedness), and myopia (nearsightedness); and determination of the need for the prescription of corrective lenses.

Description. Refraction is the process by which light rays entering the eye bend or pass obliquely over the curved surfaces of the eye (cornea, aqueous humor, lens, and vitreous humor), which have differing densities. Clear images are produced as a point of light is focused directly on the retina. The refraction vision test is only one of a series of procedures included in a full ophthalmologic eye examination. This test alone cannot diagnose eye disease.

Professional Considerations
1. Consent form NOT required.

Risks
Allergic reaction to eye drops (itching, hives, rash, tight feeling in the throat, shortness of breath, bronchospasm, anaphylaxis, death).

Contraindications
Previous allergy to mydriatic drops; narrow-angle glaucoma.

2. **Preparation:**
   A. Eye drops may be placed in both eyes to dilate the pupils and to prevent lens accommodation during the examination.
3. **Procedure:**
   A. The examiner locates the pupillary opening with a retinoscope and then assesses for stasis of the red-orange retinal reflection of the retinoscope light.
   B. Brightness, clarity, shape, size, vascularity, and uniformity of the retina are observed.
   C. A variety of lenses with varying lens powers are inserted into the client's test glasses.
   D. This process continues until the lens power that best neutralizes retinal reflex motion, produces the most clarity and brightness, and produces the most consistently correct reading of a visual chart is determined.

4. **Postprocedure care:**
   A. See *Client and family teaching.*
5. **Client and family teaching:**
   A. This is a simple eye test to determine if you do or do not need corrective lenses.
   B. Bring sunglasses to wear after the procedure.
   C. Do not drive or operate any machinery until distant vision returns.
6. **Factors that affect results:**
   A. Inadequate pupil dilatation, excessive lens accommodation, or incomplete cooperation of the client prevents accurate results.
7. **Other data:**
   A. Most clients show some degree of ametropia or refractive error.

RENAL ANGIOGRAM (RENAL ARTERIOGRAM), DIAGNOSTIC

Norm. Radiopaque iodine contrast material should circulate symmetrically and without interruption through the renal parenchyma and renal vasculature.

Usage. Visualization of the renal parenchyma and renal vasculature; assists in differentiation of renal masses; identification of renovascular abnormalities such as abscesses, aneurysms, arteriovenous fistula, hypervascularity, hypovascularity, emboli, fibrosis, infarction, intrarenal hematoma, parenchymal laceration, polyarteritis nodosa, renal artery dysplasia, stenosis, thrombolic occlusions, and accidental injury; and evaluation of chronic renal disease, renal failure, and transplant donors and recipients as well as posttransplantation evaluation of vascular flow and rejection of the donor organ.

Description. Renal angiogram is an invasive radiographic procedure involving injection of iodine radiopaque contrast material through a catheter inserted into the aorta near the bifurcation of the renal arteries or directly into the renal arteries. For clients with preexisting renal impairment, gadolinium-enhanced magnetic resonance angiography or magnetic resonance urography is a better choice than this procedure, because it is non-nephrotoxic.

Professional Considerations
1. Consent form IS required.

Risks
Embolus, hematoma, hemorrhage, infection, allergic reaction to contrast material (itching, hives, rash, tight feeling in the throat, shortness of breath, bronchospasm, anaphylaxis, death), renal toxicity from contrast medium.

Contraindications
Previous allergy to iodine, shellfish, or radiographic dye; renal insufficiency. The procedure may be contraindicated during pregnancy if iodinated contrast media is used, because of the radioactive iodine crossing the blood-placental barrier. Caution should be taken with clients who have bleeding tendencies and those with renal failure because of end-stage renal disease. Sedatives are contraindicated in clients with central nervous system depression.

2. **Preparation:**
   A. Establish intravenous access.
   B. A narcotic or sedative may be prescribed.
   C. The client should void and remove all jewelry and metal objects.
   D. Have an emergency cart readily available.
   E. Obtain local anesthetic, povidone-iodine solution, intravenous fluid, contrast material, guidewire, vascular and renal catheters, and sterile gloves.
   F. See *Client and family teaching.*
3. **Procedure:**
   A. The client is positioned supine.
   B. A peripheral intravenous infusion is started.
   C. The arterial site is cleansed and anesthetized.
   D. A catheter is introduced in accordance with the Seldinger technique into the femoral artery or into the transaxillary, transbrachial, or translumbar vessels, and advanced under fluoroscopy to the aorta. Test aortograms with a small amount of contrast material are completed.
   E. The catheter is then replaced with a renal catheter, and larger amounts of radiopaque contrast material are injected through the catheter directly into the aorta near

the bifurcation of the renal arteries or directly into the renal arteries.
   F. Rapid, serial radiographic films are then taken to record circulation of the contrast material through the renal parenchyma and vasculature.
   G. The catheter is removed, and a pressure dressing is applied over the insertion site.
4. **Postprocedure care:**
   A. If sedation was used, continue assessment of respiratory status. If deep sedation was used, follow institutional protocol for postsedation monitoring. Typical monitoring includes continuous ECG monitoring and pulse oximetry, with continual assessments (every 5-15 minutes) of airway, vital signs, and neurologic status until the client is lying quietly awake, is breathing independently, and responds to commands spoken in a normal tone.
   B. Monitor the catheter insertion site for bleeding, inflammation, or hematoma formation.
5. **Client and family teaching:**
   A. This test determines the adequacy of blood flow through both renal arteries.
   B. Fast for 8 hours before the procedure.
   C. For 5 minutes after injection of the contrast material, an urge to cough, a flushed sensation, nausea, or a salty taste may occur.
   D. It is important to lie motionless throughout the procedure. Sedation may be used to help you relax.
6. **Factors that affect results:**
   A. Interpretation of the results may be impaired by the presence of gas, feces, or contrast material such as barium in the gastrointestinal tract.
   B. Movement of the client during the procedure obscures the radiography.
   C. Calcium antagonists can cause false-positive captopril renograms.
7. **Other data:**
   A. None.

RENAL ARTERIOGRAM, DIAGNOSTIC
(see Renal angiogram, Diagnostic)

RENAL ECHOGRAM
(see Kidney ultrasonography,
Diagnostic)

RENAL FAILURE INDEX
(see Sodium, Plasma, Serum or Urine)

RENAL FUNCTION TEST, DIAGNOSTIC
(see Concentration test, Urine;
Creatinine clearance, Serum, Urine;
Diagnostic and renal indices,
Diagnostic; Inulin clearance test,
Diagnostic)

Description. The renal function test may consist of up to four tests: the urine concentration test, the phenolsulfonphthalein (PSP) test, and the creatinine clearance and insulin clearance tests. These four indices reflect glomerular filtration, tubular reabsorption, renal blood flow, and tubular secretion. Measurement of these separate kidney functions assists in the determination of the origin and degree of renal dysfunction and renal tissue destruction. These tests are limited in their scope to detect early or mild renal disorders. (See individual test listings for more information.)

RENAL INDICES (FeNa, RFI), DIAGNOSTIC

Norm. Norm not applicable. Indices are used only for clients experiencing or suspected of experiencing renal failure.

RENAL INDICES: DIFFERENTIATING CATEGORIES OF RENAL FAILURE

	Fractional Excretion of Sodium in Urine (Urine Na × Serum Creatinine × 100)/ (Serum Na × Urine Creatinine)	Urine Sodium	Renal Failure Index: Urine Na × (Plasma Creatinine/Urine Creatinine)
Prerenal and Volume Depletion	<1%	<20 mmol/L	<1%
Renal (Acute Tubular Necrosis)	>1%	>40 mmol/L	>1%
Postrenal	>4%		

Usage. Determination of the category of renal failure; ongoing monitoring during recovery from acute tubular necrosis.

Description. Both renal indices are mathematically calculated values of renal sodium handling, using laboratory measurement results. Urinary sodium levels are used in conjunction with urine and plasma or serum creatinine in two formulas that help narrow down the source of renal failure into prerenal, renal, and postrenal causes. Both the **fractional excretion of sodium in urine (FeNa)** and the **renal failure index** determine how well the kidneys are able to remove urine from the blood into the urine. They are expressed as

the percentage of serum sodium that is excreted in the urine.

Professional Considerations
1. Consent form NOT required.
2. **Preparation:**
   A. Obtain clean-catch urine container, towelettes, and a red-topped tube. For pediatric/infant collections, also obtain tape and a pediatric urine collection device/ bag.
3. **Procedure:**
   A. Obtain a clean-catch urine sample and a 3-mL blood sample.
   B. Pediatric/infant specimen collection:
      i. The child is placed in a supine position with the knees flexed

and the hips externally rotated and abducted.

ii. Cleanse, rinse, and thoroughly dry the perineal area.

iii. To prevent the child from removing the collection device/bag, a diaper may be placed over the genital area.

iv. *Females:* Tape the pediatric collection device/bag to the perineum. Starting at the area between the anus and vagina, apply the device/bag in an anterior direction.

v. *Males:* Place the pediatric collection device/bag over the penis and scrotum and tape it to the perineal area.

vi. Empty the collection bag into the refrigerated collection container after the infant or child voids.

4. **Postprocedure care:**
   A. Remove the collection device/bag by gently peeling it away from the skin.

5. **Client and family teaching:**
   A. None.

6. **Factors that affect results:**
   A. Both tests are most useful when urine output is oliguric.

7. **Other data:**
   A. None.

RENAL SCAN, DIAGNOSTIC

(see Renocystogram, Diagnostic; Kidney scan, Diagnostic)

RENAL ULTRASONOGRAPHY, DIAGNOSTIC

(see Kidney ultrasonography, Diagnostic)

RENIN ACTIVITY (PLASMA RENIN ACTIVITY, PRA), PLASMA

Norm. Norms are age-, diet-, position-, and vein-site dependent.

		SI UNITS
Normal-Sodium Diet, Upright and from the Peripheral Vein		
Age 20-39	0.6-4.3 ng/mL/h	0.6-4.3 µg/L/H
Mean	1.9 ng/mL/h	1.9 µg/L/H
Age ≥40	0.6-3.0 ng/mL/h	0.6-3.0 µg/L/H
Mean	1.0 ng/mL/h	1.0 µg/L/H
Low-Sodium Diet, Upright and from the Peripheral Vein		
Age 20-39	2.9-24 ng/mL/h	2.9-24 µg/L/H
Mean	10.8 ng/mL/h	10.8 µg/L/H
Age ≥ 40	2.9-10.8 ng/mL/h	2.9-10.8 µg/L/H
Mean	5.9 ng/mL/h	5.9 µg/L/H

Renal venous renin ratio: <15:2
Unilateral renal stenosis: Normal kidney:Affected kidney renin levels ratio > 1:1.4

	RENIN ACTIVITY	ALDOSTERONE
Primary hyperaldosteronism	Decreased	Increased
Secondary hyperaldosteronism	Increased	Increased

Note: Samples obtained during renal vein catheterization are compared with levels obtained in the inferior vena cava to obtain the renal venous renin ratio.

Increased. Addison's disease, aldosteronism (secondary), ambulatory clients (compared to clients on bedrest), Bartter's syndrome, chronic renal failure, cirrhosis, Conn's syndrome, erect posture for 4 hours (twofold increase), essential hypertension (rare), hypokalemia, hypovolemia (hemorrhage-induced), last half of menstrual cycle (twofold increase), low-sodium diet, nephropathy (sodium-losing), normal pregnancy, pheochromocytoma, renal hypertension, renin-producing renal tumors, and transplant rejection. Drugs include antihypertensives, diazoxide, estrogens, furosemide, guanethidine sulfate, hydralazine hydrochloride, minoxidil, nitroprusside sodium, saralasin, spironolactone, and thiazides.

Description. Renin is a proteolytic enzyme that is synthesized, stored, and secreted by the juxtaglomerular cells of the kidneys and is a primary catalyst in regulation of blood pressure, potassium, and fluid volume balance. Hydrolytic activity of the renin-angiotensin-aldosterone cycle results in the production of angiotensin II, a potent vasoconstrictor that stimulates the production of aldosterone in the adrenal cortex. Decreased renal blood flow stimulates renin secretion and an increased secretion of aldosterone. Blood loss and sodium depletion stimulate the release of renin. For this reason, the test may be preceded by the intake of a low-sodium diet for a several days. Hypertensive states with low plasma renin activity are suggestive of body fluid expansion imbalance. The test is an indirect measurement of the *activity* of renin through measurement of the rate of production of angiotensin I, which increases as a result of renin stimulation. Aldosterone levels are usually measured at the same time. High plasma renin activity suggests hypertension from the vasoconstrictive effects of angiotensin. The sample may be drawn peripherally or directly from the renal vain during a renal vein catheterization.

Professional Considerations
1. Consent form IS required for the renal artery catheterization procedure, if it will be done in conjunction with sample collection for renin determination.
2. **Preparation:**
   A. Preparation and cooperation of the client are critical for accurate results.
   B. The client must be assessed for medications that affect the results (estrogens can affect results for up to 6 months), and certain medications may be withheld for 2-4 hours prior to the test.

C. See *Client and family teaching.*
D. Preschedule this test with the laboratory.
E. Tube: lavender topped, ice-cold. Also obtain a container of ice.
F. A local anesthetic may be administered prior to renal vein catheterization.
3. **Procedure:**
   A. The test should be performed in the morning because renin levels exhibit a diurnal variation.
   B. Completely fill an ice-cold lavender top tube with blood. Avoid prolonged tourniquet use to avoid causing a drop in renin.
   C. Gently tilt the tube several times to mix the sample.
   D. The same procedure is used in handling blood samples obtained during renal vein catheterization.
4. **Postprocedure care:**
   A. Place the specimen immediately on ice.
   B. Send the specimen to the laboratory immediately.
   C. If a renal artery catheterization was performed, monitor vital signs, catheterization site and distal pulses every 15 minutes × 2, then every 30 minutes × 2.
5. **Client and family teaching:**
   A. This test measures one of the fluid balance controls in the body.
   B. Follow a 3 g/day sodium diet for 3-14 days prior to the test. Do not eat licorice prior to the test.
   C. If the sodium depletion renin level will be measured, follow a low-sodium diet for 3 days prior to the test. Diuretics may also be prescribed prior to the test.
   D. Fast for 8 hours prior to the test.
   E. The recumbent position test requires that your be able to lie down on your back for at least 1 hour. The upright position test requires that you be able to stand or sit upright for 2 hours.
6. **Factors that affect results:**
   A. Improper position of the client, provides unreliable results. Levels are highest when drawn with the client in an upright position.
   B. Failure to follow the dietary restrictions, or failure to withhold appropriate medications prior to the test invalidates the results.

C. Results are invalidated if the collection tube was not chilled prior to venipuncture or if the specimen was not placed on ice after collection.

D. Reject tubes incompletely filled or specimens not well-mixed.

7. Other data:

A. Renin is very unstable and samples must be handled properly.

B. The 24-hour urine sample for sodium should be indexed against renin levels.

C. A second nonfasting blood sample, with exercise, may also be prescribed.

RENOCYSTOGRAM (RENOGRAM SCAN, RENAL SCAN), DIAGNOSTIC

Norm. Radionuclide contrast material should circulate bilaterally, symmetrically, and without interruption through the renal parenchyma, ureters, and urinary bladder; 50% of radionuclide should be excreted within the first 10 minutes. The initial uptake or vascular phase occurs within 30-45 seconds after administration of the radionuclide. The transit or tubular phase follows over the next 2-5 minutes, and drainage of the radionuclide from the kidneys occurs during the excretory phase.

Captopril radiography method:

Renovascular hypertension: GFR decreases more than 20%, with a 10% difference between the left and right kidneys.

Renal artery stenosis:

The kidney shows a disproportionate reduction in perfusion after administration of captopril.

Usage. Azotemia, excretory defects, nephroureteral dilatation, renal ischemia (acute tubular necrosis), renal obstruction or mass, renal parenchymal disease, renovascular hypertension, unilateral kidney disease, and upper urinary obstruction; assessment of renal perfusion and status before transplantation and after transplantation (to differentiate between acute tubular necrosis and transplant rejection); and evaluation of hydroureteronephrosis and urinary tract patency, also used for clients hypersensitive to iodine-based contrast material used with intravenous pyelography or those in whom urethral catheterization is contraindicated.

Description. The renocystogram is a dynamic nuclear medicine study of the kidneys and ureters in which the dispersion, clearance, and excretion of a radionuclide is recorded by means of a gamma radiographic scan. Radionuclide uptake, transit, and excretion times are computed, and renogram curves are plotted on a graph for each kidney and ureter. Quantitative evaluation of renal function occurs as the external radiation detectors record vascular supply, perfusion, tubular filtration, and excretory phases. A renogram curve is produced as the radionuclide dispersion is plotted on a graph or computed. Comparison of the right and left kidney, curve shape, and relative function is calculated. Curve shapes are characteristic of certain disorders. This scan uses less radiation than an IVP or CT scan. However, IVP is better for anatomic definition, and arteriography is better for assessment of renal arterial anatomy. Renocystogram is superior to magnetic resonance imaging for medullary renogram evaluation (which must derive medullary information from a mixed study renogram), but equivalent in use for cortical renograms. When the evaluation is being done to identify the presence of renal vascularization abnormalities in hypertension and suspected renal artery stenosis, captopril radiography may be used. For suspected renal artery stenosis only, duplex ultrasound is less costly and invasive and provides similar diagnostic accuracy to captopril radiography.

Professional Considerations

1. Consent form IS required.

Risks

Allergic reaction, bleeding, infection, urinary tract obstruction.

Contraindications

During pregnancy, this test is performed only when imperative. It is contraindicated during breast-feeding, with congenital renal abnormality, clients with open flank wounds present, or with previous allergic reaction to the same radionuclide.

Precautions

During pregnancy, risks of cumulative radiation exposure to the fetus from this and other previous or future imaging studies must be weighed against the benefits of the procedure. Although formal limits for client exposure are relative to this risk:benefit comparison, the United States Nuclear Regulatory Commission requires that the cumulative dose equivalent to an embryo/fetus from occupational exposure not exceed 0.5 rem (5 mSv). Radiation dosage to the fetus is proportional to the distance of the anatomy studied from the abdomen and decreases as pregnancy progresses. For pregnant clients, consult the radiologist/radiology department to obtain estimated fetal radiation exposure from this procedure.

2. **Preparation:**
   A. Obtain the client's current weight.
   B. The client should empty the bladder. Insert an indwelling urinary catheter for pediatric clients.
   C. Establish intravenous access and infuse 500 mL of IV fluids (unless contraindicated). Unless contraindicated, the client should be well hydrated with 10 mL of water per kilogram of body weight.
   D. Have emergency equipment readily available.
3. **Procedure:**
   A. The client is positioned upright.
   B. After placement of external posterior radiation detectors over both kidneys, an intravenous injection of radionuclide ^{99m}Tc-DTPA (technetium with the chelating agent diethylenetriaminepentaacetic acid) or ^{131}I-*ortho*-iodohippurate (radioiodine hippuran) is administered. Detectors record the uptake and excretion radiation counts when gamma scanning of both kidneys is completed.
   C. The scan takes about 45 minutes.
   D. If captopril renography will be done, captopril is administered

and the scan is repeated 1 hour later. Monitor blood pressure every 15 minutes throughout the procedure.
4. **Postprocedure care:**
   A. Urine or serum blood samples may be obtained.
   B. Assess the injection site for infiltration of radionuclide analog.
   C. Observe the client carefully for up to 60 minutes after the study for a possible (anaphylactic) reaction to the radionuclide.
   D. When urine is being discarded, rubber gloves should be worn for 24 hours after the procedure. Wash the gloved hands with soap and water before removing the gloves. Wash the ungloved hands after gloves are removed.
   E. If captopril was administered, continue blood pressure measurements every 30 minutes until client meets discharge criteria. Assess for orthostatic hypotension.
5. **Client and family teaching:**
   A. This is a screening test used when it is suspected that renal blood flow is reduced.
   B. This examination takes approximately 45 minutes and involves receiving an IV line to administer the test material and some fluids.
   C. Immediately flush the toilet after each voiding after the procedure, and meticulously wash your hands with soap and water after each void for 24 hours after the procedure.
   D. There will be a small amount of radiation exposure during testing.
   E. For captopril renography, eat and drink only liquids beginning midnight before the test. Do not take milk products at all.
   F. For captopril renography, you will be given a glass of water to drink.
   G. For captopril renography, you will need to slowly change from a lying or sitting position to a standing position, in case you experience dizziness.
   H. In women who are breast-feeding, formula should be substituted for breast milk for 1 or more days after the procedure.

6. Factors that affect results:
    A. The presence of contrast material from prior diagnostic testing within 7 days interferes with accuracy.
    B. Abnormalities may be accentuated in the presence of dehydration or masked in the presence of overhydration.
    C. Injection of radiographic contrast material within 24 hours before the test invalidates the results.
7. Other data:
    A. This study records the activity of the entire kidney but does not distinguish between specific areas of disease within the kidneys.
    B. Health care professionals working in a nuclear medicine area must follow the federal standards set by the Nuclear Regulatory Commission. These standards include precautions for handling the radioactive material and monitoring of potential radiation exposure.
    C. Technetium half-life is 6 hours.
    D. Spinal fractures may be noted in the scan.

RENOGRAM SCAN, DIAGNOSTIC

(see Renocystogram, Diagnostic)

REPTILASE TIME, SERUM

Norm. 18-20 seconds.

Increased. Congenital afibrinogenemia and dysfibrinogenemia.

Decreased. Not clinically significant.

Description. Reptilase is an enzyme from Russell's viper (*Vipera russellii*, syn. *Daboia russelli*) venom used to determine blood coagulation time. It is a variation of the thrombin time used to detect the presence of adequate fibrinogen levels without interference from heparin, fibrin-fibrinogen degradation products, or increased concentrations of plasmin. Prolonged thrombin time in the presence of a normal reptilase time is confirmation that heparin, rather than low fibrinogen levels, is the cause of the coagulation defect.

Professional Considerations

1. Consent form NOT required.
2. Preparation:
    A. Tube: 2.7-mL or 4.5-mL blue topped.
    B. Specimens MAY be drawn during hemodialysis.
3. Procedure:
    A. Draw a 3-mL blood sample and discard, leaving the needle in place.
    B. Withdraw 2-mL of blood into a syringe or vacuum tube. Remove the syringe or tube, leaving the needle in place. Attach a second syringe, and draw a blood sample quantity of 2.4 mL for a 2.7-mL tube and 4.0 mL for a 4.5-mL tube.
4. Postprocedure care:
    A. None.
5. Client and family teaching:
    A. The test will measure your blood's ability to clot properly.
    B. Results are normally available within 24 hours.
6. Factors that affect results:
    A. Send specimens to the laboratory immediately.
    B. Contamination of the sample with tissue thromboplastin causes falsely elevated results. This is the reason for the double-draw technique.
7. Other data:
    A. The reptilase time may be used in place of the thrombin time in fibrinogen evaluation in clients anticoagulated with heparin.

RESERPINE, SERUM

Norm. Negative. *Serum therapeutic level:* 20 ng/mL.

Overdose Symptoms and Treatment

Symptoms. Lethargy, drowsiness, respiratory depression.

Treatment:

Note: Treatment choice(s) depend on client history and condition and episode history.
Protect airway.
Support blood pressure with vasopressors.
Monitor neurologic checks every hour.
Hemodialysis and peritoneal dialysis will NOT remove reserpine.

Increased. Parkinson's disease.

Description. Reserpine, an alkaloid of the *Rauwolfia serpentina* plant, is used primarily as an antihypertensive, sedative, or tranquilizer. It acts at adrenergic receptor sites, primarily of the central and peripheral nervous systems and heart, by interfering with the binding of serotonin. Reserpine is metabolized in the liver and excreted as an inactive metabolite in small amounts in the urine and stool. Reserpine has a very slow onset of peak action (2-3 weeks) with a prolonged effect (4-6 weeks); thus alterations in dosage occur in small increments and at 7- to 14-day intervals. Half-life is 4.5 hours, with a duration of 45-168 hours.

Professional Considerations
1. Consent form NOT required.
2. Preparation:
   A. Tube: Lavender topped.
   B. Specimens MAY be drawn during hemodialysis.
3. Procedure:
   A. Draw a 7-mL blood sample.
   B. Heelstick is acceptable, collected in a Microtainer.
4. Postprocedure care:
   A. None.
5. Client and family teaching:
   A. This test measures the level of reserpine in your body.
   B. Results are normally available within 24 hours.
   C. Know and understand the side effects of this drug, and recognize the signs of overdose (see p. 965).
   D. For intentional overdose, refer the client and family for crisis intervention.
6. Factors that affect results:
   A. Specimens collected in heparin invalidate results.
7. Other data:
   A. *Rauwolfia* alkaloids lower seizure threshold. Clients with convulsive disorders should be observed closely.

RESPIRATORY ANTIGEN PANEL (ANTIGEN DETECTION TEST, ADT, RESPIRATORY VIRUS IMMUNOFLUORESCENCE, RESPIRATORY VIRUS DIRECT STAIN PANEL), SPECIMEN

Norm. Negative for adenovirus, influenzavirus A and B, parainfluenza virus 1, 2, and 3, and respiratory syncytial virus (RSV).

Usage. Enables early and direct detection of seven common respiratory viruses so that treatment can begin while one is awaiting confirmatory cultures.

Description. The Respiratory Antigen Panel allows for direct immunofluorescence detection of respiratory viral antigens from nasopharyngeal secretions and sputum, with specificity of 97%-99% and varying sensitivities. The seven viruses that are responsible for common and severe respiratory illness are included in the panel: respiratory syncytial virus, respiratory adenovirus, and influenza viruses A and B, and parainfluenza viruses 1, 2, 3. After the virus is identified, antibodies are added, and the sample is incubated. Antigen-antibody complexes are observed under direct immunofluorescence after IgG is added to the specimen. Sensitivity for RSV is 95%-99%. Thus confirmatory culture is not needed. For all other organisms, sensitivity ranges from only 20%-50%; therefore confirmatory culture is recommended.

Professional Considerations
1. Consent form NOT required.
2. Preparation:
   A. Obtain viral transport media.
3. Procedure:
   A. Collect a 1-mL nasal aspirate, or sputum, or a throat swab. Place immediately in viral transport media.
4. Postprocedure care:
   A. Document source of specimen on the laboratory requisition and send specimen to the laboratory.
   B. Specimen is viable for 2 hours at room temperature or for 3 days when refrigerated.
5. Client and family teaching:
   A. Teach client the proper method to produce a deep cough specimen.
6. Factors that affect results:
   A. Results are invalidated if swab or specimen was allowed to dry.
   B. False positive reactions for group A streptococcus have been found in the presence of *S. milieri*.
7. Other data:
   A. None.

RESPIRATORY DISTRESS INDEX
(*see Polysomnography, Diagnostic*)

RESPIRATORY SYNCYTIAL VIRUS (RSV), CULTURE

Norm. Negative for respiratory syncytial virus (RSV).

Usage. Detection of the presence of RSV in obtained medium.

Description. RSV is an important cause of lower respiratory infections in infants. This virus, originally isolated in 1956, has become a major pathogen in children worldwide. It typically occurs seasonally during the winter months, afflicts almost all infants by 2 years of age and can be very severe and even fatal in the immunocompromised. Symptoms are most pronounced in those infants with the lowest cellular and humoral immunity. Thus, those with prematurity, congenital heart disease, and cystic fibrosis or other underlying respiratory problems are at greatest risk of having RSV. RSV risk is also increased in those infants in day care, or living in crowded conditions, as well as those exposed to passive smoke. In adults, RSV manifests itself as an upper respiratory infection. Currently, there is no antiviral medication available that will treat RSV; thus treatment is primarily supportive and includes oxygenation, hydration, and nutritional interventions.

Professional Considerations

1. Consent form NOT required.
2. Preparation:
   A. Obtain a chilled viral transport medium and a sterile wire swab in a pack.
   B. Open the transport medium, and place it in ice.
   C. Obtain assistance for restraint of the client if necessary.
3. Procedure:
   A. Explain the procedure to the client and offer reassurance.
   B. Bend the wire swab; open the pack.
   C. Restrain the client if necessary, pass the wire through one naris and into the nasopharynx, and rotate the swab quickly.
   D. Remove the swab, place it into the medium, and close.
   E. Transport to the laboratory immediately.
4. Postprocedure care:
   A. None.
5. Client and family teaching:
   A. This test is performed to try to isolate the pathogen causing the illness.

   B. Results are normally available within 48-72 hours.
6. Factors that affect results:
   A. Specimens must remain cold and do not tolerate freezing and thawing well.
   B. Inaccurate swabbing or swabbing of the wrong location.
7. Other data:
   A. Serologic isolation should also be considered.
   B. Many efforts are underway to develop vaccines, monoclonal antibodies and other prophylactic measure for RSV. RSV intravenous immune globulin and palivzumab are two products now available for immunoprophylaxis and are recommended as described below:
      i. Palivzumab monoclonal immune globulin:
         a. Prophylaxis in children <age 2 with respiratory disease requiring continuous oxygen or inhalation or steroid treatment for at least 6 months;
         b. Premature infants (born prior to week 26 of gestation).
      ii. Ribavirin inhalation
         a. High-risk infants with a severe RSV infection.
      iii. Ribavirin plus intravenous polyclonal immunoglobulin
         a. Clients (any age) after allogenic stem cell or organ transplant; and
         b. Accompanied by more than one course of treatment for transplant rejection; and
         c. Accompanied by RSV pneumonia.
   C. There is some evidence showing later development of reactive airway disease in those who had active RSV illness at an early age.

RESPIRATORY VIRUS DIRECT STAIN PANEL

(see Respiratory antigen panel, Specimen)

RESPIRATORY VIRUS IMMUNOFLUORESCENCE

(see Respiratory antigen panel, Specimen)

RETICULOCYTE COUNT, BLOOD

Norm. Constitutes 1%-2% of the total RBC count.

		SI UNITS
Adult females	0.5%-2.5%	$0.005\text{-}0.025 \times 10^{-3}$
Adult males	0.5%-1.5%	$0.005\text{-}0.015 \times 10^{-3}$
Cord blood	3.0%-7.0%	$0.030\text{-}0.070 \times 10^{-3}$
Newborn	1.1%-4.5%	$0.011\text{-}0.045 \times 10^{-3}$
Neonates	0.1%-1.5%	$0.001\text{-}0.015 \times 10^{-3}$
Infants	0.5%-3.1%	$0.005\text{-}0.031 \times 10^{-3}$
Children >6 months	0.5%-4.0%	$0.005\text{-}0.040 \times 10^{-3}$
Immature reticulocyte fraction (IRF)	0.13%-0.31%	$0.001\text{-}0.004 \times 10^{-3}$

Increased Total Reticulocyte Count. Acquired autoimmune hemolytic anemia, DiGuglielmo disease, erythemic myelosis (chronic), erythroblastosis fetalis, hemolytic anemias, hemoglobin C disease, hemorrhage (chronic), hereditary spherocytosis, infants, leukemia, malaria, metastatic carcinoma, myxoma of left heart atrium, paroxysmal nocturnal hemoglobinuria, polycythemia, posthemorrhagic anemia (acute), pregnancy, sickle cell disease, thalassemia major, thrombotic thrombocytopenic purpura, transfusion therapy, treatment of iron-deficiency anemia, and vitamin B_{12}–deficiency or folic acid deficiency.

Increased Immature Reticulocyte Fraction. Anemia (hemolytic), blood loss, bone marrow regeneration, folic acid/folate deficiency, iron deficiency, myelodysplasia, and thalassemia.

Decreased Total Reticulocyte Count. Alcoholism, anemia (aplastic, hemolytic (aplastic crisis), iron deficiency, megaloblastic, pernicious, pure red cell), anoxia, aregenerative crisis, blood loss, bone marrow regeneration, chronic infection, iron-deficiency anemias, myxedema, and radiation therapy. Drugs include carbamazepine and chloramphenicol.

Children <6 months old who were born before gestational week 26. Ribavirin inhalation treatment may be considered in high-risk infants with clinical symptoms indicating a serious course of an RSV infection. Treatment with ribavirin in combination with intravenous polyclonal immunoglobulin should be considered in patients who have received an allogenic stem cell transplantation or organ transplantation with >1 episode of rejection treatment and who have mild or moderate RSV pneumonia. Evidence-based documentation for treatment of other groups of patients is lacking.

Description. A reticulocyte is a nonnucleated red blood cell containing a basophilic network of granules or filaments characteristic of an immature cell of the erythrocyte class. Formed in the bone marrow, reticulocytes reach maturity after 1 day in the circulating blood and are an index of bone marrow function. The reticulocyte count is the number of reticulocytes per 1000 erythrocytes and is significant only when reported as a percentage of the total number of erythrocytes. This test assists in the diagnosis and differentiation of bone marrow depression from anemias, hemorrhage, hemolysis, or radiation, and in evaluation of bone marrow activity and response to therapeutic interventions. Some test results include an immature reticulocyte fraction (IRF), determined by the staining abilities of the reticulocytes. Young reticulocytes have a higher of RNA staining. Higher than normal amounts of immature reticulocytes can indicate conditions in which there is more red blood cell production, such as after erythropoietin administration. The IRF is also useful in detecting new or increasing erythropoiesis after bone marrow or stem cell transplant.

Professional Considerations
1. Consent form NOT required.
2. **Preparation:**
   A. Obtain venipuncture supplies and a lavender-topped tube or

white blood cell pipette and supravital dye (such as brilliant cresyl blue or new methylene blue).

B. Do NOT draw specimens during hemodialysis.

3. **Procedure:**
   A. Adult:
      i. Leaving the tourniquet on no more than 1 minute, draw a 4-mL blood sample without trauma.
      ii. Gently tilt or roll the specimen six to eight times to mix the anticoagulant and the blood.
   B. Infant:
      i. Draw a fresh drop of capillary blood into a white blood cell pipette and mix with an equal volume of a supravital dye.

4. **Postprocedure care:**
   A. None.

5. **Client and family teaching:**
   A. This test measures your body's ability to make adequate numbers of red blood cells.
   B. Results are normally available within 4 hours.

6. **Factors that affect results:**
   A. Reject hemolyzed specimens or specimens not thoroughly mixed with EDTA anticoagulant.
   B. Hemodilution of the sample may occur if the specimen is drawn from an extremity that is being infused with intravenous solution.
   C. False-positive results have been reported with laboratory handling of the specimen that included drying of the coverslip preparation; incorrect concentration of sodium metabisulfite; and mixture with fibrinogen, gelatin, or thrombin on the slide.
   D. After transfusion with blood containing sickle cell trait, cells with the sickle cell trait are present for 4 months.
   E. False low results may occur when the sample is drawn soon after a blood transfusion.
   F. Drugs that may cause false-positive results include antipyretics, chloroquine hydrochloride, chloroquine phosphate, corticotropin, furazolidone (in infants), hydroxychloroquine sulfate, levodopa, primaquine phosphate, pyrimeth-

amine, quinacrine hydrochloride, quinine sulfate, and sulfonamides.
   G. Drugs that may cause false-negative results include azathioprine, chloramphenicol, dactinomycin, methotrexate sodium, and sulfonamides.

7. **Other data:**
   A. Reticulocyte count corrected for abnormal hematocrit only $= $ Reticulocyte % $\times$ (Hct/45).
   B. The immature reticulocyte fraction (IRF) was formerly called the reticulocyte maturity index (RIM).

RETICULOCYTE PRODUCTION INDEX (RPI), DIAGNOSTIC

Norm. Index of 1.

Increased. Accelerated red blood cell production.

Decreased. Alcoholism; anemia (aplastic, iron deficiency, megaloblastic, pernicious, pure red cell); aregenerative crisis; aplastic crisis of hemolytic anemia; chronic infection; iron-deficiency anemias; myxedema; and radiation therapy.

Description. The reticulocyte production index (RPI) is a calculated measurement of the number of circulating reticulocytes in relation to packed cell volume of hematocrit. The raw reticulocyte count is expressed as a percentage of erythrocytes. In anemia, a 1%-2% reticulocyte count is not really normal because it is based on a lower-than-normal amount of erythrocytes. Also the normal life span of reticulocytes is 2 days, but in the presence of accelerated red blood cell production, reticulocytes are released prematurely and circulate for up to 4 days. The RPI normalizes the reticulocyte count by multiplying it by the hematocrit divided by 45 and by correcting for the increased life span of reticulocytes (based on the degree of anemia) to give a more accurate portrayal of the rate of reticulocyte production. This index is used to calculate the degree of increased erythropoietic activity associated with the premature release of reticulocytes (shift) from the bone marrow in anemia.

Professional Considerations
1. Consent form NOT required.
2. **Preparation:**
   A. See *Reticulocyte count, Blood; Hematocrit, Blood.*
   B. Do NOT draw specimens during hemodialysis.
3. **Procedure:**
   A. Obtain samples for reticulocyte count and for VPRC (volume of packed red cells, hematocrit). See *Reticulocyte count, Blood; Hematocrit, Blood.*
   B. Calculation: Reticulocyte maturation time in the circulating blood changes as follows:

Hematocrit	Reticulocyte Maturation Time
35	1.5 days
30	1.75 days
25	2.0 days
20	2.25 days
15	2.5 days

The RPI is calculated as:

$$RPI = \frac{\text{Reticulocyte percentage}}{\text{Reticulocyte maturation time (days)}}$$

$$\times \frac{\text{Client's VPRC (1/1)}}{0.45}$$

4. **Postprocedure care:**
   A. See *Reticulocyte count, Blood; Hematocrit, Blood.*
5. **Client and family teaching:**
   A. This test measures the number of immature red blood cells in your bloodstream.
   B. Results are normally available within 24 hours.
6. **Factors that affect results:**
   A. See *Reticulocyte count, Blood; Hematocrit, Blood.*
7. **Other data:**
   A. See *Reticulocyte count, Blood; Hematocrit, Blood.*

RETINOBLASTOMA CHROMOSOME ABNORMALITIES, DIAGNOSTIC

Norm:

Female Karyotype	44 autosomes + 2X chromosomes 46,XX
Male Karyotype	44 autosomes + 1X and 1Y chromosome 46,XY

Note: Retinoblastoma chromosomal defect is identified as female, 46,XX,13q–; male, 46,XY,13q–.

Usage. Screening for retinoblastoma, identification of numerical chromosomal defects, and genetic counseling.

Description. Retinoblastoma is the most frequently occurring congenital ocular tumor in children, occurring in 1 in 20,000 births. Tumor occurrence is usually bilateral and nonmetastatic and may occur up to several years later in the second eye. Clinical symptoms include strabismus, impaired vision, and the appearance of white to yellow reflex from the pupil, referred to as "cat's-eye." Left untreated, this tumor is fatal because optic nerve, subarachnoid space, and cerebral tissue invasion occurs. Heredity accounts for 40% of the incidence of retinoblastoma through autosomal dominant transmission, from an unaffected gene-carrier parent or from germinal mutation in a normal parent. The retinoblastoma gene is located on the long arm of chromosome 13, q band 14. Deletion in the q band occurs in 50% of clients with retinoblastoma. Leukocyte screening of peripheral blood is the most common technique for chromosomal abnormality detection and analysis. Tissue cultures are cultivated from the blood sample, fixed, and stained. The chromosomes are then counted, photographed, and the karyotype is arranged according to the Denver nomenclature from cut photographs. Diagnosis is confirmed by computed tomography with or without magnetic resonance imaging, and radiotherapy is a common approach to treatment. Prognosis is dependent on location, size, and the amount of ocular and extraocular involvement.

Professional Considerations

1. Consent form NOT required.
2. Preparation:
   A. See *Client and family teaching.*
   B. Tube: Green topped.
   C. Specimens MAY be drawn during hemodialysis.
3. Procedure:
   A. A morning sample is preferred. Draw a 10-mL blood sample.
4. Postprocedure care:
   A. None.
5. Client and family teaching:
   A. This test is a genetic screen.
   B. Fast for 3 hours before the blood is drawn.
6. Factors that affect results:
   A. Insufficient number of cells in sample.
7. Other data:
   A. Retinoblastoma is also associated with elevated plasma somatostatin levels.
   B. The risk for metastasis of retinoblastoma is elevated when diagnosis is delayed, when both eyes are involved, and when there is invasion to the uvea, orbit, and optic nerve.

RETROGRADE PYELOGRAPHY, DIAGNOSTIC

Norm. Bilateral, symmetric, and uniform opacification of ureters, renal calyces, and renal pelvis. Normal size and architecture of these structures. Superimposed films on inspiration and expiration normally show two outlines of the renal pelvis 2 cm apart.

Usage. Assessment of displacement, drainage, enlargement, or fixation of the structures of the renal collecting system; detection of complete or partial obstruction as a result of blood clot, calculus, perinephric abscess, inflammation, stricture, or tumor formation; assessment for integrity of the renal pelvis and ureters after blunt trauma to the ureteropelvic junction. Also used in clients with bladder tumor, severe renal insufficiency, or hypersensitivity to iodine-based contrast material, and when visualization of the renal collecting system with excretory urography is inadequate.

Description. Retrograde pyelography is an invasive radiographic (fluoroscopic) examination of the kidneys from a distal direction via the ureters. During cystoscopy, catheters are passed into the ureters, and radiopaque contrast material is injected. The mucous membrane absorbs minimal amounts of the iodine radiopaque contrast material. Thus the complications of hypersensitivity reactions or delayed excretion of the dye in renal impairment that are associated with intravenous dye injections are avoided.

Professional Considerations

1. Consent form IS required.

Risks

Bladder perforation, hemorrhage, nausea, vomiting, urinary tract infection, vasovagal response.

Contraindications

Pregnancy (because of the radioactive iodine crossing the blood-placental barrier); severe dehydration. Sedatives are contraindicated in clients with central nervous system depression.

2. Preparation:
   A. See *Client and family teaching.*
   B. The client should disrobe below the waist.
3. Procedure:
   A. If deep sedation or anesthesia is used, monitor respiratory status and ECG continuously throughout the procedure.
   B. The client is placed in a dorsal lithotomy position, and a cystoscopic examination is performed. (See *Cystoscopy, Diagnostic.*)
   C. A catheter is then advanced through the ureter(s) into the renal pelvis. After drainage of the renal pelvis, iodine radiopaque contrast material is injected through the catheter(s) into the kidney(s) and anterior, posterior, lateral, and oblique radiographic films are obtained. A small amount of contrast material may be injected into the ureters as the catheter is removed, and radiographs of the ureters may then be taken.
   D. The procedure may also be performed without cystoscopy by injection of the radiopaque contrast material into the lower ureter after wedging a bulb catheter at the distal end of the ureter.

4. Postprocedure care:
   A. A ureteral or Foley catheter may be left in place after the examination.
   B. Continue assessment of respiratory status. If deep sedation or anesthesia was used, follow institutional protocol for postsedation monitoring. Typical monitoring includes continuous ECG monitoring and pulse oximetry, with continual assessments (every 5-15 minutes) of airway, vital signs, and neurologic status until the client is lying quietly awake, is breathing independently, and responds to commands spoken in a normal tone.
   C. Monitor vital signs at the end of the procedure and then every 4 hours for 24 hours.
   D. Observe for signs of allergic reaction to the dye for 24 hours.
   E. Encourage the oral intake of fluids when not contraindicated. Monitor urinary output for quantity and hematuria for 24 hours. Notify physician for bladder distention, anuria, oliguria, or hematuria. Gross hematuria or persistent hematuria after the third voiding is abnormal.
   F. Notify the physician if there are symptoms of infection (fever, tachycardia, hypotension, chills, dysuria, flank pain).
   G. Resume previous diet.
   H. Administer analgesic as prescribed.
5. Client and family teaching:
   A. This test helps to evaluate kidney structure.
   B. Fast for 8 hours before the procedure if general anesthesia is to be administered.
   C. A laxative may be prescribed the evening before the procedure.

A cleansing enema may be prescribed to be given the morning of the procedure.
   D. A sedative may be prescribed to be given just before the procedure.
   E. After the procedure is over, save all the urine voided and report chills or pain with urination. Notify the physician if there are symptoms of infection (see above, section 4-F).
6. Factors that affect results:
   A. Views are obscured by the presence of feces, gas, or barium in the bowel.
7. Other data:
   A. Impaired renal function does not affect test results.
   B. If the renal pelves are not visualized by this exam, ureteral obstruction may be present and may be localized by antegrade pyelography (see separate test listing).

REVERSE GIEMSA, DIAGNOSTIC

(see Banding in genetic disorders, Diagnostic)

REVIEW OF PERIPHERAL BLOOD SMEAR: RED BLOOD CELL MORPHOLOGY

(see Red blood cell morphology, Blood)

RFI

(see Renal indices, Diagnostic)

Rh TYPE, BLOOD

(see ABO group and Rh type, Blood)

RHEUMATOID FACTOR (RF), BLOOD

Norm:

Qualitative	Negative
Quantitative	
Normal	<1:20
Chronic inflammatory disease	<1:40
Diagnostic for rheumatoid arthritis	1:40-1:60
Advanced rheumatoid arthritis	>1:60

Increased. Allografts (skin, renal), ankylosing rheumatoid spondylitis, cancer, cirrhosis, dermatomyositis, diabetes mellitus, diseases (of the kidney, liver, or lung), endocarditis, healthy clients over 60 years of age, hepatic neoplasms, hepatitis, hypertension, infectious mononucleosis, juvenile rheumatoid arthritis, kala-azar, leishmaniasis, leprosy, lymphomas, macroglobulinemia, malaria, mixed connective tissue disease, neuropathy, osteoarthritis, paraproteinemia, polyarteritis nodosa, pulmonary interstitial fibrosis, sarcoidosis, schistosomiasis, scleroderma, Sjögren syndrome, splenomegaly, subacute bacterial endocarditis, syphilis, systemic lupus erythematosus, transfusions (multiple), tuberculosis, vaccinations (multiple), viral infections, and yaws.

Decreased after Previous Elevations. Gold salt therapy.

Description. Rheumatoid factor is an immunoglobulin present in the serum of 50%-95% of adults with rheumatoid arthritis. It appears in the serum and synovial fluid several months after the onset of rheumatoid arthritis and is present for up to years after therapy. The antibody of the macroglobulin type produced in the synovium appears in the presence of autoimmunity, chronic infections, or connective tissue defects. This factor, though not specific for rheumatoid arthritis, is very helpful in diagnosis because high titers correlate with severe disease as compared to titers with other diseases. Analgesia and anti-inflammatory pharmacologic preparations do not affect the presence of rheumatoid factor.

Professional Considerations
1. Consent form NOT required.
2. Preparation:
   A. Tube: Red topped, red/gray topped, or gold topped.
   B. Specimens MAY be drawn during hemodialysis.
3. Procedure:
   A. Draw a 2-mL blood sample.
4. Postprocedure care:
   A. None.
5. Client and family teaching:
   A. This is a screening test for many different disorders.

B. Results are normally available within 24 hours.
6. Factors that affect results:
   A. Anticoagulant in the specimen tube invalidates the results.
7. Other data:
   A. Clients who have rheumatoid factor identified early in the course of their rheumatoid arthritis have a greater risk of developing articular destruction than those identified later.

RINNE TEST, DIAGNOSTIC
(*see Tuning fork test of Weber, Rinne, and Schwabach tests, Diagnostic*)

ROCHALIMAEA HENSELAE ANTIBODY, SERUM

Norm. Titer <1:64.

Increased. Titer >1:64 or a fourfold rise in titer between acute and convalescent sera: cat-scratch disease.

Description. A serologic test to identify antibodies to *Rochalimaea henselae* (*Bartonella* species), an organism implicated in 1992 as the causative of cat-scratch disease in humans who have been bitten or scratched by an infected cat. The disease is characterized by unexplained regional lymphadenopathy, fever, malaise, and skin lesion at the site of injury. Although the cause of cat-scratch disease is not firmly established, *R. henselae* has been found in significantly higher levels in cats owned by clients infected with the disease and recently wounded by the cat. *R. henselae* is believed to be transmitted through the saliva or other body fluids of the sick cat when biting or scratching a human. In this indirect fluorescent antibody test, a sample of the client's serum with the *R. henselae* antigen and titers of antibodies to the antigen are measured. This test is more sensitive and specific than the skin test for *Bartonella* species.

Professional Considerations
1. Consent form NOT required.
2. Preparation:
   A. Tube: Red topped, red/gray topped, or gold topped.

B. Specimens MAY be drawn during hemodialysis.
3. **Procedure:**
   A. Draw a 2-mL blood sample.
4. **Postprocedure care:**
   A. None.
5. **Client and family teaching:**
   A. Avoid traumatic contact, such as rough playing, with kittens and cats because this disease may be transmitted through bites and scratches from the animals.
   B. Results are normally available within 24 hours.
6. **Factors that affect results:**
   A. None found.
7. **Other data:**
   A. Fleas have also been suspected as transmission sources for this disease.
   B. Most cases resolve spontaneously. Many antibiotics are not effective against *R. henselae* infections. Aminoglycosides have been found to be bactericidal against the organism.

ROCKY MOUNTAIN SPOTTED FEVER (RMSF) SEROLOGY, SERUM

Norm. Negative.
Indirect fluorescent antibody assay (most sensitive): Diagnostically significant: titer >128 in a single specimen, or fourfold rise in paired serum titers, or any positive titer for IgM.
Latex agglutination test: Active Rocky Mountain spotted fever: titer >128.
Complement fixation for rickettsial infection: >1:160 or fourfold increase in paired samples within 7 days.
Weil-Felix agglutination reaction for rickettsial disease (least sensitive test): Strong agglutination response to *Proteus* Ox-19++++ is suggestive of rickettsial disease.

Positive. High titers occur with continuous exposure to bacterial, *Proteus,* or rickettsial infection and recent vaccinations.

Negative. Normal finding. Low titers occur with antibiotic therapy (early in the disease course), and in symptomatic clients who are unable to produce antibodies during active infection (immunodeficiency disorders).

Description. Rocky Mountain spotted fever (RMSF) is an infectious disease caused by the parasite *Rickettsia rickettsii* transmitted to man by the bite of an infected tick (usually the wood tick, *Dermacentor andersoni;* the dog tick, *Dermacentor variabilis;* and occasionally the Lone Star tick, *Amblyomma americanum*). Although believed to exist in the Western Hemisphere, this disease can occur anywhere that the vector is present. Symptoms include the sudden onset of fever lasting 2-3 weeks and the appearance of a rash spreading from the palms of the hands and soles of the feet to the entire body. Death may occur if RMSF is diagnosis is delayed or the disease is left untreated or treated only with chloramphenicol and not tetracycline. Other factors placing the client at higher risk of death include elderly age, absence of classic symptoms, and lack of noted tick bite.

Professional Considerations
1. Consent form NOT required.
2. **Preparation:**
   A. Tube: Red topped, red/gray topped, or gold topped.
   B. Specimens MAY be drawn during hemodialysis.
3. **Procedure:**
   A. Draw a 5-mL blood sample, without trauma.
   B. An acute sample should be drawn with the onset of symptoms.
   C. Draw a convalescent sample 7 days later.
4. **Postprocedure care:**
   A. Send specimens to the laboratory immediately.
5. **Client and family teaching:**
   A. This is a screening test to determine exposure to certain bacteria, including *Rickettsia.*
   B. Return in 1 week to have a convalescent sample drawn. This will help determine if the disease is responding to treatment.
6. **Factors that affect results:**
   A. Weil-Felix false-positive reactions have been reported in *Borrelia* infection, *Proteus* infection, endemic typhus, leptospirosis, and liver disease (severe) and in clients who have been recently vaccinated.
   B. Weil-Felix false-negative reactions have been reported when antibiotic therapy is started before the first specimen is drawn.

ROTAVIRUS ANTIGEN, STOOL **975**

C. The latex agglutination test is useful only during active infection.

7. **Other data:**
   A. The Weil-Felix test is able to establish titers but does not use the causal agent as the reactive antigen. It is useful in screening for rickettsial infections but is unable to distinguish murine typhus from spotted fever. Indirect fluorescent antibody testing can be used for specific identification of RMSF.
   B. If the Weil-Felix agglutination test is positive, the possibility of a *Proteus* urinary tract infection should be considered.

ROENTGENOGRAPHY
(see Radiographic and Radiography)

ROSE BENGAL SCAN
(see Liver ^{131}I-scan, Diagnostic)

ROTAVIRUS ANTIGEN, BLOOD

Norm. Negative antigen screen.

Positive. Presence of rotavirus antibodies and postviral lactase deficiency.

Negative. Normal finding. Also disaccharidase deficiencies.

Description. Rotavirus is a sporadic, acute, infectious, diarrheal disease of the Reoviridae viral class, in which five serographs have been identified. It replicates exclusively in the epithelial cells of the small intestine during the winter or cooler months. This virus is the major cause of sporadic acute enteritis in infants and epidemic acute gastroenteritis in small children. Occurrence in the young is presumed to be due to the absence of a well-developed immune system. Rotavirus is presumed to be transmitted by the fecal-oral route and is detectable only during the first 7-8 days of illness. Symptoms in children start with vomiting and progress to fever, diarrhea, and abdominal cramping. Radioimmunoassay and complement-fixing antibody titers are used for rotavirus detection.

Professional Considerations
1. Consent form NOT required.
2. **Preparation:**
   A. Tube: Red topped, red/gray topped, or gold topped.
   B. Specimens MAY be drawn during hemodialysis.
3. **Procedure:**
   A. Draw a 5-mL blood sample without trauma.
   B. Heelstick is acceptable, collected in a Microtainer.
4. **Postprocedure care:**
   A. None.
5. **Client and family teaching:**
   A. These clients are most often children; therefore emotional support and comfort measures should be offered during blood draws.
   B. Results are normally available within 24 hours.
   C. Parents should maintain enteric precautions during the client's diarrheal symptoms.
6. **Factors that affect results:**
   A. Hemolysis of the specimen invalidates the results.
7. **Other data:**
   A. Clients with the rotavirus may be free of symptomatic illness.
   B. There is no specific treatment for rotavirus. Fluid and electrolyte balance should be supported to prevent severe dehydration.
   C. Rectal swabs and stool samples should be examined for the presence of rotavirus antigen. (See *Rotavirus antigen, Stool.*)
   D. Rotavirus should be suspected, when the symptoms of diarrhea, vomiting, and fever occur together in children.
   E. In 1998, a vaccine for rotavirus was made available, and subsequently removed from use by the FDA due to an increase in incidence of intestinal intussusception. Although the risk of intussusception was subsequently estimated to be 1:2500, the manufacturer is not planning a reintroduction of the vaccine.

ROTAVIRUS ANTIGEN, STOOL

Norm. Negative. The presence of rotavirus in neonates under 2 weeks of age is inconclusive.

Usage. Directly detects the rotavirus antigen that is shed in large amounts in the stool.

Description. Rotavirus illness is a diarrheal disease of the Reoviridae viral family, in which five serogroups have been identified. It replicates exclusively in the epithelial cells of the small intestine and is pathogenic primarily in infants and children during the winter or cooler months. Rotavirus is presumed to be transmitted by the fecaloral route. Rotavirus antigen in the stool is detected by direct visualization with electron microscopy or by the more common enzyme-linked immunosorbent assay (ELISA) screen. Also see *Rotavirus antigen, Blood.*

Professional Considerations

1. Consent form NOT required.
2. **Preparation:**
   A. Obtain a clean, dry, preservative-free, covered cardboard specimen container or a tube with a screw-topped cap, and a larger container of ice; or obtain a sterile culture swab and a closed, sterile container.
   B. The client should disrobe below the waist for rectal swab collection.
3. **Procedure:**
   A. *Stool collection:*
      i. Obtain 5 mL or 5 g of liquid stool in a closed container or soiled diaper as soon as possible after evacuation from the bowel.
   B. *Rectal swab collection:*
      i. Place the client in the left lateral position with knees and hips flexed and draped.
      ii. Gently insert a sterile cotton-tipped swab at least 2.5-3.0 cm into the rectum. Rotate the swab from side to side and leave it in place for a few seconds to allow absorption of rectal flora.
      iii. Place the swab into a sterile container without preservatives and cover tightly.
4. **Postprocedure care:**
   A. The stool container should be placed on ice and transported promptly to the laboratory.
   B. The rectal swab container should be labeled with the site and time

of collection, packed in ice, and sent promptly to the laboratory.
5. **Client and family teaching:**
   A. These clients are most often children; therefore supportive measures should be offered if collection occurs by rectal swabbing.
   B. Results are normally available within 24 hours.
   C. Parents should maintain enteric precautions during the client's diarrheal symptoms.
6. **Factors that affect results:**
   A. Reject specimens placed in preservatives or those not placed on ice.
   B. Prolonged rotaviral shedding has been found in clients with immunosuppression.
7. **Other data:**
   A. Clients with the rotavirus may be free of symptomatic illness.

RPR, DIAGNOSTIC
(see Rapid plasma reagin test, Diagnostic)

RUBELLA SEROLOGY, SERUM AND SPECIMEN

Norm. Negative titer. A fourfold rise in titer of paired titer or a sample positive for rubella-specific IgG or IgM is diagnostic of exposure to rubella.

Hemagglutination Inhibition Test:

Susceptibility to rubella infection	<1:8
Immunity uncertain	1:8
Immunity from prior infection or vaccination	>1:8
Resistance to rubella infection	>1:64

Fluorescent Antibody Test:

Susceptibility to rubella infection	<1+
Positive for rubella antibodies	>1+

Time-Resolved Fluorometric Immunoassay for Rubella Antibody

Low levels of antibody	15 IU/mL

Usage. Determination of rubella immune status. Differentiation of

R

rubella, measles, scarlet fever, erythema infectiosum, and exanthema subitum during pregnancy.

Description. Rubella, also known as "German measles," is an acute viral communicable disease of children and young adults. This infection is caused by the togavirus and produces a discrete red or pink macular rash that desquamates and vanishes in 2-3 days. It is transmitted client to client by direct contact with the discharges of infected clients or droplet-spray inhalation. Symptoms include rash, arthritis, and mild fever. Rubella is most common in underdeveloped countries, but outbreaks have occurred in well-developed countries secondary to suboptimal uptake of the vaccine. This test is useful when a pregnant woman is exposed to the rubella virus or an illness similar to rubella. Apparent or nonapparent transplacental fetal infection during the first trimester of pregnancy can result in spontaneous abortion or fetal congenital defects such as cataracts, cardiac lesions, congenital heart defects, deafness, encephalitis, hepatitis, growth and mental retardation, microcephaly, ocular lesions, pulmonary stenosis, radiolucencies of long bones, or retinopathy. This test measures rubella antibody levels to determine the existence of active disease or active immunity. The oral fluid test measures rubella antibodies from fluid taken from around the gum line.

Professional Considerations
1. Consent form NOT required.
2. **Preparation:**
   A. Tube: Red topped, red/gray topped, or gold topped. For oral fluid specimens obtain a sponge oral fluid collection device.
   B. Specimens MAY be drawn during hemodialysis.
3. **Procedure:**
   A. Draw a 3-mL blood or umbilical cord blood sample. Heelstick is acceptable, collected in a Microtainer.
   B. Collect oral fluid by saturating well the sponge device around the gum line.
   C. An acute sample should be drawn as soon as possible after symptoms appear.
   D. The convalescent sample should be drawn at least 7-14 days after the acute sample and preferably 14-21 days after the onset of symptoms.
4. **Postprocedure care:**
   A. None.
5. **Client and family teaching:**
   A. This test will reveal exposure to togavirus, the causative virus of rubella.
   B. If pregnant, avoid anyone known to have rubella.
   C. Return in 7-14 days for repeat testing.
   D. A negative test result in the mother rules out infection in the fetus.
   E. Rubella is highly communicable from adults for a week before and 4 days after the appearance of rash. Infants may transmit the virus in feces for up to 6 months.
6. **Factors that affect results:**
   A. Rubella antibodies remain present and static for many years.
   B. The antibody levels decline with age.
   C. The incidence of false-negative tests increases with age.
7. **Other data:**
   A. Confirmation of congenital infection requires that samples be drawn from the mother and the infant.
   B. Saliva samples are increasingly being used as an alternative to serum for detection of rubella virus. Oral samples are stable for 7 days.
   C. Several studies have demonstrated NO association of the measles, mumps, rubella (MMR) vaccine with autism.
   D. The MMR vaccination is recommended to be done twice, first between 12 and 15 months of age, and repeated between 4 and 6 years of age. It should NOT be given during pregnancy or within 28 days before becoming pregnant.

RUBEOLA SEROLOGY, SERUM

Norm. Negative. The presence of antibodies 1 week after the onset of symptoms is indicative of susceptibility to rubeola infection. Recent exposure to the virus shows a fourfold or greater increase in antibody titers in two consecutive samples (acute and convalescent) drawn 1-4 weeks apart with use of hemagglutination inhibition or complement fixation methods.

Usage. Diagnosis of measles.

Description. Rubeola is an acute, contagious, viral, communicable disease caused by the measles virus of the Paramyxoviridae family. It is transmitted by direct contact with or inhalation of the infected oral or nasal secretions of infected clients. Rubeola is characterized by the appearance of a blotchy red facial rash appearing 3 days after a fever, with progression to a generalized rash lasting about 1 week. Other symptoms include Koplick's spots in the mouth, rose-colored maculopapular skin eruptions, photosensitivity, and catarrhal symptoms. Uncomplicated cases are usually self-limiting, but death may occur from complications and in undernourished children.

Professional Considerations
1. Consent form NOT required.
2. Preparation:
   A. Tube: Red topped, red/gray topped, or gold topped.
   B. Specimens MAY be drawn during hemodialysis.
3. Procedure:
   A. Draw a 2-mL blood sample.
   B. Heelstick is acceptable, collected in a Microtainer.
4. Postprocedure care:
   A. None.
5. Client and family teaching:
   A. This test can reveal exposure to the Paramyxoviridae, which includes measles.
   B. Results are normally available within 24 hours.
6. Factors that affect results:
   A. Hemolysis or contamination alters the results.
7. Other data:
   A. ELISA assay is 20 times more sensitive than the complement fixation test and the hemagglutination inhibition test and is the assay of choice.

RUBIN'S TEST (UTEROTUBAL INSUFFLATION), DIAGNOSTIC

Norm. Bilaterally patent fallopian tubes.
Normal patency: Pressure rises to 80-100 mm Hg and then decreases as carbon dioxide passes through the fallopian tubes.
Partial patency: Pressure rises to between 120 and 130 mm Hg.
Occlusion of tubes: Pressure rises above 200 mm Hg.

Usage. Diagnosis of obstruction, stenosis, or stricture of the fallopian tubes; and detection of spasm of the uterine end of the fallopian tubes.

Description. Rubin's test involves transuterine fallopian tube insufflation with carbon dioxide. A flowmeter and pressure gauge are attached to the source of the carbon dioxide. Changes in pressure are recorded on a kymograph. Displacement of adhesions and removal of debris from the tubes may occur during the procedure.

Professional Considerations
1. Consent form NOT required.

Risks
Air embolism, hemorrhage, infection, and referred shoulder pain.

Contraindications
Infections of the cervix, fallopian tubes, or vagina; in suspected pregnancy; and with uterine bleeding.

2. Preparation:
   A. See *Client and family teaching.*
   B. An analgesic may be given 1 hour before the procedure to minimize tubal spasm from anxiety or discomfort.
   C. Obtain povidone-iodine solution, a vaginal speculum, cervical swabs, and a cervical cannula.
   D. The client should void.
3. Procedure:
   A. The client is placed in the dorsal lithotomy position, and the perineal area is cleansed with 1% povidone-iodine solution.
   B. The physician introduces a vaginal speculum and exposes the cervix.
   C. The cervix is swabbed.

D. A sterile cannula with a rubber tip is inserted into the cervical canal.

E. The cannula tip is pressed tightly against the cervical os to seal the opening and is secured with a tenaculum.

F. A rest period of approximately 2 minutes permits relaxation of the fallopian tubes.

G. 60 cc/minute of carbon dioxide (never air because of the risk of embolism) is administered into the uterus, and pressures are recorded by means of a kymograph.

H. During insufflation, a swishing sound may be heard with a stethoscope as the carbon dioxide passes through the tubes.

I. Shoulder pain caused by gas-induced subphrenic pneumoperitoneum is an indication of patency of at least one fallopian tube.

4. **Postprocedure care:**
   A. Nausea, vomiting, cramping, dizziness, and pain associated with carbon dioxide gas absorption may be reduced by having the client rest for 2-3 hours with the pelvis elevated.

5. **Client and family teaching:**
   A. This test will determine the patency of the fallopian tubes.
   B. Rubin's test takes approximately 30 minutes and is performed on an ambulatory care basis.
   C. You may be prescribed a laxative to take the night before the exam-

ination or may be given a suppository or enema before the procedure.

D. Shoulder-top pain may be felt with insufflation.

E. You may rest with the pelvis elevated for several hours to reduce discomfort secondary to gas absorption.

6. **Factors that affect results:**
   A. Anxiety can cause fallopian tube spasm.

7. **Other data:**
   A. This test is performed 4-5 days after the last day of menstruation.
   B. Because Rubin's test can ensure only that at least one fallopian tube is patent, it is of limited value.
   C. See also *Hysterosalpingography, Diagnostic.*

RUMPEL-LEEDE TOURNIQUET TEST, DIAGNOSTIC

(see Capillary fragility test, Diagnostic)

SAECG, DIAGNOSTIC

(see Signal-averaged electrocardiography, Diagnostic)

SAHARA CLINICAL BONE ULTRASONOMETRY

(see Bone ultrasonometry, Diagnostic)

SALICYLATE (ASPIRIN, ACETYLSALICYLIC ACID), BLOOD

Norm. Negative.

		SI UNITS
Analgesia therapeutic level	<100 μg/mL	0.72 mmol/L
Anti-inflammatory therapeutic level	100-200 μg/mL	1.09-1.45 mmol/L
Panic level	>50 μg/dL	3.62 mmol/L

Overdose Symptoms and Treatment

Symptoms. Acidemia, alkalosis, convulsions, dizziness, hyperactivity, hyperglycemia, hyperpnea, hyperthermia, ketosis, nausea, respiratory arrest, tinnitus, vomiting.

Treatment:

Note: Treatment choice(s) depend on client history and condition and episode history.

Early emptying of the stomach is important; use ipecac syrup if the client is conscious.

Monitor salicylate levels with serial serum draws.

Oral activated charcoal should be considered as vomiting ceases. The *Position Statement and Practice Guidelines on the Use of Multi-Dose Activated Charcoal in the Treatment of Acute Poisoning* from the American Academy of Clinical Toxicology, European Association of Poisons Centres and Clinical Toxicologists (1999) indicates that data are insufficient to recommend the use of charcoal therapy for salicylate poisoning. One animal study and two of four human studies did not show increased clearance with charcoal therapy.

Urine alkalinization to pH >7.5 with bicarbonate and fluids. Measure urine pH every hour.

Fluid resuscitation may be necessary. This may be orally in mild cases, intravenously in severe cases.

A single dose of vitamin K may be given for the rare case of hypoprothrombinemia.

In the case of renal failure, dialysis is indicated. Both hemodialysis and peritoneal dialysis WILL remove acetylsalicylic acid.

4. **Postprocedure care:**
   A. Assess for tinnitus and dizziness, signs of mild salicylate toxicity.
5. **Client and family teaching:**
   A. Watch for and seek medical attention for signs of toxicity, such as tinnitus and dizziness.
   B. If activated charcoal was given for elevated levels, the client should drink 4-6 glasses of water each day for 2 days to prevent constipation. The activated charcoal will cause stools to be black for a few days.
   C. For intentional overdose, refer client and family for crisis intervention.
6. **Factors that affect results:**
   A. Negative result found in ketoacidosis.
   B. False high values have been found in infants with hyperbilirubinemia.
   C. Sodium azide increases results.
   D. An herbal or natural remedy that increases results is *Ginkgo biloba*.
   E. Urine alkalinization (as by antacids) speeds renal excretion.
7. **Other data:**
   A. Salicylate poisoning may include alkalemia, followed by acidemia, ketosis, and hyperglycemia.
   B. Salicylate hepatitis can occur at blood concentrations of 20-25 mg/dL.

Usage. Monitoring for salicylate toxicity during salicylate therapy or when overdose is suspected.

Description. Salicylates are a group of nonnarcotic drugs with analgesic, antipyretic, anti-inflammatory, and platelet aggregation–inhibiting (aspirin only) effects. Salicylates are absorbed in the gastrointestinal tract, metabolized in the liver, and excreted in the urine, with a half-life of 2-3 hours in short-term use and 15-30 hours in chronic use.

Professional Considerations
1. Consent form NOT required.
2. **Preparation:**
   A. Optimal sampling time for blood is 2-6 hours after salicylate ingestion.
   B. Tube: Red topped, red/gray topped, or gold topped.
   C. Do NOT draw specimens during hemodialysis.
3. **Procedure:**
   A. Draw a 1-mL blood sample.
   B. Heelstick is acceptable, collected in a Microtainer.

SALMONELLA TITER, BLOOD

Norm. Less than a fourfold rise in titer between acute and convalescent specimens.

Positive. Fever of undetermined origin and salmonellosis.

Description. *Salmonella* is a complex genus of gram-negative, non–spore-forming rods that are facultatively anaerobic. There are four subgenera of *Salmonella* (*S. typhi*, *S. choleraesuis*, *S. enteritidis*, and *S. arizonae*) as well as 1500 serotypes. *Salmonella* causes salmonellosis; typhoid fever; paratyphoid fever; septicemia; and sometimes inflammations of the joints and organs. The mode of transmission is through the fecal-oral route, most commonly by ingestion of food contaminated with the feces of infected clients or animals. *Salmonella* organisms enhance their own uptake into the intestinal epithelium of the host. This test uses cellular (O) antigens and flagellar (H) antigens to detect the presence of *Salmonella* antibodies in a sample of serum.

Professional Considerations
1. Consent form NOT required.
2. Preparation:
   A. Specify for *Salmonella* antigens of groups A, B, C, or D on the laboratory requisition.
   B. Tube: Red topped, red/gray topped, or gold topped.
   C. Specimens MAY be drawn during hemodialysis.
3. Procedure:
   A. Draw a 7-mL blood sample. Label the specimen as the acute sample.
   B. Repeat the test in 3-5 days and label the tube as the convalescent sample.
   C. Heelstick is acceptable, collected in a Microtainer.
4. Postprocedure care:
   A. None.
5. Client and family teaching:
   A. Thoroughly cook food, and avoid ingesting raw eggs or foods that have been sitting at room temperature for more than 2 hours.
   B. In addition to standard precautions, practice enteric precautions

with the clothing and linen of infected clients.
6. Factors that affect results:
   A. Hemolysis or insufficient volume invalidates the results.
   B. Titers on a single specimen are not diagnostically significant.
   C. False-positive results may occur because of cross-reacting bacterial antibodies.
   D. Antibiotic treatment may cause false-negative results.
7. Other data:
   A. Stool culture is the definitive technique for diagnosing bacterial diarrhea.
   B. The use of fluoroquinolones in animals has contributed to increasing emergence of strains of *Salmonella* resistant to these drugs. For this reason, this class of drugs is recommended to be restricted to use in humans only.

SaO$_2$, BLOOD
(see Blood gases, Arterial, Blood)

SCA GENE TEST, DIAGNOSTIC

Norm. Normal repeat numbers range from 15 to 29.

CYTOSINE ADENOSINE GUANINE REPEAT RANGE					
	SCA1	**SCA2**	**SCA3**	**SCA6**	**SCA7**	**SCA12**
Normal	6-39	14-31	12-41	7-18	7-17	Not found
Pathologic	41-81	35-64	40-84	21-27	38-130	Not found

Wilmot and Warren (1998).

Usage. Genetic testing determines diagnosis, course of disease, and likelihood of transmission of disease from generation to generation.

Description. SCA gene testing identifies autosomal dominant neurodegenerative spinocerebellar ataxia (SCA) genes found in Machado-Joseph disease (MJD) and other ataxias. SCA 1, SCA2, SCA3, SCA6, SCA7, and SCA12 members of a group known as "triplet repeat

diseases" or "CAG repeat diseases" (cytosine, adenine, and guanine). In CAG repeat diseases, the trinucleotide sequence repeats abnormally within the gene coding sequence. At least 8 genes have been identified as causative for the cerebellar ataxias. MJD, one of the most common ataxias, is characterized by abnormalities in the SCA3 gene. It includes symptoms of progressive weakness of the extremities, spasticity, dysphagia, exophthalmos, diplopia and urinary frequency, and can occur in either mild or severe form, beginning at age 10 years. By identification of the intricate intracellular mechanisms by which SCA functions, treatments and cures for neurodegenerative diseases may eventually be found. This test involves isolating the DNA from the blood sample, then amplifying the CAG repetitions via polymerase chain reaction.

Professional Considerations

1. Consent form IS required.
2. Preparation:
   A. Tube: Lavender topped.
3. Procedure:
   A. Collect a 3.5 mL blood sample. Lavender-topped tubes need 10 to 20 mL of whole blood.
4. Postprocedure care:
   A. None.
5. Client and family teaching:
   A. Consult insurance provider or legal counsel before having test done.
   B. Persons with the disease had numbers from 35 to 59.
   C. A repeat number in the low fifties for SCA2 represents probably a severe form of the disease.
6. Factors that affect results:
   A. Less than 3 mL in EDTA tube.
   B. SCA diseases vary considerably across different ethnic groups and geographic regions.
7. Other data:
   A. None.

SCHICK TEST FOR DIPHTHERIA, DIAGNOSTIC

Norm. Negative test.

Usage. Measurement of immunity to diphtheria. To eliminate the carrier state of strains during epidemics.

Description. The Schick test is an intracutaneous skin test to determine the immunity strain for diphtheria by detecting the presence of antitoxins in the blood to this respiratory disease. One performs the test by injecting $1/50$ of the minimum lethal dose of diphtheria toxin and then observing the site for a reaction, which would indicate lack of diphtheria immunity. A negative response indicates the presence of diphtheria antitoxin in the client's bloodstream.

Professional Considerations

1. Consent form NOT required.
2. Preparation:
   A. Obtain two intradermal needles with syringes, and two alcohol pads.
3. Procedure:
   A. Cleanse the forearm sites for injection with alcohol pads and allow the areas to dry.
   B. Inject intracutaneously 0.1 mL of purified diphtheria toxin into one forearm and 0.1 mL of inactivated diphtheria toxoid into the other forearm.
   C. Observe the sites for reaction 24-48 hours (no longer than 120 hours) later. Absence of erythema, induration, and necrosis at the site is indicative of immunity to diphtheria.
4. Postprocedure care:
   A. Leave the injection sites open to air.
   B. For positive responses, inject $1/13$ U of diphtheria antitoxin to neutralize the toxin.
5. Client and family teaching:
   A. This test will indicate whether you are immune to diphtheria.
   B. The recommended schedule for active immunization of children is 2 months, 4 months, 6 months, 18 months, and 4-6 years of age.
6. Factors that affect results:
   A. Expired toxin will cause false-negative results.
7. Other data:
   A. If a client has been actively immunized but the Schick test is positive, the client is unable to produce antibodies.

SCHILLING TEST, DIAGNOSTIC

Norm. Over 10% absorption of vitamin B_{12} or $\geq 7\%$ of a 1-mg dose excreted within the first 24 hours. Clients lacking intrinsic factor will excrete <2% of the administered dose in the first 24 hours. Clients with intestinal malabsorption will excrete 3%-5% of the administered dose in the first 24 hours.

	STAGE I ABNORMAL
Stage II Normal	Pernicious anemia
	Gastrectomy or gastric bypass
	Congenital absence or abnormal
	functioning of intrinsic factor
Stage II Abnormal	Bacterial overgrowth syndrome
	Fish tapeworm
	Ileal dysfunction or resection
	Pancreatic insufficiency
	Pernicious anemia + ileal dysfunction +
	prolonged cyanocobalamin deficiency
	Renal insufficiency

Snow (1999).

Usage. Alcoholism, Crohn's disease in terminal ileum, differential diagnosis of macrocytic anemias, enteric steatorrhea, folic acid anemia, gastritis, malabsorption, megaloblastic anemia, pernicious anemia, and small intestine malabsorption.

Description. The Schilling test is a vitamin B_{12} (cyanocobalamin) absorption test that indicates if a client lacks intrinsic factor by measuring excretion of orally administered, radiolabeled cyanocobalamin (vitamin B_{12}) in a 24-hour urine sample. Vitamin B_{12} normally combines with intrinsic factor from the stomach and is absorbed in the terminal ileum. The test is based on the fact that, in normal clients, absorbed vitamin B_{12} in excess of the body's needs is excreted in the urine. Because parenteral nonradiolabeled cyanocobalamin is also administered to saturate the vitamin B_{12}-binding sites, all the radiolabeled cyanocobalamin should eventually be excreted in the urine.

Professional Considerations
1. Consent form NOT required.

Risks
Increased renal dysfunction.

Contraindications
Pregnancy, breast-feeding.

2. **Preparation:**
   A. Assess kidney function by serum urea nitrogen and creatinine levels.
   B. See *Client and family teaching*.
   C. Obtain a 3-L urine container without a preservative.
3. **Procedure:**
   A. *Stage I test:*
      i. 0.5 mCi of cyanocobalamin CO-57 is administered in capsule form, followed 2 hours later by an intramuscular injection of vitamin B_{12}.
      ii. Collect all urine over the next 24 hours in a clean container without preservatives.
   B. *Stage II test:*
      i. *The Stage II test is performed if the excretion of the radiolabeled cyanocobalamin is low (<7%) from the Stage I test.*
      ii. 3-7 days later, the procedure should be repeated with use of hog intrinsic factor given orally along with radioactive cyanocobalamin.
      iii. If this excretion is normal, the original values were attributable to intrinsic factor deficiency. However, if this second test remains abnormal, malabsorption is attributable to an intestinal disorder or renal insufficiency. A normal test after antibiotic treatment would indicate malabsorption of vitamin B_{12} caused by bacterial infection.

4. Postprocedure care:
    A. Food and drink are permitted after the intramuscular dose of vitamin B_{12}.
    B. Observe the client carefully for up to 60 minutes after injection for a possible (anaphylactic) reaction to the radionuclide.
    C. When urine is being handled, rubber gloves should be worn for 24 hours after the procedure. Wash the gloved hands with soap and water before removing the gloves. Wash the ungloved hands after gloves are removed.
    D. Send the entire specimen to the laboratory. The test is performed on an aliquot of the 24-hour specimen.
5. Client and family teaching:
    A. This test will indicate whether you lack intrinsic factor, which helps your body absorb vitamin B_{12}.
    B. The client should fast for 8-12 hours before the test.
    C. Do not take B vitamins for at least 3 days or laxatives for at least 24 hours before the test.
    D. Save all the urine voided, urinate before defecating, and avoid contaminating the urine with stool or toilet tissue. If any urine is accidentally discarded, discard the entire specimen and restart the collection the next day.
    E. Instruct the client to meticulously wash the hands with soap and water after each void for 24 hours.
6. Factors that affect results:
    A. Incomplete urine collection or stool mixed with urine invalidates the results.
    B. A radioactive scan within 7 days before the test invalidates the results.
    C. Diabetes mellitus, hypothyroidism, intestinal bacterial overgrowth by decreasing intestinal vitamin B_{12} absorption, kidney disease, liver disease, myxedema, pancreatic insufficiency.
    D. Partial gastrectomy will cause no detection of vitamin B_{12} as a result of lack of the intrinsic factor that enables vitamin B_{12} absorption.
7. Other data:
    A. At least 5 days should pass between Schilling tests.

B. Bone marrow procedures should be performed before the Schilling test.
C. Half-life of CO-57 is 270 days.

SCHIRMER TEARING EYE TEST, DIAGNOSTIC

Norm. ≥ 10 mm of moisture from each eye after 5 minutes.
Absent tear production in Sjögren syndrome.
Reduced tear production in meibomian gland dysfunction.

Usage. Aging that results in tearing, leukemia, lymphoma, Sjögren syndrome, and rheumatoid arthritis.

Description. The Schirmer test differentiates "keratoconjunctivitis sicca" from abnormal or reduced tearing of the eyes. In normal eyes, both basic and reflex tearing keep the eyes moist. Basic tearing occurs throughout the day supplying basic essential nutrients and lubricants to the eyes, and reflex tearing occurs in response to eye irritation. Either or both types of tearing capability may be absent or reduced in different disorders and lead to ocular surface damage. The Schirmer tearing eye test involves the simultaneous testing of the tearing ability of both eyes to assess the function of the lacrimal glands. The amount of moisture accumulating on filter paper held against the conjunctival sac is evaluated. Filter paper that remains dry for 15 minutes indicates insufficient tear formation.

Professional Considerations
1. Consent form NOT required.
2. Preparation:
    A. Two sterile strips of filter paper ruled in millimeters.
    B. Topical anesthetic such as proparacaine.
3. Procedure:
    A. To measure the function of accessory lacrimal glands, instill one drop of topical anesthetic into each conjunctival sac before inserting the strips.
    B. Position the client sitting upright with the head tilted back against a headrest.

C. Instruct the client to look upward and gently lower the inferior lids. Hook the folded ends of the filter paper strips over the inferior eyelids at the juncture between the middle and the lateral third.

D. After 5 minutes, remove the strips and measure the length of the moistened area in millimeters, starting from the folded ends of the strips.

E. The diagnosis of aqueous, tear-deficient dry eye is confirmed if 5 mm or less of tearing is evident on the filter paper.

4. Postprocedure care:
   A. Assess for corneal abrasion caused by rubbing the eyes before the topical anesthetic has worn off.

5. Client and family teaching:
   A. This test assesses the tearing ability of the eyes.
   B. After the test, do not rub your eyes until the topical anesthetic has worn off (usually about 30 minutes). Rubbing the eyes before this time can cause a corneal abrasion, which is painful and takes several days to heal.

6. Factors that affect results:
   A. Rubbing or squeezing the eyes increases tearing.

7. Other data:
   A. The results of the Schirmer test are not consistently reproducible. The test also is not very sensitive for detecting dry eyes. Two additional tests being developed are the tear break-up time (TBUT) test and the fluorescein meniscus time (FMT). The TBUT identifies unstable tears that contribute to dry eye, and the FMT measures how long it takes for tears to form.
   B. Drops containing sodium hyaluronidate are sometimes helpful in preventing ocular surface damage from dry eye. Punctal occlusion increases the amount of tears remaining on the eye surface by reducing the rate of tear outflow.

SCHLICHTER TEST (MBD, MAXIMUM BACTERICIDAL DILUTION, SERUM KILLING TEST), SPECIMEN

Norm. Bactericidal activity >1:8 dilution.

Usage. Endocarditis and osteomyelitis.

Description. Determination of the maximal dilution necessary to be bactericidal for 99.9% of clients with an infecting organism. The maximum inhibitory dilution (MID) is the highest dilution of the client's serum that will inhibit growth of the pathogen. The maximum inhibitory dilution (MID) is the highest dilution of the client's serum that will eradicate the organism.

Professional Considerations

1. Consent form NOT required.
2. Preparation:
   A. Obtain venipuncture supplies and a red-topped, red/gray-topped, or gold-topped tube, or a sterile tube and sterile aspiration set for body fluid testing.
   B. List any recent antibiotic therapy on the laboratory requisition.
   C. Specimens MAY be drawn during hemodialysis.
3. Procedure:
   A. Obtain both peak and trough levels: Draw a 3-mL blood sample in the blood tube or a 2-mL body fluid sample by sterile aspiration.
4. Postprocedure care:
   A. Transport to laboratory within 1 hour after collection.
5. Client and family teaching:
   A. This test evaluates the success of antibiotic treatment.
6. Factors that affect results:
   A. Specimens over 4 hours old invalidate the results.
7. Other data:
   A. It is preferred that two specimens be obtained: One before antibiotic treatment and the other 30-45 minutes after an antibiotic dose.
   B. Results take 2-3 days.

SCINTIMAMMOGRAPHY (MIRALUMA™, SESTAMIBI BREAST IMAGING, RADIONUCLIDE BREAST IMAGING), DIAGNOSTIC

Normal or Negative. No uptake, or minimal symmetric, bilateral, uniform, diffuse uptake; equal to soft-tissue uptake.

Abnormal or Positive. Malignant lesions are noted by focal areas of increased uptake of the radioisotope. The results may be graded from 1-5, reflecting the progressive probability of a malignant lesion or as equivocal, low, moderate, or high uptake of the isotope, with low, moderate, and high generally associated with malignant disease.

Usage. Follow-up or adjunct test to mammography in evaluating breast lesions in clients with an abnormal mammogram or palpable breast mass. Since the test depends on the molecular differences between cancer cells and normal cells and not on tissue density, it is useful in the further evaluation of breast lesions in women, especially if the woman has dense breast tissue (that is, fibrocystic disease, fatty tissue, or previous breast surgery, radiation therapy, chemotherapy, biopsy, breast implants, or silicone injections). It is not used for routine breast cancer screening, for confirming the presence or absence of breast cancer, or in place of biopsy. It helps the health care professional more accurately predict the chances of a breast lesion being cancerous. Research is being conducted to establish the effectiveness of the test in detecting axillary lymph node involvement in breast cancer and in the evaluation of breast tumor response to chemotherapy.

Description. A nuclear medicine planar scan in which a radioisotope, technetium-99m sestamibi, (Miraluma, ^{99m}Tc-sestamibi, ^{99m}Tc-MIBI) is used to provide pictures of breast lesions. A "trace" amount of the radioisotope is injected intravenously and accumulates in areas of increased metabolic activity, such as that found in malignant cells. Images of each breast are taken by a gamma (Anger) camera to identify any areas of focal uptake of the isotope,

indicating the possible presence of a cancerous lesion. A high-resolution method of this procedure has been shown to be more sensitive than a conventional camera for differentiating indeterminate breast lesions, but is still inferior to biopsy.

Professional Considerations
1. Consent form IS required.

Risks
Rare reports of severe hypersensitivity or seizures. Allergic reaction (itching, hives, rash, tight feeling in throat, shortness of breath, bronchospasm, anaphylaxis, death). Women of childbearing age should have minimal exposure because of the relatively high radiation dose to ovaries.
Pregnant females: No studies have been done in pregnant females; the test should be administered only if clearly needed.
Nursing mothers: Components of ^{99m}Tc-sestamibi are excreted in breast milk; therefore formula feedings should be substituted for breast feedings.
Pediatric population: Safety has not been established.

Contraindications
Previous allergic reaction to Cardiolite or Miraluma (which are the same drug) or other radioactive dyes.

2. Preparation:
   A. Have emergency equipment readily available.
   B. Assess for hypersensitivity to radioactive dyes.
   C. Ask if the female client is pregnant or nursing.
   D. Ask the client if there are any known breast lumps or other problems with the breast, a surgery or injury to the breasts, breast implants, or injections. The test should be performed before or at least 7-10 days after fine-needle aspiration, 4-6 weeks after a breast biopsy, and at least 2-3 months after breast surgery or radiotherapy. (This decreases the risk of nonspecific uptake of ^{99m}Tc-sestamibi.)
   E. No fasting is necessary. The client may eat, drink, and take prescribed medications as usual before the test.

F. Have client remove all clothing and jewelry above the waist and provide hospital gown.

G. Establish intravenous access in the arm opposite from the breast with the suspected lesion.

H. At this time there are no definite guidelines regarding the timing of the test with a specific phase of the menstrual cycle.

3. **Procedure:**
   A. The radioisotope (20-30 mCi of ^{99m}Tc-sestamibi) is injected intravenously in the arm *opposite* that of the breast in question. (This minimizes false uptake of the isotope in the ipsilateral axillary lymph nodes.) The dorsal pedal vein may be used if bilateral lesions are suspected or the client has had a mastectomy.
   B. The client is positioned in a prone position on an imaging table that has an overlay with "cutouts" that allow the breasts to hang free. Five minutes after the injection of isotope, the camera will be positioned to take a lateral view of each breast, beginning with the breast with the abnormality and followed by the contralateral breast. The client may be asked to lie supine or to sit up with hands clasped behind head to obtain additional images of each breast. Each view takes about 10 minutes. The total test time is about 45 minutes to 1 hour.

4. **Postprocedure care:**
   A. Encourage the intake of fluids to aid excretion of the radioactive medium from the body.

5. **Client and family teaching:**
   A. You may be asked to bring previous mammograms or other test results for the doctor to compare with scintimammograms.
   B. You will be asked to remove all clothing and jewelry above your waist.
   C. A venous access line will be necessary.
   D. You may experience a slight metallic taste after the injection of the isotope.
   E. You should remain still and breath normally while the images are being taken by the camera.
   F. There is no compression of the breasts during the procedure.

G. You should allow 60-90 minutes for the test.

H. Most of the radioactive material will be excreted from the body through urine and feces within 48 hours and is not harmful to other persons nearby.

I. The nuclear medical physician will interpret the test and report the results to your doctor within several days.

6. **Factors that affect results:**
   A. The sensitivity of scintimammography is decreased in lesions that are less than 1.0 cm at the largest dimension.
   B. False-positive results have been found with fibroadenomas, sclerosing adenomas, and juvenile adenomas.
   C. The uptake of ^{99m}Tc-sestamibi by the myocardium and the liver may mask overlying breast activity in certain client positions.

7. **Other data:**
   A. Other radioisotopes being evaluated for use in scintimammography include ^{99m}Tc-tetrofosmin (Myoview) and ^{99m}Tc-MDP (methylene diphosphate).
   B. Health care professionals working in a nuclear medicine area must follow federal standards set by the Nuclear Regulatory Commission. These standards include precautions for handling the reactive material and monitoring of potential radiation exposure.

SCLERODERMA ANTIBODY, BLOOD

Norm. Negative.

Positive. CREST (calcinosis, Raynaud's, esophageal dysfunction, sclerodactyly, telangiectasia) syndrome, and scleroderma.

Description. Scleroderma antibody (Scl-70) is found in the blood of clients with progressive systemic sclerosis.

Professional Considerations
1. Consent form NOT required.
2. **Preparation:**
   A. Tube: Red topped, red/gray topped, or gold topped.

B. Specimens MAY be drawn during hemodialysis.

3. Procedure:

A. Draw a 5-mL blood sample.

4. Postprocedure care:

A. Refrigerate separated serum.

5. Client and family teaching:

A. This test evaluates you for possible systemic sclerosis.

B. Results are normally available within 24 hours.

6. Factors that affect results:

A. False-positive results may be created by aminosalicylic acid, diphenyl-hydantoin, ethosuximide, isoniazid, methyldopa, penicillin, propylthiouracil, streptomycin sulfate, tetracycline, and trimethadione.

7. Other data:

A. Absence of scleroderma antibody does not exclude diagnosis.

SCOUT FILM, DIAGNOSTIC

(see Flat-plate radiography of abdomen, Diagnostic)

SECRETIN PROVOCATION TEST

(see Secretin stimulation for Zollinger-Ellison syndrome, Diagnostic)

SECRETIN STIMULATION FOR ZOLLINGER-ELLISON SYNDROME (SECRETION PROVOCATION TEST), DIAGNOSTIC

Norm. Serum gastrin: ≤200 pg/mL with no increase in production.

Increased. Gastrinoma (gastrin levels increase <100 pg/mL), and Zollinger-Ellison (ZE) syndrome (gastrin levels increase ≥110 pg/mL within 10 minutes). Drugs include amino acids, calcium, catecholamines, and insulin. Herbal or natural remedies include coffee (Coffea).

Decreased. Duodenal ulcer. G-cell hyperplasia (astral) and pancreatic dysfunction. Drugs include atropine.

Description. A stimulation test to assess for gastrinomas that can be correlated with chemical findings for diagnostic purposes. Secretin is a polypeptide secreted by the duodenal mucosa and the upper jejunum in response to gastric acidity. It acts to stimulate gastric pepsinogen, hepatic duct bicarbonate and water, pancreatic juice, bile, and intestinal fluid secretion and to inhibit gastric acid and gastrin secretion and intestinal smooth muscle contraction. ZE syndrome is a gastrointestinal disease in which elevated gastrin is formed, and pancreatic gastrinomas are present. In clients with ZE syndrome, the intravenous administration of secretin produces a paradoxical increase in serum gastrin levels. This test aids diagnosis of ZE syndrome for clients with baseline gastrin levels of 100-500 pg/mL (equivocal levels).

Professional Considerations

1. Consent form NOT required.

Risks

Allergic reaction to secretin.

Contraindications

Positive reaction to secretin skin testing.

2. Preparation:

A. See Client and family teaching.

B. Establish intravenous access.

C. Obtain secretin for intravenous administration, a tourniquet, and 7 each of alcohol wipes, needles, syringes, and red-topped tubes. Number the tubes sequentially.

D. Perform secretin skin testing to assess for allergy to the foreign protein. Inject 0.1 mL intradermally and observe 30 minutes for development of a wheal at the injection site.

3. Procedure:

A. Draw a 5-mL blood sample for the gastrin level.

B. Inject intravenously 2-3 U/kg of body weight of secretin over 30 seconds. Repeat step 3A every 5 minutes × 6 for a total of 30 minutes after injection, using the tubes in sequential order.

C. An alternative procedure is to infuse secretin 9 U/kg of body weight over 1 hour and draw blood specimens every 15 minutes. In ZE syndrome, gastrin levels peak after 45-90 minutes.

4. Postprocedure care:
   A. Label all the tubes and laboratory requisitions with the time the specimens were collected.

5. Client and family teaching:
   A. This test helps diagnose ZE syndrome.
   B. Fast from food and fluids from midnight before the test.

6. Factors that affect results:
   A. None.

7. Other data:
   A. Gastrin secretion may increase by 100-200 pg/mL (ng/L) every 5 minutes after secretin injection when gastrinoma is present.
   B. Calcium provocation tests are also sometimes performed to aid in the diagnosis of ZE syndrome.

SECRETIN TEST FOR PANCREATIC FUNCTION, DIAGNOSTIC

Norm:

DUODENAL FLUID		SI UNITS
Volume	95-235 mL/h	
Bicarbonate	74-121 mEq/L	74-121 mmol/L
Amylase	87,000-267,000 mg	
Lipase	<1.5 U/mL	<415 IU/L

Usage. Assessment of exocrine secretory ability of the pancreas for carcinoma, ductal obstruction, or chronic pancreatitis.

Description. Secretin is a polypeptide secreted by the duodenal mucosa and the upper jejunum in response to gastric acidity. Some of its actions are to stimulate pancreatic enzyme secretion and bicarbonate pancreatic juice production. This test allows an assessment of pancreatic endocrine function by assessing duodenal contents for volume, bicarbonate, amylase, lipase, and trypsin before and after pancreatic stimulation by secretin. In chronic pancreatitis and cystic fibrosis, all values are low because of pancreatic tissue destruction. In early stages of obstructive pancreatic cancer, volume may be low, with other values normal. In pancreatic pseudocyst, bicarbonate may be decreased, with other values normal. This test is usually followed by magnetic resonance cholangiopancreatography (MRCP), endoscopic ultrasound (EUS), or spiral computed tomography (spiral CT) and is replacing endoscopic retrograde cholangiopancreatography for confirming diagnosis of chronic pancreatitis.

Professional Considerations
1. Consent form IS required.

Risks
Allergic reaction to secretin. Complications of nasogastric tube insertion include bleeding, dysrhythmias, esophageal perforation, laryngospasm, and decreased mean pO_2.

Contraindications
Positive reaction to secretin skin testing.

---

2. Preparation:
   A. Obtain a double-lumen orogastric tube, pH paper, secretin, and two aspiration syringes or mechanical suction.
   B. Perform secretin skin testing to assess for allergy to the foreign protein. Inject 0.1 mL intradermally and observe 30 minutes for development of a wheal at the injection site.
   C. Establish intravenous access.
   D. See *Client and family teaching.*

3. Procedure:
   A. An orogastric tube is passed into the duodenum to the ligament of Treitz. Placement is assessed by analysis of the pH of secretions. Gastric pH is acidic, whereas duodenal secretions are alkaline.
   B. The gastric (proximal) lumen is continuously aspirated to prevent

acidic gastric secretions from contaminating duodenal contents.

C. All the duodenal fluid is aspirated from the distal portion of the lumen and placed into a sterile container. The container is labeled with the date, time, and specimen source and sent to the laboratory for baseline volume, bicarbonate, and amylase measurement.

D. Secretin, 1-2 U/kg of body weight, is administered intravenously.

E. All fluid is aspirated from the distal lumen every 20 minutes and analyzed for volume, bicarbonate, amylase, and lipase levels, as for the baseline sample.

F. Test may be followed by MRCP, EUS or spiral CT.

4. **Postprocedure care:**
A. Remove the orogastric tube.

5. **Client and family teaching:**
A. This test is one of several used to screen for pancreatic cancer or pancreatitis.
B. A nasogastric tube will be inserted through your nose into your stomach. Insertion may be uncomfortable and cause a pressure-like feeling or cause you to gag and cough. You will be asked to take sips of water and swallow to make tube insertion easier.

6. **Factors that affect results:**
A. Failure to insert the tube fully into the duodenum causes unreliable results.

7. **Other data:**
A. There is a 5.1% chance of false-positive and a 5.2% chance of false-negative results.
B. This test is somewhat out of favor because duodenal intubation is unpopular, and pancreatic disease is usually far advanced before exocrine function is appreciably reduced.
C. This test is of little help in distinguishing chronic pancreatitis from advanced pancreatic cancer.
D. Pancreozymin may be used in place of secretin for pancreatic stimulation but is more expensive.

SEDIMENTATION RATE, ERYTHROCYTE (ESR, ZETA SEDIMENTATION RATE), BLOOD

Norm:

AGE	FEMALES	MALES
Westergren, Modified Westergren Methods		
Pregnancy weeks 1-20	18-48 mm/hour	
Pregnancy weeks 21-40	30-70 mm/hour	
<50 years	20 mm/hour	15 mm/hour
50-85	30 mm/hour	20 mm/hour
>85	42 mm/hour	30 mm/hour
Children	0-10 mm/hour	0-10 mm/hour
Wintrobe Method	0.36-0.45	0.41-0.51
Zeta Sedimentation Ratio	41%-54% (41-54 arbitrary units, SI units)	

Increased. Anemia, ankylosis spondylitis, arteritis (temporal), arthritis (rheumatoid), cat-scratch disease, cholesterol, coccidioidomycosis, colon cancer, Crohn's disease, dermatomyositis, endocarditis, fever of undetermined origin, fibrinogen elevation, hemolytic anemia, hyperfibrinogenemias, industry-related diseases, infection, inflammation, macroglobulinemia, malignancy, multiple myeloma, obstructive hepatic disease, osteomyelitis, pain (acute, chronic, abdominal, pelvic), paraproteinemia, pelvic inflammatory disease, pericarditis, peritonitis, poly-clonal hyperglobulinemias, polymyalgia rheumatica, pregnancy, pulmonary embolism, sickle cell disease, sinusitis, Sjögren syndrome, subacute bacterial endocarditis, systemic lupus erythematosus, and tissue destruction. Drugs include dextran, fat emulsion, oral contraceptives, and vitamin A.

Decreased. Congestive heart failure and poikilocytosis. Drugs include albumin, corticotropin, cortisone, and lecithin.

Description. The erythrocyte sedimentation rate (ESR) is the most widely-used lab test to monitor the course of inflammatory disease, as well as infections. When a tube of well-mixed venous blood is positioned vertically, the red blood cells will tend to fall to the bottom. The rate at which they fall is the ESR. The ESR is a reflection of acute-phase reaction in inflammation and infection. A limitation of this test is that it lacks sensitivity and specificity for disease processes. Various methods are used to measure the ESR. The Westergren method is used most often because of the simplicity of the procedure. The Wintrobe method is more accurate for borderline elevations in the ESR. The zeta sedimentation ratio is a sedimentation rate calculation that provides more accurate data than the ESR in clients with anemia, requires the smallest amount of blood for testing, and provides the fastest results.

Professional Considerations
1. Consent form NOT required.
2. Preparation:
    A. Specimens MAY be drawn during hemodialysis.
    B. *Westergren method:*
        i. Obtain venipuncture supplies and a blue-topped tube, a 30-cm-long pipette with a 2.5-mm internal diameter and calibrated 0-200 mm, and a Westergren rack.
        ii. For the modified Westergren method, substitute a lavender-topped tube for the blue-topped tube.
    C. *Wintrobe method:*
        i. Obtain venipuncture supplies, a lavender-topped tube, and a Wintrobe hematocrit tube.
    D. *Zeta sedimentation ratio:*
        i. Obtain venipuncture supplies, a lavender-topped tube, and a capillary tube.
    E. Screen client for the use of herbal preparations or medicines or "natural" remedies.
3. Procedure:
    A. *Westergren method:*
        i. Draw a 4-mL blood sample in a blue-topped tube. Gently roll the tube to mix the sample.
        ii. Fill a pipette to the 0 mark with the blood sample.
        iii. Place the filled pipette vertically in the Westergren rack at room temperature.
        iv. After exactly 60 seconds, measure and record the distance to the top of the column of cells.
    B. *Modified Westergren method:*
        i. Draw a 2-mL blood sample in a lavender-topped tube.
        ii. Add 0.5 mL of 3.8% sodium citrate or 0.85% sodium chloride to the sample, and follow the steps as for the Westergren method above.
    C. *Wintrobe method:*
        i. Draw a 7-mL blood sample in a lavender-topped tube.
        ii. Fill a 7-cm-long Wintrobe capillary hematocrit tube with the blood sample, and then place the cap on the tube.
        iii. Spin the tube for 5 minutes.
    D. *Zeta sedimentation ratio:*
        i. Draw a 7-mL blood sample. Gently roll the tube to mix the sample.
        ii. Heelstick is acceptable, collected in a Microtainer.
        iii. Fill a capillary tube with 100 mL of the blood sample.
        iv. Place the capillary tube vertically into a centrifuge.
        v. Spin for cycles of 45 seconds.
        vi. Read the capillary tube like a standard hematocrit tube. The results are called the "zetacrit."
        vii. Divide the true hematocrit by the zetacrit and express the result as a percentage.

4. **Postprocedure care:**
   A. Perform the Westergren method within 2 hours, the modified Westergren method within 12 hours, the Wintrobe method within 4 hours, and the zeta method within 4 hours of collection.
5. **Client and family teaching:**
   A. This test is used in situations in which acute infection or inflammation is suspected. It is a screening test only.
   B. Results are normally available within 4 hours.
6. **Factors that affect results:**
   A. *All methods:*
      i. Conditions that counteract accelerated ESR in the conditions listed in the above *Increased* category include hypofibrinogenemia, polycythemia vera, sickle cell anemia, and spherocytosis.
      ii. Results are elevated in the presence of anemia during pregnancy.
      iii. Purified polysaccharides taken from cultures of the herb *Echinacea purpura* have been shown to slightly increase the ESR.
      iv. Hemolysis or clotting invalidates the results.
   B. *Westergren or modified Westergren method:*
      i. Heparin falsely increases the results.
      ii. Bubbles in the pipette decrease the results.
      iii. Tilting the pipette more than 3 degrees from vertical can increase the results by as much as 30%.
   C. *Wintrobe method:*
      i. Inadequate duration or speed of the centrifuge, or specimens overdiluted with EDTA, causes unreliable results.
   D. ESR results will be higher for the same client when plastic pipettes instead of glass tubes are used for the test.
7. **Other data:**
   A. ESR is often normal in clients with connective tissue disease or neoplasms.

SEGMENTED NEUTROPHILS, BLOOD

(see Differential leukocyte count, Peripheral Blood)

SELECTIVE SEROTONIN REUPTAKE INHIBITORS (SSRIs), BLOOD

Norm:

	THERAPEUTIC LEVELS	PANIC LEVEL
Citalopram	25-550 ng/mL	Not established
Desmethylcitalopram	25-750 ng/mL	Not established
Didesmethylcitalopram	25-800 ng/mL	Not established
Desmethylvenlavaxine	200-400 ng/mL	Not established
Fluoxetine	15-1,000 ng/mL	>2000 ng/mL
Fluvoxamine	50-1,000 ng/mL	Not established
Milnacipran	25-650 ng/mL	Not established
Norfluoxetine	25-500 ng/mL	>2000 ng/mL
Paroxetine	20-500 ng/mL	Not established
Sertraline	50-500 ng/mL	>500 ng/mL
Venlafaxine	25-500 ng/mL	Not established

Usage. Monitoring for therapeutic levels during drug therapy with selective serotonin reuptake inhibitors (SSRIs).

Description. SSRIs are a group of drugs that act by reducing serotonin reentry into the neurons of the brain. This leads to higher levels of serotonin and an improved mood in some clients.

SSRIs are used to treat depression, with similar efficacy to the 50%-60% improvement rate achieved by tricyclic antidepressants. SSRIs are most effective in mild depression or when taken early in a course of depression.

Professional Considerations

1. Consent form NOT required.
2. **Preparation:**
   A. Tube: red topped.
3. **Procedure:**
   A. Draw a TROUGH 5-ml blood sample.
4. **Postprocedure care:**
   A. None.
5. **Client and family teaching:**
   A. Specific to the medication.
6. **Factors that affect results:**
   A. SSRI toxicity may occur with concomitant alcohol intake.
   B. Trough levels are most consistently reproducible.
   C. Increases and decreases (see following table):
7. **Other data:**
   A. SSRIs are protein bound, so assess client serum albumin.

	DRUGS THAT MAY CAUSE INCREASED LEVELS	DRUGS THAT MAY CAUSE DECREASED LEVELS
Citalopram	Azole antifungals Cimetidine Erythromycin	Carbamazepine Omeprazole
Fluoxetine	Benzodiazepines	
Paroxetine	Cimetidine	
Sertraline	Benzodiazepines	

SEMEN ANALYSIS, SPECIMEN

Norm:

pH	pH 7.2-8.0
Appearance	Highly viscid, opaque, white, or gray-white
Odor	Musty or acrid odor
Sperm density	>20 × 10^6/L
Spermatozoa total number	>80 × 10^6/ejaculate
Sperm motility	>60% or progressive motility score of 3-4
Volume	1.5-5.0 mL (0.0015-0.005 L, SI units)
Normal spermatozoa	≥60
Defective heads	<35
Defective midpieces	≤20
Defective tails	≤20
Immature	<4

Increased. Not applicable.

Decreased Number. Cryptorchidism, hyperpyrexia, infertility, Klinefelter syndrome, testicular irradiation. Drugs include heavy tobacco smoking and heavy consumption of the herb coffee (*Coffea*), which may decrease the number of motile spermatozoa.

Decreased Motility. Drugs include chemotherapeutics, cimetidine, and ketoconazole. Herbs include St. John's wort at highly concentrated doses of 0.6 mg/mL.

Description. Semen consists of spermatozoa in seminal plasma, which provides a nutritive medium for conveying the sperm to the endocervical mucus. The components of semen are obtained from the testes, seminal vesicles, prostate, epididymis, vas deferens, bulbourethral glands, and urethral glands.

S

Because the interpretation is derived from microscopic visualization, the literature discusses common problems with interoperator reliability in interpretation of the results. Some computerized systems are being tested for semen analysis.

Professional Considerations

1. Consent form NOT required.
2. Preparation:
   A. Obtain a clean glass container.
   B. Screen client for the use of herbal preparations or medicines or "natural" remedies.
   C. See *Client and family teaching*.
3. Procedure:
   A. Collect a fresh specimen in a clean glass jar. The client may obtain the specimen at home if he is unable to masturbate or is uncomfortable with masturbation.
4. Postprocedure care:
   A. Specimens must be received within 1 hour and examined within 3 hours.
5. Client and family teaching:
   A. This test is used to estimate the number of sperm and evaluate fertility.
   B. Do not have intercourse or masturbate for 48 hours before specimen collection.
   C. Collect a fresh semen specimen in a plastic cup. The specimen may be collected by masturbation at the institution or at home, but it must be collected by masturbation. Do not use a condom or a lubricant, other than saliva.
   D. Keep track of the time the semen was collected.
   E. *For home collection:* After collecting the specimen, keep the container of semen warm by putting it in a pocket next to the body.
   F. If the specimen is collected at home, it must be delivered to the laboratory within 1 hour.
6. Factors that affect results:
   A. Temperature extremes decrease the sperm count.
   B. Reject semen specimens more than 1 hour old.
   C. Males with infertility tend to have increased semen volume, which is associated with diminished sperm count.
   D. *Herbal effects:* Several studies have shown that St. John's wort is mutagenic to sperm cells and saw palmetto induces metabolic changes in sperm. High doses of *Echinacea purpura* has been found to interfere with sperm enzyme activity.
   E. An herbal or natural remedy that has been shown to increase sperm motility in vitro is *Astragalus membranaceus*.
7. Other data:
   A. Repeat testing may be necessary because results vary with samples.
   B. Motility is graded as 0 = none, 1 = poor, 2 = moderate, 3 = good, and 4 = excellent.
   C. See also *Infertility screen, Specimen*.

SENSITIVE TSH ASSAY

(see Thyroid-stimulating hormone, Sensitive assay, Blood)

SENTINEL LYMPH NODE BIOPSY, DIAGNOSTIC

Norm. A sentinel lymph node is defined as a lymph node that stains blue or is radioactive.

Usage. Helps avoid total axillary node dissection during early breast cancer; provides staging information for operable invasive breast cancer; identifies location of sentinel node for subsequent tumor resection.

Description. Metastasis to axillary lymph nodes can be determined by identifying lymph flow from the tumor site to the primary lymph node via radio guided biopsy. The sentinel lymph node is the first lymph node in the lymphatic basin to receive lymph flow from a primary tumor. Thus it will be the first node to contain metastasis and can be identified on lymphoscintigraphy by following the blue dye to the most proximal node.

Professional Considerations

1. Consent form IS required for the biopsy portion of this procedure.

Risks

Bleeding, infection, reaction to the dye.

Contraindications

Sentinel lymph node biopsy is contraindicated in clients who have had previous breast surgery or radiation to the breast, as well as in clients who have clinically palpable nodes, locally advanced breast disease, tumors in more than one location in the breast, lymphatic problems, burns, breast reduction surgery or breast implants.

2. **Preparation:**
   A. 3-5 mL of Isosulfan blue radioactive tracer is injected subdermally around the circumference of the tumor (for palpable masses) or peritumorally or intratumorally under the guidance of ultrasound
   B. The site is then massaged for 5 minutes to promote migration of the tracer.
3. **Procedure:**
   A. 2-6 hours after tracer injection, the area of the tumor site is scanned via lymphoscintigraphy to identify the "hot spot," which is marked on the skin and later used for localization of tumor for excision. The remainder of the lymph node basin is examined for residual radioactivity.
4. **Postprocedure care:**
   A. A dry, sterile dressing is required.
   B. Assess vital signs and the site for bleeding.
5. **Client and family teaching:**
   A. Consume only clear liquids after midnight and before the biopsy.
   B. A lumpectomy is usually performed immediately after the sentinel node biopsy.
   C. Do not lift more than 10 pounds for 48 hours after the procedure.
   D. Final results may take up to a week.
   E. Observe for signs of infection and report to the physician: increasing pain, redness, swelling, drainage, or fever >101°F (38.3° C).
6. **Factors that affect results:**
   A. Surgeon's skill and frequency of performing procedure.
   B. The shine-through effect of radiocolloid from the primary site may effect localization of the sentinel node.
7. **Other data:**
   A. None.

SEROTONIN (5-HYDROXYTRYPTAMINE), SERUM OR BLOOD

Norm:

	ADULTS	SI UNITS
Whole blood, high-performance liquid chromatography (HPLC)	46-319 ng/mL or µg/L	0.26-1.81 µmol/L
Serum, HPLC	25-208 ng/mL or µg/L	0.41-1.18 µmol/L

Increased. Carcinoid syndrome, cystic fibrosis, dumping syndrome, endocarditis, metastasis, myocardial infarction, nontropical sprue, oat cell carcinoma of the lung (causing ectopic production), pain (chronic), pancreatic islet cell tumor (causing ectopic production), primary pulmonary hypertension, and thyroid medullary carcinoma (causing ectopic production). Drugs include imipramine, methyldopa, monoamine oxidase (MAO) inhibitors, reserpine, selective serotonin reuptake inhibitors SSRIs (citalopram, desmethylcitalopram, didesmethylcitalopram, fluoxe-tine, milnacipran, norfluoxetine, paroxetine, sertraline, venlafaxine), and tramodol (decreasing the serotonin reuptake).

Decreased. Depression, Down syndrome, Parkinson's disease, phenylketonuria, renal insufficiency, and teratomas (benign cystic).

Description. Serotonin is an indole amine synthesized from L-tryptophan, an essential amino acid, by the argentaffin cells of the intestinal mucosa. Serotonin is stored in and transported by platelets, but it is also found in many body tissues, including the central nervous system and gastrointestinal tract. Serotonin mediates cardiovascular integrity, neurotransmission, smooth muscle contraction (gastrointestinal motility), prolactin release, and growth hormone release and functions in hemocoagulation. This broad array of actions occurs as a result of the location of serotonin receptors throughout the body. This test is used to confirm the diagnosis of carcinoid tumors, in which the highest increases in levels are found.

Professional Considerations

1. Consent form NOT required.
2. **Preparation:**
   A. Preschedule this test with the laboratory. Clarify whether the client must follow a low-indole diet for a period of time before testing.
   B. MAO inhibitor drugs should be discontinued 1 week before the test.
   C. Avoid radionuclide scans for 7 days before the test.
   D. Tube: Chilled lavender topped, and a container of ice.
   E. Specimens MAY be drawn during hemodialysis.
3. **Procedure:**
   A. Draw a 7-mL blood sample. Place the specimen on ice.
   B. Heelstick is acceptable, collected in a Microtainer.
4. **Postprocedure care:**
   A. Send specimens to the laboratory promptly. Specimens must be transferred to a plastic container of 10 mg of EDTA and 75 mg of ascorbic acid and frozen within 4 hours of collection.
5. **Client and family teaching:**
   A. This test is used to screen for carcinoid tumors.
   B. Results are normally available within 48 hours.
6. **Factors that affect results:**
   A. Lithium either increases or decreases the level of serotonin in the brain.
   B. A radioactive scan within 7 days before this test invalidates the results of the radioimmunoassay method.
7. **Other data:**
   A. Because blood serotonin samples are unstable, urine measurements of 5-hydroxyindoleacetic acid are more commonly measured.

SERTRALINE
(see Selective serotonin reuptake inhibitors, Blood)

SERUM GLUTAMIC OXALOACETIC TRANSAMINASE (SGOT), SERUM
(see Aspartate aminotransferase, Serum)

SERUM GLUTAMIC PYRUVIC TRANSAMINASE (SGPT), SERUM
(see Alanine aminotransferase, Serum)

SERUM KILLING TEST
(see Schlichter test)

SESTAMIBI BREAST IMAGING
(see Scintimammography, Diagnostic)

SESTAMIBI-DIPYRIDAMOLE STRESS TEST AND SCAN
(see Heart scan, Diagnostic)

SESTAMIBI EXERCISE TESTING AND SCAN
(see Heart scan, Diagnostic)

SEVERE ACUTE RESPIRATORY SYNDROME (SARS)–ASSOCIATED CORONAVIRUS (COV) ANTIBODY AND REVERSE TRANSCRIPTASE POLYMERASE CHAIN REACTION (RT-PCR) TESTS, SPECIMEN

Norm. Negative.

Description. Experimental tests developed and deployed to help rapidly identify persons with Severe Acute Respiratory Syndrome (SARS). SARS, thought to be caused by a human coronavirus, first appeared in late 2002. It causes mild respiratory symptoms of cough and fever and may progress to a severe pneumonia and possibly death. SARS is thought to be transmitted by direct contact with infected droplets, but airborne transmission is also being considered.

Professional Considerations

1. Consent form IS recommended by the Centers for Disease Control and Prevention (CDC). Consent to have

the leftover specimen stored at the CDC should also be obtained.

2. **Preparation:**
    A. For aspirates, obtain NONbacteriostatic saline, plastic catheter, and sterile vial containing viral transport medium.
    B. For swabs, obtain sterile swabs made of dacron or rayon with plastic shafts and vials of viral transport medium.
    C. For blood sample: obtain a red-top or lavender-top tube with external caps and internal O-ring seals.
    D. For stool, obtain a clean container and paraffin for sealing.

3. **Procedure:**
    A. Collect acute specimens as soon as possible after illness is suspected. Collect convalescent specimens 22 days after the onset of symptoms.
    B. *Nasopharyngeal wash/aspirate* (specimen of choice): flush catheter with nonbacteriostatic saline. After instilling 1.5 mL of nonbacteriostatic saline into the nostril, aspirate from the nasopharynx. Repeat procedure through the other nostril.
    C. *Nasopharyngeal swab:* insert swab into the nostril, pressing lightly against the nasopharynx for a few seconds. Repeat in other nostril with another swab.
    D. *Oropharyngeal swab:* insert swab through the mouth, using care to avoid the tongue. Press lightly against the posterior pharynx and tonsillar area. Insert swab into vial containing viral transport medium.
    E. *Lower respiratory tract:* obtain bronchoalveolar lavage fluid. Place half of the fluid into sterile vials with external caps and internal O-ring seals. Spin the remaining fluid and fix the cell-pellet in formalin.
    F. *Blood:* collect a 5-mL blood sample in a red-top or purple-top tube. Both acute and convalescent specimens should be obtained.
    G. *Stool:* collect 10-50 mL in a clean container. Seal the lid with paraffin and place in a bag.

4. **Postprocedure care:**
    A. Label specimens with collection date, collection site, and identification numbers. Store at 4° C and ship to CDC-approved testing laboratory.
    B. If consent has been obtained for long-term storage, forward remaining specimen and client-identifying information to the CDC.

5. **Client and family teaching:**
    A. Because of the experimental nature of this test, clients should be prepared for the possibility of false-positive and false-negative results.
    B. Prepare client for the possibility of quarantine, even with negative test results.

6. **Factors that affect results:**
    A. Sensitivity and specificity of these tests is not yet known. Specimens stored with the CDC may be repeat-tested, as test methods improve.
    B. False-negative RT-PCR may occur if viral RNA is not present in the specimen at the time of collection.
    C. False-negative CoV antibody results may occur if specimen is collected earlier than 21 days or longer after the onset of illness.
    D. Use of calcium alginate swabs or swabs with wooden shafts may cause false-negative results as a result of viral inactivation or inhibition of PCR.

7. **Other data:**
    A. It is not known yet if there are other causative agents for SARS.
    B. The CDC website maintains current and ongoing updates concerning SARS testing and interpretation.

SEX HORMONE BINDING GLOBULIN

(see Testosterone, Free, Bioavailable and Total, Blood)

SFMC

(see Soluble fibrin monomer complex, Serum)

SGOT, SERUM

(see Aspartate aminotransferase, Serum)

SGPT, SERUM

(see Alanine aminotransferase, Serum)

SHAKE TEST
(see Foam stability test, Amniotic Fluid)

SHBG
(see Testosterone, Free, Bioavailable and Total, Blood)

SICKLE CELL TEST, BLOOD

Norm. Sickling test: negative, no sickled red blood cells seen, no hemoglobin S; solubility test: negative.

Positive. Pain (chronic) and sickle cell anemia.

Negative. Drugs include phenothiazines at concentrations >128 mg/mL.

Description. Sickle cell disease is an inherited disease characterized by chronic hemolytic anemia and painful episodes of "sickle cell crises," which usually require high doses of narcotics for relief. It is common in the black population, affecting 3 of every 1000 persons. Those inheriting the disease are at a higher risk for mortality and morbidity. Sickle cell disease causes pain crises, hemolytic anemia, splenic malfunction and infections. The sickle cell test is a screening test used to demonstrate the presence of hemoglobin S, which causes red blood cells to assume a sickle shape or crescent shape under reduced oxygen supply. The sickling test is positive in sickle cell anemia or trait or in combinations of other hemoglobin S abnormalities.

Professional Considerations
1. Consent form NOT required.
2. Preparation:
   A. Tube: Lavender topped, green topped, or black topped.
   B. Note whether the client received a blood transfusion within the previous 4 months because this may produce false-negative results.
   C. Specimens MAY be drawn during hemodialysis.
3. Procedure:
   A. Draw a 3-mL blood sample. Gently roll the tube to mix the specimen.
4. Postprocedure care:
   A. Observe for signs of sickle cell disease: fatigue, dyspnea, bone pain, joint swelling, and chest pain.
5. Client and family teaching:
   A. This test is used in screening for sickle cell disease.

B. Clients with sickle cell disease should avoid hypoxic situations such as high altitudes, strenuous activity, extreme cold, and traveling in an unpressurized aircraft.
   C. Refer clients with sickle cell disease for genetic counseling.
6. Factors that affect results:
   A. If hemoglobin S concentration is <25%, erythrocytes will not sickle.
   B. False-positive results may be caused by polycythemia, hemoglobin abnormalities, or high blood protein levels (such as systemic lupus erythematosus, multiple myeloma).
   C. Collection of more than 7 mL of blood may cause false-positive results.
   D. False-negative results may be caused by anemia in combination with less than 7 mL of blood drawn, blood transfusion of normal hemoglobin within the previous 4 months, phenothiazine drug therapy, concurrent iron deficiency or thalassemia, elevated hemoglobin F levels, and in infants under 6 months of age.
   E. Hemolysis, clotting, or lipemia of the specimen invalidates the results.
7. Other data:
   A. This test cannot reliably differentiate the homozygous sickle cell state from the heterozygous trait.
   B. The Sickledex Test is a trade name for the sickle cell test.

SICKLEDEX TEST, DIAGNOSTIC
(see Sickle cell test, Blood)

SIDEROCYTE STAIN, DIAGNOSTIC
(see Hemosiderin stain, Diagnostic)

SIDEROPHILIN
(see Transferrin, Serum)

SIGMOIDOSCOPY, DIAGNOSTIC

Norm. Negative.

Usage. Identify bowel obstruction, carcinoma of sigmoid colon, celiac sprue, colitis, Crohn's disease, diverticulitis, diverticulosis, and help diagnose causes of malabsorption.

Description. Sigmoidoscopy is the endoscopic visualization of the interior space and walls of the sigmoid colon, using a sigmoidoscope. A sigmoidoscope is a 50-cm fiberoptic tube with a lighted mirror lens system that illuminates the sigmoid colon for visualization The most common method for this procedure is a flexible sigmoidoscopy, in which a short, flexible tube with a light source is inserted through the rectum and advanced to the sigmoid colon. The American Cancer Society recommends screening sigmoidoscopy every 5 years for all adults over age 50, followed by a colonoscopy in those with positive results.

Professional Considerations
1. Consent form IS required.

Risks
Bowel perforation (rare), peritonitis, hemorrhage.

Contraindications
Anorectal fistula, diverticulitis, paralytic ileus, third-trimester pregnancy. Sedatives are contraindicated in clients with central nervous system depression.

2. **Preparation:**
   A. See *Client and family teaching.*
   B. Obtain sterile specimen containers if a biopsy is planned.
   C. The client should disrobe below the waist or wear a gown.
3. **Procedure:**
   A. The client is placed in the left lateral position.
   B. Monitor blood pressure, heart rate, and oxygen saturation rate by pulse oximeter before analgesic and sedative is given and then every 5 minutes during the procedure.
   C. An analgesic or sedative may be administered. Monitor respiratory status continually after sedation.
   D. The sigmoidoscope is lubricated and inserted into the anus and rectum and then slowly advanced into the sigmoid colon. Insufflation occurs to aid in visualization.

However, insufflation of CO_2 rather than air reduces abdominal pain and bowel distention after colonoscopy.
   E. During the procedure, biopsy specimens and photographs may be taken and suction used to remove excess secretions.
4. **Postprocedure care:**
   A. Assess for side effects of the sedative: hypotension, depressed respirations, and bradycardia.
   B. Continue the assessment of the respiratory status. If deep sedation was used, follow institutional protocol for postsedation monitoring. Typical monitoring includes continuous ECG monitoring and pulse oximetry, with continual assessments (every 5-15 minutes) of airway, vital signs, and neurologic status until the client is lying quietly awake, is breathing independently, and responds to commands spoken in a normal tone.
5. **Client and family teaching:**
   A. This test is performed to evaluate the colon for several different disorders.
   B. Consume a full liquid diet the evening before the test.
   C. Laxatives may be prescribed to be administered the night before the test with or without an enema or suppository 1 hour before the test, except in pregnant women. Magnesium citrate and a Fleet enema also produce excellent results.
   D. The urge to defecate as the sigmoidoscope is inserted into the rectum is normal.
   E. The procedure takes approximately 30 minutes.
   F. Resume normal activities and diet as soon as you feel ready.
   G. Call a physician if your temperature is higher than 101° F (38.3° C), or if you have trouble breathing or experience stomach pain, nausea, or bright red rectal bleeding.
6. **Factors that affect results:**
   A. Retained barium from previous studies makes visualization impossible.
   B. Fixation of bowel from previous radiation therapy or surgery may inhibit the passage of the sigmoidoscope.

7. **Other data:**
   A. Women more than men fail to comply with recommendations to have this procedure done for cancer screening. A major contributor to this decision is a low perceived risk of bowel cancer because of current health/symptom status, and lack of having a family history or colorectal cancer.

SIGNAL-AVERAGED ELECTROCARDIOGRAPHY (SIGNAL-AVERAGED ECG, SAECG), DIAGNOSTIC

Norm. No late potentials detected.

Usage. Determination of the risk for developing life-threatening dysrhythmias for the following high-risk conditions: myocardial infarction, clients with a history of reentrant dysrhythmias, survivors of sudden cardiac death, and syncope. Aids decision making about the need for further evaluation and treatment, including electrophysiologic study, drug treatment, antitachycardia pacemaker, or coronary artery bypass grafting.

Description. Signal-averaged electrocardiography (SAECG) is an inexpensive, noninvasive method for detection of late ventricular potentials (late potentials). Late potentials are low-amplitude electrical activity occurring in diastole during a normally isoelectric phase. Their presence signals slowed conduction velocity and is usually associated with disease, ischemia, or scarring of the heart muscle. The existence of late potentials is believed to indicate a potential for the development of reentrant dysrhythmias, which may lead to sudden cardiac death. Traditional electrocardiography is not sensitive enough to detect the very low-amplitude electrical activity of late potentials. Signal averaging is an electrocardiographic method that amplifies and averages up to 10,000 samples of electrical activity per second from the electrocardiographic signals of 100-1000 cardiac cycles to reduce the effect of random noise and artifact, thus allowing the detection of late potentials. The procedure may take up to 20 minutes, depending on the number of cardiac cycles averaged and the amount of elec-

trical interference present. The presence of late potentials in the SAECG is determined by examination of the duration of the QRS complex, the root mean square voltage of the last 40 msec of the QRS complex, and the duration of the terminal QRS complex that measures under 40 mV.

Professional Considerations

1. Consent form NOT required.
2. **Preparation:**
   A. Provide a private, comfortable, calm, warm environment to help the client relax skeletal muscles and avoid shivering.
   B. To minimize artifact caused by electrical interference, turn off all nonessential electrical equipment in the area. For example, run IV pumps on battery, and turn off the hypothermia machine, television, and radio. Plug the SAECG machine into an outlet different from that of essential equipment such as a ventilator or monitor.
   C. Obtain electrodes, conduction gel, and an SAECG machine.
3. **Procedure:**
   A. Position the client supine or with the head of the bed slightly elevated.
   B. For electrode placement, clip hair from the sites and then cleanse the sites with an alcohol wipe and scrape them lightly with the edge of an electrode.
   C. Lead placement varies by institutional protocol and SAECG machine manufacturer recommendations but generally involves the placement of bipolar lead sets on the anterior and posterior areas of the torso. Apply leads according to institutional protocol.
   D. Follow the manufacturer's recommendations for obtaining the SAECG. This generally involves activating the SAECG machine, which runs an electrocardiographic template of the client's common cardiac cycle and then compares it to the template, amplifies it, and averages the electrical signals from a set number of subsequent cardiac cycles.
4. **Postprocedure care:**
   A. Remove the electrodes and cleanse the skin of conductive gel.

5. **Client and family teaching:**
   A. This test is performed to determine the risk of developing life-threatening dysrhythmias in high-risk conditions. This is a special kind of electrocardiogram that takes longer than a normal electrocardiogram.
   B. It is important to lie motionless and try to relax the muscles as much as possible throughout the procedure.
6. **Factors that affect results:**
   A. Because a specific number of cardiac cycles will be averaged, the procedure will take longer than normal for bradycardia and less time than normal for tachycardia.
   B. Ectopic beats are not included in the averaging. Thus the procedure time increases for clients demonstrating a great deal of ectopy.
   C. Artifact is not included in the averaging. Thus movement or shivering of the client as well as electrical interference by nearby equipment will increase the procedure time.
7. **Other data:**
   A. SAECG has not been found useful for atrial dysrhythmias, continuously irregular rhythms, or rhythms with wide QRS complexes.

SIMS-HUHNER TEST, DIAGNOSTIC

Norm:

Mucus tenacity: stretches ≥10 cm,
Number of motile sperm: ≥6-20/HPF

Usage. Infertility testing; rape trauma.

Description. Examination of the postcoital endocervical mucus to detect its quality and the ability of the spermatozoa to penetrate the mucus. It is believed that the presence of anti-sperm antibodies in cervical mucus may, in part, explain why sperm cannot penetrate normally. This test is included in infertility work-ups when prior semen analysis results are normal.

Professional Considerations
1. Consent form NOT required, unless the specimen is being collected for medicolegal purposes.
2. **Preparation:**
   A. The test should be timed to coincide with midovulation. The male

should abstain from ejaculation for 3 days before this test. Intercourse should be performed without using a lubricant. The woman should lie recumbent for 15-30 minutes after intercourse in which male ejaculation has occurred and then arrive for testing within 1-5 hours.
   B. Obtain a glass cannula with a rubber tube, a syringe, a Petri dish, slides, and a ruler.
   C. The client should disrobe below the waist or wear a gown.
   D. Obtain a speculum and a glass slide.
3. **Procedure:**
   A. Specimen collection must be witnessed if used for medicolegal purposes.
   B. The client is placed in the dorsal lithotomy position and draped for privacy and comfort.
   C. The external cervical os is wiped clear of mucus.
   D. An endocervical mucus sample is obtained by aspiration in a glass cannula attached by a rubber tube to a syringe.
4. **Postprocedure care:**
   A. For medicolegal specimens, place the specimen in a sealed plastic bag and label it as legal evidence. All persons handling the specimen must sign a record with the date and time received.
   B. Deliver the specimen in a syringe to the laboratory, where the following occurs:
      i. After the mucus volume is measured, the specimen is placed in a Petri dish, and color and viscosity are noted.
      ii. One measures the tenacity of the mucus (*Spinnbarkeit*) by grasping a portion of the mucus and noting the distance it can be drawn before it breaks.
      iii. Next, a drop of mucus is placed on a microscope slide and covered with a coverslip, and the number of motile sperm are counted.
5. **Client and family teaching:**
   A. This test is performed to evaluate endocervical mucus as part of a fertility work-up when sperm counts have been normal.

6. Factors that affect results:
   A. Specimens collected more than 6 hours after coitus yield unreliable results.
   B. An herb that have been found to decrease sperm motility and viability is St. John's wort.
7. Other data:
   A. Mucus can also be microscopically examined for leukocytes, erythrocytes, and trichomonads.
   B. See also *Infertility screen, Specimen*.

SINGLE-PHOTON EMISSION COMPUTED TOMOGRAPHY (SPECT SCAN), BRAIN, DIAGNOSTIC

Norm. Normal brain and structures.

Usage. Evaluate AIDS, Alzheimer's disease, anoxia, cerebrovascular accident, head trauma, Parkinson's disease, evaluate mild brain injury, transient ischemic attack; helps differentiate type of dementia (Alzheimer's, focal, multi-infarct, diffuse) by allowing identification of pattern of cerebral ischemia; helps differentiate Parkinson's disease from dopa-responsive dystonia; allows identification of the focus of seizure activity. SPECT is used experimentally in psychiatry to identify patterns coinciding with individual disorders.

Description. SPECT scan is a nuclear medicine procedure that gives clinical information about organ function (versus CT and radiography, which give information about anatomy). In this scan, a radiopharmaceutical selected for its absorptive properties is injected intravenously, crosses the blood-brain barrier, decomposes, and remains for several hours in the brain tissue, where its qualitative and quantitative distribution can be detected with the SPECT camera. The camera sends images to a computer that can reproduce visual images, or "slices," of the brain along several planes. Advantages of SPECT imaging over older nuclear medicine scans are that it can identify patterns of dementia earlier in the process and allow for early intervention for potentially reversible types of dementia. This scan can be done in a three-dimensional format. In addition to imaging the brain, SPECT is used for many organs, with different radiopharmaceuticals selected, based on their absorptive properties for the organ being imaged. Newer equipment called "dual mode imaging" combines SPECT with structural imaging modalities such as Ultrafast CT or MRI for improved imaging results. See *Dual modality imaging, Diagnostic*.

Professional Considerations
1. Consent form IS required.

Risks
Allergic reaction to the radiopharmaceutical (itching, hives, rash, tight feeling in the throat, shortness of breath, anaphylaxis, death).

Contraindications
Inability to lie motionless during the scan; women who are breast-feeding; previous allergic reaction to the radiopharmaceutical agent.

Precautions
During pregnancy, risks of cumulative radiation exposure to the fetus from this and other previous or future imaging studies must be weighed against the benefits of the procedure. Although formal limits for client exposure are relative to this risk:benefit comparison, the United States Nuclear Regulatory Commission requires that the cumulative dose equivalent to an embryo/fetus from occupational exposure not exceed 0.5 rem (5 mSv). Radiation dosage to the fetus is proportional to the distance of the anatomy studied from the abdomen and decreases as pregnancy progresses. For pregnant clients, consult the radiologist/radiology department to obtain estimated fetal radiation exposure from this procedure.

2. Preparation:
   A. Remove all metal objects from the client's clothes, hair, and body.
   B. See *Client and family teaching*.
3. Procedure:
   A. The client is transported to the nuclear medicine department, positioned supine on the scanning table, and left to rest quietly for approximately 10 minutes to allow the brain to reach a basal activity level.

S

B. A radiopharmaceutical is injected intravenously and allowed to circulate and cross the blood-brain barrier.

C. The SPECT scan is then taken while the client lies motionless, with open eyes.

4. Postprocedure care:

A. See *Client and family teaching.*

5. Client and family teaching:

A. Do not drink caffeine-containing beverages for 24 hours before the scan.

B. It is important to lie motionless during this scan. If the client is confused, a family member familiar to the client may remain in the room to reassure the client during the scan.

C. The scan takes about 30 minutes.

D. For about 24 hours after the scan, meticulously wash your hands after urination to remove any radioactivity from contaminated urine.

6. Factors that affect results:

A. The presence of metal objects, such as metal eyeglasses, over the scanning area may block some views.

B. Movement of the client during imaging obscures the clarity of the images.

7. Other data:

A. The radiopharmaceutical half-life is about 6 hours.

SINUS RADIOGRAPHY, DIAGNOSTIC

Norm. Negative.

Usage. Cysts, postoperative nasal-sinus surgery, rhinitis, and sinusitis.

Description. Sinus x-rays (roentgen rays) are short electromagnetic waves that penetrate the soft sinus tissues to produce an image that is recorded on radiographic film. The sinuses are usually radiolucent because of the air content. Any deviation from total radiolucencies indicates tumor or infection.

Precautions

During pregnancy, risks of cumulative radiation exposure to the fetus from this and other previous or future imaging studies must be weighed against the benefits of the procedure. Although formal limits for client exposure are relative to this risk: benefit comparison, the United States Nuclear Regulatory Commission requires that the cumulative dose equivalent to an embryo/fetus from occupational exposure not exceed 0.5 rem (5 mSv). Radiation dosage to the fetus is proportional to the distance of the anatomy studied from the abdomen and decreases as pregnancy progresses. For pregnant clients, consult the radiologist/radiology department to obtain estimated fetal radiation exposure from this procedure.

Professional Considerations

1. Consent form NOT required.

2. Preparation:

A. Shield the pregnant uterus during x-ray exposure.

B. Remove earrings, glasses, hairpins, or other radiopaque objects from the head area.

3. Procedure:

A. The head is placed in a fixed position.

B. Radiographs of sinuses are taken from several angles.

C. The exam takes 10-15 minutes.

4. Postprocedure care:

A. Remove the lead apron.

5. Client and family teaching:

A. This test is performed to evaluate sinus cavities for signs of infection or growth.

6. Factors that affect results:

A. Movement during radiography distorts the images.

7. Other data:

A. Anaerobic organisms are the predominant pathogens of chronic sinusitis.

B. See also *Tomography of paranasal sinuses, Diagnostic.*

SJÖGREN'S ANTIBODIES (SS-A [Ro] AND SS-B [La]), BLOOD
(*see Anti-La/SS-B test, Diagnostic; Anti-Ro/SS-A test, Diagnostic*)

SKELETAL MUSCLE ANTIBODY, SPECIMEN
(*see Striational autoantibody, Specimen*)

SKIN CULTURE
(*see Culture, Skin, Specimen*)

SKIN, FUNGUS, CULTURE

Norm. Negative.

Usage. Dermatitis and fungal infections.

Description. Culture of skin scrapings, nails, scalp, hair, or debris under the nails is taken to isolate and identify fungi. A single negative culture does not rule out a fungal infection.

Professional Considerations
1. Consent form NOT required.
2. Preparation:
   A. Obtain a sterile scraper and a dermatophyte test medium or a sterile container.
3. Procedure:
   A. Place the skin or scalp scrapings, nail clippings, hair stubs, or nail debris scrapings into a dermatophyte medium or sterile container.
4. Postprocedure care:
   A. Store the specimens at room temperature.
5. Client and family teaching:
   A. Culture results for *Candida* are usually available within 1 week and for dermatophytes within 2 weeks.
   B. All negative cultures are final after 4 weeks.
6. Factors that affect results:
   A. Cotton-plugged tubes should not be used because they may cause the specimen to become trapped in the cotton and lost.
   B. Closed rubber stopper tubes should not be used because they keep the specimen moist and aid in bacterial growth.
7. Other data:
   A. None.

SKIN, *MYCOBACTERIA*, CULTURE

Norm. No growth.

Usage. Abscess, AIDS, amyloidosis, Buruli ulcers, granulomatous cutaneous lesions, and osteomyelitis.

Description. Isolation of mycobacteria on the skin as the cause of infection. Some of the common mycobacteria are *M. tuberculosis* and the nontubercular *M. avium-intracellulare, genavense,* and *marinum* found in clients with acquired immunodeficiency syndrome (AIDS) or immunosuppression.

Professional Considerations
1. Consent form NOT required.
2. Preparation:
   A. Obtain a sterile scraper and a mycobacterial culture medium.
3. Procedure:
   A. Scrape the skin or lesion (do not use a swab) and place the specimen in the mycobacterial culture medium.
4. Postprocedure care:
   A. Transport the specimen directly to the laboratory.
5. Client and family teaching:
   A. Negative cultures are reported after 9 weeks.
6. Factors that affect results:
   A. Specimens not incubated at 86°F (30°C) may not grow.
7. Other data:
   A. The yield on cultures is proportional to the amount of specimen submitted.

SKIN TEST FOR HYPERSENSITIVITY, DIAGNOSTIC

Norm. Negative.

Positive. There is no agreement on a threshold value for a positive skin test result.

Usage. Allergies and cat-scratch disease.

Description. An intradermal test using allergen extracts to determine sensitivity to various drugs, materials, and pollens that a client may react to in an allergic manner, such reaction possibly resulting in anaphylaxis. The result is based on an immediate hypersensitivity reaction.

Professional Considerations
1. Consent form NOT required.
2. Preparation:
   A. Obtain an alcohol wipe, 0.1 mL of the test substance in question, and an intradermal 26- or 27-gauge needle.
   B. Have emergency equipment and medications on hand for possible anaphylaxis.
   C. See *Client and family teaching.*
3. Procedure:
   A. Wipe the skin with an alcohol wipe and let it air-dry.

B. Intradermally inject 0.1 mL of the test substance in question in the underpart of the forearm.

4. **Postprocedure care:**
   A. Observe for redness and swelling (a wheal) at the site of the injection.
   B. Results are read 15 minutes after injection. Assess the wheal size of the skin reaction by measuring the mean wheal diameter (MWD) or the mean of the largest wheal diameter and that perpendicular to it. MWDs of skin tests may be expressed in absolute values (millimeters), or they may be related to the size of a control. An MWD >7 mm has a higher diagnostic value for symptomatic allergies. An MWD greater than or equal to a histamine control also has a greater diagnostic value.
   C. Assess for anaphylaxis symptoms for $\frac{1}{2}$ hour.

5. **Client and family teaching:**
   A. Withhold allergy medications and antihistamines for 48 hours before the test.
   B. Report drowsiness, skin rash or itching, difficulty breathing, and palpitations immediately.

6. **Factors that affect results:**
   A. A subcutaneous rather than an intradermal injection will produce a false-negative result.

7. **Other data:**
   A. Most skin tests are available in prepackaged sterile kits.

SLEEP APNEA STUDY
(*see Polysomnography, Diagnostic*)

SLEEP OXIMETRY
(*see Polysomnography, Diagnostic*)

SLEEP STUDY
(*see Polysomnography, Diagnostic*)

SLIT-LAMP VISION TEST, DIAGNOSTIC

Norm. Normal.

Usage. Detection of conjunctivitis, corneal abrasions, iritis, and opacities.

Useful after bone-marrow transplantation to monitor clients for cataracts acquired secondary to chemotherapy and radiation therapy as well as to monitor for hemorrhage secondary to thrombocytopenia.

Description. The slit lamp is a special microscopic instrument with a lighting system that allows detailed visualization of the anterior segment of the eye. Slit-lamp vision testing involves visualization of the anterior chamber, conjunctiva, cornea, crystalline lens, eyelashes, eyelids, iris, sclera, tear film, and vitreous face and evaluation of ocular fluid and tissue size and shape by using a slit-lamp light source.

Professional Considerations
1. Consent form NOT required.

Risks
Allergic reaction to eye drops (itching, hives, rash, tight feeling in the throat, shortness of breath, anaphylaxis).

Contraindications
Allergy to mydriatic eye drops; narrow-angle glaucoma.

2. **Preparation:**
   A. Remove contact lenses and glasses.
3. **Procedure:**
   A. The client is positioned sitting upright with the chin resting on a chin rest and the forehead touching the forehead bar of the slit-lamp instrument.
   B. The client is instructed to gaze into the eye of the microscope as the examiner examines the eye from the other side of the microscope.
   C. Pupillary dilatation drops may be needed, such as in iritis.
4. **Postprocedure care:**
   A. See *Client and family teaching*.
5. **Client and family teaching:**
   A. If dilatory drops are used, vision will be blurred for up to 2 hours. The client should bring sunglasses to wear after the test. The client should not drive or operate machinery during this time.
   B. The test takes 10 minutes and is painless.
6. **Factors that affect results:**
   A. Inability of the client to remain still during the examination prevents proper examination.

7. **Other data:**
   A. Three other slit-lamp procedures may be used: fluorescein staining to detect scratches on the cornea or conjunctiva; Hruby lens to better visualize the posterior vitreous and retina; and gonioscopy, where a special contact lens eliminates the corneal curve so that glaucoma testing can be performed.

SMA-6, -7, -12, -20 (CHEM-6, -7, -12, -20), BLOOD

Norm. See individual test listings.

Increased or Decreased. See individual test listings.

Description. SMA is an acronym for the sequential multiple analyzer (SMA) automated system that analyzes multiple blood values from one tube of blood.

For the blood values of an SMA-6 see *Carbon dioxide, Total content, Blood; Chloride, Serum; Creatinine, Serum; Potassium, Serum; Sodium, Plasma or Serum; Urea nitrogen, Plasma or Serum.*

For the blood values of an SMA-7 see *Carbon dioxide, Total content, Blood; Chloride, Serum; Creatinine, Serum; Glucose, Blood; Potassium, Serum; Sodium, Plasma or Serum; Urea nitrogen, Plasma or Serum.*

For the blood values of an SMA-12 see *Albumin, Serum; Alkaline phosphatase, Serum; Aspartate aminotransferase, Serum; Bilirubin, Serum; Calcium, Serum; Cholesterol, Blood; Glucose, Blood; Lactate dehydrogenase, Blood; Phosphorus, Serum; Protein, Total serum; Urea nitrogen, Plasma or Serum; Uric acid, Serum.*

For the blood values of an SMA-20 see *Alanine aminotransferase, Serum, Alkaline phosphatase, Serum; Aspartate aminotransferase, Serum; Bilirubin, Serum; Calcium, Serum; Carbon dioxide, Total content, Blood; Chloride, Serum; Cholesterol, Blood; Creatine kinase, Serum; Creatinine, Serum; Gamma-glutamyltranspeptidase, Blood; Glucose, Blood; Lactate dehydrogenase, Blood; Phosphorus, Serum; Potassium, Serum; Protein, Total serum; Sodium, Plasma or Serum; Triglycerides, Blood; Urea nitrogen, Plasma or Serum; Uric acid, Serum.* For further information, see individual test listings.

Professional Considerations
1. Consent form NOT required.
2. **Preparation:**
   A. Tube: Red topped, red/gray topped, or gold topped.
   B. Do NOT specimens draw during hemodialysis.
3. **Procedure:**
   A. Draw a 5-mL blood sample.
4. **Postprocedure care:**
   A. None.
5. **Client and family teaching:**
   A. See individual test listings.
6. **Factors that affect results:**
   A. See individual test listings.
7. **Other data:**
   A. See individual test listings and also *Basic metabolic panel, Blood,* and *Comprehensive metabolic panel, Blood.*

SMALL BOWEL SERIES, DIAGNOSTIC

Norm. No abnormalities in the small bowel contour, position, or motility.

Usage. Cancer, Crohn's disease, diarrhea, enteritis, hematemesis, Hodgkin's disease, lymphosarcoma, malabsorption syndrome, melena, polyps, ulcers, and weight loss.

Description. Fluoroscopic examination of the small intestine after ingestion of barium sulfate. The barium enters the stomach and empties into the duodenal bulb. Circular folds appear as barium enters the duodenal loop. These folds deepen in the jejunum and then lessen in the ileum. The procedure takes 2-6 hours depending on barium transit time through the small bowel.

Professional Considerations
1. Consent form NOT required.

Risks
Aspiration of contrast material, bowel obstruction, constipation.

Contraindications
In obstruction or perforation of the small intestine because the barium may intensify the obstruction or cause seeping of the barium into the abdominal cavity.

Precautions
During pregnancy, risks of cumulative radiation exposure to the fetus from this and other previous or future imaging studies must be weighed against the benefits of the procedure. Although formal limits for client exposure are relative to this risk: benefit comparison, the United States Nuclear Regulatory Commission requires that the cumulative dose equivalent to an embryo/fetus from occupational exposure not exceed 0.5 rem (5 mSv). Radiation dosage to the fetus is proportional to the distance of the anatomy studied from the abdomen and decreases as pregnancy progresses. For pregnant clients, consult the radiologist/radiology department to obtain estimated fetal radiation exposure from this procedure.

2. **Preparation:**
   A. See *Client and family teaching.*
3. **Procedure:**
   A. Preliminary radiographs are taken in supine, erect, and lateral side positions.
   B. The client is given 500 mL flavored but chalky-tasting barium orally.
   C. Radiographs are taken at 30- to 60-minute intervals with the client in supine, erect, and lateral side positions for 2-6 hours to track the barium passage through the small intestine.
4. **Postprocedure care:**
   A. Encourage fluids (4-6 glasses of water per day for 2 days when not contraindicated) to promote the passage of the barium through the intestines.
   B. A cathartic may be prescribed to prevent barium impaction.
5. **Client and family teaching:**
   A. Fast from food and fluids and refrain from smoking from midnight before the test.
   B. A cathartic may be prescribed to be administered the evening before the test.
   C. Bring reading material or other diversion to the test because the procedure is lengthy.
   D. Stool will be barium colored for up to 72 hours.
6. **Factors that affect results:**
   A. Chronic narcotic use can cause delayed motility.

7. **Other data:**
   A. Barium enema, oral cholecystography, and routine radiography should precede a small bowel series, since retained barium clouds details on the radiographs.

SMOOTH MUSCLE ANTIBODY, BLOOD
(*see Anti–smooth muscle antibody, Serum*)

S MUCOPOLYSACCHARIDE TURNOVER, DIAGNOSTIC

Norm. Normal turnover.

Usage. Glucuronidase deficiency, Hurler syndrome, Maroteaux-Lamy syndrome, mucopolysaccharidoses I-VII (except Morquio syndrome), Sanfilippo syndrome type A or B, and Scheie syndrome.

Description. The mucopolysaccharidoses form a group of inherited disorders caused by the deficiency of enzymes required for the lysosomal degradation of glycosaminoglycans. Evaluation of the rate of turnover of S-35–labeled mucopolysaccharidoses in cultures of the skin assists in their diagnosis. Skin containing fibroblasts that lack an enzyme necessary for the breakdown of mucopolysaccharides will accumulate polysaccharides.

Professional Considerations
1. Consent form NOT required.
2. **Preparation:**
   A. Obtain a 4-mm punch biopsy instrument, sterile gauze, tape, and a sterile plastic container.
3. **Procedure:**
   A. Obtain a skin biopsy using a 4-mm punch biopsy instrument.
   B. Place the specimen in the sterile plastic container.
4. **Postprocedure care:**
   A. Transport the specimen to the laboratory immediately.
5. **Client and family teaching:**
   A. Genetic counseling is necessary for clients and families undergoing genetic testing.
6. **Factors that affect results:**
   A. An inadequate amount of biopsy tissue can cause false-negative results.

7. **Other data:**
   A. The mucopolysaccharidoses, besides involving diseases of connective and vascular tissues, also secrete substantial amounts of chondroitin-6-sulfate, heparin sulfate, and keratin sulfate.

SO₂, BLOOD
(see Blood gases, Arterial, Blood)

SODIUM, PLASMA, SERUM OR URINE

Norm:

		SI UNITS
Plasma or Serum		
Adult	136-145 mEq/L	136-145 mmol/L
Umbilical cord	116-166 mEq/L	116-166 mmol/L
Infant	139-146 mEq/L	139-146 mmol/L
Child	138-145 mEq/L	138-145 mmol/L
Panic level	≤110 mEq/L	≤110 mmol/L
Urine		
Adults	75-200 mEq/24 hours	75-200 mmol/day
Hypovolemia	<20 mmol/L	
Suggestive of SIADHS	>40 mmol/L.	
Children		
Newborn	14-40 mEq/24 hours	14-40 mmol/day
6-10 years		
Female	20-69 mEq/24 hours	20-69 mmol/day
Male	41-115 mEq/24 hours	41-115 mmol/day
10-14 years		
Female	48-168 mEq/24 hours	48-168 mmol/day
Male	63-177 mEq/24 hours	63-177 mmol/day

Panic Level Symptoms and Treatment

Symptoms (Low Sodium). Impaired cognition, depressed level of consciousness, convulsions.

Treatment (Sodium ≤110 mEq/L, 110 mmol/L, SI units):

Note: Treatment choice(s) depend on client history and condition and episode history.

Measure serum osmolality by blood test or by calculated means to determine if relative or true hyponatremia. Measure urine specific gravity.

Maintain a patent airway.

Monitor for convulsions caused by brain cell edema.

Monitor hourly neurologic checks.

The use of hypertonic saline is controversial because of its association with osmotic demyelinating syndrome. The literature demonstrates uncertainty over the cause of osmotic demyelinating syndrome, with the possible causes being rapid infusions of hypertonic saline, cerebral ischemia that occurs in severely hyponatremic clients, or some other unknown cause. However, most sources agree that slow infusions are indicated when levels reach the panic (low) level above. Give hypertonic saline (3%-5%) slowly and with extreme caution. Change to a less hypertonic infusion as soon as possible. Sodium should be replaced at about the amount of time over which the loss occurred.

Increased (Hypernatremia). Congestive heart failure, Cushing's disease, dehydration, diabetes insipidus, diaphoresis, diarrhea, hyperaldosteronism, hypertension, hypovolemia, insensible water loss, ostomies, salicylate toxicity, toxemia, vomiting, and Zollinger-Ellison syndrome with diarrhea. Drugs include ACTH, androgens, carbenicillin, carbenoxolone, clonidine, corticosteroids, diazoxide, estrogens, gamma-hydroxybutyrate (GHB), guanethidine, lactulose, mannitol, methoxyflurane, methyldopa, mineralocorticoids, oral contraceptives, oxyphenbutazone, phenylbutazone, rauwolfia alkaloids, reserpine, and sodium bicarbonate. Herbal or natural remedies include licorice.

Increased Urinary Sodium Concentration. Hyponatremia as a result of renal salt losses, osmotic diuresis or renal failure with water retention. Also dehydration, fever, head trauma, hypernatremia, hyponatremia, kidney stone, nephrotic syndrome, salicylate toxicity, starvation, and syndrome of inappropriate antidiuretic hormone secretion (SIADHS). Drugs include caffeine, calcitonin, cisplatin, diuretics, dopamine, heparin, lithium, niacin, sulfates, tetracycline, and vincristine.

Decreased. (Hyponatremia) Addison's disease, adrenal insufficiency, aminoglycoside toxicity, ascites in cardiac failure, bowel obstruction, burns, cerebral palsy, chronic renal failure, cirrhosis, congenital adrenal hyperplasia, diabetes mellitus, emphysema, glomerulonephritis, hyperglycemia, hyperosmolality, hyperthermia, hypophosphatemia, hypotension, hypothyroidism, hysterectomy, malabsorption, malnutrition, meningitis, metabolic acidosis, myxedema, nephrotic syndrome, ostomies, overhydration, pain (abdominal), paracentesis, paralytic ileus, psychogenic polydipsia, pyelonephritis (chronic), renal hypertension, sigmoidoscopy, sprue, syndrome of inappropriate antidiuretic hormone secretion syndrome (SIADHS), toxemia, toxic shock syndrome, and vomiting. Drugs include aminoglutethimide, ammonium chloride, amphotericin B, carbamazepine, chlorpropamide, cisplatin, clofibrate, chlorpropamide, cyclophosphamide, diuretics (oral and mercurial), fosinopril,

heparin, miconazole, nonsteroidal anti-inflammatory agents (NSAIDs), spironolactone, tolbutamide, tricyclic antidepressants, vasopressin, and vincristine.

Decreased Urinary Sodium Concentration. Hyponatremia associated with edema or with volume depletion from extrarenal causes. Also acute renal failure, diarrhea, emphysema, fluid retention, malabsorption, pyloric obstruction, and sprue. Drugs include corticosteroids, diazoxide, epinephrine, levarterenol, and propranolol.

Description. Sodium is the major cation of extracellular fluid. Its primary function is to maintain osmotic pressures and acid-base balance and to transmit nerve impulses. It is absorbed from the small intestine and excreted in the urine in amounts dependent on dietary intake. In normal clients, the sodium content of the body remains fairly constant despite wide variations in sodium intake.

Urinary sodium levels are used in conjunction with urine and plasma or serum creatinine in two formulas that help narrow down the source of renal failure into prerenal, renal, and postrenal causes. See *Renal indices, Diagnostic,* for further explanation of the use of these formulas.

Professional Considerations
1. Consent form NOT required.
2. **Preparation:**
   A. *Serum or plasma:*
      i. Tube: Red topped, red/gray topped, or gold topped.
      ii. Do NOT draw specimens during hemodialysis.
   B. *Urine:*
      i. Obtain a clean, 3-L container without preservatives.
      ii. Write the beginning time of collection on the laboratory requisition.
3. **Procedure:**
   A. *Serum:* Draw a 1-mL blood sample.
   B. *Urine:*
      i. Discard the first morning-urine specimen.
      ii. Save all the urine voided for 24 hours in a refrigerated, clean 3-L container without preservatives. Document the quantity of urine output during the collection period.

Include the urine voided at the end of the 24-hour period. For catheterized clients, keep the drainage bag on ice and empty the urine into the collection container hourly.

4. Postprocedure care:
   A. Compare the urine quantity in the specimen container with the urinary output record for the test. If the specimen contains less urine than what was recorded as output, some of the sample may have been discarded, thus invalidating the test.
   B. Document the quantity of urine output and the ending time for the collection period on the laboratory requisition.
   C. Send the entire 24-hour urine specimen to the laboratory for testing.
5. Client and family teaching:
   A. Save all the urine voided in the 24-hour period and urinate before defecating to avoid loss of urine. If any urine is accidentally discarded, discard the entire specimen and restart the collection the next day.
   B. Routine blood results are normally available within 2 hours.
6. Factors that affect results:
   A. Drawing blood samples proximal to intravenous infusion of sodium chloride will falsely elevate the results.
   B. Herbal or natural remedy goldenseal (*Hydrastis canadensis*) causes increased renal water loss while sodium is spared. This will cause a relative increase in sodium value.
7. Other data:
   A. An average dietary intake of 90-250 mEq/day will maintain sodium balance in adults.
   B. Minimum daily requirement is 15 mEq.
   C. The rate of sodium excretion during the night is one fifth the peak rate during the day.
   D. Urinary excretion of sodium is highly dependent on dietary intake, state of hydration, and renal function.
   E. Signs of hypernatremia include dry and sticky mucous membranes, fever, thirst, and rubbery skin turgor.
   F. Signs of hyponatremia include abdominal cramping, apprehension, oliguria, and rapid weak pulse.

SOLUBLE FIBRIN MONOMER COMPLEX (SFMC), SERUM

Norm. 0-0.4 μg/mL

Positive. Indicates low-grade or chronic intravascular coagulation.

Increased. Acute thrombosis (including arterial, coronary, pulmonary, and deep vein), before disseminated intravascular coagulation, disseminated intravascular coagulation, exacerbations of chronic relapsing pancreatitis.

Decreased. Elevation slows or stops with the administration of glycoprotein IIB/IIIA inhibitors.

Description. Fibrin monomers are intermediate products formed during the proteolysis of fibrinogen by thrombin. During the intravascular coagulation, low levels of thrombin are available in the blood, but the fibrin monomers formed are not in sufficient quantities to aggregate and form a clot. Instead, they associate themselves with fibrinogen or with fibrinogen degradation products to form soluble complexes. Demonstration of soluble fibrin monomer complex (SFMC) in plasma then indicates low-grade or chronic intravascular coagulation.

Professional Considerations
1. Consent form NOT required.
2. Preparation:
   A. Red-topped tube, a buffered citrate collection tube.
3. Procedure:
   A. Draw a plain red-topped tube to remove fluid contamination. Discard this tube.
   B. Draw blood into a buffered citrate collection tube filled to the proper level (sodium citrate of 0.105M should be used). Other anticoagulants may cause invalid results.
   C. Gently invert tube 6 times to mix.
4. Postprocedure care:
   A. Deliver specimen to lab immediately. If specimen is not processed immediately, it must be frozen at −94° F (−70° C) until testing takes place.

B. Assess the client for other signs or symptoms of thrombosis, emboli, or venoocclusive disease.
5. **Client and family teaching:**
   A. Results are normally available within 24 hours.
6. **Factors that affect results:**
   A. Specimen is heat sensitive and deteriorates rapidly. Send the specimen to the lab immediately.

7. **Other data:**
   A. Studies have suggested that fibrin monomer may play a role in tumor biology. Fibrin monomers may enhance platelet adhesion to circulating tumor cells and facilitate metastatic spread.
   B. See also *Fibrinopeptide A, Blood.*

SOLUBLE TRANSFERRIN RECEPTOR ASSAY, SERUM

S

Norm:

Males	2.2-4.5 mg/L
Females	1.8-4.6 mg/L

Values are not affected by age or by inflammation.

Note: Reference ranges are not yet standardized. Results should be compared to the ranges on the individual test kit used for this test. No reference values have been established for pregnant females, and recent or frequent blood donors.

Increased. Tissue iron-deficiency states, with an increase proportional to the severity of the anemia; also hemolytic anemia, hereditary spherocytosis, megaloblastic anemia (caused by vitamin B_{12} and folate deficiency), myelodysplastic syndromes, polycythemia, and thalassemia.

Decreased. Aplastic anemia.

PARAMETER	TESTS FOR CHANGES IN	IRON-DEFICIENCY ANEMIA	ANEMIA OF CHRONIC IRON DISEASE	DEFICIENCY AND ANEMIA OF CHRONIC DISEASE
Ferritin	Iron stores	Low	High	Normal or high
TIBC	Iron status	High	Low	Normal or high
Serum FE	Iron status	Low	Low	Low
sTfR	Iron status	High	Normal	High

Usage. Helps distinguish between iron deficiency anemia and anemia of chronic disease. Assessment of body iron status and tissue iron stores in conjunction with measured serum ferritin levels; helps detect and determine the cause of iron deficiency in inflammatory states and in the anemia of chronic disease because transferrin levels are not affected by the acute phase response; may help evaluate erythropoiesis in clients receiving erythropoietin treatment; holds promise for usefulness in evaluating iron status during pregnancy because results are not affected by gestational changes. This test is NOT helpful in assessing iron status with coexisting conditions associated with greatly enhanced erythropoiesis (such as megaloblastic anemia, thalassemia.) This test is not as sensitive and specific as serum ferritin for differentiating iron-deficiency anemia from anemia of chronic disease in elderly clients with anemia.

Description. Transferrin is a beta globulin and a glycoprotein with a short (7-day) half-life. Formed in the liver, transferrin facilitates cellular iron uptake by transporting dietary iron from the intestinal mucosa to iron storage sites and hemoglobin synthesis sites in the body (bone, muscle, erythrocytes, lymphocytes). Transferrin enables iron storage by binding to two types of transferrin receptors (type 1 and type 2) at the iron storage sites. 80% of transferrin receptors are found in erythroid tissue (precursor cells of bone marrow), though these receptors are present in almost all body tissue. During transferrin receptor–mediated endocytosis in which iron is transported into the cells, a soluble form of transferrin receptor (sTfR) can be detected in serum and is closely related to erythroid transferrin receptor turnover. The major drivers of the serum transferrin receptor concentration are cellular iron demands and erythroid proliferation rate. Therefore the serum transferrin receptor level can be a sensitive identifier of early tissue iron deficiency as long as hyperplastic erythropoiesis is not also present. Serum soluble transferrin receptor increases in iron deficiency and is usually unaffected by chronic disease states. In general, to increase sensitivity and specificity, the measurement of iron transferrin receptor should be performed in combination with other tests of iron status, including ferritin, TIBC, serum FE. In this test, an enzyme-linked immunoassay measures serum transferrin receptors using monoclonal antibodies directed against the receptors.

Professional Considerations

1. Consent form NOT required.
2. Preparation:
   A. Tube: Lavender-topped, green-topped, or serum separator tube (SST). Also obtain ice.
3. Procedure:
   A. Draw a 5-mL (lavender-topped tube), 7-mL (green-topped tube), or 6 mL (SST) blood sample. Place tube immediately on ice.
4. Postprocedure care:
   A. Document the date of last blood transfusion.
   B. Separate cells from plasma within 30 minutes and freeze.
5. Client and family teaching:
   A. This test should be performed in combination with other tests.
6. Factors that affect results:
   A. Concentrations have been found to be higher in blacks than in nonblacks.
   B. Concentrations have been found to be higher in persons living at high altitudes than in persons living at sea level.
7. Other data:
   A. The serum receptors are almost identical in men and women.

SOMATOMEDIN-C, BLOOD

(see Insulin-like growth factor-I, Blood)

SOMATOSENSORY EVOKED POTENTIAL, DIAGNOSTIC

Norm. Results of the somatosensory evoked potential (SEP) are interpreted by a physician trained in neurophysiology.

Usage. Aids in the diagnosis of demyelinating diseases, including multiple sclerosis; neurodegenerative diseases, including adrenoleukodystrophy, adrenomyeloneuropathy, and Friedreich's ataxia; and spinal cord lesions. May help predict recovery prognosis in coma, especially nontraumatic coma.

Description. SEP testing uses peripheral electrical nerve stimulation to examine the conduction velocity of impulses through the somatosensory pathway along peripheral nerves to the cortex of the brain in a fashion similar to that of the electroencephalogram (EEG). The test uses sophisticated signal averaging to filter out the effect of other brain activity during testing. Of significance are conduction time for the SEP to occur after stimulation (latency) and the amplitude of the SEP waveform.

Professional Considerations

1. Consent form NOT required.
2. Preparation:
   A. Obtain EEG electrodes, an EEG machine, and electroconductive gel.
   B. Remove jewelry and metal objects from the client's head and limbs.
3. Procedure:
   A. Scalp electrodes are placed over the sensory cortex of the scalp on the side opposite that to be stimulated.
   B. Small painless electrical stimuli are administered to large sensory fibers in the median or posterior tibial nerves.
   C. The afferent volley is recorded as well as waves that reflect peripheral nerve trunk activity.
4. Postprocedure care:
   A. Remove electrodes from the scalp and cleanse scalp of electroconductive gel.
5. Client and family teaching:
   A. The hair should be clean, dry, and free of hair spray or other hair fixatives.

B. Small painless electrical stimuli are administered to peripheral nerves. The brain's response is recorded by means of scalp electrodes.

6. **Factors that affect results:**
   A. The client must be able to lie motionless during the test.
   B. Results must be compared with the norms of the laboratory performing the test because different variations of the test will be performed, depending on the client's history and the purpose of the test.
   C. Complete lesion of the spinal cord results in no SEP recording when nerves distal to the lesion are stimulated.
   D. Lesions between the stimulated nerve and the thalamus increase the latency of the SEP.
   E. Lesions of the somatosensory cortex reduce the amplitude of the SEP wave.
   F. SEPs are a useful diagnostic tool for infants and children; however,

growth and maturation of the nervous system complicate the technical application and interpretation of the results.
   G. SEP examines a restricted anatomic pathway and does not reflect general brainstem or cerebral function.

7. **Other data:**
   A. This test is unaffected by general anesthesia, medications, and metabolic abnormalities.

SOMATOSTATIN-RECEPTOR SCINTIGRAPHY, DIAGNOSTIC
(see Octreotide scan, Diagnostic)

SOMATOTROPIN, BLOOD
(see Growth hormone, Blood)

SONOMETRY
(see Bone ultrasonometry, Diagnostic)

SPECIFIC GRAVITY, URINE

Norm:

		SI UNITS
Adults	1.016-1.022	1.016-1.022
No fluids for 12 hours	1.007-1.030	1.007-1.030
No fluids for 24 hours	≥1.026 indicates normal renal concentrating ability	
Stress conditions	1.001-1.040	1.001-1.040
Newborns	1.012	1.012
Infants	1.002-1.006	1.002-1.006

Increased. Adrenal insufficiency, bactiuria, congestive heart failure, diabetes mellitus, diarrhea, fever, fluid volume deficit, glomerulonephritis, obstruction uropathy, proteinuria, syndrome of inappropriate antidiuretic hormone secretion (SIADHS), toxemia of pregnancy, and vomiting. Drugs include dextran, radiographic contrast media, and sucrose.

Decreased. Chronic renal insufficiency, diabetes insipidus, fluid volume excess, hypothermia, intracranial pressure increase, and malignant hypertension. Drugs include aminoglycosides, carbenoxolone, lithium, and methoxyflurane.

Description. Specific gravity is the ratio of the density of urine compared to the density of an equal volume of water, which has a defined density of 1.000. Specific gravity is dependent on the number, size, and weight of urine solutes (chloride, creatinine, glucose, phosphates, protein, sodium, sulfates, urea, uric acid) dissolved in solvent. Specific gravity evaluates the kidneys' ability to regulate fluid balance as well as the hydration status of the body.

Professional Considerations
1. Consent form NOT required.
2. **Preparation:**
   A. Obtain a calibrated hydrometer (urinometer) or a temperature-

compensated refractometer and a random urine specimen.

3. **Procedure:**
   A. *Urinometer procedure:*
      i. The urinometer should be clean and dry before use.
      ii. Place the urinometer on a level surface and fill it with 15 mL of urine.
      iii. Insert a glass cylinder into the urinometer, using a spinning motion.
      iv. When the spinning stops, read the base meniscus, avoiding surface bubbles.
      v. Subtract 0.001 from the reading for every 3° C room temperature below 20° C to determine the specific gravity. Alternatively, add 0.001 to the reading for every 3° C room temperature above 20° C to determine the specific gravity.
      vi. For every 1 g/dL proteinuria, subtract 0.003 from the specific gravity.
      vii. For every 1 g/dL glucosuria, subtract 0.004 from the specific gravity.
   B. *Refractometer procedure:*
      i. Clean the cover and prism with a drop of distilled water and allow them to dry.
      ii. Close the cover.
      iii. Hold the instrument horizontally.
      iv. Apply a drop of urine at the notched bottom of the cover so that the drop flows over the prism surface.
      v. Point the instrument toward a light.
      vi. Rotate the eyepiece until the scale is in focus.
      vii. Read the specific gravity between the sharp dividing line of the dark and light contrast.

4. **Postprocedure care:**
   A. Cleanse the urinometer.

5. **Client and family teaching:**
   A. Give instructions about obtaining a urine specimen.

6. **Factors that affect results:**
   A. The reading is invalid if the glass cylinder touches the sides or bottom of the urinometer while the meniscus is being read.
   B. The urine specimen must be at room temperature.

7. **Other data:**
   A. The urinometer needs to be calibrated to produce accurate readings.
   B. Dipstick methods of measuring urine specific gravity are unreliable.

SPECT SCAN, BRAIN
(see Single-photon emission computed tomography, Brain, Diagnostic)

SPECT/CT
(see Dual modality imaging, Diagnostic)

SPEECH AUDIOMETRY
(see Audiometry test, Diagnostic)

SPERM COUNT, SPECIMEN
(see Infertility screen, Specimen and semen analysis, Specimen)

SPHINGOMYELINASE, DIAGNOSTIC

Norm. 1.53-7.18 U/g

Increased. Not clinically significant.

Decreased. Colitis (chronic), Niemann-Pick disease, types A and B.

Description. Sphingomyelinase is an enzyme that acts as a catalyst in the metabolism of sphingomyelin. Sphingomyelin is a phospholipid ubiquitously distributed in all membranes of mammalian cells and in serum lipoproteins. Niemann-Pick disease is an autosomal recessive lysosome storage disease caused by sphingomyelinase deficiency. Massive tissue accumulation of sphingomyelin results. Two types of Niemann-Pick disease have been identified: type A—a severe, neurodegenerative infantile form leading to death by 4 years of age; and type B—a chronic, nonneuronopathic form. A subacute form, similar to type B but with mild neuronal involvement (retinal storage, peripheral neuropathy, mild neurologic changes, or psychiatric disorders), has also been identified. In this test, a skin biopsy is used to perform fibroblast tissue culture and fibroblast assay for sphingomyelinase activity.

Professional Considerations
1. Consent form NOT required.
2. Preparation:
   A. Obtain a skin punch-biopsy setup and a sterile plastic cup.
3. Procedure:
   A. Cleanse the biopsy site with alcohol and allow it to air-dry.
   B. Obtain a skin punch biopsy with a 4-mm punch.
4. Postprocedure care:
   A. Place the biopsy specimen in a sterile cup.
5. Client and family teaching:
   A. A mild analgesic may be used for site tenderness.
   B. Contact the physician for redness, swelling, increasing tenderness, purulent drainage, or slow healing noted at the site.
   C. Genetic counseling must be provided for individuals and families undergoing genetic testing.
6. Factors that affect results:
   A. Inadequate punch-biopsy specimen may cause false-negative results.
7. Other data:
   A. Timeliness of results depends on laboratory availability.

SPINAL PUNCTURE
(see Lumbar puncture, Diagnostic)

SPIRAL CT, DIAGNOSTIC
(see Computed tomography of the body, Diagnostic)

SPIROMETRY, DIAGNOSTIC
(see Pulmonary function test, Diagnostic)

SPLEEN ECHOGRAM
(see Spleen ultrasonography, Diagnostic)

SPLEEN SCAN, DIAGNOSTIC

Norm. Homogeneous distribution of the radiolabeled erythrocytes throughout the spleen.

Usage. Evaluation of the size, shape, and location of the spleen in suspected congenital anomalies, in cancer, or after trauma.

Description. The spleen scan is a nuclear medicine examination of the left upper quadrant of the abdomen after intravenous administration of either technetium-99m–labeled or chromium-51–labeled, heat-treated, red blood cells. Because erythrocytes are sequestered by the spleen, the radiolabeled cell accumulation in the spleen can be identified with the scinticounter.

Professional Considerations
1. Consent form IS required.

Risks
Hematoma, infection.

Contraindications
Inability to lie motionless during the scan; during pregnancy; or breast-feeding.

2. Preparation:
   A. Establish intravenous access.
   B. Have emergency equipment available for potential anaphylaxis.
3. Procedure:
   A. A 5-mL sample of the client's blood is removed with a heparinized syringe by means of venipuncture. It is heat treated and labeled with the selected radionuclide in the nuclear medicine department.
   B. The labeled blood is injected through the established intravenous access into the client.
   C. After 1 hour, scintiscans are taken of the left upper quadrant of the abdomen from anterior, posterior, left lateral, and oblique views.
   D. Scanning is repeated in 24 hours.
4. Postprocedure care:
   A. Observe the individual for 1 hour after the study for possible anaphylactic reaction to the radionuclide.
   B. General body-substance isolation precautions protect the health care professional from potential radiation exposure.
5. Client and family teaching:
   A. Technetium half-life is 6 hours. Chromium-51 half-life is 27.8 days.

B. General body-substance isolation precautions protect the client's family from potential radiation exposure.

6. **Factors that affect results:**
   A. Impaired hepatic function causes a greater-than-normal splenic uptake of the labeled cells.
   B. Hematoma, infarct, abscess, or tumor causes decreased uptake.
   C. Amyloidosis, sarcoidosis, or granulomas may cause many filling defects.

7. **Other data:**
   A. This test may be performed with a liver scan.
   B. Health care professionals working in a nuclear medicine area must follow federal standards set by the Nuclear Regulatory Commission. These standards include precautions for handling the radioactive material and monitoring of potential radiation exposure.

SPLEEN ULTRASONOGRAPHY (SPLEEN ECHOGRAM, SPLEEN ULTRASOUND), DIAGNOSTIC

Norm. Proper size, shape, and position of the spleen. Negative for abscess, cyst, tumor, or splenomegaly. Spleen tissue stipples with fine, homogeneous, low-level echoes. Spleen is not visualized until the transducer reaches 9-11 cm above the umbilicus.

Usage. Assessment of status after trauma; detection or differentiation of splenic abnormalities such as abscess or cyst; ongoing monitoring of the spleen during medical therapy; guidance for splenic needle biopsy.

Description. Evaluation of the spleen's size, shape, and position by the creation of an oscilloscopic picture from the echoes of high-frequency sound waves passing over the abdominal area (acoustic imaging). The time required for the ultrasonic beam to be reflected back to the transducer from differing densities of tissue is converted by a computer to an electrical impulse displayed on an oscilloscopic screen to create a three-dimensional picture of the spleen. The echomorphology of splenic lesions assists in the diagnosis of the

lesion and can be described as iso-echogenic, hyperechogenic, hypoechogenic, or complex in comparison to the normal spleen echogenicity. The differing tissue densities of specific lesions assists in the diagnosis of the lesion. However, spleen ultrasonography can not definitively localize a splenic tumor, due to close proximity of other organs in the area.

Professional Considerations
1. Consent form NOT required.
2. **Preparation:**
   A. This test should be performed before intestinal barium tests or after the barium is cleared from the system.
   B. Obtain ultrasonic gel or paste.
   C. See *Client and family teaching.*
3. **Procedure:**
   A. The client is positioned supine in a bed or on a procedure table.
   B. The skin overlying the spleen is covered with ultrasonic gel, and a lubricated transducer is passed slowly and firmly over the left upper quadrant of the abdomen at various angles and at specific intervals 1-2 cm apart. The transducer is passed between rather than over the ribs. This may be performed with the client in several positions. The right lateral decubitus position provides the best information. Higher-frequency linear ultrasound probes are selected for clients who are thin.
   C. Photographs are taken of the oscilloscopic display.
4. **Postprocedure care:**
   A. Wipe the ultrasonic gel from the skin.
5. **Client and family teaching:**
   A. Fast from food and fluids overnight (when possible), and abstain from smoking for several hours before the test.
   B. The procedure is painless and carries no risks.
   C. The procedure takes less than 30 minutes.
6. **Factors that affect results:**
   A. Dehydration interferes with adequate contrast between organs and body fluids.
   B. Intestinal barium, food, or gas (particularly in the supine position) obscures the results by pre-

venting the proper transmission and deflection of the high-frequency sound waves.

7. **Other data:**
   A. Further testing may include computed tomography or magnetic resonance imaging.

SPLEEN ULTRASOUND
(see Spleen ultrasonography, Diagnostic)

SPLENOPORTOGRAPHY, DIAGNOSTIC

Norm. Splenic pulp pressure: 50-180 mm H_2O, or 3.5-13.5 mm Hg. Smooth flow of dye through the splenic venous system without obstruction or diversion. Timely flow of the dye through the hepatic portal system without evidence of collateral veins.

Usage. Cirrhosis, hepatocellular carcinoma, and portal hypertension.

Description. Splenoportography is the radiographic examination of the venous system of the spleen and portal system of the liver after injection of contrast medium directly into the splenic vein or splenic parenchyma. The measurement of splenic pulp pressure before dye injection helps detect portal hypertension.

Professional Considerations
1. Consent form IS required.

Risks
Allergic reaction to contrast media (itching, hives, rash, tight feeling in the throat, shortness of breath, anaphylaxis); renal toxicity from contrast medium; hemorrhage requiring blood transfusion or splenectomy, or both.

Contraindications
Previous allergy to iodine, shellfish, or radiographic contrast media; pregnancy (if iodinated media is used, because of the radioactive iodine crossing the blood-placental barrier); renal insufficiency; ascites, coagulation disorders, impaired hepatic or renal function, or splenic infection. Sedatives are contraindicated in clients with central nervous system depression.

2. **Preparation:**
   A. Establish intravenous access.
   B. Assess platelet count, prothrombin time (PT), activated partial thromboplastin time (aPTT), urea nitrogen, creatinine, and liver enzymes.
   C. Administer a sedative and an analgesic, as prescribed, 30 minutes before the test.
   D. Obtain antiseptic, sterile drapes, 1-2% lidocaine (Xylocaine) local anesthetic, a percutaneous injection tray, a manometer, contrast medium, and material for a dry, sterile dressing.
   E. See *Client and family teaching.*

3. **Procedure:**
   A. The client is positioned supine with the left hand under the head.
   B. The left sides of the thorax and abdomen are washed with an antiseptic.
   C. The spleen is located by means of fluoroscopy.
   D. The puncture site is marked, usually the ninth or tenth intercostal space at the mid- or postaxillary line.
   E. After local anesthesia is injected around the puncture site, a sheathed needle is inserted percutaneously into the spleen. The needle is removed, and the sheath is connected to a spinal manometer for splenic pulp pressure measurement.
   F. After sheath placement is verified, radiographic contrast medium is injected through the splenic parenchyma into the splenic vein, and cineradiographic films are taken to record splenic venous system filling.
   G. The needle is removed, and a dry, sterile dressing is applied to the puncture site.
   H. The procedure takes less than 1 hour.

4. **Postprocedure care:**
   A. Assess vital signs every 15 minutes × 4, then every 30 minutes × 4, then hourly × 4, and then every 4 hours until 24 hours after the procedure.
   B. Observe for bleeding and swelling at the puncture site each time vital signs are taken.

5. **Client and family teaching:**
   A. Fast from food and fluids from midnight before the test.

B. A sensation of warmth or flushing after the dye injection is normal and will be transient.

C. Immediately report any left upper quadrant pain.

D. The client must assume a left-side lying position for 24 hours.

E. The client may resume previous diet after the procedure. The oral intake of fluids, where not contraindicated, is encouraged.

6. Factors that affect results:

A. Cirrhosis causes delayed emptying of the intrahepatic radicles.

B. Portal hypertension causes elevated splenic pulp pressure and evidence of the development of collateral veins.

7. Other data:

A. The newer computed tomographic percutaneous transsplenic portography (CT-PTSP) utilizes thinner needles for splenic puncture and CT rather than cineradiography. The use of thinner needles decreases the amount of pain and the risk of hemorrhage associated with the procedure. CT has a high-contrast resolution and can thus detect a low dose of contrast dye. CT-PTSP thus decreases the length of time that the client must be monitored and be on bed rest after the procedure and allows the procedure to be performed on an outpatient basis.

B. CT during arterial portography (CTAP) is an alternative method of visualizing the portal venous system.

SpO₂
(see Oximetry, Diagnostic)

SPONDEE THRESHOLD SPEECH TEST, DIAGNOSTIC

Norm. 0-20 dB (decibels) in adults, 0-15 dB children.

Usage. Evaluates the ability to hear conversational speech and provides more specific evaluation after abnormal pure-tone audiometry results.

Description. Spondees are two-syllable words (such as "baseball," "airplane") presented to a client through earphones to measure the lowest level at which the client repeats 50% of the words. This test measures degree of hearing loss and is often performed after audiometric testing.

Professional Considerations

1. Consent form NOT required.

2. **Preparation:**

A. Obtain a speech audiometer, earphones, and a recorded spondee list.

3. **Procedure:**

A. Explain to the client that a series of two-syllable words in decreasing loudness will be transmitted through the earphones. The client should repeat these words when he or she hears them to the best of his or her ability.

4. **Postprocedure care:**

A. A client with abnormal results should be referred to an audiologist.

5. **Client and family teaching:**

A. The earphones are placed over the client's ears, and testing proceeds as described above, with only one ear tested at a time.

6. **Factors that affect results:**

A. Unfamiliarity with the language or words used may make the results unreliable.

B. This test is unreliable in young children who do not yet have fully developed speech.

7. **Other data:**

A. See also *Audiometry test, Diagnostic.*

SPUTUM, FUNGUS, CULTURE

Norm. No growth.

Usage. AIDS, actinomycosis, aspergillosis, candidiasis, coccidioidomycosis, fungal infections, histoplasmosis, neoplastic disease, and pneumonia.

Description. Fungi are slow-growing, eukaryotic organisms that can grow on living and nonliving organic materials and are subdivided into yeasts and molds. Only a few fungi species infect humans. Normal host defense mechanisms limit the damage these fungi cause superficially. When inhaled or inoculated deep into tissues or when acquired by an immunocompromised client, fungi can cause serious infections.

Professional Considerations

1. Consent form NOT required.
2. Preparation:
   A. A first morning specimen is preferred because it represents overnight secretions of the tracheobronchial tree.
   B. Obtain a sterile plastic container or a sputum trap.
3. Procedure:
   A. Obtain 1-3 mL of sputum in a sterile container and cover it with a lid, or obtain a specimen in a sputum trap.
4. Postprocedure care:
   A. Refrigerate the specimen or deliver it to the laboratory within 1 hour.
   B. Preliminary reports will be available in 48-72 hours and negative reports after 4 weeks.
5. Client and family teaching:
   A. Cough deeply and expectorate 5-10 mL of sputum into a sterile plastic container and then cap it tightly. Deep coughs are necessary to produce sputum, rather than saliva. To produce the proper specimen, take several breaths in, without fully exhaling each, and then expel sputum with a "cascade cough."
6. Factors that affect results:
   A. A contaminated specimen cup invalidates the results.
7. Other data:
   A. Pathogenic fungi include *Alternaria, Aspergillus, Blastomyces dermatitidis, Candida, Coccidioides immitis, Cryptococcus, Histoplasma capsulatum, Monilia* (now called *Candida*), *Mucor, Penicillium, Rhizopus, Scopulariopsis,* and *Sporothrix schenckii.*
   B. A single negative culture does not rule out a fungal infection.

SPUTUM, GRAM STAIN, DIAGNOSTIC

(*see Gram stain, Diagnostic*)

SPUTUM, MYCOBACTERIA, CULTURE AND SMEAR

Norm. No growth.

Usage. Acquired immunodeficiency syndrome, hemoptysis, mycobacteria, splenomegaly, and tuberculosis.

Description. Mycobacteria are rod-shaped, aerobic bacteria that resist decolorizing chemicals after staining, hence "acid fast." Many new species of nontuberculous mycobacteria (or new components of species complexes) as well as multiple drug-resistant isolates of *M. tuberculosis* have been recognized. *Mycobacterium* species are capable of producing human disease characterized by destructive granulomas that can necrose, ulcerate, and cavitate. *M. tuberculosis* is transmitted by the airborne route, most commonly to the lungs, where it survives well, causes areas of granulomatous inflammation, and, if not dormant, causes cough, fever, and hemoptysis. In this test, an acid-fast bacteria (AFB) culture and stain of sputum are performed to detect mycobacteria. The smear is followed by a confirmatory culture. Sputum cultures for *M. tuberculosis* obtains a higher yield and is more cost effective than blood cultures are. Newer methods of testing for tuberculosis include polymerase chain reaction and

Professional Considerations

1. Consent form NOT required.
2. Preparation:
   A. A first morning specimen is preferred because it represents an accumulation of overnight secretions of the tracheobronchial tree.
   B. Obtain a sterile plastic cup with a lid.
   C. For clients who are inpatients, waiting until the morning after admission to obtain sputum samples produces a less false-negative result.
3. Procedure:
   A. Sputum may be induced by inhalation of hypertonic saline aerosol.
   B. Laryngeal swabs and gastric isolates may also be useful in individuals unable to produce sputum or cooperate with induction procedures.
4. Postprocedure care:
   A. Refrigerate the specimens if not delivered to the laboratory within an hour.
   B. A preliminary report is available in 72 hours, the final report in 4-6 weeks.
5. Client and family teaching:
   A. Cough deeply and expectorate 5-10 mL of sputum into a sterile

plastic container and then cap it tightly. Deep coughs are necessary to produce sputum, rather than saliva. To produce the proper specimen, take several breaths in, without fully exhaling each, and then expel sputum with a "cascade cough."

B. Repeat the procedure for three consecutive mornings.

6. Factors that affect results:
A. Contamination of the specimen invalidates the results.
B. An insufficient sputum amount may cause false-negative results.
C. Repeated induction of sputum increases the yield via the polymerase chain reaction.

7. Other data:
A. Because 5-10 mL of sputum are required, the specimen may be collected over a 2-hour period. However, a 24-hour period is unacceptable.
B. Bronchial washings often do not contain enough sputum because they are diluted with anesthetics and irrigating fluid.

SPUTUM, ROUTINE, CULTURE
(see Culture, Routine, Specimen)

SPUTUM ACID-FAST BACTERIA (AFB), CULTURE
(see Acid-fast bacteria, Culture and Stain)

SPUTUM CULTURE AND SENSITIVITY (C & S), SPECIMEN
(see Culture, Routine, Specimen)

SPUTUM CYTOLOGY, SPECIMEN
(see Cytologic study of respiratory tract, Diagnostic)

SPUTUM FOR *HAEMOPHILUS* SPECIES, CULTURE

Norm. No *Haemophilus* species isolated.

Positive. Chronic bronchitis, epiglottitis, *Haemophilus influenzae*, meningitis, otitis media, and pneumonia.

Negative. Viral pulmonary disease.

Description. The gram-negative *Haemophilus* coccobacillus is the leading cause of pediatric otitis, meningitis, epiglottitis, and adult pneumonia.

Professional Considerations
1. Consent form NOT required.
2. Preparation:
A. A first morning specimen is preferred because it represents overnight secretions of the tracheobronchial tree.
B. Obtain a sterile plastic cup with a lid.
3. Procedure:
A. Obtain 3-5 mL of sputum in a sterile container and cover it with a lid, or obtain a specimen in a sputum trap.
4. Client and family teaching:
A. Cough deeply and expectorate 3-5 mL of sputum into a sterile plastic container and then cap it tightly.
5. Postprocedure care:
A. Refrigerate the specimen within 2 hours of collection.
B. Results are normally available within 24 hours, the final report within 48 hours.
6. Factors that affect results:
A. Specimens over 2 hours old and not refrigerated may cause false-negative results.
7. Other data:
A. 5%-15% of *H. influenzae* pathogens produce penicillinase and therefore are resistant to treatment with ampicillin.

SPUTUM HEMOSIDERIN PREPARATION, SPECIMEN

Norm. Negative.

Usage. Blood in the alveolar space.

Description. Hemosiderin are iron-storage granules normally found in the liver cytoplasm, spleen, and bone marrow. Hemosiderin is also a by-product of macrophage degradation of erythrocytes. This test uses Prussian blue stain on a smear of sputum to detect the presence of hemosiderin in the lungs, representing previous alveolar hemorrhage (AH). AH has a variety of causes, including anti–basement-membrane–

mediated diseases, pulmonary infection, and vasculitis. AH can also occur in immunocompromised people with invasive fungal pneumonia and thrombocytopenia and in people who have undergone heart transplantation for chronic congestive heart failure.

Professional Considerations
1. Consent form NOT required.
2. Preparation:
   A. Obtain a sterile plastic sputum cup, a sterile container with a lid, glass slides, and a cytologic sputum fixative.
3. Procedure:
   A. Obtain a sputum specimen in a sterile plastic container.
4. Postprocedure care:
   A. Smear sputum on a glass slide and apply cytologic fixative. Place the slide in a sterile container and cap it tightly.
5. Client and family teaching:
   A. Cough deeply and expectorate 3-5 mL of sputum into a sterile plastic container. Deep coughs are necessary to produce sputum, rather than saliva. To produce the proper specimen, take several breaths in, without fully exhaling each, and then expel sputum with a "cascade cough."
6. Factors that affect results:
   A. Failure to "fix" the specimen invalidates the results.
7. Other data:
   A. Results are available within hours but require interpretation with other clinical data.

SQUAMOUS CELL CARCINOMA ANTIGEN
(see Tumor antigen 4 and sub-fraction SCC antigen, Blood and Specimen)

SSRI
(see Selective serotonin reuptake inhibitors, Blood)

ST. LOUIS ENCEPHALITIS VIRUS SEROLOGY, SERUM

Norm. A less than fourfold rise in titer between acute and convalescent samples.

Usage. Hemagglutination titer <1:10. Complement fixation titer <1:8.

Description. St. Louis encephalitis virus is a group B arbovirus, a member of Flaviviridae, that is transmitted to humans by the bite of infected mosquitoes, with the donor host being birds. This virus causes inflammation of the tissues of the central nervous system. Symptoms may range from mild headache and fever to encephalitis and death. This virus occurs in the western, central, and southern United States and in Jamaica, Panama, Brazil, and Trinidad.

Professional Considerations
1. Consent form NOT required.
2. Preparation:
   A. Tube: Red topped, red/gray topped, or gold topped.
   B. Specimens MAY be drawn during hemodialysis.
3. Procedure:
   A. Draw a 7-mL blood sample as soon as possible after symptoms appear, and label it as the acute sample.
   B. Repeat the test in 10-14 days, and label the tube as the convalescent sample.
4. Postprocedure care:
   A. See *Client and family teaching.*
5. Client and family teaching:
   A. Return in 10-14 days to have a convalescent sample drawn, which is necessary to interpret the results of the acute sample.
6. Factors that affect results:
   A. Failure to collect a convalescent sample.
   B. False-positive results may occur in clients recently vaccinated for yellow fever.
7. Other data:
   A. 10%-15% of clients with St. Louis encephalitis do not develop complement fixation antibodies.
   B. There is no specific treatment for this disease.
   C. Standard precautions and vector-control practices are adequate to prevent spread of this disease.

STABLE FACTOR, BLOOD
(see Factor VII, Blood)

STEMLINE DNA ANALYSIS, SPECIMEN
(see DNA ploidy, Specimen)

STEREOTACTIC BREAST BIOPSY, DIAGNOSTIC

Negative. Benign.

Positive. Atypical or malignant cells.

Description. Stereotactic breast biopsy is a radiograph-guided method of localizing and sampling nonpalpable breast lesions that are discovered on mammography and considered to be suspicious for malignancy. The position of the lesion in the breast can be calculated relative to a fixed grid and a needle placed within the lesion with direct confirmation of its position on a stereotactic radiograph. The placement is accurate to within 2 mm. Stereotactic breast biopsy can be performed by means of fine-needle aspiration cytology or core needle histology.

Professional Considerations
1. Consent form IS required.

Risks
Bruising, infection at needle aspiration site, vasovagal reaction.

Contraindications
Large abnormal breast tissue area.

Precautions
During pregnancy, risks of cumulative radiation exposure to the fetus from this and other previous or future imaging studies must be weighed against the benefits of the procedure. Although formal limits for client exposure are relative to this risk: benefit comparison, the United States Nuclear Regulatory Commission requires that the cumulative dose equivalent to an embryo/fetus from occupational exposure not exceed 0.5 rem (5 mSv). Radiation dosage to the fetus is proportional to the distance of the anatomy studied from the abdomen and decreases as pregnancy progresses. For pregnant clients, consult the radiologist/radiology department to obtain estimated fetal radiation exposure from this procedure.

2. Preparation:
   A. This procedure is performed by a radiologist with mammographic experience.
   B. Equipment is assembled according to the type of biopsy (fine-needle aspiration or core needle) and the radiologist's preference.
   C. The client is assessed for any allergies, use of anticoagulants or antiplatelet agents, or bleeding disorders.
3. Procedure:
   A. The client is positioned prone on the x-ray table with the breasts hanging down for the mammogram films and biopsy. An upright seated position with lateral arm support may also be used, but is associated with a higher incidence of vasovagal reactions.
   B. The skin is prepared according to the radiologist's preference and institutional policy.
   C. A local anesthetic is injected into the biopsy site.
   D. A small incision is made at the site of needle insertion.
   E. The needle (either a 14-gauge automated needle or a 11- to 14-gauge vacuum-assisted biopsy probe) is inserted percutaneously into the lesion with placement confirmed by radiography.
   F. Multiple samples are taken from different positions in the lesion. At least 12 samples are required for best diagnostic accuracy. The first sample is usually taken from the core of the lesion, followed by samples taken from the periphery.
   G. Metallic clips may be placed within the breast to mark the biopsy site for easy identification should later biopsy be needed.
   H. The specimen obtained from core needle biopsy is placed in formalin and sent immediately to the laboratory.
   I. The specimen obtained from fine-needle aspiration is fixed on cytology slides and sent immediately to the lab.
4. Postprocedure care:
   A. Place Steri-Strips and a pressure dressing over the site.
   B. If metal clips were placed, two orthogonal planes should be taken via mammogram to con-

firm clip location for later comparison.
5. **Client and family teaching:**
   A. The client may eat or drink as usual.
   B. The procedure generally takes 1 hour.
   C. Most individuals are able to return to their usual routine, including driving or work, after the procedure.
   D. The dressing may be removed the next day.
   E. There may be some tenderness, swelling, bruising, or slight bleeding at the site. An ice pack or nonaspirin pain reliever will help to relieve the above.
   F. If the biopsy diagnosis is benign, routine mammograms should be continued.
6. **Factors that affect results:**
   A. Core needle biopsy yields better diagnostic results than does fine needle aspiration. All specimens taken must be examined to avoid false negative results.
   B. Needle placement can be inaccurate and yield a false-negative result if the breast tissue is displaced during biopsy.
   C. Physician experience with at least 5-14 prior biopsies of this type significantly improve the diagnostic accuracy of the procedure.
7. **Other data:**
   A. If inadequate tissue was obtained or if a malignancy is suspected but not confirmed, an open surgical biopsy is recommended. Open surgical biopsy is also recommended if atypical cells are identified.
   B. Although complications from this procedure may include infection and hematoma, the complication rate is low.
   C. Results from either fine-needle aspiration or core needle biopsy are available within 24 hours.
   D. A one-year follow-up mammography is recommended for benign lesions.

STOOL CULTURE, ROUTINE, STOOL

Norm. Negative for pathogens; no growth other than normal flora.

Usage. Coccidioidomycosis, dysentery, enteric fever, failure to thrive (fat, ova, and parasite), gastroenteritis, salmonellosis, typhoid with *Salmonella*, and ulcerative colitis.

Description. To screen for common pathogens such as *Helicobacter, Salmonella, Shigella, Campylobacter, Vibrio, Yersinia,* or *Clostridium difficile.* This test may be indicated in clients with persistent or bloody diarrhea accompanied by fever or recent out-of-country travel (to a third-world country), in clients with a history of recent antibiotic usage, or in clients known to be exposed to enteric pathogens.

Professional Considerations
1. Consent form NOT required.
2. **Preparation:**
   A. Obtain a bedpan or a plastic toilet-seat specimen hat, a wooden tongue blade, and a sterile container with a lid.
3. **Procedure:**
   A. Using a wooden tongue blade, place a fresh stool sample 1 inch in diameter in a sterile container and cap it tightly.
4. **Postprocedure care:**
   A. Send the specimen to the laboratory immediately.
   B. If there will be a 2- or 3-hour delay before testing, place the specimen in a transport medium such as buffered saline-glycol or alkaline peptone water.
5. **Client and family teaching:**
   A. Defecate in a bedpan or toilet-seat specimen hat, and avoid contaminating the stool with urine, toilet tissue, soap, or water.
6. **Factors that affect results:**
   A. Refrigerate the specimens if they are not sent to the laboratory immediately.
   B. Barium or mineral oil inhibit bacterial growth.
   C. Keep the specimens free of toilet tissue, bismuth, soap, water, or urine, because these speed up deterioration of ova.
7. **Other data:**
   A. Rectal swabs can be used, but they are less likely to yield positive results.
   B. *Vibrio parahaemolyticus,* a marine bacterium, causes gastrointestinal symptoms as a result of improperly

S

refrigerated crab, lobster, or shrimp.

C. *Vibrio cholerae*, rice-watery in appearance with a fishy odor, causes both epidemic and environmental cholera.

D. *Helicobacter pylori* has been cultured from the diarrheal stools of infected individuals in developing countries. Immigration is responsible for the development of isolated areas of high prevalence in some Western countries.

E. The optimal specimen for the diagnosis of *C. difficile*–associated diarrhea is a watery or loose stool.

F. Results are normally available in 48 hours.

STOOL, FUNGUS, CULTURE

Norm. Negative for fungus; no growth.

Usage. Fungal infections and immunosuppressed clients.

Description. Fungi are slow-growing, eukaryotic organisms that can grow on living and nonliving organic materials and are subdivided into yeasts and molds. Only a few fungi species infect humans. Normal host defense mechanisms limit the damage these fungi cause superficially. This is a screening test performed on a sample of stool to determine the presence of fungi in clients at risk for fungal infection (those on antibiotic therapy, parenteral nutrition, and those who are immunocompromised).

Professional Considerations
1. Consent form NOT required.
2. **Preparation:**
   A. Obtain a bedpan or a plastic toilet-seat specimen hat, a wooden tongue blade, and a sterile container with a lid.
3. **Procedure:**
   A. Using a wooden tongue blade, place a fresh stool sample 1 inch in diameter in a sterile container and cap it tightly.
4. **Postprocedure care:**
   A. Refrigerate the specimen if it is not sent to the laboratory immediately.
5. **Client and family teaching:**
   A. Defecate in a bedpan or toilet-seat specimen hat, and avoid contam-

inating the stool with urine, toilet tissue, soap, or water.
6. **Factors that affect results:**
   A. Dried specimens are not acceptable.
7. **Other data:**
   A. Negative cultures are reported after 1 week. Results may take 4 weeks if a systemic fungal infection is indicated.
   B. Fungi in stool may be *Aspergillus, Candida, Cryptococcus, Geotrichum, Histoplasma, Rhodotorula,* or *Torulopsis* species.

STREPTODORNASE, SERUM
(*see Antideoxyribonuclease B titer, Serum*)

STREPTOZYME, BLOOD

Norm. Titer <166 Todd units or <100 streptozyme units.

Positive. Bacterial endocarditis, glomerulonephritis, pharyngitis, reactive arthritis, recent streptococcal infection, rheumatic and connective tissue diseases, rheumatic fever, scarlet fever, and upper respiratory infections.

Negative. Hematuria.

Description. A nonspecific screening test for the detection of antibodies to multiple exoenzymes of various species of streptococci using a commercial reagent containing erythrocytes coated with streptococcal antigens (DNase, streptokinase, streptolysin O, and hyaluronidase). This test can determine current or recent streptococcal infection earlier than the ASO titer can, but it cannot determine the location or type of streptococcal infection. In a positive test, antibodies begin rising by week 3 after infection and decrease by week 10.

Professional Considerations
1. Consent form NOT required.
2. **Preparation:**
   A. Tube: Red topped, red/gray topped, or gold topped.
   B. Specimens MAY be drawn during hemodialysis.
3. **Procedure:**
   A. Draw a 1-mL blood sample as soon as possible after symptoms

appear, and label it as the acute sample.
4. **Postprocedure care:**
   A. Repeat testing in 10 days, and label the tube as the convalescent sample.
   B. Subsequent samples, taken biweekly for the next 4-6 weeks, are recommended.
5. **Client and family teaching:**
   A. Serial testing is recommended.
6. **Factors that affect results:**
   A. Antibiotic therapy may cause decreased results.
7. **Other data:**
   A. Serial testing over a period of weeks is more significant than a single determination.
   B. This test is not as sensitive in children as it is in adults.
   C. See also *Antistreptolysin-O titer, Blood*

STRESS/EXERCISE TEST, DIAGNOSTIC

Norm. Negative.
Client reaches and maintains 85% of his/her target heart rate, without cardiac symptoms.
Test results usually include the following information:
ECG: baseline and during test, including the presence of changes
Estimate of exercise capacity
Any cardiac symptoms occurring during the test
Criteria used for ending the test: determination of whether the maximal heart rate was attained.
Blood pressure and any arrhythmias occurring during the test

Usage. Coronary artery disease; evaluation of cardiopulmonary fitness and exercise tolerance; preoperative screening for clients at high risk for surgical cardiovascular compromise; assessment of the efficacy of interventions such as coronary artery bypass graft, coronary angioplasty, medications, and cardiac rehabilitation; dysrhythmias; and valvular competence.

Description. Stress testing measures the efficiency of the heart during a period of physical stress on a treadmill or on a stationary bicycle. The effects of exercise on cardiac output and myocar-

dial oxygen consumption are evaluated by concurrent monitoring of electrocardiograms, blood pressure, and oxygen consumption. An advantage of exercise testing is that it can identify (in a safe environment) individuals prone to cardiac ischemia during activity, when resting electrocardiograms are normal.

Professional Considerations
1. Consent form IS required.

Risks
Cardiac ischemia, including myocardial infarction, dysrhythmias, hypotension, hypertension, dizziness.

Contraindications
Cardiac contraindications: Active unstable angina, aortic stenosis (hemodynamically significant), chest pain, cardiac inflammation (endocarditis, myocarditis, pericarditis), congestive heart failure (acute), coronary insufficiency syndrome, digitalis toxicity, electrolyte abnormalities (severe), heart blocks (2°, 3°), hypertension (SBP >200 mm Hg, or DBP >110 mm Hg), left bundle branch block or other uncontrolled dysrhythmias, left ventricular hypertrophy, myocardial infarction (recent), obesity (weight higher than capacity of equipment-usually 350 pounds), pacemaker (fixed-rate), recent significant changes in ECG, thromboembolic processes (active).
Other contraindications: Alcohol intoxication, asthma (severe) or chronic obstructive pulmonary disease, infection (acute), pulmonary embolism (recent), thrombophlebitis; also inability to walk on a treadmill or pedal a bicycle.

2. **Preparation:**
   A. Have emergency equipment readily available.
   B. See *Client and family teaching.*
3. **Procedure:**
   A. The stress test is performed by specially trained (that is, ACLS-certified) nurses, exercise physiologists, and physical therapists. The American Association of Cardiovascular and Pulmonary Rehabilitation has recommended direct physician supervision of all initial stress tests and tests for individuals considered at high risk for complications.

B. Attach electrocardiogram leads and a blood pressure cuff.

C. While the client is on a treadmill, stationary bicycle, or stair stepper, computerized electrocardiographic recordings and blood pressure readings are obtained. Oxygen consumption may be measured by having the client breathe through a special mouthpiece during exercise.

D. The client is stressed in stages by increases in miles per hour and the percentage grade of elevation of the treadmill.

E. The test is terminated when any of the following occurs:

    i. Signs of ischemia are present (ST-segment depression of ≤1-2 mm for a duration >0.06 second, or ST-segment elevation).

    ii. Maximum effort has been achieved.

    iii. A predetermined target has been achieved.

    iv. Dyspnea, hypertension >250 mm Hg systolic blood pressure.

    v. Tachycardia >200 minus the client's age.

    vi. New dysrhythmias, new conduction disturbances (that is, heart block), or increasing ectopy.

    vii. Chest pain with or without ECG changes.

    viii. Faintness, weakness, dizziness, or confusion.

    ix. Blood pressure fails to rise as body exercise stress increases.

    x. Extreme fatigue, or request by the client that the test be stopped.

4. **Postprocedure care:**

A. The client should be monitored at rest until the heart rate, blood pressure, and electrocardiogram are at baseline values.

B. Remove the electrodes and the blood pressure cuff.

5. **Client and family teaching:**

A. Wear flat walking or tennis shoes and comfortable attire.

B. According to physician preference and instructions, gradually discontinue beta-blocker drugs before the test.

C. Fast from food and fluids and refrain from smoking and caffeine usage for 4 hours before the test.

D. Clients may take all their medications as usual.

E. During the test, immediately report to the technician any chest pain, dizziness, light-headedness, nausea, or discomfort you experience.

F. After the test, rest for a few hours at home.

6. **Factors that affect results:**

A. False-positive electrocardiogram responses are caused by anemia, digitalis, diuretics, estrogen, hypertension, hypoxia, Lown-Ganong-Levine syndrome, syndrome X in women, or valvular heart disease.

B. False-positive results may be caused by the following baseline EKG abnormalities.

    i. 1 mm or more elevation or depression of the ST segment

    ii. Right or left ventricular hypertrophy

    iii. T-wave inversions in multiple leads due to old injury

    iv. Abnormal conduction, such as increased QT interval, ST-T changes, and right or left bundle branch blocks

C. False-positive results occur more frequently in women than in men.

D. False-negative tests occur when individuals with known significant CAD fail to demonstrate exercise-induced ST-segment depression.

E. Conditions that may affect performance include lung disease, muscle pain, and electrolyte imbalances.

7. **Other data:**

A. Ischemic ST-segment displacement >0.1 mm of 80-msec duration during exercise but not found at rest means a five times greater risk of coronary heart disease in males.

B. Exertional hypotension may indicate left coronary artery disease, myocardial ischemia, or left ventricular dysfunction.

C. The exercise stress test may also be performed with radionuclide (thallium) or radiopharmaceutical (sestamibi) perfusion studies. See *Heart scan, Diagnostic.*

D. Schulman et al. (1997) found that exercise testing is useful for identifying evidence of the presence of significant coronary lesions: "Having either ST-segment depression or a normalized exercise time <1 during exercise had a 95% sensitivity, 71% specificity, and 86% predictive accuracy in identifying abnormal coronary flow reserve (CFR)."

E. See also *Stress test, Pharmacologic, Diagnostic.*

STRESS TEST, PHARMACOLOGIC, DIAGNOSTIC

Norm. Negative.

Usage. Coronary artery disease; detection of ischemia and assessment of myocardial viability; evaluation of left ventricular function; preoperative cardiac risk stratification; and valvular competence.

Description. Pharmacologic stress testing is used to evaluate individuals with suspected or proven coronary artery disease who are unable to perform satisfactory levels of exercise to reach 85% of their maximal heart rate. A pharmacologic agent is used to elevate heart rate and blood pressure and cardiac response is examined through an imaging technique. The *dobutamine echocardiographic stress test* induces pharmacologic stress by the infusion of dobutamine, a synthetic amine that increases myocardial contractility. Dobutamine directly stimulates cardiac alpha$_1$- and beta$_1$-adrenergic receptors thereby increasing oxygen demand. When this occurs in the presence of an impaired oxygen supply, echocardiography can directly visualize myocardial wall motion abnormalities in individuals with fixed coronary artery stenosis. The *adenosine pharmacologic stress test* is a potent vasodilator that mimics the effect of exercise on the heart. Use of adenosine is preferred over dobutamine due to adenosine's short duration of action and the fact that reversal agents are not needed.

Professional Considerations
1. Consent form IS required.

Risks of Dobutamine Infusion
Cardiac ischemia, including myocardial infarction and dysrhythmias, dizziness, flushing, hypotension, hypertension, and palpitations.

Contraindications for Adenosine
Active bronchospasm, asthma history, atrioventricular block (high-degree).

Drugs include methylxanthines such as theophylline, aminophylline, caffeine or cafergot, and oral dipyridamole.

Contraindications for Dobutamine
Tachyarrhythmias (atrial, ventricular). Drugs include beta blockers.

2. **Preparation:**
   A. Have emergency equipment readily available.
   B. Establish intravenous access.
   C. See *Client and family teaching.*
3. **Procedure:**
   A. The stress test is performed by specially trained (that is, ACLS-certified) nurses and echocardiographers. The American Association of Cardiovascular and Pulmonary Rehabilitation has recommended direct physician supervision of all initial stress tests and tests for individuals considered at high risk for complications.
   B. Attach electrocardiogram leads and a blood pressure cuff.
   C. Obtain a baseline 12-lead ECG and blood pressure.
   D. The individual is placed in the best position to obtain echocardiographic images (usually left lateral decubitus), and baseline images are obtained.
   E. Dobutamine is diluted according to institutional policy and procedure and administered by means of an infusion pump at an initial rate of 5 mg/kg/minute.
   F. The infusion rate is increased every 3 minutes to 10, 20, and a maximum of 40 mg/kg/minute unless end points develop.
   G. Heart rate and ECG rhythm strip are monitored continuously, and blood pressure and 12-lead ECG are recorded at each stage of drug infusion.
   H. Continuous echocardiography is also performed. Direct recordings of images are made at rest, at mid-infusion, at peak infusion, and at 1-2 minutes after infusion.
   I. The test is terminated when any of the following occurs:
      i. Signs of ischemia are present (ST-segment depression of <1-2 mm for a duration >0.06 second, or ST-segment elevation).
      ii. Heart rate >75-85% of predicted maximum for age.

iii. Development of new wall motion abnormality.
iv. Hypertension >210-260 mm Hg systolic blood pressure or diastolic blood pressure >100 mm Hg.
v. New dysrhythmias.
vi. Chest pain with or without ECG changes.
vii. Symptomatic hypotension or blood pressure decrease more than 20 mm Hg.
viii. Heart rate decrease more than 20 beats per minute.
ix. Prespecified dosage of dobutamine has been reached or target heart rate has been reached.
x. The client requests to terminate test.

4. **Postprocedure care:**
A. The client should be monitored until the heart rate, blood pressure, and electrocardiogram are at baseline value.
B. Remove the electrodes and the blood pressure cuff.

5. **Client and family teaching:**
A. The entire procedure lasts approximately 60 minutes.
B. According to physician preference and instructions, gradually discontinue beta-blocker drugs before the test. Antianginal agents may also be discontinued 24-48 hours before testing to maximize test sensitivity.
C. Fast from food and fluids and refrain from smoking and caffeine usage for 4 hours before the test.
D. Clients may take all their medications as usual.
E. The administration of dobutamine is associated with mild side effects such as chest tightness, dyspnea, flushing, nausea, headache, paresthesias, chills, anxiety, or palpitations. Individuals are instructed to immediately report any side effects they experience to the technician. Side effects generally subside quickly after the dobutamine is discontinued.
F. Do not take caffeine-containing foods, herbs, or drinks for 24 hours before the test. These include coffee, colas and chocolate.

6. **Factors that affect results:**
A. Chest wall deformities, emphysema, and severe obesity limit visualization of the heart with transthoracic probes.

7. **Other data:**
A. The half-life of dobutamine is 2 minutes.
B. Side effects may be treated with intravenous beta-adrenergic blockers.
C. Abnormalities of ventricular contraction detected by echocardiography precede ECG signs or symptoms of ischemia.
D. The adenosine or dipyridamole stress tests also induce pharmacologic cardiac stress that is examined through radionuclide (thallium, sestamibi) imaging. See also *Heart scan, Diagnostic.*
E. See also *Stress/exercise test, Diagnostic.*

STRIATIONAL AUTOANTIBODY, SPECIMEN

Norm. Negative, titer <60.

Positive. Autoimmune liver disorders, Lambert-Eaton myasthenic syndrome, myasthenia gravis, myopathic disorders, and small cell lung carcinoma. Recipients of D-penicillamine and bone marrow allographs may have positive titers.

Description. Striational autoantibodies are immunoglobulins that react to contractile elements of skeletal muscle. They are detected by enzyme-linked immunoassay or immunofluorescence microscopy. Striational autoantibodies are a valuable marker of myasthenia gravis in the adult and are associated with thymoma. Their prevalence increases with the age of onset of myasthenia gravis. They are rarely positive at ages under 20 years.

Professional Considerations
1. Consent form NOT required.
2. **Preparation:**
A. Tube: Red topped, red/gray topped, or gold topped.
B. Specimens MAY be drawn during hemodialysis.
3. **Procedure:**
A. Draw a 7-mL blood sample.
4. **Postprocedure care:**
A. None.
5. **Client and family teaching:**
A. Results are normally available in 1 week.
6. **Factors that affect results:**
A. None found.

7. **Other data:**
   A. Titer rarely positive in adolescence.

STUART-PROWER FACTOR, BLOOD
(see Factor X, Blood)

SUCROSE HEMOLYSIS TEST, DIAGNOSTIC

Norm. <5% hemolysis, or negative.

Usage. Screening for paroxysmal nocturnal hemoglobinuria (PNH).

Description. Paroxysmal nocturnal hemoglobinuria is an acquired anemia characterized by the production of abnormal hemopoietic cells, red blood cells with an abnormal sensitivity to complement, and erythrocyte hemolysis. Symptoms include leukopenia or thrombocytopenia as well as nocturnal hemoglobinuria, chronic anemia, and thrombosis. Symptom severity is related to the degree of red blood cell sensitivity to complement and varies from client to client. In this test, sucrose provides a medium of low ionic strength that promotes the binding of complement to red blood cells. Blood from clients with PNH demonstrates the results of excessive lysis.

Professional Considerations
1. Consent form NOT required.
2. **Preparation:**
   A. Tube: Blue topped.
   B. Specimens should NOT be drawn during hemodialysis.
3. **Procedure:**
   A. Draw a 5-mL blood sample.
   B. Mix the washed red blood cells with ABO-compatible normal serum and 10% isotonic sucrose.
   C. Incubate the tube 30 minutes at room temperature.
   D. Centrifuge the tube.
   E. Read the percentage of hemolysis that results.
4. **Postprocedure care:**
   A. None.
5. **Client and family teaching:**
   A. Results are normally available within 2 hours of the test.

6. **Factors that affect results:**
   A. Hemolysis or clotting of the specimen invalidates the results.
   B. False-positive results occur with megaloblastic anemia, autoimmune hemolytic anemias, dyserythropoietic anemia, lymphoma, adenocarcinoma of the colon, eosinophilia, renal failure, or bronchogenic carcinoma.
   C. False-negative results may occur in clients who have received recent blood transfusions or if the specimen has been collected in a lavender-topped tube containing EDTA or a green-topped tube containing heparin.
7. **Other data:**
   A. Recent advances in the diagnosis of PNH include direct identification of affected cells by flow cytometry, detection of impaired synthesis of GPI anchor, and cytogenic analysis of the abnormal expression of the PIG-A gene.

SUDAN BLACK B STAIN, DIAGNOSTIC

Norm. Lymphocytes do not stain; granulocytes do stain.

Usage. Differentiation of acute leukemias; lipid and phospholipid staining.

Description. The microscopic examination of a sample of bone marrow or blood stained with Sudan black stain, a fat-soluble dye. This stain differentiates acute granulocytic leukemia (which accepts the stain) from acute lymphocytic leukemia (which does not accept the stain).

Professional Considerations
1. Consent form NOT required.
2. **Preparation:**
   A. Obtain a bone marrow biopsy tray or a red-topped tube.
   B. Blood samples MAY be drawn during hemodialysis.
3. **Procedure:**
   A. After a bone marrow biopsy or venipuncture, place the aspirate or blood on a slide.
   B. Place the Sudan black stain on the slide and examine it under a microscope.

4. Postprocedure care:
   A. Apply a pressure bandage to the bone marrow aspiration site.
5. Client and family teaching:
   A. Bone marrow aspiration is painful but only briefly. The client may receive premedication and an analgesic to ease the pain.
   B. The bone marrow aspiration site may be sore and bruised for several days after the biopsy.
6. Factors that affect results:
   A. Inadequate specimen amounts may produce inaccurate results.
7. Other data:
   A. Lymphocytes, plasma cells, and lymphoblasts, because they do not hold the Sudan black stain, are called "sudanophilic cells."
   B. Myeloblasts, though they do not stain with Wright's stain, may stain with Sudan black stain.

SUDS

(see Acquired immunodeficiency syndrome evaluation battery, Diagnostic)

SUGAR WATER TEST SCREEN, DIAGNOSTIC

(see Sucrose hemolysis test, Diagnostic)

SUPREME BG, DIAGNOSTIC

(see Glucose monitoring machines, Diagnostic)

SWAN-GANZ CATHETER PULMONARY WEDGE PRESSURE, DIAGNOSTIC

(see Pulmonary artery catheterization, Diagnostic)

SWEAT TEST, DIAGNOSTIC

(see Chloride, Sweat, Specimen)

SYNOVIAL FLUID ANALYSIS, SPECIMEN

(see Body fluid analysis, Specimen)

SYNOVIAL FLUID MUCIN TEST, DIAGNOSTIC

(see Mucin clot test, Specimen)

SYPHILIS, SERUM

(see Microhemagglutination Treponema pallidum (MHA-TP) test, Serum)

TAG 72

(see CA 72-4, Blood)

T- AND B-LYMPHOCYTE SUBSET ASSAY (LYMPHOCYTE [T & B] ASSAY, LYMPHOCYTE SUBSET TYPING, LYMPHOCYTE MARKER STUDIES), BLOOD

Norm:

T-cells	60-80% of total lymphocyte count
B-cells	5-15% of total lymphocyte count

T-CELL AND B-CELL LYMPHOCYTE SUBSET PERCENTAGES AND COUNTS				
	CD3+		CD19+	
AGE (YEARS)	% (MEDIAN)	COUNT × 10⁹/L	% (MEDIAN)	COUNT × 10⁹/L
18-39	57%-82% (70)	0.66-2.40	6%-26% (13)	0.09-0.57
40-69	57%-83% (71)	0.57-2.21	6%-27% (14)	0.08-0.50
70-79	47%-82% (65)	0.60-2.82	3%-31% (11)	0.06-0.79
80-89	47%-88% (67)	0.51-2.62	2%-26% (8)	0.04-0.57
≥90	40%-91% (67)	0.44-2.43	3%-24% (8)	0.03-0.58

Adapted from McNerlan et al. (1999).

T-CELL AND B-CELL LYMPHOCYTE SUBSET PERCENTAGES AND COUNTS—cont'd				
	CD3+ CD4+		**CD3+ CD8+**	
AGE (YEARS)	**% (MEDIAN)**	**COUNT × 10⁹/L**	**% (MEDIAN)**	**COUNT × 10⁹/L**
18-39	28%-57% (43)	0.34-1.70	16%-38% (24)	0.22-0.88
40-69	30%-60% (46)	0.34-1.54	12%-47% (26)	0.15-0.98
70-79	18%-53% (35)	0.28-1.77	11%-65% (25)	0.17-1.75
80-89	21%-60% (40)	0.31-1.48	8%-70% (25)	0.11-1.73
≥90	16%-63% (39)	0.26-1.44	9%-57% (24)	0.10-1.34

Adapted from McNerlan et al. (1999).

Usage. Acquired immunodeficiency syndrome, autoimmune diseases, DiGeorge syndrome, Graves disease, Hodgkin's disease, humoral immunodeficiency, leukemia, lymphoma, multiple myeloma, systemic lupus erythematosus, Waldenström's macroglobulinemia, and X-linked agammaglobulinemia.

Description. Quantification of T and B cells as a percentage of total peripheral blood lymphocytes to determine immunodeficiency states. Lymphocyte stem cells are produced in the bone marrow and released into the peripheral circulation. The tissue that traps the lymphocyte stem cells determine whether they mature into a T or B lymphocyte. T lymphocytes mature in the thymus gland or the precortical areas of lymph nodes and are responsible for cell-mediated immunity. B lymphocytes mature in the tonsils, spleen, germinating centers of the lymph nodes, and nodules of the intestinal tract and are responsible for antibody-mediated immunity. This test is performed by use of flow cytometry and monoclonal antibody technology.

Professional Considerations
1. Consent form NOT required.
2. Preparation:
   A. Tube: Two EDTA-anticoagulated, lavender-topped tubes.
   B. Do NOT draw specimens during hemodialysis.
3. Procedure:
   A. Draw two 7-mL blood samples.
4. Postprocedure care:
   A. Keep the specimens at room temperature and process them within 3 hours.
5. Client and family teaching:
   A. Explain the rationale for the test and explain the results, which should be available the same day.
6. Factors that affect results:
   A. Drugs that may increase lymphocytes include steroids and immunosuppressives.
   B. Refrigerating or freezing blood decreases lymphocyte counts.
   C. Some lymphocyte subset counts vary with age. See *Norms*.
7. Other data:
   A. Fresh tissue, bone marrow, and suspensions of lymph node or spleen can also be used for analysis.
   B. This test is also useful for monitoring clients on chemotherapy or immunosuppressive agents.
   C. CD4 is commonly used to monitor progression of and response to treatment of HIV infection.
   D. See also *Acquired immunodeficiency syndrome evaluation battery, Diagnostic*, when applicable.

T_3 OR T_4 THYROID TEST, BLOOD
(*see Thyroid test: Thyroxine, Blood, or Thyroid test: Triiodothyronine, Blood*)

T_3 RESIN UPTAKE TEST, DIAGNOSTIC
(*see Thyroid test: Thyroid hormone binding ratio, Blood*)

TA90 IMMUNE COMPLEX ASSAY (TA90 IC), SERUM

Norm. Negative or ≤1.

Usage. Identifies subclinical metastasis of early–stage malignant melanoma;

Helps predict the risk of recurrence of melanoma; Helps guide decisions about treatment after surgery. Significant predictor of survival for Stage II and III clients.

Description. Detects the presence of an immune complex of a 90-kDa tumor-associated antigen and its antibody, which are found in the sera of clients with malignant melanoma. When found in the sera of patients who have had removal of a malignant melanoma, this test has a sensitivity of 70% and specificity of 85% for predicting recurrence of the disease.

Professional Considerations
1. Consent form NOT required.
2. Preparation:
   A. Tube: Red topped, red/gray topped, or gold topped.
3. Procedure:
   A. Draw a 2-mL blood sample.
4. Postprocedure care:
   A. Write the collection time and date on the laboratory requisition.
5. Client and family teaching:
   A. Results are normally available within 2 days.
6. Factors that affect results:
   A. Reject specimens received more than 1 hour after collection.
7. Other data:
   A. None.

TANGENT SCREEN TEST, DIAGNOSTIC

Norm. Normal, no loss of visual field.

Usage. Detection and monitoring of central visual field loss.

Description. A screening test that measures central vision. It is often used in the diagnosis of optic neuritis. The test involves having the client indicate when an object moving across a visual field of concentric circles can be seen.

Professional Considerations
1. Consent form NOT required.
2. Preparation:
   A. The client should wear corrective lenses during the test.
3. Procedure:
   A. Have the client sit 1 meter from the target screen.

B. Occlude one eye and perform the tangent screen test.
C. Repeat the procedure with the other eye occluded.
4. Postprocedure care:
   A. If the test is positive, the client should be referred to a neuro-ophthalmologist.
5. Client and family teaching:
   A. The client should fixate on a central target.
   B. The examiner will move an object into the client's visual field at 30-degree intervals while he or she remains fixated on a central target.
   C. The client will signal when he or she sees the object come into view.
6. Factors that affect results:
   A. The client must be able to cooperate with signaling when the object enters his or her visual field.
   B. Central visual boundaries vary with object size, brightness, contrast background, pupil size, and the client's age.
7. Other data:
   A. Abnormal results warrant further examination with a perimeter to measure peripheral visual fields.

TARTRATE-RESISTANT ACID PHOSPHATASE (TRAP), BLOOD

Norm. Negative.

Positive (Leukocytes are not inhibited by L-tartrate): Hairy cell leukemia, lymphoma, mononucleosis, and prolymphocytic leukemia.

Description. Tartrate-resistant acid phosphatase (TRAP) is an enzyme produced by osteoclasts and contained in hairy cells. The presence of tartrate resistance to acid phosphatase is diagnostic for hairy cell leukemia (leukemic reticuloendotheliosis), a chronic form of leukemia characterized by distinctive cells called "hairy cells," which have many fine, cytoplasmic projections. Thus this test is used to help diagnose hairy cell leukemia and assess response to treatment and is a marker for the rate of bone resorption. Newer research has found that TRAP is produced by some osteoclasts, but the significance of this is not yet known.

Professional Considerations
1. Consent form NOT required.
2. Preparation:
   A. Obtain four glass microslides for smears and fixative (glutaraldehyde-acetone).
   B. Specimens MAY be drawn during hemodialysis.
3. Procedure:
   A. Draw a 2-mL blood sample in a heparinized syringe.
   B. Place two drops of blood on each of the four slides.
4. Postprocedure care:
   A. Spray fixative on the slides immediately.
5. Client and family teaching:
   A. Results are normally available in 1-2 days.
6. Factors that affect results:
   A. Rare false-negative results occur.
   B. Results should be interpreted with caution in jaundiced patients because hyperbilirubinemia skews the accuracy of the results.
   C. Abnormal erythrocyte or platelet levels will affect results.
7. Other data:
   A. Serum levels of acid phosphatase isoenzyme 5 may also be elevated in hairy cell leukemia.

TAU TEST (hTAU ANTIGEN), CSF

Norm. <200 pg/mL^{-1}.
Note: (Tapiola, 2001) used a cutoff of <380 pg/mL and found that the combination of the Tau Test and the Beta-*Amyloid Protein 40/42, CSF* test had a specificity of 95% to differentiate Alzheimer's disease from control subjects and 85% to differentiate Alzheimer's disease from those with other dementias.

Usage. Biologic marker for Alzheimer's disease; helps differentiate causes of cognitive impairment; evaluation of disease progression; evaluating response to treatment for Alzheimer's disease. This test is not used alone but is compared to the Ab42 test in determining consistency with a diagnosis of Alzheimer's disease. Increased levels of Tau with corresponding decreased levels of Ab42 in cerebral spinal fluid would consistent with Alzheimer's disease.

Description. While there are no definitive tests to diagnosis Alzheimer's disease, there some tests that may be used to assist in the complex diagnosis. Alzheimer's disease, the most common form of dementia, is characterized by the presence of senile plaques and neurofibrillary tangles containing abnormal masses of cytoplasmic proteins. The neurofibrillary tangles of Alzheimer's disease contain mainly the Tau protein in a (abnormal) hyperphosporylated state. Elevated levels of the abnormal Tau proteins can be detected in the cerebrospinal fluid in more than 90% of clients with Alzheimer's disease, even before the dementia symptoms appear. Levels also correlate with elevated Apolipoprotein E (see *Apolipoprotein E,4 genotyping, Plasma*), a known risk factor for Alzheimer's disease. This test is sometimes performed in conjunction with beta-amyloid protein 40/42 (see *Beta-amyloid protein 40/42, Specimen*), which is often decreased when the Tau test is elevated. There are 6 isoforms of the Tau protein, which can be detected by monoclonal antibodies. The AT8 monoclonal antibody is highly specific for the most common abnormal isoform of the Tau protein found in Alzheimer's disease and can detect its presence even before the neurofibrillary tangles appear. This test is an enzyme-linked immunosorbent assay using monoclonal antibodies for the detection of Tau proteins in cerebrospinal fluid (CSF).

Professional Considerations
1. Consent form IS required for the procedure used to obtain the specimen.

Risks
See *Lumbar puncture, Diagnostic.*

Contraindications
See *Lumbar puncture, Diagnostic.*

2. Preparation:
   A. See *Lumbar puncture, Diagnostic.*
   B. Obtain a sterile container for CSF.
3. Procedure:
   A. Collect a 1 mL sample of CSF during the lumbar puncture procedure.
4. Postprocedure care:
   A. See *Lumbar puncture, Diagnostic.*
5. Client and family teaching:
   A. See *Lumbar puncture, Diagnostic.*

6. Factors that affect results:
   A. Levels increase as the number of neurofibrillary tangles increase.
   B. The use of this test in the diagnosis of Alzheimer's disease must also be correlated to both physical and neurologic testing of the client being evaluated for diagnosis of dementia.
   C. Having one of these markers (Tau or beta-amyloid protein 40/42) be abnormal without a corresponding change in the other would help to rule out Alzheimer's disease.
7. Other data:
   A. The trade name of the monoclonal antibody test is INNOTEST hTAU Antigen, manufactured by Immunogenetics N.V.
   B. Tau antigen testing can be performed on nasal secretions to detect CSF leakage.

TB TEST, DIAGNOSTIC
(see Mantoux skin test, Diagnostic)

TBUT
(see Schirmer tearing eye test, Diagnostic)

TEAR BREAK-UP TIME
(see Schirmer tearing eye test, Diagnostic)

TEE
(see Transesophageal ultrasonography, Diagnostic)

TEICHOIC ACID ANTIBODY, BLOOD

Norm. Titer ≤1:2 or less than a fourfold rise in titer between acute and convalescent samples.

Increased. Endocarditis, infections caused by Staphylococcus aureus, osteomyelitis, and subacute bacterial endocarditis.

Description. Teichoic acid is a macromolecule present on the cell wall of gram-positive bacteria. Antibodies to teichoic acid can be seen in some infections, such as prolonged exposure to Staphylococcus endocarditis. Monitoring teichoic acid antibody levels may be helpful in assessing response to therapy in clients with gram-positive infections. Although sensitivity of all methods for measuring teichoic acid is low, the enzyme-linked immunosorbent assay (ELISA) method is the most sensitive.

Professional Considerations
1. Consent form NOT required.
2. Preparation:
   A. Tube: Red topped, red/gray topped, or gold topped.
   B. Specimens MAY be drawn during hemodialysis.
3. Procedure:
   A. Draw a 5-mL sample as soon as possible after symptoms appear or diagnosis is suspected, and label the tube as the acute sample.
   B. Repeat the test in 14 days, and label the tube as the convalescent sample.
   C. Serial testing may also be performed.
4. Postprocedure care:
   A. See Client and family teaching.
5. Client and family teaching:
   A. The client must return in 2 weeks for convalescent sample testing.
6. Factors that affect results:
   A. Technical variability.
7. Other data:
   A. The clinical significance of this test has not been fully established.

TELOMERASE ENZYME MARKER, BLOOD, SPUTUM OR URINE

Norm. Negative for the presence of active telomerase enzyme.

Usage. Early marker for detection of cancers.

Description. Approximately 80-90% of cancer cells have an active ribonucleoprotein telomerase enzyme preventing their telomeres (chromosome ends) from wearing out, and such prevention allows them to divide indefinitely. This is in contrast to noncancerous cells in which telomerase is repressed, causing the telomeres to shorten with each division. The detection of the active telomerase enzyme in a person's blood, sputum or urine can serve as an early marker for the presence of cancer. It is believed that if drugs can be developed that will selectively inactivate telomerase this may stop the growth or even destroy cancer cells.

Professional Considerations
1. Consent form NOT required.
2. **Preparation:**
   A. Tube: Gold topped. For urine study (used in evaluating bladder cancer), obtain a clean-catch container.
3. **Procedure:**
   A. Draw a 2-3 mL blood sample, or obtain a urine clean-catch specimen if urine sample is to be studied.
4. **Postprocedure care:**
   A. None
5. **Client and family teaching:**
   A. For urine collection, teach clean-catch technique.
6. **Factors that affect results:**
   A. None found.
7. **Other data:**
   A. None.

TEMAZEPAM
(see Benzodiazepines, Plasma and Urine)

TENSILON TEST, DIAGNOSTIC

Positive. Unequivocal improvement in a single weakened muscle.

Negative. Equivocal or no improvement in a weakened muscle. False-negative tests are fairly common, and repeated tests are of use.

Usage. Diagnosis of myasthenia gravis.

Description. Myasthenia gravis is an autoimmune neuromuscular disease characterized by fatigue of the limb, facial, bulbar, and ocular muscles with repetitive activity and by improvement with rest. Respiratory muscle fatigue can also occur. It is caused by circulating antibodies directed toward the skeletal muscle acetylcholine receptor. The factors that trigger the autoimmune response are unknown. In the Tensilon (edrophonium chloride) test, a short-acting anticholinesterase is administered intravenously, and muscle response is observed. The test is most useful if improvement in ptosis or the strength of an extraocular muscle is demonstrated because of the objective nature of this response. After intravenous administration of Tensilon, muscle strength will improve quickly in clients with myasthenia gravis.

Professional Considerations
1. Consent form NOT required.
2. **Preparation:**
   A. Assess for use of medications that affect muscle function, allergies, and respiratory disease.
   B. Establish intravenous access with a butterfly needle or an infusion of 5% dextrose in water or 0.9% saline.
   C. Obtain baseline vital signs.
   D. Have emergency respiratory support equipment and atropine available for use in the event of complications.
3. **Procedure:**
   A. Determine the muscle to observe for response.
   B. An initial test dose is administered because some people may be sensitive to Tensilon and may experience bradycardia or bronchospasm. These individuals should not receive additional Tensilon.
   C. Administer an initial dose of Tensilon intravenously as follows:
      i. Adults: 2 mg.
      ii. Children weighing >75 pounds: 2 mg.
      iii. Children weighing <75 pounds: 1 mg.
      iv. Infants: 0.5 mg.
   D. Muscle strength may improve within 45 seconds. If no improvement is noted, additional Tensilon should be infused as follows:
      i. Adults: up to 8 mg over 30 seconds.
      ii. Children weighing >75 pounds: up to 8 mg at a rate of 1 mg/30-45 seconds.
      iii. Children weighing <75 pounds: up to 5 mg at a rate of 1 mg/30-45 seconds.
      iv. Infants: Do not administer further Tensilon.
   E. Flush the IV access line between doses to ensure that the medication has infused.
   F. Be prepared for possible respiratory distress because Tensilon may stimulate a cholinergic crisis that causes extreme muscle weakness. If this occurs, up to 1 mg of intravenous atropine should be administered promptly.

G. Atropine may be administered during the test to clients with respiratory diseases, such as asthma, to minimize the side effects of Tensilon.

H. Once an unequivocal response is noted, the test is complete, and Tensilon administration should be stopped.

4. Postprocedure care:
   A. Monitor vital signs every 5 minutes × 4.

5. Client and family teaching:
   A. Instruct the client on the procedure and on the potential side effects of Tensilon.

6. Factors that affect results:
   A. Prednisone delays the effect of Tensilon.
   B. Quinidine and anticholinergics inhibit the action of Tensilon.
   C. Skeletal muscle relaxants may mask the effect of Tensilon.

7. Other data:
   A. The side effects of Tensilon include abdominal cramps, bradycardia, diaphoresis, diarrhea, hypotension, incontinence, pupillary constriction, respiratory distress, and salivation.

TERMINAL DEOXYNUCLEOTIDYLTRANSFERASE (TdT), BLOOD OR BONE MARROW

Norm:

	BLOOD	BONE MARROW
Adult	0-4 TdT U/10 cells or 0-0.67 pU/cell	0-5.7 TdT U/10 cells or 0-0.95 pU/cell
Child	0-3.5 TdT U/10 cells or 0-0.58 pU/cell	2.9-8.9 TdT U/10 cells or 0.48-1.49 pU/cell

Usage. Acute lymphoblastic leukemia, blast crisis, Hodgkin's disease, lymphoma, and myelogenous leukemia.

Description. Terminal deoxynucleotidyltransferase (TdT) is an intracellular protein that is a biochemical marker that aids in the diagnosis and classification of acute leukemias. It acts as a catalyst in the polymerization of deoxynucleotide triphosphates in the absence of a template. Approximately 1-5% of normal mononuclear cells express TdT in normal peripheral blood and bone marrow.

Professional Considerations

1. Consent form NOT required for blood sample. Consent form IS required for bone marrow aspiration. See *Bone marrow aspiration analysis, Specimen,* for procedural risks and contraindications.

2. Preparation:
   A. Contact the laboratory to determine if the test must be prescheduled.
   B. Tube: Lavender topped for blood sample. Container of formalin for bone marrow specimen.
   C. Blood specimens should NOT be drawn during hemodialysis.
   D. See *Bone marrow aspiration analysis, Specimen,* for bone marrow specimen.

3. Procedure:
   A. Draw a 10-mL blood sample.
   B. For bone marrow sample, see *Bone marrow aspiration analysis, Specimen.*

4. Postprocedure care:
   A. For bone marrow sample, see *Bone marrow aspiration analysis, Specimen.*

5. Client and family teaching:
   A. Results are normally available in 1-2 days.
   B. See *Bone marrow aspiration analysis, Specimen.*

6. Factors that affect results:
   A. Heparin in the blood tube may decrease the results.
   B. Insufficient bone marrow may produce indeterminate results

7. Other data:
   A. Some children with acute lymphoblastic leukemia have low TdT activity.
   B. TdT-positive leukemics that relapse can show a change in phenotype and can then be TdT-negative.

TESTOSTERONE, FREE (BIOAVAILABLE) AND TOTAL, BLOOD

Norm:

	MALE		FEMALE	
TOTAL TESTOSTERONE	ng/dL	SI UNITS nmol/L	ng/dL	SI UNITS nmol/L
Adult	300-1200	10.4-41.6	30-95	1.0-3.3
Prepubertal Values				
Cord blood	13-55	0.45-1.91	5-45	0.17-1.56
Premature infant	37-198	1.28-6.87	5-22	0.17-0.76
Newborn	75-400	2.6-13.9	20-64	0.69-2.22
1-5 months	1-177	0.03-6.14	1-5	0.03-0.17
6-11 months	2-7	0.07-0.24	2-5	0.07-0.17
12 months-5 years	2-25	0.07-0.87	2-10	0.07-0.35
6-9 years	3-30	0.10-1.04	2-20	0.07-0.69
Pubertal Values—Tanner Stage				
1	2-23	0.07-0.80	2-10	0.07-0.35
2	5-70	0.17-2.43	5-30	0.17-1.04
3	15-280	0.52-9.72	10-30	0.35-1.04
4	105-545	3.64-18.91	15-40	0.52-1.39
5	265-800	9.19-27.76	10-40	0.35-1.39

FREE TESTOSTERONE	pg/mL	SI UNITS (pmol/L)	PERCENTAGE OF TOTAL TESTOSTERONE
Male Values			
Adults	50-210	174-729	1.0-2.7
Children			
Cord blood	5-22	17.4-76.3	2.0-4.4
Newborn	1.5-31.0	5.2-107.5	0.9-1.7
4 weeks-3 months	3.3-8.0	11.5-62.5	0.4-0.8
3-5 months	0.7-14.0	2.4-48.6	0.4-1.1
5-7 months	0.4-4.8	1.4-16.6	0.4-1.0
6-9 years	0.1-3.2	0.3-11.1	0.9-1.7
10-11 years	0.6-5.7	2.1-19.8	1.0-1.9
12-14 years	1.4-156	4.9-541	1.3-3.0
15-17 years	80-159	278-552	1.8-2.7
Female Values			
Adults	1.0-8.5	3.5-29.5	0.5-1.8
Children			
Cord blood	4.0-16.0	13.9-55.5	2.0-3.9
Newborn	0.5-2.5	1.7-8.7	0.8-1.5
4 weeks-3 months	0.1-1.3	0.3-4.5	0.4-1.1
3-5 months	0.3-1.1	1.0-3.8	0.5-1.0
5-7 months	0.2-0.6	0.7-2.1	0.5-0.8
6-9 years	0.1-0.9	0.3-3.1	0.9-1.4
10-11 years	1.0-5.2	3.5-18.0	1.0-1.9
12-14 years	1.0-5.2	3.5-18.0	1.0-1.9
15-17 years	1.0-5.2	3.5-18.0	1.0-1.9

T

1038 TFI, DIAGNOSTIC

Increased Total Testosterone. Adrenal hyperplasia, adrenal tumor, arrhenoblastoma, central nervous system lesions, hirsutism (idiopathic), hyperthyroidism, ovarian tumor (virilizing), testicular feminization, testicular tumor, virilizing luteoma, and virilization. In women, idiopathic hirsutism, cystic ache, polycystic ovary syndrome, adrenogenic alopecia, abnormal menstruation, anovulation, adrenogenital syndrome with virilization, ovarian tumor, and Stein-Leventhal syndrome with virilization. Drugs include anticonvulsants, atrial natriuretic hormone (long-acting), barbiturates, cimetidine, clomiphene, estrogens, gonadotropin (males), kaliuretic hormone, oral contraceptives, and vessel dilator hormone.

Increased Free Testosterone. Androgen resistance, hirsutism, polycystic ovary syndrome, tumor (virilizing). See also *Increased total testosterone.*

Decreased Total Testosterone. Anemia, cirrhosis, cryptorchidism, Down syndrome, gynecomastia, hypogonadism (mate), hypopituitarism, impotence, Klinefelter syndrome, male climacteric, obesity, and orchiectomy. Drugs include androgens, cyproterone, dexamethasone, diethylstilbestrol, digoxin (males), digitalis, estrogens (males), ethyl alcohol (ethanol), glucose, glucocorticoids, gonadotropin-releasing hormone analogs, halothane, ketoconazole, metoprolol, metyrapone, phenothiazines, spironolactone, and tetracycline.

Decreased Free Testosterone. Hypogonadism, P-450$_{c17}$ enzyme deficiency. See also *Decreased total testosterone.*

Description. Testosterone is the dominant androgen found in the adrenal glands, brain, ovary, pituitary, skin, kidney, and testes. It circulates both freely and is bound to plasma proteins (sex hormone–binding globulin [SHBG]). Testosterone promotes the growth and development of the male sexual organs and increases body mass and hair replacement. This test measures total testosterone levels in clients with normal SHBG levels. *Free testosterone* is that portion of circulating testosterone that is not bound to the *sex hormone–binding globulin (SHBG) plasma protein.* Free testosterone is a better indicator of clinical status than total testosterone level

is. The Free Testosterone test is used to differentiate true abnormal testosterone levels from those caused by abnormally low or high amounts of circulating SHBG. Some conditions that increase SHBG are hyperthyroidism and low estrogen-production states (pregnancy; taking oral contraceptives or anticonvulsant drugs). Some conditions that decrease SHBG include excess androgen states, hypothyroidism, and obesity. Free testosterone may be measured directly, or calculated after total testosterone and SHBG levels are known.

Professional Considerations
1. Consent form NOT required.
2. **Preparation:**
   A. Tube: Green topped (plasma) or red topped, red/gray topped, or gold topped (serum).
   B. Specimens MAY be drawn during hemodialysis.
3. **Procedure:**
   A. Because of the diurnal pattern of testosterone secretion, several morning specimens or pooled specimens should be tested.
   B. Draw a 1.5-mL blood sample.
4. **Postprocedure care:**
   A. None.
5. **Client and family teaching:**
   A. Discuss the test results and the implications thereof with the physician.
   B. Results may not be available for several days.
6. **Factors that affect results:**
   A. In adult men, serum testosterone levels peak in the early morning and after exercise and decrease after glucose loading and immobilization. Because of this diurnal rhythm of circulating testosterone levels, the blood is generally drawn in the morning.
   B. Results are invalidated if the client has undergone a radioactive scan within the previous 7 days.
   C. During pregnancy, free testosterone values are lower because estradiol occupies space on the sex hormone–binding globulin sites.
7. **Other data:**
   A. None.

TFI, DIAGNOSTIC
(see Pulse volume recording of peripheral vasculature, Diagnostic)

THALLIUM, SERUM OR 24-HOUR URINE

Norm:

		SI UNITS
Serum	<10 ng/mL	<49 nmol/L
Urine		
Adult	<2 μg/L	<9.8 μmol/L
	or <10 μg/24 hours	
Panic level	>2 μg/L	>9.8 μmol/L

Panic Level Symptoms and Treatment

Symptoms. Abdominal pain, alopecia, ataxia, constipation, coma, delirium, diaphoresis, hypertension, intractable insomnia, optic neuritis, pulmonary edema, rash, tachycardia, and vomiting.

Treatment:
Note: Treatment choice(s) depend on client history and condition and episode history.
Give syrup of ipecac by nasogastric tube. Prussian blue (ferric ferrocyanide) is then given because it binds to thallium and prevents absorption in the gastrointestinal tract. The dose is 125 mg/kg in 50 mL of 15% mannitol twice daily by nasogastric tube. Continue this until excretion of thallium is <0.5 mg/day. Neither chelating agents nor hemodialysis seems beneficial. Hemoperfusion may be helpful.

Increased. Metal poisoning.

Description. Thallium is an extremely toxic heavy metal used in manufacturing and found in chlorinated chemicals, cosmetics, dyes, fireworks, jewelry, medications, pesticides, photoelectric cells, rat poison, and semiconductors. Thallium accumulates in the bone, kidney, liver, and muscle tissue. Thallium poisoning may cause blindness, liver damage, paralysis, paresthesia, peripheral neuropathy, and renal damage. This test helps identify clients who have acquired abnormal body amounts of thallium through ingestion or inhalation or through skin absorption.

Professional Considerations
1. Consent form NOT required.

2. **Preparation:**
   A. *Serum:*
      i. Tube: Metal-free green topped.
      ii. Specimens MAY be drawn during hemodialysis.
   B. *Urine:*
      i. Obtain a 3-L, metal-free urine collection container.
      ii. Provide a plastic, metal-free urinal or bedpan for specimen collection.
3. **Procedure:**
   A. *Serum:* Draw a 5-mL blood sample in a metal-free, green-topped tube.
   B. *Urine:*
      i. Collect all the urine voided in a 24-hour period in a plastic, metal-free bedpan or urinal.
      ii. The urine is mixed with 0.4% sodium bismuth in 20% nitric acid and 10% sodium iodine. If thallium is present, a red precipitate forms.
4. **Postprocedure care:**
   A. Observe the client for symptoms of thallium poisoning.
5. **Client and family teaching:**
   A. For urine collection, urinate before defecating and avoid contaminating the specimen with stool or toilet tissue. If any urine is accidentally discarded, discard the entire specimen and restart the collection the next day.
   B. Blood and urine thallium levels tend to decrease rapidly after exposure.
6. **Factors that affect results:**
   A. Urine or blood allowed to come into contact with metal will falsely elevate results.
7. **Other data:**
   A. Poisoning occurs 1-10 days after exposure. A lethal dose is 1 g or 8-12 mg/kg.
   B. The urine of a client with thallium poisoning will also show proteinuria, increased red cells,

casts, eosinophils, lymphocytes, or polymorphonuclear leukocytes.

THALLIUM EXERCISE SCINTIGRAPHY, DIAGNOSTIC
(see Heart scan, Diagnostic)

THALLIUM-DIPYRIDAMOLE STRESS TEST AND SCAN
(see Heart scan, Diagnostic)

THALLIUM IMAGING, DIAGNOSTIC
(see Heart scan, Diagnostic)

THEOPHYLLINE (AMINOPHYLLINE), BLOOD

Norm. Note: Measurement should be a peak specimen, after steady state has been reached.

	PEAK	SI UNITS
Therapeutic	10-20 μg/mL	55-111 μmol/L
Toxic level	>25 μg/mL	>137 μmol/L
Panic level	>30 μg/mL	>165 μmol/L

Panic Level Symptoms and Treatment. 75% of persons with levels over 25 μg/mL have toxic symptoms.

Symptoms. Dysrhythmias, gastrointestinal bleeding, headache, hypotension, nausea, restlessness, seizures, syncope, tachycardia, and vomiting.

Treatment:

Note: Treatment choice(s) depend on client history and condition and episode history.
Maintain a patent airway.
Withhold theophylline.
Perform gastric lavage if it can be done within 6 hours of ingestion.
Induce vomiting with syrup of ipecac.
Give activated charcoal.
Provide hydration.
Give diazepam for convulsions.
Provide continuous ECG monitoring for dysrhythmias.
Monitor theophylline levels every 2 hours.
Monitor and treat electrolyte imbalance.
Administer charcoal hemoperfusion for severe overdose.
40% of theophylline may be removed by hemodialysis. A higher clearance rate can be achieved with hemoperfusion but is associated with more complications. Peritoneal dialysis will NOT remove theophylline.

Increased. Congestive heart failure, chronic obstructive pulmonary disease, liver dysfunction, and overdose. Drugs that may cause increased levels include allopurinol, cimetidine, ciprofloxacin, clindamycin, erythromycin, lincomycin, oral contraceptives, and probenecid.

Decreased. Smoking. Drugs that may cause decreased levels include barbiturates, carbamazepine, furosemide, isoniazid, nortriptyline, phenytoin, and rifampin. An herbal or natural remedy is St. John's wort (Hypericum perforatum).

Description. Theophylline is a methylxanthine drug that decreases breakdown of intracellular cyclic adenosine monophosphate (cAMP), which in turn stimulates dilatation of the smooth muscles of the bronchial airways and relaxation of the pulmonary blood vessels. However, this therapeutic effect does not occur until levels are at or near the top of the therapeutic range. At lower levels, theophylline exhibits anti-inflammatory properties, enabling the sparing of steroid medication. It is for the latter reason that there has been a return to use of intravenous theophylline for acute exacerbation of obstructive pulmonary disease. Theophylline is 60% plasma protein bound, with a half-life of 6-10 hours in adults and 2-5 hours in children (half-life is reduced 40% in cigarette smokers); 90% of theophylline is metabolized in the liver. Steady-state levels occur in 15-20 hours in adults and in 5-40 hours in children.

Professional Considerations
1. Consent form NOT required.
2. **Preparation:**
   A. Tube: Red topped, red/gray topped, or gold topped.
   B. The client should not ingest substances that contain xanthene for 12 hours before the test. The substances to avoid include chocolate, cocoa, coffee, cola, and tea.
   C. Do NOT draw specimens during hemodialysis.
3. **Procedure:**
   A. Draw a 3-mL PEAK blood sample. Obtain serial measurements at the same time each day.
4. **Postprocedure care:**
   A. Refrigerate the specimen. Do not freeze it.
5. **Client and family teaching:**
   A. Explain the significance of therapeutic drug levels and the periodic monitoring thereof.
   B. If activated charcoal was given for elevated levels, the client should

drink 4-6 glasses of water each day for 2 days to prevent constipation. The activated charcoal will cause stools to be black for a few days.
   C. For intentional overdose, refer client and family for crisis intervention.
   D. Referrals to appropriate rehabilitation centers and therapeutic community programs should be offered to all addicted clients who may be interested.
6. **Factors that affect results:**
   A. Peak levels with oral dosing occur 1-3 hours after uncoated or liquid preparations and 4-7 hours after enteric-coated or extended-release preparations.
   B. Ingestion of xanthines within 12 hours before the test may elevate levels.
7. **Other data:**
   A. A minor metabolite of theophylline is caffeine.

THIAMINE, SERUM
(see Vitamin B$_1$, Serum)

THIOCYANATE, BLOOD OR URINE

Norm:

		SI UNITS
Serum		
Nonsmokers	1-4 µg/mL	0.02-0.07 mmol/L
Smokers	3-12 µg/mL	0.05-0.21 mmol/L
Pediatric	≤0.1 µg/mL	≤0.02 mmol/L
Nitroprusside therapy	6-29 µg/mL	0.10-0.51 mmol/L
Panic level	>35 µg/mL	>0.63 mmol/L
Urine		
Nonsmokers	1-4 mg/24 hours	
Smokers	7-17 mg/24 hours	
Panic levels	>0.2 mg/dL	>0.03 mmol/L

Poisoning Symptoms and Treatment

Symptoms. Agitation, confusion, focal brain damage, hyperreflexia, hypotension, metabolic acidosis, myocardial damage, psychotic behavior, thrombophlebitis, and thyroid enlargement.

Treatment:
Note: Treatment choice(s) depend on client history and condition and episode history.

Perform gastric lavage.
Administer intravenous fluids at 3 L/day (if normal renal function is present) to maintain adequate output.
Monitor amyl nitrate inhalation.
Give sodium nitrite and sodium thiosulfate infusions.
Both hemodialysis and peritoneal dialysis WILL remove thiocyanate.
Increased. Poisoning from nitroprusside; smoking.

Description. Thiocyanate is a major metabolite of the drug nitroprusside and is the important gauge of nitroprusside-induced toxicity during prolonged administration or with unusually high rates of infusion (see also *Cyanide, Blood*, which has a more important role in early toxicity of nitroprusside). Both sodium and potassium thiocyanate depress the metabolic activities of all cells but mostly those of the brain and heart. Half-life is 7 days. Formerly this drug was used to treat hypertension by producing peripheral vasodilatation. More recently this measure has been studied for detection of smoking deceivers in smoking-cessation programs.

Professional Considerations
1. Consent form NOT required.
2. Preparation:
   A. Tube: Red topped, red/gray topped, or gold topped.
   B. Obtain a sterile plastic container for urine sample.
   C. Do NOT draw specimens during hemodialysis.
3. Procedure:
   A. *Blood:* Draw a 2-mL blood sample.
   B. *Urine:* Obtain a 20-mL, fresh urine sample in a sterile plastic cup.
4. Postprocedure care:
   A. Tighten the top of the plastic urine container.
5. Client and family teaching:
   A. The treatment for poisoning will take at least 1 week.
   B. Death is possible from thiocyanate poisoning.
6. Factors that affect results:
   A. Eating cabbage or smoking cigarettes can falsely increase blood and urine results.
   B. Concurrent use of salicylates make results unreliable.
7. Other data:
   A. It takes 1 week to reduce thiocyanate by 50% if normal kidney function is present.
   B. Some clients show a temporary improvement for several days, only to relapse and die as long as 2 weeks later.

THIORIDAZINE
(see Phenothiazines, Blood)

THORACENTESIS, DIAGNOSTIC

Norm:

Amount	<20 mL
Color	Clear
Specific gravity	<1.016
pH	Equal to serum level
Protein	<3 g/dL
Fibrinogen	None
Cells	Few lymphocytes, few red blood cells
Lactate dehydrogenase	Equal to serum level
Glucose	Equal to serum level
Amylase	Equal to serum level

Usage

Therapeutic: relieves dyspnea because of pleural effusion.
Diagnostic: evaluates underlying cause of pleural effusion. Abnormal accumulation of fluid in the pleural space may be classified as either transudate or exudate.

	TRANSUDATE	EXUDATE
Color	Clear	Cloudy, turbid
Specific gravity	<1.016	>1.016
pH	Equal to serum level	<7.3
Protein	<3 g/dL	>3 g/dL
Fibrinogen	None or may be present	Present
Cells	Few lymphocytes	Many; may be a few red blood cells or purulent
Lactate	Equal to serum level	May be >lactate dehydrogenase, serum
Glucose	Equal to serum level	May be <serum
Amylase	Equal to serum level	May be >serum

Description. Thoracentesis is the removal of fluid or air from the pleural space by transthoracic aspiration. It is performed to determine the nature or cause of an effusion, to relieve dyspnea caused by an effusion, or to obtain fluid for testing.

Professional Considerations
1. Consent form IS required.

Risks
The risk of pneumothorax as a complication is small if the needle is withdrawn immediately. Also air embolism, bradycardia, hypertension, pulmonary edema.

Contraindications
Bleeding disorders or anticoagulated state, uncontrolled coughing.

2. Preparation:
   A. The procedure may be preceded by ultrasonography or chest radiography.
   B. Identify the upper border of the effusion by the loss of fremitus and the presence of flat percussion. The thoracentesis will be performed in the interspace below this level and 5-10 cm lateral to the spine.
   C. Obtain sterile gloves, injectable lidocaine, a thoracentesis tray, collection bottles with heparin, sterile 4 × 4-inch gauze pads, tape, a container of ice and povidone-iodine solution.
   D. Obtain baseline vital signs.
   E. List any recent antibiotic therapy on the laboratory requisition.
3. Procedure:
   A. The client is positioned sitting upright, often in the orthopneic position, with arms and head supported by a table at the bedside. Clients who cannot sit up are placed in the lateral decubitus position, lying on the side of the effusion, near the edge of the bed. This procedure can be performed on those who are ventilator dependent.
   B. The skin is cleansed with povidone-iodine solution.
   C. The underlying tissue at the previously identified effusion site is anesthetized.

D. A 20-gauge or larger needle is placed immediately above the superior aspect of the lower rib and advanced until the parietal membrane is penetrated and no more than 1 L of fluid is aspirated.
E. At least 50 mL of fluid is needed for diagnostic studies. Place syringe on ice for transport to the laboratory.
4. Postprocedure care:
   A. Apply a pressure dressing and assess the puncture site for bleeding and crepitus every 5 minutes × 6.
   B. Assess vital signs every 30 minutes × 4.
   C. A follow-up chest radiograph should be taken within several hours of the procedure, or immediately if respiratory distress is exhibited.
5. Client and family teaching:
   A. Describe the procedure and the usual sensations the client may expect related to the test.
   B. Do not cough, breathe deeply, or move during the procedure.
6. Factors that affect results:
   A. Complications that affect results include an air embolism, a hemothorax, a pneumothorax, and a pulmonary edema.
   B. Transudate in the pleural space may be caused by ascites, cirrhosis (hepatic), congestive heart failure, hypertension (pulmonary, systemic), nephritis, and nephrosis.
   C. Exudate in the pleural space may be caused by blocked lymphatic drainage, empyema, esophageal rupture, infarction (pulmonary), infection, neoplasm, pancreatitis, rheumatoid arthritis, systemic lupus erythematosus, thoracic duct disruption, accidental injury, and tuberculosis.
   D. Allowing fluid to stand for a prolonged period before processing may cause deterioration and artifacts.
7. Other data:
   A. If the thoracentesis is performed below the tenth intercostal space, care should be taken to avoid laceration of the spleen or liver or penetration of the diaphragm (ipsilateral shoulder pain is a sign of diaphragmatic penetration).

B. Malignant cells cannot be recovered from all fluids for clients with malignancies.

C. Increased amylase levels in the effusion are associated with pancreatitis, lung cancer, and esophageal perforation.

D. The most common pathogens found in pleural effusions are *Mycobacterium tuberculosis, Staphylococcus aureus, Streptococcus pneumoniae,* and *Haemophilus influenzae.*

THROAT CULTURE FOR *CANDIDA ALBICANS*, CULTURE

Norm. Negative, no growth.

Usage. Immunosuppressive diseases, stomatitis, and thrush.

Description. *Candida albicans* is an opportunistic fungus that occurs in the aged, debilitated, newborns, and clients with acquired immunodeficiency syndrome (AIDS) or cancer who are immunosuppressed. Steroid use is also a causative factor. This fungus occurs mostly on the buccal mucosa, tongue, palate, and mucous membranes. It appears as patches or plaques that are white to gray in color.

Professional Considerations
1. Consent form NOT required.
2. Preparation:
   A. Obtain a sterile cotton swab, a sterile container, and a tongue blade.
3. Procedure:
   A. Swab suspicious lesions and place the swab in a sterile container.
4. Postprocedure care:
   A. List the specific site of the specimen on the laboratory requisition.
   B. Deliver the swab to the laboratory immediately or refrigerate the sample immediately.
5. Client and family teaching:
   A. The turnaround time for results is normally 3-7 days.
6. Factors that affect results:
   A. Dry swab or insufficient specimen volume.
7. Other data:
   A. A Gram stain or potassium hydroxide (KOH) preparation

may be prescribed to obtain a more rapid diagnosis.

B. Other *Candida* species (*C. tropicalis, C. glabrata, C. kruei*) are being reported in individuals after lengthy imidazol or triazole antifungal therapy. These species are less susceptible to treatment.

THROAT CULTURE FOR *CORYNEBACTERIUM DIPHTHERIAE*, CULTURE

Norm. Negative.

Positive. Diphtheria.

Description. *Corynebacterium* is an anaerobic, gram-positive, non-acid fast, motile bacteria that does not produce endospores. *C. diphtheriae* liberates a cytotoxin that causes diphtheria, an acute infection of the oropharynx, larynx, nose, and other mucous membranes characterized by a patchy gray pseudomembrane over a lesion surrounded by reddened, inflamed tissue. The mode of transmission is usually direct contact with the discharges from lesions of an infected client. Culture of the throat is taken for incubation and study of the appearance and growth patterns of bacteria as well as the microscopic appearance and staining properties to identify the presence or absence of *Corynebacterium*.

Professional Considerations
1. Consent form NOT required.
2. Preparation:
   A. See *Client and family teaching.*
   B. Obtain a tongue blade, sterile swab, and Culturette.
   C. Call the laboratory so that it can have on hand the special culture medium for *C. diphtheriae.*
3. Procedure:
   A. With the client's head tilted back and mouth opened, depress the tongue with the tongue blade. Have the client say "ah" to elevate the uvula and expose the infective lesions.
   B. Shine a light into the oropharynx to locate the characteristic gray lesions. Remove the patchy gray pseudomembrane by rubbing it firmly with a sterile swab.

C. Press a sterile Culturette swab firmly against the lesion for a few seconds. For asymptomatic clients, culture the tonsillar fossae, the posterior pharynx, and the retrouvular areas.

D. Remove the swab, taking care to avoid touching any area except the infected site.

4. Postprocedure care:
   A. Return the swab to the Culturette tube and crush the ampule of the medium.
   B. Transport the specimen to the laboratory immediately. The specimen should be refrigerated if it is not tested immediately.

5. Client and family teaching:
   A. Antiseptic gargles or mouthwashes before the procedure may prevent bacterial growth. Avoid using these products for 8 hours before the test.
   B. Erythromycin is used to treat this disease.
   C. If started on empiric therapy, you should continue taking the prescribed drug(s) unless and until the test results are found to be negative.
   D. Results are normally available within 4 days.

6. Factors that affect results:
   A. Obtain cultures before starting the client on antibiotics.

7. Other data:
   A. Diphtheria is communicable for up to 4 weeks from the appearance of the bacilli in the lesions.
   B. A positive throat culture may also indicate a carrier state.
   C. Cultures of the nose and the pseudomembrane are also helpful in making a positive diagnosis.
   D. Toxic strains of this disease have recently been found in Russia, and nontoxogenic strains have been isolated with increasing frequency in the United Kingdom, France, and Australia.
   E. Treatment includes beta-lactam and aminoglycoside antibiotics though 20% of strains are rifampin resistant.
   F. Low protection rate against diphtheria correlates with female gender and latest vaccination within 3 years of life.

THROAT CULTURE FOR GROUP A BETA-HEMOLYTIC STREPTOCOCCI, CULTURE

Norm. Negative, no growth.

Usage. Glomerulonephritis, pharyngitis, scarlet fever, strep throat, and tonsillitis.

Description. Group A beta-hemolytic streptococci is a bacteria usually introduced into the respiratory tract whose incubation period is 3-5 days. The onset of streptococcal sore throat is sudden, with frank chills, headache, malaise, fever, throat soreness, and exudative gray-white patches on the tonsils or pharynx.

Professional Considerations
1. Consent form NOT required.
2. Preparation:
   A. Obtain a sterile cotton swab or Culturette, and a tongue blade.
   B. Obtain the specimen before initiating antibiotic therapy.
3. Procedure:
   A. Depress the tongue and take a swab of the throat and pharynx (both tonsils). Avoid swabbing the tongue, saliva, buccal mucosa, or the lips.
   B. Place the swab in a sterile container, or return the swab to the Culturette tube and crush the distal end to release the ampule of medium.
4. Postprocedure care:
   A. Send the specimen to the laboratory within 2 hours or refrigerate the specimen.
5. Client and family teaching:
   A. It is important to obtain the specimen before beginning antibiotics. Strep throat remains contagious until 24 hours after antibiotic therapy is started.
   B. If there is no improvement within 2 days, return to the health professional for further examination.
   C. Place a cool mist humidifier in the bedroom to relieve any tight, dry feeling in the throat. A sore throat may be relieved with salt water gargle (1 cup of warm water + 1 teaspoon of salt).
   D. For a schoolchild with positive culture, wait 24 hours after antibiotics have been started

before letting the child return to school.

E. Call the physician if developing a rash or coughing up green, yellow, or bloody sputum.

6. **Factors that affect results:**
   A. Technical proficiency is required to avoid false-positive and false-negative results.
   B. Previous antibiotic therapy may cause false-negative results. Up to 10% of clients who deny the use of antibiotics have been shown to have taken unprescribed antibiotics before contact with the health professional.
   C. The use of antibacterial gargles may cause false-negative results.

7. **Other data:**
   A. For a faster diagnosis, the swab can be incubated for 2 hours and then examined for fluorescent organisms; a rapid strep test for direct antigen detection can obtain results in 7-20 minutes (the highest sensitivity with high colony counts); however, results should be confirmed with a throat culture.
   B. Left untreated, symptoms usually subside within 3-5 days. Treatment will not shorten this time frame, but will reduce the risk of future rheumatic fever. Penicillin is the treatment of choice, but erythromycin and clindamycin are also effective.

THROAT CULTURE FOR *NEISSERIA GONORRHOEAE*, CULTURE

Norm. Negative; no *Neisseria gonorrhoeae* isolated.

Usage. Gonococcal infection of pharynx, gonorrhea, and pharyngitis.

Description. *N. gonorrhoeae* is a pyogenic, gram-negative, oxidase-positive cocci that is an obligate parasite of humans. It is the causative organism of the sexually transmitted infection gonorrhea. *N. gonorrhoeae* inhabits the mucous membranes of the genital tract and may also be found in the oral mucosa of clients who engage in oral sex (gonococcal pharyngitis). Left

untreated, gonorrhea leads to skin lesions, arthritis, meningitis, and reproductive problems.

Professional Considerations
1. Consent form NOT required.
2. **Preparation:**
   A. Obtain a Thayer-Martin culture medium, sterile cotton swabs, and a tongue blade.
3. **Procedure:**
   A. Depress the tongue and swab from the tonsilar regions and the posterior pharynx.
   B. Place the specimen immediately onto the Thayer-Martin medium and incubate it in a carbon dioxide environment.
4. **Postprocedure care:**
   A. Transport the specimen to the laboratory within 2 hours.
5. **Client and family teaching:**
   A. Gonorrhea infection is treatable with antibiotics.
   B. Evaluate the client's knowledge of safe sex practices and review appropriate measures.
   C. If the results are positive, provide the client with the appropriate information on sexually transmitted diseases.
      i. Notify all sexual partners from the previous 90 days to be tested for gonorrhea infection.
      ii. Do not have sexual relations until the physician confirms that the infection is gone.
6. **Factors that affect results:**
   A. Refrigerating the specimen invalidates the culture.
7. **Other data:**
   A. Preliminary reports are available within 24 hours and the final report within 48 hours.
   B. For a faster diagnosis, the swab can be incubated for 2 hours and then examined for fluorescent organisms.
   C. Penicillin is the treatment of choice (plus probenecid), but erythromycin and clindamycin are also effective.
   D. For positive results, the client should also be serologically tested for syphilis. Consider also testing for AIDS.
   E. Positive results must usually be reported to the local health department.

THROAT CULTURE, ROUTINE, CULTURE
(see Culture, Routine, Specimen)

THROAT CULTURE, SWAB, DIAGNOSTIC
(see Culture, Routine, Specimen)

THROMBIN TIME, SERUM

Norm:

Within 2 seconds of 9-second to 13-second control value; or
Within 5 seconds of 15-second to 20-second control value; or
<1.5 times control value.

Increased. Acute leukemia, afibrinogenemia, amyloidosis, cirrhosis, disseminated intravascular coagulation (DIC), dysfibrinogenemia, epistaxis, factor deficiency, fibrinopenia, lymphoma, obstetric complications, polycythemia vera, shock, and stress. Drugs include asparaginase, fibrin degradation products, heparin, streptokinase, tissue plasminogen activator (TPA), uremia, and urokinase.

Decreased. Thrombocytosis.

Description. Thrombin is an enzyme that functions in the release of fibrin from fibrinogen in the final stage of the clotting cascade. This test measures the clotting time of a sample of plasma to which thrombin has been added. Thrombin time is longer than normal when abnormalities in the conversion of fibrinogen into fibrin are present.

Professional Considerations
1. Consent form NOT required.
2. Preparation:
   A. Tube: 2.7-mL blue-topped or 4.5-mL blue-topped tube and a control tube, and a waste tube or syringe.
3. Procedure:
   A. Withdraw 2 mL of blood into a syringe or vacuum tube. Remove the syringe or tube, leaving the needle in place. (From a heparinized line, discard an amount equal to the volume of the tubing prime.) Attach a second syringe, and draw a blood sample volume of 2.4 mL for a 2.7-mL tube and 4.0 mL for a 4.5-mL tube.
   B. Gently tilt the tube five or six times to mix the sample.
4. Postprocedure care:
   A. Send the sample to the laboratory within 2 hours.
   B. Refrigerate the sample. The plasma should be frozen if it is not tested promptly.
5. Client and family teaching:
   A. Results can be available within an hour.
6. Factors that affect results:
   A. Hemolyzed specimens invalidate the results.
   B. Failure to discard the first 1-2 mL of blood may result in specimen contamination with tissue thromboplastin.
   C. Heparin therapy within 2 days before the test increases the results. Collecting a sample from a heparinized line without discarding the first blood withdrawn can falsely prolong results.
   D. A recent blood or plasma transfusion will invalidate the results.
7. Other data:
   A. The test is used as a rapid screening device to detect profound fibrinogen deficiency.
   B. This test is not reliable to monitor heparin therapy in clients with DIC.
   C. This test will NOT differentiate primary fibrinolysis from DIC.

THROMBOPLASTIN TIME, ACTIVATED PARTIAL, DIAGNOSTIC
(see Activated partial thromboplastin time and partial thromboplastin time, Plasma)

THYMIDYLATE SYNTHASE, SPECIMEN

Norm. Negative. *Note:* No definite norms have been established for this test.

Immunoreactivity Grades:

Grade 1	Negative to weakly positive
Grade 2	Moderately positive
Grade 3	Positive
Grade 4	Strongly positive

Usage. Evaluation of colorectal, gastric, cervical, and other epithelial cancers.

Description. Thymidylate synthase is an enzyme that acts as a catalyst in the thiamine DNA conversion. Cells that are producing DNA need larger amounts of thymidylate synthase to fuel the DNA production. In the cell cycle more thymidylate synthase (20% more) is produced during S and G2 phase because this is the phase when most the rapid cell proliferation takes place. In some cancers, such as those of the gastrointestinal tract such as gastric and rectal, thymidylate synthase is being studied as a possible tumor marker. Normal gastrointestinal tract cells are rapid proliferators, and tumors in these tissues can be very rapid in growth, elevating thymidylate synthase expression. Research is also being done to examine chemotherapeutics to block thymidylate synthase and therefore to promote a slowdown or to deny altogether tumor cell reproduction in some cancers. Immunohistochemical staining is used on a sample of tissue, and thymidylate synthase reactivity is observed and graded. This test involves staining specimens and identifying the amount of immunoreactivity in the specimen.

Professional Considerations
1. Consent form NOT required for this test but IS required for the procedure used to obtain the specimen.
2. Preparation:
   A. See *Biopsy, Site-specific, Specimen.*
3. Procedure:
   A. See *Biopsy, Site-specific, Specimen.*
4. Postprocedure care:
   A. See *Biopsy, Site-specific, Specimen.*
5. Client and family teaching:
   A. See *Biopsy, Site-specific, Specimen.*
6. Factors that affect results:
   A. None found.
7. Other data:
   A. Low reactivity is associated with better colorectal cancer and bladder cancer 5-year survival rates than high reactivity is.

THYROCALCITONIN, SERUM
(see Calcitonin, Plasma or Serum)

THYROID ANTIMICROSOMAL ANTIBODY, BLOOD
(see Thyroid peroxidase antibody, Blood)

THYROID ANTITHYROGLOBULIN ANTIBODY, SERUM

Norm. Negative, or titer <1:100.

Positive or Increased. Anemia (autoimmune hemolytic, pernicious), goiter (nontoxic nodular), granulomatous thyroiditis, Graves disease, Hashimoto's (chronic) thyroiditis, hyperthyroidism, hypothyroidism, myxedema, rheumatoid arthritis, Sjögren syndrome, systemic lupus erythematosus, thyroid cancer, and thyrotoxicosis. Drugs include lithium.

Description. Thyroid antiglobulin antibody is an autoantibody directed against the antigen thyroglobulin, a thyroid glycoprotein that functions in the synthesis of triiodothyronine (T_3) and thyroxine (T_4). This antibody may be present in inflammation of the thyroid gland or may be the cause of hypothyroidism secondary to thyroid-tissue destruction. The test is also helpful in identifying thyroid autoimmunity in clients who have other autoimmune diseases.

Professional Considerations
1. Consent form NOT required.
2. Preparation:
   A. Tube: Red topped, red/gray topped, or gold topped.
3. Procedure:
   A. Draw a 7-mL blood sample.
4. Postprocedure care:
   A. None.
5. Client and family teaching:
   A. Results are normally available within a few days.
6. Factors that affect results:
   A. Antibody may be present in a small number of clients with no disease symptoms.
7. Other data:
   A. The thyroid antimicrosomal antibody test should also be performed to eliminate other causes of thyroiditis.

THYROID ECHOGRAM
(see Thyroid ultrasonography, Diagnostic)

THYROID FUNCTION TESTS, BLOOD

Norm:

			SI UNITS
Free Thyroxine Index		**Mean**	
Puberty through adulthood	4.2-13.0	8.0	
Cord blood	6.0-13.2	9.8	
First 72 hours	9.9-17.5	13.9	
7 days	7.5-15.1	11.2	
4-52 weeks	5.0-13.0	8.4	
1-3 years	5.4-12.5	8.1	
3-10 years	5.7-12.8	8.2	
Thyroxine (T$_4$) Radioimmunoassay			
Adults	4.5-12.0 µg/dL		58.5-155 nmol/L
Pregnant >14 weeks	9.1-14.0 µg/dL		117-181 nmol/L
Elderly (>60 years)			
Female	5.5-10.5 µg/dL		71-135 nmol/L
Male	5.0-10.0 µg/dL		65-129 nmol/L
Children			
Cord blood	7.4-13.0 µg/dL		95-168 nmol/L
First 72 hours	11.8-22.6 µg/dL		152-292 nmol/L
7-14 days	9.8-16.6 µg/dL		126-214 nmol/L
4-16 weeks	7.2-14.4 µg/dL		93-186 nmol/L
4-12 months	7.8-16.5 µg/dL		101-213 nmol/L
12 months-5 years	7.3-15.0 µg/dL		94-194 nmol/L
5-10 years	6.4-13.3 µg/dL		83-172 nmol/L
10-15 years	5.6-11.7 µg/dL		72-151 nmol/L
Triiodothyronine (T$_3$) Radioimmunoassay			
Adults	80-230 ng/dL		1.2-3.5 nmol/L
Children			
Cord blood	15-75 ng/dL		0.23-1.16 nmol/L
First 72 hours	32-216 ng/dL		0.49-3.33 nmol/L
7-14 days	Average 250 ng/dL		Average 3.85 nmol/L
2-4 weeks	160-240 ng/dL		2.46-3.70 nmol/L
4-16 weeks	117-209 ng/dL		1.80-3.22 nmol/L
16-52 weeks	110-280 ng/dL		1.70-4.31 nmol/L
1-5 years	105-269 ng/dL		1.62-4.14 nmol/L
5-10 years	94-241 ng/dL		1.45-3.71 nmol/L
10-15 years	83-213 ng/dL		1.28-3.28 nmol/L
Thyroid-Stimulating Hormone (TSH)			
Adults	0.4-4.7 µU/mL		0.4-4.7 mU/L
>60 years			
Female	2.0-16.8 µU/mL		2.0-16.8 mU/L
Male	2.0-7.3 µU/mL		2.0-7.3 mU/L
Newborn (1-3 days)	3.0-20.0 µU/mL		3.0-20.0 mU/L
Premature infant	0.5-29.0 µU/mL		0.5-29.0 mU/L

Usage. Work-up of suspected thyroid disorder and differentiation of primary thyroid disease from secondary causes and from abnormalities in thyroid-binding globulin levels.

Description. Thyroid function testing involves performing several measurements on one sample of blood. These tests have largely been replaced by the third-generation thyroid-stimulating hormone assay. Tests included are as follows: *Thyroid test: Free thyroxine index, Serum; Thyroid test: Thyroid-stimulating hormone, Blood and sensitive assay; Thyroid test: Thyroxine, Blood; and Thyroid test: Triiodothyronine, Blood.* See individual test listings for further description. Many clients are found to have subclinical thyroid disease as described below, which may or may not be treated. Subclinical hypothyroidism is more common than subclinical hyperthyroidism.

SUBCLINICAL THYROID DISEASE FINDINGS				
	IMAGING FINDINGS	SENSITIVE TSH	THYROXINE	TRIIODO-THYRONINE
Subclinical hyperthyroidism	Asymptomatic abnormalities	Suppressed	Normal	Normal
Subclinical hypothyroidism	Asymptomatic abnormalities	Mildly elevated	Normal	

CONDITIONS CAUSING CHANGES IN THYROID FUNCTION TESTS			
	Low Free T3 or Free T4	Normal Free T3 or Free T4	High Free T3 or Free T4
High TSH	**Endogenous Causes** Amyloid goiter Iodine organification defect Iodine transport abnormalities Reidel's thyroiditis Thyroglobulin synthetic defect Thyroid dysgenesis Thyroiditis (chronic autoimmune) Thyroiditis (transient, hypothyroid phase) TSH-receptor defects TSH-resistance TTF2 mutations	**Endogenous Causes** Pendred's syndrome Heterophile antibody Subclinical autoimmune hypothyroidism State of recovering from non-thyroid illness TSH receptor defects TSH-resistance	**Endogenous Causes** Anti-TPO antibodies Familial Dysalbuminaemic hyperthyroxinaemia Pituitary tumor that secretes TSH Psychiatric illness (acute) Thyroid hormone resistance
	Exogenous Causes Amiodarone therapy Lithium therapy Interferon therapy Interleukin therapy After radioiodine treatment After neck radiation therapy Iodine deficiency Iodine-excess goiter Post-thyroidectomy	**Exogenous Causes** Amiodarone therapy Cholestyramine therapy Intermittent T4 therapy Sertraline therapy	**Exogenous Causes** Amiodarone therapy Intermittent T4 Therapy
Normal TSH			Same as above

CONDITIONS CAUSING CHANGES IN THYROID FUNCTION TESTS

	Low Free T3 or Free T4	Normal Free T3 or Free T4	High Free T3 or Free T4
Low TSH	**Endogenous Causes** Congenital deficiency Hypothyroidism (secondary) Nonthyroidal illness TSH suppression secondary to recent treatment for hyperthyroidism	**Endogenous Causes** Hyperthyroidism (subclinical) Nonthyroidal illness	**Endogenous Causes** Activating germline TSH-receptor mutation Graves' disease Hydatidiform mole Hyperthyroidism (Primary) Iodine excess* Multinodular goiter Pregnancy-Thyrotoxicosis with hyperemesis gravidarum or familial gestational hyperthyroidism Presence of ectopic thyroid tissue* Thyroiditis (lymphocytic)* Thyroiditis (postpartum)* Thyroiditis (postviral)* Thyroiditis (transient)* Toxic nodule
		Exogenous Causes Thyroxine ingestion Dobutamine therapy Dopamine therapy Steroid therapy	**Exogenous Causes** Amiodarone therapy* Thyroxine ingestion*

*Accompanied by low radioiodine uptake.
Adapted from Dayan (2001).

Professional Considerations
1. Consent form NOT required.
2. **Preparation:**
   A. Tube: Red topped, red/gray topped, or gold topped.
3. **Procedure:**
   A. Completely fill the tube with venous blood.
4. **Postprocedure care:**
   A. None.
5. **Client and family teaching:**
   A. Results are normally available within a few days.
6. **Factors that affect results:**
   A. Results are invalidated if the client has undergone a radionuclide scan within 7 days before the test.
   B. Basbug et al, (1999) found that "moderate decreases in thyroid hormones with concomitant increases in TSH levels in maternal serum correlated with severity of preeclampsia or eclampsia and high levels of endothelin."
   C. Abnormal thyroid test findings often found in critically ill patients should be repeated after the critical nature of the condition is resolved.
   D. The production, circulation, and disposal of thyroid hormone are altered throughout the stages of pregnancy
   E. An herb or botanical that may interfere with success of thyroid replacement therapy is kelp, which contains iodine.
7. **Other data:**
   A. Many illness affect thyroid test values, but are not indicative of thyroid disease. For this reason, routine thyroid testing of hospitalized patients is not recommended.
   B. An herbal or natural remedy that interferes with thyroid medication is kelp.

THYROID HORMONE BINDING RATIO, BLOOD

Norm:

			SI UNITS
T$_3$ Uptake			
Adults >60 years	24-39%		24-39 Arb units
Female	22-32%		22-32 Arb units
Male	24-32%		24-32 Arb units
Neonates	25-37%		25-37 Arb units
Thyroid Hormone Binding Ratio			
Adults ≤50 Years	0.85-1.14		0.85-1.14 Arb units
Adults >50 Years			
Female	0.80-1.04		0.80-1.04 Arb units
Male	0.87-1.11		0.87-1.11 Arb units
Children			
Cord blood	0.75-1.05		0.75-1.05 Arb units
First 72 hours	0.90-1.40		0.90-1.40 Arb units
7-14 days	0.82-1.15		0.82-1.15 Arb units
4-16 weeks	0.75-1.05		0.75-1.05 Arb units
1-15 years	0.88-1.12		0.88-1.12 Arb units
Free Thyroxine Index		Mean	
Puberty Through Adulthood	4.2-13.0	8.0	
Infants and Children			
Cord blood	6.0-13.2	9.8	
First 72 hours	9.9-17.5	13.9	
7 days	7.5-15.1	11.2	
4-52 weeks	5.0-13.0	8.4	
1-3 years	5.4-12.5	8.1	
3-10 years	5.7-12.8	8.2	

"Arb" means "arbitrary."

Increased T$_3$ Uptake and THBR. Decreased TBG (from genetic deficiency or other causes), hyperandrogenic state, hyperthyroidism, hypoproteinemia, liver disease (severe), malnutrition, metastasis, nephrosis, nephrotic syndrome, protein loss, and thyrotoxicosis factitia. Drugs include adrenocorticotropic hormone, androgens, barbiturates, corticosteroids, glucocorticoids, furosemide, penicillin (large doses), phenylbutazone, phenytoins, salicylates (high doses), thyroid extract, and thyroxine.

Decreased T$_3$ Uptake and THBR. Cretinism, endocrine-secreting tumors, hepatitis (acute), hypothyroidism, increased TBG (from congenital excess or other causes), and pregnancy. Drugs include chlorpromazine, estrogens, heroin, lithium carbonate, methadone, oral contraceptives, perphenazine (long-term use), and propylthiouracil.

Description. This test measures the amount of unbound thyroid hormone binding sites on thyroxine-binding globulin (TBG), a major protein carrier of thyroid hormones. The measurement is obtained by measurement of the amount of radiolabeled T$_3$ bound by a T$_3$-binding resin (T$_3$ uptake) after all TBG-binding sites in a client's blood sample are saturated. The number of sites available is dependent on the amount of thyroxine (T$_4$) present because it is present in greater quantities than triiodothyronine (T$_3$) has a greater affinity for TBG than T$_3$ has. The greater the number of TBG-binding sites available, the lower will be the T$_3$

uptake by the resin. The greater the amount of T_4 present, the smaller will be the proportion of unbound TBG-binding sites, and the greater will be the T_3 uptake by the resin. T_3 uptake is used to calculate the thyroid hormone binding ratio (THBR) as follows:

$$THBR = \frac{(\% \ T_3 \ uptake)}{(Mean \ \% \ T_3 \ uptake \ of \ reference \ serum)}$$

THBR compared to T_4 level is useful in determining whether thyroid hormone changes are attributable to thyroid disease or to abnormalities in TBG. If the values show parallel changes, a problem in thyroid function is indicated. However, if the results show opposite changes, an abnormality in the amount of TBG is more likely. Use of these results in a further calculation provides an indirect measurement of free T_4 in the bloodstream by multiplication of the T_3 uptake by the client's T_4 level to obtain the free thyroxine index (FTI).

Professional Considerations
1. Consent form NOT required.
2. **Preparation:**
   A. Tube: Red topped, red/gray topped, or gold topped.
3. **Procedure:**
   A. Draw a 7-mL blood sample.
4. **Postprocedure care:**
   A. Refrigerate specimens until tested. Freeze specimens at −20° C if the test is not performed within 1 week after collection.
5. **Client and family teaching:**
   A. Results are normally available within 72 hours.
6. **Factors that affect results:**
   A. THBR results may be falsely increased in acidosis (severe) and atrial fibrillation.
   B. Drugs that cause falsely elevated results include dicumarol, heparin, phenytoin, and salicylates.
   C. Because thyroid hormone is bound to proteins, protein levels should be considered when interpreting the results.
7. **Other data:**
   A. "THBR" replaces nomenclature of "T_3 uptake."
   B. See also *Thyroid test: Thyroxine, Blood; Thyroid test: Triiodothyronine, Blood.*

THYROID PEROXIDASE (TPO, ANTIMICROSOMAL ANTIBODY, ANTITHYROID MICROSOMAL ANTIBODY) ANTIBODY, BLOOD

Norm. 0.0-2.0 IU/mL

Usage. Lends evidence for thyroid disease in clients with concomitant illnesses, which can affect other thyroid tests. Helps predict the progression of chronic thyroiditis.

Increased. Graves' disease, hypothyroidism (idiopathic), thyroiditis (Hashimoto's, postpartum). Others include anemia (pernicious), lupus erythematosus, rheumatoid arthritis, and Sjögren's syndrome.

Decreased. Not applicable.

Description. Thyroid peroxidase (TPO) is now known to be the thyroid microsomal antigen. TPO is a membrane-bound enzyme essential for the synthesis of thyroid hormones thyroxine (T_4) and triiodothyronine (T_3). Thyroid peroxidase autoantibodies are autoimmune antibodies that inhibit the synthesis of the thyroid hormones and can also cause cytotoxic cell changes. TPO antibodies are present in 90% of clients with autoimmune diseases of the thyroid. This test has replaced the *thyroid antimicrosomal antibody test* because it is a more sensitive indicator of thyroid cells' antimicrosomal component.

Professional Considerations
1. Consent form NOT required.
2. **Preparation:**
   A. Tube: red topped.
3. **Procedure:**
   A. Draw a 5-mL blood sample.
4. **Postprocedure care:**
   A. None.
5. **Client and family teaching:**
   A. None.
6. **Factors that affect results:**
   A. Reject hemolyzed or anticoagulated specimen.
7. **Other data:**
   A. TPO antibodies may be present in up to 10% of all clients and up to 30% of healthy elderly clients.
   B. One study found that women with TPO antibodies present during pregnancy had almost three times

the risk for postpartum depression as compared with the average pregnancy. Another supplementation with thyroxin during pregnancy had no impact on the incidence of postpartum depression.

THYROID PROFILE, BLOOD
(see Thyroid function tests, Blood)

THYROID SCAN, DIAGNOSTIC

Norm. Homogeneous uptake of radioactive tracer and normal size, shape, and position of the thyroid gland.

Usage. Differentiation of hyperfunctioning nodule and of thyroid tissue hyperplasia; of help in diagnosing thyroid cancer; evaluation of thyroid in client with history of irradiated head and neck; monitoring of the thyroid gland during therapy; used for clients with differentiated thyroid carcinoma to screen for recurrence or persistence.

Description. A thyroid scan is a nuclear medicine scan of the thyroid after injection of a radioactive tracer (^{123}I, ^{125}I, ^{131}I, or ^{99m}Tc) for the purpose of detecting areas of increased or decreased tracer uptake by thyroid and surrounding area tissue. Hyperfunctioning thyroid nodules, which are usually nonmalignant, cause areas of increased uptake, labeled as "hot nodules." "Cold nodules" are nodules that do not take up the tracer (that is, tissue is not functioning as normal thyroid tissue) and are more likely to be malignant. For detection of metastatic thyroid cancer, whole body scanning with ^{131}Iodine in conjunction with levothyroxine withdrawal or stimulation with recombinant human TSH is done.

Professional Considerations
1. Consent form NOT required.

Risks
Allergic reaction to tracer (itching, hives, rash, tight feeling in the throat, shortness of breath, anaphylaxis).

Contraindications
Previous allergy to iodine, shellfish, or radioactive tracer; pregnancy (because of the radioactive iodine crossing the blood-placental barrier); breast-feeding.

2. **Preparation:**
   A. See *Client and family teaching.*
   B. Have emergency equipment readily available.
   C. Jewelry and metal objects near the head or neck area should be removed before scanning.
3. **Procedure:**
   A. Oral radioactive tracer is administered 6 hours before scanning. Intravenous radioactive tracer is administered ½ hour before scanning.
   B. The client is positioned supine, with a pillow, rolled towel, or sponge beneath the shoulder blades, and the neck hyperextended.
   C. The thyroid gland is scanned with a gamma camera that moves over one or more sections of the thyroid gland.
   D. Scan takes ½ hour.
4. **Postprocedure care:**
   A. Resume previous diet 2 hours after oral radioactive tracer administration.
   B. Observe the client carefully for up to 60 minutes after the study for a possible (anaphylactic) reaction to the radionuclide.
   C. Rubber gloves should be worn by health care providers when discarding urine for 24 hours after the procedure. Wash the gloved hands with soap and water before removing the gloves. Wash the ungloved hands after the gloves are removed. An incontinent client requires special handling of any soiled linen or disposable pads. These should be placed in special storage for a few weeks before cleaning or discarding. Consult with your radiation safety officer for details.
5. **Client and family teaching:**
   A. Drugs that may be discontinued up to 21 days before the scan include anticoagulants, antihistamines, corticosteroids, cough syrup, radiopaque dyes (28-42 days), phenothiazines, salicylates, thyroxine (10 days), triiodothyronine (3 days), iodides, vitamins, and antithyroid medica-

tions such as propylthiouracil or methimazole (Tapazole) (3 days).

B. Foods that should not be ingested for 14-21 days before the test include shellfish and salt or salt substitutes containing iodine.

C. Fast from food and fluids for 4 hours before and 1 hour after if radioactive tracer will be administered orally.

D. There is no discomfort with this test.

E. Describe the procedure and expected sensations.

F. Meticulously wash your hands with soap and water after each void for 24 hours. The toilet should be flushed 2-3 times after each voiding.

6. **Factors that affect results:**

A. If a radioactive iodine tracer is used, uptake may be increased in clients on a diet with subnormal iodine levels or those on phenothiazine therapy.

B. Ingestion of drugs listed under *Client and family teaching* within 2-3 weeks before the test may cause decreased tracer uptake.

C. Gastroenteritis may interfere with absorption of orally administered radioactive tracer.

D. Receipt by the client of intrathecal or intravenous contrast material within 21 days before the scan invalidates the results.

7. **Other data:**

A. Health care professionals working in a nuclear medicine area must follow federal standards set by the Nuclear Regulatory Commission. These standards include precautions for handling the radioactive material and monitoring of potential radiation exposure.

B. Technetium half-life is 6 hours. Iodine-131 half-life is 8 days. Iodine-123 half-life is 13.3 hours.

THYROID ULTRASONOGRAPHY (THYROID ECHOGRAM, THYROID ULTRASONOGRAM), DIAGNOSTIC

Norm. Proper size, shape, and position of the thyroid gland. Negative for cyst or tumor. Thyroid tissue demonstrates an even mixture of medium-level echoes. Suspicious for malignancy: Hypoechogenicity, poorly defined irregular margins, and microcalcifications.

Usage. Differentiation between cyst and tumor not distinguishable by other studies, guidance for aspiration of thyroid cyst or suspected thyroid tumor, monitoring of thyroid nodules during pregnancy, and ongoing monitoring of size and density of thyroid during radioactive therapy; with color-flow Doppler, provides information about vascular flow and velocity.

Description. High-frequency B-mode sonography and color-power Doppler are used to evaluate the thyroid gland size, shape, and positions. Ultrasound creates an oscilloscopic picture from the echoes of high-frequency sound waves passing over the neck area (acoustic imaging). The time required for the ultrasonic beam to be reflected back to the transducer from differing densities of tissue is converted by a computer to an electrical impulse displayed on an oscilloscopic screen to create a three-dimensional picture of the thyroid gland. The differing tissue densities of cysts and tumors enable the ultrasonogram to be helpful in determining which is present. Cysts are clearly demarcated by smooth borders and do not demonstrate internal echoes. Adenoma appearances vary but usually demonstrate halo. Multinodular goiter may also demonstrate a halo. In thyroiditis, the gland appears enlarged, with a greater than normal amount of low-level echoes. Ultrasound is a cost-effective procedure for screening for thyroid cancer because thyroid tissue has a high echogenicity. Thyroid cancer is usually poorly defined, with low-level echoes and without a halo. Advantages of this test are that it is safe for use during pregnancy because it does not use radiation, it can visualize the entire area of the anterior neck, it can detect smaller nodules (2 mm) than can a nuclear scan, it can differentiate cysts from solid nodules (which a nuclear scan cannot), and it can improve the sensitivity of fine-needle aspiration biopsy.

Professional Considerations

1. Consent form NOT required.

2. **Preparation:**
  A. Remove any metallic objects or jewelry from the head and neck area
  B. Obtain ultrasonic gel.
3. **Procedure:**
  A. The client is positioned supine, with a towel roll, pillow, or sponge beneath the shoulder blades, and the neck hyperextended, with the head turned away from the side of the thyroid gland being scanned. This permits better transducer access to the area because the mandible is moved out of the scanning area.
  B. The neck area is covered with ultrasonic gel, and a lubricated transducer is passed slowly and firmly over the thyroid gland and neck at specific intervals. Each lobe of the thyroid gland is examined separately and completely, beginning with transverse scanning followed by longitudinal scanning. Finally the isthmus is scanned transversely.
  C. Photographs are taken of the oscilloscopic display.

D. The procedure takes less than 20 minutes.
4. **Postprocedure care:**
  A. Remove ultrasonic gel from the skin.
  B. If thyroid cyst aspiration is performed under ultrasonogram guidance, see separate test listing, *Needle aspiration, Diagnostic.*
5. **Client and family teaching:**
  A. The procedure is painless.
6. **Factors that affect results:**
  A. Thyroid volume is larger in males than in females, and varies with body surface area.
7. **Other data:**
  A. Ultrasound alone should not be relied on for diagnosis of malignant thyroid nodules. Aspiration biopsy cytologic examination is necessary to confirm or add to the diagnosis.

THYROID-STIMULATING HORMONE, BLOOD
(see Thyroid stimulating hormone, Sensitive assay, Blood)

THYROID-STIMULATING HORMONE, FILTER PAPER, BLOOD

Norm:

NEWBORN		SI UNITS
At birth, peak occurs up to	30 µU/mL	30 mU/L
3 days old	<20 µU/L	<20 mU/L
10 days old	<10 µU/mL	<10 mU/L

Usage. Newborn screening for congenital hypothyroidism. May also be used to follow children known to have congenital hypothyroidism. Must be interpreted in light of T$_4$ levels.

Description. See also *Thyroid test: Thyroid-stimulating hormone (TSH), Blood.* Thyroid screening is recommended for all newborns from birth to up to 4 weeks. With congenital hypothyroidism, TSH will be elevated. Test kits developed in the late 1980s are considered specific enough to use for screening purposes. Early detection of congenital hypothyroidism enables treatment and prevents complications, which include mental retardation and subnormal growth patterns.

Professional Considerations
1. Consent form NOT required.
2. **Preparation:**
  A. Obtain alcohol wipe, lancet, and TSH filter paper card.
  B. Prewarming the heel is not necessary.
3. **Procedure:**
  A. Cleanse the lateral curvature of the infant's heel with alcohol and allow it to dry.
  B. Puncture the lateral heel curvature with a lancet.
  C. Saturate a spot on the TSH filter paper card with heelstick blood.
  D. Allow the blood spot to dry before sending the sample to the lab.

4. **Postprocedure care:**
   A. Apply pressure to the puncture site until the bleeding stops. Let the site air-dry.
5. **Client and family teaching:**
   A. Results are normally available immediately.
6. **Factors that affect results:**
   A. The test must be repeated if the blood amount is not enough to completely saturate a spot on the card.
   B. Touching the filter paper or exposure to extremes of heat and light can cause errors in the results.
7. **Other data:**
   A. None.

THYROID-STIMULATING HORMONE, SENSITIVE ASSAY (SENSITIVE TSH ASSAY, SENSITIVE THYROTROPIN ASSAY), BLOOD

Norm:

		SI UNITS
Adults	0.4-4.2 µU/mL	0.4-4.2 mIU/L
Adults >80 years	0.4-10 µU/mL	0.4-10 mIU/L
Newborn by day 3	<20 µU/mL	<20 mU/mL
Diagnostic Values		
Borderline hyperthyroidism	0.1-0.29 µU/mL	0.1-0.29 mIU/L
Primary hyperthyroidism	<0.1 µU/mL	<0.1 mIU/L
Borderline hypothyroidism	5.1-7.0 µU/mL	5.1-7.0 mIU/L
Probable hypothyroidism	>7.0 µU/mL	>7.0 mU/L
Desired level when receiving thyroxine therapy	0.5-3.5 µU/mL	0.5-3.5 mU/L

Increased. Addison's disease (primary), anti-TSH antibodies, eclampsia, euthyroid goiter (with enzyme defect), fasting state, goiter (iodine-deficiency type), hyperpituitarism, hypothyroidism (primary), hypothermia, pituitary adenoma (that secretes thyrotropin), postoperatively (subtotal thyroidectomy), preeclampsia, psychiatric illness (acute), status after therapy with radioactive iodine, and thyroiditis. Drugs include amiodarone, benserazide, clomiphene, iopanoic acid, ipodate, lithium, methimazole, metoclopramide, morphine, propylthiouracil, radiographic dye, SSKI, and thyroid-releasing hormone.

Decreased. Hashimoto's thyroiditis, hyperthyroidism, hypothyroidism (secondary, tertiary) (sometimes), and organic brain syndrome. Drugs include ASA, heparin, ketoconazole, T_3, and TSH. Drugs that decrease TSH function include dopamine, glucocorticoids, and octreotide.

Description. Serum TSH assay is an ultrasensitive indicator that has largely replaced all the other tests used to screen for and diagnose hypothyroidism and monitor treatment. Third-generation TSH sensitive assay is considered to be the most appropriate initial test when thyroid disorder is suspected. If the assay is normal, further testing is not indicated. If the assay is abnormal, a T_4 assay should be prescribed. Clients are considered to have subclinical hypothyroidism if the sensitive thyrotropin level is elevated but the free thyroxine level is normal. Subclinical hyperthyroidism is diagnosed when serum thyrotropin level is low in association with normal free thyroxine and triiodothyronine levels. There is a two-step assay that uses monoclonal antibodies directed against TSH.

Professional Considerations
1. Consent form NOT required.
2. **Preparation:**
   A. Tube: Red topped, red/gray topped, or gold topped.
   B. MAY be drawn during hemodialysis.
3. **Procedure:**
   A. Draw a 1-mL blood sample.

4. **Postprocedure care:**
   A. None.
5. **Client and family teaching:**
   A. Results are normally available within 24 hours.
   B. Samples may be stored up to 4 days refrigerated, or at room temperature.
6. **Factors that affect results:**
   A. Levels are elevated temporarily when the client is recovering from illness, but they return to normal after recovery.
   B. Previous treatment with corticosteroid therapy may result in lower TSH levels while thyroid hormone levels are normal. Therefore thyroid hormones should also be measured in clients who have had previous corticosteroid therapy for chronic conditions such as rheumatoid arthritis.
   C. Because TSH levels are often low in early pregnancy, further testing for abnormal results should include free thyroid hormones and thyroid releasing hormone measurements
   D. The National Cholesterol Education Program found that ingestion of 90 mg of soy isoflavones per day resulted in a small, but insignificant increase in the TSH level in post-menopausal women.
   E. Conditions in which the results of this test should not be evaluated in isolation include recent treatment for thyrotoxicosis, disease of the pituitary gland including TSH-secreting tumor, non-thyroidal illness, and resistance to thyroid hormone. (Dayan, 2001)
7. **Other data:**
   A. Sensitive TSH measurement has been found to be accurate for detection of neonatal thyroid disease.
   B. Clients over 60 years of age with sensitive TSH $\leq$0.1 mIU/L are at risk for atrial fibrillation.
   C. The test takes several hours to complete.

THYROID STIMULATION BLOCKING ANTIBODY, BLOOD
(see Thyroid receptor antibody, Blood)

THYROID RECEPTOR ANTIBODY (TRab, THYROID-STIMULATING IMMUNOGLOBULINS, TSI), BLOOD

Norm. Negative.

ACTIVITY LEVELS OF TRAB SUB-TYPES	NORMAL	ELEVATED AND PREDOMINANT IN
Stimulating TRab	<130% basal activity	Autoimmune Graves' disease
Blocking TRab, TSBab	<10% inhibition	Autoimmune hypothyroidism
Binding TRab (TBII)	<10% inhibition	

Usage. Helps differentiate Graves'-disease from non-autoimmune hyperthyroid disorders. When a client with hyperthyroidism has a positive thyroglobulin antibody test, this test can confirm the diagnosis of Graves' disease.

Description. Thyroid receptor antibody, also called, "thyroid-stimulating immunoglobulin" is an autoimmune antibody that can be stimulatory, blocking or binding. Stimulating TRab stimulates cyclic adenosine monophosphate production, which in turn causes thyroxine (T_4) and triiodothyronine (T_3) release and subsequent symptoms of hyperthyroidism. Blocking TRab (thyroid stimulation blocking antibody, TSBab) prevents thyroid-stimulating hormone (TSH) from binding to its receptor sites, resulting in hypothyroidism. Binding TRab binds to or near the TSH receptor on thyroid cells, interfering with TSH activity at the TSH receptor site. Thus TRab can be present in several types of autoimmune thyroid diseases. The predominant type of TRab helps differentiate which type of disease is present.

Professional Considerations
1. Consent form NOT required.
2. Preparation:
   A. Tube: Red topped, red/gray topped, or gold topped.
3. Procedure:
   A. Draw a 7-mL blood sample.
4. Postprocedure care:
   A. Separate and freeze the serum.
5. Client and family teaching:
   A. Results are normally available within days.
6. Factors that affect results:
   A. Up to 4% of results may be false positive due the presence of TSH, T_4 and T_3 autoantibodies.

B. Levels may be elevated in autoimmune thyroiditis or nonspecific goiter.
C. Administration of radioactive iodine within 48 hours of this test may increase autoimmune antibodies.
D. Stimulating TRab also binds, and so can affect the binding TRab level.
7. Other data:
   A. Neonates born from mothers with high levels of thyroid-stimulating immunoglobulins are at risk for thyrotoxicosis due to transplacental passage of the immunoglobulins.

THYROID TEST: FREE THYROXINE INDEX (FT$_4$I, T$_7$), SERUM

Norm:

		MEAN
Puberty Through Adulthood	4.2-13.0	8.0
Infants and Children		
Cord blood	6.0-13.2	9.8
First 72 hours	9.9-17.5	13.9
7 days	7.5-15.1	11.2
4-52 weeks	5.0-13.0	8.4
1-3 years	5.4-12.5	8.1
3-10 years	5.7-12.8	8.2
T Uptake:	32.0-48.4%	

Increased. Dysalbuminemia, hyperthyroxinemia, hyperthyroidism, and psychiatric illness (acute). Drugs include amiodarone, furosemide, propranolol, radiographic dyes, and thyroxine.

Decreased. Anorexia nervosa, heparin, hypothyroidism, and illness (severe). Drugs include carbamazepine and diphenylhydantoin.

Description. Thyroxine (T_4) is a hormone produced in the thyroid gland from iodide and thyroglobulin in a multistep process. Less than 0.05% of thyroxine circulates freely and is thus biologically active. Biologically active T_4 stimulates the basal metabolic rate, including usage of carbohydrates and lipids, protein synthesis, bone calcium release, and vitamin metabolism. In infants, T_4 plays an important role in central nervous system growth and development. Circulating T_4 levels affect the release of thyroid-stimulating hormone (TSH) and hypothalamic thyroid-releasing hormone (TRH) through a negative-feedback mechanism. Because of the tiny quantity of free T_4 normally present, direct measurement is difficult and expensive. An alternative, the free thyroxine index (FT$_4$I), is derived from a calculation and provides an indirect measurement of free T_4 levels, based on total T_4 levels and thyroid uptake (T-uptake) expressed as the percentage of hormone unbound to the thyroid binding protein. T-uptake measures the binding sites that are saturated with thyroxine, and then is used in a calculation with the total serum T_4 level to determine the amount of thyroxine circulating freely in the blood. This is done in clients with conditions that can alter the number of thyroxine binding sites, which leads to misleading free T_4 values alone. The calculation is as follows:

$$FT_4I = \frac{\text{T-Uptake \%}}{T_4 \times \text{Mean TU\%}}$$

This calculation takes into account both the quantity of total T_4 and the availability of thyroxin-binding globulin binding sites.

Professional Considerations
1. Consent form NOT required.
2. **Preparation:**
   A. Tube: Red topped, red/gray topped, or gold topped.
3. **Procedure:**
   A. Draw a 5-mL blood sample.
4. **Postprocedure care:**
   A. None.
5. **Client and family teaching:**
   A. Results are normally available in 72 hours.

6. **Factors that affect results:**
   A. Results are invalidated if the client has undergone a radionuclide scan within 7 days before the test. Schedule any needed scans after the thyroid profile tests.
   B. During pregnancy, both T_4 and THBR are elevated, but the FT_4I is normal.
   C. The value may be normal in hypothyroid clients receiving phenytoin or salicylate therapy.
   D. The National Cholesterol Education Program found that ingestion of 56 mg of soy isoflavones per day resulted in a small, but insignificant increase in the free thyroxine index in postmenopausal women.
7. **Other data:**
   A. See also *Thyroid test: Thyroxine, Blood; Thyroid test: Thyroid hormone binding ratio, Blood.*
   B. Older methods calculated the FT_4I by multiplying total T_4 and T_3 uptake.
   C. An herbal or natural remedy that interferes with thyroid medication is kelp.

THYROID TEST: THYROXINE (T_4), BLOOD

Norm:

		SI UNITS
Radioimmunoassay		
Adults	5-12 µg/dL	65-155 nmol/L
Pregnant >14 weeks	9.1-14.0 µg/dL	117-181 nmol/L
Elderly >60 years		
Female	5.5-10.5 µg/dL	71-135 nmol/L
Male	5.0-10.0 µg/dL	65-129 nmol/L
Children		
Cord blood	7.4-13.0 µg/dL	95-168 nmol/L
First 72 hours	11.8-22.6 µg/dL	152-292 nmol/L
7-14 days	9.8-16.6 µg/dL	126-214 nmol/L
4-16 weeks	7.2-14.4 µg/dL	93-186 nmol/L
4-12 months	7.8-16.5 µg/dL	101-213 nmol/L
12 months-5 years	7.3-15.0 µg/dL	94-194 nmol/L
5-10 years	6.4-13.3 µg/dL	83-172 nmol/L
10-15 years	5.6-11.7 µg/dL	72-151 nmol/L
Whole Blood Newborn Screening (Filter Paper Method)		
Infants		
First 5 days	>7.5 µg/dL	>97 nmol/L
6 days	>6.5 µg/dL	>84 nmol/L
Panic Levels		
Thyroid storm possible	>20 µg/dL	>257 nmol/L
Myxedema possible	<2.0 µg/dL	<26 nmol/L

Panic Level Symptoms and Treatment

Thyroid Storm Symptoms. Hyperthermia, diaphoresis, vomiting, dehydration, and shock.

Thyroid Storm Treatment:
Note: Treatment choice(s) depend on client history and condition and episode history.
Supportive treatment for shock.
Fluid and electrolyte replacement for dehydration.
Antithyroid drugs (propylthiouracil and Lugol's solution).

Myxedema Symptoms. Hypothermia, hypotension, bradycardia, hypoventilation, CO_2 narcosis, lethargy, and coma.

Myxedema Treatment:
Support airway and blood pressure.
Monitor neurologic checks every hour.
Administer thyroid hormone (levothyroxine) intravenously.

Increased. Acute intermittent porphyria, cirrhosis (primary biliary), congenital excess of thyroxine-binding globulin, excess dietary iodine intake, familial dysalbuminemic hyperthyroxinemia, goiter (toxic multinodular, uninodular), Graves' disease, hyperemesis gravidarum, hyperthyroidism, liver disease (early stage), lymphoma, newborn infants, obesity, pregnancy, psychiatric disorder (acute), subacute thyroiditis (first stage), and thyrotoxicosis. Drugs include amiodarone (within the previous 4 months), amphetamines, Betadine, clofibrate, dextrothyroxine, dinoprost tromethamine, estrogens (within the previous 4 weeks), floraquin, furosemide, 5-fluorouracil, halothane, heparin, heroin, iodinated radiographic contrast dyes, iodinated vaginal suppositories (within the previous 4 weeks), iodothiouracil (within the previous several weeks), iopanoic acid, ipodate, levarterenol, levodopa, methadone, Metrecal, oral contraceptives, perphenazine (long-term use, occasional increase), phenylbutazone (first few days of therapy), progesterone, beta-blockers, thyroid extract (within the previous 6 weeks), thyroid-

releasing hormone, thyrotropin, thyroxine (within the previous 4 weeks), and Vioform (clioquinol).

Decreased. Acromegaly, cirrhosis, cretinism, eclampsia, exercise (strenuous), genetic deficiency of thyroxine-binding globulin, goiter (some), Hashimoto's thyroiditis (chronic thyroiditis), hypoproteinemia, hypothyroidism (primary, secondary), iodide deficiency (severe), liver disease (chronic), malnutrition, myxedema, nephrosis, nephrotic syndrome, pancreatic malabsorption, panhypopituitarism, postoperatively (caused by stress), preeclampsia, radioactive iodine therapy, Sheehan syndrome, Simmonds' disease, subacute thyroiditis (third stage), thyroidectomy, thyroid gland agenesis, and tumor (pituitary). Drugs include adrenal corticoids (within the previous 2 weeks), adrenocorticotropic hormone (within the previous 2 weeks), amiodarone (rare), androgens (within the previous 3 weeks), anabolic steroids, antithyroid drugs, asparaginase, barbiturates, carbamazepine, chlorpromazine, corticotropin, cortisone (long-term use), danazol, diphenylhydantoin, ethionamide, fenclofenac, furosemide (high doses), gold salts (within the previous several weeks), iodides, isoniazid (long-term use), isotretinoin, lithium carbonate, l-triiodothyronine (within the previous 4 weeks), methimazole (within the previous 7 days), oxyphenbutazone, penicillin, phenobarbital, phenytoin (within the previous 10 days), prednisone, propranolol, propylthiouracil (within the previous 7 days), reserpine, rifampicin, salicylates, somatotropin, SSKI (early in therapy), sulfonamides, and thiocyanate (within the previous 3 weeks).

Description. Thyroxine (T_4) is a hormone produced in the thyroid gland from iodide and thyroglobulin in a multistep process. Production occurs in response to the effects of pituitary thyroid-stimulating hormone (TSH) on the thyroid gland. T_4 is the major hormone synthesized by the gland and the hormone from which triiodothyronine (T_3) is derived. When released from the thyroid gland, almost all (99.96%) of T_4 is bound to protein (thyroxine-binding globulin, thyroxine-binding prealbumin, and albumin). The remainder of T_4

(0.04%) is called "free thyroxine" and is the only portion of this hormone that is biologically active. Biologically active T_4 stimulates the basal metabolic rate, including usage of carbohydrates and lipids, protein synthesis, bone calcium release, and vitamin metabolism. In infants, T_4 plays an important role in central nervous system growth and development. Circulating T_4 levels affect the release of TSH and hypothalamic thyroid-releasing hormone (TRH) through a negative-feedback mechanism. This test measures total T_4 (protein-bound and free).

Professional Considerations
1. Consent form NOT required.
2. Preparation:
   A. Tube: Red topped; or for whole blood newborn screening, obtain an alcohol wipe, a lancet, and filter paper for T_4 testing.
   B. The most accurate picture of T_4 levels is obtained when the client has been free of thyroid medications for 1 month.
   C. Newborn screening for hypothyroidism should be performed at least 72 hours after birth and after newborn has been taking feedings containing protein for at least 24 hours.
3. Procedure:
   A. Draw a 1-mL blood sample.
   B. Do NOT draw specimens during hemodialysis.
   C. Whole-blood newborn screening:
      i. Prewarming the heel is not necessary.
      ii. Cleanse the lateral curvature of the heel with an alcohol wipe, and allow the area to dry.
      iii. Puncture the lateral curvature of the heel with a lancet until free flow of blood is obtained.
      iv. Completely saturate all test circles on the filter paper with heelstick blood. The circles should be completely filled.
      v. Place the filter paper in a light-protected container for delivery to the laboratory.
      vi. Cord blood may also be used.
4. Postprocedure care:
   A. Let the heelstick site air-dry.
   B. Indicate pregnancy status on the laboratory requisition.
5. Client and family teaching:
   A. Results are normally available within 72 hours.
6. Factors that affect results:
   A. Results are invalidated if the client has undergone a radionuclide scan within 14 days before the test.
   B. Results are invalidated in hemolyzed or lipemic specimens.
   C. With the double-antibody testing method, results may be increased in the presence of antithyroxine antibodies.
   D. With the single-antibody testing method, results may be decreased in the presence of antithyroxine antibodies.
   E. Cord blood levels are lower in premature infants than in full-term infants.
   F. The following iodine contrast media may increase test results:
      i. *Cholecystography:* Telepaque within the previous 6 weeks; Orografin.
   G. Lukinác et al. (1996) found levels reduced after hemodialysis.
   H. The National Cholesterol Education Program found that ingestion of 56 mg of soy isoflavones per day resulted in a small, but insignificant increase in the thyroxine level in postmenopausal women.
7. Other data:
   A. Test results are usually evaluated in conjunction with free T_4 and TSH levels.
   B. An herbal or natural remedy that interferes with thyroid medication is kelp.

THYROID TEST: THYROXINE BY RIA, BLOOD
(*see Thyroid test: Thyroxine, Blood*)

THYROID TEST: THYROXINE FREE (FT₄), SERUM

Norm. Norms vary among newer test kits and should be compared with those from the manufacturer.

RADIOIMMUNOASSAY		SI UNITS
Adults	0.58 to 1.64 ng/dL	7.48-18.06 pmol/L
Premature Infants		
25 to 30 weeks	0.5-3.3 ng/dL	6.4-42.5 pmol/L
31 to 36 weeks	1.3-4.7 ng/dL	16.7-60.5 pmol/L
Full-Term Infants		
0-1 mo	0.8-2.2 ng/dL	10.32-28.38 pmol/L
1-6 mo	0.8-1.8 ng/dL	10.32-23.22 pmol/L
≥6 mo	0.8-1.6 ng/dL	10.32-20.64 pmol/L
1-12 yr	0.9-1.4 ng/dL	11.61-18.06 pmol/L
≥12 yr	0.8-1.5 ng/dL	10.32-19.35 pmol/L

Increased. Hyperthyroidism and psychiatric illness (acute). Drugs include amiodarone, heparin, propranolol, radiographic dyes, and thyroxine.

Decreased. Anorexia nervosa, hypothyroidism, illness (severe), and pregnancy. Drugs include carbamazepine, phenylbutazone (after the first few days of therapy), heparin, rifampicin, and thiocyanate.

Description. Thyroxine (T_4) is a hormone produced in the thyroid gland from iodide and thyroglobulin in a multistep process. Less than 0.05% of thyroxine circulates freely and is thus biologically active. Biologically active T_4 stimulates the basal metabolic rate, including usage of carbohydrates and lipids, protein synthesis, bone calcium release, and vitamin metabolism. In infants, T_4 plays an important role in central nervous system growth and development. Circulating T_4 levels affect the release of thyroid-stimulating hormone (TSH) and hypothalamic thyroid-releasing hormone (TRH) through a negative-feedback mechanism. Because of the tiny quantity of free T_4 normally present, direct measurement is difficult and expensive. Equilibrium dialysis is the common standard used for measuring free T_4. Radioimmunoassay is often used but is subject to the influence of the serum albumin and lipid levels. Newer testing kits are being developed to improve the accuracy and ease of direct measurement of free T_4.

Professional Considerations
1. Consent form NOT required.
2. **Preparation:**
   A. Tube: Red topped, red/gray topped, or gold topped.
   B. Do NOT draw specimens during hemodialysis.
3. **Procedure:**
   A. Draw a 1-mL blood sample.
4. **Postprocedure care:**
   A. The serum should be separated within 48 hours after collection.
5. **Client and family teaching:**
   A. Results are normally available within 72 hours.
6. **Factors that affect results:**
   A. RIA results are invalidated if the client has undergone a radionuclide scan within 14 days before the test.
   B. Value may be normal in hypothyroid clients receiving phenytoin or salicylate therapy.
   C. Lukinac et al. (1996) found levels reduced after hemodialysis.
   D. Because thyroxin is affected by protein binding, findings may be altered (lower) in pregnancy when hemodilution occurs.
7. **Other data:**
   A. van Wassenaer et al. (2002) found that "in untreated infants, low FT_4 values during the first 4 weeks after birth in infants born at <30 weeks' gestation are associated with worse neurodevelopmental outcome at 2 and 5 years. In T_4-treated infants, high FT_4 is not associated with worse outcome."

B. An herbal or natural remedy that interferes with thyroid medication is kelp.

C. See also *Thyroid test: Thyroxine, Blood; Thyroid test: Thyroid hormone binding ratio, Blood.*

THYROID TEST: TRIIODOTHYRONINE (T$_3$), BLOOD

Norm:

		SI UNITS
Adults	80-230 ng/dL	1.2-3.5 nmol/L
Children		
Cord blood	7.4-13.0 µg/dL	95-168 nmol/L
First 72 hours	32-216 ng/dL	0.49-3.33 nmol/L
7-14 days	Avg. 250 ng/dL	Avg. 3.85 nmol/L
2-4 weeks	160-240 ng/dL	2.46-3.70 nmol/L
4-16 weeks	117-209 ng/dL	1.80-3.22 nmol/L
16-52 weeks	110-280 ng/dL	1.70-4.31 nmol/L
1-5 years	105-269 ng/dL	1.62-4.14 nmol/L
5-10 years	94-241 ng/dL	1.45-3.71 nmol/L
10-15 years	83-213 ng/dL	1.28-3.28 nmol/L

Increased. Congenital excess of thyroxine-binding globulin, familial dysalbuminemic hyperthyroxinemia, fasting state, Graves' disease, high altitudes, hyperthyroidism, pregnancy, psychiatric illness (acute), and T$_3$ thyrotoxicosis. Drugs include amiodarone (rarely), antithyroid medications, dextrothyroxine, dinoprost tromethamine, estrogens, heroin, lithium, l-triiodothyronine, methadone, oral contraceptives, rifampicin, terbutaline, and thyroxine.

Decreased. Anorexia nervosa, eclampsia, elderly, genetic deficiency of thyroxine-binding globulin, goiter (caused by iodine deficiency), hepatic cirrhosis, iodine deficiency (severe), myxedema, obesity, postoperatively (caused by stress), preeclampsia, radioactive iodine therapy, renal failure, starvation, and thyroidectomy. Drugs include amiodarone, androgens, antithyroid drugs, asparaginase, cimetidine, dexamethasone, fenclofenac, fenoprofen, iodinated radiographic contrast dyes, iopanoic acid, ipodate, isotretinoin, lithium compounds, phenytoin, propranolol, propylthiouracil, radiographic dyes, salicylates, and valproic acid.

Description. Triiodothyronine (T$_3$) is a hormone produced primarily in peripheral tissues from conversion of thyroxine (T$_4$) but also is produced in small amounts by the thyroid gland; 99.96% of T$_3$ is bound to protein (thyroxine-binding globulin, thyroxine-binding prealbumin, and albumin); and the remainder is the biologically active form. About four times as much T$_3$ as T$_4$ circulates freely, partly because of its lower affinity for serum proteins. Additionally, T$_3$ has a shorter half-life than T$_4$. Biologically active T$_3$ stimulates the basal metabolic rate, including usage of carbohydrates and lipids, protein synthesis, bone calcium release, and vitamin metabolism. In infants, T$_3$ plays an important role in central nervous system growth and development. Circulating T$_3$ levels affect the release of thyroid-stimulating hormone (TSH) and hypothalamic thyroid-releasing hormone (TRH) through a negative-feedback mechanism. T$_3$ levels are used to confirm a diagnosis of hyperthyroidism when T$_4$ levels are borderline high and to help diagnose T$_3$ thyrotoxicosis. This test is a radioimmunoassay measurement of total T$_3$ levels.

Professional Considerations
1. Consent form NOT required.
2. **Preparation:**
   A. Tube: Red topped, red/gray topped, or gold topped.
   B. List the dose and administration time of any thyroid drugs on the laboratory requisition
   C. Do NOT draw specimens during hemodialysis.

3. **Procedure:**
   A. Draw a 1-mL blood sample. Cord blood may be used.
4. **Postprocedure care:**
   A. Indicate pregnancy status on the laboratory requisition.
5. **Client and family teaching:**
   A. Results are normally available within 72 hours.
6. **Factors that affect results:**
   A. Results are invalidated if the client has undergone a radionuclide scan within 14 days before the test.
   B. Results are invalidated in hemolyzed or lipemic specimens.
   C. With the double-antibody testing method, results may be increased in the presence of antithyroxine antibodies.
   D. With the single-antibody testing method, results may be decreased in the presence of antithyroxine antibodies.
   E. Lukinác et al. (1996) found levels reduced after hemodialysis.
7. **Other data:**
   A. Results are normally evaluated in conjunction with T_4 and TSH levels.

THYROID TEST: TRIIODOTHYRONINE BY RIA, BLOOD
(*see Thyroid test: Triiodothyronine, Blood*)

THYROXINE, BLOOD
(*see Thyroid test: Thyroxine, Blood*)

TILT TABLE TEST (HEAD-UP TILT TABLE TEST), DIAGNOSTIC

Norm. Negative or absence of hypotension or bradycardia with position changes.

Usage. Evaluation of recurrent idiopathic syncope once cardiac causes have been ruled out. Vasovagal syncope (also known as vasodepressor, neurodepressor, dysautonomia, or neurogenic syncope) is a sudden, short-term loss of consciousness caused by malfunction in the regulatory mechanisms between the nervous and cardiac systems.

Description. The head-upright table, by sudden assumption of an upright position, can produce passive orthostatic stress, which induces syncope in individuals affected by vasovagal syncope. Administration of an intravenous isoproterenol (Isuprel) infusion increases sensitivity of the tilt table test for those susceptible to vasovagal syncope by producing the elevation of circulating catecholamines associated with this type of event.

Professional Considerations
1. Consent form IS required.

Risks
Dizziness, dysrhythmias, hypotension, tachycardia.

Contraindications
Gradual loss of more than 500 mL of blood, hypertension, hypotension.

2. **Preparation:**
   A. See *Client and family teaching.*
   B. Start an IV at KO (keep-open) rate for administration of isoproterenol or emergency medication.
3. **Procedure:**
   A. The test can be run while the client is medicated or unmedicated.
   B. Baseline monitoring of heart rate (HR), rhythm (ECG), blood pressure (BP), with the client in a supine resting state every 5 minutes for 15-30 minutes.
   C. The table is then tilted up to 90 degrees for usually 5-7 minutes (up to 30 minutes). *Note:* Duration of the tilt has been found to be a more important variable than tilt angle. Duration of the tilt should be determined based on the suspected cause of the orthostatic intolerance: approximately 5 minutes to document orthostatic hypotension, approximately 10 minutes to identify orthostatic tachycardia, or neurally mediated syncope (Khurana et al. 1996).
   D. BP and HR are monitored and documented every minute for 25-45 minutes by automatic cuff or arterial line and ECG.
   E. The test is terminated, and the client is returned to the supine position when presyncopal

hypotension and bradycardia or full syncope develop.

F. Isoproterenol provocation may be added if no symptoms are produced during the unmedicated test.

   i. Return the client to the supine position for 5 to 10 minutes for the recovery period.

   ii. Isoproterenol may then be added as a single stage (1 µg/minute for 5 minutes) or as a multistage protocol (repeated 3 times with progressively increasing doses of 1, 2, and 3 µg/minute).

   iii. The table is tilted 60-80 degrees after each stage, and the test proceeds as previously described.

4. **Postprocedure care:**

A. Monitor the vital signs for 15 minutes.

B. Full return to consciousness and baseline BP and HR is usually rapid when the client is placed in the supine position.

C. Normal intake and activity can be resumed immediately after the test.

D. Occasionally temporary residual pallor, weakness, headache, and bradycardia (rarely) last up to 30 minutes.

5. **Client and family teaching:**

A. Any medication known to cause orthostatic hypotension or bradycardia should be stopped at least 3 days before the test. Your physician will tell you which drugs to stop.

B. Fast from food and fluids for 4-8 hours before the test.

C. Describe the procedure and the usual sensations the client can expect related to the tilt table test (see under *Procedure*). With the medicated test, mild stomach cramping, salty taste in the mouth, and minor vision changes are not unusual. Increased heart rate and light-headedness are common.

D. An IV line will be inserted before the test.

E. The goal of the test is to reproduce syncope or near-syncope in a carefully controlled environment in which the client will not fall.

F. Usual testing time takes 1-2 hours.

G. Normal diet and activity may be resumed after the test is complete.

H. If you develop chest pain after the procedure, call 911. Do not drive yourself to the hospital.

I. Call the doctor if you experience shortness of breath, a fainting spell, a severe headache or dizziness, or pain in your back.

6. **Factors that affect results:**

A. The positive effect of the isoproterenol-tilt table declines with age.

7. **Other data:**

A. Abrupt infusion of 5 g of isoproterenol may cause intolerable changes in HR and BP.

B. This test is up to 75% effective in reproducing vasovagal syncope.

TISSUE PATHOLOGY
(*see Histopathology, Specimen*)

TISSUE TYPING, BLOOD
(*see Human leukocyte antigen typing, Blood*)

T-LYMPHOCYTES, BLOOD

Norm:

	SI UNITS
500-2400/mm³ or 500-2400/µL	500-2400 cells × 10⁶/L
45%-85% of total lymphocytes	0.45-0.85 fraction of total lymphocytes
75%-80% of circulating lymphocytes	0.75-0.80 fraction of total circulating lymphocytes

Increased. Autoimmune disease, delayed hypersensitivity reactions, and Graves' disease. Herbal or natural remedies include *Astragalus mongholicus*, *Acanthopanax senticosus*, and *Panax ginseng*.

Decreased. Agammaglobulinemia (sex-linked, Swiss-type), AIDS, antibody to human T-cell lymphotropic virus, ataxia telangiectasia, chronic mucocutaneous candidiasis, Hodgkin's disease, immunosuppression, leukemia (chronic lymphocytic), lepromatous leprosy, lymphoma, Nezelof syndrome, systemic lupus erythematosus, thymic hypoplasia, transplant rejection, and Wiskott-Aldrich syndrome. Drugs include immunosuppressives and steroids.

Description. T lymphocytes are white blood cells with a long life span that are produced by and receive an antigenic imprint in the thymus gland. T lymphocytes are responsible for a cell-mediated type of immunity and control of the immune system response. Subsets of T lymphocytes secrete lymphokines such as interferon, chemotaxin, and macrophage migration–inhibition factor that function in cell-mediated immune response to varying antigens. Three of the T-lymphocyte subsets are "helper T cells" (OKT-4 cells), which help B cells produce certain antibodies; "suppressor T cells" (OKT-8 cells), which prevent unnecessary formation of antibodies; and "cytotoxic killer T cells," which have the ability to cause lysis of specific targeted cells such as those containing viral antigens. Overall,

T lymphocytes function in both good and bad ways. The T-cell characteristics that are beneficial by helping provide resistance to tumor and immunoresistance to bacterial and viral antigens can also harm the body via delayed hypersensitivity reactions, autoimmune responses, and rejection of transplanted tissue. This test is used to type and classify lymphocytic leukemias and lymphomas as well as define immunodeficient states such as AIDS. Identification of T lymphocytes is accomplished by the "rosette technique," in which sheep erythrocytes gather around T cells to form a rosette pattern.

Professional Considerations
1. Consent form NOT required.
2. **Preparation:**
   A. Tube: Heparinized green-topped tube.
   B. Do NOT draw specimens during hemodialysis.
3. **Procedure:**
   A. Draw a 5-mL blood sample.
4. **Postprocedure care:**
   A. Send specimens to the laboratory for processing within 2 hours.
5. **Client and family teaching:**
   A. Results are normally available within 24 hours.
6. **Factors that affect results:**
   A. Prolonged refrigeration decreases levels of helper T cells (OKT-4 cells).
7. **Other data:**
   A. See also *Acquired immunodeficiency syndrome evaluation battery, Diagnostic; T- and B-lymphocyte subset assay, Blood.*

TOBRAMYCIN, SERUM

Norm. Negative.

TOBRAMYCIN THERAPY		SI UNITS
Trough		
Therapeutic	0.5-2 µg/mL	1-4 µmol/L
Serious infection	0.5-1 µg/mL	1-2 µmol/L
Life-threatening infection	1-2 µg/mL	2-4 µmol/L
Peak		
Therapeutic	4-10 µg/mL	8-12 µmol/L
Serious infection	6-8 µg/mL	12-17 µmol/L
Life-threatening infection	8-10 µg/mL	17-21 µmol/L

Panic Level Symptoms and Treatment. Both sustained high peak and trough levels can be toxic.

Symptoms. Ototoxicity, nephrotoxicity, neuromuscular toxicity.

Treatment:
Note: Treatment choice(s) depend on client history and condition and episode history.
Hydrate to keep urine output ≥3 mL/kg/hour.
Hemodialysis may be helpful.
The use of activated charcoal has not been shown to increase elimination of tobramycin.

Usage. Monitoring for therapeutic and safe levels during tobramycin therapy.

Description. Tobramycin is an aminoglycoside antibiotic used to treat infections caused by certain gram-negative bacilli that are resistant to gentamicin. It causes misreading of the genetic code to prevent protein synthesis by the bacterial ribosome. Tobramycin is minimally metabolized, with most of it being excreted in the urine, with a half-life of 2 hours and peak levels reached within 30 minutes (IV doses) or 30-60 minutes (IM doses). Nephrotoxicity (probably reversible) and ototoxicity (probably irreversible) are possible at levels only slightly above the therapeutic peak and trough levels. Therefore it is very important to monitor tobramycin levels during its usage. Clients with any degree of preexisting renal failure are at higher risk for toxicity because of impaired ability to clear the drug from the body.

Professional Considerations
1. Consent form NOT required.
2. **Preparation:**
   A. Tube: Red topped, red/gray topped, or gold topped.
   B. Do NOT draw specimens during hemodialysis.
3. **Procedure:**
   A. Draw trough levels just before the dose. Draw peak levels 30 minutes after the last intravenous

dose or 30 minutes to 3 hours after the last intramuscular dose.
   B. Draw a 1-mL blood sample. Label the specimen as "trough" or "peak."
4. **Postprocedure care:**
   A. Record the collection time on the laboratory requisition.
5. **Client and family teaching:**
   A. The information is needed to make sure the safe and effective dose of tobramycin is being given.
   B. Drink 2-3 liters of water each day when taking tobramycin.
   C. Results are normally available within 4 hours.
6. **Factors that affect results:**
   A. In clients with normal renal function, 24-36 hours are required before steady-state levels are reached.
   B. Hyperlipidemia may cause falsely elevated results.
   C. Cross-reactivity may occur from clients cotreated with gentamicin or netilmicin.
   D. For aerosolized tobramycin delivery, use of a holding chamber results in greater delivery of the medication than use of a T-piece does.
7. **Other data:**
   A. Renal function (creatinine, beta$_2$-microglobulin, muramidase, albumin) and hearing should be monitored throughout therapy with tobramycin.
   B. A once-daily dosing regimen has been shown to be safe and effective for mother and fetus during pregnancy.
   C. An every-6-hour dosing regimen with a larger daily dosage administered has been shown in one study to provide better pulmonary function and longer time of wellness in clients with cystic fibrosis than an every-8-hour dosing regimen.
   D. Usual methods of continuous peritoneal dialysis (CAPD) result in relatively low drug clearance during any specific dialysate exchange, but cumulative drug removal may necessitate dosage supplementation with increased flow rates. Tobramycin added to

the peritoneal dialysate is absorbed into the bloodstream.

E. Aminoglycosides are inactivated when used concomitantly with antipseudomonal penicillins in the treatment of gram-negative infections in the client with renal failure.

TOLBUTAMIDE TOLERANCE TEST (TTT), DIAGNOSTIC

Norm:

RESPONSE TO TOLBUTAMINDE ADMINISTRATION			
Serum Glucose Level			Serum Insulin Level
30 Minutes G_{30}	90-120 Minutes G_{90-120}	180 Minutes G_{180}	
Normal 50% below baseline	80-100% of baseline	Baseline	Remains ≤150 µIU/mL
Abnormal	40-64% of baseline		Rapid serum insulin increase above baseline at 10, 20, and 30 minutes. >150 µIU/mL at 60 minutes
Fasting hypogly- cemia	<55 mg/dL (lean persons) <62 mg/dL (obese persons)		

Usage. Helps diagnose insuloma; Also used in the differential diagnose of types of hypoglycemia.

Description. There are primarily three types of hypoglycemia; one type that involves an insulin-secreting tumor of the pancreas known as "insulinoma," one that that is the result of hyperactive islet cells, and a third type that is result of liver disease. Insulinomas secrete disproportionately high levels of insulin in response to blood glucose levels, causing frequent hypoglycemic episodes. Insulinoma can be diagnosed through this indirect test that administers intravenous tolbutamide, a sulfonylurea, which stimulates the pancreas to produce insulin. When administered to a person with insulinoma, there is an exaggerated response, causing abnormally rapid and high insulin levels and abnormally prolonged hypoglycemic response.

Professional Considerations
1. Consent form IS required.

Risks
Acute hypoglycemic reaction.

Contraindications
In pediatric or pregnant clients or in clients with baseline glucose levels less than 60 mg/dL.

2. Preparation:
   A. Tubes: Red topped, red/gray topped, or gold topped. Also obtain ice for the blood sample for insulin measurement.
   B. Obtain baseline blood samples for glucose and insulin levels. Evaluate results before beginning tolbutamide infusion.
   C. Due to the risk of acute hypoglycemia during this test, have oral glucose/rapid-acting carbo-

hydrate and/or 50% dextrose in water available for emergency treatment.

D. Establish patent intravenous access.

3. Procedure:
   A. Draw a 3-mL baseline blood sample immediately before tolbutamide injection for glucose in a red-topped tube.
   B. Draw a 7-mL blood sample for insulin immediately before tolbutamide injection in a red topped, red/gray topped or gold topped tube. Place tube immediately on ice.
   C. Administer tolbutamide 1 g (or 25-40 mg/kg) IV push over 2-3 minutes.
   D. Client should rest comfortably over the next 2 hours while being monitored closely for signs of acute hypoglycemia.
   E. Draw serial glucose and insulin samples at 0, 2, 10, 20, 30, 60, 90, 120, 150, and 180 minutes after the tolbutamide infusion is completed.

4. Postprocedure care:
   A. Client should eat a meal containing rapid-acting carbohydrates.

5. Client and family teaching:
   A. Eat a high-carbohydrate meal for each of the three days before this test. Then fast after midnight the night before the test or for at least 8 hours, if the test is not done in the early morning.
   B. This test can take up to 3 hours.

6. Factors that affect results:
   A. Concurrent beta adrenergic blockers will diminish response to the test.
   B. Response to tolbutamide may be altered in clients taking MAO inhibitors, sulfonylureas (oxyphenbutazone, phenylbutazone), probenecid, and salicylates.

7. Other data:
   A. The treatment for the insulinoma is surgical removal, while the others can often be managed medically.

TOMOGRAPHY OF PARANASAL SINUSES, DIAGNOSTIC

Norm. Negative for foreign body, fracture, tumor or anatomic anomalies.

Usage. Adjunct to conventional radiography for clients with suspected fracture (status posttrauma), bony tumor invasion of the paranasal sinus area, or foreign-body introduction into the paranasal sinus area; evaluation of the extent and location of sinus disease; detection of anatomic abnormalities before surgery. Improves planning and safety of paranasal sinus surgery by providing a map of the area.

Description. Computed tomography (CT) of the paranasal sinuses is a radiographic scan that reconstructs an image of the paranasal sinus area based on differing densities and composition of the tissues. A detector records the intensity of the x rays from multiple angles as they are transmitted through the paranasal sinus area. A computer then reconstructs the differing intensities into pixels, which appear in differing shades for differing tissues and represent "slices" across the plane of the area. This test may provide additional information that standard radiography cannot because it can portray boundaries between tissues that are normally indistinguishable by traditional radiography. In particular, CT provides a sensitive display of the deep air passages and posterior ethmoid and sphenoid sinuses, which are difficult to reach by nasal endoscopy. By providing the landmarks necessary to recognize hazardous anatomy and pathologic conditions, tomography of the paranasal sinuses can increase the safety and efficacy of paranasal sinus surgery. This procedure also offers the advantage of superior visibility of the ethmoid sinus over plain films of the paranasal sinuses. See also *Computed tomography of the body, Diagnostic* for a further description of the types of CT technology available.

Professional Considerations
1. Consent form NOT required.

Risks
None.

Contraindications
Clients who are unable to lie motionless.

Precautions
During pregnancy, risks of cumulative radiation exposure to the fetus from this

and other previous or future imaging studies must be weighed against the benefits of the procedure. Although formal limits for client exposure are relative to this risk:benefit comparison, the United States Nuclear Regulatory Commission requires that the cumulative dose equivalent to an embryo/fetus from *occupational* exposure not exceed 0.5 rem (5 mSv). Radiation dosage to the fetus is proportional to the distance of the anatomy studied from the abdomen and decreases as pregnancy progresses. For pregnant clients, consult the radiologist/radiology department to obtain estimated fetal radiation exposure from this procedure

---

2. **Preparation:**
   A. Remove radiopaque objects such as jewelry, eyeglasses, or hairpins from the head area.
3. **Procedure:**
   A. The client is positioned supine, with the head secured in a hyperextended position on a headrest (coronal imaging) or prone, resting on chin with head hyperextended (axial imaging) on a motorized handling table.
   B. The client must lie motionless as the table slowly advances through the circular opening of the scanner. The CT scanner sends a narrow beam of x-rays across the area to be imaged in a linear fashion.
   C. Imaging in both axial and coronal planes is completed.
4. **Postprocedure care:**
   A. Replace radiopaque objects that were removed before the scan.
5. **Client and family teaching:**
   A. It is necessary to lie motionless during the scan. Because this can be a frightening test, it should be carefully described before the client enters the CT room.
6. **Factors that affect results:**
   A. Radiopaque objects left in place obscure visualization.
   B. Increase in size of the maxillary sinus is normal in aging but often not found in aging in persons with cystic fibrosis.
7. **Other data:**
   A. Further testing may include magnetic resonance imaging (MRI), which is more sensitive than CT for identification of neoplasm.

MRI is replacing CT of the paranasal sinuses as the study of choice for oropharyngeal and paranasal sinus lesions.
   B. Anatomic anomalies, such as paradoxical middle turbinates, are common findings in persons with chronic sinusitis.

TONOMETRY TEST FOR GLAUCOMA, DIAGNOSTIC

Norm:
10-22 mm Hg; mean 16 mm Hg with standard deviation of 3 mm Hg.
Warning: 22-28 mm Hg. More testing required.
Normal values of 21 or less can occur in a condition known as normal or low tension glaucoma.
Major concern: >38 mm Hg
Panic levels: There is lack of definitive intraocular pressure cutoff level for glaucoma.

Usage. Screening for glaucoma. Ongoing monitoring for clients with glaucoma.

Description. In glaucoma, intraocular pressure increases either because of blocked drainage or excessive production of aqueous humor. Tonometry testing involves measurement of intraocular pressure using a tonometer, an instrument that is lightly pressed directly against the anesthetized eye. The tonometry test can be conducted in any of three ways. In *contact tonometry*, in which the instrument touches the eye, the Schiøtz method, the Goldmann applanation method, commonly known as the "blue light" test or a handheld method with small penlike tonometer may be used. Contact tonometers make an indentation in the eye with a specific amount of weight and records the amount of resistance to the indentation, which is then converted to an intraocular pressure. In noncontact (indentation) tonometry, pneumotonometry or "air" tonometry may be used. Noncontact tonometry measures eye pressure indirectly. Noncontact has been found to improve compliance with testing in children, and there has been improvement in the accuracy of the hand-held units. Pneumotonometry is the gentlest method and preferred for clients after LASIK surgery. Overall, tonometry is superior to *digital tension*, which tends to underestimate pressure, for obtaining intraocular pressure in young children. The Goldmann applanation method is considered the criterion standard for this procedure.

Professional Considerations
1. Consent form NOT required.

Risks
Corneal abrasion or infection.

Contraindications
Corneal infection or ulcer, unless absolutely necessary. It is also contraindicated in clients who may be unable to hold very still during the test (that is, those with persistent coughing or sneezing).

2. Preparation:
   A. Remove contact lenses and loosen any jewelry or clothing (tie, tight collar, necklace) around the neck area.
   B. All methods except the noncontact methods: Anesthetic eye drops are instilled bilaterally.
   C. Schiøtz method: Obtain sterile tonofilms for the contact tonometer.
3. Procedure:
   A. Schiøtz method:
      i. The client is positioned supine.
      ii. One eye is tested at a time. After the tonometer is zeroed, the eyelids are held open as the tonometer is placed against the eyeball. The tonometer is pressed against the eye with a specific amount of weight, and the tonometer scale reflects a number that is converted to millimeters of mercury (mm Hg) for an intraocular pressure (IOP) reading.
   B. Goldmann applanation method:
      i. A fluorescein-stained paper is touched against the surface of the eye and removed.
      ii. The slit-lamp is advanced until the tonometer touches the eye surface.
      iii. A digital measurement of the pressure required to flatten a

small portion of the eye surface is recorded.
   C. Handheld tonometer method:
      i. A small, penlike handheld tonometer is lightly pressed against the surface of the eye and a digital measurement of the eye pressure is taken.
   D. Non-contact "air puff" method (indentation tonometry):
      i. The client's head is positioned on a chin rest and the equipment is aligned to the eye. As a calibrated puff of air is expelled from the equipment against the eye surface, this causes an indentation in the eye surface and a photoelectric cell measures the amount of corneal deformity indicated by changing reflections back to the light source from the corneas.
   E. Noncontact pneumotonometry method:
      i. A handheld pneumotonometer connected to a long tube is placed against the cornea. A stream of air flows through the tube and is directed into the sensing tip, where ocular pressure, standard deviation, and ocular pulse pressure are measured and displayed on a screen.
4. Postprocedure care:
   A. Eyeglasses may be worn in place of contact lenses.
   B. See *Client and family teaching.*
5. Client and family teaching:
   A. Provide a thorough explanation of the procedure, emphasizing that the client must cooperate by keeping the eyes open during testing.
   B. Contact lenses must be removed. Bring eyeglasses to wear, if needed, after the test.
   C. Avoid rubbing the eyes or replacing contact lenses until the local anesthesia has worn off (about 2 hours). Rubbing the eyes before this time can cause corneal abrasion, which is painful and takes several days to heal.
6. Factors that affect results:
   A. It may be necessary to adjust the weight placed against the eyeball to obtain a consistent pressure reading.

7. **Other data:**
   A. IOP evaluation in the detection of glaucoma has approximately 50% specificity.
   B. Pneumotonometry is another specialized method of measuring IOP and is used in cases of irregular corneas or after keratoplasty when the applanation tonometer cannot be used.
   C. For abnormal findings, the client should have a full ophthalmologic examination, including cup-to-disk ratio and field studies.

TORCH, BLOOD
(see Toxoplasmosis, Other, Rubella, Cytomegalovirus, Herpes virus serology, Blood)

TOTAL BODY SCAN, DIAGNOSTIC
(see Bone scan, Diagnostic)

TOTAL IRON-BINDING CAPACITY (TIBC), SERUM
(see Iron and total iron-binding capacity/transferrin, Serum)

TOURNIQUET TEST, DIAGNOSTIC
(see Capillary fragility test, Diagnostic)

TOXICOLOGY, DRUG SCREEN, BLOOD OR URINE

Norm. Negative.

Overdose Symptoms and Treatment. (See individual test listings.)

Treatment of Overdose. (See individual test listings.)

Usage. Monitor toxic, overdose, or newly comatose situations, or screen for drug abuse. Determine causes for agranulocytosis, impotence, and pruritus. Screening for substance use in on-the-job injuries.

Description. Toxicology drug screening is normally done with a urine test via immunoassay for several drugs. Positive results are confirmed by gas chromatography and additional blood testing may be requested. Common drugs included in this test are acetaminophen, alcohol, amphetamines, barbiturates, benzodiazepines, cannabinoids, cocaine metabolite, hypnotics, methadone, methaqualone, narcotics, opiates, organic bases, phencyclidine, phenothiazines, phenytoins, propoxyphene, salicylates, and tricyclic antidepressants. Drugs NOT detected by this rapid test method include clonidine, calcium-channel blockers, beta-adrenergic blockers, and albuterol. (See also *Toxicology: Volatiles group by GLC, Blood or Urine,* and many are also in individual test listings.)

Professional Considerations
1. Consent form NOT required unless results may be used for legal purposes.
2. **Preparation:**
   A. *Blood:* Tube: Red topped, red/gray topped, or gold topped or lavender topped.
   B. *Urine:* Obtain a clean container with a tight-fitting lid.
3. **Procedure:**
   A. If the specimen may be used as legal evidence, have the specimen collection witnessed.
   B. *Blood:* Draw a 2-mL blood sample in a red-topped, red/gray-topped, or gold-topped tube, or draw a 5-mL blood sample in a lavender-topped tube.
   C. *Urine:* Obtain a 50-mL random urine specimen in a clean container. Tightly cap the container.
4. **Postprocedure care:**
   A. Specify suspected drug(s) on the requisition.
   B. If the specimen may be used for legal purposes, write the client's name, date, exact time of collection, and specimen source on the laboratory requisition. Sign and have the witness sign the laboratory requisition. Transport the specimen to the laboratory immediately in a sealed plastic bag marked as legal evidence. All clients handling the specimen should sign and mark the time of

receipt on the laboratory requisition.

C. Assess for possible signs of drug withdrawal.

5. **Client and family teaching:**
   A. Results are normally not available for days.
   B. If activated charcoal was given for elevated levels, the client should drink 4-6 glasses of water each day for 2 days to prevent constipation. The activated charcoal will also cause stools to be black for a few days.
   C. For intentional overdose, refer the client and family for crisis intervention and offer resource information for counseling.
   D. Referrals to appropriate rehabilitation centers and therapeutic community programs should be offered to all addicted clients who may be interested.

6. **Factors that affect results:**
   A. Failure to maintain a clear chain of custody may invalidate results for legal purposes.

B. Failure to tightly cap the specimen container may cause falsely decreased results for volatiles.

7. **Other data:**
   A. The test provides only qualitative detection of drugs. Any drug identified in a screening should be confirmed by a test specific to that drug.
   B. The blood drug screening is usually performed with urine drug screening.
   C. Barbiturates coingested with other substances have the highest incidence of mortality out of all cases of sedative-hypnotic overdose
   D. The AdultaCheck 4 Test Strip can be used to identify if a urine specimen has been tampered with or adulterated.
   E. See also individual listings of specific drugs or classes of drugs for therapeutic ranges and panic levels.

TOXICOLOGY, VOLATILES GROUP BY GLC, BLOOD OR URINE

Norm. Negative for acetone, ethyl alcohol (ethanol), ethylene glycol, isopropanol, and methyl alcohol (methanol).

Positive. Ingestion of substances.

		SI UNITS
Blood Panic Levels		
Acetone	>20 mg/dL	>3.44 mmol/L
Ethyl alcohol (ethanol)	>100 mg/dL	>21.7 mmol/L
Ethylene glycol	>20 mg/dL	>3.2 mmol/L
Lethal level	>30 mg/dL	>4.8 mmol/L
Isopropanol	>400 mg/L	>6.64 mmol/L
Methanol	>200 mg/L	>6.24 mmol/L
Urine Panic Levels		
Acetone	>27 mg/dL	>4.65 mmol/L
Ethyl alcohol (ethanol)	>100 mg/dL	>21.7 mmol/L
Ethylene glycol	Presence of oxalate crystals in urine	Presence of oxalate crystals in urine
Isopropanol (isopropyl alcohol)	>500 μg/mL	>8.32 mmol/L
Methanol	>50 mg/L	>1.56 mmol/L

Overdose Symptoms and Treatment

Note: Treatment choice(s) depend on client history and condition and episode history.

Acetone panic level symptoms:

Coma, hypotension, respiratory depression.

Acetone panic level treatment:

Support airway, breathing, and circulation.

Monitor hourly neurologic checks.

Administer blood glucose, monitor serum and urine acetone levels, and provide arterial pH monitoring.

Hemodialysis WILL remove acetone. Hemoperfusion will NOT remove acetone.

Ethyl alcohol (ethanol) poisoning symptoms:

<50 mg/dL	Muscular incoordination
50-100 mg/dL	Worsening incoordination of movement
100-150 mg/dL	Mood and behavior changes
150-200 mg/dL	Delayed reactions
200-300 mg/dL	Ataxia, double vision, nausea, vomiting
300-400 mg/dL	Amnesia, dysarthria, hypothermia
400-700 mg/dL	Respiratory failure coma, death possible

Ethyl alcohol poisoning treatment:

Support oxygenation and breathing.

Consider NG aspiration and rapid lavage if within 4 hours of ingestion. Do NOT use gastric lavage.

Hemodialysis WILL remove ethanol but is seldom necessary unless levels rise >300 mg/dL. During hemodialysis, levels drop an average of 62 mg%/hour.

Isopropanol panic level symptoms. Coma, confusion, dizziness, headache, hypotension, nausea, oliguria initially followed by diuresis, respiratory depression, stupor, uncoordinated movement, vomiting. Death is possible.

Isopropanol panic level treatment:

Implement aspiration precautions and support airway.

Administer vasopressors for hypotension.

Hemodialysis is usually indicated when levels exceed 400 mg/dL. Peritoneal dialysis is minimally effective in removing isopropanol. Hemodialysis will not remove isopropanol but will remove its acetone metabolite.

Monitor electrolytes and treat imbalance.

Monitor for hepatic or renal damage.

Monitor closely for central nervous system depression. Administer thiamine and D5W if client is obtunded.

Methanol poisoning symptoms. Eight to 36 hours after ingestion: headache, weakness, abdominal and back pain, nausea and vomiting, dizziness, hallucinations and confusion, metabolic acidosis, possible blindness, respiratory depression, and coma; death is possible.

Methanol poisoning treatment (within 2 hours of ingestion):

Support airway, breathing, and circulation.

Consider NG aspiration and rapid lavage if within 4 hours of ingestion.

Administer ethyl alcohol (ethanol) IV or PO to block breakdown of methanol into its toxic metabolites. Adjust infusion rate to maintain blood ethanol level of 100-150 mg/dL (may need higher doses in alcoholics). Remeasure ethanol levels frequently. Continue this treatment until methanol level is <20 mg/dL.

As an alternative to ethanol, fomepizole has been found to be effective as an antidote to methanol, and can eliminate the need for dialysis, but not in clients with renal problems or levels above 50 mg/dL. Administer IV loading dose of

Continued

Methanol poisoning treatment—cont'd
15 mg/kg followed by
maintenance dose of 10 mg/kg
every 12 hours × 4, followed by
15 mg/kg every 12 hours to reach
therapeutic fomepizole level >8.6
mg/mL. Continue until methanol
concentrations are undetectable.
Dosing frequently must be
increased if dialysis is also used.
Dialyze to eliminate methanol and
its toxic formic acid metabolites.
Use forced diuresis is dialysis is
not available. Indications for
hemodialysis include methanol
level >50 mg/dL, or pH <7.20, or
renal failure, or presence of visual
symptoms.
Correct acidemia with $NaHCO_3$ if
pH is <7.20.
Keep environment dark to reduce
stress on vision.
Consider using folic acid
(leucovorin) in clients with folic
acid deficiency. Give leucovorin
50 mg IV every 4 hours for several
days. Folic acid potentiates
metabolism of formic acid into
carbon dioxide and water.

Usage. Evaluation for poisoning; monitoring response to treatment for poisoning. This test is frequently routine for clients who are newly unconscious with unknown cause.

Description. The toxicologic volatiles screen tests for the presence of acetone, ethyl alcohol (ethanol), ethylene glycol, isopropanol, and methanol in a blood sample.

Acetone level helps identify isopropyl alcohol (isopropanol, rubbing alcohol) ingestion or toxicity because, when ingested, isopropanol is converted to acetone.

Isopropanol is a portion of rubbing alcohol (70% isopropanol), perfumes, aftershaves, and antifreeze that is metabolized to acetone, carbon dioxide, and water in the blood and urine. This alcohol is readily absorbed by the gastrointestinal tract, having a half-life of 30-180 minutes, and produces central nervous system depression. Isopropanol is often ingested in desperation by alcoholics.

Ethyl alcohol, also known as grain alcohol (ethanol), is a substance, often abused, that depresses the central nervous system and may lead to coma progressing to death at levels above the panic level listed above.

Ethylene glycol is the main compound contained in antifreeze and is also found in other automotive products that, when ingested and metabolized, causes toxicity to humans. Ethylene glycol may be ingested as an inexpensive substitute for alcohol. Methanol and isopropanol may be ingested by alcoholics accustomed to taking ethyl alcohol (ethanol) when ethyl alcohol is unavailable. After ingestion, oxalic acid is excreted by the kidneys, causing oxalate crystals in the urine, acidosis, tetany, and renal failure. The minimum lethal dose is approximately 100 mL, but any amount ingested may produce toxic symptoms. Half-life is 3 hours without treatment, 2.5 hours with dialysis, and 17 hours with concomitant orally administered ethyl alcohol.

Methyl alcohol, also known as wood alcohol (methanol), is an alcohol produced in the distillation process and is sometimes found in improperly prepared alcohols, such as moonshine. It is also an ingredient in antifreeze, some varnishes, paints, paint thinners, windshield washer fluid, and camp stove fluid.

Both blood and urine levels of these substances are important. Although blood levels reflect the most recently ingested substance(s), urine levels may reflect substances ingested over a longer period. This test is frequently routine for clients who are newly unconscious with unknown cause.

Professional Considerations
1. Consent form NOT required unless results may be used as legal evidence.
2. **Preparation:**
   A. Tube: Gray topped (contains glycolytic inhibitor) for the blood sample.
   B. Obtain a clean container with a tight-fitting lid, and a container of ice for the urine sample.
   C. Do NOT draw specimens during hemodialysis.

3. Procedure:
   A. Specimen collection should be witnessed if it may be used as legal evidence.
   B. *Blood sample:* Do NOT use alcohol for venipuncture. Instead, cleanse the site with a povidone-iodine wipe and allow the area to dry. Draw a 5-mL blood sample. Tightly cap the tube.
   C. *Urine sample:* Obtain a 50-mL random urine specimen in a clean container. Tightly cap the container. Transport it on ice.
4. Postprocedure care:
   A. Place the urine specimen on ice.
   B. Write the client's name, the date, the contents of the tube, and the exact time of specimen collection, along with your signature and the signature of the witness, on the tube label and laboratory requisition if the specimen may be used as legal evidence. Transport the specimen on ice to the laboratory in a sealed plastic bag labeled as legal evidence.
   C. Store the blood or urine sample at 4°C.
   D. Monitor for panic level symptoms.
5. Client and family teaching:
   A. Results may be available within hours.
   B. For intentional overdose, refer client and family for crisis intervention.
   C. Referrals to appropriate rehabilitation centers and therapeutic community programs should be offered to all addicted clients who may be interested.
6. Factors that affect results:
   A. Failure to tightly cap the specimen container may cause false low results.
   B. Failure to maintain a clear chain of custody may invalidate the results for legal purposes.
7. Other data:
   A. Because of the low molecular weight of these volatiles, an osmolar gap results. See *Osmolality, Calculated tests, Blood.*
   B. Ethylene glycol can also be detected in gastric secretions.
   C. The highest known ethylene glycol concentration in which a person survived is 1889 mg/dL.

TOXOPLASMOSIS, OTHER, RUBELLA, CYTOMEGALOVIRUS, HERPESVIRUS SEROLOGY (TORCH), BLOOD

Norm. Negative for all diseases.

Usage. Maternal and infant screening.

Description. This serologic test is performed to detect the congenitally acquired diseases of toxoplasmosis, rubella, cytomegalic inclusion disease, herpes, and others such as syphilis and varicella infections in infants who manifest symptoms of viral or other infections during the first year of life. The test may also be performed on the mother during pregnancy to screen for diseases that are likely to cause birth defects. The literature discounts the value of *routine* TORCH screening and discusses the value of various methods of testing. TORCH screening IS recommended in HIV-infected pregnant women who have not had previous TORCH screening. One study recommends enzyme immunoassay to document past infection. IgM enzyme-linked immunosorbent assay (ELISA) is recommended to detect recent toxoplasmosis or rubella. Finally, several studies relate that culture is required to confirm herpes or cytomegalovirus infection.

Professional Considerations
1. Consent form NOT required.
2. Preparation:
   A. Tube: Red topped, red/gray topped, or gold topped.
3. Procedure:
   A. Draw a 3-mL blood sample.
4. Postprocedure care:
   A. Any individual positive test or higher-than-normal titer should be repeated in 7-10 days to observe for changing titer.
5. Client and family teaching:
   A. Return in 7-10 days for repeat testing if the results are positive.
6. Factors that affect results:
   A. See individual test listings.
7. Other data:
   A. For positive tests, genetic counseling may be indicated.
   B. See individual test listings for full descriptions.
   C. TORCH test sera should be held in the laboratory for a year in the event repeat testing is necessary.

TOXOPLASMOSIS SEROLOGY, SERUM

Norm:

Immunofluorescence

Adults	IgM titer <1:64
	IgG titer <1:1024
Neonates	IgM undetectable

Indirect Hemagglutination

No previous infection	Titer <1:4
Probable past infection	Titers >1:4 and <1:256
Suggestive of recent infection	Titer >1:256

Increased. Current or past infection with *Toxoplasma gondii*.

Decreased. Not applicable.

Description. Toxoplasmosis is a systemic, parasitic disease caused by the protozoa *T. gondii*. It is transmitted to humans by ingestion of the undercooked meat of infected animals or often by the ingestion of oocysts acquired from handling cat litter containing contaminated cat feces. It may also be transmitted to a fetus through the placenta of an infected mother. After ingestion, this parasite travels to various body tissues and is found grouped together in oocysts. Acquired toxoplasmosis often causes no symptoms in clients with intact immune systems. In immunosuppression, it may cause hyperpyrexia, lymphadenopathy, lymphocytosis, and in some cases, encephalitis, pneumonitis, myocarditis, myositis, and possible death. Fetal congenital toxoplasmosis can cause severe birth defects, including blindness, hydrocephalus, and mental retardation, and may lead to fetal or postnatal death. Serologic testing for *T. gondii* antibody titer is recommended for all pregnant females. If antibody titer is low positive, indicating past infection, there is no risk to the fetus. However, the fetus is at risk for birth defects if the disease is acquired during pregnancy. Thus, if antibody titer is initially high (indicative of current active infection) or initially negative, the test should be repeated at each prenatal checkup throughout the first 5 months of pregnancy and just before delivery. Toxoplasmosis occurs in advanced AIDS.

Professional Considerations
1. Consent form NOT required.
2. **Preparation:**
   A. Assess whether the woman has handled cat feces during pregnancy.
   B. Assess whether the client has eaten any raw or undercooked meat.
   C. Tube: Red topped, red/gray topped, or gold topped.
3. **Procedure:**
   A. Draw a 3-mL blood sample as soon as pregnancy is known or as soon as possible after symptoms appear. Label the specimen as the acute sample. Repeat the test in 7-14 days to detect rising antibody titer and label the tube as the convalescent sample. For pregnancy, repeat the test as described under *Description,* above.
4. **Postprocedure care:**
   A. None.
5. **Client and family teaching:**
   A. Cat owners who are pregnant or who have AIDS must feed the cat commercially prepared or well-cooked food and prevent the cat from roaming and scavenging. Avoid handling the cat litter if possible. Cat litter should be handled (preferably by another household member) with gloved hands and discarded every day, with daily disinfection of the litter container by being rinsed with boiling water. If you must handle the cat litter or litter box, avoid touching anything else afterward until you have performed meticulous handwashing. Also avoid handling other cats and avoid gardening (where you may come

into contact with contaminated cat feces).

B. Thoroughly cook any meat to be ingested.

6. **Factors that affect results:**
   A. None found.
7. **Other data:**
   A. Except for placental-fetal transfer, toxoplasmosis is not communicable between clients.
   B. When toxoplasmosis is acquired early in pregnancy, abortion may be recommended.
   C. Pyrimethamine and sulfonamides are used to treat toxoplasmosis.

TOXOPLASMOSIS SKIN TEST, DIAGNOSTIC

Norm. Negative.

Positive. Current or past infection with *Toxoplasma gondii*.

Description. Toxoplasmosis is a systemic, parasitic disease caused by the protozoon *T. gondii*. It is transmitted to humans by ingestion of the undercooked meat of infected animals or often by the ingestion of oocysts acquired from handling cat litter containing contaminated cat feces. It may also be transmitted to a fetus through the placenta of an infected mother. After ingestion, this parasite travels to various body tissues and is found grouped together in oocysts. Acquired toxoplasmosis often causes no symptoms in clients with intact immune systems. In immunosuppression, it may cause hyperpyrexia, lymphadenopathy, lymphocytosis, and in some cases encephalitis, pneumonitis, myocarditis, myositis, and possible death. Fetal congenital toxoplasmosis can cause severe birth defects, including blindness, hydrocephalus, and mental retardation, and may lead to fetal or postnatal death.

Professional Considerations
1. Consent form NOT required.
2. **Preparation:**
   A. Assess whether a pregnant woman has handled cat feces during her pregnancy.
   B. Assess whether the client has eaten any raw or undercooked meat.

C. Obtain an alcohol wipe, a 1-mL syringe, an intradermal needle, *Toxoplasma* antigen, and a control.

3. **Procedure:**
   A. Cleanse the forearm injection site with an alcohol wipe, and allow the area to dry.
   B. Inject *Toxoplasma* antigen intradermally and record the site of injection. Inject the control in the other arm, and record the site of injection.
   C. Read the skin test in 24-48 hours. A positive test is indicated by redness and induration >10 mm in diameter.
4. **Postprocedure care:**
   A. See *Toxoplasmosis serology, Serum,* for pregnancy precautions and precautions for persons with AIDS.
5. **Client and family teaching:**
   A. After the injection, return in 24-48 hours for a skin-test reading.
6. **Factors that affect results:**
   A. None found.
7. **Other data:**
   A. Many clients may be infected with *T. gondii* but are free of symptoms. Therefore any pregnant woman should be tested for the presence of antibodies to *T. gondii*. See *Toxoplasmosis serology, Serum.*

TRab
(see *Thyroid receptor antibody, Blood*)

TRACER, DIAGNOSTIC
(see *Glucose monitoring machines, Diagnostic*)

TRANSCRANIAL DOPPLER ULTRASONOGRAPHY, DIAGNOSTIC
(see *Doppler ultrasonographic flow studies, Diagnostic*)

TRANSESOPHAGEAL ECHOCARDIOGRAM
(see *Transesophageal ultrasonography, Diagnostic*)

T

TRANSESOPHAGEAL ULTRASONOGRAPHY (TRANSESOPHAGEAL ECHOCARDIOGRAM, TEE), DIAGNOSTIC

Norm. Negative or normal structure or function and absence of a pathologic condition.

Usage. Transesophageal echocardiogram (TEE) is especially indicated for examination of prosthetic heart valves, detection of mitral valve regurgitation, aortic dissection (site and extent), congenital heart disease of the adult, cardiac tumors and masses, embolic or thrombotic disorders (particularly of the left atrium), vegetative endocarditis, and intraoperative guide to left ventricular function and for clients with conditions making standard transthoracic echocardiograms unreliable: obesity, chest deformities, chronic lung disease, or intubation; provides guidance for pericardiocentesis in cardiac tamponade; helps evaluate for transvenous pacemaker malposition; newer use in ruling out the presence of atrial thrombus before cardioversion as an alternative to anticoagulation.

Description. Ultrasound uses high-frequency sound waves to induce vibrations that echo or reflect from the solid structures within the body. These echoes create images from which chamber and valve size, function, and pericardial effusion can be determined. A specially adapted flexible gastroscope is fitted with a high-frequency transducer to send, receive, and translate the reflected vibrations. This tube, when swallowed or advanced into the esophagus, is positioned behind the heart and related structures. It can be rotated anteriorly, laterally, or posteriorly to allow an unimpeded route for sound-wave reflection off the heart chambers, walls, and valves. Abnormalities that are missed by standard diagnostic techniques can be displayed. Only the upper aortic view is limited by the interference of the left mainstem bronchus. The newest echocardiographic equipment includes three-dimensional capabilities, which can provide many views of the heart structures.

Professional Considerations
1. Consent form IS required.

Risks

Vasovagal bradycardia and drug-induced tachycardia are likely dysrhythmias; esophageal perforation; bleeding; transient hypoxemia; oversedation.

Contraindications

Esophageal obstructions, stenosis, fistula, or dysphagia; history of radiation therapy to the esophagus or surrounding area (mediastinum); acute penetrating chest injuries. Neonates and young children are not candidates because of the unavailability of specially sized TEE scopes. Sedatives are contraindicated in clients with central nervous system depression. Clients who can not tolerate lying flat.

2. **Preparation:**
   A. See *Client and family teaching.*
   B. Obtain a chest radiograph, ECG, and laboratory work, including CBC, electrolytes, PT, and PTT.
   C. Start an IV infusion at KVO (keep-vein-open) rate for administration of sedation or emergency medications.
   D. Remove dentures and glasses. Have the client void before the procedure.
   E. A drying agent is typically given to reduce secretions (that is, glycopyrrolate 0.1 to 0.2 mg IV). Some clients require a small IV dose of an antianxiety agent (such as midazolam or diazepam). Prophylactic antibiotics are usually given if the client has a prosthetic valve.

3. **Procedure:**
   A. The client is monitored continuously: heart rate and rhythm by cardiac monitor, blood pressure by noninvasive monitor, and O_2 by pulse oximetry.
   B. Position the client in the left lateral decubitus position.
   C. Topical anesthesia per physician preference is used to numb the throat and suppress the gag reflex. This may be repeated several times during the procedure.
   D. The client should be awake enough to follow commands but drowsy. This procedure may also be performed on a fully anesthetized or intubated client.
   E. The client is asked to open the mouth and flex the neck forward in a chin-to-chest position.

F. The lidocaine-lubricated probe is inserted, and the client is asked to swallow.

G. Over the next 5-20 minutes the probe is gently withdrawn, and cardiac images are viewed or recorded at different levels.

H. The nurse remains with the client to monitor respiratory status, vital signs, and cardiac rhythm and to assess the need for further sedation or suctioning.

4. **Postprocedure care:**

A. Continue assessment of respiratory status. If deep sedation was used, follow institutional protocol for postsedation monitoring. Typical monitoring includes continuous ECG monitoring and pulse oximetry with continual assessments (every 5-15 minutes) of airway, vital signs, and neurologic status until client reaches level 3, 2, or 1 on the Ramsay Sedation Scale.

B. Once the gag reflex has returned the client can resume fluids. Full diet is not recommended until 3 hours after procedure.

5. **Client and family teaching:**

A. Fast for 6-8 hours before the test. Medications may be taken with a small amount of water as directed by the physician. You will have to remove your dentures and eyeglasses, but you should keep your hearing aid on so that you can hear the physician's instructions.

B. You will be given a sedative for the procedure. You should arrange for someone to drive you home because you may be drowsy after the procedure and will not be permitted to drive.

C. Do not eat or drink for 4-6 hours before the procedure. Take any prescription medications with a small sip of water.

D. This procedure lets the physician look at your heart and its major blood vessels from the back, without the lungs blocking the view. A flexible tube about the thickness of a pen is inserted into the mouth and moved down into the esophagus. The tip of the tube produces sound waves that bounce off the heart and are changed into pictures on a video screen.

E. Breathe through the nose and swallow during introduction of the probe, and breathe through the mouth for the remainder of the procedure, which takes about 30 minutes.

F. The tongue and throat may feel swollen after the topical anesthetic; the mouth and lips will feel sticky and dry if a drying agent is used. Do not eat or drink after the procedure until the numbness is gone.

G. The doctor must review the videotape of the procedure before discussing the test results.

H. Home-going instructions: Promptly report persistent sore throat, dysphagia, stiff neck, and epigastric, and substernal or abdominal pain that worsens with breathing or movement.

6. **Factors that affect results:**

A. See the description of the test.

7. **Other data:**

A. None.

TRANSFER FACTOR
(*see Diffusing factor carbon monoxide, Diagnostic*)

TRANSFER FUNCTION INDEX
(*see Pulse volume recording of peripheral vasculature, Diagnostic*)

TRANSFERRIN, CARBOHYDRATE-DEFICIENT (CDT), SERUM

Norm. Quantitative: <6 units %; qualitative: not detected.

QUANTITATIVE TEST	% OF TRANSFERRIN
Pentasialo-	13% to 23%
Tetrasialo-	38% to 49%
Trisialo-	17% to 31%
Disialo-	2% to 15%
Monosialo-	0% to 5%

Usage. Used sometimes with MCV and GGTP to detect recent heavy alcohol consumption; monitoring for relapse after alcohol rehabilitation; helps diagnose carbohydrate-deficient glycoprotein syndromes. Also used to detect carbohydrate-deficient glycoprotein syndromes, rare autosomal recessive genetic traits in which levels of transferrin, haptoglobin, thyroxine-binding globulin, antithrombin II, and protein C are reduced, causing multisystemic symptoms such as skeletal problems and muscular weakness, ataxia, peripheral neuropathy, psychomotor or mental retardation, lipodystrophy, and problems with sight or vision.

Increased. Alcohol abuse, heavy intake. Iron-depletion treatment.

Decreased. Carbohydrate-deficient glycoprotein syndrome. Drugs include iron compounds.

Description. Carbohydrate-deficient transferrin (CDT) is transferrin with less than the normal amount of sugar chains. CDT is a sensitive and specific biologic marker for alcohol abuse in persons with normal iron states. The mechanism by which CDT increases in response to alcohol consumption is not yet well understood. Heavily influenced by mean alcohol consumption within 30 days before testing, CDT is elevated in clients who have had high alcohol consumption (>50-60 g/day) during this time. Many studies have found moderate sensitivity and specificity (80%-90%), but newer tests using lecithin-affinity chromatography have sensitivities and specificity close to 100%. CDT is equal in sensitivity but more specific than gamma glutamyltranspeptidase for detection of long-term heavy alcohol consumption.

Professional Considerations
1. Consent form NOT required.
2. **Preparation:**
   A. *Qualitative test:* Tube: Red topped. Also obtain dry ice.
   B. *Quantitative test* (used for infants): Obtain alcohol wipe, capillary tube, lancet, and filter paper.
3. **Procedure:**
   A. *Quantitative test:* Obtain a 2-mL blood sample. Place tube on dry ice.

B. *Qualitative test:*
   i. Cleanse the lateral curvature of the infant's heel with alcohol and allow it to dry.
   ii. Puncture the lateral heel curvature with a lancet.
   iii. Collect blood in capillary tube and completely saturate two spots on the filter paper card with heelstick blood.
   iv. Allow the blood spot to dry before sending the sample to the lab.
4. **Postprocedure care:**
   A. Apply pressure to the puncture site until the bleeding stops. Let the site air-dry.
   B. Test is usually performed at a reference laboratory.
5. **Client and family teaching:**
   A. 5-14 days may be required for testing.
   B. Offer resources for alcoholism treatment or genetic counseling if appropriate.
6. **Factors that affect results:**
   A. The test must be repeated if the blood amount is not enough to completely saturate both spots on the filter paper card.
   B. Touching the filter paper or exposure to extremes of heat and light can cause errors in the results.
   C. When test is used to monitor for relapse after treatment, results should be compared to initial baseline specimen values.
   D. Unexplained false-positive and false-negative results have been found in several studies. Iron overload accounts for some false-negative results. Therefore a negative result does not exclude the possibility of alcohol consumption.
   E. Concomitant liver diseases reduces the specificity of this test.
7. **Other data:**
   A. None.

TRANSFERRIN, SERUM

Norm:

		SI UNITS
Adult	200-400 mg/dL	2-4.0 g/L
Maternal (term)	305 mg/dL	3.0 g/L
Fetal	190 mg/dL	1.9 g/L
Newborn	130-275 mg/dL	1.3-2.8 g/L

Increased. Iron-deficiency states with normal protein levels and pregnancy. Drugs include oral contraceptives.

Decreased. Congenital absence of transferrin (hereditary atransferrinemia), hemolytic states, hepatic disease (acquired), inflammation (chronic), iron overload, low iron states combined with protein malnutrition, neoplasm, proteinuria (severe) and other protein-losing states, and renal disease.

Description. Transferrin is a beta globulin and glycoprotein with a short (7-day) half-life. Formed in the liver, transferrin transports dietary iron from the intestinal mucosa to iron-storage sites and hemoglobin-synthesis sites in the body (bone, muscle, erythrocytes, lymphocytes). Transferrin enables iron storage by binding to transferrin receptors at the iron-storage sites. Transferrin is capable of binding more than its own weight in iron. That is, 1 g of transferrin can carry 1.43 g of iron. Normally, iron saturation of transferrin (transferrin saturation) is between 20% and 45%. Because of its short half-life, values will decrease more quickly in protein malnutrition states than albumin will. Thus transferrin is sometimes used to evaluate nutritional status. Transferrin also has growth-stimulating properties that are separate from its iron-transport properties.

Professional Considerations
1. Consent form NOT required.

2. **Preparation:**
    A. See *Client and family teaching.*
    B. Tube: Red topped, red/gray topped, or gold topped.
3. **Procedure:**
    A. Draw the specimen during the morning hours if it is to be used to evaluate transferrin saturation because a diurnal pattern with a morning peak exists.
    B. Draw a 1-mL blood sample.
4. **Postprocedure care:**
    A. None.
5. **Client and family teaching:**
    A. Fast from food and fluids (except water) for 12 hours before the test.
    B. Results are normally available within 24 hours.
6. **Factors that affect results:**
    A. None found.
7. **Other data:**
    A. Transferrin is also called "siderophilin" and "iron-binding protein."
    B. See also *Iron and total iron binding capacity/transferrin, Serum; Soluble transferrin receptor assay, Serum; Transferrin, Carbohydrate deficient, Serum.*

TRANSFERRIN, SOLUBLE RECEPTOR, SERUM
(see Soluble transferrin receptor assay, Serum)

TRANSFUSION REACTION WORK-UP, DIAGNOSTIC

Norm. Not applicable.

TRANSFUSION REACTION SYMPTOMS AND TREATMENT

Note: Treatment choice(s) depend on client history and condition and episode history.

Mild Febrile Reaction

Symptoms
- Slight, nonsustained temperature rise <1° C
- Urticaria, rash, or hives
- Headache
- Malaise
- Mild chills

Treatment
- Slow the transfusion rate. Verify that the information on the client's blood band, hospital bracelet, blood bag, and blood transfusion requisition all correspond properly and notify the physician.

Continued

Mild Febrile Reaction—cont'd

Treatment

If all information matches properly, possible courses of action available to the physician include:

- Continue the transfusion while monitoring the recipient closely for further development of hemolytic or nonhemolytic reaction.
- Add a microaggregate filter to filter the blood if not already being used.
- Administer antipyretic and antihistamine and continue the transfusion while monitoring the client closely for further development of hemolytic or nonhemolytic reaction.
- Stop the transfusion, and return the blood to the blood bank.
- Stop the transfusion, and complete the transfusion-reaction blood work and urine tests as described below.

Hemolytic Reaction

Symptoms

Early signs:
- Sustained rise in temperature >1° C
- Nausea or vomiting
- Pronounced chills and shivering
- Palpitations
- Pain in the chest or back
- Apprehension
- Infusion-site tenderness and warmth

Progressive signs:
- Shock
- Oliguria
- Hemoglobinuria
- Bleeding tendencies (disseminated intravascular coagulation)
- Acute renal failure
- Anaphylaxis

Treatment

- Stop the transfusion immediately, and leave a normal saline infusion at a keep-open rate. Notify the physician immediately.
- Monitor vital signs every 5-15 minutes.
- Completely fill a red-topped tube and a lavender-topped tube with a blood sample.
- Obtain a 50-mL random, fresh urine sample in a clean container.
- Document pretransfusion and posttransfusion vital signs on the blood bank requisition.
- Return the blood bank requisition, laboratory requisition for the transfusion reaction work-up, the bag of blood, the urine specimen, and the red-topped and lavender-topped tubes to the blood bank promptly.
- If DIC is suspected, additional testing should include fibrinogen level, fibrin split products, platelet count, PT/PTT, and thrombin time.

Acute Nonimmune Febrile Reaction

Symptoms
- Sustained rise in temperature >1° C
- Hematemesis
- Diarrhea
- Hypotension
- Tachycardia
- Shock
- Sepsis

Treatment

In addition to following the procedures above for a hemolytic reaction:
- Draw blood for aerobic and anaerobic culture and Gram stain.

Anaphylactic Reaction

Symptoms
- Tachycardia
- Dyspnea, wheezing (bronchospasm and upper airway edema)
- Apprehension
- Flushing
- Urticaria, hives
- Angioedema
- Shock
- Circulatory collapse
- Bowel spasm, with diarrhea

Treatment

In addition to following procedures above for a hemolytic reaction:
- Have an emergency cart readily available.
- Maintain a patent airway and blood pressure.
- Administer epinephrine intravenously as follows:
  a. Bolus with epinephrine 0.2-0.5 mg of 1:1000 dilution mixed in 10-mL of 0.9% saline over 5-10 minutes.
  b. Follow the bolus with a continuous infusion of epinephrine at 1-4 mg/minute.
- Other drugs used to treat anaphylaxis may include aminophylline, atropine (for brady-cardia), cimetidine, diphen-hydramine, and hydrocortisone.
- Use IgA-deficient blood or plasma-deficient blood for future transfusions.

Usage. Helps determine the cause of transfusion reaction.

Description. An acute transfusion reaction work-up is indicated whenever an unexpected reaction to transfusion of blood products is noted. Symptoms are most likely to occur within the first 15-30 minutes of transfusion and may be stimulated by as little as 10 mL of incompatible blood. Recombinant erythropoietin should be considered as an alternative to transfusion for anemic clients with nonmyeloid cancers.

Mild febrile reactions and urticaria may occur in clients who have been immunized to blood-protein constituents through past receipt of donor blood or past pregnancies. A microaggregate filter used with transfusion can minimize the transfusion of such blood constituents.

Hemolytic transfusion reaction: With correctly administered blood, a hemolytic transfusion reaction may be attributable to recipient antibodies reacting to donor antigens not identified during type-and-crossmatch or type-and-screen procedures. Reactions are more likely to occur in clients who have had recent transfusions of blood because new antibodies to past donor blood may have developed since the last type and crossmatch was performed. In blood administered incorrectly (that is, to the wrong recipient), a transfusion reaction is most likely caused by ABO incompatibility or antigen-antibody reactions. An incompatible or contaminated transfusion may cause fatal hemolytic reactions and disseminated intravascular coagulation. Thus it is important to observe recipients closely for early signs of reaction, so that the transfusion may be promptly stopped and complications minimized.

Acute nonimmune febrile reactions may be caused by bacterial contamination of the donor blood. This type of reaction may cause fever and erythrocyte hemolysis and may progress to shock and sepsis.

Anaphylactic transfusion reactions may occur in clients with subnormal immunoglobulin A (IgA) who have a history of recurrent infections. The receipt of IgA in donor blood stimulates an antibody response to IgA that causes anaphylaxis.

Delayed transfusion reactions include delayed hemolytic reactions, graft-versus-host disease, purpura, and hemosiderosis. Delayed hemolytic reactions usually are caused by recipient anti-Rh antibodies, anti-Duffy antibodies, and anti-Kidd antibodies that were not detected during type-and-crossmatch procedures. A transfusion of blood containing these antigens causes delayed hemolysis and continued anemia. Graft-versus-host disease is usually fatal and occurs in immunosuppressed clients whose immune systems are unable to provide resistance against donor lymphocytes. Purpura with thrombocytopenia may develop about 7 days after transfusion in clients deficient in and who have developed antibodies to platelet antigen PLA-1. Hemosiderosis (iron overload) may occur in clients receiving multiple transfusions over a short period of time.

Laboratory procedures for an acute transfusion-reaction work-up include direct Coombs' testing; repeated type and crossmatch on original recipient and donor samples; type and crossmatch on postreaction recipient sample with donor sample; hemoglobin and hematocrit level; serum haptoglobin; urea nitrogen, plasma or serum; recipient and donor blood culture and Gram stain; and urine measurement of bilirubin, hemoglobin, urobilinogen, and hemosiderin.

Professional Considerations

1. Consent form NOT required.
2. **Preparation:**
   A. Assess the client during the transfusion for signs of a transfusion reaction listed above.

3. **Procedure:**
   A. Follow procedures described under *Treatment*.
4. **Postprocedure care:**
   A. Continue monitoring vital signs every 5-15 minutes until they are stable.
5. **Client and family teaching:**
   A. Complete results may take several days.
   B. See *Other data* and provide information appropriate to the type of reaction that occurred.
6. **Factors that affect results:**
   A. See individual test listings.
7. **Other data:**
   A. For delayed transfusion reactions, the following should be performed if future transfusions are needed:
      i. *Delayed hemolytic reactions:* The client should be advised to carry the information in writing that any blood transfusions received must be negative for Rh (c and E), Duffy, and Kidd antigens.
      ii. *Graft-versus-host disease:* If the client survives this complication, future donor blood should be irradiated before transfusion.
      iii. *Purpura:* The client should be advised to carry the information in writing that any blood transfusions received must be PLA-1 negative.
      iv. *Hemosiderosis:* Hemosiderosis may be fatal. The risk for developing this complication may be minimized in clients who need multiple transfusions by performing lead chelation therapy.
   B. Card or slide hemagglutination or dipstick methods are available for use in ABO blood grouping at the bedside just before transfusion.

TRANSRECTAL ULTRASONOGRAPHY, DIAGNOSTIC

(see *Prostate ultrasonography, Diagnostic*)

TRANSTHYRETIN (TTR, PREALBUMIN, PA, TRYPTOPHAN-RICH PREALBUMIN), SERUM

Norm:

		SI UNITS
Adult	10-40 mg/dL	100-400 mg/L
Male	(mean) 21.5 mg/dL	(mean) 215 mg/L
Female	(mean) 18.2 mg/dL	(mean) 182 mg/L
Maternal	17-18.6 mg/dL	170-186 mg/L
Children		
Cord blood	(mean) 13 mg/dL	(mean) 130 mg/L
Newborn	10.4-11.4 mg/dL	104-114 mg/L
12 months	(mean) 10 mg/dL	(mean) 100 mg/L
24-36 months	16-28.1 mg/dL	160-281 mg/L

Increased. Adrenal hyperfunction, Hodgkin's disease, shigellosis. Drugs include corticosteroids (high dose) and NSAIDs (high dose).

Decreased. Abdominal peritoneal dialysis, cirrhosis, chronic illness (with concomitant subnormal nutritional status), cystic fibrosis, diabetes mellitus, disseminated malignant disease, epithelial ovarian carcinoma, hereditary amyloidosis, protein and calorie malnutrition. Drugs include amiodarone, estrogens, and oral contraceptives (containing estrogen).

Description. Transthyretin is a transport protein, synthesized in the liver that carries thyroid hormone and retinol in the body. Transthyretin is a precursor of albumin, and its half-life of 2-4 days makes it a much more sensitive marker for nutritional status and for liver dysfunction than albumin, which has a half-life of 22 days. Because transthyretin reflects changes in nutritional status more quickly than albumin does, it is frequently used to evaluate nutritional needs in postoperative and critically ill clients. Transthyretin mutations have been associated with many familial amyloidosis diseases, autosomal dominant disorders in which amyloid deposits accumulate in peripheral nerves, resulting in neuropathy.

Professional Considerations
1. Consent form NOT required.
2. Preparation:
   A. Tube: Red topped, red/gray topped, or gold topped.
   B. Do NOT draw specimens during hemodialysis.
3. Procedure:
   A. Draw a 1-mL blood sample without hemolysis.
4. Postprocedure care:
   A. None.
5. Client and family teaching:
   A. Results are normally available within 24 hours.
6. Factors that affect results:
   A. Hemolyzed or lipemic specimens interfere with the nephelometric testing method.
7. Other data:
   A. None.

TRANYLCYPROMINE
(see Amphetamines, Blood)

TRAP
(see Tartrate-resistant acid phosphatase, Blood)

TRAZODONE
(see Tricyclic antidepressants, Plasma or Serum)

TRIAZOLAM
(see Benzodiazepines, Plasma and Urine)

TRICHINOSIS SEROLOGY, SERUM

Norm. Negative or titer <1:16. Possible current or past infection: titer >1:5.

Positive. A fourfold rise in titer is diagnostic for trichinosis.

Description. Trichinosis is a parasitic disease caused by the larva of *Trichinella spiralis,* a roundworm acquired in humans by ingestion of raw or poorly cooked pork or other animals it inhabits (cats, dogs, swine, and some wild animals such as walrus and bear). The ingested worm larvae mature and reproduce in the intestinal tract and then migrate through the lymphatic system and bloodstream to other sites in the body. Those reaching muscle tissue become encapsulated as cysts, causing inflammation and necrosis. The symptoms of trichinosis are progressive. Soon after ingestion, hyperpyrexia, gastrointestinal upset, eosinophilia, and muscle edema occur. These symptoms are followed by muscle soreness and may progress to neurotoxicity and myocarditis. Clients with chronic trichinosis may experience myalgia, eye burning, headache, and easy fatigability. This test detects the presence of *T. spiralis* antibodies by mixing of serial dilutions of the client's serum with *T. spiralis* antigen and observation for antigen-antibody reactions. Titers may be negative soon after symptoms appear but begin rising about 21 days after infection. Levels peak about 60 days after infection and then slowly return to higher-than-baseline levels until about 2 years later.

Professional Considerations
1. Consent form NOT required.
2. Preparation:
   A. Tube: Red topped, red/gray topped, or gold topped.
   B. Assess for history of recent ingestion of raw pork or poorly cooked pork or other susceptible animals.
   C. The test may need to be prescheduled with the laboratory.
   D. Specimens MAY be drawn during hemodialysis.
3. Procedure:
   A. Draw a 5-mL blood sample. Repeat the test every 3-5 days to detect rising titer.
4. Postprocedure care:
   A. None.
5. Client and family teaching:
   A. Before eating it, thoroughly cook pork or meat from other susceptible animals until it turns gray.

   B. Serial testing is necessary to confirm *T. spiralis* infection.
6. **Factors that affect results:**
   A. Titers may be negative in the presence of infection if drawn during the first 3 weeks after exposure.
7. **Other data:**
   A. Other tests used to diagnose trichinosis include skin testing, muscle biopsy, or examination of cerebrospinal fluid for *T. spiralis.*
   B. Trichinosis has been treated with thiabendazole (intestinal phase), mebendazole (muscular stage), and corticosteroids.

TRICHINOSIS SKIN TEST, DIAGNOSTIC

Norm. Negative.

Positive. Current or past infection with *T. spiralis.*

Description. Trichinosis is a parasitic disease caused by the larva of *Trichinella spiralis,* a roundworm acquired in humans by ingestion of raw or poorly cooked pork or other animals it inhabits (cats, dogs, swine, and some wild animals such as walrus and bear). The ingested worm larvae mature and reproduce in the intestinal tract and then migrate through the lymphatic system and bloodstream to other sites in the body. Those reaching muscle tissue become encapsulated as cysts, causing inflammation and necrosis. The symptoms of trichinosis are progressive. Soon after ingestion, hyperpyrexia, gastrointestinal upset, eosinophilia, and muscle edema occur. These symptoms are followed by muscle soreness and may progress to neurotoxicity and myocarditis. This test is based on an immediate hypersensitivity reaction. The presence of *T. spiralis* antibodies is indicated when intradermal injection of the killed larvae of *T. spiralis* produces signs of an antigen-antibody reaction.

Professional Considerations
1. Consent form NOT required.
2. Preparation:
   A. Obtain an alcohol wipe, a 1-mL syringe with an intradermal needle, *T. spiralis* antigen, and a control.

B. Assess for history of recent ingestion of raw pork or poorly cooked pork or other susceptible animals.
3. **Procedure:**
   A. Cleanse the forearm site for injection with an alcohol wipe and allow the area to dry.
   B. Inject *T. spiralis* antigen intradermally. Inject the control into the site in the opposite forearm. Record the sites of injection.
   C. 20 minutes later, observe the injection site for a blanched wheal with surrounding erythema, a symptom of a positive reaction.
4. **Postprocedure care:**
   A. None.
5. **Client and family teaching:**
   A. Before eating it, thoroughly cook pork or meat from other susceptible animals until it turns gray.
   B. In positive tests, the wheal and redness should disappear within a few hours.
6. **Factors that affect results:**
   A. Positive results may also indicate past trichinosis infection.
7. **Other data:**
   A. Injected corticosteroids may help mediate an excessive reaction to the skin test.
   B. See also *Trichinosis serology, Serum.*

TRICHOMONAS PREPARATION, SPECIMEN

Norm. Negative. No *Trichomonas* identified.

Negative. No *Trichomonas* identified.

Positive. Trichomoniasis.

Description. Trichomoniasis is a sexually transmitted protozoan infection of the genitourinary tract. This infection causes considerable foamy, yellow drainage as well as petechiae and vaginal burning and itching in females and a persistent, white urethral discharge or frequently no symptoms in males. The causative organism, *Trichomonas vaginalis*, is transmitted by direct contact with the vaginal and urethral fluids of infected individuals. Diagnosis of trichomoniasis is made by direct microscopic examination of a wet mount of the secretions of infected individuals.

Professional Considerations
1. Consent form NOT required.
2. **Preparation:**
   A. Obtain a speculum, a pipette, a sterile tube to which 1 mL of sterile nonbacteriostatic 0.9% saline has been added, and a sterile swab approved for microbiologic use.
   B. See *Client and family teaching.*
   C. The client should disrobe below the waist for the collection of a vaginal, cervical, or urethral swab.
3. **Procedure:**
   A. *Female: vaginal, cervical, or urethral specimen:*
      i. Place the client in the dorsal lithotomy position and drape her for comfort and privacy.
      ii. For the vaginal specimen, collect it by pipette aspiration from the vaginal pool or by swabbing the circumference of the vagina with a sterile swab. Express the secretions into the sterile tube of saline and cover the tube.
      iii. For the cervical swab, place the speculum over the cervical os and gently express secretions onto the sterile swab. Alternatively, aspirate endocervical secretions through a pipette. Transfer the secretions to the sterile tube of saline and cover the tube.
   B. *Male or female: urethral specimen:*
      i. Insert the cotton-tipped end of sterile swab into the urethral meatus. Rotate the swab and hold it in place for 10 seconds to allow absorption of secretions. Transfer the secretions to the sterile tube of saline and cover the tube.
   C. *Male: prostatic specimens.* Provide privacy for the client.
      i. Instruct the client to stimulate ejaculation by masturbation. The semen should be collected into a clean container. If the client is uncomfortable with masturbation or unable to collect the specimen, it may be collected into a plastic condom at home and brought in within 1 hour. The client should be instructed to empty the condom into a

clean container and cover it tightly to prevent the specimen from drying out.

D. *Urine collection for examination of sediment:*

  i. Instruct the client to cleanse the area surrounding the urethral meatus with four soapy sponges and then to rinse and dry the area.

  ii. While holding the labia open or the foreskin back, the client should void about 20 mL of urine into a clean container and then stop the stream and cap the container.

4. **Postprocedure care:**

A. Write the specimen source and the collection time on the laboratory requisition.

B. Send the specimen to the laboratory immediately.

C. Do not refrigerate the specimen.

5. **Client and family teaching:**

A. For vaginal or cervical specimens, avoid douching for 72 hours.

B. If results are positive, notify any sexual contacts to be tested. Do not have sexual relations until your physician confirms that follow-up testing is negative.

C. Assess the client's knowledge of and teach safe sex practices.

6. **Factors that affect results:**

A. Results are invalidated if the specimen dries before microscopic examination.

B. The test is less sensitive for asymptomatic females. Wet mounts are negative in 30-50% of females positive for *Trichomonas*. Unfortunately, negative microscopy results give false reassurance.

7. **Other data:**

A. Trichomoniasis may be treated with metronidazole.

B. Consider testing for *Chlamydia* and *Neisseria gonorrhoeae* with positive results.

TRICYCLIC ANTIDEPRESSANTS, PLASMA OR SERUM

Norm. Negative.

TRICYCLIC ANTIDEPRESSANT	THERAPEUTIC TROUGH LEVELS	SI UNITS
Amitriptyline	100-250 ng/mL	360-900 nmol/L
Panic level	>400 ng/mL	>1275 nmol/L
Amoxapine	20-100 ng/mL	64-319 nmol/L
Panic level	>500 ng/mL	>1594 nmol/L
Desipramine	150-300 ng/mL	563-1126 nmol/L
Panic level	>400 ng/mL	>1500 nmol/L
Doxepin	50-200 ng/mL	180-720 nmol/L
Panic level	>400 ng/mL	>1440 nmol/L
Imipramine	75-250 ng/mL	279-890 nmol/L
Panic level	>400 ng/mL	>1440 nmol/L
Maprotiline	150-400 ng/mL	541-1442 nmol/L
Panic level	>1000 ng/mL	>3605 nmol/L
Nortriptyline	50-150 ng/mL	190-570 nmol/L
Panic level	>200 ng/mL	>760 nmol/L
Protriptyline	50-150 ng/mL	190-570 nmol/L
Panic level	>400 ng/mL	>1520 nmol/L
Trazodone	300-2500 ng/mL	1000-6000 nmol/L
Panic level	>4000 ng/mL	>9600 nmol/L

Overdose Symptoms and Treatment

Symptoms. Confusion, agitation, hallucinations, seizures, coma, dysrhythmias, hyperthermia, flushing, and dilatation of the pupils; death may occur. Sodium-channel blockade manifesting as early prolonged QRS interval, rightward axis of 40 msec, presence of an R-wave in aV$_R$ lead and an S-wave in leads I and

aV_L. Life-threatening cardiac toxicity or seizures are seen if concentrations are over 1000 ng/mL.

Treatment:

Note:Treatment choice(s) depend on client history and condition and episode history.

Give activated charcoal (multi-dose).

Give bicarbonate 1-2 mmol/kg IV for delayed cardiac conduction or ventricular dysrhythmias, hypotension, reduced level of consciousness, or convulsion. Adjust the dose according to arterial pH and correction of symptoms. Alternatively, hypertonic saline may be used for hypotension.

Administer IV fluids for hypotension. Follow with vasopressor, if needed.

Monitor cardiac pattern for QRS elongation, dysrhythmias, and conduction abnormalities for 72 hours (adults) or 96 hours (children).

Hemodialysis and peritoneal dialysis will NOT remove amitriptyline, desipramine, doxepin, imipramine, nortriptyline, or protryptiline. No information is available on the effectiveness of dialysis in removing amoxapine, maprotiline, and trazodone.

Hemoperfusion will remove amitriptyline.

Provide supportive intervention for lethargy, confusion, hallucinations, urinary retention, hypertension, hyperpyrexia, respiratory depression, and declining level of consciousness.

Usage. Monitoring for therapeutic or toxic levels during tricyclic antidepressant therapy or for toxic levels in attempted suicide.

Description. "Tricyclic antidepressants" is a term describing a group of drugs with similar cyclic chemical structures, frequently used to treat depression on a long-term basis. These drugs act by blocking norepinephrine and serotonin reuptake in the central nervous system and have anticholinergic properties. They are metabolized in the liver, with a variable half-life and peak levels occurring 4-8 hours after an oral dose. Because certain drugs of this group are metabolized to others in the group, the levels of all of them should be measured and considered when one is evaluating clinical symptoms. Therapeutic blood monitoring is important, both because the drugs have a narrow window of therapeutic effectiveness and levels have been shown to correlate poorly with clinical effectiveness. Thus toxicity is a risk when doses are increased to improve clinical symptoms.

Professional Considerations

1. Consent form NOT required.
2. **Preparation:**
   A. Draw specimen 1 week after drug therapy starts in order to assure that the drug has reached steady state.
   B. Tube: Red topped, red/gray topped, or gold topped (for serum); green topped (for plasma).
   C. Samples for amitriptyline, desipramine, doxepin, imipramine, nortriptyline, or protryptiline levels MAY be drawn during hemodialysis. Do NOT draw samples for amoxapine, maprotiline, or trazodone during hemodialysis.
   D. Write the name of the drug ingested (if known) on the laboratory requisition.
3. **Procedure:**
   A. Draw TROUGH blood 10-12 hours after the previous dose. Obtain serial measurements at the same time each day.
   B. Draw a 7-mL blood sample in a syringe. Remove the stopper from either a red-topped, red/gray-topped, or gold-topped tube (for serum), or from a green-topped tube (for plasma), and eject the blood into the tube. Replace the stopper. For a plasma specimen, gently roll the tube several times to mix the blood with the anticoagulant.
4. **Postprocedure care:**
   A. Send the specimen to the laboratory promptly. The serum should be separated within 2 hours, and the sample should be frozen or

refrigerated if not tested promptly.

B. If concurrent monoamine oxidase inhibitors have been ingested, monitor the client for hyperpyrexia and provide convulsion precautions.

5. **Client and family teaching:**

A. It will take 7-21 days of therapy for a steady state to be reached.

B. For overdose, intensive care may be required.

C. For an intentional overdose, refer the client and family for crisis intervention and offer resource information for counseling.

D. Referrals to appropriate rehabilitation centers and therapeutic community programs should be offered to all addicted clients who may be interested.

E. If activated charcoal was given for elevated levels, the client should drink 4-6 glasses of water each day for 2 days to prevent constipation. The activated charcoal will also cause stools to be black for a few days.

F. Cardiac deaths have occurred up to 6 days after an overdose.

6. **Factors that affect results:**

A. Drugs that may cause increased levels include barbiturates, bupropion, cimetidine, corticosteroids, methylphenidate, neuroleptics, oral contraceptives, selective serotonin reuptake inhibitors SSRIs (citalopram, desmethylcitalopram, didesmethylcitalopram, fluoxetine, milnacipran, norfluoxetine, paroxetine, sertraline, venlafaxine), and valproic acid.

B. Drugs that may cause decreased levels include barbiturates, chloral hydrate, glutethimide, nicotine (cigarette smoking), and phenobarbital.

C. Levels for black clients may be as much as 50% higher than that for white clients taking the same-dosage regimen.

D. Toxicity occurs more readily and at lower levels with advancing age as a result of slowed metabolism and also with concomitant phenothiazines

7. **Other data:**

A. Tricyclic antidepressants cause serum glucose to increase and glucose tolerance to decrease. Monitor diabetics for hyperglycemia when using these drugs.

B. Neurotoxicity and cardiotoxicity are less likely to occur with trazodone than with other drugs of this group.

C. Children are more sensitive than adults to toxic effects.

D. When tricyclic antidepressants are taken concurrently with the herb *Pausinystalia yohimbe*, the risk for hypertension is increased.

TRIFLUOPERAZINE
(*see Phenothiazines, Blood*)

TRIGLYCERIDES, BLOOD

Norm:

		SI UNITS
Serum Values		
Adult Females		
20-29 years	10-100 mg/dL	0.11-1.13 mmol/L
30-39 years	10-110 mg/dL	0.11-1.24 mmol/L
40-49 years	10-122 mg/dL	0.11-1.38 mmol/L
50-59 years	10-134 mg/dL	0.11-1.51 mmol/L
>59 years	10-147 mg/dL	0.11-1.66 mmol/L
Adult Males		
20-29 years	10-157 mg/dL	0.11-1.77 mmol/L
30-39 years	10-182 mg/dL	0.11-2.05 mmol/L
40-49 years	10-193 mg/dL	0.11-2.18 mmol/L
50-59 years	10-197 mg/dL	0.11-2.22 mmol/L
>59 years	10-199 mg/dL	0.11-2.24 mmol/L

		SI UNITS
Children		
Female: 1-19 years	10-121 mg/dL	0.11-1.36 mmol/L
Male: 1-19 years	10-103 mg/dL	0.11-1.16 mmol/L

Note: Plasma values are lower by about 3%.

Classification of Triglyceride Levels

Borderline high	200-400 mg/dL	2.3 mmol/L
High	400-1000 mg/dL	4.5-11.3 mmol/L
Very high	>1000 mg/dL	>11.3 mmol/L

Increased. Alcoholism, aortic aneurysm, aortitis, arteriosclerosis, diabetes mellitus, diet (recent high-carbohydrate, prolonged high-fat), familial hypertriglyceridemia, fat embolism, glycogen storage diseases, gout, hepatic cholesterol ester storage disease, hypercholesterolemia, hyperlipoproteinemia, hypothyroidism, metabolic syndrome, myocardial infarction (for up to 1 year), myxedema, nephrotic syndrome, obesity, pancreatitis, pregnancy, renal insufficiency (chronic), starvation (early), stress, Tangier disease, and von Gierke's disease. Tobacco use. Drugs include cholestyramine, corticosteroids, estrogens, ethyl alcohol (ethanol), miconazole (intravenous), oral contraceptives, and spironolactone.

Decreased. Abetalipoproteinemia, acanthocytosis, cirrhosis (portal), chronic obstructive pulmonary disease, hyperalimentation, hyperthyroidism, malabsorption, and malnutrition. Drugs include ascorbic acid, asparaginase, clofibrate, dextrothyroxine, gemfibrozil, heparin, lovastatin, metformin, niacin, phenformin, pravastatin, and sulfonureas. Herbal or natural remedies include *Cordyceps sinensis,* garlic (aged extract taken over time), and soy.

Description. Also known as "fat," triglyceride is a compound consisting of fatty acid or glycerol ester that constitutes a major part (up to 70%) of very-low-density lipoproteins (VLDL) and a small part (<10%) of low-density lipoproteins (LDL) in fasting serum samples. Dietary triglycerides are carried as part of chylomicrons through the lymphatic system and bloodstream to adipose tissue, where they are released for storage. Triglycerides are also synthesized in the liver from fatty acids and from protein and glucose

above the body's current needs and then stored in adipose tissue. They may be later retrieved and formed into glucose through gluconeogenesis when needed by the body. Triglyceride levels are taken into consideration with total cholesterol, high-density lipoprotein cholesterol, and chylomicron levels when categorizing a client's serum into lipoprotein phenotypes that represent genetic lipoprotein abnormalities. Treatments differ for the different phenotypes.

Professional Considerations
1. Consent form NOT required.
2. **Preparation:**
   A. Tube: Red topped, red/gray topped, or gold topped; or lavender topped.
   B. A fasting specimen is preferred.
   C. See *Client and family teaching.*
3. **Procedure:**
   A. Draw a 1-mL blood sample.
4. **Postprocedure care:**
   A. None.
5. **Client and family teaching:**
   A. Avoid variations in diet and weight for 21 days; avoid alcohol and refined carbohydrates for 3 days.
   B. Fast 12 hours before the test. Water is permitted.
6. **Factors that affect results:**
   A. Drugs that may cause falsely elevated results include cholestyramine, estrogens, furosemide, miconazole, and oral contraceptives.
   B. Triglyceride levels for black clients have been demonstrated to be lower than those for white clients.
7. **Other data:**
   A. The "Summary of the second report of the National Cholesterol Education Program (NCEP)

expert panel report on detection, evaluation and treatment of high blood cholesterol in adults," *JAMA* 269:3015-3023, 1993, provides good summary of triglycerides in context with other lipids as well as lipid phenotyping.

B. Metabolic syndrome consists of a group of findings occurring together: general obesity, central obesity, elevated triglycerides, low levels of high-density lipoprotein cholesterol, hyperglycemia and hypertension. This condition is becoming more prevalent and is associated with an increased risk of developing cardiovascular disease and type 2 diabetes.

C. Low-density lipoproteins become morphologically smaller and more dense in the presence of hypertriglyceridemia. This change is associated with an increased risk of atherogenesis.

TRIIODOTHYRONINE, BLOOD
(see Thyroid test: Triiodothyronine, Blood)

TROPONIN I and TROPONIN T (cTnI OR cTnT), SERUM

Norm:

		SI UNITS
Troponin I		
Negative	<0.4 ng/mL	<0.4 µg/L
Indeterminate or suspicious for injury to myocardium	0.5-2.3 ng/mL	0.5-2.3 µg/L
Positive for myocardial injury	>2.3 ng/mL	>2.3 µg/L
Troponin T	<0.1 ng/L	<0.1 µg/L

Ranges vary according to the specific method and technology used.

Usage. Confirmation of acute myocardial infarction, including extent; Indicator of reperfusion after treatment with thrombolytic therapy.

Increased Troponin I. Acute myocardial infarction, angina, coronary syndromes, electrical countershock, myocarditis.

Increased Troponin T. Acute myocardial infarction, angina, heart failure, muscle damage, renal failure. A hypothesis exists in the literature that increases may possibly be a marker for ruptured plaques and severe coronary artery disease.

Description. Cardiac troponin I is a subunit of the actin-myosin complex contractile protein of the myofibril manufactured only in the myocardium. Troponin-T and cardiac-specific troponin-I are two isoforms that leak into the bloodstream during myocardial necrosis. Because of the low-to-undetectable values in the serum of healthy people and the quick elevation (detectable within 1 hour after myocardial cell injury), these ultrasensitive markers have been praised for their usefulness in the early diagnosis of acute myocardial infarction (MI), especially in the detection of silent MIs and microinfarctions and in the case of chest pain not accompanied by typical electrocardiogram changes. Both tests show similar accuracy in identifying acute myocardial injury. Some studies have found an even correlation between the degree of elevation of troponin I and T and the severity and extent of coronary lesions, angina, and ECG changes, and thus these values may be useful in predicting outcome for cardiac conditions. Some research has found that troponin levels are predictive of later intracoronary thrombus and obstruction in the distal microvasculature. Troponin-T has been found to be an independent predictor of outcome for chronic hemodialysis patients. Newer ultrasensitive tests for measurement of both types of troponin are available.

Professional Considerations
1. Consent form NOT required.
2. **Preparation:**
   A. Tube: Red topped, green topped, or lavender topped.
3. **Procedure:**
   A. Draw a 5-mL blood sample.
4. **Postprocedure care:**
   A. None.
5. **Client and family teaching:**
   A. Results are normally available within 4 hours.
6. **Factors that affect results:**
   A. It is not yet known definitively whether troponins can also be found in myocardial ischemia or strain, but levels have been found to be elevated in the absence of myocardial necrosis when other diseases, such as septic shock, renal failure, pulmonary embolism, and arterial hypertension are present.
7. **Other data:**
   A. The only FDA-approved test has a 90-minute turnaround time, a bit slow for triage purposes in an emergency room.
   B. The troponin-I assay costs less than the troponin-T assay.
   C. The American College of Emergency Physicians recommends that the cause of acute myocardial infarction should not be ruled out for chest pain unless a repeat CK-MB taken 6-10 hours after the onset of symptoms and a repeat troponin I and T taken 8-12 hours after the onset of symptoms are both negative.

TRUS
(see Prostate ultrasonography, Diagnostic)

TRYPANOSOMIASIS SEROLOGIC TEST (CHAGAS' DISEASE SEROLOGIC TEST), BLOOD

Norm. Negative titer.

Positive. American trypanosomiasis (Chagas' disease).

Description. American trypanosomiasis, also known as "Chagas' disease," is endemic in Latin America, and whose cause is thought to be either autoimmune or parasitic. Symptoms may include central nervous system (CNS) changes, CNS lesions in immunocompromised clients, and meningoencephalitis in children. The course of the disease may run months to years and is frequently fatal. Serologic testing is useful after the acute stage of the disease, when blood films are not very sensitive. Serologic tests have good sensitivity but lack specificity for detection of Chagas' disease. Newer molecular assays based on the polymerase chain reaction hold promise for more specific testing.

Professional Considerations
1. Consent form NOT required.
2. **Preparation:**
   A. Tube: Red topped, red/gray topped, or gold topped.
   B. Obtain a container of ice.
   C. Specimens MAY be drawn during hemodialysis.
3. **Procedure:**
   A. Draw a 5-mL blood sample. Place the tube on ice.
4. **Postprocedure care:**
   A. Write the name of the suspected parasite and the place and date of recent travel on the laboratory requisition.
5. **Client and family teaching:**
   A. Results may not be available for several days because testing is performed by the Centers for Disease Control and Prevention (Atlanta) or sent to a parasitology laboratory.
6. **Factors that affect results:**
   A. Reject specimens that are not frozen.
7. **Other data:**
   A. Transmission of American trypanosomiasis is possible by transfusion of contaminated blood to immunocompromised clients.
   B. Drugs used for treatment of Chagas' disease include nitrofurans and nitroimidazoles. For clients with immunosuppression, the nitroimidazoles benznidazole has been used.
   C. Staging of Chagas' disease is done via examination of cerebrospinal fluid 2, after serologic diagnosis has been confirmed.
   D. See also *African trypanosomiasis, Blood; Parasite screen, Blood.*

TRYPSIN, PLASMA OR SERUM

Norm:

BEHRINGWERKE ANTIBODY METHOD

Young adult 18-36 years	185-272 µg/L
Middle adult 37-66 years	185-272 µg/L
Older adult >66 years	147-1438 µg/L

IMMUNOREACTIVE (CATIONIC) TRYPSIN BY RIA METHOD

Adults	16.7-32.3 µg/L

RIA DOUBLE-ANTIBODY (GEOKAS'S) METHOD

Adults	22.2-44.4 µg/L
Children	
Cord	21.4-25.2 µg/L
<6 months	25.9-36.7 µg/L
6-12 months	30.2-44.0 µg/L
1-3 years	28.0-31.6 µg/L
3-5 years	25.1-31.5 µg/L
5-7 years	32.1-39.3 µg/L
7-10 years	32.7-37.1 µg/L

SORIN ANTIBODY METHOD

Adults	5.0-85.0 µg/L
Children	11.1-51.3 µg/L

Increased. Beta-thalassemia, chronic renal failure, cystic fibrosis (initial years), hepatic disease, malnutrition (acute), pancreatitis (acute), pancreatic viral infection, peptic ulcer disease, and recent endoscopic retrograde cholangiopancreatography. Drugs include bombesin, cerulein, cholecystokinin, and secretin.

Decreased. Beta-thalassemia, cystic fibrosis (advanced), diabetes mellitus, malnutrition (chronic), pancreatic cancer, and pancreatitis (chronic).

Description. Trypsin is a proteolytic enzyme produced in the pancreas in the precursor form of inactive trypsinogen. Trypsinogen is converted to trypsin in the duodenum by enterokinase. Trypsin exists in several forms in the bloodstream. One form includes a trypsinogen that is bound to alpha-antitrypsin, another to alpha-macroglobulin, and a third as free trypsin. During the initial years of cystic fibrosis, serum trypsin levels are elevated as a result of pancreatic cell destruction and liberation of trypsin into the bloodstream. Over time, pancreatic insufficiency leads to abnormally low trypsin levels. Because of the possibility of overlap with normal values as pancreatic function declines, the value of this test is limited when one is diagnosing cystic fibrosis. Elevations reflect either pancreatic damage or impairment or organs involved in its clearance. Trypsin is believed to play a role in activating the complement cascade.

Professional Considerations
1. Consent form NOT required.
2. Preparation:
   A. Tube: Red topped, red/gray topped, or gold topped (serum sample), or green topped (plasma sample).
   B. Specimens MAY be drawn during hemodialysis.
   C. See *Client and family teaching.*
3. Procedure:
   A. Draw a 7-mL blood sample.
4. Postprocedure care:
   A. Transport the specimen to the laboratory and refrigerate it at 4° C or freeze it at −20° C until testing.

5. **Client and family teaching:**
   A. Fast from food for 8 hours before the test.
6. **Factors that affect results:**
   A. Levels are elevated in nonfasting samples.
   B. Trypsin levels demonstrate a diurnal variation, with the highest levels occurring during the late evening.
   C. Because of the problem of wide variability in trypsin norms, values should be compared to the norms of the laboratory performing the test.
   D. Values are not affected by hemodialysis.
7. **Other data:**
   A. Sensitivity is 90%; false-negative rate is approximately 7%.
   B. For elevated immunoreactive trypsin levels, refer clients for confirmatory sweat testing.

TRYPSIN, STOOL

Norm. Positive.

Gelatin digestion	2+ to 4+
≤1 year	Positive at dilutions >1:80
>1 year	Positive at dilutions >1:40
Cystic fibrosis	Negative at dilutions >1:10

Negative. Cystic fibrosis (advanced), insufficiency, and malabsorption in children, pancreatic (chronic).

Description. Trypsin is a proteolytic enzyme produced in the pancreas in the precursor form of inactive trypsinogen. Trypsinogen is converted to trypsin in the duodenum by enterokinase. Trypsin is present in the stool of young children but amounts lessen in older children and adults as a result of intestinal bacterial destruction of trypsin. In clients with pancreatic insufficiency, stool trypsin tests are negative. One performs this test by observing the digestive activity of serial dilutions of stool or duodenal fluid on the gelatin of unexposed radiographic film after incubation. A negative result necessitates test repetition on at least two more stool samples.

Professional Considerations
1. Consent form NOT required.
2. **Preparation:**
   A. Obtain a tongue blade and a clean container.
   B. See *Client and family teaching.*
3. **Procedure:**
   A. Obtain a dime-sized sample of stool and place it in a covered, dry, clean container.
4. **Postprocedure care:**
   A. Send the specimen to the laboratory promptly. The specimen must be tested within 2 hours.
5. **Client and family teaching:**
   A. Defecate in a bedpan. For infants the stool sample may be taken from a diaper.
   B. Avoid laxatives or barium procedures the week before the specimen collection.
6. **Factors that affect results:**
   A. The stool from constipated samples may produce false-negative results because of the extended time allowed for intestinal bacteria to destroy trypsin.
   B. False-positive results may be caused by the presence of bacterial proteases in the sample.
7. **Other data:**
   A. See also *Trypsin, Serum.*

TRYPSINOGEN-2, URINE

Norm. Negative or <50 ng/mL.

Positive (≥50 ng/mL). Possible pancreatitis.

Description. Trypsinogen is a pancreatic proteinase with two main isoenzymes, 1 and 2. The pancreas secretes these in high concentrations in pancreatic fluid, with much smaller concentrations appearing in the serum. Trypsinogens, being small in size, are usually readily filtered through the glomeruli. The kidney has a much higher reabsorption of trypsinogen 1, thus leaving trypsinogen-2 concentration higher in the urine. In people with acute pancreatitis the trypsinogen-2 level in the urine will dramatically increase. This test can be used as a rapid screening of patients with possible acute pancreatitis, thus avoiding a costly acute abdomen work-up.

Professional Considerations

1. Consent form NOT required.
2. Preparation:
   A. See *Client and family teaching*.
   B. Obtain a clean container for urine sample.
3. Procedure:
   A. Obtain a 5-10 mL clean-catch or catheter urine sample.
4. Postprocedure care:
   A. Send specimen to the laboratory within 1 hour.
5. Client and family teaching:
   A. Instruct client on proper technique for clean-catch specimen.

B. Test is a quick 3-minute dipstick test, and so results will be immediately available.
C. Clients with positive results will likely be referred for further testing.

6. Factors that affect results:
   A. Extremely high concentrations of trypsinogen-2 in the urine might result in a false-negative reading.
   B. Trypsinogen-2 is present in the epithelium cells of the bile ducts and peribiliary glands. Inflammation in these structures may cause a positive result that is attributable not to pancreatitis but to cholangitis.
7. Other data:
   A. Dipstick kits for point-of-care testing are available.

TRYPTOPHAN, PLASMA

Norm:

		SI UNITS
Adults	0.51-1.49 mg/dL	25-73 μmol/L
Infants (First Day of Life)		
Premature	0.32-0.92 mg/dL	15-45 μmol/L
Full-term	0.51-1.49 mg/dL	25-73 μmol/L

Increased. Sepsis and tryptophanuria.

Decreased. Blue-diaper syndrome (tryptophan malabsorption syndrome), carcinoid syndrome, Hartnup's disease, hypothermia, kwashiorkor, and postoperative abdominal surgery (first 48 hours). Drugs include alclofenac, aspirin, glucose, and indomethacin.

Description. Tryptophan is an essential amino acid that functions as a precursor for serotonin and niacin. Some tryptophan also occurs naturally in the body. Tryptophan metabolism involves action by the enzyme tryptophan pyrrolase. Tryptophanuria is an inherited, X-linked trait in which an enzyme, tryptophan pyrrolase, is deficient. The resulting accumulation of nonmetabolized tryptophan results in elevated serum levels as well as tryptophan excretion in the urine after renal reabsorption sites for tryptophan become

saturated. Symptoms of tryptophanuria include dwarfism, photosensitivity, and ataxia. In blue-diaper syndrome, an autosomal recessive trait, intestinal absorption of tryptophan is impaired. Dietary tryptophan is broken down into indoles and excreted in the stool, where they are hydrolyzed to the blue-tinged pigment indigo blue. Other symptoms of blue-diaper syndrome include hypercalcemia, growth defects, nephrocalcinosis, and frequent infections. This test aids diagnosis of these two genetic traits.

Professional Considerations

1. Consent form NOT required.
2. Preparation:
   A. Tube: Heparinized, green-topped tube.
   B. Obtain a container of ice water.
   C. Specimens MAY be drawn during hemodialysis.
   D. See *Client and family teaching*.

3. **Procedure:**
   A. Draw a 7-mL blood sample. Place the tube immediately in a container of ice water.
4. **Postprocedure care:**
   A. Send specimens to the laboratory promptly. Plasma should be separated and frozen within 60 minutes of collection.
5. **Client and family teaching:**
   A. Fast for 8 hours before the test.
6. **Factors that affect results:**
   A. A delay in sample separation and freezing over 1 hour invalidates the results.
7. **Other data:**
   A. Dietary supplementation of tryptophan is associated with an eosinophilia-myalgia syndrome, which includes myalgia, arthralgia, fatigue, rash, hair loss, edema, impaired motion of the joints, muscle cramping, and paresthesias as well as several laboratory value abnormalities.
   B. Tryptophan levels have been found to be higher, and serotonin levels have been found to be lower, in the plasma of violent offenders.

TRYPTOPHAN-RICH PREALBUMIN
(see Transthyretin, Serum)

T-SCAN
(see Mammography, Diagnostic)

TSBab
(see Thyroid receptor antibody, Blood)

TSH ASSAY
(see Thyroid-stimulating hormone, Sensitive assay, Blood)

TTR
(see Transthyretin, Serum)

T-TUBE CHOLANGIOGRAPHY, POSTOPERATIVE, DIAGNOSTIC

Norm. Even filling of the biliary ductal system. Absence of strictures, obstruction, calculi, abnormal pathways, or delays in emptying.

Usage. Evaluation of biliary ducts after gallbladder surgery or liver transplantation.

Description. T-tube cholangiography is the instillation of radiographic contrast medium through a T-tube (percutaneously inserted, T-shaped, bile duct drainage tube), followed by fluoroscopic examination of the biliary ducts. Use of intraoperative cholangiography minimizes the number of biliary calculi remaining after surgery, but up to 3% of surgeries miss some calculi, and bile duct damage, resulting in strictures, can result. Because of this possibility, T-tube cholangiography is usually performed 7-10 days after exploratory gallbladder or duct surgery or cholecystectomy for the purpose of evaluating duct patency and identifying any remaining stones or further ductal obstruction. Biliary duct obstruction or anastomotic leakage is also possible after liver transplantation, thus a T tube is also placed after this type of surgery. If retained stones are identified, the T tube is left in place because this is the route of choice for removal of the remaining stones. Four to 6 weeks are required for the sinus tract surrounding the T tube to be well healed before percutaneous removal of remaining stones.

Professional Considerations
1. Consent form IS required.

Risks
Allergic reaction to dye (itching, hives, rash, tight feeling in the throat, shortness of breath, anaphylaxis, death); renal toxicity from contrast medium.

Contraindications
Previous allergy to iodine, shellfish, or radiographic dye; pregnancy (because of the radioactive iodine crossing the blood-placental barrier); renal insufficiency.

2. **Preparation:**
   A. A cleansing enema may be prescribed.
   B. Have emergency equipment readily available.

C. The T tube may be clamped for 24 hours before the procedure.

D. See *Client and family teaching.*

3. **Procedure:**
   A. The client is positioned supine.
   B. Local anesthesia may be injected around the T-tube site if the site is inflamed and painful.
   C. After the T tube is cleansed with 70% alcohol, radiographic contrast medium is instilled through the tube via a large-caliber catheter.
   D. Fluoroscopic radiographs are taken in a variety of positions to track dye progress through the biliary duct system. Upright films are taken to detect inadvertent injection of air through the T tube.
   E. The procedure is concluded with films of contrast medium emptying into the duodenum. Delays in emptying prolong the procedure, which normally takes less than ½ hour.
   F. If findings are normal, the T tube is removed, and a dry, sterile dressing is applied to the site.

4. **Postprocedure care:**
   A. If the T tube has been removed, assess the site for redness, edema, pain, or drainage every hour × 4 and then every 4 hours until 24 hours after removal. A T tube left in place should be reconnected to drainage.
   B. Assess for allergic reaction to the dye (listed above) for 24 hours.
   C. Resume previous diet.

5. **Client and family teaching:**
   A. Fast from food and fluids for 6 hours before the procedure.

6. **Factors that affect results:**
   A. Inadvertent injection of air may cause bubbles that look like biliary calculi. One may differentiate these by observing for movement when the client is positioned upright. Calculi move down with gravity, whereas air bubbles rise.

7. **Other data:**
   A. This procedure uses a low-dilution or high-dilution iodine contrast medium. A low-dilution medium requires longer x-ray exposure than a high-dilution medium does.
   B. The administration of morphine sulfate 0.05 mg/kg intravenously preoperatively may result in spasm of the ampulla of Vater and

duodenum, resulting in improved quality of cholangiography.

C. Routine antibiotic prophylaxis after procedure is not necessary under selected conditions.

D. See also, *Magnetic resonance cholangiopancreatography, Diagnostic.*

TUBERCULIN SKIN TEST (TB), DIAGNOSTIC
(see Mantoux skin test, Diagnostic)

TUBERCULOSIS TEST
(see Mantoux skin test, Diagnostic)

TULAREMIA AGGLUTININS, SERUM

Norm. <1:40. Current or past tularemia infection: >1:80.

Positive. A fourfold rise in titer is considered diagnostic of *Francisella tularensis* infection.

Negative. Normal finding. May also occur the first few days after infection.

Description. Tularemia is a highly-contagious, serious infectious disease caused by the organism *F. tularensis,* which inhabits wild animals such as rabbits, muskrats, beavers, and some domestic animals such as cats as well as ticks and deerflies. The pneumonic aerosolized form of disease is considered a biological weapon and can cause respiratory collapse and death. The mode of transmission is through direct contact of human skin or mucous membranes with the blood, tissue, or lesions of infected animals; ingestion of poorly cooked, infected animal meat; or through the bite of infected ticks. Airborne transmission is also possible from contaminated dust. Tularemia infection causes ulceration, lymph node edema, headache, pharyngeal inflammation, or pneumonia in humans 2-10 days after exposure. After infection, antibody levels begin rising within 7-21 days, peak in 60-90 days, and then decline over several months to higher-than-normal levels. Titers at peak antibody levels are as high as 1:640. This test is a febrile agglutinin test.

Professional Considerations
1. Consent form NOT required.
2. Preparation:
   A. Tube: Red topped, red/gray topped, or gold topped.
   B. This test should be drawn before skin testing for tularemia.
3. Procedure:
   A. Draw a 5-mL blood sample without hemolysis. Draw the first sample about 1 week after suspected exposure, and repeat the test every 3-5 days to observe for rising titers.
4. Postprocedure care:
   A. None.
5. Client and family teaching:
   A. If routinely handling wild animals (such as skinning rabbits), wear gloves and goggles during contact, and thoroughly cook any wild animal meat to be ingested.
   B. Serial testing is required to interpret the results.
6. Factors that affect results:
   A. Hemolysis of the specimen invalidates the results.
   B. False-positive results may occur in the presence of *Brucella abortus* or *Proteus vulgaris* (OX-19) with the Weil-Felix agglutination test.
   C. False-negative results may occur when the specimen is drawn early in the infective process.
   D. False-positive results may occur if skin testing for tularemia has been performed within the previous 7 days.
   E. Microagglutination testing has been shown to be more specific and faster than traditional tube agglutination testing for tularemia serodiagnosis.
7. Other data:
   A. Avoid contact with open lesions of clients suspected of having tularemia.
   B. If present, lesions should be cultured for *F. tularensis.*
   C. Streptomycin, tetracyclines, gentamicin, and chloramphenicol are used to treat tularemia.

TULAREMIA SKIN TEST, DIAGNOSTIC

Norm. Negative. No redness, induration, or wheal.

Positive. Current or past infection with *Francisella tularensis.*

Negative. Normal finding. May also occur the first few days after infection.

Description. Tularemia is an infectious disease caused by the organism *F. tularensis,* which inhabits wild animals such as rabbits, muskrats, beavers, squirrels, and some domestic animals as well as ticks and deerflies. The mode of transmission is through direct contact of human skin or mucous membranes with the blood, tissue, or lesions of infected animals; ingestion of poorly cooked, infected animal meat; or through the bite of infected ticks. Airborne transmission is also possible from contaminated dust. Tularemia infection causes ulceration, lymph node edema, headache, pharyngeal inflammation, or pneumonia in humans 2-10 days after exposure. After infection, antibody levels begin rising within 7-21 days, peak in 60-90 days, and then decline over several months to higher-than-normal levels. After recovery, lifetime immunity exists. The Foshay skin test for tularemia is based on a delayed hypersensitivity reaction. Results will be positive for clients with current infection of at least 7 days or for up to 5 years after recovery.

Professional Considerations
1. Consent form NOT required.
2. Preparation:
   A. Obtain a 1-mL syringe with an intradermal needle and purified *F. tularensis* antigen.
3. Procedure:
   A. Cleanse the forearm site for injection with an alcohol wipe and allow the area to dry.
   B. Inject *F. tularensis* antigen, derived from culture, intradermally.
   C. Record the site of injection.
   D. Inspect the injection site in 48 hours. Reaction is positive if redness and induration of >5 mm diameter are present at the site.
4. Postprocedure care:
   A. Let the site air-dry.
5. Client and family teaching:
   A. If routinely handling wild animals (such as skinning rabbits), wear gloves and goggles during contact, and thoroughly cook any wild animal meat to be ingested.

B. Return in 48 hours to have the injection site viewed and the skin test interpreted.
6. **Factors that affect results:**
   A. False-negative results may occur during the first week after infection as a result of insufficient antibody formation. If tularemia is suspected, the test should be repeated in 1 week.
7. **Other data:**
   A. If serum testing for tularemia agglutinins is to be done, it should be performed before this test.

TUMOR ANTIGEN 4 (TA-4) AND SUB-FRACTION SCC-ANTIGEN, BLOOD AND SPECIMEN

Norm. TA-4 norms not available. Consult reference range provided with test results.

Sub-fraction SCC-antigen Norm. SCC-antigen range from 1.5-2.5 ng/mL.

Usage. Levels correlate with certain squamous cell carcinoma disease progression and response to treatment, and also as a prognostic indicator for the disease.

Increased TA-4. Squamous cell carcinomas (cervix, esophagus, lungs, head, neck, penis).

Increased Sub-Fraction SCC-Antigen. Higher levels of SCC-antigen after treatment (especially 8 ng/mL or above) indicate progression of the carcinoma.

Increased Sub-Fraction SCC-Antigen. Cervical squamous cell carcinoma.

Decreased Sub-Fraction SCC-Antigen. Decreasing levels of previously-elevated SCC antigen are evident after irradiation.

Description. A glycoprotein eutopic antigen present in squamous epithelium that is related to squamous cell differentiation. TA-4 is not released in high amounts by normal squamous epithelium, but is secreted in progressively increasing amounts by squamous cell

carcinomas as they develop. Research studies have indicated that the release of TA-4 antigen into the serum is greatly influenced by the infiltrative growth, the size of the mass, and the degree of histologic differentiation of the tumor. A sub-fraction, sometimes referred to as the "squamous cell carcinoma antigen" (SCC-antigen), is specific for cervical cancer. This carbohydrate antigen is produced and released from the CaSki cell line of an epidermoid uterine cervix carcinoma. TA-4 can help pinpoint cancer via detection in biopsies, and can also be measured from the bloodstream as more TA-4 circulates when cancer progresses.

Professional Considerations
1. Consent form NOT required.
2. **Preparation:**
   A. Tube: Red topped or serum separator (red/gray or gold topped)
3. **Procedure:**
   A. Collect a 3-mL blood sample.
   B. Refrigerate specimen.
4. **Postprocedure care:**
   A. None.
5. **Client and family teaching:**
   A. This test is not used for early screening for SCCs.
   B. This test is mainly used to evaluate the extent or prognosis of the disease and effectiveness of the treatments. Results may also indicate early recurrent disease after a period of time following initial treatment.
   C. Results are normally available within 3-7 working days.
6. **Factors that affect results:**
   A. Levels are higher when the cancer is well differentiated than earlier in the disease course.
   B. Two methods can be used to detect serum TA-4: conventional radioimmunoassay (RIA) using a polyclonal antibody approach or the immunoradiometric assay (IRMA) using two monoclonal antibodies. Both methods provide essentially the same results but the IRMA appears to have a greater sensitivity and accuracy in detecting TA-4 in SCC of all organs, thus decreasing the level of false positives in healthy tissues.
   C. Due to the origin of TA-4 antigen, interference with the reliability of

the antigen as a tumor marker for SCC can occur with preexisting inflammatory skin disease or hyperkeratosis skin disease with an inflammatory component.

7. **Other data:**
A. Survival rate or prediction of a disease-free state in those individuals who have levels of TA-4 greater than or equal to 15 µU/mL was worse compared to lower levels. Prognosis was particularly poor in individuals who had TA-4 levels of ≥15 µU/mL; coupled with a lymphocyte percentage of ≤30. Researchers strongly suggested the usefulness of simultaneously determining serum TA-4 levels and lymphocyte percentages in predicting the prognosis of cervical squamous cell carcinoma.

TUMOR-ASSOCIATED GLYCOPROTEIN 72, BLOOD
(see CA 72-4, Blood)

TUNING FORK TEST, OF WEBER, RINNE, AND SCHWABACH TESTS, DIAGNOSTIC

Norm:
Weber's test: The tone is heard equally well in both ears.
Rinne's test: The tone is heard twice as long by air conduction (AC) as by bone conduction (BC).
Schwabach's test: The tone is heard for the same length of time by both the client and the examiner.

Usage. Assists in the differential diagnosis of conduction and perceptive or sensorineural hearing loss, hearing disorders, and tinnitus.

Description. The Weber, Rinne, and Schwabach tests are three simple tuning-fork hearing tests.
Weber's test helps determine whether hearing loss is the result of conductive or sensorineural causes. In clients with normal hearing, a vibrating tuning fork positioned midline on the skull is heard equally well by both ears. However, in conductive hearing loss, the tone seems loudest in the affected ear, but, in sensorineural hearing loss, the tone seems loudest in the unaffected ear.

Rinne's test also helps differentiate conductive from sensorineural hearing loss by comparing the duration of tone perception by bone conduction to the duration of tone perception by air conduction. In a client with normal hearing, a vibrating tuning fork that can no longer be heard by bone conduction can still be heard by air conduction for twice as long. Conductive hearing loss may be secondary to blocked pathways of sound conduction in the middle or external ear, thus bone conduction will be longer than air conduction (BC > AC). Perceptive or sensorineural loss may be secondary to inner ear disease or vestibulocochlear (eighth cranial nerve) disorders; thus air conduction will be longer than bone conduction (AC > BC) but not so high as the 2:1 ratio expected in normal clients.

The *Schwabach test* helps evaluate bone conduction by comparing the length of time the client hears a tuning fork placed against his or her mastoid process with the length of time it is heard by a client with normal hearing.

Professional Considerations
1. Consent form NOT required.
2. **Preparation:**
A. Obtain a low-frequency tuning fork of 256-512 Hz.
B. The test should take place in a quiet room, free of noise and visual distractions.
3. **Procedure:**
A. *Weber's test:*
i. The examiner sets the tuning fork into light vibration by pinching the prongs between the thumb and index finger or by tapping it on his or her own knuckles.
ii. The tuning fork is placed on the skull at the midpoint or on the maxillary incisors.
iii. The client is asked to state whether the sound can be heard better in one ear than the other and, if so, to state which ear hears the tone more loudly.
B. *Rinne's test:*
i. The examiner sets the tuning fork into light vibration by pinching the prongs between the thumb and index finger or

by tapping it on his or her own knuckles.

ii. The ear not being tested should be masked from detecting sound by bone conduction by providing a sound stimulus into it during step B-iii.

iii. The vibrating fork is held by its stem on the mastoid process of the ear until vibration is no longer heard by the client.

iv. The fork is then held close to the external auditory meatus (within 2.5 cm of the pinna). If the client still hears the vibrations, this is called a positive Rinne's test. If the fork is not heard by air conduction, the test is repeated, but air conduction is first tested until the sound is no longer heard, and then the stem of the fork is placed on the mastoid process of the ear. If the sound is still heard, this is called a negative Rinne's test.

C. Schwabach's test:

i. The examiner sets the tuning fork into light vibration by pinching the prongs between the thumb and index finger or by tapping it on his or her own knuckles.

ii. The ear not being tested should be masked from detecting sound by bone conduction by providing a sound stimulus into it during step C-iii.

iii. The vibrating fork is held by its stem on the mastoid process of the client, who is instructed to indicate whether the tone is heard. Each time he or she hears the tone, the tuning fork is quickly transferred to the mastoid process of the examiner, who listens for the tone. This process continues back and forth between the client and the examiner until the tone is no longer heard by one of them, and the results are recorded. The process is then repeated in the other ear.

4. **Postprocedure care:**
   A. None.

5. **Client and family teaching:**
   A. Testing is noninvasive and can take up to 15 minutes.
   B. Thorough audiologic testing is indicated if results are abnormal.

6. **Factors that affect results:**
   A. The examiner should strike the tuning fork with equal intensity for each repetition of the tests.
   B. For the Schwabach test, the examiner must have normal hearing for the results to be meaningful.

7. **Other data:**
   A. None.

TUTTLE TEST
(see Esophageal acidity test, Diagnostic)

TYPE-AND-CROSSMATCH, BLOOD

Norm. Recipient blood type is determined to be either type A, B, O, or AB, and either Rh positive or Rh negative. Antibodies present in the recipient sample and donor blood are identified. Recipient and donor samples are mixed and observed for antigen-antibody reactions.

Usage. Determination of compatibility of recipient and donor blood before blood-product transfusion.

Description. The type-and-crossmatch technique includes a series of procedures designed to identify donor blood that may be potentially safe to transfuse into a particular recipient with the lowest possible risk of causing a hemolytic reaction. The ABO group and Rh type of the recipient's blood sample is first determined. Donor blood of the same ABO blood group and Rh type is then chosen for further testing before transfusion. General antibody screening (indirect Coombs' testing) is then performed on both recipient and donor blood. If antibody screening is positive, more specific antibody identification is performed to determine the specific nature of irregular antibodies, which may cause a transfusion reaction. One identifies the exact antibody by combining the recipient or donor serum with a panel of red blood cell samples, each containing a known antigen, and observing for antigen-antibody reactions. Finally, recipient and donor blood samples are combined (crossmatched) and observed for antigen-antibody reactions that may cause a transfusion reaction. Newer techniques substitute a computerized crossmatch procedure. If no such reaction occurs, the donor blood is considered to be compatible for transfusion into the recipient. Absence of antigen-antibody reaction during crossmatching decreases but does not completely eliminate the possibility of a hemolytic transfusion reaction.

Professional Considerations
1. Consent form NOT required.
2. **Preparation:**
   A. Tube: Red topped, red/gray topped, or gold topped AND lavender topped. Also obtain a 30-mL syringe; a blood band (if required); two labels, stamped with the client's addressograph plate; and blood.
   B. Note the client's age, medications, past transfusions of blood products, and number of pregnancies on the laboratory requisition.
   C. Consult institutional protocol for any additional requirements.
   D. Do NOT draw specimens during hemodialysis.
3. **Procedure:**
   A. The entire procedure should be performed by the person who performs the venipuncture.
   B. Ask the client to state his or her full name and social security number. Verify that this information matches the client's wrist identification band and addressograph stamp on the blood bank requisition and labels.
   C. Some institutions use blood bands as an extra precaution to validate the proper recipient:
      i. Write the client's name, social security number, and hospital number and the date on the blood band, and place the band on the client's wrist, cutting off the distal end of the number stickers.
      ii. Write the blood band number on both addressograph labels, and place a label on each tube. Alternatively, place addressograph labels on each

tube, and place a number sticker from the blood band on each tube.
      iii. Place a blood band number sticker on the blood bank requisition.
   D. Do NOT draw specimens from an extremity into which blood or dextran is infusing. Draw a 25-mL blood sample, without hemolysis, in a 30-mL syringe. Completely fill the red-topped tube and the lavender-topped tube with the sample.
   E. The caregiver performing this procedure should initial the following after drawing the blood: the blood band (if used), the label on each tube, and the blood bank requisition.
   F. Staple the remaining blood band number stickers (if used) to the requisition.
4. **Postprocedure care:**
   A. Send both tubes with the requisition and blood band number stickers (if used) to the blood bank.
   B. Testing must be performed within 48 hours of specimen collection.
5. **Client and family teaching:**
   A. Screening for antibodies may take longer, up to several hours, if initial screening is positive.
   B. Type-and-crossmatches are good for only 72 hours because of the possibility of the recipient developing irregular antibodies in response to a recent blood transfusion.
   C. A type-and-crossmatch takes approximately 1 hour to complete.
6. **Factors that affect results:**
   A. Hemolysis of the specimen invalidates the results.
   B. Drugs causing a false-positive Rh test include levodopa, methyldopa, and methyldopate hydrochloride.
7. **Other data:**
   A. A type-and-screen involves only the ABO group and Rh-type determinations and the general antibody screening. It is sometimes prescribed instead of a type-and-crossmatch if there is only a small possibility of the client needing blood or if the blood must be transfused in an emergency. Donor blood should

not be transfused if the general antibody screen is positive.

B. Identification of cold-reacting antibodies reactive at 30°C may require the use of a blood warmer during transfusion.

C. See also *ABO group and Rh type, Blood; Antibody identification, Red blood cell, Blood; Coombs' test, Indirect, Serum.*

TYPHUS TITER, BLOOD
(see Bacterial serology, Blood and Weil-Felix agglutinins, Blood)

TZANCK SMEAR, SPECIMEN

Norm. Absence of multinucleated giant cells.

Usage. Helps diagnose viral infections in which blistering vesicles are present.

Description. The Tzanck smear is a rapid and sensitive inexpensive staining technique that can confirm the presence of herpes simplex virus or varicella zoster virus by examination of the morphology of cells present in fluid from the vesicles. Both viruses contain multinucleated giant cells, which can be seen under a microscope with this staining technique. The Tzanck smear cannot differentiate the type of virus present.

Professional Considerations
1. Consent form NOT required.
2. Preparation:
   A. Obtain scalpel blade, matches, and 3-4 glass slides.
3. Procedure:
   A. Using a scalpel, carefully and gently rupture the surface of the vesicle. Using the curved edge of the scalpel blade, scrape the soft (mushy) epidermis from the base of the vesicle and smear it onto a glass slide.
   B. Light a match and hold it under the slide for about 10 seconds to "fix" the specimen. Repeat on 2-3 additional vesicles.
   C. Add Giemsa, PAP or Wright's stain to the slide. Wait 1 minute, and then rinse under water.

D. Add immersion oil and a cover slip and examine under microscope.
4. Postprocedure care:
   A. Gently blot vesicle with sterile gauze. Leave site open to air.
5. Client and family teaching:
   A. The test may cause mild discomfort, but it will be brief.
   B. It is important to prevent transferring the virus to others when vesicles are present. Keep your hands away from the vesicles, use careful handwashing, and avoid skin-to-skin contact with other people when vesicles are present or moist or draining.
6. Factors that affect results:
   A. Several samples may be needed to locate the multinucleated giant cells.
7. Other data:
   A. Tzanck smear staining can also identify noninfectious pustular eruptions by the presence of eosinophils and neutrophils.

UBT
(see Urea breath test, Diagnostic)

UDS
(see Toxicology, Drug screen, Urine)

UFP, DIAGNOSTIC
(see Papanicolaou smear, Ultrafast and Fine-needle aspiration, Diagnostic)

UGI, DIAGNOSTIC
(see Upper gastrointestinal series, Diagnostic)

UGP, URINE
(see Urinary chorionic gonadotropin peptide, Urine)

ULCERATIVE LESIONS, CULTURE
(see Body fluid, Routine, Culture; Culture, Routine, Specimen)

ULTRA, DIAGNOSTIC
(see Glucose monitoring machines, Diagnostic)

ULTRAFAST COMPUTED TOMOGRAPHY, DIAGNOSTIC
(*see Computed tomography of the body, Diagnostic*)

ULTRASONOGRAPHY, ABDOMINAL AORTA, DIAGNOSTIC
(*see Abdominal aorta ultrasonography, Diagnostic*)

ULTRASONOGRAPHY, BONE, DIAGNOSTIC
(*see Breast ultrasonography, Diagnostic*)

ULTRASONOGRAPHY, BRAIN, DIAGNOSTIC
(*see Brain ultrasonography, Diagnostic*)

ULTRASONOGRAPHY, BREAST, DIAGNOSTIC
(*see Breast ultrasonography, Diagnostic*)

ULTRASONOGRAPHY, CAROTID ARTERY, DIAGNOSTIC
(*see Carotid Doppler, Diagnostic*)

ULTRASONOGRAPHY, COLOR DUPLEX, DIAGNOSTIC
(*see Color duplex ultrasonography, Diagnostic*)

ULTRASONOGRAPHY, COMPRESSION, DIAGNOSTIC
(*see Compression Ultrasonography, Diagnostic*)

ULTRASONOGRAPHY, CORONARY, DIAGNOSTIC
(*see Coronary intravascular ultrasonography, Diagnostic*)

ULTRASONOGRAPHY, ENDOSCOPIC, DIAGNOSTIC
(*see Endoscopic ultrasonography, Diagnostic or Transesophageal ultrasonography, Diagnostic*)

ULTRASONOGRAPHY, EYE AND ORBIT, DIAGNOSTIC
(*see Eye and orbit ultrasonography, Diagnostic*)

ULTRASONOGRAPHY, GALLBLADDER, DIAGNOSTIC
(*see Gallbladder and biliary system ultrasonography, Diagnostic*)

ULTRASONOGRAPHY, GYNECOLOGIC, DIAGNOSTIC
(*see Gynecologic ultrasonography, Diagnostic*)

ULTRASONOGRAPHY, HEART, DIAGNOSTIC
(*see Echocardiogram, Diagnostic*)

ULTRASONOGRAPHY, KIDNEY, DIAGNOSTIC
(*see Kidney ultrasonography, Diagnostic*)

ULTRASONOGRAPHY, LIVER, DIAGNOSTIC
(*see Liver ultrasonography, Diagnostic*)

ULTRASONOGRAPHY, OBSTETRIC, DIAGNOSTIC
(*see Obstetric ultrasonography, Diagnostic*)

ULTRASONOGRAPHY, PANCREAS, DIAGNOSTIC
(*see Pancreas ultrasonography, Diagnostic*)

ULTRASONOGRAPHY, PELVIC, DIAGNOSTIC
(*see Gynecologic ultrasonography, Diagnostic*)

ULTRASONOGRAPHY, PROSTATE, DIAGNOSTIC
(*see Prostate ultrasonography, Diagnostic*)

U

ULTRASONOGRAPHY, SPLEEN, DIAGNOSTIC
(see Spleen ultrasonography, Diagnostic)

ULTRASONOGRAPHY, THYROID, DIAGNOSTIC
(see Thyroid ultrasonography, Diagnostic)

ULTRASONOGRAPHY, TRANSCRANIAL, DIAGNOSTIC
(see Doppler ultrasonographic flow studies, Diagnostic)

ULTRASONOGRAPHY, TRANSESOPHAGEAL, DIAGNOSTIC
(see Transesophageal ultrasonography, Diagnostic)

ULTRASONOGRAPHY, TRANSRECTAL, DIAGNOSTIC
(see Prostate ultrasonography, Diagnostic)

ULTRASONOGRAPHY, TRANSVAGINAL, DIAGNOSTIC
(see Gynecologic ultrasonography, Diagnostic; Obstetric ultrasonography, Diagnostic; or Urinary bladder ultrasonography, Diagnostic)

ULTRASONOGRAPHY, URINARY BLADDER, DIAGNOSTIC
(see Urinary bladder ultrasonography, Diagnostic)

UPPER GI ENDOSCOPY, DIAGNOSTIC
(see Esophagogastroduodenoscopy, Diagnostic)

UPPER GASTROINTESTINAL (UGI) SERIES, DIAGNOSTIC

Norm. Mucosa is smooth and regular and free of lesions, polyps, narrowing, or filling defects. Barium fills smoothly and does not leak into the abdominal cavity. The passage of barium progresses at a normal rate, and there is no reflux into the esophagus (indicating hiatal hernia or incompetent cardiac sphincter). Gastric folds measure approximately 5 mm in the antrum and body of the stomach and are slightly wider near the fundus than near the esophagus.

Usage. Investigation of abnormal gastrointestinal symptoms. Allows fluoroscopic visualization of the esophagus, stomach, and duodenum; helps evaluate organ size, lumen size, outline, and position of the examined areas; and detection of strictures, scarring, varices, ulcers, tumors, hiatal hernia, or inflammation of the upper gastrointestinal tract.

Description. Upper gastrointestinal series (UGI) involves examining the upper gastrointestinal tract under fluoroscopy after the client drinks barium sulfate. Barium sulfate is a chalky substance of "milkshake" consistency that has radiopaque properties. Films of specific portions of the tract are taken as the barium passes through and outlines the structures. Barium-swallow studies of the esophagus with or without a small bowel series may be performed with this test. (See Barium swallow, Diagnostic; Small bowel series, Diagnostic.)

Professional Considerations
1. Consent form NOT required.

Risks
Aspiration of contrast material, bowel obstruction, constipation.

Contraindications
Suspected ileus, obstruction, or gastrointestinal perforation.

Precautions
During pregnancy, risks of cumulative radiation exposure to the fetus from this and other previous or future imaging studies must be weighed against the benefits of the procedure. Although formal limits for client exposure are relative to this risk:benefit comparison, the United States Nuclear Regulatory Commission requires that the cumulative dose equivalent to an embryo/fetus from occupational exposure not exceed 0.5 rem (5 mSv). Radiation dosage to

the fetus is proportional to the distance of the anatomy studied from the abdomen and decreases as pregnancy progresses. For pregnant clients, consult the Radiologist/Radiology Department to obtain estimated fetal radiation exposure from this procedure.

2. **Preparation:**
   A. Notify the physician before preparation if the client is pregnant.
   B. When it is possible, medications that affect the motility of the gastrointestinal tract should be withheld for 24 hours before the study.
   C. If this test is to be followed by a small bowel series for a bowel cleansing routine, see also *Small bowel series, Diagnostic.*
   D. The client should disrobe and put on a gown. All jewelry and metal objects should be removed.
   E. Obtain 8 ounces of barium sulfate solution.
   F. See *Client and family teaching.*
3. **Procedure:**
   A. The client is positioned supine on the fluoroscopic tilt table and strapped into place. The hydraulic table is then moved into a vertical position.
   B. Baseline fluoroscopic radiographs are taken of the area to be studied.
   C. The client is then given 8 ounces of barium sulfate solution and is instructed to drink portions of it at specified intervals as the table is tilted to various angles.
   D. Initial films are taken of the esophagus as the barium travels downward.
   E. Stomach films are taken as barium mixed with air enters the stomach. The lower esophagus is examined for reflux of the barium from the stomach or for free-flowing barium between the stomach and the esophagus, both of which conditions indicate hiatal hernia.
   F. As the client finishes ingesting the barium, the filled stomach and the emptying of the barium into the duodenum are radiographed from several angles. Gastric folds are examined for

thickening, indicated by a rugal pattern that is not obliterated by filling of the stomach with barium sulfate.
   G. The test takes less than 1 hour.
4. **Postprocedure care:**
   A. Resume previous diet.
   B. See *Client and family teaching.*
5. **Client and family teaching:**
   A. Fast from food and fluids, and do not chew gum or smoke overnight before the study.
   B. A laxative or suppository may be prescribed to be taken the night before the study.
   C. If this test is to be followed by a small bowel series, bring something to read, if desired, because the procedure time may increase to 4-6 hours.
   D. After swallowing a chalky barium solution, you will be asked to move to several positions and at times to hold your breath while the radiographs are taken.
   E. Drink 6-8 glasses of water or other fluids each day for 2 days after the test to help pass the barium through the gastrointestinal system.
   F. Observe stools for passage of barium for 1-3 days. This will make the stools look chalky white.
   G. Call the physician if unable to defecate. A mild laxative may be prescribed prophylactically, or cathartics or enemas may be prescribed as needed if pending impaction is suspected.
6. **Factors that affect results:**
   A. The client must be able to cooperate in swallowing the barium sulfate.
7. **Other data:**
   A. *Helicobacter pylori* infection should be suspected if isolated thickened gastric folds are found.

UREA
(see *Urea nitrogen, Plasma or serum*)

UREA BREATH TEST (UBT, ^{13}C-UBT, ^{14}C-UBT), DIAGNOSTIC

Norm. Negative for *Helicobacter pylori.*

Usage. Diagnosis of gastric *H. pylori* colonization; Confirmation of eradication of *H. pylori* infection after treatment

Description. *H. pylori* infection is an underlying cause found in most cases of gastritis and peptic ulcer. *H. pylori* infection is thought to be acquired in childhood, with the highest rates of seroconversion occurring in those aged 4-5 years. The source of infection is thought to be direct person-to-person transmission, but isolates have inconsistently been found in water, food, or animals. The urea breath test detects exhaled labeled carbon dioxide absorbed into the bloodstream from the stomach when the urease enzyme produced by *H. pylori* breaks down ingested radiolabeled urea. The labeled carbon dioxide (CO_2), known as ^{13}C or ^{14}C, is present in exhalations within 10-30 minutes. After the radiolabeled urea is ingested, a test meal is given to delay emptying from the stomach so as to allow the urease enzyme to act. The addition of citric acid to the test meal improves the sensitivity and specificity of the urea breath test. The difference between the ^{13}C and ^{14}C tests is that the ^{14}C is radioactive, is inexpensive, and can be interpreted using a liquid scintillation counter, widely available in radiology settings. The ^{13}C test is not radioactive and may be performed in any setting, but is much more expensive, and the mass spectrometer equipment needed for interpretation is not widely available.

This test is useful in pediatrics and is a sensitive indicator of *H. pylori* eradication 4-6 weeks after treatment with antibiotics.

Professional Considerations

1. Consent form NOT required for the ^{13}C test. Consent form IS required for the ^{14}C test.

Risks

There is a very small amount of radiation with the ^{14}C test.

Contraindications

Pregnancy.

2. **Preparation:**
   A. Obtain 200 mL of test drink for client ingestion.

B. Remove dentures, if present, to avoid trapping of the mixture under them.
C. See *Client and family teaching.*

3. **Procedure:**
   A. ^{14}C test:
      i. The client must rinse his/her mouth before drinking the mixture.
      ii. A baseline breath is taken by having the client blow into a solution that contains an acid/base indicator.
      iii. The client drinks a mixture or ingests a pill of radiolabeled ^{14}C-urea. A standard meal may be given.
      iv. Breath samples are measured at frequent intervals (e.g., 6, 12, 20, and 30 minutes) after ingestion.
      v. Alternatively, the client will blow into a balloon 10 minutes after urea ingestion and the balloon contents are transferred to a trapping solution for analysis.
   B. ^{13}C test:
      i. The client drinks a mixture of radiolabeled ^{13}C-urea or ^{14}C-urea. A standard meal may be given.
      ii. Breath samples are taken by being blown into a bag or balloon.
      iii. In the ^{13}C test, breath samples are measured at 0 and at 30 minutes after ingestion of the urea mixture.

4. **Postprocedure care:**
   A. The client may resume eating and drinking and all medications.

5. **Client and family teaching:**
   A. Do not take antibiotics (except vancomycin, nalidixic acid, trimethoprim, amphotericin B) or bismuth mixtures (e.g., Pepto-Bismol) within 1 month before the test.
   B. Do not take omeprazole, lansoprazole, or pantoprazole within 14 days before the test.
   C. Do not take cimetidine, famotidine, nizatidine or ranitidine within 24 hours before the test.
   D. Do NOT eat or drink for at least 6 hours before the test.
   E. The test takes about 30 minutes.
   F. ^{13}C test only: There is no radioactivity exposure from this test.

G. *¹⁴C test only:* The radioactivity received from this test is much less than that received from a regular chest radiograph and less than what you normally receive from a natural day of radiation.

6. **Factors that affect results:**
   A. A fatty meal profoundly affects results by increasing values at 30-, 40-, 50-, 60, 90-, and 120-minute intervals.
   B. Taking antibiotics or Pepto-Bismol for 1 month or Prilosec or Carafate for 1 week before the test can cause false-negative results.
   C. Taking drugs which inhibit bacterial growth, such as antibiotics,

within 1 month before the test can cause false-negative results.
   D. Antacids may produce falsely low results.
   E. Substituting orange juice for citric acid reduces diagnostic accuracy (specificity) of this test. Citric acid has 100% specificity, but orange juice has only 88% specificity.

7. **Other data:**
   A. *H. pylori* infection is treated with a 7 day cycle of tetracycline, metronidazole, and bismuth subsalicylate.
   B. See also *Campylobacter-like–organism test, Specimen; and Helicobacter pylori, Quick office serology, Serum and Titer, Blood*

UREA NITROGEN, PLASMA OR SERUM

U

Norm:

		SI UNITS
Young adult <40 years	5-18 mg/dL	1.8-6.5 mmol/L
Adult	5-20 mg/dL	1.8-7.1 mmol/L
Elderly >60 years	8-21 mg/dL	2.9-7.5 mmol/L
Mild azotemia	20-50 mg/dL	7.1-17.7 mmol/L
Children		
Cord blood	21-40 mg/dL	7.5-14.3 mmol/L
Premature infant, first 7 days	3-25 mg/dL	1.1-7.9 mmol/L
Full-term newborn	4-18 mg/dL	1.4-6.4 mmol/L
Infant	5-18 mg/dL	1.8-6.4 mmol/L
Child	5-18 mg/dL	1.8-6.4 mmol/L
Panic Level	>100 mg/dL	>35.7 mmol/L

Panic Level Symptoms and Treatemt

Symptoms. Acidemia, agitation, coma, confusion, fatigue, nausea, stupor, and vomiting.

Treatment:

Note: Treatment choice(s) depend on client history and condition and episode history.
Correct the cause.
Administer sodium bicarbonate IV for severe acidemia.
Prescribe a low-protein diet.
Hemodialysis and peritoneal dialysis WILL remove urea nitrogen.
Avoid or reduce drug usage of long-acting barbiturates, narcotics,

sulfonamides, anticoagulants, and antibiotics such as vancomycin, kanamycin, and polymycin.

Increased. Addison's disease, allergic purpura, amyloidosis, analgesic abuse, blood transfusions, cachexia, cardiac failure, congenital hypoplastic kidneys, dehydration, diabetes mellitus, diabetic ketoacidosis, diet (high-protein), Fanconi syndrome, fluid therapy (excessive), gastrointestinal bleeding, glomerulonephritis, Goodpasture syndrome, gout, heavy-metal poisoning, hemoglobinurias, infection, intestinal obstruction, multiple myeloma, myocardial infarction (acute), nephritis, nephropathy (hypercalcemic, hypokalemic), nephrosclerosis, pancreatitis, peritonitis, pneumonia, polyarteritis nodosa, polycystic disease, postoperative state, protein intake (excessive), pyelonephritis, renal artery stenosis or thrombosis, renal cortical necrosis, renal hypoperfusion states, renal malignancy, renal tuberculosis, renal vein thrombosis, scleroderma, sepsis, shock, sickle cell anemia, starvation, stress, subacute bacterial endocarditis, suppuration, systemic lupus erythematosus, thyrotoxicosis, tumor necrosis, uremia, and urinary tract obstruction. Drugs include acetohexamide, acetone, alkaline antacids, aminophenol, ammonium salts, amphotericin B, anabolic steroids, androgens, antimony compounds, arginine, arsenicals, ascorbic acid, asparaginase, bacitracin, calcium salts, capreomycin, captopril, carmustine, carbutamide, cephaloridine, chloral hydrate, chloramphenicol, chlorobutanol, chlorothiazide sodium, chlorthalidone, clonidine, colistimethate sodium, dextran, dextrose infusions, disopyramide phosphate, doxapram, ethacrynic acid, fluorides, fluphenazine, fosinopril, furosemide, guanethidine sulfate, gentamicin sulfate, guanachlor, guanethidine analogs, hydroxyurea, indomethacin, kanamycin, Lipomul (maize oil, corn oil emulsion), lithium carbonate, marijuana, meclofenamate sodium, mephenesin, mercury compounds, mercurial diuretics, methicillin, methoxyflurane, methsuximide, methyldopa, methylprednisolone sodium succinate, methysergide, metolazone, metoprolol tartrate, minoxidil, mithramycin, morphine, nalidixic acid, naproxen sodium, neomycin, nitrofurantoin, paramethasone, pargyline, polymyxin B, propranolol, salicylates, spectinomycin, streptodornase, streptokinase, sulfonamides, tetracycline, thiazide diuretics, tolmetin sodium, triamterene, and vancomycin.

Decreased. Acromegaly, alcohol abuse, amyloidosis, celiac disease, cirrhosis, diet (inadequate protein), fluid intake (excessive), hemodialysis, hepatitis, infancy, liver destruction, malnutrition, nephrosis, plasma volume expansion, and pregnancy (late). Drugs include streptomycin and thymol. Herb or natural remedy is *Cordyceps sinensis*.

Description. Commonly referred to as BUN (blood urea nitrogen), this measurement is actually performed on plasma or serum. Plasma or serum levels of urea nitrogen are about 12% higher than BUN levels, resulting from the relatively higher percentage of protein contained in erythrocytes. Urea nitrogen is the nitrogen portion of urea, a substance formed in the liver through an enzymatic protein-breakdown process. Urea is normally freely filtered through the renal glomeruli, with a small amount reabsorbed in the tubules and the remainder excreted in the urine. Elevated urea nitrogen in the bloodstream is called "azotemia." However, the value is nonspecific as to cause and thus may be a result of either prerenal, renal, or postrenal causes. Prerenal causes may be grouped under factors that result in inadequate renal circulation or conditions resulting in abnormally high levels of blood protein. Renal causes are those of impaired renal filtration and excretion of urea nitrogen. Postrenal causes are lower urinary tract obstructive conditions that result in diffusion of urea nitrogen in dormant urine back into the bloodstream through the tubules. "Uremia" is a term used to describe symptoms occurring at very high elevations of urea in the bloodstream and may occur at urea nitrogen levels of about 200 mg/dL (>70 mmol/L). Also of significance are low urea nitrogen levels in severe hepatic disease. A damaged liver that is unable to synthesize urea from protein results in a buildup of blood ammonia (NH_3), causing hepatic encephalopathy.

Professional Considerations
1. Consent form NOT required.
2. Preparation:
   A. Tube: Red topped, red/gray topped, or gold topped.
   B. Do NOT draw specimens during hemodialysis.
3. Procedure:
   A. Draw a 1-mL blood sample without hemolysis.
4. Postprocedure care:
   A. None.
5. Client and family teaching:
   A. This test result alone is of little diagnostic value but must be compared to itself over time or used with other test results.
6. Factors that affect results:
   A. Falsely elevated results may occur in hemolyzed specimens.

B. Values are somewhat affected by hemodilution.

C. In contrast to creatinine level, dietary protein intake does influence the urea nitrogen level.

7. **Other data:**

A. Both creatinine levels and urea nitrogen levels should be considered when evaluating renal function.

URETHROGRAPHY, RETROGRADE, DIAGNOSTIC

Norm. Negative for congenital anomaly, diverticula, fistula, obstruction, or stricture. Normal size, shape, and position of the urethra and prostate gland.

Usage. Aids in the diagnosis of urethral abnormalities and anomalies, including diverticula, fistula, obstruction, and strictures; and evaluation of status after urethral or radical prostate surgery; helps identify the precise anatomic location of the prostate for prostate radiotherapy.

Description. Retrograde urethrography is a procedure in which radiographs are taken as radiopaque contrast medium is instilled into the urethra. Autourethrography, in which the client performs the instillation (injection) of the contrast medium, has been found to enhance the client's tolerance, cause less anxiety, and decrease the instance of extravasation of contrast medium outside of the urethra. In addition, the radiologist does not have to remain with the client during x-ray exposure. Retrograde urethrography is primarily performed in males. A double-balloon catheter can be used for retrograde urethrography in women to diagnose a urethral diverticulum. Retrograde urethrography is inferior to magnetic resonance urography if abnormalities in the periurethral tissues is suspected. (See *Magnetic resonance urography, Diagnostic*.)

Professional Considerations

1. Consent form IS required.

Risks

Bladder infection, allergic reaction to contrast (itching, hives, rash, tight feel-ing in the throat, shortness of breath, anaphylaxis), renal toxicity from contrast medium (very unlikely).

Contraindications

Pregnancy, previous allergic reaction to radiographic contrast; renal insufficiency. Sedatives are contraindicated in clients with central nervous system depression.

Precautions

During pregnancy, risks of cumulative radiation exposure to the fetus from this and other previous or future imaging studies must be weighed against the benefits of the procedure. Although formal limits for client exposure are relative to this risk:benefit comparison, the United States Nuclear Regulatory Commission requires that the cumulative dose equivalent to an embryo/fetus from occupational exposure not exceed 0.5 rem (5 mSv). Radiation dosage to the fetus is proportional to the distance of the anatomy studied from the abdomen and decreases as pregnancy progresses. For pregnant clients, consult the Radiologist/Radiology Department to obtain estimated fetal radiation exposure from this procedure.

2. **Preparation:**

A. Have emergency equipment readily available.

B. Obtain sterile towels, a balloon urinary catheter, 10- and 60-mL syringes, and contrast medium.

C. An analgesic or sedative may be prescribed. Monitor respiratory status continually if sedation is used.

D. Record baseline vital signs.

E. The client should disrobe below the waist.

F. If autourethrography is to be performed, the client must be instructed about the dye-instillation technique.

3. **Procedure:**

A. With the client positioned supine, baseline radiographs of the lower urinary tract structures are taken.

B. A catheter filled with radiopaque contrast connected to a special occluding clamp is advanced into the urethra just proximal to the urethral meatus. Alternatively a catheter filled with radiopaque contrast is advanced into the urethra until the balloon is just proximal to the meatus and then the balloon is partially inflated with air.

C. Standard or fluoroscopic radiographs are taken as dye is injected by the radiologist or the client (autourethrography) through the catheter, with the client in various positions.

D. The clamp-and-catheter apparatus or the catheter is removed after balloon deflation.

E. The client is instructed to urinate to expel the contrast medium.

4. Postprocedure care:

A. Monitor vital signs at the end of the procedure. If deep sedation was used, follow institutional protocol for postsedation monitoring. Typical monitoring includes continuous ECG monitoring and pulse oximetry, with continual assessments (every 5-15 minutes) of airway, vital signs, and neurologic status until the client is lying quietly awake, is breathing independently, and responds to commands spoken in a normal tone.

B. Administer analgesic as prescribed.

C. See *Client and family teaching.*

5. Client and family teaching:

A. Expect some discomfort with contrast instillation, but this will be relieved when the radiographs are completed and the catheter is removed.

B. Observe for signs of allergic reactions to the contrast (listed above) for 24 hours. Call the physician in the event of itching or hives. Go to the nearest emergency room or call an ambulance for shortness of breath.

C. Save all the urine voided. Inspect the urine for quantity and hematuria (pink or red color) for 24 hours. Notify the physician for no urine in 8 hours, less than 1 ounce (30 mL) of urine per hour, or pain with urination.

D. Drink 6-8 glasses of water or other fluids during the next 24 hours (when not contraindicated).

E. Notify the physician for symptoms of infection: fever, fast heart rate, hypotension (feeling faint, weak, or dizzy), chills, dysuria, or flank pain.

6. Factors that affect results:

A. Urethral obstruction will block the flow of contrast through the urethra.

7. Other data:

A. This test is often combined with voiding cystourethrography.

URIC ACID, SERUM

Norm:

		SI UNITS
Adult Females	2.4-6.0 mg/dL	143-357 µmol/L
Adult Males	3.4-7.0 mg/dL	202-416 µmol/L
Children	2.5-5.5 mg/dL	119-327 µmol/L
Panic Level	>12 mg/dL	>714 µmol/L

Panic Level Symptoms and Treatment

Symptoms. Painful swelling of great toe, hypertension, arthritis.

Treatment:

Note: Treatment choice(s) depend on client history and condition and episode history.

Acute phase: allopurinol, colchicine, indomethacin, or phenylbutazone, orally; or corticotropin (ACTH) intramuscularly; also analgesics for severe pain.

Chronic phase: allopurinol, probenecid, or sulfinpyrazone, orally.

Increased. Alcoholism, anemia (hemolytic, pernicious, sickle cell), arteriosclerosis, arthritis, berylliosis (chronic), Blackfoot Indians, body size (larger than average), calcinosis universalis and circumscripta, congestive heart failure, dehydration, diabetes mellitus, diet (high protein, excess nucleoproteins), Down syndrome, eclampsia, exercise, fasting, Filipinos, glomerulonephritis (chronic), Graves' disease, gout, hemolysis (prolonged), hepatic disease, hypertension or hypertensive vascular damage, hyperuricemia, hypoparathyroidism, hypothyroidism, infections (acute), intestinal obstruction, ketoacidosis, ketosis, lead poisoning, Lesch-Nyhan syndrome, leukemia, lipoproteinemia (type III), lymphoma, maple syrup urine disease, mononucleosis (infectious), multiple myeloma, neoplasm (disseminated), nephritis, nephropathy, New Zealand Maoris, Pima Indians (Akimel O'odham), pneumonia (resolving), polycystic kidneys, polycythemia vera, pregnancy (onset of labor), psoriasis, renal failure, sarcoidosis, starvation, stress, toxemia of pregnancy, uremia, urinary obstruction, and von Gierke's disease. Drugs include acetazolamide, asparaginase, busulfan, chlorothiazide sodium, chlorthalidone, corticosteroids, cyclophosphamide, dactinomycin, daunorubicin hydrochloride, dextran, diazoxide, diuretics (except spironolactone, mercurials, and ticrynafen), epinephrine, ethacrynic acid, ethambutol, ethyl alcohol (ethanol), fructose, furosemide, gentamicin sulfate, glucose, hydralazine, hydrocortisone, hydroxyurea, ibufenac, levodopa, mecamylamine, mechlorethamine hydrochloride, 6-mercaptopurine, methicillin, methotrexate, methyldopa, metoprolol tartrate, niacin, nicotinic acid (large doses), nitrogen mustards, norepinephrine, phenothiazines, probenecid, propranolol, propylthiouracil, pyrazinamide, quinethazone, rifampin, salicylates (low doses), theophylline, thiazide diuretics, 6-thioguanine, triamterene, and vincristine.

Decreased. Acromegaly, bronchogenic carcinoma, celiac disease, Dalmatian dog mutation, Fanconi syndrome, Hodgkin's disease, myeloma, pernicious anemia, Wilson's disease, yellow atrophy of liver, and xanthinuria. Drugs include acetohexamide, ACTH, allopurinol, anticoagulants, azlocillin, azothioprine, bacitracin, benziodaron, chlorine, chlorpromazine hydrochloride, chlorprothixene, chlorthalidone, cincophen, corticosteroids, corticotropin, cortisone, coumarins, dicumarol, ethacrynic acid, glyceryl guaiacolate, lithium carbonate, mannitol, marijuana, oxyphenbutazone, phenothiazines, phenylbutazone, piperazine, potassium oxalate, probenecid, radiographic dyes, salicylates (long-term, large doses), saline infusions, sodium oxalate, sulfinpyrazone, thyroid hormone, and triamterene. Herbal or natural remedies include products containing aristolochic acids (*Akebia* spp., *Aristolochia* spp., *Asarum* spp., birthwort, *Bragantia* spp., *Clematis* spp., *Cocculus* spp., *Diploclisia* spp., Dutchman's pipe, *Fang chi, Fang ji, Fang chi, Guang fang ji, Kan-Mokutsu, Menispernum* spp., *Mokutsu, Mu tong, Sinomenium* spp., and *Stephania* spp.)

Description. Uric acid (lithic acid) is formed as the purines adenine and guanine are continuously metabolized during the formation and degradation of ribonucleic acid (RNA) and deoxyribonucleic acid (DNA) and from metabolism of dietary purines. After synthesis in the liver triggered by the action of xanthine oxidase, part of the uric acid is excreted in the urine. Elevated amounts of serum uric acid (uricemia) become deposited in joints and soft tissues and cause gout, an inflammatory reaction to the urate crystal deposition. Conditions of both fast cell turnover and slowed renal excretion of uric acid may cause uricemia. Elevated amounts of urinary uric acid precipitate into urate stones in the kidneys.

Professional Considerations
1. Consent form NOT required.
2. **Preparation:**
   A. Tube: Red topped, red/gray topped, or gold topped.
   B. See *Client and family teaching.*
3. **Procedure:**
   A. Draw a 1-mL blood sample.
4. **Postprocedure care:**
   A. None.
5. **Client and family teaching:**
   A. Fast for 8 hours before sampling.
   B. Foods high in purines that can contribute to gout include caffeine-containing beverages,

legumes, mushrooms, organ meats, spinach, gravies, and baker's and brewer's yeast.

C. Switching from a normal diet to a low-purine diet may potentially decrease urine uric acid levels by half.

6. **Factors that affect results:**
   A. Drugs that may cause falsely elevated results include aminophylline, caffeine, and vitamin C.

7. **Other data:**
   A. Mortality for women with ischemic heart disease increases fivefold if their uric acid level is ≥7 mg/dL (416 mmol/L).

URIC ACID, URINE

Norm:

		SI UNITS
Adult female	250-750 mg/24 hours	1.5-4.5 mmol/day
Adult male	250-800 mg/24 hours	1.5-4.8 mmol/day

Usage. Determines whether renal calculi may be the result of hyperuricosuria.

Description. Uric acid (lithic acid) is formed as the purines adenine and guanine are continuously metabolized during the formation and degradation of ribonucleic acid (RNA) and deoxyribonucleic acid (DNA) and from metabolism of dietary purines. After synthesis in the liver triggered by the action of xanthine oxidase, part of the uric acid is excreted in the urine. Elevated amounts of serum uric acid (uricemia) become deposited in joints and soft tissues and cause gout, an inflammatory reaction to the urate crystal deposition. Conditions of both fast cell turnover and slowed renal excretion of uric acid may cause uricemia. Elevated amounts of urinary uric acid precipitate into urate stones in the kidneys.

Professional Considerations
1. Consent form NOT required.
2. **Preparation:**
   A. Obtain a 3-L container to which 10 mL of 12.5 M sodium hydroxide solution has been added.
   B. Write the beginning time of collection on the laboratory requisition.
3. **Procedure:**
   A. Discard the first morning-voided urine.
   B. Save all the urine voided for the next 24 hours in a 3-L container to which 10 mL of 12.5 M sodium hydroxide solution has been

added. For specimens collected from an indwelling urinary catheter, empty the urine into the collection container hourly. Document the quantity of urinary output during the collection period. Do not refrigerate the specimen.

4. **Postprocedure care:**
   A. Write the ending time on the laboratory requisition.
   B. Compare the quantity of urine with the urinary output record for the collection. If the specimen contains less than what was recorded as output, some urine may have been discarded, thus invalidating the test.

5. **Client and family teaching:**
   A. Save all the urine voided during the collection period, urinate before defecating, and avoid contaminating the specimen with stool or toilet tissue. If any urine is accidentally discarded, discard the entire specimen and restart the collection the next day.
   B. Foods high in purines that can contribute to gout include caffeine-containing beverages, legumes, mushrooms, organ meats, spinach, gravies, and baker's and brewer's yeast.
   C. Switching from a normal diet to a low-purine diet may potentially decrease urine uric acid levels by half.

6. **Factors that affect results:**
   A. Drugs that increase the rate of uric acid excretion include ascor-

bic acid, cytotoxics, probenecid, radiographic dyes, salicylates (long-term, large doses), and sulfinpyrazone.

B. Drugs that slow uric acid excretion include diuretics and insulin.

C. Trauma has been shown to increase the rate of urinary uric acid excretion.

7. Other data:

A. Herbal or natural remedies that can cause Fanconi's syndrome and increased uric acid in the urine include products containing aristolochic acids (*Akebia* spp., *Aristolochia* spp., *Asarum* spp., birthwort, *Bragantia* spp., *Clematis* spp., *Cocculus* spp., *Diploclisia* spp., Dutchman's pipe, *Fang chi, Fang ji, Fang chi, Guang fang ji, Kan-Mokutsu, Menispernum* spp., *Mokutsu, Mu tong, Sinomenium* spp., and *Stephania* spp.).

URINALYSIS (UA), URINE

Norm:

Albumin	Negative
Appearance	Clear to faintly hazy
Bilirubin	Negative
Color	Yellow
Glucose or reducing substances	Negative
Ketones	Negative
Nitrite	Negative
Occult blood	Negative
Odor	Faint (not fruity, musty, fishy, or fetid)
pH	4.5-8.0
Protein	Negative
Specific gravity	1.003-1.030
Urobilinogen	Negative or 0.1-1 Ehrlich U/dL

Cells

Erythrocytes	<3 cells/HPF
Leukocytes	≤4 cells/HPF

Urinary Tract Epithelium

≤10 cells/HPF

Casts	Moderate clear protein casts
Crystals	Small amount
Bacteria or fungi	None or <1000/mL
Parasites	None

Increased or Decreased. For specific causes of increased or decreased values of constituents, see individual test listings as follows: *Albumin, 24-Hour urine; Bilirubin, Urine; Glucose, Qualitative, Semiquantitative, Urine; Ketone, Semiquantitative, Urine; Nitrite, Bacteria screen, Urine; Occult blood, Urine; pH, Urine; Protein, Urine; Specific gravity, Urine; Urobilinogen, Urine.*

Changes in Urine Color. A variety of substances may alter urine color as follows:

COLOR	POSSIBLE CAUSE
Black	Ferrous sulfate, homogentisic acid, indicans, indigo carmine dye used in renal function tests and cystoscopy, levodopa, melanin, methemoglobin, phenols, urobilinogen. Herbal or natural remedies include cascara sagrada (*Rhamnus purshiana*).
Blue	Amitriptyline, some diuretics, methylene blue, nitrofurans, *Pseudomonas*
Brown	Acid hematin, Addison's disease, bile pigment, furazolidone, levodopa, metronidazole, myoglobin, nitrofurantoin, porphyrinuria, renal disease, some sulfonamides

Continued

COLOR	POSSIBLE CAUSE
Dark yellow to amber	Bilirubin, chlorpromazine, food (carrots), nitrofurantoin, phenacetin, quinacrine, riboflavin, urobilinogen. Herbal or natural remedies include cascara sagrada (*Rhamnus purshiana*).
Green	Bacterial infection, biliverdin, some diuretics, vitamins
Light	Diuresis caused by alcohol ingestion or diuretics, diabetes insipidus, glycosuria
Orange	Bile pigment, chlorzoxazone, dehydration, fever, fluorescein sodium, jaundice, some oral anticoagulants, phenazopyridine, phenothiazines, pyridium, rifampin, sulfasalazine
Red	Deferoxamine mesylate, foods (beets, rhubarb, senna), hemoglobin, malaria, myoglobin, porphobilinogen, phenolphthalein, phenolsulfonphthalein, porphyrins, renal injury, rifampin, sulfobromophthalein

Automated Microscopy. >2 white blood cell (WBC)/hpf indicates urinary tract inflammation causing pyuria.

Description. A frequently performed screening test that gives a general indication of the client's overall state of health as well as the health of the urinary tract. The dipstick reagent strip method is commonly used to measure pH, ketones, protein, sugars, and other reducing substances. Additional reagent strips are available to measure bilirubin and urobilinogen levels. The sample is also centrifuged, with the sediment then examined microscopically for determination of the presence and type of cells, casts, crystals, and organisms such as bacteria or fungi. Urine color should correlate with specific gravity. That is, dilute urine with low specific gravity should be almost colorless, and concentrated urine with high specific gravity should be dark yellow. Glucose content should also correlate positively with specific gravity. pH should correlate inversely with ketone (acetone) level. A sweet or fruity urine odor indicates the presence of ketones in the sample. A fish or fetid odor indicates urinary tract infection. An odor of maple syrup may indicate maple syrup urine disease. A musty urine odor may be caused by recent ingestion of asparagus. An increase in epithelial cells may signal an inflammatory process in the kidneys. Erythrocytes present in the urine signal damage to the renal glomeruli. Elevated leukocyte levels indicate inflammation or infection in the urinary tract and indicate the need for urine culture. Both erythrocytes and leukocytes, if present, will appear trapped in casts and can be observed microscopically. Crystals may form at room temperature in voided urine before being tested or may be caused by a variety of drugs. More detailed descriptions of other aspects of urine analysis may be found under individual test listings described above under *Increased or Decreased.*

Professional Considerations
1. Consent form NOT required.
2. **Preparation:**
   A. Obtain a soapy sponge and a clean specimen container.
   B. If bilirubin or urobilinogen results are of specific interest, the specimen container should be wrapped in foil to protect it from light.
3. **Procedure:** A first morning void is preferred.
   A. *Female:* Instruct the client to wash the area surrounding the urethral meatus with soap and water. Then, while holding the labia open, position the specimen container beneath the urethral meatus and void into the container, filling it about half full (about 50 mL). Also see *Client and family teaching.*
   B. *Male:* Instruct the client to retract the foreskin if present. Then wash the distal end of the penis surrounding the urethral meatus with soap and water. The client should then void into the specimen container, filling it about half full (about 50 mL).

4. **Postprocedure care:**
   A. Write the collection method, date, and time on the laboratory requisition.
   B. Send the specimen to the laboratory promptly and refrigerate it until testing. The best results are obtained if testing is performed within 2 hours.
5. **Client and family teaching:**
   A. Urinate before defecating and avoid contaminating the specimen with vaginal or perineal secretions or stool.
   B. Menstruating females should insert a tampon into the vagina before cleansing and voiding.
6. **Factors that affect results:**
   A. First morning-voided specimens provide the most accurate reflection of the presence of bacteria and formed elements such as casts and crystals.
   B. A delay in testing after collection may cause falsely decreased glucose, ketone, bilirubin, and urobilinogen values. Delayed testing with specimens left at room temperature may cause falsely elevated bacteria levels because of bacterial overgrowth. Delays also inhibit microscopic clarity because of the dissolution of urates and phosphates.
   C. For detailed listings of factors that affect results, see individual test listings described under *Increased or Decreased.*
7. **Other data:**
   A. Abnormal results should be confirmed by more specific, or quantitative, follow-up testing.

URINALYSIS, FRACTIONAL, URINE

Norm. *Sugars:* negative. *Acetone:* negative. Calculated albumin excretion rate (nephorimetric [combined nephelometric, calorimetric] method).

		SI UNITS
Adult		
At rest	2-80 mg/24 hours	0.03-0.08 g/day
Ambulatory	<150 mg/24 hours	<0.15 g/day
Child <10 years	<100 mg/24 hours	<0.10 g/day

Usage. Monitoring for clients with diabetes mellitus (infrequently used). Assessment of urinary albumin excretion rate.

Description. A fractional urine involves testing up to four timed urine collections within a 24-hour period for the presence of sugars, acetone, or albumin, all of which are abnormal. Glucose results are reflective of the level of serum glucose levels because levels above the renal threshold for glomerular glucose reabsorption into the bloodstream are excreted in the urine. Acetone levels are an indication of the state of fatty acid metabolism in diabetics. The detection of microalbuminuria in an aliquot of a fractional specimen has been demonstrated to be predictive of diabetic nephropathy at an early and potentially reversible stage. This test used to be performed more frequently for diabetics. However, as studies demonstrated that renal thresholds for glucose reabsorption vary from client to client, this test is no longer considered the most accurate reflection of insulin needs. Routine daily blood glucose monitoring has replaced fractional urine analysis for ongoing diabetic monitoring. Fractional urine testing is more often used to measure the excretion rate of albumin.

Professional Considerations
1. Consent form NOT required.
2. **Preparation:**
   A. Obtain four clean 1-L specimen containers to which toluene preservative has been added (for glucose measurement) or without preservative (for albumin measurement) and reagent strips, or Clinitest and Acetest tablets.
   B. Number the containers sequentially.

3. **Procedure:**
   A. Specimens for albumin measurement should be refrigerated.
   B. *First collection period:*
      i. The first morning void, 1 hour before breakfast, is discarded.
      ii. The client should drink 8 ounces of water.
      iii. One-half hour later, the client should void and test the specimen for sugar and acetone, then transfer the specimen to container 1, and record the results as well as the beginning time of the collection period.
      iv. The client should eat breakfast.
      v. All additional urine voided until 1 hour before the midday meal should be added to container 1, and the ending time of the collection period should be recorded.
   C. *Second collection period:*
      i. The client should drink 8 ounces of water 1 hour before the midday meal.
      ii. One-half hour later, the client should void and test the specimen for sugar and acetone, then transfer the specimen to container 2, and record the results as well as the beginning time of the collection period.
      iii. The client should eat the midday meal and an afternoon snack.
      iv. All additional urine voided until 1 hour before the evening meal should be added to container 2, and the ending time of the collection period should be recorded.
   D. *Third collection period:*
      i. The client should drink 8 ounces of water 1 hour before the evening meal.
      ii. One-half hour later, the client should void and test the specimen for sugar and acetone, then transfer the specimen to container 3, and record the results as well as the beginning time of the collection period.
      iii. The client should eat the evening meal.
      iv. All additional urine voided until 1 hour before the bedtime snack should be added to container 3, and the ending time of the collection period should be recorded.
   E. *Fourth collection period:*
      i. The client should drink 8 ounces of water 1 hour before the bedtime snack.
      ii. One-half hour later, the client should void and test the specimen for sugar and acetone, then transfer the specimen to container 4, and record the results as well as the beginning time of the collection period.
      iii. The client should eat a bedtime snack.
      iv. All additional urine voided until 1 hour before breakfast the next day should be added to container 4.
      v. The client should include the void at 1 hour before breakfast in container 4, and record the time ended.

4. **Postprocedure care:**
   A. Send all four containers to the laboratory.

5. **Client and family teaching:**
   A. Collect specimens according to the procedure above.
   B. All testing should be performed on freshly voided urine with reagent strips (Keto-Diastix, Multistix) or Clinitest and Acetest tablets according to manufacturer's directions. Compare the results with the color chart on the container.

6. **Factors that affect results:**
   A. Expired reagent strips, Clinitest tablets, Acetest tablets, or those that have had prolonged exposure to air or moisture should not be used because the results will be invalid.
   B. Many drugs and factors affect the accuracy of the test media used. For detailed information, see the specific test listing for the method used as follows: *Acetone, Urine; Albumin, 24-Hour urine;* or *Glucose, Qualitative, Semiquantitative, Urine.*

7. **Other data:**
   A. None.

URINARY BLADDER ULTRASONOGRAPHY (URINARY BLADDER ECHOGRAM, URINARY BLADDER ULTRASONOGRAM), DIAGNOSTIC

Norm. Negative for tumor, cyst, overdistention, or residual urine. Proper size, shape, and position of the urinary bladder.

Usage. Assessment for residual urine in or for volume of or overdistention of the bladder; search for radiolucent stones; evaluation of large diverticulae; confirmation of suspicious filling defects seen on other imaging studies; guidance for suprapubic placement of needles and catheter in the bladder; evaluation of the size, shape, and position of the urinary bladder; helps diagnose, localize, monitor, and stage bladder tumors and evaluate hemorrhagic cystitis after bone marrow transplantation as well as detect urinary bladder involvement in Crohn's disease; differentiation of superficial from deep infiltrative bladder tumors (transurethral ultrasonography); and measurement of urinary bladder volumes (transrectal ultrasonography or transvaginal ultrasonography).

Description. Evaluation of the urinary bladder size, shape, and position by the creation of an oscilloscopic picture from the echoes of high-frequency sound waves passing over the bladder area (acoustic imaging) by the transabdominal or transurethral route. The time required for the ultrasonic beam to be reflected back to the transducer from differing densities of tissue is converted by a computer to an electrical impulse displayed on an oscilloscopic screen to create a three-dimensional picture of the urinary bladder. Additionally, transvaginal or transrectal endosonography can provide an advantage in evaluating the neck of the bladder, the bladder base, and the urethra in females. Because ultrasonography cannot confirm diagnosis of lesions found, when these lesions are found they should be followed by urinary bladder biopsy via cystoscopy.

Professional Considerations

1. Consent form NOT required for transabdominal method. Consent form IS required for transrectal, transurethral, and transvaginal methods.

Risks
Transabdominal procedure: none.
Transvaginal procedure: vaginal infection.

Contraindications
Transabdominal procedure: none.
Transvaginal procedure: third-trimester pregnancy.

2. **Preparation:**
   A. The client should disrobe below the waist or wear a gown.
   B. Obtain ultrasonic gel or paste.
   C. For transrectal ultrasonography an enema may be prescribed.
   D. See *Client and family teaching.*
3. **Procedure:**
   A. *Transabdominal ultrasonography:*
      i. The client is positioned supine.
      ii. Ultrasonic gel or paste is applied to the skin overlying the bladder.
      iii. A lubricated transducer is placed firmly against the skin over the bladder area and moved slowly back and forth at intervals 1-2 cm apart. The oscilloscope displays a three-dimensional image of the full bladder.
      iv. The client is instructed to void, and the procedure is repeated to check for the presence of residual urine.
      v. Photographs are taken of the oscilloscopic display.
      vi. The procedure takes less than 30 minutes.
   B. *Transvaginal ultrasonography:*
      i. After uroflowmetry studies are completed, 0.9% saline solution is instilled through a urethral catheter to fill the bladder.
      ii. A transducer probe is inserted into an ultrasonic gel–filled condom. The condom is covered with a sterile lubricant.
      iii. The probe is inserted into the vagina by the client or the examiner and moved to touch the vesicourethral area.
      iv. The bladder and urethral are identified by sonography.

U

Pictures are taken of the oscilloscopic display, with the client at rest, or during micturition.
C. *Transrectal ultrasonography:*
   i. The client is positioned supine, and short transabdominal ultrasonography is performed to evaluate for kidney distention.
   ii. The rectum is examined digitally for obstruction.
   iii. The client is assisted to a knee-elbow, lateral decubitus, or sitting position.
   iv. The probe is covered with an air-free, sterile, transparent cover or condom. The condom is then coated with a sterile lubricant, and the probe is slowly inserted into the rectum.
   v. After the probe is inserted into the rectum, the condom is inflated with 20-60 mL of deaerated water.
   vi. The probe is angled anteriorly, and ultrasonography of the bladder is performed.
   vii. Photographs of the oscilloscopic display are taken.
D. *Transurethral ultrasonography:*
   i. The bladder is filled with sterile 0.9% saline solution.
   ii. The probe is covered with an air-free, sterile, transparent cover and inserted into the bladder through a cystoscope.
   iii. The probe is rotated within the bladder as transverse sectional scans are taken.
   iv. Oscilloscopic images may be recorded on videotape or photographs.
4. **Postprocedure care:**
   A. Remove the gel from the skin.
   B. Sterilize the endosonography probes by soaking in glutaraldehyde solution for 10 minutes.
5. **Client and family teaching:**
   A. This test should be performed before intestinal barium tests or else after the barium is cleared from the system.
   B. Drink three to four 8-ounce glasses of fluid within 2 hours before the test (where not contraindicated because the purpose of the test is to evaluate the bladder when full), and refrain from voiding.

C. The transabdominal procedure is painless and carries no risks.
6. **Factors that affect results:**
   A. Dehydration interferes with adequate contrast between organs and body fluids.
   B. Lower intestinal barium contrast medium obscures results by preventing proper transmission and deflection of the high-frequency sound waves.
   C. The more lower abdominal fat present, the greater is the attenuation (reduction in sound-wave amplitude and intensity), which interferes with the clarity of the transabdominal picture.
7. **Other data:**
   A. Computed tomography is preferred to ultrasonography for staging and measuring urinary bladder tumors.

URINARY CHORIONIC GONADOTROPIN PEPTIDE (UGP, URINARY GONADOTROPIN FRAGMENT, UGF), URINE

Norm. <0.2 ng/mL or <5 fmol/mg creatinine.

Increased. Down syndrome, gynecologic cancers (cervical, endometrial, ovarian, and vulvovaginal), pregnancy, recurrence of gynecologic cancer, transitional cell carcinoma of the bladder.

Decreased. Survival rate from gynecologic cancer is increased, nonpregnant.

Description. Urinary chorionic gonadotropin (CG) peptide (UGP), is a betasubunit core fragment that is found in pregnancy and is also known to originate from cancer tissue itself. It is elevated in gynecologic cancers, especially when the disease is advanced. UGP is secreted into the circulation and rapidly cleared and is generally not detected in the serum. The urine test uses immunohistochemical staining to identify the CG-beta expression at the level of messenger RNA.

Professional Considerations
1. Consent form NOT required.
2. **Preparation:**
   A. Obtain a soapy sponge and a clean specimen container.

3. **Procedure:**
   A. Wash the area around the meatus with a soapy sponge.
   B. Hold the labia open, and position the specimen container beneath the urethral meatus.
   C. Void into the container at least 10 mL of urine. A first morning specimen is preferred.
4. **Postprocedure care:**
   A. Write the collection date and time and the suspected diagnosis on the laboratory requisition.
   B. Send the specimen to the laboratory within 2 hours.
   C. Freeze the specimen.
5. **Client and family teaching:**
   A. This test shows sensitivity as a survival and prognostic indicator for cancers of the cervix, ovary, and vulvovaginal area.
6. **Factors that affect results:**
   A. The sensitivity of the test is increased when results are corrected for urinary concentration.
7. **Other data:**
   A. Use of UGP alone, or together with serum CA-125 levels, as a test for ovarian cancer, at the time or at annual Pap smear test, or in women with benign pelvic masses, should be carefully evaluated.
   B. False-positive results have been detected in 2% of healthy postmenopausal women.
   C. A past history of gynecologic malignancy does not falsely increase UGP levels.

URINE, ANAEROBIC CULTURE, SUPRAPUBIC PUNCTURE, CULTURE
(see Body fluid, Routine, Culture)

URINE, CULTURE AND SENSITIVITY (C & S), URINE
(see Culture, Routine, Specimen)

URINE, FUNGUS, CULTURE
(see Body fluid, Fungus, Culture)

URINE, MYCOBACTERIA, CULTURE
(see Body fluid, Mycobacteria, Culture)

URINE CULTURE, ROUTINE, CATHETERIZED, URINE
(see Body fluid, Routine, Culture)

URINE CULTURE, ROUTINE, CLEAN-CATCH, URINE
(see Body fluid, Routine, Culture)

URINE CULTURE, ROUTINE, SUPRAPUBIC PUNCTURE, URINE
(see Body fluid, Routine, Culture)

URINE CULTURE, ROUTINE, URINE
(see Body fluid, Routine, Culture)

U

URINE CULTURE AND NUCLEIC ACID AMPLIFICATION TESTS FOR *NEISSERIA GONORRHOEAE*, URINE

Norm. Negative. No *Neisseria gonorrhoeae* isolated.

Positive. Gonorrhea.

Description. Gonorrhea is a sexually transmitted disease caused by the organism *N. gonorrhoeae*. *N. gonorrhoeae* is a gonococcus transmitted from client to client by direct contact with exudates from the mucous membranes of infected clients. This disease causes purulent urethral discharge within 7 days of infection. Other symptoms may include rectal pruritus, cervicitis, endometritis, epididymitis, salpingitis, pelvic peritonitis, or vulvovaginitis. A culture is performed on the sediment of centrifuged urine. Although cultures are considered the criterion standard for diagnosis of cervical infections due to their specificity, it can take 48 hours or longer for growth to occur. Newer nucleic acid amplification tests (NAATs) and antigen/antibody detection methods are becoming available that can detect the organisms in a urine specimen.

Professional Considerations
1. Consent form NOT required.
2. **Preparation:**
   A. Obtain four soapy sponges and a sterile specimen container.

3. **Procedure:**
   A. Instruct the client to void and discard the urine.
   B. Cleanse the penis or vulva × 4 with the soapy sponges, moving distally to proximally or front to back, discarding each sponge after one use.
   C. Collect the first 10 mL of the first morning-voided urine in a sterile container; OR collect the entire first morning void in a sterile container; OR at least 2 hours after the previous void, collect the first 10 mL of urine voided in a sterile container.
4. **Postprocedure care:**
   A. Write the collection date and time, any recent antibiotic therapy, and the suspected diagnosis on the laboratory requisition.
   B. Send the specimen to the laboratory within 1 hour. Do not refrigerate it.
5. **Client and family teaching:**
   A. At least 2 days are required for results.
   B. Gonorrhea is a reportable disease in the United States.
   C. The follow-up culture should be performed 7-10 days after treatment.
   D. Gonorrhea infection is treatable with antibiotics.
   E. If results are positive, provide the client with the appropriate information on sexually transmitted diseases.
      i. Notify all sexual partners from the previous 90 days to be tested for gonorrhea infection.
      ii. Do not have sexual relations until your physician confirms that the infection is gone.
   F. Do not use feminine hygiene sprays or douche during treatment.
   G. Wear underpants and pantyhose that have a cotton lining in the crotch.
   H. Take showers instead of tub baths until the infection is gone.
6. **Factors that affect results:**
   A. False-negative results may occur for some strains of N. gonorrhoeae when Thayer-Martin or Martin-Lewis growth medium is used (because of vancomycin content of the medium).
   B. Specimen contamination with other genital flora may result in overgrowth of normal flora.
7. **Other data:**
   A. Gonorrhea is treated with aqueous procaine penicillin G (remember that penicillin-resistant strain has been reported) or ampicillin or spectinomycin or tetracycline or ciprofloxacin (remember that ciprofloxacin-resistant gonococci have been reported).
   B. The client should also be tested for syphilis.
   C. Dipstick methods are available for purposes of screening for N. gonorrhoeae.

URINE CYTOLOGY, URINE
(see Cytologic study of urine, Diagnostic)

URINE DRUG SCREEN
(see Toxicology, Drug screen, Urine)

UROBILINOGEN, URINE

Norm:

		SI UNITS
24-hour specimen	0.5-4.0 mg or 0.5-4.0 Ehrlich units	0.9-7.2 μmol
2-hour specimen		
Female	0.1-1.1 mg or 0.1-1.1 Ehrlich units	0.2-1.9 μmol
Male	0.3-2.1 mg or 0.3-2.1 Ehrlich units	0.5-3.6 μmol

RANDOM SPECIMEN (DIPSTICK METHOD)	EHRLICH UNITS/DL	COLOR
Normal or negative	0.1-1	Yellow to yellow-green
Positive	0.2-4	Yellow-orange
	0.8-12	Orange-brown

Increased. Anemia (hemolytic, pernicious), bananas eaten within 48 hours before the test, cholangitis, cirrhosis, congestive heart failure causing hepatic dysfunction, Dubin-Johnson syndrome, hepatic parenchymal damage, hemolytic processes, hepatitis (early), idiopathic pulmonary hemosiderosis, infectious mononucleosis, jaundice (hemolytic), lead poisoning, malaria, polycythemia vera, portal hypertension, pulmonary infarction, sickle cell disease, thalassemia major, and tissue hemorrhage. Drugs include sodium bicarbonate.

Decreased. Carcinoma of the head of the pancreas, cholelithiasis, complete common bile duct obstruction, diarrhea (severe), inflammation (severe), and renal insufficiency. Drugs include antibiotics that suppress the normal flora of the intestine such as chloramphenicol, cholestatics, and vitamin C.

Description. Urobilinogen is a reduction product formed by the action of bacteria on conjugated bilirubin in the gastrointestinal tract. The majority of urobilinogen is excreted in the stool. A small portion is reabsorbed by the enterohepatic pathway and reexcreted in bile. The remainder is excreted in the urine. A random dipstick check for urine bilinogen is normally negative because of its rapid oxidation to urobilin. An increase in urine urobilinogen indicates that some type of hemolytic process or hepatic dysfunction is occurring in the body. Urine urobilinogen levels are usually the highest in early to midafternoon. Thus, when reagent strips test positive, a 2-hour urine collection between 1 and 3 PM is indicated.

Professional Considerations
1. Consent form NOT required.
2. **Preparation:**
   A. *Dipstick method:*
      i. A dipstick method should not be used for clients taking the drug phenazopyridine.
      ii. Obtain a container of Bili-Labstix, Multistix, Urobilistix, or other reagent strip for urine urobilinogen testing, and a clean container.
   B. *2-hour specimen:*
      i. Obtain a light-protected, 1- to 2-L urine collection container without preservatives, a cup for drinking, and a pitcher of water (500 mL).
   C. *24-hour specimen:*
      i. Obtain a light-protected, 3-L urine collection container without preservative.
      ii. Instruct the client to save all the urine voided for the next 24 hours, to urinate before defecating, and to avoid contaminating urine with stool or toilet tissue.
      iii. Write the beginning time of collection on the container and the laboratory requisition.
      iv. Plan collection so that the test ends during laboratory open hours.
   D. See *Client and family teaching.*
3. **Procedure:**
   A. *Dipstick method:*
      i. Obtain a 20-mL random urine sample in a clean plastic container.
      ii. Immediately dip the reagent strip into the specimen and slide the strip along the edge of the container to remove excess urine.
      iii. Hold the strip horizontally next to the color chart on the container, and time the reading according to the manufacturer's directions (most are 45-60 seconds).
      iv. When the timing is completed, compare the color of the reagent pad for the urobilinogen measurement to the color chart, and record the measurement as follows:

B. *2-hour specimen:*
  i. Collect the specimen during early to midafternoon.
  ii. Instruct the client to void and to discard the urine.
  iii. Instruct the client to drink all the 500 mL of water in the pitcher over the next 10 minutes.
  iv. Save all the urine voided over the next 2 hours in a refrigerated, light-protected, urine collection container. The urine must be transferred into the container *immediately* after each void.
C. *24-hour specimen:*
  i. Discard the first morning-void urine.
  ii. Save all the urine voided in a refrigerated, light-protected, 3-L container without preservatives. For specimens collected from an indwelling urinary catheter, keep the foil-covered drainage bag on ice, and empty the urine into the light-protected collection container hourly. Document the quantity of urinary output during the collection period.
4. **Postprocedure care:**
A. *2-hour collection:*
  i. Send the specimen to the laboratory immediately for prompt measurement.
B. *24-hour collection:*
  i. Write the ending time of collection on the laboratory requisition.
  ii. Compare the urine quantity in the container with the urinary output record for the test. If the container has less urine than what was recorded as output, some of the urine may have been discarded, thus invalidating the test. The test must be restarted.
  iii. Send valid specimens to the laboratory immediately for prompt measurement.
5. **Client and family teaching:**
A. Avoid eating bananas for 2 days before the test.
B. Collect specimens according to the appropriate procedure, as described above.
6. **Factors that affect results:**
A. Drugs that may cause falsely increased results include acetazolamide, aminosalicylic acid, antipyrine, aspirin, chlorpromazine, 5-hydroxyindoleacetic acid, phenazopyridine, phenothiazines, sulfobromophthalein (Bromsulphalein), and sulfonamides. Herbal or natural remedies include cascara sagrada (*Rhamnus purshiana*).
B. Urine alkalinization increases the excretion rate of urine urobilinogen. Urine acidification decreases the excretion rate of urine urobilinogen.
C. Dipstick methods can detect only abnormally high levels, not abnormally low levels.
D. The level may be normal in clients with incomplete common bile duct obstruction.
E. False-positive or falsely increased results may occur in porphyria.
7. **Other data:**
A. None.

UROFLOWMETRY, DIAGNOSTIC

Norm. Normal uroflow curve, with normal peak and normal voiding time for quantity voided.

	VOLUME	RATE (Q[max])	
		FEMALE	**MALE**
Postvoid residual amount			
Normal		≤50 mL	≤50 mL
Equivocal		100-200 mL	100-200 mL
Abnormal		>200 mL	>200 mL

		RATE (Q[max])	
	VOLUME	FEMALE	MALE

Adults

Young <45 years	≥150 mL	18 mL/second	21 mL/second
Middle 46-65 years	≥150 mL	15 mL/second	15 mL/second
Older >65 years	>150 mL	10-15 mL/second	10-15 mL/second
	1100-2000 mL/24 hr		

Children

Younger < 8 years	≥100 mL	10 mL/second	10 mL/second
Older 8-13 years	≥100 mL	15 mL/second	12 mL/second

Usage. Part of diagnostic evaluation for voiding abnormalities (e.g., evaluating cystourethrocele, identifying postvoiding residual volumes, voiding speed as an indicator of obstruction).

Description. Uroflowmetry involves measuring the voiding duration, amount, and rate of urine voided into a funnel with a urine flowmeter that records the above information in a graphic format. The Q[max] is the maximum number of milliliters of urine per second. A Q[max] of less than 12 mL/second is associated with a higher risk for urinary retention than those with normal flow rates. This simple, noninvasive test is usually performed with other tests such as cystometry and voiding cystourethrography.

Professional Considerations
1. Consent form NOT required.
2. **Preparation:**
   A. Provide a private environment for voiding.
3. **Procedure:**
   A. Several types of urine flowmeters are available. The exact procedure depends on the type of flowmeter used and should be followed according to the manufacturer's instructions and institutional protocol.
   B. In general, the flowmeter is activated just before the void, as described above. The client voids while standing to avoid straining pressure effects on urine volume. The volume voided and the rate, pattern, and duration of voiding are analyzed and displayed graphically by the urine flowmeter. A uroflow curve displays the changes in the urine flow rate throughout the void.
   C. Serial recordings of each void over 2-3 days may be performed to provide the most accurate evaluation of the client's urine flow patterns. This helps correct for aberrancies such as hesitancy as a result of nervousness, or single voided specimens of extremely small or large volume.
   D. The client's position during each void and the amount and route of fluid intake throughout testing should be recorded.
4. **Postprocedure care:**
   A. None.
5. **Client and family teaching:**
   A. Do not void for several hours before the test. Drink several glasses of water at least an hour before the test so that your bladder is full and you are feeling like you have to urinate.
   B. When the urge to void is felt, assume a standing voiding position and perform a normal void, completely emptying the bladder urine into the funnel of the flowmeter. The void should be performed without straining and while the rest of the body is held as motionless as possible. Urinate before defecating, and do not allow stool or toilet tissue to enter the funnel.
6. **Factors that affect results:**
   A. The quantity of urine voided affects the flow rate. Optimal amounts for evaluation of bladder function are between 150 and 400 mL. Quantities over 400 mL cause deterioration of bladder detrusor muscle function.
   B. Recent urethral instrumentation may cause decreased flow rates.

U

C. Age affects the flow rate (Drach et al, 1979).

7. Other data:
A. None.

UROGRAPHY, EXCRETORY, DIAGNOSTIC
(see Intravenous pyelography, Diagnostic)

UTEROSALPINGOGRAPHY, DIAGNOSTIC
(see Hysterosalpingography, Diagnostic)

UTEROTUBAL INSUFFLATION, DIAGNOSTIC
(see Rubin's test, Diagnostic)

VAGINAL ASPIRATE FOR MOTILE/NONMOTILE SPERM, SPECIMEN
(see Sims-Huhner test, Diagnostic)

VAGINAL CULTURE
(see Genitals, Routine, Culture)

VAGINAL CYTOLOGY
(see Hormonal evaluation, Cytologic, Specimen)

VALPROIC ACID, BLOOD

Norm. Negative.

VALPROIC ACID THERAPY	TROUGH	SI UNITS
Therapeutic level	50-100 µg/mL	350-690 µmol/L
Toxic level	>100 µg/mL	>690 µmol/L
Panic level	>200 µg/mL	>1380 µmol/L

Panic Levels Symptoms and Treatment

Symptoms. Burning feet paresthesia, numbness, tingling, weakness, mental changes.

Treatment:
Note: Treatment choice(s) depend on client history and condition and episode history.
Naloxone.
Hemodialysis and peritoneal dialysis will NOT remove valproic acid.
The use of activated charcoal did NOT enhance valproic acid elimination in animal studies.

Usage. Monitoring for therapeutic levels during valproic acid therapy.

Description. Valproic acid is an anticonvulsant effective against myoclonus and grand mal, petit mal, and complex partial seizures, and also used for long-term control of manic episodes in bipolar disorders. It is being used experi-mentally for panic disorders, and migraine treatment. Newer research has found that it has a role in resistance to cancer activity by suppressing tumor growth. After oral or rectal administration, it is metabolized by the liver and excreted in the urine, with a half-life of 6-8 hours and elimination half-life of 15-20 hours.

Professional Considerations
1. Consent form NOT required.
2. **Preparation:**
   A. Tube: Red topped, red/gray topped, or gold topped (for serum level), or green topped (for plasma level).
   B. Specimens MAY be drawn during hemodialysis.
3. **Procedure:**
   A. Draw a 1-mL blood sample. Draw the trough level immediately before dose administration. Draw the peak level 1-3 hours after dose administration.
4. **Postprocedure care:**
   A. Specimens must be kept in a tightly capped tube until testing to prevent evaporation of valproic acid from the sample.

5. **Client and family teaching:**
   A. Long-term use of this drug may result in hepatotoxicity.
   B. Overdose of this drug can cause neurotoxicity.
   C. For an intentional overdose, refer the client and family for crisis intervention and offer resource information for counseling.
6. **Factors that affect results:**
   A. Absorption is slowed by the presence of food in the gastrointestinal tract; thus peak levels occur later for doses given on a full stomach than for doses given on an empty stomach.
   B. Valproic acid reaches steady-state levels in about 96 hours.

C. Drugs that may decrease valproic acid half-life include carbamazepine, fluoxetine, phenobarbital, phenytoin, and primidone.
D. Hepatic failure may cause elevated results.
E. Concurrent administration of methsuximide decreases valproic acid levels.
7. **Other data:**
   A. Periodic liver function tests should be performed throughout valproic acid therapy.
   B. Valproic acid increases serum levels of phenobarbital.
   C. A case has been reported of fatal acute pancreatitis caused by valproic acid.

VANCOMYCIN, SERUM

Norm. Negative.

		SI UNITS
Trough		
Therapeutic	5-10 µg/mL	3-7 µmol/L
Nephrotoxicity	>10 µg/mL	>7 µmol/L
Panic level	>15 µg/mL	>10 µmol/L
Peak		
Therapeutic	30-40 µg/mL	20-27 µmol/L
Ototoxicity	>40 µg/mL	>27 µmol/L
Panic level	>60 µg/mL	>41 µmol/L

Panic Levels Symptoms and Treatment

Symptoms. Hypotension, leukopenia or neutropenia (agranulocytosis, granulocytopenia); exfoliative dermatitis, lacrimation, thrombocytopenia, dermatitis, tubular necrosis, deafness, colitis. Ototoxicity (prolonged levels >30 mg/mL).

Treatment:
Note: Treatment choice(s) depend on client history and condition and episode history.
Ipecac (within 30 minutes) or gastric lavage (within 60 minutes).
Supportive therapy for hypotension. The use of activated charcoal orally has NOT been shown to enhance the elimination of vancomycin. (See American Academy of Clinical Toxicology, 1999.)

Hemodialysis, hemofiltration, and peritoneal dialysis WILL remove vancomycin. Charcoal hemoperfusion will NOT remove vancomycin.

Usage. Monitoring for therapeutic (and safe) levels during vancomycin therapy.

Description. Vancomycin is an aminoglycoside antibiotic that inhibits cell wall synthesis of gram-positive bacteria. It is frequently used in the treatment of infections caused by methicillin-resistant *Staphylococcus aureus* (MRSA) and in treatment for pseudomembranous colitis. Vancomycin is metabolized in the liver, with 80% excreted through the kidneys and a small amount in bile. Oral doses are primarily excreted in the feces. Vancomycin half-life is very dependent on renal glomerular function. Rapid infusions of this drug have been associated with histamine release causing "redman syndrome," in which the skin becomes flushed, erythematous, and pruritic.

Professional Considerations
1. Consent form NOT required.
2. **Preparation:**
   A. Tube: Red topped, red/gray topped, or gold topped.
   B. Specimens MAY be drawn during hemodialysis.
3. **Procedure:**
   A. Draw the trough level just before dose. Draw the peak level 30 minutes after intravenous administration.
   B. Draw a 1-mL blood sample.
4. **Postprocedure care:**
   A. Send the sample to the laboratory promptly. Serum should be separated and frozen within 4 hours.
5. **Client and family teaching:**
   A. Overdoses can cause renal failure and hearing loss.
   B. Slowing the rate of drug infusion can decrease feelings of the skin being flushed, red, and itchy.
6. **Factors that affect results:**
   A. Minimum inhibitory concentration (MIC) of vancomycin varies

for different organisms and will affect the therapeutic trough level needed. MIC should be included in sensitivity testing results. In general, an average peak vancomycin level that is two to four times higher than the MIC is considered adequate for control of the organism. See *Minimum inhibitory concentration, Specimen.*
   B. Clients with impaired glomerular renal function will have elevated levels if dosages are not adjusted accordingly.
7. **Other data:**
   A. Renal function and hearing should be assessed before and throughout vancomycin therapy. Clients that demonstrated increased nephrotoxicity in one study were those also receiving another aminoglycoside concurrently, those who received vancomycin for over 3 weeks, and those who had trough levels >10 mg/L.
   B. Vancomycin administered intravenously over 2 hours, as compared to 1 hour, has been shown to reduce the occurrence of redman syndrome.

VANILLYLMANDELIC ACID (VMA), URINE

Norm:

	µg/mg Creatinine	µg/g of Body Weight	SI UNITS mmol/mol of Creatinine
Adults	≤7	<150	4.0
Children			
Birth-11 months	15-27	<180	15.4
12-23 months	<18	<230	10.3
2-4 years	11-13	<150	7.4
5-9 years	<8.5	<150	4.9
10-14 years	<7	<150	4.0
15-18 years	<5	<150	2.9l

NORMS	µG/24 HOURS	SI UNITS
Adults	7-9 mg/24 hours	35-45 µmol/day
Children		
≤12 months	≤1.8 mg/24 hours	≤9 µmol/day
12 months-4 years	≤3 mg/24 hours	≤15 µmol/day
4-15 years	≤4 mg/24 hours	≤20 µmol/day

Increased. Ganglioblastoma, ganglioneuroma, neuroblastoma, and pheochromocytoma. Drugs include aspirin, aminosalicylic acid, epinephrine, glyceryl guaiacolate, levodopa, lithium carbonate, mephenesin, methocarbamol, nalidixic acid, norepinephrine, oxytetracycline, penicillin, phenazopyridine, phenosulfonphthalein, salicylates, sulfobromophthalein (Bromsulphalein), and sulfonamides.

Decreased. Familial dysautonomia (Riley-Day syndrome). Drugs include chlorpromazine, clofibrate, clonidine, guanethidine analogs, imipramine, levodopa, methyldopa, monoamine oxidase (MAO) inhibitors, reserpine, and salicylates.

Description. Vanillylmandelic acid (VMA) occurs as an end product of epinephrine and norepinephrine metabolism and is freely excreted in the urine. This test aids in the diagnosis and monitoring for clients with catecholamine-secreting tumors.

Professional Considerations
1. Consent form NOT required.
2. Preparation:
   A. Withhold drugs that may cause increased or decreased results (listed above) for 72 hours before the test. Diuretics, antihypertensives, and sympathomimetics (including nonprescriptive cold and allergy medications) must be withheld for 5-14 days.
   B. Obtain a clean, 3-L container with hydrochloric acid (HCl) or acetic acid preservative.
   C. Write the starting time of collection on the laboratory requisition and container.
   D. See *Client and family teaching.*
3. Procedure:
   A. Discard first morning urine specimen.
   B. Save all the urine voided for a 24-hour period in a refrigerated, clean, 3-L plastic container to which HCl or acetic acid preservative has been added. For specimens collected from indwelling urinary catheters, keep the drainage bag on ice and empty urine into the collection container hourly. Add preservative as

needed to maintain pH at about 3.0 (range, 2.0 to 4.0). Document the quantity of urine output throughout the collection period.
4. Postprocedure care:
   A. Compare the urine quantity in the container with the record of urine output during the collection period. If the container contains less urine than what was documented as output, some may have been discarded, invalidating the test.
5. Client and family teaching:
   A. Avoid the following foods for 72 hours before the test: avocados, bananas, beer, cheese (aged), Chianti wines, chocolate, citrus fruits, cocoa, fava beans, grains, tea, vanilla, walnuts, and wine. Also avoid the herb coffee (*Coffea*) for 72 hours before the test.
   B. Save all the urine voided for 24 hours, urinate before defecating, and avoid contaminating urine with stool or toilet tissue. If any urine is accidentally discarded, discard the entire specimen and restart the collection the next day.
   C. Avoid stress, strenuous exercise, and smoking of tobacco before and throughout the urine collection period.
6. Factors that affect results:
   A. Drugs that cause decreased results in normal clients may not suppress levels to below normal level in clients with catecholamine-secreting tumors.
7. Other data:
   A. Consistency in results has been demonstrated between random, 6-hour, 12-hour, and 24-hour specimens.

VARICELLA-ZOSTER VIRUS SEROLOGY, SERUM

Norm. Less than a fourfold increase in titer between acute and convalescent samples.

Increased. Chickenpox and herpes zoster (shingles).

Description. Varicella-zoster virus, also known as human herpesvirus 3, is the causative agent of chickenpox and shingles, which are time-limited viral infections that produce skin lesions or vesicles. The mode of transmission is directly from client to client, airborne spread of infected respiratory secretions or vesicle fluid, or indirectly through contact with contaminated secretions on inanimate objects. The virus multiplies in the respiratory tract and then spreads through the bloodstream to the skin and internal organs. After causing chickenpox in childhood, the latent virus may reemerge to cause shingles in the elderly. In this test, complement fixation, indirect immunofluorescence, or agglutination methods are used to detect the antibody to the varicella-zoster virus.

Professional Considerations
1. Consent form NOT required.
2. Preparation:
   A. Tube: Red topped, red/gray topped, or gold topped.
3. Procedure:
   A. Draw a 3-mL blood sample as soon as possible after symptoms appear. Label the tube as the "acute sample." Repeat the test in 10-14 days and label the tube as the "convalescent sample."
4. Postprocedure care:
   A. None.
5. Client and family teaching:
   A. Return for convalescent sampling in 10-14 days.
6. Factors that affect results:
   A. None found.
7. Other data:
   A. Chickenpox and shingles are contagious for up to 6 days after lesions or vesicles appear. Immunocompromised clients may be contagious for longer periods of time.
   B. For clients exposed to varicella-zoster, varicella-zoster immune globulin from zoster-convalescent clients or human immune globulin given within 4 days may limit or prevent symptoms.
   C. The incidence of varicella in children under age 4 years is increasing. Since maternal antibody protection lasts only about 1 year after birth, the varicella vaccine is recommended to be given between the ages of 12 and 18 months.

VASOACTIVE INTESTINAL POLYPEPTIDE (VIP), BLOOD

Norm. Adults and children: <50 pg/mL (<50 ng/mL, SI units).

Increased. Achlorhydria (WDHA) syndrome, ectopic islet cell tumor, hypokalemia, islet cell hyperplasia, islet cell tumor, laxative abuse, pancreatic cholera syndrome, tachycardia, Verner-Morrison syndrome, vipoma, and watery diarrhea.

Decreased. Asthma exacerbation.

Description. Vasoactive intestinal polypeptide (VIP) is a gastrointestinal hormone produced by neuroendocrine cells in the small and large intestine, pancreas, brain, and peripheral nervous system. Its actions include stimulating watery pancreatic secretions with a high pH, stimulating glycogenolysis, inhibiting stomach secretions, stimulating the release of insulin and glucagon, causing peripheral vasodilatation, slowing gastric motility, stimulating intestinal chloride secretion, and inhibiting intestinal sodium absorption. Clients with vipoma neoplasms have symptoms of watery diarrhea that is high in potassium and bicarbonate. VIP is also found abundantly in the human lung and is thought to cause bronchodilation.

Professional Considerations
1. Consent form NOT required.
2. Preparation:
   A. When possible, medications should be withheld for 1-2 days.
   B. Observe clients with watery diarrhea closely for symptoms of dehydration during the 12-hour preparation fast.
   C. Preschedule this test with the laboratory, and verify collection instructions with the laboratory performing the test.
   D. Obtain a chilled plastic syringe to which 1.2 mg of EDTA has been added.
   E. See *Client and family teaching.*
3. Procedure:
   A. Draw a 7-mL blood sample.
4. Postprocedure care:
   A. Transport the specimen to the laboratory immediately.

B. The specimen must be separated and transferred to a special VIP container and then frozen.

5. **Client and family teaching:**
   A. Fast from food and fluids for 12 hours before the test.

6. **Factors that affect results:**
   A. Results are invalidated if the client has undergone a radioactive scan within 1 week before the test.

7. **Other data:**
   A. None.

VDRL, SERUM
(see Venereal Disease Research Laboratory test, Serum)

VECTORCARDIOGRAM, DIAGNOSTIC

Norm. Requires interpretation by an expert. P, QRS, and T loops are evaluated for direction, magnitude, and inscription.

Usage. Identification and classification of myocardial infarction; evaluation of risk for myocardial infarction progression to complete heart block; and helps in the diagnosis of ventricular preexcitation and localization of ventricular bypass tracts.

Description. A vectorcardiogram (VCG) is a spatial representation of the sequence of changes in the heart's electrical activity measured three-dimensionally along the x-(horizontal, transverse, left-to-right) axis, y-(vertical, head-to-foot) axis, and z-(sagittal, anteroposterior) axis. A vector represents the heart's electrical potential with respect to specific direction and magnitude. The vectorcardiograph simultaneously records two lead axes at a time to represent the frontal plane vector (x, y), the horizontal plane vector (x, z), and the sagittal plane vector (y, z) and provides a screen display or graphic recording of P, QRS, and T vector loops that move in the same direction as the heart's electrical activity. The literature demonstrates controversy regarding the ability of VCG to better detect and classify myocardial infarction than ECG. This expensive procedure is infre-

quently performed in clinical settings but is used as a teaching tool.

Professional Considerations
1. Consent form NOT required.
2. **Preparation:**
   A. Obtain a vectorcardiogram machine, electrodes, and conductive gel.
3. **Procedure:**
   A. The client is positioned supine.
   B. Conductive electrodes are applied according to institutional protocol (usually to the anterior and posterior upper torso, left lower extremity, and the forehead or nape of the neck).
   C. The machine is activated, and the vectorcardiogram is completed in about 10 minutes.
4. **Postprocedure care:**
   A. Remove the electrodes. Cleanse the skin of conductive gel.
5. **Client and family teaching:**
   A. It is important to relax, breathe normally, and lie very still throughout the recording.
6. **Factors that affect results:**
   A. The client's sex, age, medications, and clinical picture must be considered when one is interpreting the results.
   B. One study recommends that respiratory status be identical for serial vectorcardiograms from the effect of respiration and ventilation on the results.
7. **Other data:**
   A. The vectorcardiogram is most useful when evaluated in combination with an electrocardiogram.

VENEREAL DISEASE RESEARCH LABORATORY TEST (VDRL), SERUM

Norm. Negative. Nonreactive.

Positive. Treponemal disease: bejel, pinta, syphilis, yaws.

Description. Syphilis is a complex sexually transmitted disease characterized by a wide range of symptoms that imitate other diseases. It is caused by the organism *Treponema pallidum*. The Venereal Disease Research Laboratory test (VDRL) is a sensitive screening test for the presence of reagin, the antibody specific for the treponemal spirochete. In this test, the sample is heat inactivated and then mixed with an antigen (cardiolipin phospholipid derived from beef heart in complex with lecithin and coated on particles of cholesterol) to reagin. The mixture is then examined microscopically to detect flocculation of the cholesterol particles, indicating a positive test. The VDRL is more sensitive than the rapid plasma reagin (RPR) test for primary syphilis. The test becomes reactive during primary-stage syphilis (about 14 days after a chancre is visible) and is reactive in virtually all cases of secondary-stage syphilis. Results will revert to negative with treatment or by the tertiary stage. Many biologic false-positive results are possible; thus specificity is low. A newer test, the VDRL enzyme-linked immunosorbent assay (ELISA) is being studied for possible replacement of this cardiolipin test for large-scale screening for syphilis.

Professional Considerations

1. Consent form NOT required.
2. Preparation:
   A. Tube: Red topped, red/gray topped, or gold topped.
3. Procedure:
   A. Draw a 3-mL blood sample.
4. Postprocedure care:
   A. None.
5. Client and family teaching:
   A. Syphilis is a sexually transmitted disease; information regarding sexual partners is necessary for control of the disease.
   B. If testing positive for syphilis and diagnosis is confirmed:
      i. Notify all sexual contacts from the previous 90 days (if early stage) to be tested for syphilis.
      ii. Syphilis can be cured with antibiotics. These may worsen the symptoms for the first 24 hours.
      iii. Do not have sex for 2 months and until after repeat testing has confirmed that the syphilis is cured. Use condoms after that for 2 years. Return for repeat testing every 3-4 months for the next 2 years to make sure the disease is cured.
      iv. Do not become pregnant for 2 years because syphilis can be transmitted to the fetus.
      v. If left untreated, syphilis can damage many body organs, including the brain, over several years.
6. Factors that affect results:
   A. Refrigeration destroys *Treponema* spirochetes in 72 hours.
   B. Conditions that may cause false-positive results include active immunization in children, antinuclear antibodies, blood loss (with multiple transfusions), brucellosis, chancroid, chickenpox, cirrhosis, the common cold, diabetes mellitus, fever (relapsing), first week of life, hepatitis (infectious), hypergammaglobulinemia, leprosy, leptospirosis (Weil's disease), Lyme disease, lymphogranuloma venereum, lymphoma, infection (chronic), malaria, measles, mononucleosis (infectious), mycoplasmal pneumonia, nonsyphilitic treponemal diseases (bejel, pinta, yaws), periarteritis nodosa, pneumococcal pneumonia, pneumonia, pregnancy, rat-bite fever, rheumatic fever, rheumatic heart disease, rheumatoid arthritis, scarlet fever, scleroderma, senescence, subacute bacterial endocarditis, systemic lupus erythematosus, tuberculosis (advanced pulmonary), treponematosis, trypanosomiasis, tuberculosis, typhus fever, and vaccinia.
7. Other data:
   A. Suspected biologic false-positive tests necessitate the fluorescent treponemal antibody-absorbed double stain test.
   B. The greatest risk for transmission of syphilis occurs in freshly drawn blood products that must be administered immediately (platelets) or those not refrigerated for 72 hours before infusion.
   C. Syphilis is treated with penicillin.

VENEREAL DISEASE RESEARCH LABORATORY (VDRL) TEST, CEREBROSPINAL FLUID, SPECIMEN

Norm. Nonreactive.

Usage. The only test approved for cerebrospinal fluid testing for neurosyphilis.

Description. Syphilis is a complex, sexually transmitted disease characterized by a wide range of symptoms that imitate other diseases. It is caused by the organism *Treponema pallidum*. The venereal disease research laboratory test (VDRL) is a screening test for the presence of reagin, the antibody specific for the treponemal spirochete. In this test, the sample is heat inactivated and then mixed with an antigen (cardiolipin phospholipid derived from beef heart in complex with lecithin and coated on particles of cholesterol) to reagin. The mixture is then examined microscopically to detect flocculation of the cholesterol particles, indicating a positive test. Unlike serum results, cerebrospinal fluid (CSF) results may remain positive long after treatment; thus this test is not useful for monitoring response to therapy.

Professional Considerations
1. Consent form NOT required for the test but IS required for the procedure used to obtain the specimen. For procedural risks and contraindications, see *Lumbar puncture, Diagnostic*.
2. Preparation:
   A. See *Lumbar puncture, Diagnostic*.
3. Procedure:
   A. Obtain a 5-mL sample of CSF in a sterile, capped vial by lumbar puncture, or from the ventricles of the brain during special procedures (see *Lumbar puncture, Diagnostic*).
4. Postprocedure care:
   A. See *Lumbar puncture, Diagnostic*.
5. Client and family teaching:
   A. Syphilis is a sexually transmitted disease; information regarding sexual partners is necessary for control of the disease.
   B. See also *Venereal Disease Research Laboratory test, Serum*, for additional teaching related to syphilis.
6. Factors that affect results:
   A. False-negative results may occur in clients with tabes dorsalis.
7. Other data:
   A. Serial testing is recommended for clients with AIDS who are suspected of having syphilis but have a negative VDRL test.

VENEZUELAN EQUINE ENCEPHALITIS VIRUS SEROLOGY, SERUM

Norm.
A less than fourfold rise in titer between acute and convalescent samples.

Usage. Confirmation of diagnosis of Venezuelan equine encephalitis.

Description. Venezuelan equine encephalitis is caused by a group A arbovirus (arthropod-borne virus) that results in fever and mild, flu like symptoms (most commonly) but may progress to severe encephalitis symptoms of disorientation, convulsions, paralysis, coma, and death in children. Occurrence is primarily in South America, Central America, Mexico, and the United States. Mode of transmission to humans from horses is through the bite of an infected mosquito. Identification of the virus is performed through viral neutralization, complement fixation, hemagglutin inhibition, fluorescent antibody, and agar gel precipitation. There is no vaccine for Venezuelan equine encephalitis, but there is some literature suggesting antiviral therapy with VEEV-specific human or "humanized" monoclonal antibodies may help protect those exposed from developing the symptoms.

Professional Considerations
1. Consent form NOT required.
2. Preparation:
   A. Tube: Red topped, red/gray topped, or gold topped.
3. Procedure:
   A. Draw a 7-mL blood sample as soon as possible after symptoms appear and label it as the "acute sample." Repeat the test in 10 days and label the sample as the "convalescent sample."
4. Postprocedure care:
   A. None.
5. Client and family teaching:
   A. The mode of transmission is a mosquito bite.
   B. Hypertension can be a result of this viral infection.
6. Factors that affect results:
   A. None found.
7. Other data:
   A. Testing may also be performed on cerebrospinal fluid.

B. Venezuelan equine encephalitis is not transmitted client to client.
C. There is no specific treatment for this illness.

VENLAFAXINE
(see Selective serotonin reuptake inhibitors, Blood)

VENOGRAPHY (PHLEBOGRAPHY), DIAGNOSTIC

Norm. Negative. Normal finding. Absence of thrombosis. No obstructions to flow or filling defects identified.

Positive. Abnormal finding. An intraluminal filling defect in the deep venous contrast column indicates deep venous thrombosis (DVT). An abrupt cutoff of a deep vein with the development of collateral circulation may also indicate the presence of DVT.

Usage. Detection of site and presence of venous thrombosis of the lower extremities; radiographic guidance for insertion of peripherally inserted central catheter (PICC); used with magnetic resonance imaging for the detection and evaluation of arteriovenous malformations and vascular venous lesions.

Description. Venography is an invasive, radiographic, or nuclear medicine procedure whereby radiopaque dye or a radionuclide is injected intravenously and the lower extremities are radiographed for the DVT. Although considered to be the criterion standard for detection of deep venous thromboses, venography is similar in accuracy to newer ultrasonographic techniques for symptomatic clients. In asymptomatic clients, however, it remains superior in accuracy but higher in risk to ultrasonography for the detection of DVT. For initial detection of proximal DVT, venography has largely been replaced by the use of compression ultrasonography (CUS) and color duplex ultrasonography. Venography is more often reserved for detection of calf DVT, and for further testing for repeat symptoms during the first 6 months after an acute DVT.

Professional Considerations
1. Consent form IS required.

Risks
Allergic reaction to dye (itching, hives, rash, tight feeling in the throat, shortness of breath, anaphylaxis), bacteremia, cellulitis (onset 2-12 hours; peak 12-24 hours), congestive heart failure, embolism, renal toxicity from contrast medium, thrombophlebitis, vasospasm, venous thrombosis, venipuncture-site infection.

Contraindications
Severe congestive heart failure, severe pulmonary hypertension, previous allergy to radiographic dye, iodine or shellfish, pregnancy (because of the radioactive iodine crossing the blood-placental barrier), renal insufficiency.

2. **Preparation:**
   A. This test is normally performed in a Radiology department.
   B. Have emergency equipment readily available.
   C. Obtain radiographic dye, heparin and saline flush solution, and a tourniquet.
3. **Procedure:**
   A. The client is positioned or semiupright on the fluoroscopic table, with the weight placed on the nonexamined extremity.
   B. A tourniquet may be placed on the extremity to control the speed of blood flow.
   C. After intravenous access is established in a foot vein, radiographic dye is injected, and several rapid, sequential radiographs are taken of the extremity as the dye flows in the bloodstream. Alternatively one may conduct a nuclear medicine study whereby a radionuclide is injected, followed by scintigraphic scanning of the extremity.
   D. The intravenous access site is flushed with heparin/saline solution, and the access is removed.
4. **Postprocedure care:**
   A. Assess injection site for symptoms of dye infiltration (redness, edema, warmth, tenderness).
   B. Assess vital signs; peripheral pulses; and color, motion, temperature, and sensation of lower

extremities every 15 minutes × 4, then every 30 minutes × 4, then hourly × 4, and then every 4 hours until 24 hours after the procedure.

5. Client and family teaching:
   A. A feeling of warmth around the neck and face is normally felt after the injection.
   B. Procedure time is 1-1½ hours.
6. Factors that affect results:
   A. None.
7. Other data:
   A. Limitations of this procedure include poor visualization when a client has previously had a DVT in the affected extremity, intra-limb contrast material dilution, and difficulties obtaining pedal venous access secondary to client characteristics.

VENTILATION/PERFUSION LUNG SCAN, DIAGNOSTIC
(see Lung scan, Perfusion and ventilation, Diagnostic)

VENTRICULOGRAPHY, DIAGNOSTIC

Norm. Normal cardiac ventricular structure; lack of disease process.

Usage. Noninvasive test to detect changes in the heart function, assess for cardiac damage and evaluate heart-wall motion and pumping function. Conditions include atrial septal defect, cardiomyopathy, heart failure, Lyme disease (secondary), mitral stenosis, and superior vena cava obstruction. May be used before coronary angiography to detect those clients with severe coronary artery disease who are at risk for angiographic procedural complications.

Description. Ventriculography is a noninvasive nuclear medicine test that allows for the heart chambers and major blood vessels to be outlined. A small dose of a radioactive isotope is injected in the person's veins. The isotope attaches itself to red blood cells that then pass through the heart. Special scanners or cameras can track the radioactive isotopes as they flow through the heart. The image is often synchronized with an electrocardio-gram. Frequently the test is given in two stages: one at rest, one with exercise.

Professional Considerations
1. Consent form MAY be required.

Risks
Small exposure to radiation from the radioactive isotopes. With exercise testing, potential for cardiac ischemia, myocardial infarction, dysrhythmias, blood pressure changes.

Contraindications
Clients unable to lie motionless for the scan, previous allergy to radioisotope.

Precautions
During pregnancy, risks of cumulative radiation exposure to the fetus from this and other previous or future imaging studies must be weighed against the benefits of the procedure. Although formal limits for client exposure are relative to this risk:benefit comparison, the United States Nuclear Regulatory Commission requires that the cumulative dose equivalent to an embryo/fetus from *occupational* exposure not exceed 0.5 rem (5 mSv). Radiation dosage to the fetus is proportional to the distance of the anatomy studied from the abdomen and decreases as pregnancy progresses. For pregnant clients, consult the Radiologist/Radiology Department to obtain estimated fetal radiation exposure from this procedure.

2. Preparation:
   A. Have emergency equipment available.
   B. Obtain baseline ECG.
   C. Review for history of allergic type of responses to radiographic dyes.
3. Procedure:
   A. Insert a intravenous access device.
   B. Inject the isotope.
   C. A scanner will be placed over the chest area.
   D. Imaging takes place; depending on the type of test, the patient may have a resting image, a resting and then an exercise image, or an exercise and then a resting image.
4. Postprocedure care:
   A. Assess for any chest pain or discomfort.
   B. For scans that involved exercise, monitor the patient until vital signs return to baseline values.

C. Proper disposal of any radioactive waste.
5. **Client and family teaching:**
   A. Do not take caffeine or any stimulants for 3-6 hours before the test.
   B. Because this test may take some time, bring items to occupy yourself while waiting.
   C. Wear comfortable clothing.
   D. In women who are breast-feeding, formula should be substituted for breast milk for 1 or more days after the procedure.
6. **Factors that affect results:**
   A. Client's ability to lay still for the scan.
   B. Drugs that alter cardiac contractility.
   C. Recent MI (within 24 hours).
   D. Recent previous exposure to radioactive tracers may interfere with the quality of the scan.
   E. The decrement of the R-wave amplitude changes can indicate clients with 3-vessel disease at risk of angiographic complications.
   F. Standard volumes of contrast material are often associated with ventricular ectopy, which makes the readings uninterpretable. Reducing the volume of contrast material from 15 mL/second for 3 seconds to 15 mL/second for 1 second has been shown to reduce ectopy without affecting results.
7. **Other data:**
   A. Abnormal findings in the scan may indicate the need for more extensive studies.
   B. Health care professionals working in a nuclear medicine area must follow federal standards set by the Nuclear Regulatory Commission. These standards include precautions for handling the radioactive material and monitoring potential radiation exposure.

VIDEO-ASSISTED MEDIASTINOSCOPY

(see Mediastinoscopy, Diagnostic)

VIRAL CULTURE, SPECIMEN

Norm. Negative. No virus isolated.

Positive. Acquired immunodeficiency syndrome, adenovirus, chickenpox, conjunctivitis, cytomegalovirus, enteroviruses, herpes simplex, herpes zoster, keratitis, mumps virus, parainfluenza, pneumonia (viral), respiratory syncytial virus, rhinovirus, shingles, and varicella-zoster virus.

Description. Viruses are the tiniest known infectious agents and are made up of a single type of deoxyribonucleic acid (DNA) or ribonucleic acid (RNA) surrounded by an envelope of protein (proteinaceous coat). Viruses are parasites in that they reproduce with the aid of the enzymes of their living host. Thus they will not grow on artificial (nonliving) media. Viruses must be inoculated onto special viral culture media consisting of growing cells. The availability of viral culture methodology allows the rapid diagnosis and treatment of viral illnesses, as well as pattern tracking for outbreaks of viral illnesses.

Professional Considerations
1. Consent form NOT required.
2. **Preparation:**
   A. Blood cultures MAY be drawn during hemodialysis.
   B. Clarify specific instructions with the laboratory performing the test.
   C. Obtain the proper supplies, as listed below, depending on the site to be cultured.
      Blood: Chilled, heparinized green-topped tube.
      Biopsy: Biopsy tray and sterile container.
      Conjunctivae: Virocult or Culturette swab, or sterile spatula and viral transport medium.
      Cerebrospinal fluid: Sterile vial with cap.
      Lesion: Virocult or Culturette swab, and 1-mL syringe with intradermal needle.
      Pharynx: Virocult or Culturette swab.
      Rectal swab: Virocult or Culturette swab.
      Stool: Clean, dry container.
      Urine: Sterile specimen container.
   D. Obtain ice for packing around specimens to be cultured for influenzavirus or cytomegalovirus.
3. **Procedure:**
   A. *Blood:* Draw a 5-mL blood sample as soon as possible after symp-

toms appear. Label the tube as the acute specimen. Repeat the test in 14-28 days, and label the sample as the convalescent specimen.

B. *Biopsy:* Using a sterile technique, collect an individual tissue sample into a cold, sterile container. Label it with the collection site and date.

C. *Conjunctivae:* Gently pull the lower eyelid down. Firmly swab the lower conjunctival border back and forth several times with a sterile swab. Place the swab in a chilled viral transport medium. Alternately, gently but firmly scrape the conjunctiva with a sterile spatula and smear the sample onto a chilled viral transport medium.

D. *Cerebrospinal fluid:* Obtain a 5-mL sample of cerebrospinal fluid by lumbar puncture into a chilled, sterile vial.

E. *Lesion:* Aspirate fluid from the vesicle with an intradermal needle and a 1-mL syringe. Eject the fluid into 1-2 mL of chilled viral transport medium. Firmly swab the base of the opened lesion and place the swab into a chilled viral transport medium.

F. *Pharynx:* With the client's head tilted back and the mouth open, have him or her say "ah" to elevate the uvula. Firmly swab any visible lesions as well as the posterior surface of the nasopharyngeal area. Place the swab into a chilled viral transport medium.

G. *Rectal swab:* Insert a sterile swab into the rectum about 2-4 inches. Leave the swab in place for 10 seconds to allow absorption of fluid. Firmly rub the swab several times around the circumference of the rectum. Remove the swab and place it in a chilled viral transport medium.

H. *Stool:* Place a marble-sized stool sample in a clean, dry container.

I. *Urine:* Obtain a midstream, clean-catch urine specimen in a sterile container. See clean-catch collection instructions in the test *Body fluid, Routine, Culture.*

4. **Postprocedure care:**

A. Keep the specimen cold (not frozen) and transport it to the laboratory immediately. Speci-mens for influenzavirus or cytomegalovirus culture should be transported in an ice bath.

B. Write the client's name, age, specimen source, recent antibiotic therapy, symptoms, and suspected diagnosis on the laboratory requisition.

5. **Client and family teaching:**

A. The convalescent blood sample is needed 14-28 days after the first blood sample.

B. Results may take up to 4 weeks, but prophylactic antibiotics are normally started immediately.

6. **Factors that affect results:**

A. Failure to keep the specimen cold after collection invalidates the results.

7. **Other data:**

A. None.

VISCOSITY, SERUM

Norm. 1.4-1.8 relative to water.

Increased. Arthritis (rheumatoid), dysproteinemias, hyperfibrinogenemia, hyperviscosity syndrome, myeloma (IgA), systemic lupus erythematosus, and Waldenström's macroglobulinemia.

Decreased. An herb or natural remedy is *Cordyceps sinensis.*

Description. "Serum viscosity" is a term describing a physical property of fluid related to the resistance to flow generated by friction. Low-viscosity fluids flow freely, whereas high-viscosity fluids flow more slowly. In hyperviscosity syndrome, of which most cases occur in clients with Waldenström's macroglobulinemia, death can occur as a results of the impact of high serum viscosity. Sequelae include retinal hemorrhage, bleeding, pulmonary hypertension, congestive heart failure, and neurologic deficits.

In this test, the viscosity of serum is compared to that of water at room temperature. Serum is normally more viscous than water.

Professional Considerations

1. Consent form NOT required.

2. **Preparation:**

A. Tubes: Two red topped, red/gray topped, or gold topped. For

evaluation of polycythemia vera and neonatal hyperviscosity syndrome, whole-blood viscosity should be measured. Draw the specimen in a heparinized, green-topped tube.
3. **Procedure:**
   A. Completely fill two tubes with blood.
4. **Postprocedure care:**
   A. None.

5. **Client and family teaching:**
   A. Clinical symptoms do not correlate well with test results.
6. **Factors that affect results:**
   A. None.
7. **Other data:**
   A. Increased viscosity may cause dilatation of the retinal veins, causing fundus changes in clients.

VISUAL ACUITY TESTS, DIAGNOSTIC

Norm:

	DISTANCE VISION
Snellen Chart	
Adults	20/20 (near vision, 14/14)
Children	
<4 years	20/40 or better
4-7 years	20/30 or better
>7 years	20/20
Allen Cards	
3 years	15/30
4 years	20/30
Infant testing for optokinetic nystagmus	Present at 2 months of age
Strabismus	Absent
Stereopsis	Present
Color vision	Present bilaterally
Peripheral vision	Intact bilaterally

Usage. Part of routine ophthalmologic examination; community health screening for vision testing.

Description. Visual acuity testing involves testing a client's ability to read a standard Snellen chart of symbols (usually letters) at a specified distance to test distance vision, and a Jaeger card to test near vision. A Snellen chart consists of numbered rows of letters that progressively decrease in size from top to bottom. A Jaeger card contains text in progressively decreasing size. For young children and infants, substitute testing in place of the Snellen chart is performed as described below. Children are tested for distance vision, nystagmus, strabismus, stereopsis, color vision, and peripheral vision. The tests may be performed with and without current corrective lenses. For unsatisfactory tests, they will be repeated with new combinations of corrective lenses,

until the best possible vision correction is obtained.

Professional Considerations
1. Consent form NOT required.
2. **Preparation:**
   A. Obtain charts, a hand-held eye-occluder wand, an eye patch for children, and glasses for testing for stereopsis.
3. **Procedure:**
   A. The client is positioned sitting 20 feet away from the Snellen chart.
   B. Each eye is tested separately as follows:
      i. The eye not being tested is occluded.
      ii. The client is instructed to read the line closest to the bottom of the chart that he or she can read and then to attempt to read one line lower.
      iii. The fractionated visual acuity is recorded as follows: The distance in feet the client is

positioned away from the chart is the numerator (that is, 20), and the number of the lowest line read correctly is the denominator. If the client can read one symbol of a line farther down, the results are recorded as:

20/Number of the lowest line read perfectly +
Number of symbols read correctly on the line below

For example, "20/100 + 1" means the client, at a distance of 20 feet, read the line at which a normal eye could read at 100 feet, plus 1 symbol on the line below. A passing score for a line requires that the client read the entire line with no more than one error.

C. *Near-vision testing:*
   i. The client is instructed to read a Jaeger card at normal reading distance. The numerator score is the distance at which the card was read, and the denominator score is the line number of the smallest-sized letters read correctly.
D. *Testing in young children:*
   i. For young children, the "E" chart is substituted for the Snellen chart. The child must indicate which direction the letter E is pointing. Pictures of familiar objects may be placed above, below, left, and right of the chart for the child to use in identification of direction. The test is performed for each eye separately.
   ii. Other substitutes for young children are Allen cards, which contain pictures of objects familiar to children. The numerator score is the distance at which three of the objects can be recognized by the child, and the denominator is 30. The eyes are tested separately.
   iii. *Strabismus testing:* A light is shined into the child's eyes from 16 inches away, and the bilateral reflection of the light in the eyes is observed. Strabismus causes an off-center

reflection in one eye. A second test involves occluding one eye at a time, as the child gazes at an object 1 foot away, and observing for inward or outward movement of the uncovered eye, which indicates strabismus.
   iv. *Stereopsis testing:* Wearing stereoscopic glasses, the child is shown a stereo picture and asked if the object is on the page or in front of the page. With intact stereopsis, the child should be able to see a three-dimensional object that appears to be in front of the page. Without stereopsis, the object appears flat on the page.
   v. *Color-vision testing:* The child is asked to identify objects made of specifically patterned colored dots fused into gray dots.
   vi. *Peripheral-vision testing:* As the child gazes ahead, he or she is asked to indicate on which side of the visual field an object is appearing.
E. *Testing of infants:*
   i. One test infants for optokinetic nystagmus by passing a bright object back and forth in front of the eyes and observing whether nystagmus occurs.
   ii. The infant is also assessed for the ability to follow a lighted object moved in front of the visual field.
   iii. *Peripheral-vision testing:* As the child is distracted, a bright object is moved into the peripheral visual field, and the child's response to the object is noted.
4. **Postprocedure care:**
   A. None.
5. **Client and family teaching:**
   A. Young children may cooperate best if testing is practiced at home before this test.
   B. Eye exercises may be prescribed for very young children with strabismus. Simple exercises that can be performed at home involve using small pictures pasted on Popsicle sticks to strengthen the muscle. The child holds the stick

at arm's length in front of the visual field. While focusing on the picture, he or she slowly and steadily moves the stick in toward the eyes and attempts to maintain single vision. When double vision occurs, the child restarts the exercise.

6. Factors that affect results:
A. The client must be able to follow directions.

7. Other data:
A. Client questionnaires are also used to assess the client's subjective functional impact of visual impairments. Three that are often used include the Activities of Daily Vision Scale, the National Eye Institute Visual Function Questionnaire, and the Visual Function Index.

VISUAL EVOKED POTENTIAL, DIAGNOSTIC

Norm. P-100 is of normal latency. Latency is equivalent bilaterally (test results require expert interpretation).

Usage. Diagnosis or monitoring of demyelinating diseases, glaucoma, maculopathy, migraine headaches, nitrous oxide toxicity (chronic), papilledema, Parkinson's disease, pressure on the optic pathway as a result of tumors or granulomas, pseudotumor cerebri, retinal diseases of the optic nerve, toxic optic neuropathies, and vitamin B deficiency. Also used intraoperatively during eye surgery to provide early warning of potential optic nerve damage.

Description. Visual evoked potential (VEP) is a low-amplitude, electrical waveform representation of the brain's response to a visual stimulus. Because the amplitude is too low to be noted on a traditional electroencephalogram (EEG), sophisticated computer signal-averaging techniques are used to average out the effect of other brain activity during testing. The test involves placing repetitive, patterned stimuli such as a striped, checkerboard, or dotted pattern in the visual field while VEP waveforms are recorded and the amount of time taken for the VEP to occur is measured. Variations of the technique include

varying the pattern size, intensity, and visual field size as well as alternating the pattern itself in an effort to selectively stimulate portions of the visual field. Results are analyzed according to an algorithm and are related to the "P-100" wave. The P-100 wave occurs at about 100 milliseconds after each stimulus in normal clients. Of significance is the amount of time required for the VEP to occur after stimulation (latency) and a comparison of latency measurements of both eyes. Factors that affect latency include head size, electrode location, visual field position of the stimulus, and integrity of the visual nerve pathways.

Professional Considerations
1. Consent form NOT required.
2. Preparation:
A. See *Client and family teaching.*
B. Obtain EEG electrodes, a machine and cap, and electroconductive gel.
C. Remove jewelry and metal objects from the client's head.
3. Procedure:
A. The client is positioned sitting with his or her eyes located about 1 meter away from the screen. One eye is patched.
B. Scalp electrodes are placed in occipital, parietal, and midline locations.
C. The client is instructed to focus the eyes on the screen.
D. The chosen pattern(s) is (are) displayed in a rapid, flashing sequence as the client gazes at the screen, and a recording of VEPs is made. A computer signal average of the brain's electrical activity at a specifically chosen time after each stimulus is displayed.
E. The other eye is patched, and the test is repeated on the opposite eye.
4. Postprocedure care:
A. Remove the electrodes and cleanse the scalp of electroconductive gel.
5. Client and family teaching:
A. The client must gaze continuously at a lighted screen of flashing patterns.
B. Hair should be shampooed the night before the examination and should be free of hair spray or other hair fixatives.

C. The test may take more than 1 hour.

6. **Factors that affect results:**
   A. Results must be compared with the norms of the laboratory performing the test, as different patterns and variations of the test will be performed, depending on the client's history and the purpose of the test.
   B. Cataracts or a miotic pupil may increase the latency of the response.

C. Female P-100 latency has been shown to be shorter than that of male latency.

D. After 50 years of age, latency increases by about 2 milliseconds every 10 years.

E. The client must be able to concentrate on the test. Breaking the gaze on the screen hinders the usefulness of the results.

7. **Other data:**
   A. An acute migraine attack produces prolonged peak latency.

VITAMIN A (RETINOL), SERUM

Norm:

		SI UNITS
Normals in clients older than 1 month	30-65 µg/dL 125-150 IU/dL	1.05-2.27 µmol/L
Borderline deficiency in clients older than 1 month	11-20 µg/dL	0.38-0.70 µmol/L
Deficiency in clients older than 1 month	<10 µg/dL	<0.35 µmol/L

Toxic Level Symptoms and Treatment
Note: the dose estimated to be toxic is 25,000 IU/kg.

Symptoms of acute toxicity. Long bone tenderness, neurologic changes similar to increased intracranial pressure.

Symptoms of chronic toxicity. Anemia, alopecia, ataxia, benign intracranial hypertension, brittle nails, cheilitis, conjunctivitis, diplopia, edema, erythema, exanthema, hepatic cirrhosis, hepatosplenomegaly, hyperostosis, neuritis (peripheral), papilledema, petechiae, premature closure of epiphyses, skin desquamation.

Treatment of toxicity:
Note: Treatment choice(s) depend on client history and condition and episode history.
Treatment is primarily supportive:
   Observation, particularly neurologic status.
   Hydrate if dehydrated or hypercalcemic.
   Discontinue vitamin A supplements.

Symptoms of deficiency. Changes in vision, including night blindness, Bitot's spots, reduced growth, dry skin, and weak dental enamel.

Treatment of deficiency:
High-dose vitamin A replacement. Consult medication guidelines reference.

Increased. Excessive supplementary or dietary intake.

Decreased. Celiac disease, cystic fibrosis of the pancreas, infectious hepatitis, intestinal worms, jaundice (obstructive), low prealbumin, malabsorption, nephritis (chronic), night blindness, and protein-calorie malnutrition.

Description. Vitamin A is a fat-soluble vitamin obtained from animal-based foods and the carotenes of dietary plants and stored in the liver. It is absorbed from the intestines in the presence of bile and lipase, transported to the liver in the form of chylomicrons, and stored there as retinyl ester. Vitamin A is necessary for mucous-membrane epithelial-cell integrity, proper growth, and proper night vision. Vitamin A deficiency is more common in children from lower socioeconomic groups.

Professional Considerations

1. Consent form NOT required.
2. Preparation:
   A. Tube: Red topped, red/gray topped, or gold topped, and a paper bag.
   B. See *Client and family teaching.*
3. Procedure:
   A. Draw a 5-mL blood sample without hemolysis. Place the tube in the paper bag to protect it from light.
4. Postprocedure care:
   A. None.
5. Client and family teaching:
   A. Fast from food and fluids (except for water) overnight before the test.
   B. Do not drink alcohol for 24 hours before sampling.
6. Factors that affect results:
   A. Hemolysis or prolonged exposure of the specimen to light invalidates the results.
   B. Vitamin A levels may be low in the third trimester for about 30% of pregnant clients.
   C. Levels less than 10 μg/dL (μmol/L, SI units) are common from birth to 30 days of age.
7. Other data:
   A. None.

VITAMIN B$_1$ (THIAMINE), SERUM OR URINE

Norm. *Serum:* 5.3-7.9 μg/dL
Urine: 100-200 μg/24 hours

Increased. Excessive supplemental intake.

Decreased. Alcoholism (chronic), beriberi, chronic fatigue syndrome, chronic renal failure clients receiving dialysis, diarrhea (chronic), hyperthyroidism, pregnancy, and Wernicke-Korsakoff syndrome (cerebral beriberi). Drugs include diuretics (long-term use).

Description. Vitamin B$_1$ is a water-soluble vitamin of particular salt compounds. It is found widely in foods, especially organ meats, yeast, and whole grains. Vitamin B$_1$ is absorbed in the duodenum in the presence of folic acid and excreted in the urine. This vitamin acts as an enzyme in alpha-ketoacid decarboxylation, connects the glycolytic cycle to the Krebs cycle, and activates the guanylate cyclase–cyclic guanosine monophosphate system. Deficiency of B$_1$ causes three types of beriberi. "Wet" beriberi is characterized by congestive heart failure. "Dry" beriberi is characterized by peripheral neuritis, muscle paralysis and atrophy, myelin sheath degeneration, weakness, and confusion. "Cerebral" beriberi (Wernicke-Korsakoff syndrome) occurs in chronic alcoholics and is characterized by encephalopathy, ataxia, ocular disturbances, and ocular neuropathy.

Professional Considerations

1. Consent form NOT required.
2. Preparation:
   A. Tube: Red topped, red/gray topped, or gold topped (for serum level), and a paper bag.
   B. For urine level, obtain a clean, brown, 3-L container. Write the beginning time of collection on the laboratory requisition.
   C. Do NOT draw specimens during hemodialysis.
   D. See *Client and family teaching.*
3. Procedure:
   A. *Serum level:*
      i. Draw a 5-mL blood sample. Place the sample immediately in a paper bag to protect it from light.
   B. *24-hour urine collection:*
      i. Discard the first morning void.
      ii. Save all the urine voided in a 24-hour period in a refrigerated, clean, light-protected, 3-L container without preservatives. For catheterized specimens, keep the drainage bag on ice and empty the urine into the collection container hourly. Document the quantity of urine output during the collection period.
4. Postprocedure care:
   A. Send the serum specimen to the laboratory immediately.
   B. For urine collections, write the ending time and total 24-hour urine output quantity on the laboratory requisition. Send the

specimen to the laboratory and refrigerate it.
5. **Client and family teaching:**
   A. Fast overnight before blood draw.
   B. For the urine test, save all the urine voided, void before defecating, and avoid contaminating the specimen with stool or toilet tissue. Empty each void into the refrigerated, light-protected collection container. If any urine is accidentally discarded, discard the entire specimen and restart the collection the next day.
6. **Factors that affect results:**
   A. Prolonged exposure of the specimen to light invalidates the results.
   B. Clients who consume a diet high in freshwater fish or tea made from tea leaves may have low levels because these foods contain thiamine antagonists.
   C. Hemodialysis will reduce vitamin B_1 levels.
   D. An increase in the percent of carbohydrates in the diet has been shown to reduce vitamin B_1 levels.
7. **Other data:**
   A. None.

VITAMIN B₆ (PYRIDOXINE, PYRIDOXAL, AND PYRIDOXAMINE), PLASMA

Norm. Norms are method dependent.

	SI UNITS
25-80 ng/mL	122-389 nmol/L
>50 ng/mL	>243 nmol/L

Increased. Pyridoxine megavitaminosis caused by excessive dietary supplementation.

Decreased. Alcoholism (chronic), anemia (sideroblastic), diabetes (gestational), inadequate dietary intake, lactation, malabsorption, malnutrition, pregnancy, and small bowel inflammatory disease. Drugs include cycloserine, disulfiram, hydralazine, isoniazid, levodopa, oral contraceptives, penicillamine, and pyrazinoic acid.

Description. Vitamin B_6 is a term that collectively refers to three water-soluble vitamins: pyridoxine, pyridoxal, and pyridoxamine. After absorption, pyridoxine is converted to the active forms of pyridoxal and pyridoxamine phosphates. These vitamins are found in many foods, including meats, egg yolk, fish, fowl, whole grains (such as wheat germ, rye meal, soybean meal), and vegetables such as barley, soybeans, brown rice). The B vitamins are important in heme synthesis and function as coenzymes in amino acid metabolism and glycogenolysis. Because vitamin B_6 is partially destroyed by heat, overheating of infant formula makes infants particularly prone to vitamin B_6 deficiency. A sign of vitamin B_6 deficiency include peripheral neuropathy.

Professional Considerations
1. Consent form NOT required.
2. **Preparation:**
   A. Obtain a lavender-topped tube and a paper bag.
3. **Procedure:**
   A. Draw a 7-mL blood sample. Place the sample immediately in a paper bag to protect it from light.
   B. Write the collection time on the laboratory requisition.
4. **Postprocedure care:**
   A. Send the specimen to the laboratory within 30 minutes.
   B. The plasma must be quickly separated and frozen.
5. **Client and family teaching:**
   A. Symptoms of B_6 deficiency may include colic, enhanced startle reflex, convulsions, and irritability.
6. **Factors that affect results:**
   A. Prolonged exposure of the specimen to light invalidates the results.
   B. Reject specimens received more than 30 minutes after collection.
   C. Plasma levels of vitamin B_6 tend to decrease with age, but no age-related norms have been established.
7. **Other data:**
   A. Concurrent testing recommended for evaluation of vitamin B_6 status includes plasma 5′-phosphate, plasma pyridoxal, and urinary 4-pyridoxic acid.
   B. Vitamin B_6 may be measured indirectly by tryptophan loading and measurement of subsequent xanthurenic acid in the urine.

C. Low levels are associated with increased risk for vascular disease in some studies.
D. Low levels are associated with elevated plasma homocysteine levels.

VITAMIN B$_6$ (4-PYRIDOXIC ACID), URINE

Norm. 0.5-1.3 mg/dL (2.7-7.1 μmol/day, SI units).

Increased. Pyridoxine megavitaminosis caused by excessive dietary supplementation; renal insufficiency.

Decreased. Anemia, asthma, carpal tunnel syndrome, chronic alcoholism, gestational diabetes, industrial exposure to hydrazine compounds, lactation, malnutrition, pellagra, peripheral neuritis, peritoneal dialysis, and vitamin B$_6$ deficiency. Drugs include amiodarone, anticonvulsants, cyclosporin A, disulfuram, ethyl alcohol (ethanol), hydralazine, isoniazid, oral contraceptives, penicillamine, pyrazinoac acid, and tricyclic antidepressants.

Description. Urinary 4-pyridoxic acid is a major metabolite of vitamin B$_6$ and can be used to evaluate vitamin B$_6$ deficiency. As a coenzyme, vitamin B$_6$ aids in the synthesis and breakdown of amino acids; aids in the synthesis of unsaturated fatty acids from essential fatty acids; essential for conversion of tryptophan to niacin; involved in formation of the precursor to porphyrin compound.

Professional Considerations
1. Consent form NOT required.
2. **Preparation:**
   A. Obtain a clean, 3-L container that is free of preservative. For pediatric/infant collections, also obtain tape and a pediatric urine collection device/bag.
   B. Write the beginning time of the 24-hour collection on the laboratory requisition.
3. **Procedure:**
   A. Early morning is the preferred time to begin a 24-hour collection.
   B. Discard the first morning urine specimen.

C. Save all the urine voided for 24 hours in a refrigerated, clean, 3-L container that is free of preservatives. Document the quantity of urine output during the specimen collection period. Include the urine voided at the end of the 24-hour period. For catheterized clients, keep the drainage bag on ice and empty the urine into the refrigerated collection container hourly.
D. Pediatric/infant specimen collection:
   i. The child is placed in a supine position with the knees flexed and the hips externally rotated and abducted.
   ii. Cleanse, rinse, and thoroughly dry the perineal area.
   iii. To prevent the child from removing the collection device/bag, a diaper may be placed over the genital area.
   iv. *Females:* Tape the pediatric collection device/bag to the perineum. Starting at the area between the anus and vagina, apply the device/bag in an anterior direction.
   v. *Males:* Place the pediatric collection device/bag over the penis and scrotum and tape it to the perineal area.
   vi. Empty the collection bag into the refrigerated collection container after each void.
4. **Postprocedure care:**
   A. Compare the urine quantity in the specimen container with the urinary output record for the test. If the specimen contains less urine than what was recorded as output, some of the sample may have been discarded, thus invalidating the test.
   B. Document the urine quantity and ending time on the laboratory requisition.
   C. Isoniazid (INH) is a pyridoxal antagonist. Observe if the client is using the drug.
5. **Client and family teaching:**
   A. Save all the urine voided in a 24-hour period, urinate before defecating to avoid loss of urine, and avoid contamination of the specimen with stool, toilet tissue, or prostatic or vaginal secretions. If any urine is accidentally dis-

carded, discard the entire specimen and restart the collection the next day.
B. Inform the client of the possible need for a vitamin B$_6$ supplement during pregnancy and lactation or with the use of oral contraceptives.

6. **Factors that affect results:**
   A. None.
7. **Other data:**
   A. Recommended daily requirements of vitamin B$_6$ are complicated by differences in protein intake and the use of alcohol and oral contraceptives.

B. Daily allowances for vitamin B$_6$ generally are 1.6-2.0 mg.
C. Foods rich in vitamin B$_6$ include yeast, wheat germ, pork, glandular meats, whole grain cereal, legumes, potatoes, bananas, and oatmeal.
D. Urinary testing of 4-pyridoxic acid is not widely used and is of limited value. Plasma values are preferred.

VITAMIN B$_9$
(see Folic Acid, Serum)

VITAMIN B$_{12}$ (CYANOCOBALAMIN, CBL, EXTRINSIC FACTOR), SERUM

Norm:

		SI UNITS
Low	<100 pg/mL	<74 pmol/L
Indeterminate	100-200 pg/mL	74-147 pmol/L
Normal	200-1100 pg/mL	147-810 pmol/L
High	>1100 pg/mL	>810 pmol/L

Increased. Chronic obstructive pulmonary disease, congestive heart failure, diabetes, hepatic cellular damage, leukemia (chronic granulocytic), obesity, polycythemia vera, and renal failure (chronic).

Decreased. Anemia (pernicious), atrophic gastritis, bacterial overgrowth syndromes, congenital deficiency of transcobalamin II, Crohn's disease, fish tapeworm infestation, gastrectomy or gastric bypass (with removal of parietal cells), hepatitis (alcoholic), ileal disease or resection, inflammatory bowel disease, intestinal tapeworm, intrinsic factor deficiency (pernicious anemia), protein-bound cobalamin malabsorption, malnutrition, pancreatic insufficiency, sickle cell anemia, and (strict) veganism. Drugs include p-aminosalicylic acid, antibacterials (neomycin), antigout agents (colchicine), and omeprazole.

Description. Vitamin B$_{12}$ (cyanocobalamin) is a water-soluble vitamin obtained from dietary animal sources that is necessary for proper deoxyribonucleic acid (DNA) synthesis. It can be absorbed from the gastrointestinal tract only when intrinsic factor glycoprotein secreted from the stomach parietal cells is present. Although the body stores up to 12 months' worth of this vitamin in the liver, kidneys, and heart, rapid growth states or conditions causing rapid turnover of cells increase the body's need for it. Symptoms of vitamin B$_{12}$ deficiency include anemia, a smooth red painful tongue (glossitis), and neurologic abnormalities of extremity paresthesias.

Professional Considerations
1. Consent form NOT required.
2. **Preparation:**
   A. This test should be performed before the Schilling test.
   B. Hold blood transfusion or B$_{12}$ administration until blood is drawn, when possible.
   C. Ascertain baseline hematocrit.
   D. Tube: Red topped, red/gray topped, or gold topped, and a paper bag.
   E. See *Client and family teaching.*
3. **Procedure:**
   A. Draw a 1-mL blood sample. Place the tube immediately in a paper bag to protect it from light.

4. Postprocedure care:
   A. Send the specimen to the laboratory immediately. Samples must be quickly spun, with serum separated, frozen, and protected from light.
5. Client and family teaching:
   A. Fast overnight before the test.
6. Factors that affect results:
   A. Hemolysis or prolonged exposure of the specimen to light invalidates the results.
   B. Administration of radiographic dyes within 7 days before the test invalidates the results.
   C. Falsely normal results may occur in myeloproliferative disorders such as chronic myelogenous leukemia and polycythemia vera, and in hepatic disease, congenital transcobalamin II deficiency, overgrowth of intestinal bacteria.
   D. Falsely decreased results may occur during pregnancy and in clients with folic acid deficiency, multiple myeloma or congenital deficiency of serum haptocorrins.
   E. Drugs that may cause falsely decreased results include oral contraceptives.
7. Other data:
   A. See also *Schilling test, Diagnostic; Vitamin B$_{12}$, Unsaturated binding capacity, Serum.*

VITAMIN B$_{12}$, UNSATURATED BINDING CAPACITY (UBC), SERUM

Norm. 870-2000 pg/mL (640-1473 pmol/L, SI units).

Increased. Hepatoma, leukemia (chronic myelogenous), myeloproliferative state, polycythemia vera, pregnancy, and reactive leukocytosis. Drugs include oral contraceptives.

Decreased. Hypoproteinemia.

Description. Vitamin B$_{12}$ (cyanocobalamin) is a water-soluble vitamin obtained from dietary animal sources that is necessary for proper deoxyribonucleic acid (DNA) synthesis. It is absorbed from the gastrointestinal tract only when bound by intrinsic factor glycoprotein secreted from the stomach parietal cells. After absorption, it is transported in the bloodstream by transcobalamin-binding proteins, primarily transcobalamin I. In this test, intrinsic factor is added to a mixture of the client's serum and radiolabeled vitamin B$_{12}$. The mixture is incubated, and then the fraction of bound radiolabeled vitamin B$_{12}$ is measured by a scintillation counter after removal of the unbound vitamin. The results are an indication of the level of transcobalamin-binding proteins, which are known to be elevated in certain conditions (listed above).

Professional Considerations
1. Consent form NOT required.
2. Preparation:
   A. Preschedule this test with the laboratory.
   B. Tube: Red topped, red/gray topped, gold topped, or lavender topped (depending on laboratory requirements).
3. Procedure:
   A. Draw a 7-mL blood sample.
4. Postprocedure care:
   A. Send the specimen to the laboratory immediately or else refrigerate it.
5. Client and family teaching:
   A. Results are normally available within 48 hours.
6. Factors that affect results:
   A. Clotting of the specimen may cause elevated results.
   B. Falsely elevated results may occur if intrinsic factor that is not highly purified is used.
7. Other data:
   A. See also *Vitamin B$_{12}$, Serum; Schilling test, Diagnostic.*

VITAMIN C (ASCORBIC ACID), PLASMA OR SERUM

Norm:

		SI UNITS
Normal level	0.6-2 mg/dL	34-114 μmol/L
Possible deficiency	<0.3 mg/dL	<17 μmol/L
Deficiency	<0.2 mg/dL	<11 μmol/L

Increased. Drugs that include ascorbic acid.

Decreased. Alcoholism, hyperthyroidism, malabsorption, pregnancy, renal failure, scurvy, and in smokers.

Description. Vitamin C is a water-soluble vitamin found in citrus fruits and leafy (raw) vegetables and tomatoes. It is absorbed from the diet through the small intestine and stored in the adrenal glands, kidney, spleen, liver, and leukocytes. Excess amounts of the vitamin are excreted in the urine. Vitamin C is important in cellular structure, collagen synthesis, capillary integrity, wound healing, intestinal iron absorption, and resistance to infection.

Professional Considerations

1. Consent form NOT required.
2. **Preparation:**
   A. Clarify the type of tube needed with the testing laboratory because requirements vary.
   B. Tube: CHILLED green topped, red topped, red/gray topped, gold topped, lavender topped, or black topped.

C. Obtain a container of ice.
D. See *Client and family teaching.*
3. **Procedure:**
   A. Draw a 10-mL blood sample according to specific laboratory requirements. Use a chilled tube.
   B. Place the specimen immediately on ice.
4. **Postprocedure care:**
   A. Send the specimen to the laboratory immediately. Serum or plasma must be promptly separated and frozen.
5. **Client and family teaching:**
   A. Fast overnight before the test.
   B. Results are normally available within 24 hours.
6. **Factors that affect results:**
   A. Chronic tobacco smoking decreases levels.
7. **Other data:**
   A. For clients ingesting inadequate vitamin C, scurvy can develop in about 90 days.
   B. Signs of vitamin C deficiency include petechiae, corkscrew hairs, and perifollicular petechiae.

VITAMIN D (CHOLECALCIFEROL), PLASMA OR SERUM

Norm. Norms vary according to the test method used.

		SI UNITS
Serum vitamin D_3 (1,25-dihydroxy-)	25-45 pg/mL	60-108 nmol/L
Plasma vitamin D_3 (25-hydroxy-)		
Summer	15-80 ng/mL	37-200nmol/L
Winter	14-42 ng/mL	35-105 nmol/L

Increased. Hyperparathyroidism, hypervitaminosis D, and sarcoidosis.

Decreased. Hepatic failure, hypoparathyroidism, malabsorption, osteomalacia, pseudohypoparathyroidism, renal failure, renal osteodystrophy, and rickets. Drugs include anticonvulsants and isoniazid.

Description. Vitamin D is a fat-soluble vitamin found as a dietary supplement in milk and synthesized by the body forming cholesterol in conjunction with exposure to sunlight. Vitamin D becomes biologically active through

hepatic hydroxylation to 25-hydroxyvitamin D and then to 1,25-dihydroxyvitamin D through renal hydroxylation. It works in conjunction with calcitonin and parathyroid hormone and is necessary for proper dietary calcium absorption from the intestinal tract, for regulation of skeletal calcium resorption, and for release of parathyroid hormone.

Professional Considerations

1. Consent form NOT required.
2. **Preparation:**
   A. Tube: Red topped, red/gray topped, or gold topped (for serum); or green topped (for plasma).

B. See *Client and family teaching.*
3. Procedure:
   A. Draw a 3-mL blood sample.
4. Postprocedure care:
   A. None.
5. Client and family teaching:
   A. Fast overnight before the test.
   B. Results are normally available within 24 hours.
6. Factors that affect results:
   A. Insufficient dietary phosphorus intake causes decreased 1,25-dihydroxyvitamin D.

B. Clients who have no exposure to sunlight may have decreased levels.
7. Other data:
   A. Concurrent measurement of parathyroid hormone is recommended.
   B. Hypervitaminosis D may be nephrotoxic.

VITAMIN E (ALPHA-TOCOPHEROL), SERUM

Norm:

		SI UNITS
In general	0.8-1.5 mg/dL	19-35 μmol/L
Adults	5-20 μg/mL	11.6-46.4 μmol/L
Children	3-15 μg/mL	7.0-34.8 μmol/L

Increased. Excessive intake of supplemental vitamin E.

Decreased. Chronic alcoholism, brown-bowel syndrome, certain neurologic degenerative diseases, and malabsorption caused by intestinal bile deficiency (biliary atresia, cystic fibrosis).

Description. Vitamin E is a fat-soluble vitamin found widely in foods such as green vegetables, grains, eggs, oils, liver, chicken, and fish. This vitamin prevents oxidation of vitamin A, deoxyribonucleic acid (DNA), and cell-membrane phospholipids by free radicals. It is necessary for proper reproductive function, muscle growth and development, and hemolytic resistance of red blood cell membranes. Deficiency of vitamin E causes hemolytic anemia and neurologic abnormalities.

Professional Considerations
1. Consent form NOT required.
2. Preparation:
   A. Tube: Red topped, red/gray topped, or gold topped, and a paper bag.
3. Procedure:
   A. Draw a 10-mL blood sample. Label the tube, and place it promptly in a paper bag to protect it from light.

4. Postprocedure care:
   A. Send the specimen to the laboratory.
   B. Serum must be separated within 2 hours of collection.
5. Client and family teaching:
   A. Results are normally available within 72 hours.
6. Factors that affect results:
   A. Prolonged exposure of the specimen to light invalidates the results.
7. Other data:
   A. The specimen is stable at room temperature or refrigerated for 14 days, or frozen for up to a year.

VOLATILE SCREEN, BLOOD OR URINE
(see Toxicology, Volatiles group by GLC, Blood or Urine)

VON WILLEBRAND FACTOR ANTIGEN (vWF Ag, FACTOR VIII R:Ag, FACTOR VIII–RELATED ANTIGEN), BLOOD

Norm. 45%-185% of control sample activity.

Usage. Differentiation between hemophilia A (classical hemophilia) and von

Willebrand's disease when bleeding time tests are inconclusive.

Description. Von Willebrand's disease is an autosomal dominantly transmitted factor VIII defect. It is a coagulation disorder that results in varying degrees of bleeding abnormalities. Coagulation factor VIII has three properties, namely, procoagulant activity (circulating Von Willebrand factor is newly recognized as initiating platelet adhesion), antigenic activity, and von Willebrand factor activity. In this test, factor VIII antigenic activity is determined by measurement of von Willebrand factor antigen (vWF Ag). In hemophilia A, vWF Ag activity is normal, but in von Willebrand's disease, vWF Ag is characteristically low (that is, <40% of control sample activity).

Professional Considerations
1. Consent form NOT required.
2. **Preparation:**
   A. Preschedule this test with the laboratory.
   B. Tube: 2.7-mL or 4.5-mL blue-topped tube and a control tube, and a waste tube or syringe.
3. **Procedure:**
   A. Withdraw 2 mL of blood into a syringe or vacuum tube. Remove the syringe or tube, leaving the needle in place. Attach a second syringe, and draw a blood sample of 2.4 mL for a 2.7-mL tube or 4.0 mL for a 4.5-mL tube.
   B. Gently roll the tube several times to mix the blood with the anticoagulant.
4. **Postprocedure care:**
   A. Send the specimen to the laboratory immediately and refrigerate it until it is tested.
5. **Client and family teaching:**
   A. Results are normally available within 72 hours.
6. **Factors that affect results:**
   A. Hemolysis invalidates the results.
   B. Contamination of the specimen with tissue thromboplastins invalidates the results. This is the reason for the double-draw technique.
   C. Results are invalidated if the specimen is received by the laboratory more than 2 hours after collection.

7. **Other data:**
   A. To establish a diagnosis of von Willebrand's disease, plasma factor VIII levels and von Willebrand factor assay are used in conjunction with this test.
   B. See also *von Willebrand factor assay, Blood; Factor VIII, Blood.*

VON WILLEBRAND FACTOR ASSAY, BLOOD

Norm. Aggregation occurs after addition of ristocetin to the sample.

Usage. Helps differentiate between hemophilia A (classical hemophilia) and von Willebrand's disease.

Description. Von Willebrand's disease is an autosomal dominantly transmitted factor VIII defect. It is a coagulation disorder that results in varying degrees of bleeding abnormalities. Coagulation factor VIII has three properties, namely, procoagulant activity (low or absent in hemophilia A), antigenic activity, and von Willebrand factor activity. The von Willebrand factor activity of factor VIII enhances the formation of platelet plugs. In this test, the von Willebrand factor activity of factor VIII is measured by use of a modified platelet aggregation test. In normal clients or those with hemophilia A, the antibiotic ristocetin induces platelet aggregation on a test sample. In clients with von Willebrand's disease, however, addition of ristocetin to the client's serum does not result in platelet aggregation.

Professional Considerations
1. Consent form NOT required.
2. **Preparation:**
   A. Preschedule this test with the laboratory.
   B. Tube: 2.7-mL or 4.5-mL blue-topped tube and a control tube, and a waste tube or syringe.
3. **Procedure:** The blood draw is best performed by a laboratory technician.
   A. Withdraw 2 mL of blood into a syringe or vacuum tube. Remove the syringe or tube, leaving the needle in place. Attach a second syringe, and draw a blood sample of 2.4 mL for a 2.7-mL tube or 4.0 mL for a 4.5-mL tube.

B. Gently roll the tube several times to mix the blood with the anticoagulant.
C. Serum should be immediately separated into a plastic vial and frozen before it is sent to the laboratory.
4. Postprocedure care:
   A. Send the specimen to the laboratory immediately and refrigerate it until it is tested.
5. Client and family teaching:
   A. Results are normally available within 72 hours.
6. Factors that affect results:
   A. Hemolysis or clotting of the specimen invalidates the results.
   B. Contamination of the specimen with tissue thromboplastins invalidates the results. This is the reason for the double-draw technique.
   C. Results are invalidated if the specimen is received by the laboratory more than 2 hours after collection.
7. Other data:
   A. To establish a diagnosis of von Willebrand's disease, plasma factor VIII levels and von Willebrand factor antigen measurements are used in conjunction with this test.
   B. See also *von Willebrand factor antigen, Blood; Factor VIII, Blood.*

V/Q SCAN, DIAGNOSTIC
(see Lung scan, Perfusion and ventilation, Diagnostic)

VULVA SMEAR, DIAGNOSTIC
(see Pap smear, Diagnostic)

WASHING CYTOLOGY, SPECIMEN
(see Bronchial washing, Specimen, Diagnostic)

WATER DEPRIVATION TEST FOR VASOPRESSIN DEFICIENCY, DIAGNOSTIC
(see Concentration test, Urine)

WATER LOADING TEST, DIAGNOSTIC

Norm. ≥500-mL urine output over 4 hours after water ingestion.

Urine osmolality < Serum osmolality or <180 mOsm/kg by 5 hours after water ingestion

Usage. Diagnosis of syndrome of inappropriate antidiuretic hormone secretion (SIADHS).

Description. The water loading test involves administering a large quantity of water and then comparing the osmolality of timed urine and serum collections. In a normal client, increased fluid intake increases urine output and decreases urine osmolality. In clients with SIADHS, however, excess secretion of antidiuretic hormone causes a lower-than-normal urine output in response to the water loading and a urine osmolality that does not decrease below serum osmolality.

Professional Considerations
1. Consent form NOT required.

Risks
Fluid overload, congestive heart failure. Complications of nasogastric tube insertion include bleeding, dysrhythmias, esophageal perforation, laryngospasm, and decreased mean pO_2.

Contraindications and Precautions
Perform with extreme caution in clients with a history of congestive heart failure.

2. Preparation:
   A. The baseline serum sodium level should be at least 125 mEq/L before this test is started.
   B. Withhold diuretics for 12 hours before the test.
   C. Tube: Six red topped, red/gray topped, or gold topped.
   D. Also obtain six clean plastic specimen containers.
   E. Insert a nasogastric tube if the client will be unable to drink 1 L of water over a short period of time.
3. Procedure:
   A. Draw a 1-mL blood sample for the baseline serum osmolality. Obtain a 20-mL random urine sample in a clean plastic container for baseline urine osmolality.
   B. Have the client drink 1 liter of water, or 20 mL/kg of body

weight over 15-20 minutes, or instill it through a nasogastric tube.

C. Document the quantity of urine output, starting with the time of water ingestion and ending 5 hours later.

D. Obtain samples for serum and urine osmolality as in step A every hour for 5 hours. Label each tube sequentially, and write the collection time on the label.

4. Postprocedure care:
A. Refrigerate the serum samples if they are not tested within 4 hours.
B. Refrigerate all urine samples until they are tested.

5. Client and family teaching:
A. The client will be asked to drink or have instilled at least 1 liter of water within 20 minutes.

6. Factors that affect results:
A. Diuretics administered within 12 hours before the test invalidate the results.

7. Other data:
A. None.

WEBER TEST, DIAGNOSTIC
(see *Tuning fork test of Weber, Rinne, and Schwabach tests, Diagnostic*)

WEIL-FELIX AGGLUTININS, BLOOD

Norm. A less than fourfold rise in titer between acute and convalescent samples; or titer <1:160.

Usage. Helps in the diagnosis of rickettsial infections.

Description. A test performed for the purpose of detecting and differentiating rickettsial antibodies in the serum. Rickettsial organisms cause Rocky Mountain spotted fever, Q fever, Brill-Zinsser disease, epidemic typhus, murine typhus, scrub typhus, and rickettsialpox. Three *Proteus* antigens are known to cross-react in specific relationships with rickettsial antibodies. The test is performed by mixture of serial dilutions of test serum with suspensions of *Proteus* strains OX-2, OX-19, and OX-K and observation for agglutination. A single titer >1:320 or a fourfold rise in titer between acute and convalescent samples is considered diagnostic.

Professional Considerations
1. Consent form NOT required.
2. Preparation:
A. Tube: Red topped, red/gray topped, or gold topped.
B. Specimens MAY be drawn during hemodialysis.
3. Procedure:
A. Draw a 10-mL blood sample and label it as the "acute sample." Repeat the test every 3-5 days. Draw a final sample in 10-14 days, and label it as the "convalescent sample."
4. Postprocedure care:
A. None.
5. Client and family teaching:
A. Return for serial sampling as prescribed and then in 10-14 days for final follow-up testing.
6. Factors that affect results:
A. Hemolysis invalidates the results.
B. Immunosuppressed clients may be infected but have low or negative titers.
C. Antibiotic therapy causes low initial titers.
7. Other data:
A. Because the test is based on a known cross-reaction, caution must be used in interpreting the results. Although differentiation between Rocky Mountain spotted fever and typhus fever is not possible with this test, interpretation of results can rule out certain rickettsial infections.
B. See also *Febrile agglutinins, Serum*.

WESTERGREN SEDIMENTATION RATE
(see *Sedimentation rate, Erythrocyte, Blood*)

WESTERN BLOT
(see *Acquired immunodeficiency syndrome evaluation battery, Diagnostic*)

W

WESTERN EQUINE ENCEPHALITIS VIRUS SEROLOGY, SERUM

Norm. Negative. A less than fourfold rise in titer between acute and convalescent samples; HI (hemagglutination inhibition) antibody titer <1:10; no IgM antibody detected.

Positive. Aseptic meningitis and meningoencephalitis.

Description. Western equine encephalitis is caused by a group A arbovirus (arthropod-borne virus), specifically, togavirus, which results in inflammation of parts of the brain, meninges, and spinal cord in horses and humans. Occurrence is primarily in the Western Hemisphere and in summer to early fall. Mode of transmission to humans is from small birds and mammals through the bite of an infected mosquito. Symptoms are short in duration and may range from mild to fatal (10%) encephalitis symptoms (stiff neck, lethargy, sore throat, vomiting, stupor, coma, paralysis in children). Identification of the virus is performed through viral neutralization, complement fixation, hemagglutin inhibition, fluorescent antibody, and agar gel precipitation.

Professional Considerations
1. Consent form NOT required.
2. **Preparation:**
   A. Tube: Red topped, red/gray topped, or gold topped.
3. **Procedure:**
   A. Draw a 7-mL blood sample as soon as possible after symptoms appear, and label it as the "acute sample." Repeat the test in 14 days, and label it as the "convalescent sample."
4. **Postprocedure care:**
   A. None.
5. **Client and family teaching:**
   A. The mode of transmission is by a mosquito bite. Wear insect-repellant spray or lotion on skin when outdoors.
   B. Return in 2 weeks for follow-up testing.
6. **Factors that affect results:**
   A. Cross-reactions may occur with eastern equine encephalitis virus, another group A togavirus.

7. **Other data:**
   A. Testing may also be performed on cerebrospinal fluid.
   B. Western equine encephalitis is not transmitted client to client.

WHITE BLOOD CELL COUNT DIFFERENTIAL, BLOOD
(see Differential leukocyte count, Peripheral blood)

WHITE BLOOD COUNT (WBC), BLOOD
(see Differential leukocyte count, Peripheral, Blood)

WHOLE-BLOOD CLOTTING TIME
(see Clot retraction, Blood)

WHOLE-BODY SCAN, DIAGNOSTIC
(see Bone scan, Diagnostic)

WINTROBE SEDIMENTATION RATE, BLOOD
(see Sedimentation rate, Erythrocyte, Blood)

WOUND CULTURE
(see Culture, Routine, Specimen)

WOUND, FUNGUS, CULTURE
(see Biopsy, Fungus, Culture; Body fluid, Fungus, Culture)

WOUND, MYCOBACTERIA, CULTURE
(see Biopsy, Mycobacteria, Culture; Body fluid, Mycobacteria, Culture)

XEROMAMMOGRAM
(see Mammography, Diagnostic)

X-RAY
(see Radiographic and Radiography; various types of radiography)

XYLOSE, BLOOD
*(see D-Xylose absorption test,
Diagnostic)*

XYLOSE, URINE
*(see D-Xylose absorption test,
Diagnostic)*

D-XYLOSE ABSORPTION TEST (XYLOSE TOLERANCE TEST), DIAGNOSTIC, SERUM OR URINE

Norm:

		SI UNITS
Serum		
Adults	25-40 mg/dL between 1 and 2 hours after ingestion of D-xylose	1.67-2.66 mmol/L
Children >10 years	10-33% of dose ingested, or >30 mg/dL >16% of 25-g dose	2.01 mmol/L
Urine		
Adults	4 g of xylose excreted in 5 hours	
Children	16-33% excreted in 5 hours	

Increased. Disaccharidase deficiencies, Hodgkin's disease, malabsorption, status post gastrectomy, radiation side effects of small intestine, and scleroderma.

Decreased. Amyloidosis, celiac disease, cystic fibrosis, diarrhea, massive bacterial overgrowth in small bowel, short bowel syndrome, Whipple's disease, and any other jejunal mucosal disease.

Description. D-Xylose is a pentose (sugar) that is not metabolized by the body and is normally absorbed by the proximal portion of the small bowel and excreted unchanged by the kidney into the urine. The test is used to distinguish malabsorption from maldigestion.

Professional Considerations
1. Consent form NOT required.
2. **Preparation:**
   A. See *Client and family teaching.*
   B. Obtain a large brown urine container and three red-topped, marble-topped, or gold-topped tubes.
   C. Assess renal function laboratory data (BUN, creatinine).
3. **Procedure:**
   A. At 0800 (8 AM), instruct the client to void and discard the sample.
   B. Draw a fasting blood sample.
   C. Give 25 g of D-xylose dissolved in 250 mL water by mouth. Give a smaller weight-based amount to children.
   D. Follow with 500 mL of water orally.
   E. No further fluids or food should be given until the test is completed.
   F. Collect all the urine voided for 5 hours after ingestion of D-xylose in a refrigerated container.
   G. Draw 7-mL blood specimens for D-xylose levels 60 and 120 minutes after ingestion of D-xylose.
4. **Postprocedure care:**
   A. Resume fluids and diet as prescribed.
5. **Client and family teaching:**
   A. Adults must fast for 8 hours and children for 4 hours before drinking prescribed D-xylose.
   B. Do not eat foods containing pentose: fruits, jams, jellies, and pastries.
   C. The test involves specifically timed specimens.
   D. The test takes several hours. Bring reading material or other diversions to the test.
6. **Factors that affect results:**
   A. Drugs that will increase absorption in the intestines include aspirin, atropine, and indomethacin.
   B. Poor renal function will decrease urinary output, and vomiting will decrease the amount of D-xylose consumed or absorbed.
   C. The urine output of D-xylose may be decreased by dehydration, renal insufficiency, third spacing

of fluid, and hypothyroidism, but these will not affect the serum levels.

D. Massive bacterial overgrowth in the small bowel may decrease the amount of D-xylose available for absorption by the small bowel and therefore decrease the serum and urine levels.

7. Other data:

A. Since an abnormal D-xylose test is suggestive of small bowel mucosal disease, a biopsy should be performed as the next step.

XYLOSE TOLERANCE TEST, DIAGNOSTIC

(see D-Xylose absorption test, Diagnostic)

YERSINIA ENTEROCOLITICA ANTIBODY, BLOOD

Norm. <1:160. A fourfold increase between acute and convalescent specimens (such as convalescent titer 1:1280) is diagnostic for yersiniosis.

Increased. Gastroenterocolitis or endocarditis caused by Yersinia (yersiniosis) and terminal ileitis.

Decreased. Titers decrease to normal levels 2-6 months after recovery from Yersinia infections.

Description. Yersinia enterocolitica is a bacterium found in animal carriers and bodies of water that is transmitted to humans by the fecal-oral route or by ingestion of food or water contaminated with the organism. Y. enterocolitica causes gastroenterocolitis accompanied by diarrhea, anorexia, fever, vomiting, headache, arthritis, and abscesses and may progress to septicemia. Incidence is more common in children and teens than in adults. In this test, an indirect Coombs' test is performed to identify the presence of the antibody to Y. enterocolitica.

Professional Considerations
1. Consent form NOT required.
2. Preparation:
A. Tube: Red topped, red/gray topped, or gold topped.

3. Procedure:
A. Draw a 7-mL blood sample as soon as possible after symptoms appear. Label the sample as the acute specimen.
B. Repeat the test in 2-3 weeks and label

4. Postprocedure care:
A. None.

5. Client and family teaching:
A. Return in 2-3 weeks for a convalescent blood sample.
B. Because Yersinia infection is transmitted from stool to other persons, avoid contaminating your hands with stool and wash your hands vigorously for 15 seconds with antibacterial soap after each defecation. Cleanse the toilet seat with disinfectant after each defecation until the physician confirms that you are no longer contagious.
C. Yersinia infection may be treated with amphotericin B.

6. Factors that affect results:
A. Results may not be elevated in clients who are infected with Yersinia but who are immunosuppressed or receiving antifungal therapy.

7. Other data:
A. Diagnosis should be confirmed by blood culture.
B. Standard precautions are adequate for preventing transmission of Yersinia infection to others. Use strict Standard Precautions when handling feces of infected clients because fecal shedding of Yersinia occurs throughout the period of active symptoms.
C. Reactive arthritis may be triggered by Yersinia.

ZETA SEDIMENTATION RATE, BLOOD

(see Sedimentation rate, Erythrocyte, Blood)

ZETA SEDIMENTATION RATIO (ZSR), BLOOD

(see Sedimentation rate, Erythrocyte, Blood)

ZINC, BLOOD

Norm:

		SI UNITS
All ages	70-120 µg/dL	10.7-18.4 µmol/L
Zinc deficiency	<70 µg/dL	<10.7 µmol/L

Toxic Level Symptoms and Treatment

Note: Treatment choice(s) depend on client history and condition and episode history.

Symptoms of zinc toxicity. Cough, chest discomfort, tachycardia, hypertension, gastrointestinal irritation, nausea, vomiting, diarrhea, and metallic taste in the mouth.

Treatment of zinc toxicity: Eliminate dietary zinc or reduce zinc additives to hyperalimentation. Peritoneal dialysis WILL remove excess zinc.

Symptoms of zinc deficiency. May progress from decreased weight, low sperm count, and impaired wound healing to alopecia, hypogonadism, ataxia, tremors, and impaired resistance to infection.

Treatment of zinc deficiency: Zinc replacement through diet, medication, or hyperalimentation.

Increased. Anemia, arteriosclerosis, coronary heart disease, dietary intake of acidic food or beverages from galvanized containers, industrial exposure to zinc (welding), and primary osteosarcoma of bone. Drugs include cisplatin, corticosteroids, estrogens, interferon, oral contraceptives (containing estrogen), phenytoin, and thiazides.

Decreased. Acrodermatitis enteropathica, alopecia, alcoholism, anemia (hemolytic), celiac sprue, cirrhosis, diarrhea, gallbladder disease, hepatic metastasis, hypoalbuminemia, hypogonadal dwarfism, infection (acute), leukemia, lymphoma, malabsorption, myocardial infarction, poor dietary intake, pregnancy (third trimester), receiving parenteral nutrition, renal failure (chronic), stress (acute), thalassemia major, typhoid fever, and tuberculosis (pulmonary). Drugs include antimetabolites, chlorthalidone, cisplatin, diuretics, estrogens, histidine, and penicillamine.

Description. Zinc is a nutritional trace metal important for cellular growth and metabolism. Both zinc toxicity and serious zinc deficiency are possible (see symptoms listed above), Zinc levels are usually measured as part of a heavy-metal screen for suspected zinc toxicity. Routine levels are measured for clients receiving parenteral nutrition and to monitor progress during replacement for zinc deficiency.

Professional Considerations
1. Consent form NOT required.
2. **Preparation:**
   A. Obtain a stainless steel needle and a metal-free, navy blue–topped BD Vacutainer tube from the laboratory.
   B. Do NOT draw specimens during hemodialysis.
3. **Procedure:**
   A. Draw a 1-mL blood sample without hemolysis directly into the tube through a stainless steel needle.
4. **Postprocedure care:**
   A. Send the specimen to the laboratory promptly for spinning and separation of the serum into a metal-free container.
5. **Client and family teaching:**
   A. Results are normally available within 72 hours.
6. **Factors that affect results:**
   A. Collecting the specimen in a regular, rubber-topped tube other than that specified above invalidates the results.
   B. Hemolysis invalidates results.
7. **Other data:**
   A. None.

ZSR, BLOOD
(see Sedimentation rate, Erythrocyte, Blood)

Bibliography

Adamek RJ, Wegener M, Wienbeck M et al: Long-term esophageal manometry in healthy subjects: evaluation of normal values and influence of age, *Dig Dis Sci* 39(10):2069-2073, 1994.

Adelusi B, al-Twaijiri MH, al-Meshari A et al: Correlation of smoking and coffee drinking with sperm progressive motility in infertile males, *Afr J Med Sci* 27(1-2):47-50, 1998.

Akhund IA, Alvi IA, Ansari AK, et Al. A study of relationship of ABO blood groups with myocardial infarction and angina pectoris, *J Ayab Medical College, Abbottabad: JAMC* 13(4): 25-26, 2001.

Alexander M, Baker L, Clark C, McDonald KM, Rowell R, Saynina O, Hlatky MA: Management of ventricular arrhythmias in diverse populations in California, *Am Heart J* 144(3): 431-439, 2002.

Al-Fozan H, Tulandi T: Safety and risks of laparoscopy in pregnancy, *Curr Opin Obstet Gynecol* 14:375-379, 2002.

American Academy of Clinical Toxicology, European Association of Poisons Centres and Clinical Toxicologists: Position statement and practice guidelines on the use of multi-dose activated charcoal in the treatment of acute poisoning, *J Toxicol Clin Toxicol* 37(6):731-751, 1999.

American College of Obstetricians and Gynecologists: Guidelines for diagnostic imaging during pregnancy, Committee Opinion No. 158, *ACOG Comm Opin* Sept No. 158, 1995.

Anker P, Lefort F, Vasioukhin V et al: K-ras mutations are found in DNA extracted from the plasma of patients with colorectal cancer, *Gastroenterology* 112(4):1114-1120, 1997.

Asaka M, Kimura T, Meguro T et al. Alteration of aldolase isozymes in serum and tissues of patients with cancer and other diseases, *J Clin Laboratory Analysis* 8(3):144-148, 1994.

Basbug M, Aygen E, Tayyar M et al: Correlation be-tween maternal thyroid function tests and endothelin in preeclampsia-eclampsia, *Obstet Gynecol* 94(4):551-555, 1999.

Baud JM, Mas D, Pichot O et al. Criteria for quantification and characterization of aneurysms of the abdominal aorta using ultrsonography. The AFFCA study. French Association of Continuous Educa-tion in Angiology, *J des Maladies Vasculaires* 229(50): 313-20, 1997.

Chan WS, Ray JG, Murray S et al: Suspected pulmonary embolism in pregnancy: clinical presentation, results of lung scanning, and subsequent maternal and pediatric outcomes, *Arch Intern Med* 162(10):- 1170-1175, 2002.

Cockrell JR, Folstein MF, Mini-Mental State Examination (MMSE), *Psychopharm Bull* 24:689-692, 1988.

Cohen R, Woods H: *Clinical and biochemical aspects of lactic acidosis*, Oxford, 1976, Blackwell Scientific Publications.

Cole TJ, Henry DA, Jolles H, et al: Normal and abnormal vascular structures that simulate neoplasms on chest radiographs: clues to the diagnosis, *Radiographics* 15(4):867-891, 1995.

Conference Report: *Endoscopic Ultrasonography: the state of the art*, 13th International Symposium on Endoscopic Ultrasonography, New York, NY, 2002, The Symposium.

Cros N, Muller J, Bouju S et al: Upregulation of M-creatine kinase and glyceraldehyde-3-phosphate dehydrogenase: two markers of muscle disuse, *Am J Physiol* 276(2 Pt 2):R308-R316, 1999.

Crowther MA, Douketis JD, Schnurr T et al: Oral vitamin K lowers the international normalized ratio more rapidly than subcutaneous vitamin K in the treatment of warfarin-associated coagulopathy. A randomized, controlled trial, *Ann Intern Med* 137(4):139, 2002.

Cruickshanks KJ, Wiley TL, Tweed TS et al: Prevalence of hearing loss in older adults in Beaver Dam, Wisconsin. The Epidemiology of Hearing Loss Study, *Am J Epidemiol* 148(9): 879-886, 1998.

Cummings DE , Weigle DS, Frayo RS et al. Plasma ghrelin levels after diet-induced weight loss or gastric bypass surgery, *NEJM* 346(21):1623-1630, 2002.

Dayan CM: Interpretation of thyroid function tests, *Lancet* 357:619-624, 2001.

Drach GW, Layton TN, Binard LNJ: Male peak urinary flow rate: relationships to volume voided and age, *J Urol* 122:210-214, 1979.

Elder JS, Longenecker R: Premedication with oral midazolam for voiding cystrouethrography in children: safety and efficacy, *Am J Roentgenol* 164(5):1229-1232, 1995.

Elixhauser A, Weinick RM, Betancourt JR et al: Differences between hispanics and non-hispanic whites in use of hospital procedures for cerebrovascular disease, *Ethnicity & Disease* 12(1):29-37, 2002.

Folstein MF, Folstein SE, McHugh PR: "Mini-mental state" a practical method for grading the cognitive state of patients for the clinician, *J Psychiatr Res* 12:189-198, 1975.

Frankenburg WK, Dodds J, Archer P et al: The Denver II: a major revision and restandardization of the Denver Developmental Screening Test, *Pediatrics* 89(1): 91-97, 1992.

Friedrich MG, Hellstern A, Hautmann SH et al: Clinical use of urinary markers for the detection and prognosis of bladder carcinoma: a comparison of immunocytology with monoclonal antibodies against Lewis X and 486p3/12 with the BTA STAT and NMP22 tests, *J Urol* 168(2):470-4, 2002.

Green DM, Ropper AH, Kronmal RA et al: Serum potassium level and dietary potassium intake as risk factors for stroke, *Neurology* 59:314-320, 2002.

Gruber B, Burton BK: Oromandibular-limb hypogenesis syndrome following chorionic villus sampling, *Int J Pediatr Otorhinolaryngol* 29(1):59-63, 1994.

Hankinson SE, Willett WC, Michaud DS et al: Plasma prolactin levels and subsequent risk of breast cancer in postmenopausal women, *J Natl Cancer Inst* 91(7):629-634, 1999.

Harvey SM, Sturgeon J, Dassey DE: Botulism due to *Clostridium baratii* type F toxin, *J Clin Microbiol* 40(6): 2260-2262, 2002.

Hasegawa BH, Iwata K, Wong K H et al: Dual-modality imaging of function and physiology, *Acad Radiol* 9: 1305-1321, 2002.

Haugen TB, Grotmol, T: pH of human semen, *Int J Androl* 21(2): 105-108, 1998.

Helbig JH, Uldum SA Bernander S et al: Clinical utility of urinary antigen detection for diagnosis of community-acquired, travel-associated, and nosocomial Legionnaire's disease, *J Clin Microbiol* 41: 838-840, 2003.

Henry MJ, Major CA, Reinsch S: Accuracy of self-monitoring of blood glucose: impact on diabetes management decisions during pregnancy, *Diabetes Educator* 27(4): 521-529, 2001.

Itoh T, Itoh H, Kikuchi T: Five cases of MRSA-infected patients with cerebrovascular disorder and in a bedridden condition, for whom bu-zhong-yi-qi-tang (hochu-ekki-to) was useful, *Am J Chin Med* 28:401-408, 2000.

Khurana RK, Nicholas EM: Head-up tilt table test: how far and how long? *Clin Auton Res* 6(6):335-341, 1996.

Kiuru MJ, Pihlajamaki HK, Hietanen HJ et al: MR imaging, bone scintigraphy, and radiography in bone stress injuries of the pelvis and the lower extremities, *Acta Radiologica* 43(2): 207-212, 2002.

Lidstone V, Janes S, Stross P: INR: Intervals of measurement can safely extend to 14 weeks, *Clin Lab Haematol* 22(5):291-293, 2002.

Lokeshwar VB, Schroeder GL, Selzer MG et al: Bladder tumor markers for monitoring recurrence and screening comparisons of hyaluronic acid-hyaluronidase and BTA-Stat tests, *Cancer* 95(1):61-72, 2002.

Lolekha PH, Vanavanan S, Teerakarnjana N et al: Reference ranges of electrolytes and anion gap on the Beckman E4A, Beckman Synchron CX5, Nova CRT, and Nova Stat Profile Ultra, *Clinical Chimica Acta* 307(1-2):87-93, 2001.

Lopez JB, Royan GP, Lakhwani MN et al: CA 72-4 compared with CEA and CA 19-9 as a marker of some gastrointestinal malignancies, *Int J Biol Markers* 14(3):172-177, 1999.

Lukinác L, Kusíc Z, Kes P et al: Effect of chronic hemodialysis on thyroid function tests in patients with end-stage renal disease, *Acta Med Croatica* 50(2):65-68, 1996.

Lundstrom E, Wilczek B, von Palffy Z et al: Mammographic breast density during hormone replacement therapy: differences according to treatment, *Am J Obstet Gynecol* 181(2):348-352, 1999.

Matuura H, Hakomori S: The oncofetal domain of fibronectin defined by monoclonal antibody FDC-6: its presence in fibronectins from fetal and tumor tissues and its absence in those from normal adult tissues and plasma, *Proc Natl Acad Sci USA* 82(19):6517-6521, 1985.

McNerlan SE, Alexander HD, Rea IM: Age-related reference intervals for lymphocyte subsets in whole blood of healthy individuals, *Scand J Clin Lab Invest* 59(2):89-92, 1999.

Mendelssohn DC, Cole EH: Outcomes of percutaneous kidney biopsy including those of solitary native kidneys, *Am J Kidney Dis* 26(5):580-585, 1995.

Michiels JJ, Kasbergen H, Oudega R et al: Exclusion and diagnosis of deep vein thrombosis in outpatients by sequential noninvasive tools, *Int Angiol* 21:9-19, 2002.

Miller MA, Hyland M, Ofber-Agostini M et al: Morbidity, mortality, and healthcare burden of nosocomial Clostridium difficile-associated diarrhea in Canadian hospitals. *Infect Cont Hosp Epidemiol* 23(930):137-140, 2002.

Miller V, Phillips AN, Clotet B et al. Association of virus load, CD4 cell count, and treatment with clinical progression in human immunodeficiency virus-infected patients with very low CD4 cell counts, *J Infect Dis* 186(2):189-197, 2002.

Morcos NC: Modulation of lipid profile by fish oil and garlic combination, *J Natl Med Assoc* 89(10):573-578, 1997.

Oakley KL, Moore CB, Denning DW: In vitro activity of the echinocandin antifungal agent LY303,366 in comparison with itraconazole and amphotericin B against *Aspergillus* spp., *Antimicrob Agents Chemother* 42(10):2726-2730, 1998.

Oyama J, Shimokawa H, Morita S et al: Elevated interleukin-1 beta in pericardial fluid of patients with ischemic heart disease, *Coronary Heart Disease* 12(7): 567-571, 2002.

Ozcakir HT, Goker EN, Terek MC, et al: Relationship of follicle number, serum estradiol level, and other factors to clinical pregnancy rate in gonadotropin-induced intrauterine insemination cycles, *Arch Gynecol Obstet* 266(1):18-20, 2002.

Petrick AT, Meterissian S, Steele GD et al: Desialylation of human colorectal carcinoma cells facilitates binding to Kupffer cells, *Clin Exp Metastasis* 12:108-116, 1994.

Richmond S, Reay G, Abu Harb M: Routine pulse oximetry in the asymptomatic newborn, *Arch Dis Child Fetal Neonatal Ed* 87:F83-F88, 2002.

Roger A, Pena M, Botey J, et al: The prick test and specific IgE (RAST and MASTCLA) compared with the oral challenge test with milk, eggs and nuts, *J Investig Allergol Clin Immunol* 4(4):178-181, 1994.

Rudrapatna JS, Kumar V, Sridhar H: Intestinal parasitic infections in patients with malignancy, *J Diarrhoeal Dis Res* 15(2): 71-74, 1997.

Sabbe LJ, Van De Merwe D, Schouls L et al: Clinical spectrum of infections attributable to the newly described *Actinomyces* species *A. turicensis, A. radingae,* and *A. europaeus, J Clin Microbiol* 37(1):8-13, 1999.

Schneir AB, Ly BT, Clark RF: A case of withdrawal from GHB precursors gamma-butyrolactone and 1,4-butanediol, *J Emerg Med* 21(1):31-33, 2001.

Schulman DS, Lasorda D, Farah T et al: Correlations between coronary flow reserve measured with a Doppler guide wire and

exercise testing, *Am Heart J* 134(1): 99-104, 1997.

Sexena AK, Panhotra BR, Naguib M: Sudden irreversible sensory-neural hearing loss in a patient with diabetes receiving amikacin as an antibiotic-heparin lock, *Pharmacotherapy* 22(1):105-108, 2002.

Shire N: Effects of race, ethnicity, gender, culture, literacy, and social marketing on public health, *J Gend Spec Med* 5(2):48-54, 2002.

Smith NL, Barzilay JI, Shaffer D et al: Fasting and 2-hour postchallenge serum glucose measures and risk of incident cardiovascular events in the elderly: the Cardiovascular Health Study, *Arch Intern Med* 162(2):209-216, 2002.

Smyth CM, Stead RJ: Survey of flexible fibreoptic bronchoscopy in the United Kingdom, *Eur Respir J* 19(3): 458-463, 2002.

Snow CF: Laboratory Diagnosis of Vitamin B_{12} and Folate Deficiency, *Arch Intern Med* 159:1289-1298, 1999.

Stein M, Lubetkin D, Taub HC et al: The effects of intraurethral lidocaine anesthetic and patient anxiety on pain perception during cystoscopy, *J Urol* 151(6): 1518-1521, 1994.

Su M, Lu SM, Tian DP et al. Relationship between ABO blood groups and carcinoma of esophagus and cardia in Chaoshan inhabitants of China, *World J Gastroenterol* 7(5):657-661, 2001.

Summary of the second report of the National Cholesterol Education Program (NCEP) expert panel report on detection, evaluation and treatment of high blood cholesterol in adults, *JAMA* 269:3015-3023, 1993.

Tapiola T: Biological markers for Alzheimer's disease (with special emphasis on cerebrospinal fluid ß-amyloid and tau), *Report No 57*, Kuopio, Finland, 2001, University of Kuopio Department of Neurology.

Thompson BF, Arguedas MR, Wilcox CM: Antibiotic prophylaxis prior to endoscopic retrograde cholangiopancreatography in patients with obstructive jaundice: is it worth the cost? *Alim Pharmacol Ther* 16(4): 727-734, 2002.

United States Nuclear Regulatory Commission: Instruction concerning prenatal radiation exposure, *Regulatory Guide* 8:13, 1999.

van Crevel H, Hijdra A, de Gans J: Lumbar puncture and the risk of herniation: when should we first perform CT? *J Neurol* 249:129-137, 2002.

van Wassenaer AG, Briet JM, van Baar A et al: Free thyroxine levels during the first weeks of life and neurodevelopmental outcome until the age of 5 years in very preterm infants, *Pediatrics* 110:534-539, 2002.

Vashi AR, Oesterling JE: Percent of free prostate-specific antigen: entering a new era in the detection of prostate cancer. *Mayo Clin Proc* 72:337-344, 1997.

Wakefield B, Mentes J, Diggelmann L et al: Monitoring hydration status in elderly veterans, *West J Nurs Res* 24:132-142, 2002.

Wang SE, Lara PN Jr, Lee-Ow A et al: Acetaminophen and diphenhydramine as premedication for platelet transfusions: a prospective randomized double-blind placebo-controlled trial, *Am J Hematol* 70(3):191-194, 2002.

Wells PS, Hirsh J, Anderson DR et al: Accuracy of clinical assessment of deep-vein thrombosis, *Lancet* 345:1326-1330, 1995.

WHO Wilmot GR, Warren ST: A new mutational basis for disease. In Wells, RD, Warren, ST, editors: *Genetic instabilities and hereditary neurological diseases,* San Diego, 1998, Academic Press.

World Health Organization: AIDS epidemic update, Geneva, Switzerland, December 2002, World Health Organization.

Appendix

Reportable Diseases

Reportable Disease (in many areas)	Report Immediately?	Quarantine Required?	Sexually Transmitted?
AIDS	No	No	**Yes**
Amebiasis	No	No	No
Anthrax	No	No	No
Blastomycosis	No	No	No
Botulism	**Yes**	No	No
Brucellosis	No	No	No
Campylobacteriosis	No	No	No
Chancroid	No	No	**Yes**
Chickenpox	No	No	No
Chlamydia infections	No	No	No
Cholera	**Yes**	**Yes**	No
Ciguatera	No	No	No
Creutzfeldt-Jakob disease	No	No	No
Cryptosporidiosis	No	No	No
Cyclosporosis	No	No	No
Cytomegalovirus	No	No	No
Dengue	No	No	No
Diphtheria	**Yes**	No	No
Disease outbreaks	**Yes**	**Possibly**	Not usually of public concern
Encephalitis	No	No	No
Escherichia coli infection	No	No	No
Giardiasis (acute)	No	No	No
Gonococcal infection	No	No	**Yes**
Granuloma inguinale	No	No	**Yes**
Group A streptococcal infection (invasive)	No	No	No
Guillain-Barré syndrome	No	No	No
Haemophilus influenzae (invasive)	No	No	No
Hansen's disease (leprosy)	No	No	No
Hantavirus pulmonary syndrome	**Yes**	No	No
Hemolytic-uremic syndrome	No	No	No
Hemorrhagic fever	No	No	No
Hepatitis (A; B; non-A, non-B; unspecified)	No	**Yes**	No
Herpes	No	No	No
Histoplasmosis	No	No	No
Influenza (report by number of cases)	No	No	No
Kawasaki disease/syndrome	No	No	No
Lead poisoning (>10 mg/dL)	No	No	No
Legionnaires' disease	No	No	No
Leptospirosis	No	No	No
Listeriosis	No	No	No
Lyme disease	No	No	No
Lymphogranuloma venereum	No	No	**Yes**
Malaria	No	No	No
Measles (rubella)	**Yes**	No	No

Reportable Disease (in many areas)	Report Immediately?	Quarantine Required?	Sexually Transmitted?
Measles (rubeola)	No	No	No
Meningitis (aseptic and bacterial)	No	No	No
Meningococcal infections other)	No	No	No
Mucocutaneous lymph node syndrome	No	No	No
Mumps	No	No	No
Mycobacterial disease	No	No	No
Nosocomial infections	No	No	No
Paralytic shellfish poisoning	No	No	No
Parvovirus (B19)	No	No	No
Pediculosis	No	No	No
Pertussis (whooping cough)	No	No	No
Pesticide poisoning	No	No	No
Plague	**Yes**	**Yes**	No
Poliomyelitis	**Yes**	No	No
Psittacosis	No	No	No
Rabies (human) or bite from animal that may be rabid	**Yes**	No	No
Relapsing fever	No	No	No
Reye syndrome	No	No	No
Rheumatic fever	No	No	No
Rocky Mountain spotted fever	No	No	No
Rubella (German measles)	**Yes**	No	No
Salmonellosis	No	No	No
Scabies	No	No	No
Shigellosis	No	No	No
Sporotrichosis	No	No	No
Streptococcal disease, invasive group A	No	No	No
Streptococcal B disease in newborn	No	No	No
Streptococcal pneumonia	No	No	No
Syphilis	No	No	**Yes**
Tetanus	No	No	No
Toxic shock syndrome	No	No	No
Toxoplasmosis	No	No	No
Trichinosis	No	No	No
Tuberculosis	No	No	No
Tularemia	No	No	No
Typhoid fever (*Salmonella typhi*)	No	No	No
Vancomycin-resistant enterococcal disease	No	No	No
Vibriosis	No	No	No
Waterborne diseases	No	No	No
Yellow fever	**Yes**	No	**Yes**
Yersiniosis	No	No	No

Index